Metabolic Syndrome

Rexford S. Ahima
Editor

Metabolic Syndrome

A Comprehensive Textbook

Second Edition

With 89 Figures and 107 Tables

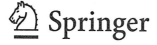 Springer

Editor
Rexford S. Ahima
Division of Endocrinology, Diabetes and Metabolism Department of Medicine
Johns Hopkins University School of Medicine
Baltimore, USA

ISBN 978-3-031-40115-2   ISBN 978-3-031-40116-9 (eBook)
https://doi.org/10.1007/978-3-031-40116-9

This Springer imprint is published by the registered company Springer Nature Switzerland AG.
The registered company address is: Gewerbestrasse 11, 6330 Cham, Switzerland

Paper in this product is recyclable.

To know nothing is bad...To learn nothing is worse
(African proverb)

To Ohenewaa, Osei, Opare, Dedaa, Grace, and FAS, who make it worthwhile.

Preface to the Second Edition

This comprehensive reference work presents an up-to-date survey of the current scientific understanding of the metabolic syndrome, as well as an overview of the most significant advances in the field. The book offers a thorough reference for obesity and the metabolic syndrome and will prove an indispensable resource for clinicians, researchers, and students. The obesity epidemic has generated immense interest in recent years due to the wide-ranging and significant adverse health and economic consequences that surround the problem. Much attention has been focused on excessive consumption of energy-dense food, sedentary lifestyle, and other behaviors that contribute to the pathogenesis of obesity. However, obesity is a highly complex condition that is influenced by genetic as well as environmental factors. The metabolic syndrome comprises of central obesity, hyperglycemia, hypertension, and dyslipidemia. The incidence of metabolic syndrome is growing worldwide, affecting more than one-third of adults in some countries. The metabolic syndrome increases the risk of developing coronary artery disease and stroke, and it is closely associated with fatty liver, dementia, cancer, sleep apnea, kidney failure, and other diseases. This reference work covers the full range of scientific and clinical aspects of obesity and metabolic syndrome: epidemiology, genetics, environmental factors, pathophysiology, and diseases associated with obesity, pediatric obesity, and clinical management.

Baltimore, USA
February 2024

Rexford S. Ahima

Preface to the First Edition

This comprehensive reference work presents an up-to-date survey of the current scientific understanding of the metabolic syndrome, as well as an overview of the most significant advances in the field. The book provides a thorough reference for obesity and the metabolic syndrome and will prove an indispensable resource for clinicians and researchers at all levels. The obesity epidemic has generated immense interest in recent years due to the wide ranging and significant adverse health and economic consequences that surround the problem. Much attention has been focused on excessive consumption of energy-dense food, sedentary lifestyle, and other behaviors that contribute to the pathogenesis of obesity. However, obesity is a highly complex condition that is influenced by genetic as well as environmental factors. The metabolic syndrome comprises of central obesity, impaired glucose tolerance or diabetes, hypertension, and dyslipidemia. The incidence of metabolic syndrome is growing worldwide, affecting more than one-third of adults in some countries. The metabolic syndrome increases the risk of developing coronary artery disease and stroke, and it is also closely associated with fatty liver, dementia, cancer, sleep apnea, kidney failure, infertility, and other diseases. This reference work covers the full range of scientific and clinical aspects of obesity and metabolic syndrome: epidemiology, genetics, environmental factors, pathophysiology, diseases associated with obesity, and clinical management.

Acknowledgments

This book would not have been possible without the knowledge that my teachers, colleagues, and students shared with me over the past four decades. I am indebted to the patients across continents dealing with obesity, diabetes, and other metabolic diseases, for sharing valuable insights and providing guidance for research and discovery. My thanks go to the national and private organizations for providing generous support to the diverse authors who contributed a wide range of chapters to this book. I greatly appreciate the help of Shobana Lenin, production editor at Straive; Kristopher Spring, senior editor, and Lillie Gaurano, editor, at Springer Nature; and the book production team at Straive. Finally, I thank my dear family and friends for sharing this exciting journey of discovery and service.

Contents

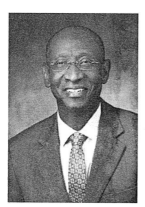

Rexford S. Ahima is a Professor of Medicine, Public Health, and Nursing, Bloomberg Distinguished Professor of Diabetes, and Director of the Division of Endocrinology, Diabetes and Metabolism at the Johns Hopkins University. He did intercalated BSc research training in Endocrinology at the Middlesex Hospital Medical School, University of London, and received MD from the University of Ghana and PhD in Neuroscience from Tulane University in New Orleans, Louisiana. He did his internship and residency training in Internal Medicine at the Jacobi Medical Center and Weiler Hospital, Albert Einstein College of Medicine, in the Bronx, New York, and clinical and research fellowship in Endocrinology, Diabetes and Metabolism at the Beth Israel Deaconess Medical Center and Harvard Medical School in Boston. Dr. Ahima has been elected to the National Academy of Medicine, the American Academy of Arts and Sciences, the American Association for the Advancement of Science, the American Society for Clinical Investigation, the Association of American Physicians, the American College of Physicians, the Interurban Clinical Club, the American Clinical and Climatological Association, and the Obesity Society. He is a former editor-in-chief of the *Journal of Clinical Investigation*, and associate editor of *Gastroenterology*, *Molecular Endocrinology*, and *Endocrine Reviews*, and current editor of the New York Academy of Sciences' *The Year in Diabetes and Obesity*. Dr. Ahima has served on various committees of the National Institutes of Health, the Endocrine Society, and other health and scholarly organizations. His research is focused on central and peripheral regulation of energy homeostasis and the pathophysiology of obesity, diabetes, and related diseases. He is board certified in Endocrinology, Diabetes, and Metabolism, and is the leader of the Johns Hopkins Diabetes Initiative.

Contributors

Alison H. Affinati Department of Internal Medicine, University of Michigan, Ann Arbor, MI, USA

Grace Frempong Afrifa-Anane Department of Environment and Public Health, University of Environment and Sustainable Development, Somanya, Ghana

Alexander B. Agyekum National Cardiothoracic Center, Korle Bu Teaching Hospital, Accra, Ghana

Charles Agyemang Department of Public & Occupational Health, Amsterdam University Medical Centers, University of Amsterdam, Amsterdam, The Netherlands

Rexford S. Ahima Department of Medicine, Division of Endocrinology, Diabetes and Metabolism, Johns Hopkins University School of Medicine, Baltimore, MD, USA

Kelly C. Allison Department of Psychiatry, Perelman School of Medicine, University of Pennsylvania, Philadelphia, PA, USA

Martin A. Alpert Division of Cardiovascular Medicine, University of Missouri School of Medicine, Columbia, MO, USA

John A. Batsis Department of Nutrition, Gillings School of Global Public Health, University of North Carolina, Chapel Hill, NC, USA

Division of Geriatric Medicine, School of Medicine, University of North Carolina, Chapel Hill, NC, USA

Center for Aging and Health, University of North Carolina, Chapel Hill, NC, USA

Salman Zahoor Bhat Department of Medicine, Division of Endocrinology, Diabetes and Metabolism, Johns Hopkins University School of Medicine, Baltimore, MD, USA

Regien Biesma Department of Epidemiology and Public Health Medicine, Royal College of Surgeons in Ireland, Dublin, Ireland

Vincent Boima Department of Medicine and Therapeutics, University of Ghana Medical School, College of Health Sciences, University of Ghana, Accra, Ghana

Carrie Burns Division of Endocrinology, Diabetes, and Metabolism, Perelman School of Medicine, Department of Medicine, University of Pennsylvania, Philadelphia, PA, USA

Stefania Carobbio Centro de Investigacion Principe Felipe, Valencia, Spain

Fernando Carrasco Departamento de Nutrición. Facultad de Medicina, Universidad de Chile, Santiago, Chile

Department of Nutrition, Clínica Las Condes, Santiago, Chile

Etienne Challet Institute of Cellular and Integrative Neurosciences, UPR3212, CNRS, University of Strasbourg, Strasbourg, France

Ray Cheever Department of Nutrition, Gillings School of Global Public Health, University of North Carolina, Chapel Hill, NC, USA

Stanley M. Chen Cardenas Johns Hopkins University School of Medicine, Department of Medicine, Division of Endocrinology, Diabetes & Metabolism, Baltimore, MD, USA

Jang Hyun Choi Department of Biological Sciences, Ulsan National Institute of Science and Technology, Ulsan, Republic of Korea

Víctor Cortés Departamento de Nutrición, Diabetes y Metabolismo, Escuela de Medicina, Pontificia Universidad Católica de Chile, Santiago, Chile

Ama de-Graft Aikins Regional Institute for Population Studies, University of Ghana, Legon, Ghana

Jacques Demongeot AGEIS Laboratory, UGA, La Tronche, France

Nicolette R. den Braver Epidemiology and Data Science, Amsterdam University Medical Centers location Vrije Universiteit Amsterdam, Amsterdam, The Netherlands

Health Behaviours and Chronic Diseases Programme, Amsterdam Public Health Institute, Amsterdam, The Netherlands

Upstream Team, Amsterdam University Medical Centers location Vrije Universiteit Amsterdam, Amsterdam, The Netherlands

Jenny Pena Dias Department of Medicine, Division of Endocrinology, Diabetes and Metabolism, Johns Hopkins University School of Medicine, Baltimore, MD, USA

Roshan Dinparastisaleh College of Medicine, Division of Pulmonary and Critical Care, University of Florida, Jacksonville, FL, USA

Daisy Duan Department of Medicine, Division of Endocrinology, Diabetes and Metabolism, Johns Hopkins University School of Medicine, Baltimore, MD, USA

Justin B. Echouffo-Tcheugui Department of Medicine, Division of Endocrinology, Diabetes, and Metabolism, School of Medicine, Johns Hopkins University, Baltimore, MD, USA

Augustus K. Eduafo Wright State University Boonshoft School of Medicine, Transplant Nephrology, Dayton, OH, USA

Carol F. Elias Department of Molecular and Integrative Physiology, University of Michigan, Ann Arbor, MI, USA

Department of Obstetrics and Gynecology, University of Michigan, Ann Arbor, MI, USA

Ana Elena Espinosa de Ycaza Universidad de Panama. Facultad de Medicina. Endocrinologia, Panama City, Panama

Nnenia Francis Division of Endocrinology, Diabetes and Metabolism, Department of Medicine, University of Kentucky, Lexington, KY, USA

Jose E. Galgani Departamento Ciencias de la Salud, Carrera de Nutrición y Dietética, Facultad de Medicina, Pontificia Universidad Católica de Chile, Santiago, Chile

Departamento de Nutrición, Diabetes y Metabolismo, Escuela de Medicina, Pontificia Universidad Católica de Chile, Santiago, Chile

Pennington Biomedical Research Center, Baton Rouge, LA, USA

Struan F. A. Grant Center for Spatial and Functional Genomics, Divisions of Human Genetics and Endocrinology & Diabetes, Children's Hospital of Philadelphia; Department of Genetics, Department of Pediatrics, Institute of Diabetes, Obesity and Metabolism, Perelman School of Medicine, University of Pennsylvania, Philadelphia, Pennsylvania, USA

Rajvarun S. Grewal California Health Sciences University – College of Osteopathic Medicine (CHSU-COM), Clovis, CA, USA

Edith Grosbellet Institute of Cellular and Integrative Neurosciences, UPR3212, CNRS, University of Strasbourg, Strasbourg, France

Danae C. Gross Department of Nutrition, Gillings School of Global Public Health, University of North Carolina, Chapel Hill, NC, USA

Jeffrey Guo Department of Nutrition, College of Agriculture and Life Sciences, Texas A&M University, College Station, TX, USA

Shaodong Guo Department of Nutrition, College of Agriculture and Life Sciences, Texas A&M University, College Station, TX, USA

Alycia Hancock Johns Hopkins University, Baltimore, Maryland, Division of Endocrinology, Diabetes & Metabolism, The Johns Hopkins University School of Medicine, Baltimore, MD, USA

Mark Hanson Institute of Developmental Sciences, Faculty of Medicine, University of Southampton, Southampton, UK

Talia A. Hitt Division of Endocrinology and Diabetes, Department of Pediatrics, Johns Hopkins University School of Medicine, Baltimore, MD, USA

Yumi Imai Division of Endocrinology and Metabolism, Department of Internal Medicine, University of Iowa, Iowa City, IA, USA

Fraternal Order of Eagles Diabetes Research Center, University of Iowa, Iowa City, IA, USA

Iowa City Veterans Affairs Medical Center, Iowa City, IA, USA

Mariem Jelassi RIADI Laboratory, ENSI, Manouba University, La Manouba, Tunisia

Laundette P. Jones Department(s) of Pharmacology & Epidemiology and Public Health, University of Maryland School of Medicine, Baltimore, MD, USA

Jonathan C. Jun Division of Pulmonary and Critical Care, Department of Medicine, Johns Hopkins University School of Medicine, Baltimore, MD, USA

Rita R. Kalyani Johns Hopkins University, Baltimore, Maryland, Division of Endocrinology, Diabetes & Metabolism, The Johns Hopkins University School of Medicine, Baltimore, MD, USA

Natraj Katta Bryan Heart, Lincoln, NE, USA

Elaine B. Kennedy University College Dublin, Dublin, Ireland

Houssem Ben Khalfallah RIADI Laboratory, ENSI, Manouba University, La Manouba, Tunisia

Sara Atiq Khan Division of Endocrinology, Diabetes, & Metabolism, Department of Medicine, University of Maryland School of Medicine, Baltimore, MD, USA

Mee Kyoung Kim Division of Endocrinology and Metabolism, Department of Internal Medicine, Yeouido St. Mary's Hospital, College of Medicine, The Catholic University of Korea, Seoul, South Korea

Sangwon F. Kim Division of Endocrinology, Diabetes, and Metabolism, Johns Hopkins University School of Medicine, Baltimore, MD, USA

Sandra Boatemaa Kushitor Department of Community Health, Ensign Global College, Kpong, Ghana

Centre for Sustainability Transitions and Department of Food Science, Stellenbosch University, Stellenbosch, South Africa

Dalal El Ladiki Division of Endocrinology and Metabolism, Department of Internal Medicine, University of Iowa, Iowa City, IA, USA

Fraternal Order of Eagles Diabetes Research Center, University of Iowa, Iowa City, IA, USA

Jeroen Lakerveld Epidemiology and Data Science, Amsterdam University Medical Centers location Vrije Universiteit Amsterdam, Amsterdam, The Netherlands

Health Behaviours and Chronic Diseases Programme, Amsterdam Public Health Institute, Amsterdam, The Netherlands

Upstream Team, Amsterdam University Medical Centers location Vrije Universiteit Amsterdam, Amsterdam, The Netherlands

Thao Minh Lam Epidemiology and Data Science, Amsterdam University Medical Centers location Vrije Universiteit Amsterdam, Amsterdam, The Netherlands

Health Behaviours and Chronic Diseases Programme, Amsterdam Public Health Institute, Amsterdam, The Netherlands

Upstream Team, Amsterdam University Medical Centers location Vrije Universiteit Amsterdam, Amsterdam, The Netherlands

Carl J. Lavie John Ochsner Heart and Vascular Institute, New Orleans, LA, USA

Ochsner Clinical School-The University of Queensland School of Medicine, New Orleans, LA, USA

Michelle H. Lee Department of Medicine, Yong Loo Lin School of Medicine, National University of Singapore, Singapore, Singapore

Junxiu Liu Department of Population Health Science and Policy, Icahn School of Medicine at Mount Sinai, New York, NY, USA

Sheela N. Magge Division of Endocrinology and Diabetes, Department of Pediatrics, Johns Hopkins University School of Medicine, Baltimore, MD, USA

Noemi Malandrino Department of Medicine, Division of Endocrinology, Diabetes and Metabolism, Johns Hopkins University School of Medicine, Baltimore, MD, USA

Sara N. Malina Division of Endocrinology and Diabetes, Department of Pediatrics, Johns Hopkins University School of Medicine, Baltimore, MD, USA

Laura E. Matarese Department of Internal Medicine, Division of Gastroenterology, Hepatology and Nutrition, Brody School of Medicine, East Carolina University, Greenville, NC, USA

Maeve A. McArdle University College Dublin, Dublin, Ireland

John C. McLenithan Department of Medicine, University of Maryland School of Medicine, Baltimore, MD, USA

Alexander R. Moschen Department of Internal Medicine 2 and Christian Doppler Laboratory for Mucosal Immunology, Faculty of Medicine, Johannes Kepler University, Linz, Austria

Martin G. Myers Jr Department of Internal Medicine, University of Michigan, Ann Arbor, MI, USA

Department of Molecular and Integrative Physiology, University of Michigan, Ann Arbor, MI, USA

Zlatko Nikoloski London School of Economics, London, UK

Nora L. Nock Department of Epidemiology and Biostatistics, Case Western University School of Medicine, Cleveland, OH, USA

Elise Tirza A. Ohene-Kyei Department of Pediatrics, Johns Hopkins University School of Medicine, Baltimore, MD, USA

David P. Olson Department of Molecular and Integrative Physiology, University of Michigan, Ann Arbor, MI, USA

Department of Pediatrics, University of Michigan, Ann Arbor, MI, USA

Albert Danso Osei Department of Medicine, MedStar Union Memorial Hospital, Baltimore, MD, USA

Hyeong-Kyu Park Department of Internal Medicine, Soonchunhyang University College of Medicine, Seoul, South Korea

Yong-Moon Mark Park Department of Epidemiology, Fay W. Boozman College of Public Health, University of Arkansas for Medical Sciences, Little Rock, AR, USA

Spencer J. Peachee Division of Endocrinology and Metabolism, Department of Internal Medicine, University of Iowa, Iowa City, IA, USA

Fraternal Order of Eagles Diabetes Research Center, University of Iowa, Iowa City, IA, USA

Vanessa Pellegrinelli Wellcome-MRC Institute of Metabolic Science and Medical Research Council Metabolic Diseases Unit, University of Cambridge, Cambridge, UK

Helen M. Roche University College Dublin, Dublin, Ireland

Prasanna Santhanam Division of Endocrinology, Diabetes, & Metabolism, Department of Medicine, Johns Hopkins University School of Medicine, Baltimore, MD, USA

Narjes Bellamine Ben Saoud RIADI Laboratory, ENSI, Manouba University, La Manouba, Tunisia

David B. Sarwer Department of Social and Behavioral Sciences and Center for Obesity Research and Education, College of Public Health, Temple University, Philadelphia, PA, USA

Leah M. Schumacher Department of Kinesiology and Center for Obesity Research and Education, College of Public Health, Temple University, Philadelphia, PA, USA

John R. Speakman State Key Laboratory of Molecular Developmental Biology, Institute of Genetics and Developmental Biology, Chinese Academy of Sciences, Beijing, People's Republic of China

Institute of Biological and Environmental Sciences, University of Aberdeen, Aberdeen, Scotland, UK

Herbert Tilg Department of Internal Medicine I, Gastroenterology, Endocrinology & Metabolism, Medical University Innsbruck, Innsbruck, Austria

Sue-Anne Toh Department of Medicine, Yong Loo Lin School of Medicine, National University of Singapore, Singapore, Singapore

NOVI Health, Singapore, Singapore

Regional Health System Office, National University Health System, Singapore, Singapore

Antonio Vidal-Puig Wellcome-MRC Institute of Metabolic Science and Medical Research Council Metabolic Diseases Unit, University of Cambridge, Cambridge, UK

Centro de Investigacion Principe Felipe, Valencia, Spain

Ivana Vucenik Department of Medical and Research Technology, University of Maryland School of Medicine, Baltimore, MD, USA

Department of Pathology, University of Maryland School of Medicine, Baltimore, MD, USA

Katie L. Wasserstein Division of Endocrinology and Diabetes, Department of Pediatrics, Johns Hopkins University School of Medicine, Baltimore, MD, USA

Angela Yang Johns Hopkins University, Baltimore, Maryland, Division of Endocrinology, Diabetes & Metabolism, The Johns Hopkins University School of Medicine, Baltimore, MD, USA

Wanbao Yang Department of Nutrition, College of Agriculture and Life Sciences, Texas A&M University, College Station, TX, USA

Overview of Metabolic Syndrome

1

Rexford S. Ahima

Abstract

The diagnosis of metabolic syndrome is based on the presence of central (abdominal) obesity, increased blood pressure, elevated glucose and triglycerides, and low high-density lipoprotein cholesterol (HDL-C) levels. The prevalence of metabolic syndrome has increased globally mainly due to excessive intake of energy-dense food and reduced physical activity. Metabolic syndrome increases the risk of developing type 2 diabetes (T2D), cardiovascular diseases, nonalcoholic fatty liver disease (NAFLD), chronic kidney disease, cancer and other diseases. The purpose of this book is to highlight the epidemiology, pathophysiology, clinical features, and treatment of metabolic syndrome. We are hopeful the chapters will provide valuable current insights as well as critical questions to guide future research.

Keywords

Metabolic syndrome · Obesity · Hypertension · Cholesterol · Glucose · Diabetes · Cardiovascular

R. S. Ahima (✉)
Department of Medicine, Division of Endocrinology, Diabetes and Metabolism, Johns Hopkins University School of Medicine, Baltimore, MD, USA
e-mail: ahima@jhmi.edu

© Springer Nature Switzerland AG 2023
R. S. Ahima (ed.), *Metabolic Syndrome*,
https://doi.org/10.1007/978-3-031-40116-9_1

The term "metabolic syndrome" was first used in the National Cholesterol Education Program (NCEP) Adult Treatment Panel III (ATP III) to describe the co-occurrence of obesity, dyslipidemia, hypertension, and abnormal glucose metabolism (Expert Panel on Detection and Treatment of High Blood Cholesterol in [29]). However, the association of metabolic disorders and cardiovascular risk factors had been recognized for many decades [5, 68]. In his American Diabetes Association Banting lecture in 1988, Reaven [65] used the term "syndrome X" to describe the relationship of insulin resistance, hypertension, type 2 diabetes (T2D), and cardiovascular diseases. Other investigators have referred to the clustering of metabolic and cardiovascular risk factors as the "insulin resistance syndrome" [27, 37].

Various organizations have proposed different criteria to describe the relationship of cardiovascular and metabolic diseases (Table 1). In 1998, the World Health Organization (WHO) proposed a working definition for metabolic syndrome focusing on the presence of insulin resistance, impaired glucose tolerance (IGT), or T2D, as well as two of the following conditions: dyslipidemia (reduced HDL-C and increased triglycerides), hypertension, and microalbuminuria [1]. The European Group for the Study of Insulin Resistance (EGIR) criteria for metabolic syndrome were similar to those of the WHO but did not include microalbuminuria [9]. The NCEP ATP III defined the metabolic syndrome based on

Table 1 Definitions of the metabolic syndrome

Organization	Obesity	Blood glucose	High TG	Low HDL-C	High blood pressure	Diagnostic criteria
WHO (1998)	Waist/hip ratio > 0.9 in men or > 0.85 in women or BMI > 30 kg/m²	IGT, IFG, or T2D	TG ≥150 mg/dL	HDL-C < 40 mg/dl in men or HDL-C < 50 mg/dl in women	≥140/90 mmHg	IGT, IFG, T2D, or reduced insulin sensitivity plus any two of the criteria
EGIR (1999)	WC >37 inches in men or > 32 inches in women	IFG or IGT		<39 mg/dL in men and women	≥140 mmHg systolic and ≥ 90 mmHg diastolic or on treatment for HTN	Three or more criteria, one of which should be insulin resistance
NCEP ATPIII (2001)	WC ≥102 cm in men or ≥ 88 cm in women	≥100 mg/dL (including T2D)	TG ≥150 mg/dl or on therapy lowering TG	<40 mg/dL in men or < 50 mg/dL in women or therapy increasing HDL-C	≥130/85 mmHg or on treatment for HTN	Three or more criteria
AACE (2003)	BMI ≥25 kg/m²	IGT or IFG	≥150 mg/dL	<40 mg/dL in men or < 50 mg/dL in women	≥130/85 mmHg	IGT or IFG plus any of the criteria
IDF (2005)	Population-specific increased WC cutoffs	IFG or on treatment for hyperglycemia or has T2D diagnosis	≥150 mg/dL or on TG lowering treatment	<40 mg/dL (men) or < 50 mg/dL (women) or on HDL treatment	≥130 mmHg systolic and/or ≥ 85 mmHg diastolic or on treatment for HTN	Three or more criteria, one of which should be central obesity
IDF (2009)	Population- and country-specific WC cutoffs	≥100 mg/dL	TG ≥150 mg/dL	<40 mg/dL in men or < 50 mg/dL in women	≥130/85 mmHg or on treatment for HTN	Three or more criteria
AHA/ NHLBI (2009)	Central obesity WC > 40 inches in men or > 35 inches in women	IFG or on treated with diabetes drug or T2D diagnosis	≥150 mg/dL or treated with lipid lowering drug	<40 mg/dL in men or < 50 mg/dL in women or on treatment	≥130 mmHg systolic and/or ≥ 85 mmHg diastolic or on treatment for HTN	Three or more criteria

Abbreviations: *IFG*, impaired fasting glucose, defined as fasting plasma glucose ≥110 mg/dL in 2001, and as ≥100 mg/dL in 2004; *IGT*, impaired glucose tolerance, defined a 2-hour plasma glucose >140 mg/dL. The World Health Organization (WHO) defined insulin resistance as the presence of IFG, IGT or insulin resistance. *EGIR*, European Group for the Study of Insulin Resistance, defined insulin resistance as plasma insulin levels >75th percentile. *AACE*, American Association of Clinical Endocrinologists; *AHA*, American Heart Association; *HTN*, hypertension; *IDF*, International Diabetes Federation; *NECP ATPIII*, National Cholesterol Education Program Adult Treatment Panel III; *NHBLI*, National Heart, Lung, and Blood Institute; *TG*, triglyceride; *WC*, waist circumference

increased waist circumference (WC), lipids, blood pressure, and fasting glucose levels [35, 52]. The International Diabetes Federation (IDF) characterized the metabolic syndrome as symptoms and physical or biochemical findings coexisting more often than could be explained by chance alone [3]. In order to account for population differences, the IDF proposed specific racial/ethnic cutoffs [13, 36]. Moreover, the subsequent IDF metabolic syndrome criteria focused on fasting plasma glucose concentration and not insulin resistance [2, 4]. The American Diabetes Association (ADA) acknowledged the clustering of clinical and laboratory features in metabolic syndrome but questioned the utility of insulin

resistance as a biomarker for cardiovascular risk [44]. The American Association of Clinical Endocrinologists' (AACE) definition of the metabolic syndrome focused on the presence of insulin resistance and not diabetes. These definitions of metabolic syndrome will change over time, given our evolving knowledge of the pathogenesis of obesity, T2D, and related diseases. Future criteria for metabolic syndrome may need to consider the contributions of adipokines, pro-inflammatory cytokines, and other factors linked to insulin resistance, diabetes, and cardiovascular diseases.

Figures 1, 2, 3, 4, and 5 illustrate global patterns of body mass index (BMI), elevated glucose, cholesterol and blood pressure, and mortality rate

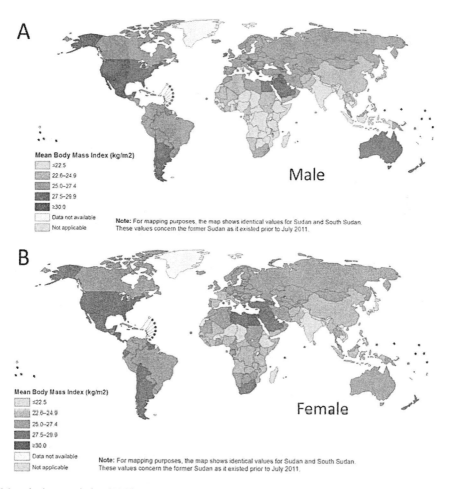

Fig. 1 Mean body mass index (BMI), ages 18 years or older, age standardized. (Adapted from the World Health Organization Global Health Observatory Map Gallery https://www.who.int/data/gho/map-gallery-search-results? &maptopics=1a7eb31d-4803-42d1-9c92-2890bf9b2c48)

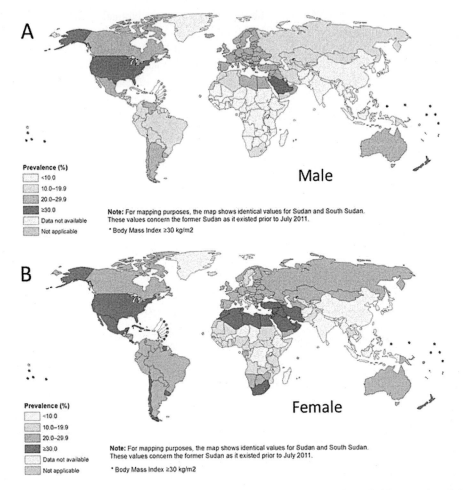

Fig. 2 Prevalence of obesity, ages 18 years or older, in 2016. (Adapted from the World Health Organization Global Health Observatory Map Gallery https://www.who.int/data/ gho/map-gallery-search-results?&maptopics=1a7eb31d-4803-42d1-9c92-2890bf9b2c48)

due to non-communicable diseases. As described in the obesity epidemiology chapters and other chapters, prevalences of obesity, metabolic syndrome and associated diseases have increased worldwide, and these trends are influenced by age, sex, race/ethnicity, low physical activity, other lifestyle factors, and genetics [17, 31, 39, 40, 42, 43, 49, 50, 53–55, 80]. The prevalence of metabolic syndrome in youth also varies according to the definition, age, and population under study [11, 21, 22, 24, 26, 47, 64, 74, 78]. Studies suggest that metabolic syndrome in youth is a strong predictor of future risk for diabetes and cardiovascular disease [11, 47, 56, 64]. The high global prevalence of metabolic

syndrome has been attributed to overconsumption of energy-dense foods, sedentary lifestyle, low socioeconomic status, and rapid urbanization [1, 35, 73]. An inverse association between the level of education and the risk of metabolic syndrome has been described [16, 51, 62, 69, 76]. In developing countries, the prevalence of metabolic syndrome is higher in urban compared to rural areas [17, 39, 42, 50, 79, 80].

A hallmark of the metabolic syndrome is insulin resistance, a pathological condition in which high insulin concentrations fail to produce a normal response in target tissues. Insulin resistance is commonly associated with abdominal (central) obesity [34, 63], though some insulin-resistant

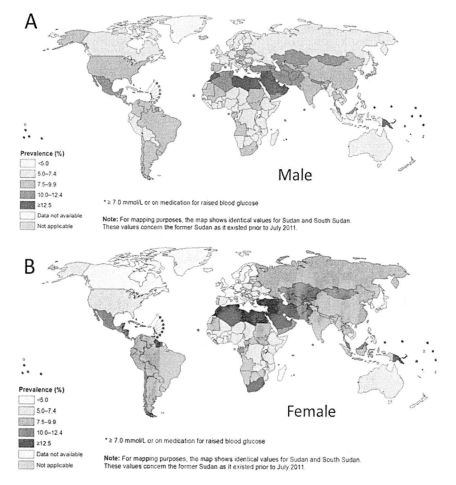

Fig. 3 Prevalence of raised fasting blood glucose (≥ 7 mmol/L or on diabetes medication), ages adults 18 years or older, (age standardized estimate) in 2014. (Adapted from the World Health Organization Global Health Observatory Map Gallery https://www.who.int/data/gho/map-gallery-search-results?&maptopics=1a7eb31d-4803-42d1-9c92-2890bf9b2c48)

individuals who are not obese may have ectopic fat accumulation in the liver and muscle [41, 48]. In adipose tissue, insulin resistance attenuates the anti-lipolytic effect of insulin which leads to elevated fatty acid levels. Insulin resistance in the muscle disrupts insulin-mediated glucose uptake and decreases glycogen biosynthesis. Insulin resistance in the liver impairs the ability of insulin to suppress glucose production. Insulin resistance is very common in obesity, and this metabolic setting increases the demand for pancreatic β-cells to synthesize and secrete more insulin. Hyperinsulinemia in obesity promotes lipogenesis and steatosis, salt retention and hypertension. A defective function of pancreatic β-cells leads to insufficient insulin production, elevated fasting glucose, glucose intolerance, and ultimately T2D [34, 63].

The metabolic syndrome is associated with low-grade inflammation and oxidative stress, partly mediated by adipokines, nutrients, and other factors [25, 30]. Inflammation is marked by elevated cytokine, chemokine and C-reactive protein (hs-CRP) levels [30, 38, 46]. Other biomarkers, including fibrinogen, apolipoprotein B, uric acid, and adhesion molecules, are associated with metabolic syndrome [58–60, 66]. Atherogenic dyslipidemia in the metabolic syndrome

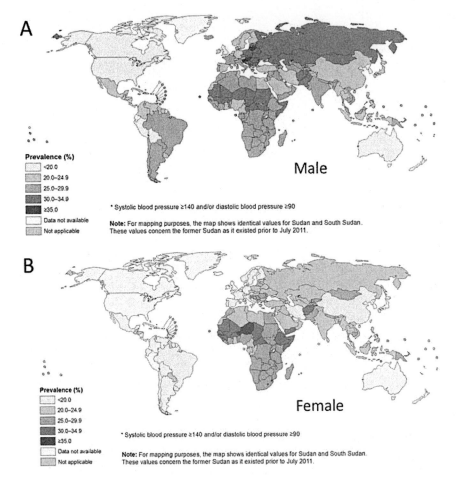

Fig. 4 Prevalence of raised blood pressure, ages 18 years or older, (age standardized), in 2015. (Adapted from the World Health Organization Global Health Observatory Map Gallery https://www.who.int/data/gho/map-gallery-search-results?&maptopics=1a7eb31d-4803-42d1-9c92-2890bf9b2c48)

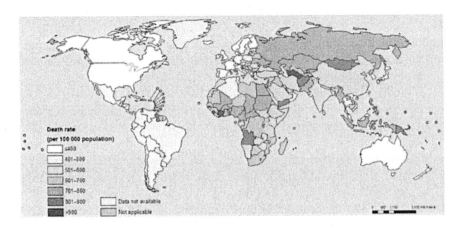

Fig. 5 Deaths due to non-communicable diseases: age-standardized death rate (per 100,000 population), in 2015. (Adapted from the World Health Organization Global Health Observatory Map Gallery https://www.who.int/data/gho/map-gallery-search-results?&maptopics=1a7eb31d-4803-42d1-9c92-2890bf9b2c48)

manifested by high triglycerides and low HDL-C levels is associated with inflammation and oxidative stress [57, 67]. Activation of the renin-angiotensin-aldosterone system (RAAS) in obesity has been linked to insulin resistance, inflammation, oxidative stress, ectopic fat accumulation, and hypertension [32].

Although obesity is often associated with metabolic dysfunction that increases the risks for T2D and cardiovascular diseases, some individuals with obesity do not have metabolic abnormalities or may transition to unhealthy status at a slower rate. The concept of "metabolically healthy obesity" (MHO) versus "metabolically unhealthy obesity" (MUO) is debated because there are no universally defined criteria [72]. Some studies have defined MHO as having two or fewer metabolic syndrome criteria, i.e. large waist circumference, high fasting blood glucose, high blood pressure, elevated triglycerides or low HDL-C, while others have defined MHO as having one or fewer metabolic syndrome components, excluding a large waist circumference [72]. MHO and MUO may be classified on the basis of clinical, laboratory or research parameters (Table 2). Some reports suggest MHO is not truly healthy state, but rather, it progresses over time to MUO [10, 28].

Despite the controversies surrounding the definitions of MUO and MHO, there is little doubt about the close association of metabolic syndrome components and excess cardiovascular risk in most individuals [33]. Hence, interventions to ameliorate obesity, hyperglycemia, dyslipidemia, and hypertension are likely to decrease the risk of developing cardiovascular diseases and other complications of metabolic syndrome. Successful weight loss from dietary management, adequate physical activity, pharmacotherapy, and surgery is highly recommended for metabolic syndrome patients. Available weight loss drugs in the United States include phentermine, extended release phentermine/topiramate, orlistat, sustained release bupropion/naltrexone, and the glucagon-like peptide (GLP)-1 receptor agonists [6, 7, 12, 23, 70, 71, 75]. Metformin improves insulin sensitivity in patients with impaired glucose tolerance or T2D. GLP-1 agonists and sodium glucose

Table 2 Comparison of metabolically unhealthy versus metabolically healthy obesity

	MUO	MHO
Clinical	Metabolic syndrome; central obesity; hypertension; T2D; dyslipidemia; NAFLD; CKD; cardiovascular disease; sleep apnea; hypoventilation	Obesity; healthy
Laboratory	BP > 130/85; fasting plasma glucose > 100 mg/dL; 2-hour oral glucose tolerance test >140 mg/dL; fasting TG > 95 mg/dL; HDL-C < 40 mg/dL in men, <50 mg/dL in women	BP < 130/85; fasting plasma glucose <100 mg/dL; 2-hour oral glucose tolerance test <140 mg/dL; fasting TG < 95 mg/dL; HDL-C > 40 mg/dL in men, > 50 mg/dL in women
Diet & physical activity	Unhealthy diet; low physical activity; sedentary	Healthy diet; high physical activity
Body composition	Visceral > subcutaneous adipose Hepatic steatosis Sarcopenia	Subcutaneous > visceral adipose Normal liver fat Normal muscle
Adipose, liver, muscle	Visceral adipocyte hypertrophy and hyperplasia, inflammation, hypoxia, fibrosis, oxidative stress NAFLD Intra- and extramyocellular fat	Subcutaneous adipocyte hyperplasia Normal liver Normal muscle
Adipokines, inflammatory markers	Reduced adiponectin: leptin ratio; elevated CRP, inflammatory cytokines	High adiponectin: leptin ratio; low CRP and inflammatory markers
Insulin sensitivity	Reduced	Normal

co-transporter 2 (SGLT2) inhibitors improve glycemic control in T2D without increasing body weight and adiposity [14, 61]. Statins are drugs of choice for atherogenic dyslipidemia, and fibrates can be used to decrease triglycerides and increase HDL-C [8, 18, 20, 45]. Antihypertensive drugs, especially RAAS blockers, are crucial for reducing blood pressure and cardiac complications [15, 19, 77, 81].

This comprehensive reference book presents an up-to-date survey of the current scientific understanding of the metabolic syndrome, as well as an overview of the most significant advances in the field over the decades. The references provide thorough information for obesity and metabolic syndrome and will prove an indispensable resource for clinicians, researchers, and students. The book covers a full range of scientific and clinical aspects: epidemiology, genetics, environmental factors, pathophysiology, diseases associated with obesity, and evidence-based management of metabolic syndrome.

Acknowledgments Supported by National Institutes of Health grants R01DK135751 and RF1 AG059621, American Heart Association Cardiometabolic and Type 2 Diabetes SRFN, and American Heart Association Obesity SFRN.

References

1. Alberti KG, Zimmet PZ. Definition, diagnosis and classification of diabetes mellitus and its complications. Part 1: diagnosis and classification of diabetes mellitus provisional report of a WHO consultation. Diabet Med. 1998;15(7):539–53. https://doi.org/10.1002/(SICI)1096-9136(199807)15:7<539::AID-DIA668>3.0.CO;2-S.
2. Alberti KG, Zimmet P, Shaw J, Group IDFETFC. The metabolic syndrome – a new worldwide definition. Lancet. 2005;366(9491):1059–62. https://doi.org/10.1016/S0140-6736(05)67402-8.
3. Alberti KG, Zimmet P, Shaw J. Metabolic syndrome – a new world-wide definition. A consensus statement from the international diabetes federation. Diabet Med. 2006;23(5):469–80. https://doi.org/10.1111/j.1464-5491.2006.01858.x.
4. Alberti KG, Eckel RH, Grundy SM, Zimmet PZ, Cleeman JI, Donato KA, Fruchart JC, James WP, Loria CM, Smith SC Jr, International Diabetes Federation Task Force on E, Prevention, Hational Heart L, Blood I, American Heart A, World Heart F, International Atherosclerosis S, International Association for the Study of O. Harmonizing the metabolic syndrome: a joint interim statement of the international diabetes federation task force on epidemiology and prevention; National Heart, Lung, and Blood Institute; American Heart Association; world Heart federation; international atherosclerosis society; and International Association for the Study of obesity. Circulation. 2009;120(16):1640–5. https://doi.org/10.1161/CIRCULATIONAHA.109.192644.
5. Albrink MJ, Krauss RM, Lindgrem FT, von der Groeben J, Pan S, Wood PD. Intercorrelations among plasma high density lipoprotein, obesity and triglycerides in a normal population. Lipids. 1980;15(9):668–76.
6. Apovian CM, Aronne L, Rubino D, Still C, Wyatt H, Burns C, Kim D, Dunayevich E, Group C-IS. A randomized, phase 3 trial of naltrexone SR/bupropion SR on weight and obesity-related risk factors (COR-II). Obesity. 2013;21(5):935–43. https://doi.org/10.1002/oby.20309.
7. Apovian CM, Aronne LJ, Bessesen DH, et al. Pharmacological management of obesity: an Endocrine Society clinical practice guideline. J Clin Endocrinol Metab. 2015;100(2):342–62.
8. Baigent C, Keech A, Kearney PM, Blackwell L, Buck G, Pollicino C, Kirby A, Sourjina T, Peto R, Collins R, Simes R, Cholesterol Treatment Trialists C. Efficacy and safety of cholesterol-lowering treatment: prospective meta-analysis of data from 90,056 participants in 14 randomised trials of statins. Lancet. 2005;366(9493):1267–78. https://doi.org/10.1016/S0140-6736(05)67394-1.
9. Balkau B, Charles MA. Comment on the provisional report from the WHO consultation. European Group for the Study of insulin resistance (EGIR). Diabet Med. 1999;16(5):442–3.
10. Bell JA, Hamer M, Sabia S, Singh-Manoux A, Batty GD, Kivimaki M. (1999). The natural course of healthy obesity over 20 years. J Am Coll Cardiol. 2015;65(1):101–2.
11. Berenson GS, Srinivasan SR, Bao W, Newman WP 3rd, Tracy RE, Wattigney WA. Association between multiple cardiovascular risk factors and atherosclerosis in children and young adults. The Bogalusa Heart study. N Engl J Med. 1998;338(23):1650–6. https://doi.org/10.1056/NEJM199806043382302.
12. Billes SK, Sinnayah P, Cowley MA. Naltrexone/bupropion for obesity: an investigational combination pharmacotherapy for weight loss. Pharmacol Res. 2014;84:1–11. https://doi.org/10.1016/j.phrs.2014.04.004.
13. Bloomgarden ZT. American Association of Clinical Endocrinologists (AACE) consensus conference on the insulin resistance syndrome: 25–26 August 2002, Washington, DC. Diabetes Care. 2003;26(4):1297–303.
14. Bolinder J, Ljunggren O, Kullberg J, Johansson L, Wilding J, Langkilde AM, Sugg J, Parikh S. Effects

of dapagliflozin on body weight, total fat mass, and regional adipose tissue distribution in patients with type 2 diabetes mellitus with inadequate glycemic control on metformin. J Clin Endocrinol Metab. 2012;97 (3):1020–31. https://doi.org/10.1210/jc.2011-2260.

15. Borghi C, Santi F. Fixed combination of lercanidipine and enalapril in the management of hypertension: focus on patient preference and adherence. Patient Prefer Adherence. 2012;6:449–55. https://doi.org/10.2147/PPA.S23232.

16. Brunner EJ, Marmot MG, Nanchahal K, Shipley MJ, Stansfeld SA, Juneja M, Alberti KG. Social inequality in coronary risk: central obesity and the metabolic syndrome. Evidence from the Whitehall II study. Diabetologia. 1997;40(11):1341–9. https://doi.org/10.1007/s001250050830.

17. Chien KL, Lee BC, Hsu HC, Lin HJ, Chen MF, Lee YT. Prevalence, agreement and classification of various metabolic syndrome criteria among ethnic Chinese: a report on the hospital-based health diagnosis of the adult population. Atherosclerosis. 2008;196(2): 764–71. https://doi.org/10.1016/j.atherosclerosis.2007.01.006.

18. Cholesterol Treatment Trialists C, Mihaylova B, Emberson J, Blackwell L, Keech A, Simes J, Barnes EH, Voysey M, Gray A, Collins R, Baigent C. The effects of lowering LDL cholesterol with statin therapy in people at low risk of vascular disease: meta-analysis of individual data from 27 randomised trials. Lancet. 2012;380(9841):581–90. https://doi.org/10.1016/S0140-6736(12)60367-5.

19. Chrysant SG, Chrysant GS, Chrysant C, Shiraz M. The treatment of cardiovascular disease continuum: focus on prevention and RAS blockade. Curr Clin Pharmacol. 2010;5(2):89–95.

20. Colhoun HM, Betteridge DJ, Durrington PN, Hitman GA, Neil HA, Livingstone SJ, Thomason MJ, Mackness MI, Charlton-Menys V, Fuller JH, Investigators C. Primary prevention of cardiovascular disease with atorvastatin in type 2 diabetes in the collaborative atorvastatin diabetes study (CARDS): multicentre randomised placebo-controlled trial. Lancet. 2004;364(9435):685–96. https://doi.org/10.1016/S0140-6736(04)16895-5.

21. Cook S, Weitzman M, Auinger P, Nguyen M, Dietz WH. Prevalence of a metabolic syndrome phenotype in adolescents: findings from the third National Health and nutrition examination survey, 1988–1994. Arch Pediatr Adolesc Med. 2003;157(8):821–7. https://doi.org/10.1001/archpedi.157.8.821.

22. Cook S, Auinger P, Li C, Ford ES. Metabolic syndrome rates in United States adolescents, from the National Health and nutrition examination survey, 1999–2002. J Pediatr. 2008;152(2):165–70. https://doi.org/10.1016/j.jpeds.2007.06.004.

23. Coomans CP, Geerling JJ, van den Berg SA, van Diepen HC, Garcia-Tardon N, Thomas A, Schroder-van der Elst JP, Ouwens DM, Pijl H, Rensen PC, Havekes LM, Guigas B, Romijn JA. The insulin

sensitizing effect of topiramate involves KATP channel activation in the central nervous system. Br J Pharmacol. 2013;170(4):908–18. https://doi.org/10.1111/bph.12338.

24. Cruz ML, Weigensberg MJ, Huang TT, Ball G, Shaibi GQ, Goran MI. The metabolic syndrome in overweight Hispanic youth and the role of insulin sensitivity. J Clin Endocrinol Metab. 2004;89(1):108–13. https://doi.org/10.1210/jc.2003-031188.

25. Dandona P, Aljada A, Bandyopadhyay A. Inflammation: the link between insulin resistance, obesity and diabetes. Trends Immunol. 2004;25(1):4–7.

26. de Ferranti SD, Gauvreau K, Ludwig DS, Neufeld EJ, Newburger JW, Rifai N. Prevalence of the metabolic syndrome in American adolescents: findings from the third National Health and nutrition examination survey. Circulation. 2004;110(16):2494–7. https://doi.org/10.1161/01.CIR.0000145117.40114.C7.

27. DeFronzo RA, Ferrannini E. Insulin resistance. A multifaceted syndrome responsible for NIDDM, obesity, hypertension, dyslipidemia, and atherosclerotic cardiovascular disease. Diabetes Care. 1991;14(3):173–94.

28. Echouffo-Tcheugui JB, et al. Natural history of obesity subphenotypes: dynamic changes over two decades and prognosis in the Framingham Heart study. J Clin Endocrinol Metab. 2019;104(3):738–52.

29. Expert Panel on Detection E, Treatment of High Blood Cholesterol in A. Executive summary of the third report of the National Cholesterol Education Program (NCEP) expert panel on detection, evaluation, and treatment of high blood cholesterol in adults (adult Treatment panel III). JAMA. 2001;285(19):2486–97.

30. Festa A, D'Agostino R Jr, Howard G, Mykkanen L, Tracy RP, Haffner SM. Chronic subclinical inflammation as part of the insulin resistance syndrome: the insulin resistance atherosclerosis study (IRAS). Circulation. 2000;102(1):42–7.

31. Ford ES, Giles WH, Dietz WH. Prevalence of the metabolic syndrome among US adults: findings from the third National Health and nutrition examination survey. JAMA. 2002;287(3):356–9.

32. Frigolet ME, Torres N, Tovar AR. The renin-angiotensin system in adipose tissue and its metabolic consequences during obesity. J Nutr Biochem. 2013;24 (12):2003–15. https://doi.org/10.1016/j.jnutbio.2013.07.002.

33. Galassi A, Reynolds K, He J. Metabolic syndrome and risk of cardiovascular disease: a meta-analysis. Am J Med. 2006;119(10):812–9. https://doi.org/10.1016/j.amjmed.2006.02.031.

34. Gill H, Mugo M, Whaley-Connell A, Stump C, Sowers JR. The key role of insulin resistance in the cardiometabolic syndrome. Am J Med Sci. 2005;330 (6):290–4.

35. Grundy SM, Brewer HB Jr, Cleeman JI, Smith SC Jr, Lenfant C, American Heart A, National Heart L, Blood I. Definition of metabolic syndrome: report of the National Heart, Lung, and Blood Institute/American Heart Association conference on scientific issues related

to definition. Circulation. 2004;109(3):433–8. https://doi.org/10.1161/01.CIR.0000111245.75752.C6.

36. Grundy SM, Cleeman JI, Daniels SR, Donato KA, Eckel RH, Franklin BA, Gordon DJ, Krauss RM, Savage PJ, Smith SC Jr, Spertus JA, Costa F, American Heart A, National Heart L, Blood I. Diagnosis and management of the metabolic syndrome: an American Heart Association/National Heart, Lung, and Blood Institute scientific statement. Circulation. 2005;112(17):2735–52. https://doi.org/10.1161/CIRCULATIONAHA.105.169404.

37. Haffner SM, Valdez RA, Hazuda HP, Mitchell BD, Morales PA, Stern MP. Prospective analysis of the insulin-resistance syndrome (syndrome X). Diabetes. 1992;41(6):715–22.

38. Han TS, Sattar N, Williams K, Gonzalez-Villalpando C, Lean ME, Haffner SM. Prospective study of C-reactive protein in relation to the development of diabetes and metabolic syndrome in the Mexico City diabetes study. Diabetes Care. 2002;25(11):2016–21.

39. Harzallah F, Alberti H, Ben Khalifa F. The metabolic syndrome in an Arab population: a first look at the new international diabetes federation criteria. Diabet Med. 2006;23(4):441–4. https://doi.org/10.1111/j.1464-5491.2006.01866.x.

40. Ilanne-Parikka P, Eriksson JG, Lindstrom J, Hamalainen H, Keinanen-Kiukaanniemi S, Laakso M, Louheranta A, Mannelin M, Rastas M, Salminen V, Aunola S, Sundvall J, Valle T, Lahtela J, Uusitupa M, Tuomilehto J, Finnish Diabetes Prevention Study G. Prevalence of the metabolic syndrome and its components: findings from a Finnish general population sample and the diabetes prevention study cohort. Diabetes Care. 2004;27(9):2135–40.

41. Jensen MD, Haymond MW, Rizza RA, Cryer PE, Miles JM. Influence of body fat distribution on free fatty acid metabolism in obesity. J Clin Invest. 1989;83(4):1168–73. https://doi.org/10.1172/JCI113997.

42. Jeppesen J, Hansen TW, Rasmussen S, Ibsen H, Torp-Pedersen C, Madsbad S. Insulin resistance, the metabolic syndrome, and risk of incident cardiovascular disease: a population-based study. J Am Coll Cardiol. 2007;49(21):2112–9. https://doi.org/10.1016/j.jacc.2007.01.088.

43. Jorgensen ME, Bjerregaard P, Gyntelberg F, Borch-Johnsen K, Greenland Population S. Prevalence of the metabolic syndrome among the Inuit in Greenland. A comparison between two proposed definitions. Diabet Med. 2004;21(11):1237–42. https://doi.org/10.1111/j.1464-5491.2004.01294.x.

44. Kahn R, Buse J, Ferrannini E, Stern M, American Diabetes A, European Association for the Study of D. The metabolic syndrome: time for a critical appraisal: joint statement from the American Diabetes Association and the European Association for the Study of diabetes. Diabetes Care. 2005;28(9):2289–304.

45. Koo BK. Statin for the primary prevention of cardiovascular disease in patients with diabetes mellitus.

Diabetes Metab J. 2014;38(1):32–4. https://doi.org/10.4093/dmj.2014.38.1.32.

46. Laaksonen DE, Niskanen L, Nyyssonen K, Punnonen K, Tuomainen TP, Valkonen VP, Salonen R, Salonen JT. C-reactive protein and the development of the metabolic syndrome and diabetes in middle-aged men. Diabetologia. 2004;47(8):1403–10. https://doi.org/10.1007/s00125-004-1472-x.

47. Li S, Chen W, Srinivasan SR, Bond MG, Tang R, Urbina EM, Berenson GS. Childhood cardiovascular risk factors and carotid vascular changes in adulthood: the Bogalusa Heart study. JAMA. 2003;290(17):2271–6. https://doi.org/10.1001/jama.290.17.2271.

48. Lim S, Meigs JB. Links between ectopic fat and vascular disease in humans. Arterioscler Thromb Vasc Biol. 2014;34(9):1820–6. https://doi.org/10.1161/ATVBAHA.114.303035.

49. Lim S, Shin H, Song JH, Kwak SH, Kang SM, Won Yoon J, Choi SH, Cho SI, Park KS, Lee HK, Jang HC, Koh KK. Increasing prevalence of metabolic syndrome in Korea: the Korean National Health and nutrition examination survey for 1998–2007. Diabetes Care. 2011;34(6):1323–8. https://doi.org/10.2337/dc10-2109.

50. Lorenzo C, Serrano-Rios M, Martinez-Larrad MT, Gonzalez-Sanchez JL, Seclen S, Villena A, Gonzalez-Villalpando C, Williams K, Haffner SM. Geographic variations of the international diabetes federation and the National Cholesterol Education Program – Adult Treatment Panel III definitions of the metabolic syndrome in nondiabetic subjects. Diabetes Care. 2006;29(3):685–91.

51. Lucove JC, Kaufman JS, James SA. Association between adult and childhood socioeconomic status and prevalence of the metabolic syndrome in African Americans: the Pitt County study. Am J Public Health. 2007;97(2):234–6. https://doi.org/10.2105/AJPH.2006.087429.

52. Marchesini G, Forlani G, Cerrelli F, Manini R, Natale S, Baraldi L, Ermini G, Savorani G, Zocchi D, Melchionda N. WHO and ATPIII proposals for the definition of the metabolic syndrome in patients with type 2 diabetes. Diabet Med. 2004;21(4):383–7. https://doi.org/10.1111/j.1464-5491.2004.01115.x.

53. Mattsson N, Ronnemaa T, Juonala M, Viikari JS, Raitakari OT. The prevalence of the metabolic syndrome in young adults. The cardiovascular risk in young Finns study. J Intern Med. 2007;261(2):159–69. https://doi.org/10.1111/j.1365-2796.2006.01752.x.

54. Mozumdar A, Liguori G. Persistent increase of prevalence of metabolic syndrome among U.S. adults: NHANES III to NHANES 1999–2006. Diabetes Care. 2011;34 (1):216–219:216. https://doi.org/10.2337/dc10-0879.

55. Nestel P, Lyu R, Low LP, Sheu WH, Nitiyanant W, Saito I, Tan CE. Metabolic syndrome: recent prevalence in east and southeast Asian populations. Asia Pac J Clin Nutr. 2007;16(2):362–7.

56. Noubiap JJ, Nansseu JR, Lontchi-Yimagou E, Nkeck JR, Nyaga UF, Ngouo AT, Tounouga DN, Tianyi FL, Foka AJ, Ndoadoumgue AL, Bigna JJ. Global, regional, and country estimates of metabolic syndrome burden in children and adolescents in 2020: a systematic review and modelling analysis. Lancet Child Adolesc Health. 2022;6(3):158–70. https://doi.org/10.1016/S2352-4642(21)00374-6. Epub 2022 Jan 17. PMID: 35051409

57. Onat A, Hergenc G. Low-grade inflammation, and dysfunction of high-density lipoprotein and its apolipoproteins as a major driver of cardiometabolic risk. Metab Clin Exp. 2011;60(4):499–512. https://doi.org/10.1016/j.metabol.2010.04.018.

58. Onat A, Uyarel H, Hergenc G, Karabulut A, Albayrak S, Sari I, Yazici M, Keles I. Serum uric acid is a determinant of metabolic syndrome in a population-based study. Am J Hypertens. 2006;19(10):1055–62. https://doi.org/10.1016/j.amjhyper.2006.02.014.

59. Onat A, Can G, Hergenc G, Yazici M, Karabulut A, Albayrak S. Serum apolipoprotein B predicts dyslipidemia, metabolic syndrome and, in women, hypertension and diabetes, independent of markers of central obesity and inflammation. Int J Obes. 2007;31(7):1119–25. https://doi.org/10.1038/sj.ijo.0803552.

60. Onat A, Ozhan H, Erbilen E, Albayrak S, Kucukdurmaz Z, Can G, Keles I, Hergenc G. Independent prediction of metabolic syndrome by plasma fibrinogen in men, and predictors of elevated levels. Int J Cardiol. 2009;135(2):211–7. https://doi.org/10.1016/j.ijcard.2008.03.054.

61. Orchard TJ, Temprosa M, Goldberg R, Haffner S, Ratner R, Marcovina S, Fowler S, Diabetes Prevention Program Research G. The effect of metformin and intensive lifestyle intervention on the metabolic syndrome: the diabetes prevention program randomized trial. Ann Intern Med. 2005;142(8):611–9.

62. Park MJ, Yun KE, Lee GE, Cho HJ, Park HS. A cross-sectional study of socioeconomic status and the metabolic syndrome in Korean adults. Ann Epidemiol. 2007;17(4):320–6. https://doi.org/10.1016/j.annepidem.2006.10.007.

63. Petersen KF, Shulman GI. Etiology of insulin resistance. Am J Med. 2006;119(5 Suppl 1):S10–6. https://doi.org/10.1016/j.amjmed.2006.01.009.

64. Raitakari OT, Juonala M, Kahonen M, Taittonen L, Laitinen T, Maki-Torkko N, Jarvisalo MJ, Uhari M, Jokinen E, Ronnemaa T, Akerblom HK, Viikari JS. Cardiovascular risk factors in childhood and carotid artery intima-media thickness in adulthood and the cardiovascular risk in young Finns study. JAMA. 2003;290(17):2277–83. https://doi.org/10.1001/jama.290.17.2277.

65. Reaven GM. Banting lecture 1988. Role of insulin resistance in human disease. Diabetes. 1988;37(12):1595–607.

66. Rubin D, Claas S, Pfeuffer M, Nothnagel M, Foelsch UR, Schrezenmeir J. S-ICAM-1 and s-VCAM-1 in healthy men are strongly associated with traits of the metabolic syndrome, becoming evident in the postprandial response to a lipid-rich meal. Lipids Health Dis. 2008;7:32. https://doi.org/10.1186/1476-511X-7-32.

67. Ruotolo G, Howard BV. Dyslipidemia of the metabolic syndrome. Curr Cardiol Rep. 2002;4(6):494–500.

68. Sarafidis PA, Nilsson PM. The metabolic syndrome: a glance at its history. J Hypertens. 2006;24(4):621–6. https://doi.org/10.1097/01.hjh.0000217840.26971.b6.

69. Silventoinen K, Pankow J, Jousilahti P, Hu G, Tuomilehto J. Educational inequalities in the metabolic syndrome and coronary heart disease among middle-aged men and women. Int J Epidemiol. 2005;34(2):327–34. https://doi.org/10.1093/ije/dyi007.

70. Smith SR, Weissman NJ, Anderson CM, Sanchez M, Chuang E, Stubbe S, Bays H, Shanahan WR, Behavioral M, Lorcaserin for O, Obesity Management Study G. Multicenter, placebo-controlled trial of lorcaserin for weight management. N Engl J Med. 2010;363(3):245–56. https://doi.org/10.1056/NEJMoa0909809.

71. Smith SM, Meyer M, Trinkley KE. Phentermine/topiramate for the treatment of obesity. Ann Pharmacother. 2013;47(3):340–9. https://doi.org/10.1345/aph.1R501.

72. Smith GI, Mittendorfer B, Klein S. Metabolically healthy obesity: facts and fantasies. J Clin Invest. 2019;129(10):3978–89. https://doi.org/10.1172/JCI129186. PMID: 31524630

73. Stefan N, Schulze MB. Metabolic health and cardiometabolic risk clusters: implications for prediction, prevention, and treatment. Lancet Diabetes Endocrinol. 2023;11(6):426–40. https://doi.org/10.1016/S2213-8587(23)00086-4. Epub 2023 May 5.PMID: 37156256

74. Sun SS, Liang R, Huang TT, Daniels SR, Arslanian S, Liu K, Grave GD, Siervogel RM. Childhood obesity predicts adult metabolic syndrome: the Fels longitudinal study. J Pediatr. 2008;152(2):191–200. https://doi.org/10.1016/j.jpeds.2007.07.055.

75. Vilsboll T, Christensen M, Junker AE, Knop FK, Gluud LL. Effects of glucagon-like peptide-1 receptor agonists on weight loss: systematic review and meta-analyses of randomised controlled trials. BMJ. 2012;344:d7771. https://doi.org/10.1136/bmj.d7771.

76. Wamala SP, Lynch J, Horsten M, Mittleman MA, Schenck-Gustafsson K, Orth-Gomer K. Education and the metabolic syndrome in women. Diabetes Care. 1999;22(12):1999–2003.

77. Watanabe S, Tagawa T, Yamakawa K, Shimabukuro M, Ueda S. Inhibition of the renin-angiotensin system prevents free fatty acid-induced acute endothelial dysfunction in humans. Arterioscler Thromb Vasc Biol. 2005;25(11):2376–80. https://doi.org/10.1161/01.ATV.0000187465.55507.85.

78. Weiss R, Dziura J, Burgert TS, Tamborlane WV, Taksali SE, Yeckel CW, Allen K, Lopes M, Savoye M, Morrison J, Sherwin RS, Caprio

S. Obesity and the metabolic syndrome in children and adolescents. N Engl J Med. 2004;350(23):2362–74. https://doi.org/10.1056/NEJMoa031049.

79. Weng X, Liu Y, Ma J, Wang W, Yang G, Caballero B. An urban–rural comparison of the prevalence of the metabolic syndrome in eastern China. Public Health Nutr. 2007;10(2):131–6. https://doi.org/10.1017/S1368980007226023.

80. Zabetian A, Hadaegh F, Azizi F. Prevalence of metabolic syndrome in Iranian adult population, concordance between the IDF with the ATPIII and the WHO definitions. Diabetes Res Clin Pract. 2007;77(2): 251–7. https://doi.org/10.1016/j.diabres.2006.12.001.

81. Zreikat HH, Harpe SE, Slattum PW, Mays DP, Essah PA, Cheang KI. Effect of renin-angiotensin system inhibition on cardiovascular events in older hypertensive patients with metabolic syndrome. Metab Clin Exp. 2014;63(3):392–9. https://doi.org/10.1016/j.metabol.2013.11.006.

Obesity and Metabolic Syndrome in the United States

2

Albert Danso Osei, Elise Tirza A. Ohene-Kyei, and Justin B. Echouffo-Tcheugui

Contents

A. D. Osei
Department of Medicine, MedStar Union Memorial Hospital, Baltimore, MD, USA

E. T. A. Ohene-Kyei
Department of Pediatrics, Johns Hopkins University School of Medicine, Baltimore, MD, USA

J. B. Echouffo-Tcheugui (✉)
Department of Medicine, Division of Endocrinology, Diabetes, and Metabolism, School of Medicine, Johns Hopkins University, Baltimore, MD, USA
e-mail: jechouf1@jhmi.edu

Abstract

The prevalence of obesity is increasing in the United States with resultant morbidity and mortality. In this chapter, we examine the epidemiology of obesity and metabolic syndrome, as well as the associated sociodemographic correlates. The health implications of obesity are enormous, and we address the multisystemic health manifestations of obesity. We highlight the importance of lifestyle

© Springer Nature Switzerland AG 2023
R. S. Ahima (ed.), *Metabolic Syndrome*,
https://doi.org/10.1007/978-3-031-40116-9_55

intervention, as well as medical and surgical options for obesity management. Additionally, we discuss childhood obesity and available treatment options and strategies. The field of obesity medicine is rapidly evolving, and we discuss avenues for research into novel therapies.

Keywords

Obesity · Metabolic syndrome · Diabetes · Cardiovascular · Pharmacotherapy

Introduction

The prevalence of obesity has been rapidly increasing over the years, with worldwide obesity almost tripled since 1975. In 2017–2020, the prevalence of adult obesity in the United States was 41.9% among adults [1], and 19.7% in children and adolescents aged 2–19 years [1]. The increasing trend is worrying given the significant morbidity and mortality associated with obesity. Obesity is a major risk factor for diabetes, cardiovascular diseases, nonalcoholic fatty liver disease (NAFLD), sleep apnea, cancer, and other diseases, with its attendant economic, social, and mental impact on individuals, families, and nations [2]. In 2019, the estimated annual medical cost of obesity in the United States was $173 billion, with people with obesity having an annual medical cost that was $1861 higher than those of individual with a healthy weight [1]. The World Health Organization (WHO) defines overweight and obesity as excessive or abnormal fat accumulation that has the tendency to impair health [2]. The body mass index (BMI) is a practical tool used to classify overweight and obesity. The BMI is calculated by dividing a person's weight in kilograms by the square of their height in meters [3]. Overweight and obesity are defined as BMI ≥ 25.0 to 29.9 kg/m^2 and ≥ 30 kg/m^2, respectively. This WHO classification was also adopted by the National Institute of Health (NIH) and the Centers for Disease Control Prevention (CDC) [4]. Childhood obesity is defined as BMI $\geq$ 95th percentile for age and sex [5].

Obesity is associated with insulin resistance, with sequelae of elevated insulin levels, hyperglycemia, endothelial dysfunction, and vascular inflammation. These predispose individuals to diabetes mellitus, hypertension, and dyslipidemia [6, 7]. The metabolic syndrome captures a clustering of the latter conditions. The National Cholesterol Education Program ATP III criteria defines the metabolic syndrome as the presence of three or more of the following: abdominal (central) obesity, defined as a waist circumference ≥ 102 cm (40 in) in men and ≥ 88 cm (35 in) in females; serum triglycerides ≥ 150 mg/dL (1.7 mmol/L) or drug treatment for elevated triglycerides; serum high-density lipoprotein (HDL) cholesterol <40 mg/dL (1 mmol/L) in males and <50 mg/dL (1.3 mmol/L) in females or drug treatment for low HDL cholesterol; blood pressure $\geq 130/85$ mmHg or drug treatment for elevated blood pressure; fasting plasma glucose (FPG) ≥ 100 mg/dL (5.6 mmol/L) or drug treatment for elevated blood glucose [8, 9]. It is important to identify individuals with obesity and metabolic syndrome, to allow for targeted pharmacological and non-pharmacological management in order to reduce the overall risk of cardiovascular disease and mortality.

In this chapter, we address the epidemiology of obesity and metabolic syndrome in the United States. We examine the historical trends in obesity and metabolic syndrome, and the sociodemographic and geographical correlates of obesity, including environmental factors which are critical to understanding the topic. Additionally, we discuss the trends in childhood obesity, and the current guidelines for the evaluation and management of obesity in children. We also expound on the multisystemic complications and health implications of obesity. We examine various pharmacological and non-pharmacological options available for obesity management. Lifestyle modification is the foundation of obesity management, as has been emphasized by several health organizations. Finally, we discuss future directions for obesity management and for research potential.

Epidemiology of Obesity and Metabolic Syndrome in the United States

Historical Trends in Obesity

While Hippocrates linked corpulency to health and death many centuries ago, it was not until after World War II, that obesity became a well-recognized problem [10]. Before the twentieth century, obesity was less common, often associated with excessive wealth, and not considered a health crisis. Multiple factors have been associated with the rise in obesity: the shift from manual jobs to service jobs leading to an increase in sedentary lifestyle, and the shift from fresh food to energy-dense processed foods, along with other factors such as genetics, stress, and socioeconomic status [10]. These factors have all led to the unprecedented rise in obesity, and obesity-related conditions, which form part of the leading causes of premature death today. Between 1976 and 2000, the prevalence of obesity among American adults aged 20–74 years increased from 15.0% in 1976–1980 to 23.3% in 1988–1994, and 30.9% in 1999–2000 [11]. Currently, the prevalence of obesity is estimated be as high as 41.9% [1]. The metabolic syndrome prevalence between 1988 and 1994 was 25.3%, with a slight decline between 1999 and 2006 to 25.0%, and then it increased to 34.2% from 2007 to 2012 [12].

Current Obesity Burden

The United States Centers for Disease Control and Prevention (CDC) collects data on obesity using the Behavioral Risk Factor Surveillance System (BRFSS), which is a national representative survey (Fig. 1) [1].

The current prevalence of obesity in adults (2017–2020) is 41.9%, which represents a 37% increase from the 1999–2000 period. At the state level, the prevalence of obesity ranges from 24.7% in the District of Columbia to 40.6% in West Virginia according to the BRFSS data (Fig. 1). Nineteen states have an adult obesity prevalence at or above 35%; for the first time in

2021, South Dakota, North Carolina, and Nebraska had obesity rates greater than 35% [13]. Among adults older than 20 years, the obesity prevalence does not differ by sex [14].

Trends in Metabolic Syndrome

Using 2003–2012 National Health and Nutrition Examination Survey (NHANES) data, the national prevalence of metabolic syndrome in the United States was 33%, with higher prevalence in women compared to men (35.6% vs. 30.3%). Hispanics had the highest prevalence (35.4%), followed by non-Hispanic Whites (33.4%) and Blacks (32.7%) [15]. The prevalence increased from 32.9% in 2003–2004 to 34.7% in 2011–2012 [15]. Subsequent 2011–2016 NHANES data showed that the weighted prevalence of metabolic syndrome was 34.7%, and the prevalence was not different among men (35.1%) and women (34.3%) [16]. The prevalence was highest among Hispanics (36.3%) and non-Hispanic White (36.0%) [16].

Sociodemographic/Geographic Correlates

Race/Ethnic Differences

Obesity affects some groups of people more than others. According to the CDC, the age-adjusted prevalence of obesity was highest among Non-Hispanic Black adults (49.9%), followed by Hispanic adults (45.6%), Non-Hispanic White adults (41.4%), and then Non-Hispanic Asian adults (16.1%) [13, 17] (Fig. 2). Metabolic syndrome seems to follow a similar pattern.

Multiple factors account for these differences in racial/ethnic prevalence of obesity and metabolic syndrome.

Environmental/Behavioral Factors

Environmental factors play a prominent role in the occurrence of obesity and metabolic syndrome. The built environment, encompassing a location's

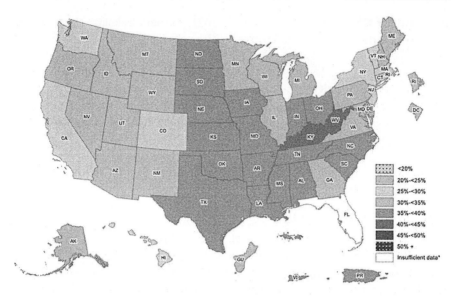

Fig. 1 Adult obesity prevalence map of the United States reported by the CDC in 2021. (Figure reproduced according to the Centers for Disease Control and Prevention (CDC))

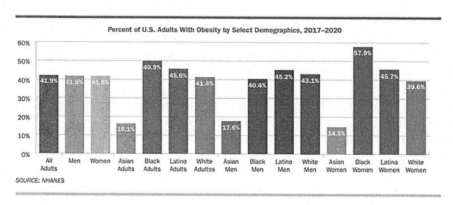

Fig. 2 Prevalence of obesity among racial/ethnic populations. (Figure reproduced according to Trust for America's Health based on NHANES data)

infrastructure that influences the quality of a neighborhood, walkability, and proximity to resources within the area, has contributed to the rising trends of obesity and metabolic syndrome [18]. The built environment influences food availability and quality. The number of vendors and types of food available in an area impact the food that residents have access to. There is evidence that fast-food restaurant density is associated with higher prevalence of obesity. A study showed that compared to older adults living in low fast-food restaurant-density neighborhoods, older adults living in high fast-food restaurant-density neighborhoods were more likely to have obesity because these adults also had increased odds of eating out more at fast foods, not meeting physical activity guidelines, and having low self-efficacy for eating healthy [19]. Furthermore, an association exists between neighborhoods that are designated as food deserts (i.e., limited access to affordable and nutritious food such as supermarkets) and obesity prevalence. High neighborhood walkability is associated with reduced obesity prevalence. Other neighborhood characteristics such as neighborhood disorder, deprivation, and crime also play a role in obesity. For example, people living in high-crime areas have decreased odds of having higher physical activity levels. Moreover, compared to urban areas, rural areas tend to have longer distances between residences and opportunities for walking and other physical activities, all of which affect the inhabitants' ability to engage in healthy habits that can prevent obesity.

Behavioral Factors

(i) **Diet** – Obesity occurs when the body's energy balance is positive (i.e., when energy intake exceeds energy expenditure). The following dietary factors that impact energy intake have been implicated in the development of obesity: increased consumption of fat and carbohydrate-dense foods; high intake of sugar-sweetened beverages and processed foods; low intake of fruits, vegetables, and fiber; irregular eating patterns; and excessive alcohol consumption [20].

(ii) **Physical activity and sedentary behavior** – Reduced energy expenditure is due to low levels of physical activity and high sedentary behavior such as prolonged watching of television and playing of video games (increased screen time) [21]. Physical inactivity and sedentary behavior are significantly associated with a high risk of obesity and metabolic syndrome. For example, in NHANES 1999–2000, adults who did not participate in moderate-to-vigorous physical activity during their leisure time had approximately twice the odds of having metabolic syndrome compared to those who reported participating in more than 150 min of moderate-to-vigorous physical activity per week [22]. Similarly, the odds of having metabolic syndrome increased for each 1 h/day increase in watching television or videos or using a computer outside of work [22].

(iii) **Sleep** – Sleep duration and quality also contribute to obesity and metabolic syndrome. Short duration of sleep is associated with obesity and metabolic syndrome risk factors and outcomes [23]. Restricted sleep time as

may be seen in individuals with night shift schedules may result in less moderate to vigorous physical activity, and increased dietary intake, particularly of high-fat foods [24–26].

Socioeconomic Factors

The prevalence of obesity varies by education and socioeconomic status. The association between obesity and education and socioeconomic status is complex and further differs by race/ethnicity and sex [27]. In the 2011–2014 NHANES, adults with high school or less education have a higher age-adjusted obesity prevalence (40.0%) compared with those with college degrees (27.8%) [27]. Considering race/ethnicity, this pattern was also observed among non-Hispanic White and Black, and Hispanic women. However, among non-Hispanic Black men, the prevalence of obesity increased as level of education increased. Finally, these differences in obesity prevalence and educational attainment were not seen in non-Hispanic Asian men and women, as well as Hispanic men. With regards to income, women in the highest income group (>350% of federal poverty level, FPL) had a lower obesity prevalence (29.7%) compared to those in the middle – defined as >130% to might d FPL (42.9%), and lower – defined as ≤130% of FPL (45.2%) income groups [27]. For women, the pattern for the association was seen among Hispanic women, non-Hispanic Asian, and White women, although it was only significant for White women. There was no difference in the prevalence of obesity and income groups among non-Hispanic Black women. However, in men, obesity prevalence was lower in the lowest (31.5%) and highest (32.6%) income groups compared to the middle-income group (38.5%) [27]. This trend was also seen among Hispanic men and non-Hispanic White even though it was not statistically significant among White men. Among non-Hispanic Black men, the pattern was reversed; obesity prevalence was greater in the highest-income group (42.7%) compared to those in the lowest-income group (33.8%). No such difference existed among non-Hispanic Asian men [27].

In 1988–2012 NHANES, those with lower educational levels had significantly increased odds of metabolic syndrome compared to those with a college education or higher [12]. This was confirmed in 1999–2018 NHANES, which showed that highly educated adults (college graduates and higher) and those with higher income (income-to-poverty ratio ≥3.5) had reduced risk for metabolic syndrome, and attributed this to the fact that adults with high income and education may have more knowledge about how to avoid metabolic risk factors [28].

Childhood Obesity

Childhood obesity is defined as a BMI of ≥95th percentile for age and sex. Children with BMI ≥120% of the 95th percentile for age and sex are classified as having severe obesity [29]. Childhood obesity is a multifactorial public health challenge with increasing prevalence over the last decade [1]. Childhood obesity prevalence rates were about 5% in mid-twentieth century but tripled between 2017 and 2018 [30]. In 2017–2020, the CDC reported that obesity prevalence in children aged 2–19 years was 19.7%, with about 14.7 million children and adolescents impacted. Hispanic children and non-Hispanic Black children were disproportionately affected with a prevalence of 26.2% and 24.8%, respectively. Obesity prevalence was 16.6% among non-Hispanic White children and 9% among non-Hispanic Asian children [1]. The trend in obesity varies across various age groups, with increasing prevalence observed with increasing age [31]. The prevalence estimates among children aged 2–5 years, 6–11 years, and 12–19 years were 13.9%, 18.4%, and 20.6%, respectively, in 2015–2016 [32]. These findings are concerning given the myriad of obesity-related health consequences and the tendency for childhood obesity to persist into adulthood.

The etiology of childhood obesity is multifactorial. Genetic predisposition has been reported with monogenic and polygenic factors identified [33]. Epigenetic factors have been associated with parental obesity, maternal weight gain during pregnancy, gestational diabetes, and maternal smoking [34]. Children with at least one parent with obesity have an increased risk of developing obesity [35, 36]. The environment also plays a crucial role in the subsequent development of obesity. Access to fresh and healthy foods, intake of sugar-sweetened beverages, sedentary lifestyle, duration of sleep, avenues for physical activity, and the presence and proximity of unhealthy food outlets, psychosocial stress, and screen time are contributory factors to childhood obesity [37–39]. Sugar-sweetened beverages can contribute a substantial portion to the total caloric intake of children [40]. There is a positive association between its intake and childhood obesity, with the American Academy of Pediatrics advocating for policy implementation to curtail consumption in children and adolescents [29, 41]. A randomized trial of sugar-sweetened beverages and adolescent body weight showed a smaller increase in BMI in those randomized to receive a 1-year intervention to decrease sugar-sweetened beverage intake (experimental group), compared to the control group. However, this was not observed at the 2-year follow-up [42]. Children currently spend more time watching television using digital devices including mobile phones and video games. This practice has been associated with obesity [43], with a greater risk of obesity associated with more than 2 h per day of television screen time [44]. Screen time reduces the time children spend being physically active and impacts the duration or quality of sleep time [45]. Additionally, there have been reports that children tend to adopt unhealthy eating habits from watching food advertisements on digital media [46]. Poor sleeping patterns including short duration of sleep have been associated with an increased risk of childhood overweight and obesity [47]. Psychosocial stress, depression, and adverse childhood experiences including a history of abuse (sexual, physical, or emotional), parental loss, dysfunctional homes, and unstable home finances have been shown to increase the risk of childhood obesity [48–51].

The clinical practice guidelines for the evaluation and treatment of children and adolescents with obesity published by the American Academy of Pediatrics provides a comprehensive framework on childhood obesity assessment and treatment options, including diet, physical activity, individual and family therapy, pharmacotherapy, and surgery [29].

Health Implications and Diseases Associated with Rising Obesity Trends

Obesity is associated with significant morbidity and mortality. A microsimulation model including the US adults between 1999 and 2016 estimated that more than 1300 excess deaths per day (almost 500,000 per year) and loss in life expectancy of about 2.4 years in 2016 were attributable to excess weight. The estimates showed that excess weight accounted for higher mortality when compared to smoking [52]. A meta-analysis of 230 cohort studies showed an increased risk of all-cause mortality in individuals with overweight or obesity [53]. Obesity is also associated with several cardiovascular diseases and risk factors including diabetes mellitus, hypertension, and dyslipidemia.

Obesity is associated with elevated blood pressure and the development of hypertension [54–56]. There is a strong association between visceral adiposity and incident hypertension [57]. Using data from Framingham Heart Study participants aged 35–75 years, with a 44-year follow-up, the age-adjusted relative risk for incident hypertension was associated with being in the overweight category was 1.46 in men versus 1.75 in women, respectively [56]. Several mechanisms have been proposed as potential explanations for the elevated blood pressure associated with obesity [58]. Obesity is associated with elevations in systemic vascular resistance and increased activation of the renin-angiotensin-aldosterone system. These factors coupled with the activation of the sympathetic nervous system, and compression of kidneys by visceral/perirenal fat, create a vicious cycle that ultimately culminates in renal injury and chronic kidney disease [58]. Insulin resistance and hyperinsulinemia, and sleep apnea may also have a contributory role in the development of hypertension in individuals with obesity [58].

Dyslipidemia and type 2 diabetes mellitus have been strongly associated with obesity. A study investigating the burden of obesity on incident diabetes mellitus in the United States from 2001 to 2016 with data from MESA and NHANES reported that approximately 30–53% of incident diabetes mellitus was attributable to obesity [59]. Obesity is associated with elevations in serum triglycerides, total cholesterol, low-density lipoprotein cholesterol, and reduced levels of high-density lipoprotein cholesterol [60].

Obesity is associated with increased risk of coronary heart disease [61]. Obesity accentuates the atherosclerotic process that usually begins in early life through inflammatory mechanisms and insulin resistance, as well as through other cardiovascular risk factors such as dyslipidemia, hypertension, and diabetes [62]. However, obesity may be independently associated with atherosclerosis, with central adiposity playing a significant role in the pathophysiology [62]. Obesity has been implicated in the development of heart failure. Using data from over 5000 participants in the Framingham Heart Study, investigators showed an increased heart failure risk of 5% for men and 7% for women for each unit increase in BMI after accounting for risk factors [63]. Obesity results in myocardial fat deposition, fibrosis, left ventricular remodeling, right ventricular dilatation, and dysfunction [62]. Alternatively, obesity leads to systolic dysfunction and heart failure through atherosclerotic heart disease. Obesity has been associated with sudden cardiac death (SCD) and increased arrhythmia risk. Obesity is commonly identified as a nonischemic etiology for SCD, and this may be related to the distribution of body fat [64, 65]. It is associated with an increased risk of arrhythmias including ventricular tachycardia, ventricular fibrillation, and atrial fibrillation [62, 66, 67]. Epicardial adiposity and subsequent scar tissue formation may drive arrhythmias and increased SCD risk [68, 69].

Obesity is strongly associated with incident atrial fibrillation, increased risk of postoperative atrial fibrillation, post-ablation atrial fibrillation, and progression of paroxysmal atrial fibrillation to permanent atrial fibrillation [70, 71]. Obesity-associated structural changes in the heart including atrial remodeling, and electrical remodeling creates an arrhythmogenic substrate. Additionally, epicardial fat deposition may be implicated in the pathophysiology of atrial fibrillation [72].

While obesity is associated with increased cardiovascular risk, individuals with established coronary heart disease or heart failure with overweight or obesity may have a better prognosis than those with coronary heart disease or heart failure at normal weight, in what is termed "the obesity paradox" [73]. This may be explained by reverse causality with patients with underweight or normal weight being sicker or the inability of BMI to distinguish between fat versus lean mass.

Obesity is associated with gastrointestinal complications including hepatobiliary disease and gastroesophageal reflux disease (GERD). Nonalcoholic fatty liver disease (NAFLD), which encompasses nonalcoholic fatty liver (NAFL) and nonalcoholic steatohepatitis (NASH), is associated with obesity and metabolic syndrome [74]. In NAFL, there is hepatic steatosis with no associated inflammation, whereas NASH is associated with inflammatory changes. NAFLD is the most common liver condition worldwide and could potentially progress to cirrhosis and hepatocellular carcinoma [75]. A systematic review and meta-analysis reported an overall prevalence of NAFLD worldwide as 32.4% [75]. The reported prevalence of NAFLD in the United States has been increasing over time. Data from NHANES indicate that the prevalence of NAFLD doubled between 2005 and 2008 (11%) when compared to the prevalence between 1988 and 1994 (5.5%). These changes corresponded to increasing prevalence of various components of the metabolic syndrome within the same time periods [76]. The prevalence of NAFLD between 1999 and 2004 was 9.8%. A two-hit hypothesis is also suggested to explain the pathophysiology of NAFLD. Insulin resistance results from liver fat accumulation, which subsequently promotes inflammatory changes, oxidative injury, and fibrosis [74]. Additionally, genomic studies have identified genetic variants including PNPLA3 (patatin-like phospholipase domain-containing protein 3), TM6SF2 (transmembrane

6 superfamily member 2), and IFNL4 (interferon lambda 4), with risk of NAFL progression to NASH [74, 77]. Increased hepatic iron and plasma leptin, decreased adiponectin, intestinal bacterial overgrowth, incretins, antioxidant deficiency, and bile acids have been implicated in the pathogenesis of NAFLD [78].

Respiratory diseases associated with obesity include obstructive sleep apnea, asthma, respiratory infections, and obesity hypoventilation syndrome. Obesity is associated with increased incidence and prevalence of asthma [79]. Asthma symptoms present similarly in obese and non-obese individuals. However, severe symptoms tend to be greater in those with obesity, with poor asthma control, and higher likelihood of needing oral steroid therapy. Additionally, individuals with obesity have a greater risk of being hospitalized for asthma exacerbation compared with those without obesity. Obesity hypoventilation syndrome (Pickwickian syndrome) is associated with severe obesity. Obesity hypoventilation syndrome has a multifactorial pathogenesis which includes disordered breathing patterns during sleep as seen with obstructive sleep apnea, increased carbon dioxide production, and impaired pulmonary dynamics or control of ventilation [80, 81]. Most patients with obesity hypoventilation syndrome have concurrent obstructive sleep apnea. Individuals with obesity have an increased risk of infections including influenza and are likely to have respiratory complications and be hospitalized during the influenza period [82]. During the coronavirus disease 2019 (COVID-19) pandemic, obesity was associated with increased risk of hospitalization including intensive care admission, intubation, and death [83–85].

Obesity is linked with an increased risk of several cancers including colorectal, biliary tract, pancreatic, breast, esophageal, and ovarian malignancies. In 2014, overweight and obesity were reported to cause about 40% of all cancers [86, 87]. In the United States, greater than 684,000 obesity-associated cancers occur yearly [87]. Overweight and obesity can also increase the likelihood of mortality from cancer. Obesity-associated breast cancer after menopause is the most common obesity-associated cancer among women, as compared to colorectal cancer among men [87]. The increased risk of obesity-associated cancer could be explained by several mechanisms including excess production of estrogen by adipose tissue which leads to increased risk of endometrial, breast, and ovarian cancers. Additionally, increased insulin and insulin-like growth factor-1 levels, chronic inflammatory changes with resultant oxidative stress, and fat cell production of adipokines may explain the association between obesity and cancer [88].

There is an increased risk of osteoarthritis and gouty arthritis with obesity. A meta-analysis showed that a BMI increase by 5 units was associated with a 35% increased risk of knee osteoarthritis (risk ratio [RR] 1.35, 95% CI 1.21, 1.51) [89]. Individuals with obesity are likely to have severe joint disease and a large proportion may need hip or knee replacement [90].

Anxiety, depression, and stigma are important psychosocial challenges associated with obesity. Individuals with obesity may experience stigma in several fields including employment, healthcare, and education [91]. Obesity and metabolic syndrome are risks factor for chronic kidney disease. Glomerular changes such as focal segmental glomerulosclerosis have been associated with severe obesity, with some reversal of changes noted with weight loss [92–94]. Obesity may pose a barrier to renal transplantation. Additionally, dialysis in patients with obesity may be fraught with challenges due to vascular access or malfunctioning of catheters [95]. The economic impact of obesity in the United States is enormous. Obesity-related medical care cost in 2019 was about $173 billion. Obesity-related absenteeism results in annual productivity costs between $3.38 billion and $6.38 billion [96].

Obesity Management

Obesity is associated with significant morbidity and mortality, which can be reduced with changes including lifestyle modification, pharmacotherapy, or surgical procedures that result in weight loss. It is important to address treatment of comorbidities

such as hypertension, diabetes mellitus, hyperlipidemia, and sleep apnea, with appropriate specialist referral as needed.

Lifestyle Modification

Patients who are overweight with no cardiovascular risk factors or coexisting comorbidities can be managed with lifestyle modification including dietary changes, behavior modification, and physical activity. A clinical trial comparing reductions in the incidence of type 2 diabetes with lifestyle modification versus metformin showed that after an average follow-up of 2.8 years, diabetes incidence was 7.8 in the metformin arm versus 4.8 cases per 100 person-years in the lifestyle group [97]. The incidence of diabetes in the placebo group was 11 cases per 100-person years. The lifestyle modification arm had reduction in diabetes incidence by 58%, compared to 31% in the metformin arm [97]. Over a longer follow-up period, there was reported reduction in CVD risk factors among those in the lifestyle modification arm [98, 99]. Subsequently, another trial in patients with type 2 diabetes mellitus investigating the effect of intensive lifestyle modification on a primary outcome of a composite of death for CVD, nonfatal myocardial infarction/stroke, or hospitalization for angina did not show a reduction in events with the lifestyle intervention arm. However, patients randomized to the intervention group had greater weight loss and reductions in glycated hemoglobin [100].

Behavioral modifications include setting a weight loss goal of 5–10% over 6 months or 0.5–1 kg weight loss per week. These goals should be SMART (specific, measurable, achievable, reasonable, and time-bound) and should be based on patient-clinician shared decision-making [101]. Important behavioral modifications include keeping food diaries, self-weighing, record of activities, portion control, environmental changes to minimize overeating, and meal planning [102, 103]. Enrolling in behavioral-based programs or commercial weight loss programs may also be beneficial [104]. Physical activity is beneficial in lowering the rates of many chronic comorbidities [105]. Programs that employ exercise in addition to moderate or severe caloric restriction showed little incremental weight loss with exercise, although it improves glycemic control and cardiopulmonary function and overall health [106, 107]. Aerobic exercises can improve functional status, systemic blood pressure, body composition, abdominal obesity, and serum lipoprotein concentrations [108]. Most health benefits of exercise, weight reduction, and weight maintenance after weight loss are achieved with at least 150 min of moderate physical activity or at 75 or more minutes of vigorous aerobic exercises weekly. In addition to routine non-exercise activity such as standing, walking, and climbing, physical activity goals can aim for 5000–10,000 daily steps [109]. More benefits are attained with increase in intensity and duration of exercise [109].

Dietary modifications to improve overall cardiovascular health include an emphasis on whole grain food, fruits and vegetables, healthy protein sources such as fish, seafood, nuts, and legumes, low fat or fat-free dairy, lean meat, poultry, and plant oils such as soybean oil. The intake of red meat, processed meats, ultra-processed food, beverages and food with added sugars, and alcoholic beverage intake should be minimized [110]. The Mediterranean diet is one with strong evidence in favor of reducing atherosclerotic cardiovascular disease [109, 111]. This dietary pattern is rich in fruits, vegetables, beans, nuts, and whole grains. Moderate intake of seafood, poultry, fermented dairy products (e.g., cheese), and alcohol forms part of this diet. Saturated fats, high amounts of red meat, and ultra-processed carbohydrates are discouraged. A very low-carbohydrate diet may be associated with short-term weight loss [109].

The Dietary Approaches to Stop Hypertension (DASH) diet has been shown to lower systolic and diastolic blood pressure [112]. The DASH diet encourages the intake of vegetables, fruits, whole grains, and fat-free or low-fat dairy products while limiting sodium (1500–2300 mg daily), total fat (about 27% of total daily calories), and saturated fat (<6% of total daily calories). The DASH diet may produce modest weight loss [109]. Carbohydrate-restricted low-calorie diets

may improve triglyceride and fasting glucose levels, in addition to modest weight loss when compared to fat-restricted diets (10–30% of total calories from fat). However, the weight reduction achieved from both diets may be comparable after about 6 months. A low-carbohydrate diet consists of about 50–150 g of carbohydrates per day, and a very low-carbohydrate diet has <50 g of carbohydrates per day. Ketogenic diet helps with weight loss and reduces hunger but may result in increased levels of low-density lipoprotein cholesterol levels [109, 113]. Ketogenic diet has less than 20 g of carbohydrate intake daily, adequate protein intake, and a higher intake of dietary fat during the induction phase. A very low-calorie diet with energy level ~ 400–800 kcal/day may promote rapid weight loss in the short-term [109], hence may be helpful for those preparing for surgical intervention. However, this dietary pattern is not sustainable in the long term.

Fasting has been used as a weight loss strategy and may range from periodic, to intermittent, to alternative day or time-restricted feeding [109]. Intermittent fasting may have variations ranging from limited food intake for 2 days and resumption of normal feeding for 5 days within the week (5:2 protocol), 1 day of limited food intake and normal food intake for 2 days (2:1 protocol), to alternating limited and full dietary intake (1:1 protocol) [109]. Food is limited to a fixed time during the day with time-restricted feeding. With periodic fasting, food is limited for more than 2 consecutive days, and this is followed by a week of normal dietary intake [109]. These dietary patterns may help weight loss but may not be sustainable in the long term. Moreover, intermittent fasting may not be appropriate for those at risk of hypoglycemia or with eating disorders [109].

Motivational Interviewing

Motivational interviewing is a patient-centered approach that allows patients and their families to identify aspects of behaviors that could be modified to improve overall health [114]. This could range from modifications in sedentary behavior patterns to improving food choices to include healthy ones. Intensive health behavior and lifestyle treatment (IHBLT) plays a pivotal role in childhood obesity management [115]. It involves a multidisciplinary approach in partnership with patients and their families which provides comprehensive health education and skill empowerment in several areas such as healthy eating habits and physical activity, which usually take place in healthcare centers or community-based settings over several months [116]. It is important for healthcare providers to promptly refer children who are overweight or obese to these programs. Other important lifestyle modifications to reinforce in patients and their families include limiting screen time [117], reduction of sugar-sweetened beverage intake [118], and moderate to vigorous physical activity (≥ 1 h/day) [119].

Pharmacotherapy for Obesity

Drugs are available for chronic weight management. It is important to combine these medications with lifestyle changes. Medications are indicated for those who are obese (BMI > 30 kg/m^2) or have BMI of 27–29.9 kg/m^2 with related health conditions, i.e., diabetes, NAFLD, sleep apnea, and cardiovascular disease.

Orlistat inhibits pancreatic lipase resulting in increased fat excretion, with demonstrable effect on weight loss [120, 121]. Orlistat is approved for children 12 years and older. It may be associated with improvement in blood pressure and lipid levels. Adverse effects with its use are predominantly gastrointestinal and include flatus, cramps, and fecal incontinence. It also lowers levels of fat-soluble vitamins (A, D, E, and K), and it is associated with oxalate-induced acute kidney injury [122]. Combination medications approved for weight loss include phentermine-topiramate, which is approved for obesity treatment in patients 12 years and older [123]. In a randomized trial, the combination therapy phentermine-topiramate showed a statistically significant reduction in BMI and improvement in lipid profile (HDL and TG) among adolescents with obesity

[124]. Topiramate, a carbonic anhydrase, acts as a central appetite suppressant. Phentermine, a norepinephrine reuptake inhibitor, is approved for short-term use (12 weeks) among adolescents 16 years and older. Longer duration of use was associated with adverse cardiovascular events including elevated heart rate and blood pressure, at the expense of modest reductions in BMI [125].

Bupropion-naltrexone is approved by the FDA for weight loss [126]. Its use can be associated with dizziness, nausea, vomiting, elevated heart rate, and transient increase in blood pressure as adverse effects. It is contraindicated in patients with a seizure disorder, uncontrolled hypertension, or eating disorders. Sympathomimetic drugs approved for short-term use include phentermine. It is associated with elevations in heart rate and blood pressure. Additionally, there is risk of abuse given its amphetamine-like effects.

The incretins, glucagon-like peptide 1 (GLP-1), and glucose-dependent insulinotropic polypeptide (GIP) have a significant role in weight loss. They stimulate glucose-dependent insulin release. GLP-1 reduces gastric emptying, blocks glucagon release, and suppresses appetite. Glucagon-like peptide-1 receptor agonists act centrally and slow gastric emptying to aid with weight loss. This class of drugs includes liraglutide, dulaglutide, exenatide, and semaglutide. Adverse events with GLP-1 receptor agonist drug are predominantly gastrointestinal (nausea and vomiting) and an increased risk of medullary thyroid cancer. Semaglutide is a once-weekly injection with demonstrable greater weight loss (change in weight -17.7 kg [95% CI -21.8 to -13.7]) in a 68-week clinical trial [127]. GLP-1 receptor agonists, semaglutide and liraglutide, which are subcutaneous injections, were approved as first-line pharmacotherapy for obesity in the United States [128]. These can be used in patients with or without diabetes. Semaglutide is a once-weekly injection as compared to liraglutide which is once daily. Semaglutide is associated with greater weight loss (-15.8% vs. -6.4%) than liraglutide as demonstrated in the STEP 8 clinical trial [128]. There is an oral formulation of semaglutide, but this is not approved yet for obesity treatment. In the STEP 1 trial, individuals randomized to 68 weeks of once-weekly subcutaneous 2.4 mg injectable semaglutide in addition to lifestyle intervention had greater mean weight loss(-15.3 vs. -2.6 kg) compared to placebo [129]. Gastrointestinal side effects including nausea, vomiting, and diarrhea were common in the treatment group (4.5 vs. 0.8%) [129]. There is risk of weight regain after discontinuing the medication [130]. Semaglutide also reduces major adverse cardiovascular events in patients with type 2 diabetes and established cardiovascular disease or chronic kidney disease [131]. Semaglutide is contraindicated in patients with history of pancreatitis or family history of medullary thyroid carcinoma or multiple endocrine neoplasia 2A or 2B [132]. It is also not to be used in pregnancy. Liraglutide is approved for obesity treatment in individuals 12 years and older, who may or may not have type 2 diabetes [133]. Liraglutide causes weight loss in patients with or without diabetes. It is also associated with reduction in major adverse cardiovascular events in patients with type 2 diabetes and cardiovascular disease [134].

The dual-acting GLP-1 and GIP receptor agonist, tirzepatide is a once-weekly injection, which is effective for obesity treatment in those with or without diabetes [135]. In a randomized trial of over 2500 adults with obesity without diabetes, weekly tirzepatide at doses of 5, 10, and 15 mg resulted in significant weight loss at 72 weeks when compared to placebo(-16.1 kg, -22.2 kg, and -23.6 kg vs. -2.4 kg) [135]. Adverse effects included nausea, constipation, and diarrhea, commonly at higher administered doses.

Bariatric Surgery

According to the recommendation of the American Society for Metabolic and Bariatric Surgery, bariatric surgery is indicated for adults with BMI ≥ 35 kg/m^2 irrespective of comorbidities, adults with BMI between 30 and 34.9 kg/m^2 with type 2 diabetes, or in the latter BMI category with no sustainable weight loss on medical and/or lifestyle interventions [136]. Bariatric surgery involves multidisciplinary assessment and preoperative preparation involving lifestyle

modifications such as smoking cessation, reducing alcohol intake, physical activity, and participation in weight loss programs geared towards dietary changes. Bariatric surgery leads to weight loss and reduces comorbidities associated with obesity, mainly diabetes for which there could be remission [137].

Pediatric bariatric surgery is a viable treatment option that provides an improvement in BMI and comorbidities [138–140]. It involves a multidisciplinary and comprehensive assessment to determine eligibility. Surgery can be considered in patients with Class 2 obesity, BMI > 35 kg/m^2 or 120% of the 95th percentile for age and sex (whichever is lower), and additionally have significant comorbidities such as diabetes, hypertension, hyperlipidemia, and obstructive sleep apnea. Alternatively, those with Class 3 obesity, BMI > 40 kg/m^2 or 140% of the 95th percentile for age and sex (whichever is lower) can be considered for surgery, with or without comorbid conditions [139].

Conclusion

The prevalence of obesity is rapidly increasing in the US and worldwide. Hence, it is important to implement preventive and therapeutic measures to address the burden of complications related to obesity. Part of this involves acknowledging obesity as a disease, as well as accounting for the associated comorbidities. Lifestyle modification involving changes in dietary patterns and increased physical activity, to prevent or address obesity, should be reinforced. Additionally, clinicians should utilize the whole range of therapies available, including GLP-1 receptor agonists and dual GLP-1 and GIP agonists. Access to medications and improved insurance coverage will lead to a higher number of patients getting access to the required prescriptions. Future studies should focus on developing newer medications such as bimagrumab to increase muscle mass, reduce fat, and improve glycemia, and triple GIP, GLP-1, and glucagon receptor agonists targeting various pathways to aid in weight loss [141, 142].

References

1. Childhood Obesity Facts|Overweight & Obesity| CDC. https://www.cdc.gov/obesity/data/childhood. html. Accessed 11 Mar 2023.
2. Obesity and overweight. https://www.who.int/news-room/fact-sheets/detail/obesity-and-overweight. Accessed 11 Mar 2023.
3. Body Mass Index (BMI)|Healthy Weight, Nutrition, and Physical Activity|CDC. https://www.cdc.gov/healthyweight/assessing/bmi/index.html. Accessed 11 Mar 2023.
4. MacMahon S, Baigent C, Duffy S, et al. Body-mass index and cause-specific mortality in 900 000 adults: collaborative analyses of 57 prospective studies. Lancet (London, England). 2009;373(9669):1083–96. https://doi.org/10.1016/S0140-6736(09)60318-4.
5. Grossman DC, Bibbins-Domingo K, Curry SJ, et al. Screening for obesity in children and adolescents us preventive services task force recommendation statement. JAMA. 2022;317(23):2417–26. https://doi.org/10.1001/JAMA.2017.6803.
6. Kon Koh K, Hwan Han S, Quon MJ, Korea S. Inflammatory markers and the metabolic syndrome insights from therapeutic interventions. J Am Coll Cardiol. 2005. https://doi.org/10.1016/j.jacc.2005.06.082.
7. Lindsay RS, Howard BV. Cardiovascular risk associated with the metabolic syndrome. Curr Diab Rep. 2004;4(1):63–8. https://doi.org/10.1007/S11892-004-0013-9.
8. Genuth S, Alberti KGMM, Bennett P, et al. Follow-up report on the diagnosis of diabetes mellitus. Diabetes Care. 2003;26(11):3160–7. https://doi.org/10.2337/DIACARE.26.11.3160.
9. Grundy SM, Cleeman JI, Daniels SR, et al. Diagnosis and management of the metabolic syndrome: an American Heart Association/National Heart, Lung, and Blood Institute Scientific Statement. Circulation. 2005;112(17):2735–52. https://doi.org/10.1161/CIRCULATIONAHA.105.169404.
10. Lewis KH, Basu S. Epidemiology of obesity in the United States. Metab Syndr. 2016;13–31. https://doi.org/10.1007/978-3-319-11251-0_2.
11. Temple NJ. The origins of the obesity epidemic in the USA–lessons for today. Nutrients. 2022;14(20):4253. https://doi.org/10.3390/NU14204253.
12. Moore JX, Chaudhary N, Akinyemiju T. Metabolic syndrome prevalence by race/ethnicity and sex in the United States, National Health and Nutrition Examination Survey, 1988–2012. Prev Chronic Dis 2019;14(3):E24. https://doi.org/10.5888/PCD14.160287.
13. State of Obesity 2022: Better Policies for a Healthier America – TFAH. https://www.tfah.org/report-details/state-of-obesity-2022/. Accessed 11 Mar 2023.
14. Overweight & Obesity Statistics – NIDDK. https://www.niddk.nih.gov/health-information/health-statistics/overweight-obesity. Accessed 11 Mar 2023.
15. Aguilar M, Bhuket T, Torres S, Liu B, Wong RJ. Prevalence of the metabolic syndrome in the United States, 2003–2012. JAMA. 2015;313(19):1973–4. https://doi.org/10.1001/JAMA.2015.4260.
16. Hirode G, Wong RJ. Trends in the prevalence of metabolic syndrome in the United States, 2011–2016. JAMA. 2020;323(24):2526. https://doi.org/10.1001/JAMA.2020.4501.
17. Stierman B, Afful J, Carroll MD, et al. National Health and Nutrition Examination Survey 2017–March 2020 prepandemic data files development of files and prevalence estimates for selected health outcomes. Natl Health Stat Rep. 2021;158. https://doi.org/10.15620/CDC:106273.
18. Lee A, Cardel M, Donahoo WT. Social and environmental factors influencing obesity. Endotext. October 2019. https://www.ncbi.nlm.nih.gov/books/NBK278977/. Accessed 11 Mar 2023.
19. Li F, Harmer P, Cardinal BJ, Bosworth M, Johnson-Shelton D. Obesity and the built environment: does the density of neighborhood fast-food outlets matter? Am J Health Promot. 2009;23(3):203. https://doi.org/10.4278/AJHP.071214133.
20. Mozaffarian D, Hao T, Rimm EB, Willett WC, Hu FB. Changes in diet and lifestyle and long-term weight gain in women and men. N Engl J Med. 2011;364(25):2392–404. https://doi.org/10.1056/NEJMOA1014296.
21. Ford ES, Li C. Physical activity or fitness and the metabolic syndrome. Expert Rev Cardiovasc Ther. 2006;4(6):897–915. https://doi.org/10.1586/14779072.4.6.897.
22. Ford ES, Kohl HW, Mokdad AH, Ajani UA. Sedentary behavior, physical activity, and the metabolic syndrome among U.S. adults. Obes Res. 2005;13(3):608–14. https://doi.org/10.1038/OBY.2005.65.
23. Cappuccio FP, Miller MA. Sleep and cardiometabolic disease. Curr Cardiol Rep. 2017;19(11):110. https://doi.org/10.1007/S11886-017-0916-0.
24. Arble DM, Bass J, Behn CD, et al. Impact of sleep and circadian disruption on energy balance and diabetes: a summary of workshop discussions. Sleep. 2015;38(12):1849–60. https://doi.org/10.5665/SLEEP.5226.
25. Markwald RR, Melanson EL, Smith MR, et al. Impact of insufficient sleep on total daily energy expenditure, food intake, and weight gain. Proc Natl Acad Sci U S A. 2013;110(14):5695–700. https://doi.org/10.1073/PNAS.1216951110.
26. Reutrakul S, Van Cauter E. Sleep influences on obesity, insulin resistance, and risk of type 2 diabetes. Metabolism. 2018;84:56–66. https://doi.org/10.1016/J.METABOL.2018.02.010.
27. Ogden CL, Fakhouri TH, Carroll MD, et al. Prevalence of obesity among adults, by household income and education – United States, 2011–2014. MMWR Morb Mortal Wkly Rep. 2017;66(50):1369–73. https://doi.org/10.15585/MMWR.MM6650A1.

28. Yang C, Jia X, Wang Y, et al. Trends and influence factors in the prevalence, intervention, and control of metabolic syndrome among US adults, 1999–2018. BMC Geriatr. 2022;22(1):1–14. https://doi.org/10.1186/S12877-022-03672-6/FIGURES/3.

29. Hampl SE, Hassink SG, Skinner AC, et al. Clinical practice guideline for the evaluation and treatment of children and adolescents with obesity. Pediatrics. 2023;151(2):e2022060640. https://doi.org/10.1542/PEDS.2022-060640/190443.

30. Products – Health E Stats – Prevalence of overweight, obesity, and severe obesity among children and adolescents aged 2–19 years: United States, 1963–1965 through 2017–2018. https://www.cdc.gov/nchs/data/hestat/obesity-child-17-18/obesity-child.htm. Accessed 11 Mar 2023.

31. Ogden CL, Fryar CD, Martin CB, et al. Trends in obesity prevalence by race and hispanic origin – 1999–2000 to 2017–2018. JAMA. 2021;324(12):1208–10. https://doi.org/10.1001/JAMA.2020.14590.

32. Hales CM, Fryar CD, Carroll MD, Freedman DS, Ogden CL. Trends in obesity and severe obesity prevalence in US youth and adults by sex and age, 2007–2008 to 2015–2016. JAMA. 2018;319(16):1723–5. https://doi.org/10.1001/JAMA.2018.3060.

33. Loos RJF, Yeo GSH. The genetics of obesity: from discovery to biology. Nat Rev Genet. 2022;23(2):120–33. https://doi.org/10.1038/S41576-021-00414-Z.

34. Larqué E, Labayen I, Flodmark CE, et al. From conception to infancy – early risk factors for childhood obesity. Nat Rev Endocrinol. 2019;15(8):456–78. https://doi.org/10.1038/S41574-019-0219-1.

35. Isganaitis E, Suehiro H, Cardona C. Who's your daddy?: paternal inheritance of metabolic disease risk. Curr Opin Endocrinol Diabetes Obes. 2017;24(1):47–55. https://doi.org/10.1097/MED.0000000000000307.

36. Whitaker RC, Wright JA, Pepe MS, Seidel KD, Dietz WH. Predicting obesity in young adulthood from childhood and parental obesity. N Engl J Med. 1997;337(13):204. https://doi.org/10.1056/NEJM199709253371301.

37. Zhou Q, Zhao L, Zhang L, et al. Neighborhood supermarket access and childhood obesity: a systematic review. Obes Rev. 2021;22(Suppl 1):e12937. https://doi.org/10.1111/OBR.12937.

38. Kim Y, Cubbin C, Oh S. A systematic review of neighbourhood economic context on child obesity and obesity-related behaviours. Obes Rev. 2019;20(3):420–31. https://doi.org/10.1111/OBR.12792.

39. Yang S, Zhang X, Feng P, et al. Access to fruit and vegetable markets and childhood obesity: a systematic review. Obes Rev. 2021;22(Suppl 1):10.1111/OBR.12980.

40. Wang YC, Bleich SN, Gortmaker SL. Increasing caloric contribution from sugar-sweetened beverages and 100% fruit juices among US children and adolescents, 1988–2004. Pediatrics. 2008;121(6):e1604. https://doi.org/10.1542/PEDS.2007-2834.

41. Luger M, Lafontan M, Bes-Rastrollo M, Winzer E, Yumuk V, Farpour-Lambert N. Sugar-sweetened beverages and weight gain in children and adults: a systematic review from 2013 to 2015 and a comparison with previous studies. Obes Facts. 2017;10(6):674–93. https://doi.org/10.1159/000484566.

42. Ebbeling CB, Feldman HA, Chomitz VR, et al. A randomized trial of sugar-sweetened beverages and adolescent body weight. N Engl J Med. 2012;367(15):1407–16. https://doi.org/10.1056/NEJMOA1203388.

43. Falbe J, Rosner B, Willett WC, Sonneville KR, Hu FB, Field AE. Adiposity and different types of screen time. Pediatrics. 2013;132(6):e1497. https://doi.org/10.1542/PEDS.2013-0887.

44. Poorolajal J, Sahraei F, Mohamdadi Y, Doosti-Irani A, Moradi L. Behavioral factors influencing childhood obesity: a systematic review and meta-analysis. Obes Res Clin Pract. 2020;14(2):109–18. https://doi.org/10.1016/J.ORCP.2020.03.002.

45. Stiglic N, Viner RM. Effects of screentime on the health and well-being of children and adolescents: a systematic review of reviews. BMJ Open. 2019;9(1):e023191. https://doi.org/10.1136/BMJOPEN-2018-023191.

46. Boyland EJ, Harrold JA, Kirkham TC, et al. Food commercials increase preference for energy-dense foods, particularly in children who watch more television. Pediatrics. 2011;128(1):e93–100. https://doi.org/10.1542/PEDS.2010-1859.

47. Ruan H, Xun P, Cai W, He K, Tang Q. Habitual sleep duration and risk of childhood obesity: systematic review and dose-response meta-analysis of prospective cohort studies. Sci Rep. 2015;5:16160. https://doi.org/10.1038/SREP16160.

48. Jackson DB, Chilton M, Johnson KR, Vaughn MG. Adverse childhood experiences and household food insecurity: findings from the 2016 National Survey of Children's Health. Am J Prev Med. 2019;57(5):667–74. https://doi.org/10.1016/J.AMEPRE.2019.06.004.

49. Chapman DP, Whitfield CL, Felitti VJ, Dube SR, Edwards VJ, Anda RF. Adverse childhood experiences and the risk of depressive disorders in adulthood. J Affect Disord. 2004;82(2):217–25. https://doi.org/10.1016/j.jad.2003.12.013.

50. Schilling EA, Aseltine RH, Gore S. Adverse childhood experiences and mental health in young adults: a longitudinal survey. BMC Public Health. 2007;7:30. https://doi.org/10.1186/1471-2458-7-30.

51. Burke NJ, Hellman JL, Scott BG, Weems CF, Carrion VG. The impact of adverse childhood experiences on an urban pediatric population. Child Abuse Negl. 2011;35(6):408–13. https://doi.org/10.1016/J.CHIABU.2011.02.006.

52. Ward ZJ, Willett WC, Hu FB, Pacheco LS, Long MW, Gortmaker SL. Excess mortality associated with elevated body weight in the USA by state and demographic subgroup: a modelling study. eClinicalMedicine. 2022;48:101429. https://doi.org/10.1016/j.eclinm.2022.101429.

53. Aune D, Sen A, Prasad M, et al. BMI and all cause mortality: systematic review and non-linear dose-response meta-analysis of 230 cohort studies with 3.74 million deaths among 30.3 million participants. BMJ. 2016;353:i2156. https://doi.org/10.1136/BMJ.I2156.

54. Shihab HM, Meoni LA, Chu AY, et al. Body mass index and risk of incident hypertension over the life course: the Johns Hopkins Precursors Study. Circulation. 2012;126(25):2983–9. https://doi.org/10.1161/CIRCULATIONAHA.112.117333.

55. Forman JP, Stampfer MJ, Curhan GC. Diet and lifestyle risk factors associated with incident hypertension in women. JAMA. 2009;302(4):401–11. https://doi.org/10.1001/JAMA.2009.1060.

56. Turpie AGG, Bauer KA, Eriksson BI, Lassen MR. Overweight and obesity as determinants of cardiovascular risk: the Framingham experience. Arch Intern Med. 2002;162(16):1867–72. https://doi.org/10.1001/ARCHINTE.162.16.1867.

57. Chandra A, Neeland IJ, Berry JD, et al. The relationship of body mass and fat distribution with incident hypertension: observations from the Dallas Heart Study. J Am Coll Cardiol. 2014;64(10):997–1002. https://doi.org/10.1016/J.JACC.2014.05.057.

58. Hall ME, Cohen JB, Ard JD, et al. Weight-loss strategies for prevention and treatment of hypertension: a scientific statement from the American Heart Association. Hypertension. 2021;78:E38–50. https://doi.org/10.1161/HYP.0000000000000202.

59. Cameron NA, Petito LC, McCabe M, et al. Quantifying the sex-race/ethnicity-specific burden of obesity on incident diabetes mellitus in the United States, 2001 to 2016: MESA and NHANES. J Am Heart Assoc. 2021;10(4):1–10. https://doi.org/10.1161/JAHA.120.018799.

60. Poirier P, Giles TD, Bray GA, et al. Obesity and cardiovascular disease: pathophysiology, evaluation, and effect of weight loss. Arterioscler Thromb Vasc Biol. 2006;26(5):89–91. https://doi.org/10.1161/01.ATV.0000216787.85457.F3.

61. Bogers RP, Bemelmans WJE, Hoogenveen RT, et al. Association of overweight with increased risk of coronary heart disease partly independent of blood pressure and cholesterol levels: a meta-analysis of 21 cohort studies including more than 300,000 persons. Arch Intern Med. 2007;167(16):1720–8. https://doi.org/10.1001/ARCHINTE.167.16.1720.

62. Powell-Wiley TM, Poirier P, Burke LE, et al. Obesity and cardiovascular disease: a scientific statement from the American Heart Association. Circulation. 2021;143(21):E984–E1010. https://doi.org/10.1161/CIR.0000000000000973.

63. Kenchaiah S, Evans JC, Levy D, et al. Obesity and the risk of heart failure. N Engl J Med. 2002;347(5):59–60. https://doi.org/10.1056/NEJMOA020245.

64. Chiuve SE, Sun Q, Sandhu RK, et al. Adiposity throughout adulthood and risk of sudden cardiac death in women. JACC Clin Electrophysiol. 2015;1(6):520–8. https://doi.org/10.1016/J.JACEP.2015.07.011.

65. Adabag S, Huxley RR, Lopez FL, et al. Obesity related risk of sudden cardiac death in the atherosclerosis risk in communities study. Heart. 2015;101(3):215–21. https://doi.org/10.1136/HEARTJNL-2014-306238.

66. Pietrasik G, Goldenberg I, McNitt S, Moss AJ, Zareba W. Obesity as a risk factor for sustained ventricular tachyarrhythmias in MADIT II patients. J Cardiovasc Electrophysiol. 2007;18(2):181–4. https://doi.org/10.1111/J.1540-8167.2006.00680.X.

67. Sabbag A, Goldenberg I, Moss AJ, et al. Predictors and risk of ventricular tachyarrhythmias or death in black and white cardiac patients: a MADIT-CRT trial substudy. JACC Clin Electrophysiol. 2016;2(4):448–55. https://doi.org/10.1016/J.JACEP.2016.03.003.

68. Jain R, Nallamothu BK, Chan PS. Body mass index and survival after in-hospital cardiac arrest. Circ Cardiovasc Qual Outcomes. 2010;3(5):490–7. https://doi.org/10.1161/CIRCOUTCOMES.109.912501.

69. Fumagalli S, Boni N, Padeletti M, et al. Determinants of thoracic electrical impedance in external electrical cardioversion of atrial fibrillation. Am J Cardiol. 2006;98(1):82–7. https://doi.org/10.1016/J.AMJCARD.2006.01.065.

70. Tsang TSM, Barnes ME, Miyasaka Y, et al. Obesity as a risk factor for the progression of paroxysmal to permanent atrial fibrillation: a longitudinal cohort study of 21 years. Eur Heart J. 2008;29(18):2227–33. https://doi.org/10.1093/EURHEARTJ/EHN324.

71. Wong CX, Sullivan T, Sun MT, et al. Obesity and the risk of incident, post-operative, and post-ablation atrial fibrillation: a meta-analysis of 626,603 individuals in 51 studies. JACC Clin Electrophysiol. 2015;1(3):139–52. https://doi.org/10.1016/J.JACEP.2015.04.004.

72. Al Chekakie MO, Welles CC, Metoyer R, et al. Pericardial fat is independently associated with human atrial fibrillation. J Am Coll Cardiol. 2010;56(10):784–8. https://doi.org/10.1016/J.JACC.2010.03.071.

73. Dramé M, Godaert L. The obesity paradox and mortality in older adults: a systematic review. Nutrients. 2023;15(7):1780. https://doi.org/10.3390/NU15071780/S1.

74. Godoy-Matos AF, Silva Júnior WS, Valerio CM. NAFLD as a continuum: from obesity to metabolic syndrome and diabetes. Diabetol Metab Syndr. 2020;12(1):1–20. https://doi.org/10.1186/S13098-020-00570-Y/TABLES/5.

75. Riazi K, Azhari H, Charette JH, et al. The prevalence and incidence of NAFLD worldwide: a systematic

review and meta-analysis. Lancet Gastroenterol Hepatol. 2022;7(9):851–61. https://doi.org/10.1016/S2468-1253(22)00165-0.

76. Younossi ZM, Stepanova M, Afendy M, et al. Changes in the prevalence of the most common causes of chronic liver diseases in the United States from 1988 to 2008. Clin Gastroenterol Hepatol. 2011;9(6):524–530.e1. https://doi.org/10.1016/J.CGH.2011.03.020.

77. Verweij N, Haas ME, Nielsen JB, et al. Germline mutations in CIDEB and protection against liver disease. N Engl J Med. 2022;387(4):332–44. https://doi.org/10.1056/NEJMOA2117872/SUPPL_FILE/NEJMOA2117872_DISCLOSURES.PDF.

78. Brunt EM, Wong VWS, Nobili V, et al. Nonalcoholic fatty liver disease. Nat Rev Dis Primers. 2015;1. https://doi.org/10.1038/NRDP.2015.80.

79. Beuther DA, Sutherland ER. Overweight, obesity, and incident asthma: a meta-analysis of prospective epidemiologic studies. Am J Respir Crit Care Med. 2007;175(7):661–6. https://doi.org/10.1164/RCCM.200611-1717OC.

80. Manuel AR, Hart N, Stradling JR. Correlates of obesity-related chronic ventilatory failure. BMJ Open Respir Res. 2016;3(1):e000110. https://doi.org/10.1136/BMJRESP-2015-000110.

81. Piper AJ. Obesity hypoventilation syndrome–the big and the breathless. Sleep Med Rev. 2011;15(2):79–89. https://doi.org/10.1016/J.SMRV.2010.04.002.

82. Karki S, Muscatello DJ, Banks E, MacIntyre CR, McIntyre P, Liu B. Association between body mass index and laboratory-confirmed influenza in middle aged and older adults: a prospective cohort study. Int J Obes. 2018;42(8):1480–8. https://doi.org/10.1038/S41366-018-0029-X.

83. Anderson MR, Geleris J, Anderson DR, et al. Body mass index and risk for intubation or death in SARS-CoV-2 infection: a Retrospective Cohort Study. Ann Intern Med. 2020;173(10):782–90. https://doi.org/10.7326/M20-3214.

84. Tartof SY, Qian L, Hong V, et al. Obesity and mortality among patients diagnosed with COVID-19: results from an integrated health care organization. Ann Intern Med. 2020;173(10):773–81. https://doi.org/10.7326/M20-3742.

85. Popkin BM, Du S, Green WD, et al. Individuals with obesity and COVID-19: a global perspective on the epidemiology and biological relationships. Obes Rev. 2020;21(11):e13128. https://doi.org/10.1111/OBR.13128.

86. Steele CB, Thomas CC, Henley SJ, et al. Vital signs: trends in incidence of cancers associated with overweight and obesity – United States, 2005–2014. MMWR Morb Mortal Wkly Rep. 2017;66(39):1052–8. https://doi.org/10.15585/MMWR.MM6639E1.

87. Obesity and Cancer|CDC. https://www.cdc.gov/cancer/obesity/index.htm. Accessed 11 Mar 2023.

88. Scappaticcio L, Maiorino MI, Bellastella G, Giugliano D, Esposito K. Insights into the relationships between diabetes, prediabetes, and cancer. Endocrine. 2017;56(2):231–9. https://doi.org/10.1007/S12020-016-1216-Y.

89. Jiang L, Tian W, Wang Y, et al. Body mass index and susceptibility to knee osteoarthritis: a systematic review and meta-analysis. Joint Bone Spine. 2012;79(3):291–7. https://doi.org/10.1016/J.JBSPIN.2011.05.015.

90. Bliddal H, Leeds AR, Christensen R. Osteoarthritis, obesity and weight loss: evidence, hypotheses and horizons – a scoping review. Obes Rev. 2014;15(7):578–86. https://doi.org/10.1111/OBR.12173.

91. Puhl RM, Himmelstein MS, Pearl RL. Weight stigma as a psychosocial contributor to obesity. Am Psychol. 2020;75(2):274–89. https://doi.org/10.1037/AMP0000538.

92. Shen WW, Chen HM, Chen H, Xu F, Li LS, Liu ZH. Obesity-related glomerulopathy: body mass index and proteinuria. Clin J Am Soc Nephrol. 2010;5(8):1401. https://doi.org/10.2215/CJN.01370210.

93. Ciardullo S, Ballabeni C, Trevisan R, Perseghin G. Metabolic syndrome, and not obesity, is associated with chronic kidney disease. Am J Nephrol. 2021;52(8):666–72. https://doi.org/10.1159/000518111.

94. Hsu CY, McCulloch CE, Iribarren C, Darbinian J, Go AS. Body mass index and risk for end-stage renal disease. Ann Intern Med. 2006;144(1):21–8. https://doi.org/10.7326/0003-4819-144-1-200601030-00006.

95. Diwan TS, Cuffy MC, Linares-Cervantes I, Govil A. Impact of obesity on dialysis and transplant and its management. Semin Dial. 2020;33(3):279–85. https://doi.org/10.1111/SDI.12876.

96. Consequences of Obesity|Overweight & Obesity|CDC. https://www.cdc.gov/obesity/basics/consequences.html. Accessed 11 Mar 2023.

97. Knowler WC, Barrett-Connor E, Fowler SE, et al. Reduction in the incidence of type 2 diabetes with lifestyle intervention or metformin. N Engl J Med. 2002;346(6):393–403. https://doi.org/10.1056/NEJMOA012512.

98. Knowler WC, Fowler SE, Hamman RF, et al. 10-year follow-up of diabetes incidence and weight loss in the Diabetes Prevention Program Outcomes Study. Lancet (London, England). 2009;374(9702):1677–86. https://doi.org/10.1016/S0140-6736(09)61457-4.

99. Nathan DM, Barrett-Connor E, Crandall JP, et al. Long-term effects of lifestyle intervention or metformin on diabetes development and microvascular complications over 15-year follow-up: the Diabetes Prevention Program Outcomes Study. Lancet Diabetes Endocrinol. 2015;3(11):866–75. https://doi.org/10.1016/S2213-8587(15)00291-0.

100. Wing RR, Bolin P, Brancati FL, et al. Cardiovascular effects of intensive lifestyle intervention in type

2 diabetes. N Engl J Med. 2013;369(2):145–54. https://doi.org/10.1056/NEJMOA1212914.

101. Obesity in adults: Behavioral therapy – UpToDate. https://www.uptodate.com/contents/obesity-in-adults-behavioral-therapy?search=obesitytreatmentadult&topicRef=5371&source=see_link#H4106436020. Accessed 11 Mar 2023.

102. Wing RR, Tate DF, Gorin AA, Raynor HA, Fava JL. A self-regulation program for maintenance of weight loss. N Engl J Med. 2006;355(15):1563–71. https://doi.org/10.1056/NEJMOA061883.

103. Teixeira PJ, Carraça EV, Marques MM, et al. Successful behavior change in obesity interventions in adults: a systematic review of self-regulation mediators. BMC Med. 2015;13(1):1–16. https://doi.org/10.1186/S12916-015-0323-6/FIGURES/1.

104. Gudzune KA, Doshi RS, Mehta AK, et al. Efficacy of commercial weight-loss programs: an updated systematic review. Ann Intern Med. 2015;162(7):501–12. https://doi.org/10.7326/M14-2238.

105. Thorogood A, Mottillo S, Shimony A, et al. Isolated aerobic exercise and weight loss: a systematic review and meta-analysis of randomized controlled trials. Am J Med. 2011;124(8):747–55. https://doi.org/10.1016/J.AMJMED.2011.02.037.

106. Goodpaster BH, DeLany JP, Otto AD, et al. Effects of diet and physical activity interventions on weight loss and cardiometabolic risk factors in severely obese adults: a randomized trial. JAMA. 2010;304(16):1795–802. https://doi.org/10.1001/JAMA.2010.1505.

107. Jakicic JM, Marcus BH, Gallagher KI, Napolitano M, Lang W. Effect of exercise duration and intensity on weight loss in overweight, sedentary women: a randomized trial. JAMA. 2003;290(10):1323–30. https://doi.org/10.1001/JAMA.290.10.1323.

108. Villareal DT, Aguirre L, Gurney AB, et al. Aerobic or resistance exercise, or both, in dieting obese older adults. N Engl J Med. 2017;376(20):1943–55. https://doi.org/10.1056/NEJMOA1616338.

109. Alexander L, Christensen SM, Richardson L, et al. Nutrition and physical activity: an Obesity Medicine Association (OMA) Clinical Practice Statement 2022. Obes Pillars. 2022;1:100005. https://doi.org/10.1016/J.OBPILL.2021.100005.

110. Lichtenstein AH, Appel LJ, Vadiveloo M, et al. 2021 Dietary guidance to improve cardiovascular health: a scientific statement from the American Heart Association. Circulation. 2021;144(23):e472–87. https://doi.org/10.1161/CIR.0000000000001031.

111. Rees K, Takeda A, Martin N, et al. Mediterranean-style diet for the primary and secondary prevention of cardiovascular disease. Cochrane database Syst Rev. 2019;3(3). https://doi.org/10.1002/14651858.CD009825.PUB3.

112. Appel LJ, Sacks FM, Carey VJ, et al. Effects of protein, monounsaturated fat, and carbohydrate intake on blood pressure and serum lipids: results of the OmniHeart randomized trial. JAMA. 2005;294(19): 2455–64. https://doi.org/10.1001/JAMA.294.19.2455.

113. Gibson AA, Seimon RV, Lee CMY, et al. Do ketogenic diets really suppress appetite? A systematic review and meta-analysis. Obes Rev. 2015;16(1):64–76. https://doi.org/10.1111/OBR.12230.

114. Resnicow K, Davis R, Rollnick S. Motivational interviewing for pediatric obesity: conceptual issues and evidence review. J Am Diet Assoc. 2006;106(12):2024–33. https://doi.org/10.1016/J.JADA.2006.09.015.

115. O'Connor EA, Evans CV, Burda BU, Walsh ES, Eder M, Lozano P. Screening for obesity and intervention for weight management in children and adolescents: evidence report and systematic review for the US Preventive Services Task Force. JAMA. 2017;317(23):2427–44. https://doi.org/10.1001/JAMA.2017.0332.

116. Liu S, Weismiller J, Strange K, et al. Evaluation of the scale-up and implementation of mind, exercise, nutrition … do it! (MEND) in British Columbia: a hybrid trial type 3 evaluation. BMC Pediatr. 2020;20(1):1–11. https://doi.org/10.1186/S12887-020-02297-1/TABLES/6.

117. Azevedo LB, Ling J, Soos I, Robalino S, Ells L. The effectiveness of sedentary behaviour interventions for reducing body mass index in children and adolescents: systematic review and meta-analysis. Obes Rev. 2016;17(7):623–35. https://doi.org/10.1111/OBR.12414.

118. Vos MB, Kaar JL, Welsh JA, et al. Added sugars and cardiovascular disease risk in children: a scientific statement from the American Heart Association. Circulation. 2017;135(19):e1017–34. https://doi.org/10.1161/CIR.0000000000000439.

119. Thivel D, Masurier J, Baquet G, et al. High-intensity interval training in overweight and obese children and adolescents: systematic review and meta-analysis. J Sports Med Phys Fitness. 2019;59(2):310–24. https://doi.org/10.23736/S0022-4707.18.08075-1.

120. Miles JM, Leiter L, Hollander P, et al. Effect of orlistat in overweight and obese patients with type 2 diabetes treated with metformin. Diabetes Care. 2002;25(7):1123–8. https://doi.org/10.2337/DIACARE.25.7.1123.

121. Kelley DE, Bray GA, Pi-Sunyer FX, et al. Clinical efficacy of orlistat therapy in overweight and obese patients with insulin-treated type 2 diabetes a 1-year randomized controlled trial. Diabetes Care. 2002;25 (6):1033–41. https://doi.org/10.2337/DIACARE.25.6.1033.

122. Weir MA, Beyea MM, Gomes T, et al. Orlistat and acute kidney injury: an analysis of 953 patients. Arch Intern Med. 2011;171(7):703–4. https://doi.org/10.1001/ARCHINTERNMED.2011.103.

123. Gadde KM, Allison DB, Ryan DH, et al. Effects of low-dose, controlled-release, phentermine plus topiramate combination on weight and associated comorbidities in overweight and obese adults

(CONQUER): a randomised, placebo-controlled, phase 3 trial. Lancet (London, England). 2011;377 (9774):1341–52. https://doi.org/10.1016/S0140-6736(11)60205-5.

124. Kelly AS, Bensignor MO, Hsia DS, et al. Phentermine/topiramate for the treatment of adolescent obesity. 2022. https://doi.org/10.1056/EVIDoa2200014.

125. Ryder JR, Kaizer A, Rudser KD, Gross A, Kelly AS, Fox CK. Effect of phentermine on weight reduction in a pediatric weight management clinic. Int J Obes. 2017;41(1):90–3. https://doi.org/10.1038/IJO.2016.185.

126. Greenway FL, Fujioka K, Plodkowski RA, et al. Effect of naltrexone plus bupropion on weight loss in overweight and obese adults (COR-I): a multicentre, randomised, double-blind, placebo-controlled, phase 3 trial. Lancet (London, England). 2010;376 (9741):595–605. https://doi.org/10.1016/S0140-6736(10)60888-4.

127. Weghuber D, Barrett T, Barrientos-Pérez M, et al. Once-weekly semaglutide in adolescents with obesity. N Engl J Med. 2022;387(24):2245–57. https://doi.org/10.1056/NEJMOA2208601.

128. Rubino DM, Greenway FL, Khalid U, et al. Effect of weekly subcutaneous semaglutide vs daily liraglutide on body weight in adults with overweight or obesity without diabetes: the STEP 8 randomized clinical trial. JAMA. 2022;327(2):138–50. https://doi.org/10.1001/JAMA.2021.23619.

129. Wilding JPH, Batterham RL, Calanna S, et al. Once-weekly semaglutide in adults with overweight or obesity. N Engl J Med. 2021;384(11):989–1002. https://doi.org/10.1056/NEJMOA2032183.

130. Rubino D, Abrahamsson N, Davies M, et al. Effect of continued weekly subcutaneous semaglutide vs placebo on weight loss maintenance in adults with overweight or obesity: the STEP 4 randomized clinical trial. JAMA. 2021;325(14):1414–25. https://doi.org/10.1001/JAMA.2021.3224.

131. Marso SP, Bain SC, Consoli A, et al. Semaglutide and cardiovascular outcomes in patients with type 2 diabetes. N Engl J Med. 2016;375(19):1834–44. https://doi.org/10.1056/NEJMOA1607141.

132. FDA Approves New Drug Treatment for Chronic Weight Management, First Since 2014|FDA. https://www.fda.gov/news-events/press-announcements/fda-approves-new-drug-treatment-chronic-weight-management-first-2014. Accessed 11 Mar 2023.

133. Kelly AS, Auerbach P, Barrientos-Perez M, et al. A randomized, controlled trial of liraglutide for adolescents with obesity. N Engl J Med. 2020;382(22):2117–28. https://doi.org/10.1056/NEJMOA1916038/

SUPPL_FILE/NEJMOA1916038_DATA-SHARING.PDF.

134. Marso SP, Daniels GH, Brown-Frandsen K, et al. Liraglutide and cardiovascular outcomes in type 2 diabetes. N Engl J Med. 2016;375(4):101. https://doi.org/10.1056/NEJMOA1603827.

135. Frías JP, Davies MJ, Rosenstock J, et al. Tirzepatide versus semaglutide once weekly in patients with type 2 diabetes. N Engl J Med. 2021;385(6):503–15. https://doi.org/10.1056/NEJMOA2107519.

136. Eisenberg D, Shikora SA, Aarts E, et al. 2022 American Society for Metabolic and Bariatric Surgery (ASMBS) and International Federation for the Surgery of Obesity and Metabolic Disorders (IFSO): indications for metabolic and bariatric surgery. Surg Obes Relat Dis. 2022;18(12):1345–56. https://doi.org/10.1016/J.SOARD.2022.08.013.

137. Sjöström L. Review of the key results from the Swedish Obese Subjects (SOS) trial – a prospective controlled intervention study of bariatric surgery. J Intern Med. 2013;273(3):219–34. https://doi.org/10.1111/JOIM.12012.

138. Olbers T, Beamish AJ, Gronowitz E, et al. Laparoscopic Roux-en-Y gastric bypass in adolescents with severe obesity (AMOS): a prospective, 5-year, Swedish nationwide study. Lancet Diabetes Endocrinol. 2017;5(3):174–83. https://doi.org/10.1016/S2213-8587(16)30424-7.

139. Inge TH, Courcoulas AP, Jenkins TM, et al. Five-year outcomes of gastric bypass in adolescents as compared with adults. N Engl J Med. 2019;380(22):2136–45. https://doi.org/10.1056/NEJMOA1813909/SUPPL_FILE/NEJMOA1813909_DISCLOSURES.PDF.

140. Inge TH, Laffel LM, Jenkins TM, et al. Comparison of surgical and medical therapy for type 2 diabetes in severely obese adolescents. JAMA Pediatr. 2018;172 (5):452–60. https://doi.org/10.1001/JAMAPEDIATRICS.2017.5763.

141. Urva S, Coskun T, Loh MT, et al. LY3437943, a novel triple GIP, GLP-1, and glucagon receptor agonist in people with type 2 diabetes: a phase 1b, multicentre, double-blind, placebo-controlled, randomised, multiple-ascending dose trial. Lancet. 2022;400 (10366):1869–81. https://doi.org/10.1016/S0140-6736(22)02033-5.

142. Heymsfield SB, Coleman LA, Miller R, et al. Effect of bimagrumab vs placebo on body fat mass among adults with type 2 diabetes and obesity: a phase 2 randomized clinical trial. JAMA Netw Open. 2021;4(1):e2033457. https://doi.org/10.1001/JAMANETWORKOPEN.2020.33457.

Obesity and Metabolic Syndrome in Latin America

3

Ana Elena Espinosa de Ycaza and Stanley M. Chen Cardenas

Contents

A. E. Espinosa de Ycaza
Universidad de Panama. Facultad de Medicina.
Endocrinologia, Panama City, Panama

S. M. Chen Cardenas (✉)
Johns Hopkins University School of Medicine,
Department of Medicine, Division of Endocrinology,
Diabetes & Metabolism, Baltimore, MD, USA
e-mail: schenca1@jhmi.edu

Abstract

Latin American populations are heterogenous with mixed genetic background and diverse cultures. From an economic standpoint, most countries in Latin America are heavily dependent on commodities, no country can be considered developed, and at least one-third of the population live in poverty, with socioeconomic inequalities widespread throughout the region. Latin America has experienced significant changes in the food environment, transitioning from small local produce markets to large super-markets with easier access to ultra-processed foods. It is the region of the world with the highest consumption of sugar-sweetened beverages. Furthermore, industrialization and urbanization have promoted sedentary lifestyle. These factors result in a high prevalence of metabolic syndrome and related diseases. Latin America is one of the regions with the steepest rise in obesity, where about 9.5% of adults have diabetes mellitus and one in three is undiagnosed. Similarly, at least one in three people with hypertension have not been identified and treated. Moreover, the double burden of undernutrition and obesity affects several Latin American countries. To mitigate this, public health interventions have been implemented in some countries to promote healthier lifestyle and reduce the burden of obesity and metabolic syndrome with varying degrees of success.

Keywords

Metabolic Syndrome · Obesity · Latin America · Hypertension · Diabetes · Hyperlipidemia

Introduction

Latin America is a group of countries that predominately speak languages derived from the Latin such as Spanish, Portuguese, and French. This linguistic concept includes from 20 to 33 countries, if the Caribbean is included. Latin America has more than 600 million people who share diverse cultures and lifestyle [1]. Hence, before discussing the metabolic syndrome in Latin America, it is important to provide a perspective of the diversity and heterogeneous populations in the region.

Data from genetic studies using single-nucleotide polymorphism genotype from 650 thousand to one million arrays in 8663 Latinos showed that those self-identified from countries such as the Dominican Republic or Puerto Rico are predominantly African descendants. Those from Argentina or Chile descend mostly from Europeans, and those from Mexico or Bolivia carry a higher proportion of the Native American ancestry [2]. A study in Brazil, evaluating mitochondrial DNA showed 33% Native American and 28% African contributions in that population [3]. In many regions of Brazil, European ancestry is predominant, representing more than 60% [4]. This mixed genetic background is also observed in Latinos living in the US, where a mixed ancestry is distributed as 65% European descendent, 18% Native American, and 6.2% African [2]. These percentages vary even within the US with more Native American to the south close to Mexico, more African ancestry in Latinos in the south by Louisiana, Midwest, and the Atlantic [2]. This admixture is the result of multiple social, political, and/or historical events that occurred over centuries including slavery, migration, and trading. It has been estimated that the admixture between Native Americans and Europeans occurred approximately 11 generations ago followed by African admixture three generations later [2]. For all the above, when analyzing studies in Latin American populations, it is essential to understand that it is not a homogenous population across the continent. Also, most of the data come from countries where there is more scientific development, focusing mainly on urban areas and less on rural and indigenous regions.

Metabolic syndrome is highly prevalent in Latinos living in the US and in Latin America. In both the US and Latin America, cardiovascular disease is the leading cause of death. Obesity has become a major public health problem as it has increased rapidly over the past decades as a consequence of urbanization and industrialization leading to changes in lifestyle (sedentarism) and nutrition transition into a more "Westernized or industrialized" dietary pattern. Similar to the rest of the world, this highlights the relevance of preventive approaches to reduce the risk of complications associated with the metabolic syndrome.

Characteristics and Metabolic Risk Factors in the Latin American Population

In some traditional regions of Latin American countries, excess weight is associated with wealth, abundance, and not infrequently believed to be a sign of good health. This belief has evolved in recent generations with better education and focus on disease prevention. Diets vary among and within different countries and cultures in Latin America. The previously mentioned nutritional transition has been observed in many countries including Chile, Brazil, and Mexico. This transition consists of a change from high prevalence of undernutrition to high prevalence of overnutrition associated with obesity and noncommunicable diseases [5]. There has been an increase in the presence of large supermarkets chains replacing smaller more traditional local markets in many areas resulting in more exposure to energy-dense and processed foods. Additionally, it is not uncommon in Latin American countries to observe marketing strategies that promote unhealthy products directed to children [1]. Also, the arrival of technology and industrialization results in more sedentarism, explaining the steep increase in rates of obesity and metabolic syndrome in the region.

Genetic factors also play an important role in the increased metabolic risk in Latin America. Studies associating genetic polymorphism with predisposition to different components of metabolic syndrome are smaller and less common than in other ethnicities. As indicated in the introduction, the diversity of ethnic and genetic backgrounds of the Latino population must be taken into account. Considering this, genome-wide association studies (GWAS) for type 2 diabetes mellitus (T2DM) performed on Mexicans and Latinos living in southern California (from the SIGMA T2D consortium) identified locus *SLC16A11* and *SLC16A13* haplotypes present at ~30% frequency in Mexicans, ~10% in East Asian, and rarely in Europeans and African Americans [6, 7]. Whole-exome sequencing studies in the same population identified a population-specific variant in the hepatic nuclear factor 1 homeobox A gene (*HNF1A*) strongly associated with T2DM in Latinos. This interesting finding results in a phenotype between MODY3 and T2DM where sulfonylureas are the preferred therapeutic option, suggesting 2% of individuals who carry this variant in Mexico might benefit from this oral agent [7, 8]. Furthermore, loss of function

variant in the insulin growth factor-2 gene present in ~17% in Mexicans and rare in other population, was associated with a 20% lower risk for T2DM [7]. In other components of the metabolic syndrome such as obesity, single-nucleotide polymorphism in the TUB (rs2272383) gene, highly expressed in the hypothalamus that encodes a transcription factor that regulates energy homeostasis has been suggested [9]. For hypertension, GWAS on the >12,000 Hispanic Community Health Study/Study of Latinos (HCHS-SOL) participants that represent different areas of Latin America, reported two loci with marginal evidence of replication, *NGF* (rs78701042) with diastolic BP, and *SLC5A8* (rs7315692) with systolic BP in Latinos [10]. In this same population, no evidence of SNP replication for lipids was found [11], reflecting the need for larger studies in Latin America to determine if these findings are universal.

Epidemiology of Obesity

Obesity is associated with increased nonmetabolic and metabolic morbidity and mortality. According to the Global Burden of Disease 2017, the regions of Latin America with the highest age-standardized deaths attributable to elevated body mass index (BMI) were in Central America and the Caribbean with 83 deaths per 100,000 habitants [12]. Nevertheless, there was only a small increase in BMI-related deaths in Latin America ranging from a decrease of 2.4% in Tropical Latin America (Brazil and Paraguay) to an increase of 20% in Andean Latin America (Bolivia, Ecuador, and Peru). Despite the significant increase in obesity rates in Latin America, the modest increase in deaths associated with BMI could be explained by a reduction in age-adjusted mortality rates from cardiovascular disease [13].

The rate at which adult obesity is rising in Latin America is one of the fastest worldwide [14], and there is no evidence of it reaching a plateau. The countries with the highest prevalence of obesity in adults are: Puerto Rico (men: 33%, women: 44%), Mexico (men: 31%, women: 40%), and Panama (men: 28%, women: 42%) [15]. More than 70% of adults in these three countries are overweight or obese [15, 16].The age-adjusted prevalence of obesity in Latin American countries is detailed in Table 1 and Fig. 1. In Mexico and Panama, the prevalence of overweight is similar in rural and urban areas, however, the prevalence of obesity is higher in urban areas [16, 17]. In Brazil, Estivaleti et al. projected obesity prevalence by 2030 using obesity trends from population national surveys that include self-reported weight and height between 2006 and 2019, concluding that obesity rates will continue to increase in all sociodemographic groups across Brazil [18].

Obesity Trends in Latin American Children and Adolescents

Latin America is one of the regions with the greatest income, socioeconomic, and health disparities. The double burden of undernutrition and obesity is notable in many Latin American countries. In 2019, the indigenous communities in Panama had the highest indicators of childhood undernutrition, underweight, and stunted growth, as well as the highest increase in obesity rates compared to other sociodemographic groups [16]. Guatemala, Honduras, Nicaragua, and Bolivia have high rates of stunting in children

Table 1 Prevalence of obesity, diabetes, and hypertension in adults in Latin America

Country	Obesity prevalence (%) age-adjusted		Diabetes prevalence (%) age-adjusted	Hypertension prevalence (%) age-adjusted[a]	
	Men	Women	All adults (20–79 years)	Men	Women
Argentina	31.4	33.4	5.4	54.0	41.2
Bolivia[b]	20.8(14.5)	31.8 (25.6)	5.5	29.4	27.2
Brazil	18.9	25.4	8.8	47.9	42.1
Chile	24.9	30.9	10.8	39.0	33.1
Colombia	13.7	21.05	8.3	31.1	30.8
Costa Rica	15.8	26.1	8.8	36.0	39.4
Cuba	14.7	30.3	7.6	40.3	39.5
Dominican Republic	21	34.1	10.5	49.0	49.2
Ecuador[b]	20.3 (14.9)	30.9 (24.7)	4.4	29.2	25.1
El Salvador	17.9	29.9	n/a	31.4	33.6
Guatemala	15.1	26.4	n/a	31.5	32.6
Guyana	10.4	27.4	n/a	38.2	41.8
Haiti	6	12.9	8.9	37.6	47.8
Honduras	15.5	28	5.1	33.2	34.4
Mexico	30.6	39.3	16.9	32.8	31.4
Nicaragua	16.9	28.9	9.3	34.5	36.9
Panama[b]	27.7 (17.8)	42.3 (27.6)	8.2	36.8	35.3
Paraguay	21.2	27.4	n/a	61.6	50.9
Perú	17.3	24.2	4.8	22.8	18.4
Puerto Rico	32.6	43.8	13.3	41.8	43.2
Uruguay	19.0	23.6	9.0	46.0	38.9
Venezuela	22.4	28.6	9.6	39.7	39.1

References: [14–16, 19, 38, 53]. n/a: not available
Bolivia obesity prevalence: STEPS Bolivia 2019
Ecuador obesity prevalence: Ecuador STEPS Survey 2018
[a]Prevalence of adults, 30–79 years
[b]Shows the unadjusted obesity prevalence of Bolivia, Panama from 2019 and Ecuador from 2018, and in parenthesis the age-adjusted prevalence from noncommunicable disease (NCD) risk factor collaboration from 2016

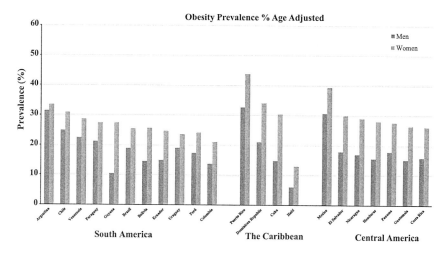

Fig. 1 Age-adjusted prevalence of obesity in Latin America

under 5 years, an indicator of chronic undernutrition. Furthermore in these countries, obesity rates in children and adults have steadily increased over the last 15 years [19].

From 1975 to 2016, the BMI has increased 1 kg/m^2 per decade in children and adolescents 5–19 years from Central America [20]. The BMI trends have started to plateau in recent years for girls from Central American and Andean countries (Bolivia, Ecuador, and Peru). Children in Mexico had the largest increase in BMI between 1984 and 2019 [21]. In Argentina, Chile, Mexico, Colombia, and Peru, 3.8 million children <5 years were classified with overweight or obesity according to the World Health Organization (WHO) classification [22]. The prevalence of obesity in school-age children in surveys from 2009 to 2012, using the cutoff points from the International Task Force on Obesity, in Mexico was 34.5% and Brazil was 33.5% [22].

Epidemiology of Metabolic Syndrome

Determining the prevalence of metabolic syndrome and comparing among the different countries in Latin America is challenging. The lack of standardized definitions for the waist circumference to define obesity in Latin Americans is an important reason. Escobedo et al. assessed the prevalence of the metabolic syndrome in seven urban Latin American populations between 2003 and 2005. This group found an overall prevalence of 22% in women and 20% in men [23]. Brazil and Mexico reported some of the highest prevalence of metabolic syndrome in the region. In Mexico, the prevalence based on a systematic review of 15 studies was 36% (NCEP/ATPIII criteria), and the overall pooled prevalence was 41% [24]. A systematic review of 26 studies in Brazil, reported a prevalence of 33%, with no significant change between 2009 and 2019. The prevalence was 31% and 37%, when defined by the NCEP/ATP III and the 2009 Joint Scientific Statement criteria, respectively [25].

There are no studies exploring the differences in prevalence of metabolic syndrome between Latin Americans living in their countries and those in the US. Nevertheless, when comparing data from Mexico City using the NCEP ATP III definition of metabolic syndrome between 2003 and 2005 to the NHANES 2003–2006 data in Mexican Americans, a prevalence of metabolic syndrome in Mexico City of 27% [23], was comparable to the prevalence of 33% for Mexican Americans [26].

Metabolic Syndrome Components

Obesity

It is accepted that central obesity, increase in waist circumference ($\geq$80 cm in women and $\geq$90 cm in men), waist/hip ratio, and body shape index are all associated with increased mortality regardless of ethnicity [27, 28]. Although, the waist circumference is the most used anthropometric measure for abdominal obesity by the (WHO) and the International Diabetes Federation (IDF), there is no clear consensus on the waist circumference cutoff for abdominal obesity for Latin Americans. The IDF suggests using, for Central and South Americans, the same cutoff as for South Asians (women $\geq$80 cm and men $\geq$90 cm). However, many studies have used the cutoff recommended for European ancestry (women $\geq$80 cm and men $\geq$94 cm) or the ATPIII cutoff (women $\geq$88 cm and men $\geq$102 cm) [29, 30].

In Latin Americans, abdominal obesity is common and has been associated with cardiovascular disease whether using the IDF or NCEP ATPIII recommended definitions. A study that included 12 Latin American countries reported a prevalence of abdominal obesity in adults (using the NCEP ATPIII definition) of 29% for men and 50% for women [31]. Similarly, but using the WHO criteria, a cross-sectional study between 2014 and 2015 assessed several anthropometric and lifestyle patterns of adolescents and adults of eight Latin American countries. Abdominal obesity defined as an elevated waist circumference was present in 33% women and 37% men. The prevalence of abdominal obesity in adults ranged from 13% in men in Colombia, to 59.9% in women from Costa Rica. An elevated waist-hip ratio (>1 in men and >0.85 in women) was found in 52% women and 51% men [32]. Reflecting that central obesity affects a high proportion of Latinos.

Since the cutoff of waist circumference to diagnose abdominal obesity in Latin America has not been established, Aschner et al., evaluated visceral adipose area by CT and waist circumference in 457 adults from five Latin American countries (Mexico, El Salvador, Colombia, Venezuela, and

Paraguay). They found a waist circumference threshold of 94 cm for men and 90–92 cm for women defined abdominal obesity [33]. However, given the relatively small sample used in the study and the heterogeneity of Latin America, these results may not be extrapolated to other countries. Neck circumference is a simple anthropometric measure that correlates with BMI; however, it has not been validated whether the neck circumference correlates with abdominal obesity [34]. Some studies showed an association between neck circumference, cardiometabolic risk, and the components of the metabolic syndrome [35, 36]. In Latin America, most studies evaluating the distribution of neck circumference and the prevalence of elevated neck circumference are from Brazil. A systematic review and meta-analysis of 14 population-based studies included five Latin American countries (Brazil, Argentina, Chile, Colombia, and Venezuela), found a mean neck circumference of 35.9 cm. The cutoff for elevated neck circumferences used in women ranged from 34 to 35 cm, and in men from 37 to 41 cm. The prevalence of elevated neck circumference was 37–57% [37]. When using cutoffs established in other populations, the prevalence of elevated waist and neck circumference is high for Latin Americans; however, additional studies to determine the optimal cutoffs to identify people at risk for metabolic complications in Latin America are needed.

Impaired Fasting Glucose, Glucose Intolerance, Prediabetes, and Diabetes

The prevalence of type 2 diabetes mellitus (T2DM) in Latin American countries has increased in parallel with obesity. Given the sharp increase in obesity over the last 15 years, diabetes is expected to continue to rise in Latin America for the next two decades. Impaired glucose tolerance (IGT), impaired fasting glucose (IFG), and HbA1c between 5.7 and 6.4% have been used to define a state of intermediate glucose metabolism abnormality or prediabetes that can result in the development of T2DM. However, there is no consensus on what is the best way to identify people at risk of T2DM that would benefit from treatment. Studies on Latin American populations have included only a few countries and have used different criteria to identify people at risk. In 2021, the age-adjusted prevalence of IFG and IGT in Central and South American adults, was 10% and 10.9% respectively [38]. Several countries did not have data available to estimate the prevalence; therefore, extrapolations from countries considered to be similar in ethnicity, language, income classification, and geographic location were made.

A study evaluated the risk of T2DM according to BMI and sociodemographic region in low- and middle-income countries in Latin America and the Caribbean (countries included: Mexico, Ecuador, Chile, Costa Rica, Guyana, and St. Vincent & the Grenadines), suggested that the optimal BMI cutoff associated with T2DM risk was 28.3 kg/m^2 for women and 25.3 kg/m^2 for men. There was a steep increase in T2DM in adults with BMI $\geq$30 kg/m^2 at age 35 and older [39].

The FINDRISC, one of the commonly used tools to assess the risk for developing T2DM has been adapted for Latin America. This tool includes demographic and easily obtained clinical data [40]. The FINDRISC was found to be a cost-effective method to identify people at risk for T2DM in Colombia and Venezuela [41]. A systematic review on diagnostic/prognostic models for diabetes in adults in Latin America that included five reports from three countries (Brazil, Mexico, and Peru) of randomly selected individuals found a high risk of bias for the analysis criterion and a discrimination performance of the models of 72% [42]. Moreover, given that only a few Latin American countries (none from Central America) have validated diabetes risk models, there is not one tool that could be used accurately in all Latin America.

The prevalence of diabetes mellitus (DM) as opposed to pre-DM has been more thoroughly assessed in Latin America. In 2017, the mean prevalence was 8.1% [43]. In 2021, according to data from IDF, 32 million adults live with DM in central and south America (A DM prevalence in adults of 9.5%), of those, one in three is undiagnosed [38]. Puerto Rico is the country with the highest prevalence (20.1%), followed by Mexico (16.9%), and the lowest prevalence was observed in Honduras (4.6%), Ecuador (4.7%), and Bolivia (5.7%) [38]. The age-adjusted prevalence of DM in Latin American countries based on IDF 2021 is presented in Table 1 and Fig. 2. These numbers could be markedly different when comparing rural and urban communities [43]. In Colombia, the prevalence of DM is 4–5 times higher in urban areas compared to rural areas. This difference could be explained by easier access to foods with higher energy density, added sugars, and ultra-processed foods in urban areas. Given the continued increase in obesity, by 2045 the number of people living with DM in Central and South America are expected to increase by 50%, and this can significantly affect the quality of life and impose a heavy burden on healthcare systems. Therefore, it is imperative to focus efforts to identify individuals at risk of DM, incentivize healthier lifestyles, and treat metabolic risk factors.

Dyslipidemia

Hyperlipidemia is highly prevalent in Latin America. Data from the Hispanic Community Health Study/Study of Latinos HCHS-SOL, a large population-based study of 16,415 self-identified Hispanic/Latinos in the US, showed that more than 60% had some form of dyslipidemia. In this cohort, there was a prevalence of about 40% of obesity and 15% of diabetes [44]. The mean LDL-C was 119.7 mg/dl, triglyceride (TG) 113.4 mg/dl, total cholesterol 194.4 mg/dl, and HDL-C 48.5 mg/dl, with 9.2% of the cohort on lipid-lowering agents. The study also reported higher prevalence of low HDL-C in women, whereas men had a higher prevalence of elevated LDL-C, TG, and mixed dyslipidemia [44]. This study included participants from different countries including Cuba, Mexico, Dominican Republic, Puerto Rico, Central, and South America. As expected, some differences were found among countries, for example, dyslipidemia was higher in Central Americans as well as in Cubans, and lowest in Dominicans. Puerto Ricans showed the highest prevalence of low HDL-C, although not

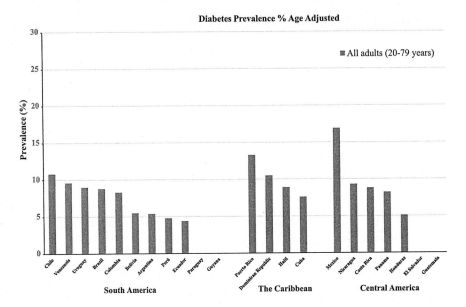

Fig. 2 Age-adjusted prevalence of diabetes mellitus in Latin America. n/a: data not available

statistically significant, and Central Americans high TG levels [44].

A systematic review of dyslipidemia in Latin America and the Caribbean that analyzed about 200 studies in this region showed that low HDL-C was the most common lipid abnormality, followed by hypertriglyceridemia, and elevated LDL-C. Additionally, the prevalence of high total cholesterol defined as ≥240 mg/dl was 20.9%, LDL-C > 160 mg/dl 19.7%, low HDL-C ≤ 40 in men and ≤ 50 in women 48.3%, TG > 200 mg/dl 20.5% [45]. Most of the studies were from Brazil [61] and Chile [21]. These results are consistent with the HCHS-SOL study [44]. Based on the data, it appears the prevalence of dyslipidemia has remained stable since 2005.

One of the challenges in many regions of Latin America is lack of awareness of the relevance of hyperlipidemia in the population that results in less treatment adherence. Using data from the HCHS-SOL, it was estimated that almost 50% of Latinos were unaware of having elevated cholesterol levels and only about 30% were receiving treatment. Men were more likely to have hyperlipidemia than women (44 vs. 41%), and tend to have lower rates of treatment (28.1 vs. 30.6%). The presence of comorbidities and higher

socioeconomic status were more likely associated with awareness of dyslipidemia [46]. Latinos born in the US were less aware than those born in Latin American countries. Although those who had lived longer in the US were more likely to receive treatment and have adequate lipid control. This trend was observed in those with health insurance. Puerto Rican or Dominican Latinos were most likely to be aware and treated. In contrast, Mexican or Central Americans were less likely to be treated for dyslipidemia. Individuals of Cuban and South American background had the lowest rates of control of dyslipidemia, whereas Puerto Ricans had the highest rate of lipid control.

In 2017, a consensus of multiple societies highlighted the relevance of understanding the characteristics of the Latin American population, particularly when addressing lifestyle changes. The overall pharmacological management of dyslipidemia is similar to other populations [47].

Hypertension

Hypertension is another highly prevalent component of the metabolic syndrome, estimated to affect more than 40% of Latin Americans

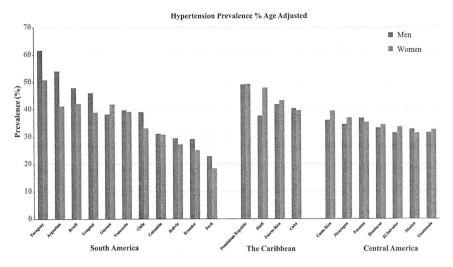

Fig. 3 Age-adjusted prevalence of hypertension in Latin America

(Table 1 and Fig. 3) [48]. Data from the HCHS-SOL cohort showed that compared to Mexicans, Dominicans, Cubans, and Puerto Ricans have highest hypertension incidence rates [49]. The incidence and prevalence of hypertension vary significantly among and within countries, and are also influenced by sex, age, and ethnicity. In Brazil, a longitudinal study, ELSA-Brazil, of 15,105 subjects reported that hypertension was more prevalent in men than women (40.1 vs. 32.2%), higher in older and in self-identified as Black 49.3% than Browns and Whites, 38.2% and 30.3%, respectively [50]. Data from a large study including more than 52,000 men and 106,000 women in Mexico are consistent with this trend, reporting that the prevalence of hypertension increases with age and varies with sex, from 26% in men and 19% in women aged 35–44, reaching 59% in men and 70% in women aged 75–84, independent of BMI [51]. A cross-sectional study that included Argentina, Chile, and Uruguay included approximately 7500 adults, reported a prevalence of hypertension of about 42.5%, i.e., 38.7% of women and 46.6% of men. Furthermore 32.5%, i.e., 36.0% of men and 29.4% women, had prehypertension [52].

In Latin America, hypertension is still vastly underdiagnosed in approximately 28% of women and 43% of men [53]. Peru reports one of the lowest rates of diagnosis of hypertension, with only 35% of men being diagnosed [54]. Of those who are diagnosed, data from South America, reported that 29–48.7% were treated [50, 52]. A review of data in Latin America reported that about 64% of women and 47% men with hypertension are treated, and in those treated only 35% of women and 23% men have their blood pressure under control [53]. This highlights the severity of the problem in the region, since hypertension is one of the most important risk factors for cardiovascular disease.

One of the problems with hypertension is that due to the asymptomatic nature of the disease, often patients are not aware of their diagnosis and will not seek medical care. In the ELSA-Brazil study, only 34% participants were aware of their diagnosis of hypertension [50]. Another study in South America reported that 63.0% of adults with hypertension, 52.5% of men and 74.3% of women, were aware of their diagnosis [52]. In addition, the lack of primary care, medications, and the use of unvalidated devices to monitor blood pressure contribute to the problem. Furthermore, in Latin America, hypertension occurs 2–3 times more frequently in people with obesity than in those with normal body weight [55].

Regional Strategies Implemented and in Development

Several public health policies have been developed and implemented in Latin American countries to address the growing epidemic of obesity. However, the double burden of obesity and undernutrition makes the creation of policies more difficult. Furthermore, the true impact of the implemented policies in Latin America is unknown.

Taxes on Sugar-Sweetened Beverages (SSBs)

SSB intake is associated with increased risk of obesity and metabolic syndrome [56]. Certain regions of Latin America have some of the highest consumption rates of SSBs, especially, the Caribbean region has the highest SSB consumption worldwide [57]. As a result, at least 21 countries in Central, South America, and the Caribbean have imposed taxes on SSBs. In 2014, Mexico imposed taxes on SSBs which resulted in reduced purchase and consumption within 2 years after implementation of the tax [58, 59].

In 2019, a study in Latin America compared different excise tax on various types of SSBs and nonalcoholic beverages. They calculated an excise tax share for the most common SSB consumed and used this metric to compare taxation across Latin America [60]. Of the 27 countries included from Latin America and the Caribbean, 17 applied excise tax on carbonated SSBs, 11 on fruit drinks, three on sweetened drink milks, 17 on energy drinks, and four on bottled water. The excise tax share for a small (355 ml) carbonated sweetened beverage ranged from 1.5% in Guatemala to 16.9% in Peru. The excise tax share for a large fruit drink (1000 ml) ranged from 1.4% in Brazil to 16.9% in Peru, for sugar-sweetened milk (1000 ml) from 5% in Panama to 16.9% in Peru, and for energy drinks from 0.6% in Honduras to 21.7% in El Salvador. Only Mexico and Dominica earmarked part of the revenue from taxation of SSBs to health and healthy lifestyle programs [60]. Despite some progress, to-date there is significant heterogeneity in taxation of SSBs. Most countries apply a very low excise tax on SSBs resulting in a small impact on retail price. Only Ecuador and Peru apply an excise tax high enough to increase retail price by at least 20% as recommended by WHO [60]. Some countries have not updated their legislations in more than 10 years [61] and in some, bottled water is also taxed.

Front of Package Labels

Most Latin American countries have mandatory inclusion of "back of the label" nutritional information; however, this information can be complex and difficult to understand for consumers. Easier and simpler front of package information has been used to aid people to understand the nutritional components of food products. The traffic light system developed in the United Kingdom has been implemented in Ecuador since 2014 [62]. The colors indicate the relative amounts of total fats, saturated fats, sugar, and sodium in processed foods. In 2016, Chile developed a mandatory Warning Octagonal Black System (WOBS) that includes labels if the product is high on saturated fats, sugars, sodium, and calories. A population survey in 2017 after the implementation of WOBS showed that 68% thought the front of package label influenced their choice of healthier foods, and 91% thought the warning labels influence their choice of food in general [63]. Following implementation of the mandatory label system in Ecuador and Chile, other Latin American countries, e.g., Mexico, Peru, Uruguay, Brazil, have adopted it [64].

Food Marketing

Food advertising directed toward children is widespread in all types of media and can influence food preferences of children [64]. Only a few Latin American countries have implemented regulations to prevent marketing of processed foods directed to children. In Chile, there were two other policies included in the law to implement the WOBS (2016): the prohibition of foods high in saturated fats, sugar, sodium, and calories in schools, and prohibition of advertisement directed toward children less than 14 years of age of foods high in saturated fats, sugars, sodium, and calories [63]. After 18 months of implementation of these policies, there was a 24% reduction in sales of beverages high on sugar, sodium, saturated fats, or calories [65].

School Food Environment

A systematic review and meta-analysis assessing food school policies on children's dietary behaviors, found positive effects on dietary patterns. Some interventions resulted in an increase in consumption of fruits and vegetables, others reduced SSB intake, and others reduced unhealthy snacks, though effects on metabolic parameters such as triglycerides, glucose, were inconsistent [66].

Most Latin American countries have a School Feeding Program often administered by the government, but only a few countries have mandatory regulations to prohibit the sale of SSBs, ultra-processed food or food high in saturated fats in schools. In Chile, after the implementation of these regulations, accessibility of the prohibited foods in schools decreased, but in Mexico and Costa Rica, vendors inside schools still offered them [64].

Physical Activity Interventions

Studies on the effectiveness of interventions to increase physical activity in Latin America are sparse. Cycle paths, Ciclovia programs, and creating more recreational spaces in urban cities have been done in Colombia and Brazil, resulting in increased physical activity and quality of life in adults [62]. Other Latin American countries have followed these efforts by increasing availability to parks and other recreational areas as well as Ciclovia programs; however, the cost-effectiveness of these interventions in most of Latin America is still unknown.

As previously discussed, the coexistence of obesity and undernutrition in several regions in Latin America needs to be considered in the development and application of public health policies. It is important to avoid interventions addressing obesity that could worsen undernutrition. The "syndemic theory," first proposed in 1996, takes into account the coexisting epidemics of undernutrition and obesity. These are not isolated entities, instead they are interrelated, have biological interactions and common social factors [67]. The syndemic approach provides a framework for intervention by focusing working on common social drivers of undernutrition and obesity that require active participation of governments, industry, medical stakeholders, organizations, and the public.

Conclusions

In Latin America, metabolic risk factors are highly prevalent. The region is facing an epidemiologic transition with rapidly increasing rates of obesity, hypertension, dyslipidemia, and diabetes. This is largely caused by a nutritional transition to less healthy diets and sedentary lifestyle affecting urban and rural areas regardless of socioeconomic status. Research is still needed to better define criteria for abdominal obesity, identify people at risk of T2DM, evaluate the effectiveness of interventions to promote healthier lifestyles, and develop programs to educate patients on dyslipidemia and hypertension screening and adherence to treatment. Although several public health interventions have been studied or applied to improve the food environment and promote physical activity, collaboration is required among all sectors of society to continue developing strategies and policies to improve healthcare access, to prevent and reduce the rates of obesity, metabolic syndrome, and its complications.

References

1. Pérez-Ferrer C, Auchincloss AH, De Menezes MC, Kroker-Lobos MF, Cardoso LDO, Barrientos-Gutierrez T. The food environment in Latin America: a systematic review with a focus on environments relevant to obesity and related chronic diseases. Public Health Nutr. 2019;22(18):3447–64.

2. Bryc K, Durand EY, Macpherson JM, Reich D, Mountain JL. The genetic ancestry of African Americans, Latinos, and European Americans across the United States. Am J Hum Genet [Internet]. 2015;96(1):37–53. https://doi.org/10.1016/j.ajhg.2014.11.010.

3. Alves-Silva J, da Silva SM, Guimarães PEM, Ferreira ACS, Bandelt HJ, Pena SDJ, et al. The ancestry of Brazilian mtDNA lineages. Am J Hum Genet. 2000;67(2):444–61.

4. Pena SDJ, di Pietro G, Fuchshuber-Moraes M, Genro JP, Hutz MH, Kehdy F de SG, et al. The genomic ancestry of individuals from different geographical regions of Brazil is more uniform than expected. PLoS One. 2011;6(2):e17063.

5. Rivera JA, Barquera S, González-Cossío T, Olaiz G, Sepúlveda J. Nutrition transition in Mexico and in other Latin American countries. Nutr Rev. 2004;62 (7 II):8–12.

6. Williams Amy AL, Jacobs Suzanne SBR, Moreno-Macías H, Huerta-Chagoya A, Churchhouse C, Márquez-Luna C, et al. Sequence variants in SLC16A11 are a common risk factor for type 2 diabetes in Mexico. Nature. 2014;506(7486):97–101.

7. Mercader JM, Florez JC. The genetic basis of type 2 diabetes in Hispanics and Latin Americans: challenges and opportunities. Front Public Health. 2017;5 (December):1–7.

8. Estrada K, Aukrust I, Bjørkhaug L, Burtt NP, Mercader JM, García-Ortiz H, et al. Association of a low-frequency variant in HNF1A with type 2 diabetes in a Latino population. JAMA. 2014;311(22):2305–14.

9. Chalazan B, Palm D, Sridhar A, Lee C, Argos M, Daviglus M, et al. Common genetic variants associated with obesity in an African-American and Hispanic/Latino population. PLoS One [Internet]. 2021;16 (5 May):1–12. https://doi.org/10.1371/journal.pone.0250697

10. Sofer T, Wong Q, Hartwig FP, Taylor K, Warren HR, Evangelou E, et al. Genome-wide association study of blood pressure traits by Hispanic/Latino background: the Hispanic community health study/study of Latinos. Sci Rep. 2017;7(1):1–12.

11. Graff M, Emery LS, Justice AE, Parra E, Below JE, Palmer ND, et al. Genetic architecture of lipid traits in the Hispanic community health study/study of Latinos. Lipids Health Dis. 2017;16(1):1–12.

12. Dai H, Alsalhe TA, Chalghaf N, Riccò M, Bragazzi NL, Wu J. The global burden of disease attributable to high body mass index in 195 countries and territories, 1990–2017: an analysis of the global burden of disease study. PLoS Med. 2020;17(7):e1003198.

13. Bank O and TW. Health at a glance: Latin America and the Caribbean 2020 [Internet]. Available from: https://www.oecd-ilibrary.org/social-issues-migration-health/cardiovascular-disease-estimated-mortality-rates-2000-and-2017-or-nearest-year_377b6d40-en

14. Afshin A, Forouzanfar MH, Reitsma MB, Sur P, Estep K, Lee A, et al. Health effects of overweight and obesity in 195 countries over 25 years. N Engl J Med. 2017;377(1):13–27.

15. Barquera S, Hernández-Barrera L, Trejo-Valdivia B, Shamah T, Campos-Nonato I, Rivera-Dommarco J. Obesity in Mexico, prevalence and trends in adults. Ensanut 2018–19. Salud Publica Mex. 2020;62(6): 682–92.

16. Instituto Conmemorativo Gorgas de Estudios de la Salud. Sistema de Información Geográfico Interactivo de la Encuesta Nacional de Salud de Panamá (ENSPA). 2019. 2019. p. https://www.gorgas.gob.pa/wp-content/uploads/external/SIGENSPA/Informe_general.htm

17. CONTINUA E. Encuesta Nacional de Salud y Nutricion 2021 [Internet]. 2021. Available from: https://www.insp.mx/resources/images/stories/2022/docs/220801_Ensa21_digital_29julio.pdf

18. Estivaleti JM, Guzman-Habinger J, Lobos J, Azeredo CM, Claro R, Ferrari G, et al. Time trends and projected obesity epidemic in Brazilian adults between 2006 and 2030. Sci Rep. 2022;12(1):12699.

19. Global Nutrition Report 2022 [Internet]. 2022. Available from: https://globalnutritionreport.org/reports/2022-global-nutrition-report/

20. NCD Risk Factor Collaboration (NCD-RisC). Worldwide trends in body-mass index, underweight, overweight, and obesity from 1975 to 2016: a pooled analysis of 2416 population-based measurement studies in 128·9 million children, adolescents, and adults. Lancet (London, England). 2017;390(10113):2627–42.

21. (NCD-RisC) NRFC. Height and body-mass index trajectories of school-aged children and adolescents from 1985 to 2019 in 200 countries and territories: a pooled analysis of 2181 population-based studies with 65 million participants. Lancet (London, England). 2020;396 (10261):1511–24.

22. Rivera JÁ, de Cossío TG, Pedraza LS, Aburto TC, Sánchez TG, Martorell R. Childhood and adolescent overweight and obesity in Latin America: a systematic review. Lancet Diabetes Endocrinol. 2014;2(4):321–32.

23. Escobedo J, Schargrodsky H, Champagne B, Silva H, Boissonnet CP, Vinueza R, et al. Prevalence of the metabolic syndrome in Latin America and its association with sub-clinical carotid atherosclerosis: the CARMELA cross sectional study. Cardiovasc Diabetol. 2009;8:52.

24. Gutiérrez-Solis AL, Datta Banik S, Méndez-González RM. Prevalence of metabolic syndrome in Mexico: a systematic review and meta-analysis. Metab Syndr Relat Disord. 2018;16(8):395–405.

25. de Siqueira Valadares LT, de Souza LSB, Salgado Júnior VA, de Freitas BL, de Macedo LR, Silva M. Prevalence of metabolic syndrome in Brazilian adults in the last 10 years: a systematic review and meta-analysis. BMC Public Health. 2022;22(1):327.

26. Ervin RB. Prevalence of metabolic syndrome among adults 20 years of age and over, by sex, age, race and

ethnicity, and body mass index: United States, 2003–2006. Natl Health Stat Rep. 2009;13:1–7.

27. Jayedi A, Soltani S, Zargar MS, Khan TA, Shab-Bidar S. Central fatness and risk of all cause mortality: systematic review and dose-response meta-analysis of 72 prospective cohort studies. BMJ. 2020;370:m3324.

28. Ross R, Neeland IJ, Yamashita S, Shai I, Seidell J, Magni P, et al. Waist circumference as a vital sign in clinical practice: a Consensus Statement from the IAS and ICCR Working Group on Visceral Obesity. Nat Rev Endocrinol. 2020;16(3):177–89.

29. Barr ELM, Zimmet PZ, Welborn TA, Jolley D, Magliano DJ, Dunstan DW, et al. Risk of cardiovascular and all-cause mortality in individuals with diabetes mellitus, impaired fasting glucose, and impaired glucose tolerance: the Australian Diabetes, Obesity, and Lifestyle Study (AusDiab). Circulation. 2007;116: 151–7.

30. Third Report of the National Cholesterol Education Program (NCEP). Expert panel on detection, evaluation, and treatment of high blood cholesterol in adults (adult treatment panel III) final report. Circulation. 2002;106(25):3143–421.

31. Aschner P, Ruiz A, Balkau B, Massien C, Haffner SM. Association of abdominal adiposity with diabetes and cardiovascular disease in Latin America. J Clin Hypertens (Greenwich). 2009;11(12):769–74.

32. Herrera-Cuenca M, Kovalskys I, Gerardi A, Hernandez P, Sifontes Y, Gómez G, et al. Anthropometric profile of latin american population: results from the ELANS study. Front Nutr. 2021;8:740361.

33. Aschner P, Buendía R, Brajkovich I, Gonzalez A, Figueredo R, Juarez XE, et al. Determination of the cutoff point for waist circumference that establishes the presence of abdominal obesity in Latin American men and women. Diabetes Res Clin Pract. 2011;93(2):243–7.

34. Pei X, Liu L, Imam MU, Lu M, Chen Y, Sun P, et al. Neck circumference may be a valuable tool for screening individuals with obesity: findings from a young Chinese population and a meta-analysis. BMC Public Health. 2018;18(1):529.

35. Zanuncio VV, Sediyama CMNO, Dias MM, Nascimento GM, Pessoa MC, Pereira PF, et al. Neck circumference and the burden of metabolic syndrome disease: a population-based sample. J Public Health (Oxf). 2022;44(4):753–60.

36. Ebrahimi H, Mahmoudi P, Zamani F, Moradi S. Neck circumference and metabolic syndrome: a cross-sectional population-based study. Prim Care Diabetes. 2021;15(3):582–7.

37. Espinoza López PA, Fernandez Landeo KJ, Pérez Silva Mercado RR, Quiñones Ardela JJ, Carrillo-Larco RM. Neck circumference in Latin America and the Caribbean: a systematic review and meta-analysis, vol. 6. England: Wellcome open research; 2021. p. 13.

38. Magliano DJ, Boyko EJ. IDF Diabetes Atlas 10th edition scientific committee. Brussels: IDF Diabetes Atlas [Internet]; 2021.

39. Teufel F, Seiglie JA, Geldsetzer P, Theilmann M, Marcus ME, Ebert C, et al. Body-mass index and diabetes risk in 57 low-income and middle-income countries: a cross-sectional study of nationally representative, individual-level data in 685 616 adults. Lancet (London, England). 2021;398(10296):238–48.

40. Lindström J, Tuomilehto J. The diabetes risk score: a practical tool to predict type 2 diabetes risk. Diabetes Care. 2003;26(3):725–31.

41. Nieto-Martínez R, González-Rivas JP, Aschner P, Barengo NC, Mechanick JI. Transculturalizing diabetes prevention in Latin America. Ann Glob Health. 2017;83(3–4):432–43.

42. Carrillo-Larco RM, Aparcana-Granda DJ, Mejia JR, Barengo NC, Bernabe-Ortiz A. Risk scores for type 2 diabetes mellitus in Latin America: a systematic review of population-based studies. Diabet Med. 2019;36(12):1573–84.

43. Sinisterra-Loaiza L, Cardelle-Cobas A, Abraham A, Calderon M, Espinoza M, González-Olivares L, et al. Diabetes in Latin America: prevalence, complications, and socio-economic impact. Int J Diabetes Clin Res. 2019;6(3):1–9.

44. Rodriguez CJ, Daviglus ML, Swett K, González HM, Gallo LC, Wassertheil-Smoller S, et al. Dyslipidemia patterns among Hispanics/Latinos of diverse background in the United States. Am J Med [Internet]. 2014;127(12):1186-1194.e1. https://doi.org/10.1016/j.amjmed.2014.07.026.

45. Carrillo-Larco RM, Benites-Moya CJ, Anza-Ramirez-C, Albitres-Flores L, Sánchez-Velazco D, Pacheco-Barrios N, et al. A systematic review of population-based studies on lipid profiles in Latin America and the Caribbean. eLife. 2020;9:1–13.

46. Rodriguez CJ, Cai J, Swett K, González HM, Talavera GA, Wruck LM, et al. High cholesterol awareness, treatment, and control among Hispanic/Latinos: results from the Hispanic community health study/study of Latinos. J Am Heart Assoc. 2015;4(7):1–10.

47. Ponte-Negretti CI, Isea-Perez JE, Lorenzatti AJ, Lopez-Jaramillo P, Wyss-Q FS, Pintó X, et al. Atherogenic dyslipidemia in Latin America: prevalence, causes and treatment: expert's position paper made by The Latin American Academy for the Study of Lipids (ALALIP) endorsed by the Inter-American Society of Cardiology (IASC), the South American society. Int J Cardiol. 2017;243(2017):516–22.

48. Ruilope LM, Chagas ACP, Brandão AA, Gómez-Berroterán R, Alcalá JJA, Paris JV, et al. Hipertensión en América Latina: perspectivas actuales de las tendencias y características. Hipertens y Riesgo Vasc [Internet]. 2017;34(1):50–6. https://doi.org/10.1016/j.hipert.2016.11.005.

49. Elfassy T, Al Hazzouri AZ, Cai J, Baldoni PL, Llabre MM, Rundek T, et al. Incidence of hypertension among us Hispanics/Latinos: the Hispanic community health study/study of Latinos, 2008 to 2017. J Am Heart Assoc. 2020;9(12):e015031.

50. Chor D, Pinho Ribeiro AL, Sá Carvalho M, Duncan BB, Andrade Lotufo P, Araújo Nobre A, et al. Prevalence, awareness, treatment and influence of socioeconomic variables on control of high blood pressure: results of the ELSA-Brasil study. PLoS One. 2015;10(6):1–14.

51. Kuri-Morales P, Emberson J, Alegre-Díaz J, Tapia-Conyer R, Collins R, Peto R, et al. The prevalence of chronic diseases and major disease risk factors at different ages among 150 000 men and women living in Mexico City: cross-sectional analyses of a prospective study. BMC Public Health. 2009;9:1–9.

52. Rubinstein AL, Irazola VE, Calandrelli M, Chen CS, Gutierrez L, Lanas F, et al. Prevalence, awareness, treatment, and control of hypertension in the southern cone of Latin America. Am J Hypertens. 2016;29(12): 1343–52.

53. Zhou B, Carrillo-Larco RM, Danaei G, Riley LM, Paciorek CJ, Stevens GA, et al. Worldwide trends in hypertension prevalence and progress in treatment and control from 1990 to 2019: a pooled analysis of 1201 population-representative studies with 104 million participants. Lancet. 2021;398(10304):957–80.

54. Regional Health – Americas TL. Latin America and Caribbean's path to improve hypertension control: time for bolder, tougher actions. Lancet Reg Heal – Am [Internet]. 2022;9:100278. https://doi.org/10.1016/j.lana.2022.100278.

55. Ruilope LM, Nunes Filho ACB, Nadruz W, Rodríguez Rosales FF, Verdejo-Paris J. Obesidad e hipertensión en Latinoamérica: perspectivas actuales. Hipertens y Riesgo Vasc [Internet]. 2018;35(2):70–6. https://doi.org/10.1016/j.hipert.2017.12.004.

56. Malik VS, Popkin BM, Bray GA, Després J-P, Willett WC, Hu FB. Sugar-sweetened beverages and risk of metabolic syndrome and type 2 diabetes: a meta-analysis. Diabetes Care. 2010;33(11):2477–83.

57. Singh GM, Micha R, Khatibzadeh S, Shi P, Lim S, Andrews KG, et al. Global, regional, and national consumption of sugar-sweetened beverages, fruit juices, and milk: a systematic assessment of beverage intake in 187 countries. PLoS One. 2015;10(8): e0124845.

58. Salgado Hernández JC, Ng SW, Colchero MA. Changes in sugar-sweetened beverage purchases across the price distribution after the implementation of a tax in Mexico: a before-and-after analysis. BMC Public Health. 2023;23(1):265.

59. Arantxa Cochero M, Rivera-Dommarco J, Popkin BM, Ng SW. In Mexico, evidence of sustained consumer response two years after implementing a sugar-sweetened beverage tax. Health Aff. 2017;36(3):564–71.

60. Roche M, Alvarado M, Sandoval RC, Gomes F da S, Paraje G. Comparing taxes as a percentage of sugar-sweetened beverage prices in Latin America and the Caribbean. Lancet Reg Heal Am. 2022;11:100257.

61. Sandoval RC, Roche M, Belausteguigoitia I, Alvarado M, Galicia L, Gomes FS, et al. Excise taxes on sugar-sweetened beverages in Latin America and the Caribbean. Rev Panam Salud Publica. 2021;45: e21.

62. Cominato L, Di Biagio GF, Lellis D, Franco RR, Mancini MC, de Melo ME. Obesity prevention: strategies and challenges in Latin America. Curr Obes Rep. 2018;7(2):97–104.

63. Ministerio de Salud de Chile. Subsecretaria de Salud Publica. Informe de evaluacion de la implementacion de la ley sobre composicion nutricional de los alimentos y su publicidad [Internet]. 2017. 2017. p. 1–97. Available from: https://www.minsal.cl/wp-content/uploads/2017/05/Informe-Implementación-Ley-20606-junio-2017-PDF.pdf

64. Duran AC, Mialon M, Crosbie E, Jensen ML, Harris JL, Batis C, et al. Food environment solutions for childhood obesity in Latin America and among Latinos living in the United States. Obes Rev an Off J Int Assoc Study Obes. 2021;22(Suppl 3):e13237.

65. Taillie LS, Reyes M, Colchero MA, Popkin B, Corvalán C. An evaluation of Chile's Law of Food Labeling and Advertising on sugar-sweetened beverage purchases from 2015 to 2017: a before-and-after study. PLoS Med. 2020;17(2):e1003015.

66. Micha R, Karageorgou D, Bakogianni I, Trichia E, Whitsel LP, Story M, et al. Effectiveness of school food environment policies on children's dietary behaviors: a systematic review and meta-analysis. PLoS One. 2018;13(3):e0194555.

67. Swinburn BA, Kraak VI, Allender S, Atkins VJ, Baker PI, Bogard JR, et al. The global syndemic of obesity, undernutrition, and climate change: the Lancet commission report. Lancet (London, England). 2019;393 (10173):791–846.

Obesity in Africa: A Silent Public Health Crisis

4

Charles Agyemang, Sandra Boatemaa Kushitor,
Grace Frempong Afrifa-Anane, and Ama de-Graft Aikins

Contents

C. Agyemang (✉)
Department of Public & Occupational Health, Amsterdam
University Medical Centers, University of Amsterdam,
Amsterdam, The Netherlands
e-mail: c.o.agyemang@amstersamumc.nl

S. B. Kushitor
Department of Community Health, Ensign Global College,
Kpong, Ghana

Centre for Sustainability Transitions and Department of
Food Science, Stellenbosch University, Stellenbosch,
South Africa

G. F. Afrifa-Anane
Department of Environment and Public Health, University
of Environment and Sustainable Development, Somanya,
Ghana

A. de-Graft Aikins
Regional Institute for Population Studies, University of
Ghana, Legon, Ghana

© Springer Nature Switzerland AG 2023
R. S. Ahima (ed.), *Metabolic Syndrome*,
https://doi.org/10.1007/978-3-031-40116-9_5

Abstract

This chapter outlines the epidemiology of overweight and obesity in Africa, their determinants, and the relationship with cardiovascular diseases (CVDs) and diabetes. The review shows that overweight and obesity rates are increasing in all African regions, with Northern and Southern African regions being the most affected. The rate of overweight and obesity is higher among women than among men and in urban areas than in rural areas although the rates in rural areas are rising rapidly. Socioeconomic status, age, parity, marital status, physical inactivity, body weight perceptions, and increased energy are powerful predictors of overweight and obesity in sub-Saharan Africa. The rapid urbanization accompanied by nutrition transition is changing the disease landscape in Africa, with CVD and its related risk factors gaining a prominent position. Some African countries have partially implemented physical activity, diet, and fiscal policies to address the risk factors of overweight and obesity. The rising levels of overweight and obesity in sub-Saharan Africa are likely to exacerbate the burden of CVD and its risk factors, such as diabetes, hypertension, and dyslipidemia if measures are not taken to curb the problem. Public health strategies focusing on a healthy food environment and diet, physical activity, weight reduction, and maintenance strategies are urgently needed in sub-Saharan African countries.

Keywords

Overweight · Obesity · Cardiovascular diseases · Diabetes · Gender · Urbanization · Sub-Saharan Africa · Africa

Introduction

Obesity is a significant contributing factor to various chronic diseases such as cardiovascular diseases (CVD), type 2 diabetes (T2D), musculoskeletal disorders, and some cancers [87]. Obesity and its related conditions lead to reduced quality of life and premature death. A meta-analysis of 97 studies, for example, showed that, compared with normal weight, being obese was associated with higher all-cause mortality for all grades of obesity combined [38]. Obesity is truly a global burden. In 2016, over 1.9 billion adults aged 18 years and older were overweight. Of these, over 650 million were obese [104].

The fundamental cause of overweight and obesity is an energy imbalance between food intake and energy expenditure. The nutrition transition, characterized by the change from diets of high nutritional quality to those in low-quality diets, is occurring globally [85]. The nutrition transition, coupled with the epidemiological and demographic transitions, has set population health toward high prevalence and incidence of obesity and related sequelae such as hypertension, diabetes, strokes, cancers, heart attacks, and other chronic noncommunicable diseases (NCDs) [34, 57, 90]. Africa is also experiencing these transitions [2, 22, 94].

In Africa, a complex coexistence of undernutrition and overnutrition has been reported. Between 1980 and 2014, the age-standardized mean BMI increased from 21.0 kg/m^2 to 23.0 kg/m^2 in men and from 21.9 kg/m^2 to 24.9 kg/m^2 in women [78]. The mean BMI increased across all regions over time. Amongst men, the highest mean BMI was recorded in northern Africa, and, for women, in northern and southern Africa, the lowest mean BMI, over time, was usually recorded in central Africa in both men and women [78]. The Mean BMI in northern and southern Africa was higher than the global average. Between 1992 and 2005, the prevalence of overweight and obesity increased by almost a third in sub-Saharan Africa [106]. Until recently, this increase was reported among women and urban residents [57]. However, data show a consistent increase in overweight and obesity among men and rural residents as well [6, 49]. The trend toward rising overweight and obesity poses health and socioeconomic challenges to individuals and the region.

Reviews examining the prevalence of overweight and obesity are needed to provide effective public health response to this health challenge. It has been recommended that such reviews can examine the risk factors of overweight and obesity and obesity-related illnesses to inform health workers, government agencies, and policy makers toward setting priorities and for designing interventions. Therefore, this chapter outlines the epidemiology of overweight and obesity in Africa. Secondly, we examined the determinants of overweight and obesity and their impact on CVDs and diabetes. The chapter finally presents policy initiatives implemented by African governments to address the challenge of overweight and obesity, and how these interventions align with the recommendations of the World Health Organization (WHO).

Box 1 Search Strategy
Three kinds of data were used for this review study: the WHO Global Infobase on overweight and obesity (https://www.who.int/data/gho), a literature on the determinants of overweight and obesity, and government policies in Africa. WHO Global Health Observatory and the Demographic and Health Surveys were used to provide prevalence estimates by sex, region, residence, and socioeconomic status and to depict trends of overweight and obesity over time in the various African regions. In addition, the determinants of overweight and obesity were reviewed in Africa using several electronic databases, including Science Direct, Ebsochost, Academic One File, elibray USA, Pubmed, Jstor, and Ajol. In webpages where the advanced search option was allowed, the search was limited to English language, human studies, and peer review journal articles. An analysis of the content of NCD policies in SSA was also conducted to identify how they align with the actions recommended by the WHO.

Measurement of Overweight and Obesity

Body mass index (BMI) is a simple weight-for-height index commonly used to classify adults as overweight and obese. It is defined as a person's weight in kilograms divided by the square of his height in meters (kg/m^2). A BMI of 25–29.9 kg/m^2 is classified as overweight, and BMI ≥ 30 kg/m^2 is classified as obesity.

Prevalence of Overweight and Obesity in Africa

Figure 1a, b shows the prevalence of overweight in 45 WHO African countries in 2016. Women, in general, had a higher prevalence of overweight (BMI $\geq$ 25 kg/m^2) than men in all countries, with the prevalence rates ranging from 28% in Guinea-Bissau to 66.1% in Algeria. Among men, the prevalence of overweight ranged from 13.4% in Algeria to 57.8% in Guinea-Bissau. The top five countries with the highest prevalence of overweight among women were Algeria (66.1%), Malawi (65.4%), Botswana (56.5%), Angola (53.7%), and Uganda (52.8%). About one in three women was overweight in the countries with the lowest rates of overweight. These countries include Guinea-Bissau (28.0%), Eswatini (28.3%), Seychelles (29.2%), Tanzania (29.2%), and Comoros (29.7%).

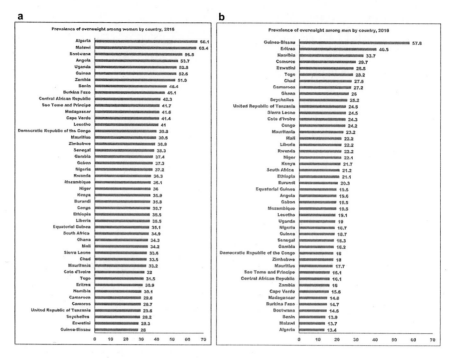

Fig. 1 (**a, b**) Estimated prevalence of overweight (BMI $\geq$ 25 kg/m^2) among adults aged 15+, 2016. (Source: WHO Global Health Observatory)

Figure 2a, b shows the prevalence of obesity in the various WHO African countries. The prevalence of obesity ranged from 1.8% in Uganda to about 20% in Algeria in men and from 6.9% in Guinea-Bissau to about 40% in Malawi in women. In men, only two countries (Algeria & South Africa) out of the 45 countries had an obesity prevalence of more than 10%. Among women, however, 36 of the 46 countries (78.3%) had a prevalence of obesity of more than 10%.

Determinants of Obesity

Urban and Rural Differences in Overweight and Obesity

Urbanization has been linked to an increased risk of overweight and obesity in Africa; therefore, most urban populations have higher overweight and obesity rates than rural populations [53]. Figure 3 displays data on the prevalence of overweight by place of residence in selected African countries based on the Demographic and Health Surveys conducted

between 2014 and 2019. In all the selected countries, the prevalence of overweight and obesity was higher in urban areas compared to rural areas. About one in every four people living in an urban area was overweight in Cameron, Ghana, Kenya, Gambia, Guinea, and South Africa.

Despite a high prevalence of overweight and obesity in urban areas, the rural areas are experiencing significant increase in the prevalence of overweight. In Table 1, obesity prevalence was higher for each survey year than the previous year. Between 2003 and 2014, the prevalence of obesity in rural areas doubled in Ghana. A similar pattern was also reported for Guinea between 2005 (1%) and 2018 (5%).

Sociodemographic Factors and Obesity

Generally, overweight and obesity rates are higher among females than males in Africa, as indicated above in Figs. 1 and 2. In 2016, for example, about 40% of women in Malawi were obese compared with 2% of men (Fig. 2a, b). The effect of

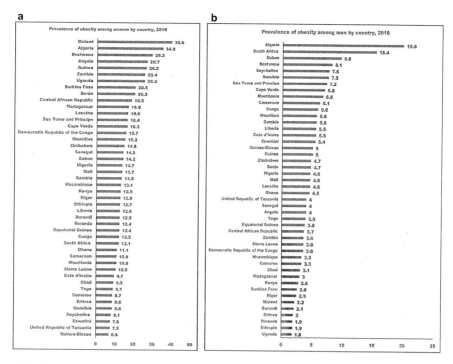

Fig. 2 (**a, b**) Estimated prevalence of obesity (BMI $\geq$ 30 kg/m^2) among adults aged 15+ in Africa, 2016. (Source: WHO Global Health Observatory)

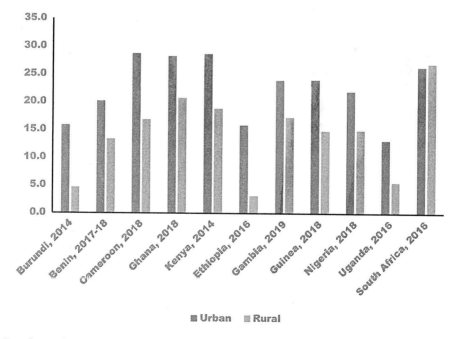

Fig. 3 Prevalence of overweight by place of residence in selected African countries

Table 1 Prevalence of obesity in selected countries in rural areas using data from demographic and health surveys

Country	1998	2003	2005	2008	2011	2014	2016	2018
Nigeria				4				5.8
Ghana		3.6		4.6		8.7		
South Africa	25.1	21					39.2	
Guinea			1.2					4.9
Cameron					4.8			6.7

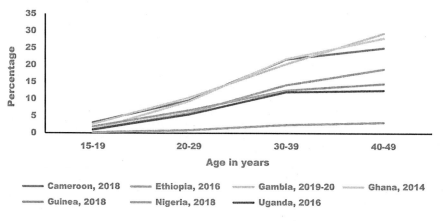

Fig. 4 Prevalence of obesity by age groups among women in selected African countries

sex on the risk of overweight and obesity has shown consistent results even when other factors like age, educational level, marital status, and employment are controlled for [12, 53].

Although body weight varies by sex, it is related to a specific stage of life. Several studies in Africa have reported a positive association between age and obesity [12, 56]. Among women of reproductive age, the prevalence of overweight and obesity has consistently increased with age (Fig. 4). In Cameroun, while 3% of women aged 15–24 years are obese, 25% of those aged 40–49 years are obese. A trend analysis of overweight and obesity prevalence by age reported a higher rate among older women between 1998 and 2017 (Fig. 4) [79].

Marital status is also an important determinant of obesity on the continent. Being married increases the likelihood of being overweight or obese. Asosega et al. [20], in a study among Ghanaian women, found that 44% of married individuals were obese compared to 30% of those who were never married. In Zimbabwe, married women were 58% more likely to be overweight and 79% more likely to be obese compared

with women who had never married [56]. In Kenya, married women were 1.73 times more likely to be overweight and obese compared to those not married [74].

Obesity also increases with parity [51]. In a systematic study of overweight and obesity among women, the prevalence of maternal obesity ranged from 6.5% in the Democratic Republic of Congo to 50.7% in Nigeria [83]. Women with one or more children were more likely to be overweight or obese than those without children [8, 30, 84].

Socioeconomic Status and Obesity

A consistent pattern is emerging among studies that examined the influence of SES on obesity. Even though the burden is concentrated among the wealthiest, obesity is increasing across both low and high SES spectrums [105]. In particular, women from medium-wealth households and those with secondary school education were more susceptible to overweight and obesity [31]. Studies that used the wealth index as a measure of SES in relation to obesity consistently found a higher prevalence of obesity as wealth increases [37, 42, 100]. In Comoros, the highest prevalence of obesity was found among women in medium households in 2012 (15%) [100]. As Fig. 5 shows, in all the selected countries, obesity rates were higher in wealthy households than in poor households. In 2016 in South Africa, the prevalence of overweight and obesity was almost similar among women from highest (49%) and middle (44%) SES households.

Regional Differences and Overweight prevalence

Figure 6 shows the time trend prevalence of overweight in various African regions. Overweight has been on the increase in all regions since 1990 although the extent of the increase has differed between regions. In 1990, the prevalence of overweight was highest in Northern African (7.5%) followed by Southern Africa (6.4%), Eastern Africa (4.5%), Middle Africa (3.7%), and Western Africa (2.6%). There has been a staggering increase of overweight in Southern Africa region since 1990 with average prevalence rate of 21% in 2015 (330% increase in the last 25 years) compared to other regions. Northern African region has also experienced rapid increase in overweight since 1990 with prevalence of 13% in 2015 (73% increase in the last 25 years). In other regions, the percentage increase in the last 25 years has been modest ranging from 9% in Eastern Africa to 70% in Western Africa.

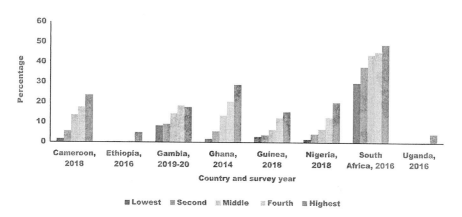

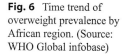

Fig. 5 Prevalence of obesity by wealth quintile among women in selected African countries

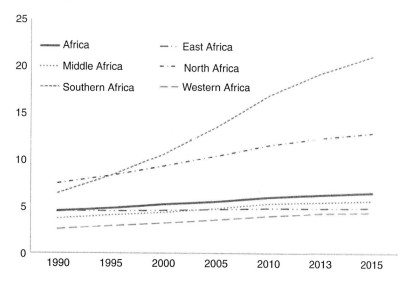

Fig. 6 Time trend of overweight prevalence by African region. (Source: WHO Global infobase)

Perceptions of Body Size and Obesity

Although, preference for a smaller body size is increasing, in most societies in sub-Saharan Africa, larger body size is socially acceptable (particularly among females) due to associated positive attributes such as wealth, good health, beauty, and fertility [7, 17, 44, 55]. For instance, in a study of body size preferences among mothers and their children in Malawi, Flax et al. 2020 reported that mothers preferred larger body sizes for themselves and their children and thus selected larger body silhouettes as healthy. Afrifa-Anane et al. [7] also found among Ghanaian urban poor residents that overweight and obese women did not want to lose weight, while those who were slim or had normal weight desired to gain weight to avoid mocking and stigmatization. The concerns about being stigmatized for weight loss compelled women to use nonprescribed medications to stimulate weight gain. Manafe et al.'s [55] study in South Africa also showed the belief that overweight individuals are healthy and that larger body size has no association with developing chronic diseases such as hypertension and diabetes. These perceptions and beliefs about larger body sizes have an impact on the obesity burden in sub-Saharan Africa [29, 86].

However, some studies have shown a changing preference for a smaller ideal body size [15, 35, 41, 61]. The change in preference from larger to smaller body size has been attributed to modernization, exposure to, and acceptance of Western cultural ideals of beauty [16]. Among adolescents in South Africa, having a normal body size was associated with respect, happiness, and being the best. At the same time, obesity was considered the unhappiest and worse body size and underweight was the weakest body size [41]. In Ghana, a study among overweight women showed that although there was admiration for some weight gain, excessive weight was abhorred by most participants. This is because fatness has negative implications such as frequent tiredness, poor self-image, declining social lifestyle, and increased disease risk [15].

Lifestyle Factors and Overweight and Obesity

Unhealthy diet, physical inactivity, smoking, and alcohol consumption are among the lifestyle factors that are associated with overweight and obesity in sub-Saharan Africa. Regarding diet, the consumption of calorie-dense foods, low intake of fruits and vegetables, and drinking of tea have been related to obesity. In Ghana, consuming fewer servings of fruit is associated with increasing the likelihood of being overweight and obese [3, 27]. On average women consume more calories than the recommended daily allowance [81]. The increased intake of ready to eat meals and sugar has also been associated with overweight and obesity [9]. Physical inactivity also has a negative effect on obesity. Individuals who engaged in vigorous activities had lower risks for obesity than those who did less rigorous activities [92]. However, most individuals do not meet the recommended levels of physical activity [43].

The association between alcohol consumption, smoking, and obesity is inconsistent [79, 98]. While some studies report a positive association, others report the inverse. Women who consumed alcohol were 1.37 times more likely to be overweight or obese than those who did not consume alcohol [8]. In Malawi, however, the proportion of current drinkers who were obese (22.9%) was less likely than nondrinkers (17.3%) to be obese [76]. In terms of smoking, obesity was high among smokers. In Malawi, smokers were 24% more likely to be obese compared to 10% of non smokers.

Relationship Between Overweight and Obesity, and CVD and Diabetes in Africa

Obese individuals develop more CVD risk factors than persons of normal weight [23, 80, 82]. Six of the papers included in the review examined the impact of obesity on CVD risk and diabetes in Africa. Among the risk factors of CVD, obesity was considered the most dominant. Overweight and obese persons had higher systolic blood pressure and diastolic blood pressure compared with normal weight persons [76]. The data suggest that the risk is higher for men than women [1, 77]. In Tanzania, a unit increase in BMI was associated with a 10% increase odds of hypertension [80]. In Nigeria, a BMI greater than 25 Kgm^2 increased the odds of hypertension by 12% [82]. In addition, the risk of diabetes was higher among obese than normal weight people [96]. In Kenya, the age- and sex-adjusted odds for diabetes increased by 3.2% among obese compared to persons of normal weight [23]. Obesity was also positively related to hypercholesterolemia. In South Africa, the total cholesterol levels of overweight women increased by 3% compared to the normal weight [96].

Obesity Interventions in Sub-Saharan Africa

To reduce the increasing prevalence of obesity and its associated consequences, the World Health Organization (WHO) proposed the 2004 Global Strategy on Diet, Physical Activity, and Health and the 2008 Action Plan on Prevention and Control of NCD. These policies aimed to change obesogenic environments to provide opportunities for healthy food choices and increased physical activity levels [101]. The global policies recommend policy actions to increase the intake of fruits and vegetables and other healthy foods, decrease the intake of sugar-sweetened beverages, and promote physical activity through multisectoral actions that target multiple settings, WHO member states were expected to provide leadership and commitment by developing multisectoral policies from the strategy for their population. This section presents an analysis of the content of NCD policies in SSA and how they align with the actions recommended by the WHO.

Promotion of Physical Activity

SSA governments have introduced several strategies to promote physical activity. Most of these

actions are in connection with the Global Strategy on Diet, Physical Activity, and Health.

One of the proposed actions for the Member States is to provide accurate and balanced information and ensure the availability of appropriate health promotion and education programs. Countries including Ghana, Botswana, South Africa, Namibia, Liberia, Ethiopia, Seychelles, Lesotho, Gambia, and Kenya have embarked on health promotion and awareness campaigns for a healthy and active life in schools, communities, and through the media to increase public awareness of the health benefits of being physically active. During these campaigns, health education materials on physical activities were distributed to increase knowledge on physical activity recommendations and benefits [63, 67, 69, 70]. South Africa proposed using role models to create awareness of the importance of regular physical activity [33]. The governments of Mauritius and Ghana specified that a culture of physical activity would be fostered particularly among people who are typically sedentary, such as drivers, market women, and secretaries, to enable them to engage in regular physical activity at home, workplace, and during recreation for at least 30 min on most days of the week [66, 68]. In Mauritius, 16 Women's Sports Associations (WSAs) were launched in the Women's Centers to address the issue of obesity and physical fitness among women. Activities including volleyball, table tennis, swimming, badminton, walking, and keep fit exercises were undertaken to promote physical activity [66].

Another recommended action by the WHO is for governments to ensure that physical environments support safe active commuting and that spaces are available for recreational activity. In Mauritius, South Africa, and Zambia, public and private physical activity clubs have been formed, and physical activity programs and organized sports activities have been developed at the national level, communities, and secondary schools to promote physical activity [33, 66, 73].

Also, the provision of and access to recreational facilities in workplaces and communities is an intervention program that has been implemented to promote physical activity in

South Africa, Mauritius, Zambia, Ghana, and Nigeria [33, 36, 66]. Access to safe walking paths, cycling lanes, and safe spaces for active play was stated in countries including Ghana, Nigeria, South Africa, Zambia, and Seychelles to promote physical activity [33, 36, 72].

Furthermore, the implementation of school-based programs that support the adoption of physical activity was a policy action recommended by the WHO. In line with the WHO resolution, promotion of physical activity in schools has been strengthened through the physical education component in the school curriculum, thus ensuring adequate opportunity for physical activity within the school environment in Ghana, Nigeria, Seychelles, South Africa, Mauritius, Kenya, and Botswana [66, 68, 72]. In Mauritius, for example, the school curriculum for Physical Education includes lessons on minor games, kids' athletics, simple physical activities, and breathing exercises. The government of Ghana also highlighted that physical education, which is more practical with outdoor and indoor games should be promoted in Basic and Senior High Schools.

Nutrition and Diet-Related Policies

To promote a healthy diet, the WHO recommends that governments develop accurate and balanced information for consumers to enable them to make well-informed, healthy choices. To increase the consumption of fruits and vegetables and other healthy diets, the governments of Zambia, Mauritius, Ethiopia, Ghana, Sierra Leone, Kenya, and Gambia highlighted the promotion of public awareness through the media, distribution of print materials, community engagement about benefits of healthy diets [63, 66, 73].

The WHO also recommends that governments should work with relevant stakeholders to develop mechanisms for promoting the responsible marketing of foods and nonalcoholic beverages to children, and address any issues of advertising. In order to promote healthy eating, countries such as Ghana, Zambia, South Africa, Mauritius, Ethiopia, Kenya, and Namibia have specified that manufacturers and the food industry will be mandated to display nutrition labeling for all prepackaged foods. This will allow customers to obtain nutritional information and make informed choices about healthy diet [33, 66, 67, 69, 73]. Countries including Ghana, Botswana, and South Africa, outlined policy actions on restricting marketing of unhealthy foods and beverages high in saturated fats, trans fats, and free sugars, particularly to children [33, 67, 68]. For instance, the government of Ghana indicated that sale of carbonated drinks like soda will be replaced with fruits such as banana, oranges, and peeled pineapples in school canteen and compounds. Students will be educated on the need to limit the intake of fats, sugar.

In addition, governments are to implement school-based programs that support the adoption of healthy diet. Therefore, there is a policy action in South Africa, Seychelles, Kenya, and Rwanda to strengthen and ensure nutritional education component in the school curriculum to promote healthy eating habits [71, 72, 95]. Also, countries including Botswana, Ghana, Mauritius, and South Africa have focused on providing healthy diets in schools. For instance, the government of Ghana underscored that school feeding program will be under the supervision of a dietician and that fruits and vegetables will form part of the meals of students in all boarding schools [63].

Also, promotion of food gardens, particularly, vegetable gardens in households, schools, and communities was highlighted in Eswatini, Lesotho, Mauritius, Rwanda, Gambia, and South Africa to increase availability and accessibility of fresh fruits and vegetables [25, 64, 70, 71]. Related to this, South Africa highlighted on establishing local markets of fruits and vegetables with the help of Department of Agriculture, Forestry, and Fisheries, Rural Development, and Land Reform. In Kenya, through the National Youth Service (NYS), the government supported an unusual form of urban farming: sack gardening in Kibera (Nairobi's largest urban poor settlement with limited space). This involves growing various crops and vegetables on the top and sides of large burlap sacks filled with soil, small stones, and manure. This approach is considered as a low-cost and healthy solution to food insecurity and access to fresh vegetables [40].

Fiscal Policies to Promote Healthy Diets

As part of the efforts to reduce the rising prevalence of obesity and noncommunicable disease, the WHO recommends fiscal policies to improve diet, particularly taxes on sugar-sweetened beverages (SSBs) and subsidies on fruits, vegetables, and/or other healthy food. SSBs refer to any beverage with added sugar or other sweetener, such as sucrose or high-fructose corn syrup, which have high levels of calories and little nutritional value [102].

Regarding taxation, the WHO recommends a minimum of 20% tax on SSBs [103]. In view of this, some SSA countries have introduced fiscal policies to promote healthier diets. However, these taxes are far below the WHO recommendation of 20%. For instance, Nigeria has adopted a sugary tax to tackle the rising prevalence of obesity and related diseases and also to increase revenue for healthcare. On 31 December 2021, the government signed into law a policy that mandates the payment of an excise duty of ten Nigerian Naira (about US$0.02) per liter on all nonalcoholic and sweetened beverages in the country [5]. In April 2018, South Africa also introduced the Health Promotion Levy (HPL) on sugary beverages (excluding fruit juices) that have more than four grams of sugar per 100 ml. A rate of 2.1cent per gram of the sugar content that exceeds four grams per 100 ml was implemented. That is, the first four grams per 100 ml are levy-free. The HPL on sugary beverages is payable by Manufacturers in the Republic of South Africa. On the other hand, subsidies on healthy foods including fruits and vegetables have been introduced to promote their intake [46]. Also, Zambia adopted 0.30 Kwacha per liter (USD 0.02) excise duty on nonalcoholic beverages at a rate of 3% in 2018 [62]. In Mauritius, there was an excise duty on soft and sugar-sweetened nonalcoholic beverages (3% per gram of sugar) at a rate of 2 Mauritian cents in 2013. This was implemented to encourage and promote alternatives such as

water, pure fruit juice, blends, vegetable juice, and dairy milk [58]. Uganda has adopted an excise duty tax of 12% (UGX 200, approx. 0.05 USD) per liter, on nonalcoholic beverages excluding fruit and vegetable juices [13]. The government of Seychelles also introduced an excise tax on drinks (including flavored milk) containing sugar contents exceeding 5 grams per 100 ml in April, 2019. This, however, excluded fresh local fruits' drinks without any additives and plain milk. Drinks exceeding 5 grams per 100 ml sugar are subject to a tax of SR4 per liter (Seychelles Revenue Commission). Rwanda has no fiscal policy, which explicitly aims at reducing SSBs consumption. However, there is a revenue-generating excise tax of 39% on both SSBs and nonsugary beverages [89].

In Botswana, Mauritius, Lesotho, Seychelles, Ghana, and Guinea, the process for fiscal policies to discourage the consumption of SSBs, fats, and salts has been initiated. For instance, in Guinea, the government stated that subsidies would be introduced to promote local production of fruits and vegetables [65]. Lesotho also proposed the exemption of fruits and vegetables from taxation to promote accessibility of fruits and vegetables [70].

Discussion

The aim of this study was to outline the epidemiology of obesity, obesity determinants, and related risks such as cardiovascular diseases and diabetes in sub-Saharan Africa. The review shows that overweight and obesity rates have been increasing in all African regions. In addition, the rate of obesity is higher among women than among men, and in urban areas than in rural areas although the rates in rural areas are increasing very fast. Sex, age, marital status and parity, socioeconomic status, body weight perceptions, and lifestyle factors are among the determinants of obesity. The review also identified that obesity increases the risk of CVDs and diabetes. This review also found that only few African countries have implemented physical activity, diet, and fiscal policies to address overweight and obesity.

The increasing prevalence of overweight and obesity in Africa over the last few decades could be explained by changes in livelihood and economic conditions. During the late 1980s, for example, (a period described as the lost decades), the continent was in economic crisis: living standards fell and deprivation increased for a growing number of citizens in affected countries [10, 18]. The first major wave of rural-urban migration occurred during this period [10]. There was a corresponding challenge of limited food availability and quality and the region recorded high prevalence of undernutrition for both children and adults. This period was also characterized by the advent of the HIV/AIDS crises [45]. During this period, the stigma attached to thinness intensified as thinness became associated not only with deprivation but also with HIV/AIDS status [50]. At the turn of the millennium, economic growth was reported in some Africa countries [97]. Globalization changed the sociocultural landscape of many countries with food market globalization playing a major role. African countries signed trade agreements that allowed increased importation of processed foods high in fat, sugar, and salt into the continent, the availability of which lessened the appeal and consumption of traditional wholesome foods [10]. The change in economic growth in combination with globalization forces, led to changes in demographic profile, urban population, weight perceptions, and lifestyle behaviors. These factors are currently fueling Africa's obesity crisis.

In demographic terms, socioeconomic status of individuals was the first affected. For example, school enrollment rates increased on the continent. Between 1999 and 2008, gross enrollment ratios increased from 19% to 27% for upper secondary and 3–6% for tertiary education [99]. This educated population contributed to the growth of the urban wealthy who had access to a globalized food economy and engaged in sedentary work patterns and lifestyles. As a result, this group may have maintained a positive energy balance over a long period of time [4, 75]. It is not surprising therefore that until recently, wealthy persons were at higher risk of obesity in Africa compared to the poor [106]. In terms of gender,

research suggests that the gap between men and women can be explained by the low levels of physical activity among women [17, 21, 88]. In urban areas, processed foods high in fat, sugar, and salt are accessible, easy to cook, and preferred to traditional meals [39, 47, 48]. As a result, there is an increase in consumption of these calorie dense foods but without the needed physical activity [32].

The positive relationship between wealth and obesity reflects the epidemiological transition in sub-Saharan Africa [10]. The pattern is generally in line with the "diffusion theory" of the epidemic of coronary heart disease (CHD) as demonstrated in high-income countries [54]. The "diffusion theory" posits that the rise of CHD starts in high socioeconomic groups, because they are the first groups who can afford diets rich in saturated fats and associated with overweight and obesity, which in turn increase the risk of CHD. With time, the disease spreads to lower socioeconomic groups as living standards improve for all. When the CHD epidemic starts to decline, the higher socioeconomic groups are once again the first groups to reap the benefit as they are the first to adopt healthy behavioral changes. Accordingly, it is expected the current socioeconomic gradient in obesity which favors the poor in sub-Saharan Africa will reverse as standards of living improve unless measures are put in place to protect the poor. Evidence from Egypt suggests that the gradient is changing in favor of the rich. In Asfaw's [19] study, poor people who had lived in urban areas for long periods were more likely than their rich peers to be obese due to their access to relatively inexpensive calorie dense foods.

In terms of perceptions of body weight, the association of fat with wealth, health, and beauty has coexisted with the stigmatization of thinness in many African countries over a long period. The HIV/AIDS pandemic intensified the stigmatization of thinness, as strong associations were made between the emaciated body and HIV/AIDS status. Yet, current evidence suggests that perceptions of body weight and of fatness, in particular, are more nuanced than originally reported. In a number of empirical studies, lay communities appear to value healthy body weight, which corresponds to a buxom rather than obese body size [24, 35]. There is also increasing awareness of the relationship between obesity and health risks including CVD and diabetes.

In some countries, policies have been implemented to address the burden of overweight and obesity. With the exception of the fiscal policies where the percent of tax implemented on SSB is lower than the recommended guideline, the nutrition and diet and physical activity strategies implemented by some countries align with WHO recommendations. In South Africa, the sugar tax has resulted in a reduction in the consumption of SSB [93]. However, gaps have been noticed by researchers in how these policies are implemented [28, 52]. Most African countries have partially implemented the policies and are below the maximum score of 18 [14]. In particular, policies on alcohol, tobacco, and unhealthy foods are the action areas where more efforts have been recommended for implementation.

Evidence shows that obesity increases the risk of CVDs and related intermediate risk factors such as hypertension, diabetes, and hypercholesterolemia in several African countries [11, 60]. The increasing burden of CVDs has increased in line with the rising levels of obesity in Africa. These conditions reduce the quality of life through disabilities and deaths [26, 59]. The increasing burden of CVD is occurring at a time when infectious diseases are still highly prevalent, placing a great

demand on the overburdened and impoverished healthcare systems in most of these countries. Given the rising numbers of urban population, accompanied by nutrition transition throughout sub-Saharan Africa [83], the prevalence of obesity and its related problems such as diabetes and hypertension are likely to increase further if measures are not taken to address the problem head-on [91]. The potential impact of the changing environment on obesity has been demonstrated among sub-Saharan African migrants in Europe. In Agyemang et al.'s study [11], the odds of overweight and obesity among Ghanaian migrant men and women in Amsterdam were 19 times and 11 times higher than their compatriots men and women living in rural Ghana (Fig. 7).

Conclusion

The rapid urbanization accompanied by nutrition transition is changing the disease landscape in Africa with CVD and its related risk factors gaining a prominent position. The rising levels of overweight and obesity in African are likely to exacerbate the burden of CVD if measures are not taken to curb the problem. Public health strategies focusing on healthy diet, physical activity, weight reduction, and maintenance strategies have been initiated in African countries, particularly in urban areas. The implementation,

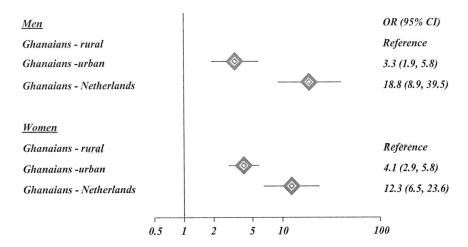

Fig. 7 Age-adjusted odds ratios (95% CI) of overweight/obesity among Ghanaians living in different locations

monitoring, and evaluation of these strategies should be strengthened with definite budget allocation and expenditure. In particular, the evaluation of these policies can examine their impact on dietary diversity, physical activity, consumption of SSBs, fats, and salt taking into account the differential effect of gender, socioeconomic, and cultural factors.

References

1. Abdelaal M, le Roux CW, Docherty NG. Morbidity and mortality associated with obesity. Ann Transl Med. 2017;5(7):1–12. https://doi.org/10.21037/atm. 2017.03.107.
2. Abubakari AR, Lauder W, Agyemang C, Jones M, Kirk A, Bhopal RS. Prevalence and time trends in obesity among adult west African populations: A meta-analysis. Obes Rev. 2008;9:297–311. https:// doi.org/10.1111/j.1467-789X.2007.00462.x.
3. Addae HY, Tahiru R, Azupogo F. Factors associated with overweight or obesity among post-partum women in the tamale Metropolis, northern Ghana: a cross-sectional study. Pan Afr Med J. 2022;41 https:// doi.org/10.11604/pamj.2022.41.238.33359.
4. Addo J, Smeeth L, Leon DA. Obesity in urban civil servants in Ghana: association with pre-adult wealth and adult socio-economic status. Public Health. 2009;123(5):365–70. https://doi.org/10.1016/j.puhe. 2009.02.003.
5. Adedeji OJ, Lucero-Prisnom E III. Taxation on beverages in Nigeria: impact and burden of the new policy. Pop Med. 2022;4:1–2. https://doi.org/10. 1136/bmj.h4047.
6. Afolabi W, Addo A, Sonibare M. Activity pattern, energy intake, and obesity among Nigerian urban market women. Int J Food Sci Nutr. 2004;55:85–90.
7. Afrifa-Anane GF, Badasu DM, Codjoe SNA, Anarfi JK. Barriers and facilitators of weight management: perspectives of the urban poor in Accra, Ghana. PLoS One. 2022;17(8):e0272274. https://doi.org/10.1371/ journal.pone.0272274.
8. Agbeko MP, Kumi-Kyereme A, Druye AA, Osei BG. Predictors of overweight and obesity among women in Ghana. Open Obes J. 2013;5:72–81. https://doi.org/10.2174/1876823701305010072.
9. Agyei A, Yorke E, Boima V. Prevalence of overweight and obesity and its relation to diet and physical activity among medical students in Accra, Ghana. Afr J Health Sci. 2022;35(2):99–113. https://www.ajol. info/index.php/ajhs/article/view/227088
10. Agyei-Mensah   S,   de-Graft   Aikins A. Epidemiological transition and the double burden of disease in Accra, Ghana. J Urban Health. 2010;87 (5):879–97. https://doi.org/10.1007/s11524-010-9492-y.
11. Agyemang C. Rural and urban differences in blood pressure and hypertension in Ghana, West Africa. Public Health. 2006;120:525–33. https://doi.org/10. 1016/j.puhe.2006.02.002.
12. Agyemang K, Pokhrel S, Victor C, Anokye NK. Determinants of obesity in West Africa: a systematic review. 2021. MedRxiv, 2021.04.27.21255462. https://www. medrxiv.org/content/10.1101/2021.04.27. 21255462v1%0Ahttps://www.medrxiv.org/content/10. 1101/2021.04.27.21255462v1.abstract%0Ahttps:// www.medrxiv.org/content/10.1101/2021.04.27. 21255462v1%0Ahttps://www.medrxiv.org/content/10. 1101/2021.04.27.212
13. Ahaibwe G, Abdool Karim S, Thow A-M, Erzse A, Hofman K. Barriers to, and facilitators of, the adoption of a sugar-sweetened beverage tax to prevent non-communicable diseases in Uganda: a policy landscape analysis. 2021; https://doi.org/10.1080/ 16549716.2021.1892307.
14. Allen LN, Wigley S, Holmer H. Implementation of non-communicable disease policies from 2015 to 2020: a geopolitical analysis of 194 countries. Lancet Glob Health. 2021;9(11):e1528–38. https://doi.org/ 10.1016/S2214-109X(21)00359-4.
15. Allison KC, Schweiger U, Pearl R, Nii R, Aryeetey O. Perceptions and experiences of overweight among women in the Ga East District, Ghana. Front Nutr. 2016;3:1. https://doi.org/10.3389/fnut.2016.00013.
16. Amenyah SD, Michels N. Body size ideals, beliefs and dissatisfaction in Ghanaian adolescents: sociodemographic determinants and intercorrelations. Public Health. 2016;139:112–20.
17. Amoah AGB. Sociodemographic variations in obesity among Ghanaian adults. Public Health Nutr. 2003;6(8):751–7. https://doi.org/10.1079/ PHN2003506.
18. Aryeetey R, Lartey A, Marquis GS, Nti H, Colecraft E, Brown P. Prevalence and predictors of overweight and obesity among school-aged children in urban Ghana. BMC Obes. 2017;4(1):1–8. https:// doi.org/10.1186/s40608-017-0174-0.
19. Asfaw A. Do government food price policies affect the prevalence of obesity? Empirical evidence from Egypt. World Dev. 2007;35:687–701. https://doi.org/ 10.1016/j.worlddev.2006.05.005.
20. Asosega KA, Adebanji AO, Abdul IW. Spatial analysis of the prevalence of obesity and overweight among women in Ghana. BMJ Open. 2021;11: e041659. https://doi.org/10.1136/bmjopen-2020-041659.
21. Averett SL, Stacey N, Wang Y. Economics and human biology decomposing race and gender differences in underweight and obesity in South Africa. Econ Hum Biol. 2014;15:23–40. https://doi.org/10.1016/j.ehb. 2014.05.003.
22. Awuah RB, Anarfi J, Agyemang C, Ogedegbe G, de-Graft Aikins A. Prevalence, awareness, treatment and control of hypertension in urban poor communities. J Hypertens. 2014;32(6):1203–10.

23. Ayah R, Joshi MD, Wanjiru R, Njau EK, Otieno CF, Njeru EK, Mutai KK. A population-based survey of prevalence of diabetes and correlates in an urban slum community in Nairobi, Kenya. BMC Public Health. 2013;13:371.

24. Benkeser RM, Biritwum R, Hill AG. Prevalence of overweight and obesity and perceptions of health and desirable body size in urban, Ghanaian Women. Ghana Med J. 2012;46(2):66–75.

25. Bergh T. Residue monitoring and control program. Department of Agriculture Forestry and Fisheries, Republic of South Africa. 2011. https://pdfs.semanticscholar.org/presentation/5394/dd36e5c4301480f1ad9719dd8be7a582bbca.pdf

26. Bertram MY, Jaswal AVS, Van Wyk VP, Levitt NS, Hofman KJ. The non-fatal disease burden caused by type 2 diabetes in South Africa, 2009. Bertram Glob Health Action. 2013;6:206–12. https://doi.org/10.3402/gha.v6i0.19244.

27. Biritwum R, Gyapong J, Mensah G. The epidemiology of obesity in Ghana. Ghana Med J. 2005;39(3):82–5.

28. Bosu WK. A comprehensive review of the policy and programmatic response to the chronic non-communicable disease in Ghana. Ghana Med J. 2012;46(2):69–78.

29. Chigbu CO, Aniebue UU, Berger U, Parhofer KG. Impact of perceptions of body size on obesity and weight management behaviour: a large representative population study in an African setting. Public Health. 2019;43(1):54–61. https://doi.org/10.1093/pubmed/fdz127.

30. Dake F, Tawiah E, Badasu DM. Sociodemographic correlates of obesity among Ghanaian women. Public Health Nutr. 2010;14(7):1285–91. https://doi.org/10.1017/S1368980010002879.

31. Daran B, Levasseur P. Is overweight still a problem of rich in sub-Saharan Africa? Insights based on female-oriented demographic and health surveys. World Dev Perspect. 2022;25:100388. https://doi.org/10.1016/J.WDP.2021.100388.

32. Delisle H, Ntandou-Bouzitou G, Agueh V, Sodjinou R, Fayomi B. Urbanisation, nutrition transition and cardiometabolic risk: the Benin study. Br J Nutr. 2012;107(10):1534–44. https://doi.org/10.1017/S0007114511004661.

33. Department of Health. Strategic plan for the prevention and control of non-communicable diseases 2013–2017; 2013.

34. Dietz WH. Reversing the tide of obesity. Lancet. 2011;378(9793):744–6. https://doi.org/10.1016/S0140-6736(11)61218-X.

35. Duda RB, Jumah NA, Hill AG, Seffah J, Biritwum R. Interest in healthy living outweighs presumed cultural norms for obesity for Ghanaian women. Health Qual Life Outcomes. 2006;4:44. https://doi.org/10.1186/1477-7525-4-44.

36. Federal Ministry of Health Nigeria. National policy and strategic plan of action on non-communicable diseases; 2013.

37. Fezeu L, Minkoulou E, Balkau B, Kengne AP, Awah P, Unwin N, Alberti GK, Mbanya JC. Association between socioeconomic status and adiposity in urban Cameroon. Int J Epidemiol. 2006;35:105–11.

38. Flegal KM, Kit BK, Orpana H. Association of all-cause. Mortality. 2013;309(1):71–82.

39. Freidberg S. French beans for the masses: A modern historical geography of food in Burkina Faso. J Hist Geogr. 2003;29(3):445–63. https://doi.org/10.1006/jhge.2002.0487.

40. Gallaher CM, WinklerPrins AMGA, Njenga M, Karanja NK. Creating space: sack gardening as a livelihood strategy in the Kibera slums of Nairobi, Kenya. J Agric Food Syst Community Dev. 2015;5(2):155–73.

41. Gitau TM, Micklesfield LK, Pettifor JM, Norris SA. Changes in eating attitudes, body esteem and weight control behaviours during adolescence in a south African cohort. PLoS One. 2014;9(10):109709. https://doi.org/10.1371/journal.pone.0109709.

42. Goetjes E, Pavlova M, Hongoro C, Groot W. Socioeconomic inequalities and obesity in South Africa—a decomposition analysis. Int J Environ Res Public Health. 2021;18(17) https://doi.org/10.3390/ijerph18179181.

43. Guthold R, Stevens GA, Riley LM, Bull FC. Worldwide trends in insufficient physical activity from 2001 to 2016: a pooled analysis of 358 population-based surveys with 1·9 million participants. Lancet Glob Health. 2018;6(10):e1077–86. https://doi.org/10.1016/S2214-109X(18)30357-7.

44. Holdsworth M, Garter A, Landais E, Marie B, Delpeuch F. Perceptions of healthy and desirable body size in urban Senegalese women. Int J Obes. 2004;28(12):1561–8.

45. Illiffe J. The African aids epidemic: a history. James Currey; 2006.

46. Jansen ADA, Stoltz E, Yu D. Improving the targeting of zero-rated basic foodstuffs under value added tax (VAT) in South Africa – an exploratory analysis (07/12; Stellenboach economic working paper, Issue May). 2012. https://www.google.co.za/url?sa=t&rct=j&q=&esrc=s&source=web&cd=6&cad=rja&uact=8&ved=0ahUKEwiv3uX0_PTXAhXGChoKHSrSB5QQFghIMAU&url=https%3A%2F%2Fwww.ekon.sun.ac.za%2Fpapers%2F2012%2Fwp072012%2Fwp-07-2012.pdf&usg=AOvVaw2ijiMXmlml2StZTXP_up9C

47. Kgaphola MS, Viljoen AT. Food habits of rural Swazi households: part 2: social structural and ideological influences on Swazi food habits. J Fam Ecol Consum Sci. 2004;32:16–25.

48. Kifleyesus A. Muslims and meals: the social and symbolic functions of foods in changing socio-economic environments. J Int Afr Inst. 2002;72(2): 245–76.

49. Kimani-Murage E, Pettifor J, Tollman S, Kipstein-Grobusch K, Norris S. Predictors of adolescent weight status and central obesity in rural South Africa. Public Health Nutr. 2011;14:1114–22.

50. Kruger HS, Puoane T, Senekal M, van der Merwe M-T. Obesity in South Africa: challenges for government and health professionals. Public Health Nutr. 2005;8(5):491–500. https://doi.org/10.1079/phn2005785.

51. Kushitor SB, Owusu L, Kushitor MK. The prevalence and correlates of the double burden of malnutrition among women in Ghana. PLoS One. 2020;15(12):1–12. https://doi.org/10.1371/journal.pone.0244362.

52. Laar A, Barnes A, Aryeetey R, Tandoh A, Bash K, Mensah K, Zotor F, Vandevijvere S, Holdsworth M. Implementation of healthy food environment policies to prevent nutrition-related non-communicable diseases in Ghana: national experts' assessment of government action. Food Policy. 2020;93:101907. https://doi.org/10.1016/j.foodpol.2020.101907.

53. Lartey ST, Magnussen CG, Si L, Boateng GO, de Graaff B, Biritwum RB, Minicuci N, Kowal P, Blizzard L, Palmer AJ. Rapidly increasing prevalence of overweight and obesity in older Ghanaian adults from 2007–2015: evidence from WHO-SAGE waves 1 & 2. PLoS One. 2019;14(8):e0215045. https://doi.org/10.1371/journal.pone.0215045.

54. Mackenbach JP, Cavelaars AE, Kunst AE, Groenhof F. Socioeconomic inequalities in cardiovascular disease mortality; an international study. Eur Heart J. 2000;21:1141–51.

55. Manafe M, Chelule PK, Madiba S. The perception of overweight and obesity among south African adults: implications for intervention strategies. Public Health. 2022;19 https://doi.org/10.3390/ijerph191912335.

56. Mangemba NT, Sebastian MS. Societal risk factors for overweight and obesity in women in Zimbabwe: a cross-sectional study. BMC Public Health. 2020;20 (103) https://doi.org/10.1186/s12889-020-8215-x.

57. Martorell R, Khan LK, Hughes ML, Grummer-Strawn LM. Obesity in women from developing countries. Eur J Clin Nutr. 2000;54(3):247–52. http://www.ncbi.nlm.nih.gov/pubmed/10713748

58. Mauritius Revenue Authority. Excise duty on sugar content of sugar sweetened products. 2015. https://www.mra.mu/index.php/customs1/more-topics/excise-tax-on-sugar-content-of-sugarsweetened-non-alcoholic-beverages. Accessed Sept 2022.

59. Mayosi BM, Flisher AJ, Lalloo UG, Sitas F, Tollman SM, Bradshaw D. The burden of non-communicable diseases in South Africa. Lancet. 2009;374(9693): 934–47. https://doi.org/10.1016/S0140-6736(09) 61087-4.

60. Medeiros F, Casanova MDA, Fraulob JC, Trindade M. How can diet influence the risk of stroke? Int J Hypertens. 2012:2–9. https://doi.org/10.1155/2012/763507.

61. Micklesfield LK, Lambert EV, Hume DJ, Chantler S, Paula R, Dickie K, Puoane T, Goedecke JH. Socio-cultural, environmental and behavioural determinants of obesity in black south African women. Cardiovasc J Afr. 2013;24(9):369–75. https://doi.org/10.5830/CVJA-2013-069.

62. Ministry of Finance. Zambia. Budget address by Honourable Margaret D. Mwanakatwe, MP, Minister of Finance, delivered to the National Assembly on Friday 28th September, 2018; Zambia: Ministry of Finance.

63. Ministry of Health. National policy for the prevention and control of chronic non-communicable diseases in Ghana (issue august). 2012. https://www.iccp-portal.org/sites/default/files/plans/national_policy_for_the_prevention_and_control_of_chronic_non-communicable_diseases_in_ghana(1).pdf

64. Ministry of Health & Social Welfare. The Gambia National Health sector strategic plan 2014–2020. 2014. https://extranet.who.int/mindbank/item/5970

65. Ministry of Health and Hygiene. National integrated program for the prevention and control of non-communicable diseases; 2010.

66. Ministry of Health and Quality of Life Mauritius. National plan of action for nutrition 2009–2010; 2009.

67. Ministry of Health and social National Services Namibia. Namibian national health policy framework; 2011.

68. Ministry of Health Ghana. National policy: non-communicable diseases. In Ministry of Health, Ghana (p. 45). 2022. https://www.moh.gov.gh/wp-content/uploads/2022/05/Ghana-NCD-Policy-2022.pdf

69. Ministry of Health Kenya. National strategy for the prevention and control of non-communicable diseases 2015–2020; 2016.

70. Ministry of Health Lesotho. National multi-sectoral integrated strategic plan for the prevention and control of non-communicable diseases (NCDS) 2014–2020; 2014.

71. Ministry of Health Rwanda. National food and nutrition policy 2013–2018; 2013.

72. Ministry of Health Seychelles. Seychelles strategy for the prevention and control of noncommunicable diseases, 2016–2025; 2016.

73. Ministry of Health Zambia. Zambian strategic plan 2013–2016. Non-communicable diseases and their risk factors; 2013.

74. Mkuu RS, Gilreath TD, Wekullo C, Reyes GA, Harvey IS. Social determinants of hypertension and type-2 diabetes in Kenya: A latent class analysis of a nationally representative sample. PLoS One. 2019;14(8):1–10. https://doi.org/10.1371/journal.pone.0221257.

75. Mogre V, Mwinlenaa PP, Oladele J, Amalba A. Impact of physical activity levels and diet on central obesity among civil servants in tamale metropolis. J Med Biomed Sci. 2012;1(2):1–9.

76. Msyamboza PK, Kathyola D, Dzowela T. Anthropometric measurements and prevalence of underweight, overweight and obesity in adult Malawians: nationwide population-based NCD STEPS survey. Pan Afr Med J. 2013;15(108) https://doi.org/10.11604/pamj.2013.15.108.2622.

77. Mufunda J, Mebrahtu G, Usman A, Nyarango P, Kosia A, Ghebrat Y, Ogbamariam A. The prevalence of hypertension and its relationship with obesity: results from a national blood pressure survey in Eritrea. J Hum Hypertens. 2006;20:59–65. https://doi.org/10.1038/sj.jhh.1001924.

78. NCD Risk Factor Collaboration (NCD-RisC) – Africa Working Group. Trends in obesity and diabetes across Africa from 1980 to 2014: an analysis of pooled population-based studies. Int J Epidemiol. 2017:1421–32. https://doi.org/10.1093/ije/dyx078.

79. Nglazi MD, Ataguba JEO. Overweight and obesity in non-pregnant women of childbearing age in South Africa: subgroup regression analyses of survey data from 1998 to 2017. BMC Public Health. 2022;22(1):1–18. https://doi.org/10.1186/s12889-022-12601-6.

80. Njelekela MA, Mpembeni R, Muhihi A, Mligiliche NL, Spiegelman D, Hertzmark E, Liu E, Finkelstein JL, Fawzi WW, Willett WC, Mtabaji J. Gender-related differences in the prevalence of cardiovascular disease risk factors and their correlates in urban Tanzania. BMC Cardiovasc Disord. 2009;9(30):1–8. https://doi.org/10.1186/1471-2261-9-30.

81. Nyakotey DA, Ananga AS, Apprey C. Assessing physical activity, nutrient intake and obesity in middle-aged adults in Akuse, lower Manya Krobo, Ghana. J Health Res. 2022;36(2):199–208. https://doi.org/10.1108/JHR-03-2020-0068.

82. Okpechi IG, Chukwuonye II, Tiffin N, Madukwe OO, Onyeonoro UU, Umeizudike TI. Blood pressure gradients and cardiovascular risk factors in urban and rural populations in Abia state south eastern Nigeria using the WHO STEPwise approach. PLoS One. 2013;8(9):4–6. https://doi.org/10.1371/journal.pone.0073403.

83. Onubi OJ, Marais D, Aucott L, Okonofua F, Poobalan AS. Maternal obesity in Africa: a systematic review and meta-analysis. J Public Health. 2015;38(3): e218–31. https://doi.org/10.1093/pubmed/fdv138.

84. Pobee RA, Owusu WB, Plahar WA. The prevalence of obesity among female teachers of child-bearing age in Ghana. Afr J Food Agric Nutr Dev Res. 2013;13(3):7804–19. http://www.ajfand.net/Volume13/No3/Shenkalwa11850.pdf

85. Popkin BM, Adair LS, Ng SW. Global nutrition transition and the pandemic of obesity in developing countries. Nutr Rev. 2012;70(1):3–21. https://doi.org/10.1111/j.1753-4887.2011.00456.x.

86. Pradeilles R, Holdsworth M, Olaitan O, Irache A, Osei-Kwasi HA, Ngandu CB, Cohen E. Body size preferences for women and adolescent girls living in Africa: a mixed-methods systematic review. Public Health Nutr. 2021;25(3):738–59. https://doi.org/10.1017/S1368980021000768.

87. Prospective Studies Collaboration. Body-mass index and cause-specific mortality in 900 000 adults: collaborative analyses of 57 prospective studies. Lancet. 2009;373(9669):1083–96. https://doi.org/10.1016/S0140-6736(09)60318-4.

88. Puoane T, Steyn K, Bradshaw D, Laubscher R, Fourie J, Lambert V, Laubscher RIA, Mbananga N. Obesity in South Africa : the south African demographic and health survey. Obes Res. 2002;10(10):1038–48.

89. Ruhara CM, Abdool KS, Erzse A, Thow AM, Ntirampeba S, Hofman KJ. Strengthening prevention of nutrition-related non-communicable diseases through sugar-sweetened beverages tax in Rwanda: a policy landscape analysis. Glob Health Action. 2021;14(1):1883911.

90. Rutter H. Where next for obesity? Lancet. 2011;378(9793):746–7. https://doi.org/10.1016/S0140-6736(11)61272-5.

91. Sanuade OA, Anarfi JK, de-Graft Aikins A, Koram KA. Patterns of cardiovascular disease mortality in Ghana: A 5-year review of autopsy cases at Korle-Bu teaching hospital. Ethn Dis. 2014;24:55.

92. Shayo GA, Mugusi FM. Prevalence of obesity and associated risk factors among adults in Kinondoni municipal district, Dar Es Salaam Tanzania. BMC Public Health. 2011;11(1):365. https://doi.org/10.1186/1471-2458-11-365.

93. Stacey NM, Edoka I, Hofman K, Swart EC, Popkin B, Ng SW. Changes in beverage purchases following the announcement and implementation of South Africa's health promotion levy: an observational study. Lancet Planet Health. 2021; https://doi.org/10.1016/S2542-5196(20)30304-1.

94. Steyn N, Mchiza Z. Obesity and the nutrition transition in sub-Saharan Africa. Ann N Y Acad Sci. 2014;1311:88–101. https://doi.org/10.1111/nyas.12433.

95. Strategy for the Prevention and Control of Obesity in South Africa 2015–2020. 2015.

96. Tibazarwa K, Ntyintyane L, Sliwa K, Gerntholtz T, Carrington M, Wilkinson D, Stewart S. A time bomb of cardiovascular risk factors in South Africa: Results from the Heart of Soweto Study "Heart Awareness Days.". Int J Cardiol. 2009;132(2):233–9. https://doi.org/10.1016/j.ijcard.2007.11.067.

97. Todaro M, Smith S. Economic development. 12th ed. Pearson Education; 2015.

98. Tumwesigye NM, Mutungi G, Bahendeka S, Wesonga R, Katureebe A, Biribawa C, Guwatudde D. Alcohol consumption, hypertension and obesity: relationship patterns along different age groups in

Uganda. Prev Med Rep. 2020;19(February):101141. https://doi.org/10.1016/j.pmedr.2020.101141.

99. UNESCO Institute for Statistics. Trends in tertiary education: sub-Saharan Africa. 2010. http://www.uis.unesco.org/FactSheets/Documents/fs10-2010-en.pdf

100. Wariri O, Alhassan JAK, Mark G, Adesiyan O, Hanson L. Trends in obesity by socioeconomic status among non-pregnant women aged 15-49 y: A cross-sectional, multi-dimensional equity analysis of demographic and health surveys in 11 sub-Saharan Africa countries, 1994-2015. Int Health. 2021;13(5):436–45. https://doi.org/10.1093/inthealth/ihaa093.

101. WHO. Global strategy on diet, physical activity and health. 2004. https://www.who.int/publications/i/item/9241592222

102. WHO. Reducing consumption of sugar-sweetened beverages to reduce the risk of childhood overweight and obesity. 2014.

103. WHO. Fiscal policies for diet and prevention of non-communicable diseases. Technical meeting report. Geneva. 2015.

104. WHO. Obesity and overweight: key facts. 2021. https://www.who.int/news-room/fact-sheets/detail/obesity-and-overweight. Accessed 10 Nov 2023.

105. Yaya S, Anjorin S, Okolie EA. Obesity burden by socioeconomic measures between 2000 and 2018 among women in sub-Saharan Africa: A cross-sectional analysis of demographic and health surveys. Obes Sci Pract. 2022:1–10. https://doi.org/10.1002/osp4.595.

106. Ziraba AK, Fotso JC, Ochako R. Overweight and obesity in urban Africa: A problem of the rich or the poor? BMC Public Health. 2009;9:1–9. https://doi.org/10.1186/1471-2458-9-465.

Zlatko Nikoloski

Contents

Abstract

The Middle East and North Africa (MENA) region encompasses 18 countries at various

Z. Nikoloski (✉)
London School of Economics, London, UK
e-mail: z.nikoloski@lse.ac.uk

levels of economic development – high-income (Qatar, Saudi Arabia), upper-middle-income (Jordan, Iraq), lower-middle-income (Egypt, Morocco), and low-income countries (Syria, Yemen). As in the rest of the world, rising obesity prevalence has also been documented in the MENA countries, with roughly one-fifth of the adult population in

© Springer Nature Switzerland AG 2023
R. S. Ahima (ed.), *Metabolic Syndrome*,
https://doi.org/10.1007/978-3-031-40116-9_6

the region considered as obese. Against this background, this chapter: (i) documents the prevalence of obesity in the region (both, from the literature and official statistical sources); (ii) identifies the major correlates of obesity; and (iii) assesses and documents the literature that links obesity with some of the most prevalent noncommunicable diseases (inter alia, diabetes, and cardiovascular diseases). We argue that the levels of obesity in the region are high and still increasing, with gender, age, income, education, nutrition patterns, and urbanization acting as the most prominent and robust correlates of obesity in the MENA region. The rates of child obesity are increasing, thus posing significant long-term health risks for the countries in the region. Finally, we argue that, in the context of MENA countries, there is robust link between obesity and certain chronic conditions (e.g., diabetes).

Keywords

Obesity · MENA · Middle East · Correlates of obesity · Overweigh · Risk factors of obesity · Diabetes · Cardiovascular diseases · Noncommunicable diseases

Introduction

The Middle East and North Africa (MENA) region encompasses 18 countries at various levels of economic development – high-income (Qatar, Saudi Arabia), upper-middle-income (Jordan, Iraq), lower-middle-income countries (Morocco, Lebanon), and low-income countries (Syria and Yemen). The global obesity epidemic has also engulfed the MENA countries with close to one-half of the adult population being considered as overweight or obese (i.e., having BMI index higher than 30) [1]. Globally, the literature has distilled a few important correlates of obesity – income, age, and gender are the most prominent ones. The fast pace of urbanization and the associated sedentary lifestyle have both played a role in exacerbating the obesity epidemic. These factors, as this literature review shows, act as

significant correlates of obesity in the MENA region as well, particularly in countries that had undergone a rapid economic growth and development due to their richness with natural resources (e.g., the Gulf countries). Finally, the rising global obesity rates are responsible for the substantial increase in the overall global burden of disease associated with noncommunicable diseases (NCD). In the MENA region, roughly 80% of the total deaths are due to noncommunicable diseases [2]. Moreover, the percentage of people living with NCDs particularly associated with obesity (e.g., diabetes, cardiovascular disease) is high. For instance, WHO reports that in some countries of the region, over 20% of adults satisfy the basic diagnostic conditions for diabetes [3].

Against this background, the aim of the literature review is to update an earlier study that took stock and synthesized the existing knowledge on obesity in the countries of the MENA region. In doing so, we have organized the review into three major parts: (i) a section that documents the overall prevalence of obesity across the countries in the region, while also paying a particular attention to the issue of rising child obesity in the region; (ii) a section that sheds light on the main correlates of obesity in the MENA region; (iii) a final section that documents the literature on the risk factors associated with obesity such as diabetes, cardiovascular diseases, stroke, and cancer.

In conducting this literature review on obesity, correlates of obesity, and obesity-related diseases, we grouped the countries of the Middle East and North Africa (MENA) region into four major groups corresponding to their level of development: low-income countries, lower-middle-income countries, upper-middle-income countries, and high-income countries. The country classifications correspond to the latest updates provided by the World Bank Research Department. Accordingly, the groups include the following countries:

(i) low-income countries (Syria and Yemen).
(ii) lower-middle-income countries (Algeria, Djibouti, Egypt, Iran, Lebanon, Morocco, the Palestinian Authority, and Tunisia).

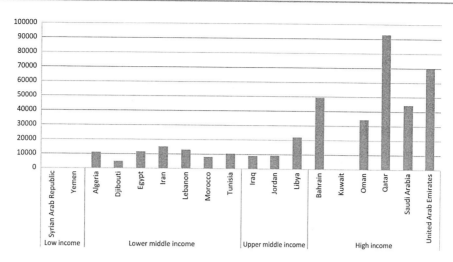

Chart 1 MENA countries: GDP per capita (international USD, constant, PPP), 2021. (Source: World Development Indicators and authors' calculations)

(iii) upper-middle-income countries (Iraq, Jordan, and Libya).

(iv) high-income countries (Bahrain, Kuwait, Oman, Qatar, Saudi Arabia, and the United Arab Emirates).

Before moving onto summarizing and discussing the literature on obesity and obesity-related diseases in the region, we present a snapshot of the economic development (as captured by GDP per capita and the Human Development Index) in the three respective country groups.

From Chart 1, we see a significant discrepancy in GDP per capita among the countries in the region, with the average per capita GDP ranging from 10,565 USD in the lower-middle-income countries, 13,383 USD in the upper-middle-income countries and 68,123 USD in the high-income countries. In order to "control" for the effect of abundance of natural resources and their impact on the overall GDP per capita in the respective countries, we also present the latest figures for the UNDP's Human Development Index (HDI). Here again, we see significant gap between the country groups in the region, with HDI ranging from 0.516 in the low-income countries, 0.697 in the lower-middle-income countries, 0.708 in the upper-middle-income

countries to 0.861 in the high-income countries (Chart 2).

Evidence on Obesity in the Middle East and North Africa Region

Evidence from Official Sources

Chart 3 captures the obesity rates per country, and it also provides the averages for the four country groups.[1] There are a few observations that stem from Chart 3. First, we see a positive correlation between level of obesity and level of economic development. Indeed, as we move up the income ladder, the obesity prevalence increases. For instance, the average prevalence of obesity in the low-income countries is 18.9%, 25.4% in the lower-middle-income countries, 36.2% in the upper-middle income countries, and close to 40% in the high-income countries. Second, in the lower-middle-income country group, there is a significant variation in the prevalence of obesity (for instance, the obesity prevalence in

---

[1] Data for Chart 3 comes from the World Health Organization (WHO) and World Obesity.

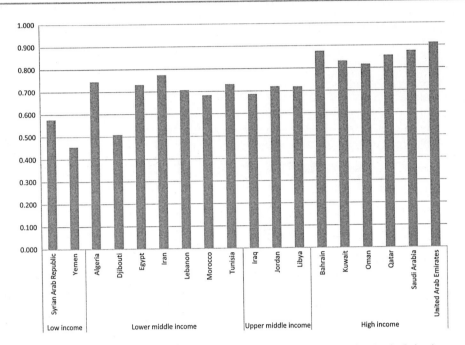

Chart 2 MENA countries: Human Development Index, 2021. (Source: UNDP and authors' calculations)

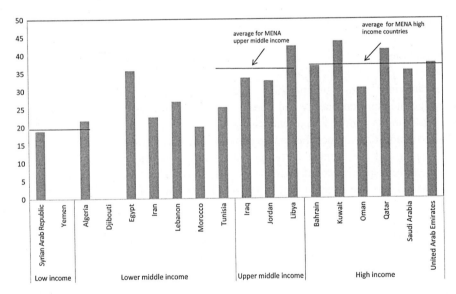

Chart 3 Selected MENA countries: % of population that is obese (BMI >30), latest. (Source: World Obesity and author's calculations)

Morocco is 20%, while it is as high as 35.7% in Egypt – almost as high as in some of the countries in the Gulf). The variation of the obesity prevalence rates is much smaller for the upper-middle-income and high-income country groups.

Evidence from the Literature

Low-Income Countries

While there is no harmonized data on prevalence of obesity in the lower-middle-income countries in MENA, isolated studies point to a rising obesity trend, especially among the urban population [4]. A study on Syria found that 43% of the population was obese [5], while the prevalence of obesity among the Palestinians has reached level of 22.1% among men and 37.2% among women [6].

Lower-Middle-Income Countries

Similar picture has also emerged in the lower-middle-income countries in the region. Obesity prevalence in some countries (e.g., Egypt and Morocco) has been rapidly increasing and risks reaching levels similar to the ones found in Gulf countries [4]. For instance, a study has found that obesity prevalence rates in Morocco are as high as 31.2% [7]. The rest of the countries in this group follow similar patterns. More specifically, prevalence of obesity has been particularly high in Algeria (30.1% among women and 9.1% among men) and Tunisia (37% among women and 13% among men) [8].

Upper-Middle-Income Countries

The existing literature also indicates that obesity rates in the upper-middle-income countries in the region are high. Overweight and obesity prevalence in the upper-middle-income countries have been reported as high as 40%. Similarly, high and alarming overweight and obesity prevalence rates are also registered among school children [4]. A recent study in Jordan has found an alarmingly high rise in the rates of overweight and obesity in the country [9].

High-Income Countries

The literature documents the high prevalence of obesity among Gulf countries, especially in Saudi Arabia [10, 11]. A recent study has reported that the obesity rates in Saudi Arabia reached 40%, with prevalence higher among women than men and among nationals than expatriates [12, 13]. Recent studies on Kuwait have documented that over 40% of adults in Kuwait meet the requirements to be considered as overweight [14, 15]. High prevalence of obesity has also been reported in Oman [16, 17] and Qatar [18].

Child Obesity in the Middle East and North Africa Region – Most Recent Evidence from the Literature

Most recently, research efforts have been targeted toward shedding light on the issue of child obesity and correlates of child obesity.

Child Obesity

In line with rising adult obesity, some of the high-income countries in the region have registered an increase in child obesity. A study in Saudi Arabia revealed that 25.7% of surveyed 20,000 adolescents in the Eastern Province were overweight or obese [19]. In Qatar, a study among 13–17-year-old adolescents showed that 23.4% of the adolescents were overweight, 19.9% were obese, and 37.6% had evidence of central obesity [20]. Finally, a study in the United Arab Emirates among adolescents revealed that one in three study participants was overweight or obese [21].

Child obesity has though also been a problem in some of the middle-income countries in the region. Osei Bonsu et al. [22] find that one in five children in Egypt is overweight or obese. Similar results were obtained from a study on primary school pupils in Egypt [23]. Similarly, a study of students aged 12–17 in Jordan revealed that 28.8% of students were overweight [24]. Child overweight and obesity have also been documented in the case of Morocco, albeit with lesser intensity [25]

Correlates of Child Obesity

This new strand of the literature has also aimed to analyze some of the correlates of child obesity. Children aged 19–37 months, those with birth weights >4 kg and those given large portions of protein foods (eggs and meat), had significant risks of overweight or obesity [22]. Existing studies have also found that mother's education and family income increase the odds of child overweight and obesity [20, 22, 24–26]. In Kuwait, a study among children aged 2–5 found that daily TV watching, for 2–3 h, increases the odds of obesity by 5.6-fold [27]. Similarly, physical inactivity has been singled out as a significant predictor of child obesity, particularly among the countries in the Gulf [21].

Correlates of Obesity in Middle East and North Africa Region

Gender

An overview of the existing literature reveals that gender is one of the main correlates of overweight and obesity, with women being more prone to being overweight and obese [11, 28]. For instance, obesity prevalence in Syria among women reached 51.8% (high prevalence has also been reported in Saudi Arabia and Bahrain, reaching levels of 80% in Bahrain) [11]. A literature review on the topic of gender and obesity has found higher prevalence of obesity among women in Algeria, Egypt, Morocco, and Tunisia [29]. Similar findings stem from a study by Zenki et al. [30]. In addition, a significant number of studies conducted in Iran have found higher obesity prevalence among women compared to men.

There are a number of reasons why prevalence of obesity is particularly high among women in the Middle East. Marriage and unemployment (which, as evidenced by the existing literature, is found to be negatively correlated to the obesity rates) are considered as the most important correlates of weight gain among women. A study on Kuwait, for instance, shows that roughly half of the unemployed women were obese, compared to only a third of the employed ones. Other significant correlates of weight gain among women include the following: higher inactivity rates and cultural factors. Due to cultural and religious reasons, the access to exercises venues for women is limited. Hence, television and Internet have become the main leisure activities among women in the region, further exacerbating the growing obesity rates. In addition, given the level of affluence in the Gulf countries and the availability of foreign workers, most of the women from affluent families in the region employ domestic helpers [4]. All of these factors lead to somewhat sedentary lifestyles and increase

in the rates of overweigh and obesity [31]. Finally, the cultural norms associated with large families, and hence, leading to multiple pregnancies is another reason why women in the region gain weight [32].

Age

Age is another important correlate of obesity and the extant literature points to a nonlinear relationship between age and obesity. A study on Morocco finds that the turning point of the inverted U curve that depicts the relationship between age and obesity occurs at year 64 for women and somewhat earlier (45–54 years) for men [32]. These findings from the Moroccan study were mirrored in other studies from Kuwait and Yemen [17, 33].

Income and Socioeconomic Class

Income (proxied, either by socioeconomic class, parents' education, or material possessions) are another important correlate of obesity in the Middle East. Higher income is associated with higher consumption, which in turn puts wealthier individuals at higher risk of becoming overweight and obese [34]. For instance, a study on Kuwait has found that affluent households in Kuwait consume more dairy products and meat, compared to the poorer households [31]. Obesity is found to increase with household wealth in both Algeria and Tunisia [8]. A positive link between income and obesity was also found in a study on Morocco [32]. A study among students in UAE has documented that students coming from richer households have higher propensity of becoming overweight and obese [35]. Given the cultural importance of housing in the Middle East, the extant literature has often proxied income by the quality of a household's housing. Using quality of housing as a benchmark for income, a study on Morocco has found that individuals living in better houses tend to have higher probability of being obese compared to those living in slums or similar poor housing conditions [32].

Education

The existing literature on global level suggests that education is negatively linked with obesity [33] and this link is resonated among countries in the MENA region. A study in Kuwait [36] noted a negative link between levels of education and the likelihood of obesity [33]. Similar findings stem from a study conducted in Morocco. The study finds that the prevalence of obesity and overweight was highest in illiterate women and lowest in women who had obtained a university degree [32]. Over time, the highest increases in prevalence of obesity were registered among women who had no education or only had primary education [37]. Similar findings were observed in the rest of the region. For instance, 28% of Syrians with university education are obese (compared to 51% of the illiterate ones). In Jordan, people with less than a high school education (less than 12 years of formal education) are roughly twice more likely to be obese compared to those who have, at least, completed a high school education. Almost identically, in Lebanon, the prevalence of obesity is negatively correlated with the years of formal education [31].

Exercise/Activity

Lack of exercise is another important correlate of obesity in the MENA region. Hot climate coupled with increased air pollution and rapidly increased urbanization and industrialization has led to a significant decrease of physical activity among the people in the region. In addition, as evidenced from the introductory part of the chapter, the rapid economic development has allowed the Gulf countries to achieve some of the highest levels of development in the world. This rapid economic development, however, brought with itself significant changes in the lifestyle, with more and more households relying on cars and mechanical appliances for work and television and the Internet for leisure, leading to sedentary lifestyle and hence increasing the prevalence of obesity in the region.

Similarly, in UAE, the inactivity rates among young urbanites are as high as 40% and as high as 70% among older residents of urban areas [38]. Among children, those with sedentary lifestyle are almost twice as likely to become obese [39]. In Morocco, the prevalence of obesity was lower among study participants who undertook at least 30 min of physical activity per day than in other individuals [32]. A study on Egypt has documented that among the leisurely activities performed on a daily basis, physical exercise was the least favorite. Low levels of physical activity have been noted in other countries in region. A study on six MENA countries has found that the inactivity rate is highest among Saudis (roughly 86%) and lowest among Syrians (33%). Similar trends on the physical activity/obesity nexus have also been documented among young people [40].

Nutrition

The changes in lifestyle marked over the last few decades and closely connected with the economic development of some of the MENA subregions have also brought with itself changes in the nutrition patterns among the countries in the region. However, as documented by the literature, the changes in the nutrition patterns have not been same across the region. Changes in nutrition patterns have been most drastic in the high-income countries, where traditional diet consisting of fiber (fruits and vegetables), milk, and limited intake of dairy products have been replaced with a diet marked by heave intake of calorific food, especially fat and carbohydrate. This has resulted to an average daily caloric intake in the Gulf countries amounting to 3000 kcal per adult individual. Interestingly, the sugar and fat combined now comprise roughly 45% of the daily energy intake of an adult living in the high-income countries in the MENA region [4]. In Saudi Arabia, for instance, a study has documented that the intake of fresh fruits and vegetables occurs only twice weekly. The consumption of fried food has been found to be relatively high [28, 41]. Changes in the caloric intake have also been noted in the upper-middle-income countries in the region [4].

Fat Intake

As evidenced from the previous section, fat intake, especially in the upper-middle-income and high-income countries in the region, has increased. In addition, studies point out that the fat intake has particularly increased in the high-income countries in the region, with fat calories increasing much more rapidly compared to the increase of the total daily caloric intake. In some of the countries in the region, the increase in the daily intake of fat calories has been as high as 50%. Moreover, a special strand of the literature has emerged that has documented the type of fat consumed by households in the MENA region. A study in Bahrain points out that almost half of the school children intake more saturated fat than they should [42].

Fiber Intake

As indicated in the previous sections in this review, one of the reasons for increased prevalence of obesity in the MENA region is the change in nutrition patterns that, inter alia, involved increase in the daily intake of fat and decrease in daily intake of fiber. Indeed, data on Saudi Arabia suggest that the average daily intake of fiber is alarmingly low averaging roughly 25 grams, with most of the daily intake coming from vegetables, cereals, and fruits. In addition, the low intake of fiber is further exacerbated by the food preparation practices, thus involving boiling and peeling of fruits and vegetables, ultimately reducing the daily average intake of fiber [43]. A cross-country survey in the region has found that the low intake (below five servings per day) of fresh fruit and vegetables (food that is high in fiber) ranged as been as high as 80% in Egypt and 96% in Syria [44]. Moreover, the intake of fiber-rich foods by children and adolescents in most Arab countries is alarmingly low. The literature documents that school children and adolescents follow similar nutrition patterns as adult individuals [4].

Urbanization

In contrast to the high income countries in the West, across the MENA region, obesity is higher among the urban population. This is connected with some of the correlates mentioned above – urbanization is highly correlated with western living and eating habits and sedentary lifestyle which significantly contributes to rising obesity rates. A study in Jordan has found that almost 60% of urban residents are obese compared to 45% in rural areas. Studies on Tunisia, Morocco, Oman, and Egypt have documented similar trends [43]. The existing research evidence points to the fact that adult urban women in UAE are more prone to being obese compared to women living in rural areas [45].

Obesity-Related Noncommunicable Diseases in the MENA Region

The rapidly increasing prevalence of overweight and obesity in the MENA region, coupled with progressively poorer diets and insufficient physical activity, has contributed to a significant transition in health risks in MENA countries [46, 47]. Over the past 30 years, the burden of noncommunicable diseases (NCD) in the region has increased substantially to overtake the disease burden from communicable diseases and maternal mortality [46, 48]. The World Development Indicators document that in 2019 almost 80% of the total deaths in the region have been due to NCDs (World Development Indicators 2019). The increased prevalence of these NCDs is partly attributable to a rise in life expectancy, but is primarily driven by an upsurge in population exposure to modifiable risk factors such as poor diet, obesity, lack of physical activity, and tobacco use [46, 47]. Excess weight remains the primary modifiable risk factor for development of NCDs in the region, with overweight and obesity estimated to be responsible for 8% of all deaths in the Eastern Mediterranean region in 2004, the fourth leading risk factor in the region after high blood pressure (15% of deaths), underweight (10%) and high blood glucose (9%). In this section, we explore the available evidence on the association between rising obesity rates in the MENA region and prevalence of a number of major obesity-related NCDs, including diabetes, cardiovascular disease, chronic kidney disease, and cancer.

Diabetes Prevalence in the MENA Region

Evidence from Official Sources

The International Diabetes Federation estimates that 73 million people aged 20–79 were living with diabetes in MENA countries in 2021 [49]. The age-standardized average prevalence of 24.5% of adults living with diabetes represents the highest regional prevalence globally.

Data from the World Development Indicators indicate a positive correlation between prevalence of diagnosed diabetes in adults aged 25 years and over and level of economic development (Chart 4). In 2021, average diabetes prevalence was 10.1% in the low-income countries, 10.2% in the lower-middle-income countries, 11.6 in the upper-

middle-income countries, and 17.4% in the high-income countries in the region. Diabetes prevalence varies widely between countries, ranging from 7.1% in Algeria to 20.9% in Egypt among lower-middle-income countries, from 8.7% in Libya to 15.4% in Jordan in the upper-middle-income group, and from 11.3% in Bahrain to 24.9% in Kuwait in the high-income country group.

Evidence from the Literature

A number of systematic reviews have been conducted on diabetes in the MENA region, with these reviews indicating that diabetes prevalence varies widely between countries and has increased substantially in the last two decades, particularly in high-income Gulf countries. For example, a meta-analysis of studies on type 2 diabetes in Arabian Gulf states found that overall estimated prevalence of diabetes was 14.9%, ranging from 5.9% in the UAE to 32.1% in Saudi Arabia [50]. Over time, the prevalence of diabetes among the Saudi population more than doubled from 12.4% in 1987 to 27.7% in 2011. Although this study found no significant difference in the prevalence of diabetes between males and females, the rate of

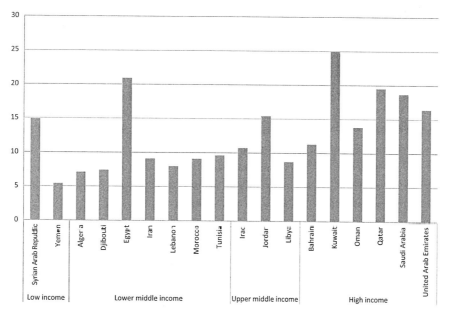

Chart 4 MENA countries: diabetes prevalence (% of population ages 20 to 79), 2021. (Source: World Development Indicators and author's calculations)

increase of diabetes prevalence was reported to be significantly higher in men than women. A further review on type 2 diabetes in the Eastern Mediterranean region also found that diabetes prevalence has increased rapidly over time [51]. In Tunisia, the prevalence of diabetes was reported to have doubled in the past 15 years, while in Jordan diabetes prevalence increased by 31.5% from 1994 to 2006. The highest prevalence of raised blood glucose in the EMR was found among Saudi men (22%) and women (21.7%). A third review found that diabetes prevalence ranged from 15.8% in Beirut, Lebanon, to 31.6% in Riyadh, Saudi Arabia [52]. High prevalence rates were also found in urban areas of Bahrain (28.1%), Kuwait (21.4%), Jordan (17.1%), and Qatar (16.7%). Over time, diabetes prevalence was shown to have increased from 2.5% in Saudi Arabia in 1982 to 31.6% in 2011.

Additional studies from low- and upper-middle-income countries show that diabetes prevalence is lower than in high-income countries, but still represents a significant health issue of concern. In Syria, a study using household survey data from 2006 showed that diabetes prevalence was 15.6% [5]. In Lebanon, prevalence of laboratory diagnosed type 2 diabetes in adults aged 25 or over was found to be 8.5% [53].

Association between Diabetes and Excess Weight in the MENA Region

The existing literature shows a strong correlation between excess weight and diabetes risk in the MENA region. In a review of diabetes in MENA countries, diabetes prevalence was found to be significantly associated with living in urban areas, older age, and lower educational attainment, but was most commonly associated with higher body mass index [52].

A Syrian study from 2006 found that although diabetes diagnosis was significantly and positively correlated with hypertension, it was not significantly related to obesity [5]. In upper-middle-income countries, the risk of having diabetes was found to be significantly and positively associated with BMI [53].

In high-income countries, overweight or obese individuals aged over 50 in Kuwait were reported to be 40% more likely to have diabetes than counterparts with a normal BMI [54]. An additional study from Kuwait further demonstrated that risk of diabetes was significantly associated with obesity prevalence [55]. In a study from Saudi Arabia, a BMI of ≥25 was associated with greater risk of diabetes, although this relationship was not significant [56]. A further study from Saudi Arabia conducted laboratory testing and found that risk of diabetes was lower in females and was significantly associated with older age and previous diagnosis of hypertension; however, obesity and physical activity were not shown to be associated with risk of developing diabetes [57]. In Qatar, diabetes risk in two studies was found to be significantly higher in individuals with BMI of ≥25 [18, 58]. Christos et al. [58] estimated that eliminating obesity and improving educational attainment could reduce diabetes cases by one-third for all Qatari residents and by 50.0% for Qatari nationals.

Cardiovascular Disease and Hypertension

Cardiovascular disease (CVD) is the leading cause of death in the MENA region, with ischemic heart disease and stroke accounting for two of the top five causes of death in all country income groups [46, 48]. WHO estimates indicate that hypertension is the primary CVD risk factor globally, accounting for 13% of global CVD deaths. The causes of the majority of hypertension cases are unknown; however, the condition has been linked to excess salt intake, lack of physical activity,overweight, and obesity [59]. Excess weight has also been shown to be an independent risk factor for CVD in general and is estimated to be the primary cause of 5% of CVD deaths globally.

Hypertension

Evidence from Official Sources

WHO estimates indicate that the global prevalence of hypertension ranges from an average of 35% in the WHO Region of the Americas to 46% in the WHO Africa Region. In the MENA region, the prevalence of hypertension is relatively low in comparison to other regions, with 31.2% of individuals aged 25 years or over estimated to have raised blood pressure (SBP >140 or DBP >90).

Evidence from the Literature

Estimates of hypertension prevalence in the MENA region varies markedly between published studies. A systematic review of CVD risk factors in Gulf countries found an estimated average hypertension prevalence of 29.5% [60]. However, a clinical study of outpatients across the region found that prevalence of hypertension was above 40.0% in a number of MENA countries, including Algeria, Egypt, Jordan, Kuwait, Lebanon, Saudi Arabia, and UAE [61]. In a study from Kuwait, prevalence of hypertension was found to be 52.0% in men and 49.0% in women, far higher than WHO estimates [54].

Hypertension was shown to be correlated with excess weight in the few studies that explored the association between these factors. A study from Kuwait found that risk of hypertension was significantly and positively related to BMI [54].

Cardiovascular Disease

The existing literature provides mixed evidence on the prevalence of CVD and its association with obesity in the MENA region. In a systematic review of CVD mortality in Syria, overall mortality ranged from 45.0% to 49.0% in included studies [62]. In a study from Kuwait, cardiac diseases were identified in 21.0% of men and 15.0% of women [54].

No clear patterns are observed in studies exploring the relationship between excess weight and CVD. In Syria, obesity was found to be the primary risk factor for CVD in the majority of individuals, with the exception of men aged over 65 years, where smoking and hypertension were the most common risk factors [62]. An Iranian study showed a significant and positive association between waist circumference and incidence of ischemic heart disease [63]. In Kuwait, one study found that being overweight or obese was not significantly associated with risk of developing cardiac disease [54]. In contrast, another Kuwaiti study found that being obese, aged over

40 years and having diabetes mellitus, a positive family history of diabetes, hypertension, or dyslipidemia was all significant, independent risk factors for developing CVD [55].

Chronic Kidney Disease

Chronic kidney disease (CKD) is a growing issue of concern in the MENA region and represents a major public health challenge. Studies on the Global Burden of Disease estimate that prevalence of CKD rose significantly between 1990 and 2010 to become one of the top ten most common causes of death in upper-middle-income and high-income MENA countries [46, 48]. Although CKD can be caused by a number of conditions such as infection, inflammation, and inherited conditions, the two principal causes of CKD globally are hypertension and diabetes [64]. Excess weight remains the primary modifiable risk factor for CKD, largely due to the increased risk of hypertension and diabetes in overweight and obese individuals [65]. However, obesity also has independent effects on CKD risk through its impact on renal physiology and metabolism, making obese people more likely to suffer CKD and end-stage renal failure [65].

Despite representing a significant and rapidly growing burden of disease, little research has been conducted on CKD in the MENA region and its association with obesity [66]. Some evidence from Iran is available, showing mixed results on the association between CKD and obesity. In one Iranian cohort study 18.0% of participants developed CKD after 9 years of follow-up [67]. Changes to waist circumference over this period was not found to be significantly associated with the risk of developing CKD in women, but a mild to moderate increase in waist circumference in men raised the risk of developing CKD by 70.0%. A further cohort study found a crude cumulative incidence of 21.8% of stage 3–5 CKD after 10 years of follow-up [68]. Age over 50 years, hypertension and known diabetes were reported to be significantly associated with raised CKD risk, but abdominal obesity was not shown to be an independent risk factor for disease development. In contrast, a cross-sectional Iranian study reported that BMI was strongly and positively correlated with risk of CKD in both men and women [69].

Cancer

Cancer represents an increasing burden of disease in the MENA region. WHO mortality statistics indicate that cancer is responsible for 270,000 deaths per year in the EMR and is the fourth leading cause of death overall. By 2035, it is predicted that the prevalence of cancer in the region will increase by between 100% and 180%. This rise is partly due to an expected increase in life expectancy but is also linked to increased prevalence of modifiable risk factors including smoking, unhealthy diets, lack of physical activity, and obesity.

Despite the growing burden of cancer in the region, evidence from published studies on the relationship between modifiable risk factors, including overweight and obesity, and cancer, in MENA countries is sparse. In one of the few studies exploring cancer risk factors, breast cancer in Iran was shown to be significantly and positively associated with BMI in both pre- and postmenopausal women, while waist circumference was significantly and positively associated with risk of breast cancer in premenopausal women only [70]. A further study on colon cancer in rapidly developing countries linked increased prevalence of the disease to rising levels of physical activity, obesity, alcohol consumption, smoking, and high consumption of red meat and fat [71].

Conclusion

Over the past 30 years, the MENA region has undergone a rapid economic transformation that has generated increased modernization and dramatic improvements in living standards. However, these changes have led to a proliferation in unhealthy behaviors linked to developed economy lifestyles; levels of physical activity have declined substantially and consumption patterns have evolved away from traditional diets containing fruit, nuts, and seeds, toward diets with a high fat, sugar, and salt content. The adoption of these behaviors has led to an alarming increase in overweight and obesity, which has become an important health threat in many countries in the region. In high-income Gulf states, obesity levels have increased substantially and many countries now rank among the most obese countries in the world. Although overall obesity prevalence is lower in low- and upper-middle-income MENA countries, rates of overweight and obesity are still high and are rapidly increasing. Across countries of all income levels, obesity is more prevalent in richer, urban areas where sedentary lifestyles and Western diets are predominant. Furthermore, in the majority of countries, the obesity epidemic disproportionately affects women as cultural factors restrict access to sports and exercise activities and employment opportunities.

The rapid increase in overweight and obesity in the region has contributed to a rising prevalence in a number of noncommunicable diseases. Available evidence strongly indicates that excess weight is the primary modifiable risk factor driving the alarming increase in diabetes in the region. Although evidence on the relationship between obesity and other NCDs is less clear, it has been linked to a considerable recent rise in the prevalence of hypertension, cancer, chronic kidney disease, and cardiovascular disease in a number of countries. These NCDs are now the leading causes of morbidity and mortality in the region and represent a critical and growing public health challenge. If the rapid upward trend in obesity prevalence in the MENA region continues, it is likely to contribute to a substantial increase in premature deaths and morbidity from these leading NCDs, generating significant costs for health systems and potentially reversing recent gains in life expectancy [48, 72]).

In order to respond appropriately to the obesity epidemic and manifest increase in NCDs, it is important that all MENA countries fully understand the epidemiology of obesity in their country. However, there is currently little evidence on the importance of excess weight on the etiology of NCDs in the MENA region. Few studies have been conducted on the relationship between overweight and obesity and the development of chronic kidney disease, CVD, and cancer. Studies that do exist are primarily concentrated on Iran and high-income Gulf states and largely neglect lower- and upper-middle-income countries. It is therefore important that more studies are available from a wider range of countries to help inform appropriate national responses to the growing obesity crisis and NCD burden. Future research should also explore how socioeconomic factors, in particular gender and education, may affect the relationship between excess weight and NCD outcomes. These research findings can be used to develop targeted prevention and outreach campaigns to reduce the disproportionate burden of obesity among women and other vulnerable groups.

Responding quickly and appropriately to the alarming rise in obesity and obesity-related NCDs is fundamentally important in MENA countries of all income levels. A significant first step to respond to the crisis in the region was taken in 2012 with the development of the Riyadh Declaration on healthy lifestyles in the Arab World and Middle East [73]. However, it is now imperative that momentum from this Declaration is continued and recommendations from the resolution are implemented. National policies targeting fat, salt, and sugar content in food and the introduction of labeling systems on fast food items should be considered in all countries. Furthermore, health education campaigns should be developed to increase awareness of the benefits of healthy diets, physical activity, and maintaining a healthy weight. Lastly, health systems should be developed to ensure that NCDs can be appropriately treated and managed [46]. Investing in effective measures to curb the rise in overweight and obesity and obesity-related NCDs will ultimately improve the health of the region and reduce long-term healthcare spending.

References

1. World Health Organization. Obesity in the Middle East and North Africa. 2019. https://www.who.int/newsroom/fact-sheets/detail/obesity-and-overweight. Accessed 1 Dec 2022

2. World Development Indicators (WDI). World Bank. 2019. https://databank.worldbank.org/source/worlddevelopment-indicators. Accessed 1 Dec 2022

3. World Health Organization, Regional Office for the Eastern Mediterranean, Alwan A, McColl K, Al-Jawaldeh A. Proposed policy priorities for preventing obesity and diabetes in the Eastern Mediterranean Region. World Health Organization. Regional Office for the Eastern Mediterranean. 2017. https://apps.who.int/iris/handle/10665/259519. License: CC BY-NC-SA 3.0 IGO.

4. Musaiger AO, Hassan AS, Obeid O. The paradox of nutrition-related diseases in the Arab countries: the need for action. Int J Environ Res Public Health. 2011;8(9):3637–71.

5. Al Ali R, Rastam S, Fouad FM, Mzayek F, Maziak W. Modifiable cardiovascular risk factors among adults in Aleppo, Syria. Int J Public Health. 2011;56(6):653–62.

6. Abu-Rmeileh NM, Husseini A, Capewell S, O'Flaherty M. Preventing type 2 diabetes among Palestinians: comparing five future policy scenarios. BMJ Open. 2013;3(12):e003558.

7. Berraho M, El Achhab Y, Benslimane A, Rhazi KE, Chikri M, Nejjari C. Hypertension and type 2 diabetes: a cross-sectional study in Morocco (EPIDIAM Study). Pan Afr Med J. 2012;11(1):52.

8. Atek M, Traissac P, El Ati J, Laid Y, Aounallah-Skhiri-H, Eymard-Duvernay S . . . Maire B. Obesity and association with area of residence, gender and socioeconomic factors in Algerian and Tunisian adults. PLoS One. 2013;8(10):e75640.

9. Ajlouni K, Khader Y, Batieha A, Jaddou H, El-Khateeb M. An alarmingly high and increasing prevalence of obesity in Jordan. Epidemiol Health. 2020;42:e2020040. https://doi.org/10.4178/epih.e2020040. Epub 2020 Jun 6.

10. Ahmed HG, Ginawi IA, Elasbali AM, Ashankyty IM, Al-hazimi AM. Prevalence of obesity in hail region, KSA: in a Comprehensive Survey. J Obes. 2014;2014:961861.

11. Mandil A, Chaaya M, Saab D. Health status, epidemiological profile and prospectus: eastern Mediterranean region. Int J Epidemiol/Global Status Epidemiol. 2013;42:616–26.

12. Al-Daghri NM, Al-Attas OS, Alokail MS, Alkharfy KM, Yousef M, Sabico SL, Chrousos GP. Diabetes mellitus type 2 and other chronic non-communicable diseases in the central region, Saudi Arabia (Riyadh cohort 2): a decade of an epidemic. BMC Med. 2011;9(1):76.

13. Amin TT, Al Sultan AI, Mostafa OA, Darwish AA, Al-Naboli MR. Profile of non-communicable disease risk factors among employees at a Saudi University. Asian Pac J Cancer Prev. 2014;15(18):7897.

14. Nikoloski Z. Determinants of diabetes in Kuwait: evidence from the World Health Survey. LSE Middle East Centre Paper Series 28 December 2019 LSE Middle East Centre Kuwait Programme Paper Series 6 August 2020. 2020. https://eprints.lse.ac.uk/106254/1/

Nikoloski_determinants_of_diabetes_in_kuwait_published.pdf

15. Oguoma VM, Coffee NT, Alsharrah S, Abu-Farha M, Al-Refaei FH, Al-Mulla F, Daniel M. Prevalence of overweight and obesity, and associations with socio-demographic factors in Kuwait. BMC Public Health. 2021;21(1):667. https://doi.org/10.1186/s12889-021-10692-1.

16. Al-Saadi R, Al-Shukaili S, Al-Mahrazi S, Al-Busaidi Z. Prevalence of uncontrolled hypertension in primary care settings in Al Seeb Wilayat, Oman. Sultan Qaboos Univ Med J. 2011;11(3):349.

17. Al-Sharafi BA, Gunaid AA. Prevalence of obesity in patients with type 2 diabetes mellitus in Yemen. International journal of endocrinology and metabolism. 2014;12(2):e13633.

18. Ali F, Nikoloski Z, Reka H, Gjebrea O, Mossialos E. The diabetes-obesity-hypertension nexus in Qatar: evidence from the World Health Survey. Popul Health Metrics. 2014;12:18.

19. Albaker W, Saklawi R, Bah S, Motawei K, Futa B, Al-Hariri M. What is the current status of childhood obesity in Saudi Arabia? Evidence from 20,000 cases in the Eastern Province: a cross-sectional study. Medicine (Baltimore). 2022;101(27):e29800. https://doi.org/10.1097/MD.0000000000029800.

20. Cheema S, Abraham A, El-Nahas KG, Abou-Amona R, Al-Hamaq AO, Maisonneuve P, Chaabna K, Lowenfels AB, Mamtani R. Assessment of overweight, obesity, central obesity, and type 2 diabetes among adolescents in Qatar: a cross-sectional study. Int J Environ Res Public Health. 2022;19(21):14601. https://doi.org/10.3390/ijerph192114601.

21. Baniissa W, Radwan H, Rossiter R, Fakhry R, Al-Yateem N, Al-Shujairi A, Hasan S, Macridis S, Farghaly AA, Naing L, Awad MA. Prevalence and determinants of overweight/obesity among school-aged adolescents in the United Arab Emirates: a cross-sectional study of private and public schools. BMJ Open. 2020;10(12):e038667. https://doi.org/10.1136/bmjopen-2020-038667.

22. Osei Bonsu E, Addo IY. Prevalence and correlates of overweight and obesity among under-five children in Egypt. Front Public Health. 2022;10:1067522. https://doi.org/10.3389/fpubh.2022.1067522.

23. Abd El-Aty NS, Osman SR, Ahmed ES, GadAllah MA. Overweight and obesity prevalence among upper Egypt primary schools' children using Egyptian and CDC growth charts. Appl Nurs Res. 2020;56:151346. https://doi.org/10.1016/j.apnr.2020.151346. Epub 2020 Aug 27.

24. Okour AM, Saadeh RA, Hijazi MH, Khalaileh HEA, Alfaqih MA. Socioeconomic status, perceptions and obesity among adolescents in Jordan. Pan Afr Med J. 2019;34:148. https://doi.org/10.11604/pamj.2019.34.148.19641.

25. Nouayti H, Bouanani NH, Hammoudi J, Mekhfi H, Legssyer A, Bnouham M, Ziyyat A. Overweight and obesity in Eastern Morocco: prevalence and associated risk factors among high school students. Rev Epidemiol Sante Publique. 2020;68(5):295–301. https://doi.org/10.1016/j.respe.2020.06.007. Epub 2020 Sep 4.

26. Hammad SS, Berry DC. The child obesity epidemic in Saudi Arabia: a review of the literature. J Transcult Nurs. 2017;28(5):505–15. https://doi.org/10.1177/1043659616668398. Epub 2016 Sep 21.

27. Alqaoud N, Al-Jawaldeh A, Al-Anazi F, Subhakaran M, Doggui R. Trend and Causes of Overweight and Obesity among Pre-School Children in Kuwait. Children (Basel). 2021;8(6):524. https://doi.org/10.3390/children8060524.

28. Salem V, AlHusseini N, Abdul Razack HI, Naoum A, Sims OT, Alqahtani SA. Prevalence, risk factors, and interventions for obesity in Saudi Arabia: a systematic review. Obes Rev. 2022;23(7):e13448. https://doi.org/10.1111/obr.13448. Epub 2022 Mar 26.

29. Bos M, Agyemang C. Prevalence and complications of diabetes mellitus in Northern Africa, a systematic review. BMC Public Health. 2013;13(1):387.

30. Al Zenki S, Al Omirah H, Al Hooti S, Al Hamad N, Jackson RT, Rao A, Al Othman A. High prevalence of metabolic syndrome among Kuwaiti adults – a wake-up call for public health intervention. Int J Environ Res Public Health. 2012;9(5):1984–96.

31. Al Nohair S. Obesity in gulf countries. Int J Health Sci. 2014;8(1):79–83.

32. El Rhazi K, Nejjari C, Zidouh A, Bakkali R, Berraho M, Barberger Gateau P. Prevalence of obesity and associated sociodemographic and lifestyle factors in Morocco. Public Health Nutr. 2011;14(1):160–7.

33. Ahmed F, Waslien C, Al-Sumaie MA, Prakash P. Secular trends and risk factors of overweight and obesity among Kuwaiti adults: National Nutrition Surveillance System data from 1998 to 2009. Public Health Nutr. 2012;15(11):2124–30.

34. Fatemeh T, Mohammad-Mehdi HT, Toba K, Afsaneh N, Sharifzadeh G. Prevalence of overweight and obesity in preschool children (2–5 year-olds) in Birjand, Iran. BMC Res Notes. 2012;5(1):529.

35. Katsaiti MS, El Anshasy AA. On the determinants of obesity: evidence from the UAE. Appl Econ. 2014;46(30):3649–58.

36. AI-Isa A. Changes in body mass index and prevalence of obesity among adult Kuwaiti women attending health clinics. Ann Saudi Med. 1997;17:307–11.

37. Aitsi-Selmi A, Chandola T, Friel S, Nouraei R, Shipley MJ, Marmot MG. Interaction between education and household wealth on the risk of obesity in women in Egypt. PLoS One. 2012;7(6):e39507.

38. Hajat C, Harrison O, Shather Z. A profile and approach to chronic disease in Abu Dhabi. Glob Health. 2012;8:18.

39. Bamoshmoosh M, Massetti L, Aklan H, Al-Karewany M, Al Goshae H, Modesti PA. Central obesity in Yemeni children: a population based cross-sectional study. World J Cardiol. 2013;5(8):295.

40. Al-Hazzaa HM, Abahussain NA, Al-Sobayel HI, Qahwaji DM, Musaiger AO. Lifestyle factors associated with overweight and obesity among Saudi adolescents. BMC Public Health. 2012;12(1):354.

41. Bazhan M, Kalantari N, Hoshyarrad A. Diet composition and risk of overweight and obesity in Iranian adolescent girls. Tehran: Department of Food Science and Technology, National Nutrition and Food Technology Research Institute, Shahid Beheshti University; 2011.

42. Gharib N, Raseed P. Energy and macronutrient intake and dietary pattern among school children in Bahrain: a cross-sectional study. Nut J. 2011;10:62.

43. Musaiger AO. Overweight and obesity in Eastern Mediterranean Region: prevalence and possible causes. J Obes. 2011;2011:407237.

44. World Health Organization. Global status report on noncommunicable diseases 2014. Geneva: World Health Organization; 2015

45. Ng SW, Zaghloul S, Ali H, Harrison G, Yeatts K, El Sadig M, Popkin BM. Nutrition transition in The United Arab Emirates. Eur J Clin Nutr. 2011;65(12):1328–37.

46. Rahim HF, Sibai A, Khader Y, et al. Non-communicable diseases in the Arab world. Lancet. 2014;383(9914):356–67.

47. World Bank. The growing danger of non-communicable diseases acting now to reverse course. Washington, DC: World Bank; 2011.

48. Global Burden of Disease Study (GBD). Global, regional, and national age–sex specific all-cause and cause-specific mortality for 240 causes of death, 1990–2013: a systematic analysis for the Global Burden of Disease Study 2013. The Lancet. 2013;385(9963):117–71.

49. International Diabetes Federation (IDF). IDF Diabetes Atlas. 2014. http://www.idf.org/diabetesatlas

50. Alharbi NS, Almutari R, Jones S, Al-Daghri N, Khunti K, de Lusignan S. Trends in the prevalence of type 2 diabetes mellitus and obesity in the Arabian Gulf States: systematic review and meta-analysis. Diabetes Res Clin Pract. 2014;106(2):30–3.

51. Musaiger AO, Al-Hazzaa HM. Prevalence and risk factors associated with nutrition-related non-communicable diseases in the Eastern Mediterranean region. Int J Gen Med. 2012;5:199–217.

52. Zabetian A, Keli HM, Echouffo-Tcheugui JB, Narayan KMV, Ali MK. Diabetes in the Middle East and North Africa. Diabetes Res Clin Pract. 2013;101(2):106–22.

53. Costanian C, Bennett K, Hwalla N, Assaad S, Sibai AM. Prevalence, correlates and management of type 2 diabetes mellitus in Lebanon: findings from a national population-based study. Diabetes Res Clin Pract. 2014;105(3):408–15.

54. Badr HE, Shah NM, Shah MA. Obesity among Kuwaitis aged 50 years or older: prevalence, correlates, and comorbidities. The Gerontologist. 2013;53(4):555–66.

55. Alarouj M, Bennakhi A, Alnesef Y, Sharifi M, Elkum N. Diabetes and associated cardiovascular risk factors in the State of Kuwait: the first national survey. Int J Clin Pract. 2013;67(1):89–96.

56. Alqurashi KA, Aljabri KS, Bokhari SA. Prevalence of diabetes mellitus in a Saudi community. Ann Saudi Med. 2011;31(1):19–23.

57. El Bcheraoui C, Basulaiman M, Tuffaha M, et al. Status of the diabetes epidemic in the Kingdom of Saudi Arabia, 2013. Int J Public Health. 2014;59(6):1011–21.

58. Christos PJ, Chemaitelly H, Abu-Raddad LJ, Ali Zirie M, Deleu D, Mushlin AI. Prevention of type II diabetes mellitus in Qatar: who is at risk? Qatar Med J. 2014;2014(2):13.

59. Kang YS. Obesity associated hypertension: new insights into mechanism. Electr Blood Pressure. 2013;11(2):46–52.

60. Tailakh A, Evangelista LS, Mentes JC, Pike NA, Phillips LR, Morisky DE. Hypertension prevalence, awareness, and control in Arab countries: a systematic review. Nurs Health Sci. 2014;16(1):126–30.

61. Alsheikh-Ali AA, Omar MI, Raal FJ, et al. Cardiovascular risk factor burden in Africa and the Middle East: The Africa Middle East Cardiovascular Epidemiological (ACE) study. PLoS One. 2014;9(8):e102830.

62. Barakat H, Barakat H, Baaj MK. CVD and obesity in transitional Syria: a perspective from the middle east. Vasc Health Risk Manag. 2012;8(1):145–50.

63. Talaei M, Sadeghi M, Marshall T, et al. Impact of metabolic syndrome on ischemic heart disease – a prospective cohort study in an Iranian adult population: Isfahan Cohort Study. Nutr Metab Cardiovasc Dis. 2012;22(5):434–41.

64. Turner JM, Bauer C, Abramowitz MK, Melamed ML, Hostetter TH. Treatment of chronic kidney disease. Kidney Int. 2012;81(4):351–62.

65. Wickman C, Kramer H. Obesity and kidney disease: potential mechanisms. Semin Nephrol. 2013;33(1):14–22.

66. Shaheen FA, Souqiyyeh MZ. Kidney health in the Middle East. Clin Nephrol. 2010;74(Suppl 1):S85–8.

67. Barzin M, Hosseinpanah F, Serahati S, Salehpour M, Nassiri AA, Azizi F. Changes in waist circumference and incidence of chronic kidney disease. Eur J Clin Investig. 2014;44(5):470–6.

68. Tohidi M, Hasheminia M, Mohebi R, Khalili D, Hosseinpanah F, et al. Incidence of chronic kidney disease and its risk factors, results of over 10 year follow up in an Iranian Cohort. PLoS One. 2012;7(9):e45304.

69. Khajehdehi P, Malekmakan L, Pakfetrat M, Roozbeh J, Sayadi M. Prevalence of chronic kidney disease and its contributing risk factors in southern Iran: a cross-sectional adult population-based study. Iran J Kidney Dis. 2014;8(2):109–15.

70. Hajian-Tilaki KO, Gholizadehpasha AR, Bozorgzadeh S, Hajian-Tilaki E. Body mass index and waist circumference are predictor biomarkers of

breast cancer risk in Iranian women. Med Oncol. 2011;28(4):1296–301.

71. Bener A. Colon cancer in rapidly developing countries: review of the lifestyle, dietary, consanguinity and hereditary risk factors. Oncol Rev. 2011;5(1):5–11.

72. Finucane MM, Stevens GA, Cowan MJ, et al. National, regional, and global trends in body-mass index since 1980: systematic analysis of health examination surveys and epidemiological studies with 960 country-years and 9·1 million participants. Lancet. 2011;377(9765):557–67.

73. Riyadh Declaration. The Riyadh Declaration. edited by International Conference on Healthy Lifestyles and Non communicable Diseases (NCDs) in the Arab World and the Middle East. Saudi Arabia. 2012.

Obesity and Metabolic Syndrome in South Asians

6

Rajvarun S. Grewal, Alycia Hancock, Angela Yang, and Rita R. Kalyani

Contents

Abstract

Obesity and the metabolic syndrome (MetS) are chronic conditions resulting from biological, environmental, cultural, and lifestyle factors.

R. S. Grewal
California Health Sciences University – College of Osteopathic Medicine (CHSU-COM), Clovis, CA, USA

A. Hancock · A. Yang · R. R. Kalyani (✉)
Johns Hopkins University, Baltimore, Maryland, Division of Endocrinology, Diabetes & Metabolism, The Johns Hopkins University School of Medicine, Baltimore, MD, USA
e-mail: rrastogi@jhmi.edu

MetS is a global health problem, particularly in South Asian countries and those of South Asian descent living across the globe. MetS, and its components including insulin resistance (IR), hypertension, and dyslipidemia, is prevalent among both non-obese and obese South Asians when using BMI cutoffs for the general population and is associated with an increased risk of developing diabetes and cardiovascular disease (CVD). Thus, Asian-specific BMI cutoffs and waist circumference (WC) criteria have been proposed. This chapter reviews the epidemiology, risk factors, pathophysiology, and

© Springer Nature Switzerland AG 2023
R. S. Ahima (ed.), *Metabolic Syndrome*,
https://doi.org/10.1007/978-3-031-40116-9_52

complications of obesity and MetS among the South Asian population. The increased prevalence of obesity and MetS among South Asians warrants both individual-level and community-level interventions to effectively manage and reduce the disease burden in this population.

Keywords

Metabolic syndrome · Obesity · Insulin resistance · Cardiovascular disease · Diabetes · Waist circumference

Introduction

South Asians, whose family origins are from the countries of Bangladesh, Bhutan, India, Nepal, Sri Lanka, Pakistan, and the Maldives, constitute one-quarter of the world's population [1]. According to the US Census, South Asians are one of the fastest-growing ethnic groups in the USA, with >5 million South Asians, comprising nearly 2% of the US population [2, 3]. A large number of South Asian individuals migrated to the United States after the implementation of the 1965 USA Immigration and Nationality Act [3]. Other notable countries with significant South Asian immigrant populations include Canada and the UK. According to the 2021 Census, approximately 7% of the Canadian population is reported to be South Asian, among which 21% migrated to Canada between 2016 and 2021, and 43.4% migrated to Canada from 2001 to 2015 [4]. According to the World Directory of Minorities and Indigenous Peoples, >5% of the UK population was reported to be South Asian in 2018 [5]. South Asian servants and seamen employed by the East India Company lived in Great Britain beginning from the seventeenth century. Indian and Pakistani men were recruited to Great Britain, mainly from Punjab, in the 1950s to help with the labor shortages post World War II. In the 1970s, family reunification increased, with which families grew their businesses in retail, manufacturing, and other services [5].

South Asian diversity stems from its cultural and religious practices, spoken and written languages, traditions, customs, food, and much more. As a result, these components can significantly impact their access to healthcare and inclusion in the healthcare system for tailored preventative measures and medical care [6]. Therefore, factors unique to South Asians must be appropriately assessed and addressed when diagnosing and managing obesity and the MetS. The increasing prevalence of MetS is multifactorial, with South Asians predisposed to a higher risk of susceptibility at similar body mass index (BMI) and lower average waist circumference (WC) levels, given a relatively greater percentage body fat compared to Caucasians at similar body weights [7]. In addition, lifestyle factors, genetic factors, urbanization, and immigration all play a significant role in increasing the risk of developing diabetes, IR, hypertension, and cardiovascular disease (CVD) complications compared to other ethnic groups. As such, identification of MetS requires early preventive measures and therapeutic interventions to prevent long-term complications in the South Asian population.

Metabolic Syndrome Definition and Epidemiology in South Asians

Definition

Metabolic syndrome (MetS) is a chronic condition characterized by a cluster of interrelated cardiometabolic risk factors, including central obesity, hypertension, hyperglycemia (impaired glucose tolerance or diabetes), and dyslipidemia [8]. These risk factors are associated with insulin resistance, hemodynamic dysfunction, oxidative stress, and low-grade pro-inflammatory states [9]. The World Health Organization (WHO) deemed that the components and associated complications of MetS including CVD, obesity, and diabetes contribute to approximately two-thirds of deaths worldwide [10]. Unique factors relevant to the South Asian population that increase their risk for MetS include migration, acculturation, urbanization, religious and cultural practices, increased caloric consumption of traditional South Asian foods, adoption of a non-traditional Western diet, sedentary activity, and genetic risk factors. These lifestyle, genetic, and environmental factors may differ depending on the migrant population around the world. Given the rapidly increasing prevalence of obesity, MetS, and its associated diseases in all populations worldwide, there is an increased consensus within the scientific community to create culturally tailored recommendations for diagnosing and potentially also management in populations that may be at higher risk, such as South Asians.

In 1988, Gerald Reaven was the first to bring attention to the pathophysiologic cluster of risk factors and coined the term "Syndrome X" [11]. In an attempt to form structured criteria, the definition of MetS has continuously evolved, with definitions proposed by various organizations such as the World Health Organization (WHO), National Cholesterol Education Program Adult Treatment Panel III (NCEP-ATP III), International Diabetes Federation (IDF), and American Heart Association/National Heart, Lung, and Blood Institute (AHA/NHLBI), each focusing on different aspects of its pathophysiology [12, 13]. In 2001, the NCEP-ATP III provided defined criteria for the definition of MetS that was later updated by the AHA/NHLBI in 2005 to help establish a clinical diagnosis. In 2009, several large organizations provided a joint statement called "Harmonizing the Metabolic Syndrome" in an attempt to offer unified criteria for diagnosis and management. It was agreed upon that waist circumference (WC) should be considered as a prominent screening tool for central adiposity with race-specific thresholds proposed, given the

higher risk of metabolic diseases in specific ethnic populations such as Asians, compared to other races and ethnicities. Recently, the recognition of MetS in clinical practice has been more widely accepted with introduction of an ICD-10 code for MetS (E88.81) [12, 14, 15].

Diagnosis of MetS based on the AHA/NHLBI guidelines requires any three of the five following major criteria:

1. *Hyperglycemia*: Fasting blood glucose greater than or equal to 100 mg/dL or pharmacological treatment for prediabetes or diabetes.
2. *Hypertension*: Elevated blood pressure ≥ 130 mmHg systolic blood pressure or ≥ 85 mmHg diastolic pressure or antihypertensive therapy in a patient with a history of hypertension.
3. *Hypertriglyceridemia*: Fasting elevated triglyceride levels ≥150 mg/dL (1.7 mmol/L) or pharmacologic treatment for hypertriglyceridemia.
4. *High-density lipoprotein (HDL cholesterol)*: HDL cholesterol levels <40 mg/DL (1.03 mmol/L) in men or < 50 mg/dL (1.3 mmol/L) in women, or pharmacologic treatment for low HDL-cholesterol.
5. *Abdominal Obesity*: In general, waist circumference ≥ 102 cm in men or ≥ 88 cm in women but with ethnic-specific criteria as listed in Table 1.

Table 1 The proposed criteria for clinical diagnosis of metabolic syndrome[a]

Criteria for diagnosis of metabolic syndrome in South Asians compared to the general population		Recommended waist circumference thresholds for abdominal obesity	
Population/country	Organization (or source)	Men	Women
Europid	IDF [14]	≥94 cm	≥80 cm
Caucasian	WHO [143]	≥94 cm (increased risk)	≥80 cm (increased risk)
		≥102 cm (still higher risk)	≥88 cm (still higher risk)
United States	AHA/NHLBI (ATP III) [142]	≥102 cm	≥88 cm
Asian (including Japanese)	IDF [14]	≥90 cm	≥80 cm
South Asian	AHA/NHLBI Revised NCEP ATP III [14]	≥90 cm	≥80 cm

[a]Adapted from "Harmonizing the Metabolic Syndrome," Joint Interim Statement of the IDF Task Force, NHLBI, AHA, World Heart Federation (WHF), International Atherosclerosis Society, and International Association for the Study of Obesity [12, 14, 142, 143]. Table 1 displays recommendations proposed by professional organizations for abdominal obesity and ethnic-specific WC thresholds for clinical diagnosis of MetS. The WHO identifies two levels of abdominal obesity in Europids: (1) an increased risk at WC ≥ 80 cm in women and ≥ 94 cm in men, and (2) risk is significantly higher at ≥88 cm in women and ≥ 102 cm in men

Research shows that South Asians are at a greater risk of developing MetS than Caucasians due to their unique body composition. Excess total adiposity, abdominal obesity, thick truncal subcutaneous fat, and fat accumulation at ectopic sites all contribute to an increased risk of MetS in South Asian populations [16]. As such, a structured approach to diagnose MetS using ethnic-specific criteria, particularly for abdominal obesity through ethnic-specific WC cutoff values, is imperative. Specifically for South Asians, the AHA/NHLBI and WHO Expert Consultation proposed ethnic-specific cutoff values for WC for Asian men at ≥ 90 cm and Asian women at ≥ 80 cm [12, 17]. However, it is important to note that there are differences in WC cutoff points in different Asian countries, for example, in Japan and China [18–20]. Table 1 provides the AHA/NHLBI (ATP III) guidelines for MetS commonly used in the USA and other ethnic-specific cutoffs for men and women and the organization referenced (adapted from the Harmonizing the Metabolic Syndrome Statement).

Epidemiology

Nationally representative studies on the prevalence of MetS from South Asian countries are sparse. However, according to the data currently available, there are regional, urbanization, socioeconomic, and cultural variations in MetS prevalence among South Asians [7]. In a systematic review of 16 studies, the mean prevalence of MetS using different definitions was 26.1% (ATP III), 29.8% (IDF), and 14% (WHO) among individuals from South Asian countries (India, Sri Lanka, Bangladesh, Pakistan, and Nepal), with a prevalence range between 8.6% and 46.1% depending on the definition being used [21].

Regional differences in MetS prevalence among South Asian countries also exist. Using the NCEP ATP III definition, the highest prevalence of MetS in South Asian countries was in Pakistan (31%), while the lowest was in Nepal (20.7%) in one study [22]. In contrast, a study in urban Karachi, Pakistan, demonstrated a prevalence rate of 34.8% and 49% according to the IDF and the NCEP ATP III criteria, respectively [23]. Other studies report that in Punjab, India, MetS prevalence was 35.8% by ATP III definitions [24]; in rural Pakistan, MetS prevalence was 40% by IDF definitions [25]; and in Colombo, Sri Lanka, MetS prevalence was 46.1% by the modified ATP III criteria [26], suggesting that MetS prevalence rates differ by South Asian country.

There are important sex differences in prevalence of MetS among South Asians. In a large study conducted in rural Andhra Pradesh, India, the prevalence of NCEP ATP III defined MetS in adults was 24.6%, with a higher prevalence among men (28.6%) than women (20.4%) [27]. MetS prevalence among urban Indian females (43.2%) was much higher than those among rural Indian females (18.4%), while similar prevalence rates were observed by urbanization status among Indian males (rural 26.9% and urban 27.7%) [24, 27].

As noted, there are differences in MetS prevalence by urbanization status. Surveys collected from large, urban cities in India show that approximately one-third of the population have MetS [28–30]. On the other hand, the rural prevalence of MetS was relatively low compared to urban prevalence. A survey in Central India revealed an overall MetS prevalence (per the ATP III criteria) of only 5% in the adult rural population [31]. Based on a population survey in semi-urban South India, MetS was 29.7% [32]. In the Chennai Urban Rural Epidemiology Study (CURES-34), the prevalence of MetS based on the definitions provided by NCEP ATP III, WHO, and IDF were 18.3%, 23.2%, and 25.8%, respectively [33]. Epidemiologic studies suggest that India has a heterogeneous population with different groups at different stages of urban transition.

Similar observations were found in studies conducted in other South Asian migrant populations across the globe, with an overall prevalence of MetS in migrant Asian Indians between 20% and 32% [7]. In another study, among migrant South Asians in the USA, the prevalence of MetS was 27% (31% males vs. 17% females). 59% had high WC levels (58% men vs. 62% women), and 47% had low HDL-C (46% men vs. 48% women) [34]. Among the migrant population in the USA, South Asians are more likely to have type 2 diabetes and MetS compared to Whites [35]. UK researchers studied Bangladeshis, Pakistanis, and Asian Indians and noted that abdominal obesity, hyperinsulinemia, and dyslipidemia in migrant South Asians were significantly higher compared to British Caucasians [36–39]. Migrant Asian Indians in Singapore have been reported to have among the highest prevalence of MetS compared to Malays and Chinese individuals [40]. While there are limited studies on the comparative prevalence of MetS in other Asian subgroups, Table 2 lists some countries with available data (adapted from [41, 42]).

Pathophysiology of the Metabolic Syndrome in South Asians

Obesity and Central Adiposity

Central to the development of MetS is the distribution of adipose tissue in the body and subsequent metabolic dysfunction that is related to an increased susceptibility to cardiovascular disease and diabetes (Fig. 1). Proinflammatory cytokines are released from adipose tissue that alters the insulin's homeostatic signaling pathway, impacting receptor and secretion function, thus contributing to insulin resistance. The distribution of body fat, particularly visceral fat, is also involved in the recruitment of proinflammatory mediators, further potentiating adverse metabolic effects [43].

The body mass index (BMI) is the most common screening tool used as a surrogate marker of total adiposity and categorized by the WHO as underweight (<18.5 kg/m^2), normal weight (18.5–24.9 kg/m^2), overweight (25–29.9 kg/m^2), and obese (>30 kg/m^2). However, BMI does not capture important differences in body composition such as the relative proportion of body fat to

lean mass, as occurs across different ethnicities or with aging [44]. Recent studies have further highlighted the importance of utilizing waist circumference (WC) to assess abdominal adiposity and visceral fat mass [45]. Compared to the BMI, the WC reflects central adipose tissue distribution in the intra-abdominal area and is related to risk of developing cardiometabolic conditions. The waist-to-hip ratio (WHR) is also used as another measure of adiposity. Guidelines from the Endocrine Society recommend that using several evidence-based measurement tools to assess adiposity is critical for optimal obesity measurement and characterizing population-level health risks and outcomes [8, 46].

The question arises as to why do South Asians have different ethnic-specific cutoffs for diagnosing MetS? South Asians are observed to have a higher prevalence of abdominal obesity with more intra-abdominal and truncal subcutaneous adiposity compared to Caucasians. Further, there is an increased accumulation of fat at ectopic sites, particularly the skeletal muscle, and liver [28]. South Asians are also at an increased risk of developing obesity-related comorbidities at lower BMI and WC levels, and have higher body fat percentage at a given BMI than Caucasians [7, 28, 47, 48, 49]. All these features lead to higher likelihood of developing insulin resistance and concomitant metabolic disorders (MetS), including atherogenic dyslipidemia. Interestingly, there are studies that point to a higher risk of developing obesity (as reflected by higher BMI levels) for South Asian immigrants with longer duration of residency in the USA, compared to the native South Asian residents [6, 50].

The CURES Study in India suggested that the optimal BMI cutoff point for presence of two cardiometabolic risk factors was 23 kg/m^2 for both Indian males and females, and a waist circumference of 87 cm for men and 82 cm for women [7, 51]. In contrast, South Asian migrants living in Canada demonstrated BMI cutoff points of 22.5 kg/m^2 for dyslipidemia and 21 kg/m^2 for hyperglycemia [52]. In 2004, a WHO consortium proposed that the proportion of South Asians with an increased risk of type 2 diabetes and CVD is

Table 2 Prevalence of MetS in South Asian countries compared to East Asian countries[a]

Country	Age	Prevalence	MetS definition used
South Asian countries			
Bangladesh [144]	≥20 years	30.9% (male) 30.5% (female) 30.7% (both)	Revised NCEP ATP III
		24.5% (both)	International Diabetes Federation (IDF)
India [24]	>20 years	39.2% (male) 50.9% (female) 45.3% (both)	NCEP ATP III
		31.8% (male) 47.2% (female) 39.5% (both)	International Diabetes Federation (IDF)
Nepal [145]	15–69 years	15.3% (male) 15.4% (female) 15.4% (both)	Revised NCEP ATP III
		13.4% (male) 18.1% (female) 15.8% (both)	International Diabetes Federation (IDF)
Pakistan [23]	≥25 years	55.6% (male) 45.9% (female) 49% (both)	Revised NCEP ATP III
Sri Lanka [146]	>18 years	31.3% (male) 36.5% (female) 34.4% (both)	World Health Organization (WHO)
East Asian countries			
South Korea [147]	20–82 years	5.2% (male) 9% (female)	NCEP ATP III
		9.8% (male) 12.4% (female)	"Asian-adapted definition"
China [148]	30–74 years	10.1% (both)	NCEP ATP III
		26.3% (both)	"Asian-adapted definition"
Singapore [40]	18–69 years	13.1% (male) 11% (female)	NCEP ATP III
		20.9% (male) 15.5% (female)	"Asian-adapted definition"
Taiwan [149]	30–92 years	11.2% (male) 18.6% (female)	NCEP ATP III
		23.8% (male) 17.7%, (female)	"Asian-adapted definition"
Hong Kong [150]	25–74 years	15.3% (male) 18.8% (female)	NCEP ATP III
		20.2% (male) 23.6% (female)	"Asian-adapted definition"
Philippines [151]	>20 years	14.3% (male) 14.1% (female)	NCEP ATP III
		18.6% (male) 19.9% (female)	"Asian-adapted definition"

Abbreviations: *IDF*, International Diabetes Federation; *WHO*, World Health Organization; *NCEP ATP III*, National Cholesterol Education Program Adult Treatment Panel III

[a]Adapted from Jayawardena et al. [41] and Nestel et al. [42]. NCEP ATP III definitions were based on those previously described [152]. Asian adaptation definition used BMI ≥ 25 kg/m^2 and waist circumference in male ≥90 cm or female ≥80 cm [40, 149, 153]

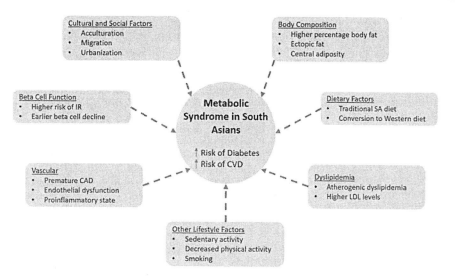

Fig. 1 Factors contributing to the metabolic syndrome in South Asians. This figure displays factors that contribute to the risk of developing MetS and related diseases among the South Asian population, such as vascular factors (premature CAD), higher risk of pancreatic beta cell dysfunction, cultural and social factors (i.e., acculturation), dietary factors (both components of the South Asian diet and conversion to Western diet), atherogenic dyslipidemia, central adiposity, and other lifestyle factors such as relatively higher sedentary activity. While there are many distinct mechanisms contributing to the pathophysiology, these factors are often interconnected and overlap clinically in South Asian individuals to increase the risk of developing metabolic syndrome, leading to a higher prevalence of diabetes and CVD compared to other ethnic populations. Abbreviations: SA = South Asian, IR = Insulin resistance, CAD = Coronary artery disease, CVD = Cardiovasular disease, LDL = Low density lipoprotein

considerably higher at BMI values lower than the existing WHO cutoff point for overweight (25 kg/m^2) [17]. This prompted revision of the WHO BMI cutoff points for the classification of overweight at 23 kg/m^2 and obesity at levels greater than or equal to 27.5 kg/m^2 in Asian populations, which are also recommend by the American Diabetes Association [17, 53, 54]. Of note, in 2009, a different consensus statement alternatively suggested that the BMI cutoff for overweight and obesity be 23 kg/m^2 and 25 kg/m^2 in India, respectively [55], which was later also recommended by the South Asian Health Foundation [45].

Cohort studies have demonstrated different BMI thresholds between Asian Americans compared to other racial groups. A BMI threshold of 25 kg/m^2 or greater for screening type 2 diabetes would only be successful at detecting 65% of cases, in other words overlooking one-third of Asian Americans diagnosed with type 2 diabetes, while lowering the BMI sensitivity to 23 kg/m^2 or greater would raise the diabetes detection rate to

more than 80% of Asian Americans [50]. Other studies have suggested that BMI thresholds are different between racial groups despite adults sharing the same BMI value and age: Caucasians with BMI valued at 25 kg/m^2 and 30 years of age translated to Asian Americans having a BMI threshold of 20 kg/m^2, Black Americans with BMI less than 18.5 kg/m^2, and Hispanic Americans with BMI of 18.5 kg/m^2 [56]. The Newcastle Heart Project conducted a cross-sectional study that found obesity levels to be higher among the Indian and Pakistan groups for BMI $>30 \text{ kg/m}^2$ compared to Bangladeshis, while the Bangladesh and Pakistan groups had greater waist-to-hip ratio than the Indian group. When data from the South Asian groups were aggregated, rates of obesity were reported greater compared to the European White population [6].

In another study, participants of South Asian descent from India underwent dual-energy X-ray absorptiometry (DXA) to identify abdominal subcutaneous fat layer boundaries and estimate the visceral fat mass. Researchers found that two or more non-anthropometric metabolic risk factors (triglycerides, HDL cholesterol, glucose, and blood pressure) were present in 55% of males and 34% of females and that optimal WC cutoffs were 92 cm for males and 79 cm for females, consistent with currently recommended ethnic-specific cutoffs for South Asians (Table 1). Visceral fat mass, as measured by DXA, had greater predictive power as reflected by higher area-under-the-curve point estimates, particularly in females, further improving MetS detection. Overall, central obesity is likely a major contributor to the differences in risk of MetS by race, particularly among South Asians [57].

Ultimately, it is important to note that since the WC may better reflect abdominal fat mass and body fat distribution compared to BMI, an increased WC is an important diagnostic tool for MetS and predictor for risk of CVD [58]. The consensus was also reached by many organizations to lower the WC in South Asians based on these ethnic-specific studies, which were adopted in the revised AHA/NHLBI Revised NCEP ATP III and IDF definitions. However, even within Asian populations, there are slight differences in the cutoff values, and hence different criteria for central obesity as shown in Table 1 [13].

Dyslipidemia

Dyslipidemia is a potentially modifiable factor that contributes to a higher risk of atherosclerosis in South Asians. It may be related to dietary choices, increased consumption of saturated fat, genetic factors, decreased physical activity, and increased BMI. One may think that a vegetarian diet would be associated with normal to low levels of total cholesterol. However, urbanization has altered the composition of vegetarian diets. Epidemiologic studies have demonstrated that both vegetarian and nonvegetarian Indian diets are associated with higher risk for coronary artery disease (CAD). The lack of an improved lipid profile on a vegetarian diet is multifactorial. One explanation is the use of high quantities of saturated fats and trans-fatty acids in the process of deep-frying vegetables in many South Asian eating patterns.

Total cholesterol may be normal or increased in South Asian populations [59]. Hypertriglyceridemia is commonly observed in MetS, as well as other conditions such as type 2 diabetes, stroke, and familial hyperlipidemia [60, 61]. Individuals with insulin resistance have been known to demonstrate an increase in production and impaired catabolism of triglyceride-rich lipoproteins, thereby leading to hypertriglyceridemia. The impaired function is correlated with low levels HDL because of impaired transport of cholesterol [62]. HDL plays a vital role in lowering the risk of coronary heart disease, On the other hand, hypertriglyceridemia has been known to be associated with an increased risk for developing coronary heart disease and MctS [63, 64]. In summary, atherogenic dyslipidemia caused by insulin resistance in MetS is common among South Asians [65].

The levels of LDL in urban India have significantly increased over time [66]. Common dyslipidemia patterns among South Asians also include low levels of HDL and high levels of triglycerides [67–70]. Multiple studies have demonstrated that the prevalence rate of hypertriglyceridemia is higher in South Asians compared to Caucasians. In some studies, it was observed that hypertriglyceridemia, defined as >150 mg/dL, was approximately 70% in the South Asian populations compared to 34% in Caucasians [71–74, 64]. Other studies represented the inverse relationship with lower HDL in which half of South Asians had levels lower than <40 mg/dL; 37% of New Delhi persons in a cross-sectional epidemiological study had HDL levels lower than 40 mg/dL. In urban Pakistan, obesity levels ranged from 46% to 68%, hypertriglyceridemia ranged from 27% to 54%, and HDL-C levels ranged from 68% to 81% [75]. Overall, hypertriglyceridemia and low HDL level are interrelated components that contribute to South Asians' development of MetS. The presence of insulin resistance-related atherogenic dyslipidemia is more severe in South Asians compared to Europeans [76]. These studies suggest that despite having relatively normal levels of LDL in comparison to other ethnic groups, atherogenic dyslipidemia and hypertriglyceridemia are more common among South Asians, which may also contribute to the elevated risks for developing coronary heart disease risk in this population [75].

Hypertension

High blood pressure is an important component of MetS, with MetS being present in up to one-third of people with hypertension in general population studies [77–79]. Epidemiologic studies conducted in the 1940s showed the prevalence of hypertension to be approximately 1.2–4.2% in India. However, its prevalence rose to a rate of 15–25% from studies published in the 1990s [80]. In a meta-analysis that examined the prevalence of hypertension across nine studies from South Asian countries, there was a weighted mean prevalence of 48.5%, with a prevalence rate ranging from 21.2% to 81.1% across the different countries included [21]. Furthermore, males and females differed in their weighted mean prevalence of hypertension at 42.3% and 38.1%, respectively. Overall, higher rates of hypertension were associated with older age for both genders. Among the South Asian populations, Pakistani women have been reported to have relatively higher rates of hypertension and Bangladeshi men and women with relatively lower rates [81]. Elevated blood pressure in Asian Indians is not confined to adults; alarmingly, children between the ages of 11 and 17 years old in urban areas have a prevalence of hypertension at 6.6%, and this trend is expected to increase if the current patterns in obesity and lifestyle behaviors continue to persist [82].

South Asians with hypertension have a higher risk of developing premature cardiovascular disease complications compared to Europeans [83]. The burden of hypertension in South Asia and its underlying mechanisms are multifactorial; however, it has been proposed that the high incidence of diabetes and IR in India plays a significant contributory role. The associated adverse effects of hypertension ultimately result in endothelial dysfunction and increased sympathetic tone. Progression of endothelial dysfunction and reduced endothelial progenitor cells, commonly seen among South Asians compared to Caucasians, can all contribute to vascular risks from hypertension [84]. This impaired vascular function in South Asians, compared to Caucasians, leads to vascular remodeling, ultimately implicated in the pathogenesis and progression of hypertension. These dysfunctions have been shown, in turn, to be associated with an increased prevalence of visceral and abdominal obesity in South Asians when compared to Caucasians [85]. Furthermore, dietary habits have been shown to play an important role in the development of hypertension in South Asians. Studies conducted at urban locations in India have demonstrated a significant increase in sodium intake over time with resultant hypertension [86]. It was found that the average daily dietary sodium intake was 8.5 g in urban India, which is significantly more than the WHO's daily recommendation of 5 g of sodium daily. Thus, blood pressure among South Asians is steadily rising, and additionally contributes to the higher risk of MetS and CVD in this population.

Hyperglycemia and Insulin Resistance in South Asians

Insulin resistance has long been recognized as an underlying mechanism in the pathogenesis of the metabolic syndrome [11, 87]. Insulin, a hormone secreted by the pancreatic beta cells, lowers glucose levels by increasing glucose uptake in skeletal muscle and adipose tissue, and suppressing hepatic glucose production. When insulin resistance develops in people with obesity, muscle glucose uptake is reduced and hepatic glucose production increases leading to chronic hyperglycemia (type 2 diabetes). The ability of insulin to inhibit lipolysis is also disrupted, causing an increase in free fatty acids (FFA), which potentiates insulin resistance by altering the insulin signaling cascade in different tissues and organs [88–90]. A hyperinsulinemic state is induced to maintain normal blood glucose levels; however, as the beta cell compensation falls over time, this process leads to relative insulin insufficiency [91]. It is important to note that visceral lipolysis increases the production of free fatty acids, underscoring that visceral fat deposits, in particular, are likely an important contributor to insulin resistance and progression to type 2 diabetes [65, 92].

South Asians with type 2 diabetes are significantly more insulin resistant than their European counterparts [93], and there is significantly lower insulin sensitivity in South Asians compared to Caucasians regardless of the total body fat levels [94]. Evidence also suggests that South Asians are at risk of developing insulin resistance, which further contributes to greater accumulation of visceral fat and glucose intolerance [95]. In addition to increased levels of insulin resistance, South Asians may also experience significantly earlier declines in beta cell function compared to other ethnic groups. Several studies in fact demonstrated that beta cell dysfunction is higher among South Asians, compared to other ethnic groups such as Caucasians, African-Americans, Chinese-Americans, and Hispanics [96]. For example, East Asians, South Asians, Caucasians, and Black individuals were compared, and despite being matched for lifestyle factors and BMI, the degree of insulin resistance in South Asian men was much greater than men of the other ethnic groups [97, 98]. Another study assessed the differences in insulin response to oral glucose load in Asian Indians compared to Europeans; among Asian Indians irrespective of diabetes status, the basal insulin levels were higher and insulin response to the load was also higher, thereby suggesting Asian Indians require increased secretion and higher levels of insulin to main euglycemia in response to the same amount of glucose load [99, 100]. Interestingly, Asian Indian vegetarians have significantly higher insulin levels than American vegetarians in fasting and oral glucose load states, suggesting that despite similar diets, Asian Indians are much more likely to develop IR [99, 101]. Asian Indian men are also more likely to develop insulin resistance than Caucasian men independent of truncal and generalized adiposity, further

supporting the notion of a genetic metabolic defect [99, 102].

Increased insulin resistance in South Asians may be explained by early fetal adaptations such as the proposed "thrifty genotype" hypothesis, which proposes that individuals can store energy during times of excess food availability, thus giving them an advantage during times of famine. However, with global migration and urbanization, this genetic advantage may predispose individuals to insulin resistance and diabetes. Its counterpart, the "thrifty phenotype" hypothesis, proposes that poor intrauterine nutrition leads to early fetal adaptations in preparation for a life of starvation, and development of insulin resistance [103]. Studies have shown that young Indian children with lower birth weights had an increased risk of developing insulin resistance [104]. In an urban South Indian population, 30–55% of adolescents were diagnosed with insulin resistance, with higher risk of developing diabetes that extends into adulthood [99].

Urbanization, Migration, and Acculturation

Urbanization and migration with corresponding changes in diet and sedentary activity have been associated with higher rates of diabetes and MetS in South Asian countries and migrant populations. For example, individuals migrating to urban areas have specifically demonstrated significant increases in BMI [28, 75]. One study demonstrated that urban residents from Moradabad, India have higher prevalence of diabetes compared to their rural residents (7.9% vs. 2.5%), which are comparable to the rates observed in South Asian migrants to the UK [99, 105, 106].

South Asian migrants to affluent countries such as the USA and the UK have a higher prevalence of metabolic disorders. For example, migrants from Gujarat to the UK had a greater dietary caloric intake, fat consumption, cholesterol, and triglycerides than nonmigrants [107–109]. In a meta-analysis, the weighted mean prevalence of MetS in urban versus rural locations was much higher by most definitions: ATPIII, 28.7

versus 21.6%; modified ATPIII, 38.8 versus 11.7%; IDF, 34.1 versus 19.2%; with the exception of WHO, 23.2 versus 30.7% [21].

The concept of acculturation – defined as the adoption of customs, practices, and beliefs of a different cultural group – is often described in the context of four acculturation strategies: integration (maintaining one's heritage while incorporating customs of a new culture), assimilation (abandoning one's heritage and fully adopting a host's culture), separation (rejecting the host culture and maintaining one's heritage), and marginalization (individual abandoning both their own and host's culture). A study of South Asians living in the USA suggests that more than half of the participants adopted the integration strategy [110]. South Asian diet typically consists of higher portions of saturated fats and carbohydrates such as vegetables, chapatis, lentils, and rice and many South Asians adopt a vegetarian diet due to religious and cultural beliefs [55, 111–113]. South Asians living in the USA relatively longer than their counterparts tend to adopt a Westernized diet by incorporating alcohol, meat, and fat, suggesting that the South Asian migrants have substituted components of their South Asian diet with components of the Western diet that may be metabolically unhealthy [114]. In fact, of all US Asians, South Asians have the highest rates of truncal obesity, which may be related to diet [115]. Two distinct dietary patterns among South Asians in the USA have been suggested: a Western pattern incorporating dairy products, fried food, pizza, and potatoes, and a vegetarian pattern incorporating high-volume snacks, rice, and sugary beverages [116].

One study analyzed diet quality by the degree of acculturation. South Asian Americans (Pakistani, Bangladesh, and Indian subjects) were divided into two groups: the Asian (less acculturated) and Western (Americanized) groups. The results showed that the less acculturated group compared to the Americanized group had a higher prevalence of MetS at 42% versus 34%, respectively, and a lower diet quality score. Furthermore, the less acculturated group had higher fatty acid component scores, while the American group had higher dairy, seafood,

and component scores. Both rates of obesity and MetS increased among the South Asian population as a result of numerous factors, including acculturation, affluence, and duration of residency in their new countries. Total calories, calories from carbohydrates, and proteins were higher for the Americanized group compared to the less acculturated group. Gender differences were evident with South Asian males having higher diet quality scores and lower levels of MetS compared to females who had lower diet quality scores and higher levels of MetS [111].

The lack of physical activity is another key contributing factor. A strong relationship exists between decreased physical activity and insulin resistance, cardiovascular disease, type 2 diabetes, and obesity [117]. South Asians, recruited from religious institutions in Illinois, USA, have significantly lowered physical activity compared with other ethnic groups, with over half of the participants not meeting the recommended guidelines as measured by accelerometer [118]. Hence, preventive measures and community-based initiatives are necessary to educate South Asians on these adverse health effects and the importance of modifying such behaviors to reduce chronic conditions of type 2 diabetes and cardiovascular disease.

Diabetes and Metabolic Syndrome in South Asians

Metabolic syndrome is associated with a higher risk of developing type 2 diabetes [46]. South Asians in the USA carry a heightened risk for type 2 diabetes, and are reported to have a higher incidence, prevalence, and underdiagnosed rates of diabetes compared to the White European population and with a faster progression rate of prediabetes to diabetes [16, 96]. In the UK Prospective Diabetes Study of people with type 2 diabetes, of whom 82% were White Caucasian, 10% Asian of Indian origin, and 8% Afro-Caribbean, Asians were significantly younger, had lower BMI and greater waist-hip ratio, were more sedentary, and had a greater prevalence of first degree relatives with known diabetes compared to the other ethnicities [119]. According to the IDF Diabetes Atlas tenth edition (2021), the number of people living with type 2 diabetes in South Asia is estimated to be over one million. The comparative prevalence of diabetes cases in South Asia versus East Asian countries in 2021 (in thousands) according to International Diabetes Federation Atlas tenth edition is shown in Table 3 [120]. Type 2 diabetes cases in South Asia are projected to reach more than 120 million in 2030 [16]. India, one of the South Asian countries with the highest diabetes prevalence is predicted to see its prevalence rise by 72%, with around 87 million people with diabetes by 2030 and 124 million by 2045 [120, 121]. In the USA, between 2011 and 2016, the National Health and Nutrition Examination Survey (NHANES) revealed that the prevalence of diabetes, adjusted for age and sex, as 23.3% for South Asians, 22.4% for Southeast Asians, and 14.0% for East Asian subpopulations [122]. Another study in the USA, which adjusted for both age and adiposity, found diabetes prevalence to be greater in South Asians (23%), versus

Table 3 Estimated number of diabetes cases in South and East Asian countries in 2021[a]

Region	Number of diabetes cases (in thousands)
South Asian countries	
India	74,194.7
Pakistan	32,964.5
Bangladesh	13,136.3
Afghanistan	1606.7
Sri Lanka	1417.6
Mauritius	250.4
Bhutan	44.8
East Asian countries	
China	140,869.6
Japan	11,005.0
Korea	3511.8
Taiwan	2457.2
North Korea	1847.1
Hong Kong	686.0
Mongolia	150.8

[a]Numbers of diabetes cases derived from the International Diabetes Federation (IDF). (Source: IDF Diabetes Atlas tenth edition [Internet]. IDF Diabetes Atlas tenth Edition. diabetesatlas.org; 2021 [accessed 03/27/23]. Available from: https://diabetesatlas.org/data/en/)

Blacks (18%), Latinos (17%), Chinese Americans (13%), and non-Hispanic Whites (6%) [6].

South Asians with recent diagnosis of type 2 diabetes have a higher prevalence of microvascular complications compared to Europeans (27.3% vs. 16.5%, $p < 0.001$), including retinopathy (17.5% vs. 7.9%, $p < 0.001$) and nephropathy (18.1% vs. 7.8%, $p < 0.001$) [123]. Diabetic neuropathy remains an exception in which South Asians have been reported to be at decreased risk possibly due to multiple factors, including lower levels of smoking and better skin microcirculation [99]. Specifically, the UK Prospective Diabetes Study group reported that Asian Indians with newly diagnosed diabetes had a lower neuropathy rate, when assessed using vibration sensation threshold, compared to the Caucasians population (4% vs. 13%, respectively) [119].

There are a growing number of diabetes screening tools, however, many do not consider health risk factors highly prevalent among South Asians. The Indian Diabetes Risk Score (IDRS) was developed to focus on various factors contributing to South Asians' unique body composition (i.e., age, sex, waist circumference, physical activity, and family history) to improve underdiagnoses rates in India [99]. Diagnostic tools that use the BMI, rather than waist circumference, which may be a less optimal indicator for estimating diabetes risk in the South Asian population. More studies and evidence-based interventions need to be done to facilitate better type 2 diabetes management at the individual to the institutional level for each respective country in South Asia and migrant countries.

Cardiovascular Disease and Metabolic Syndrome in South Asians

In the general population, people with MetS have a threefold increased risk of coronary heart disease and stroke, as well as a twofold increased risk of death from cardiac and cerebrovascular disease [41, 124]. The link between metabolic syndrome and cardiovascular disease (CVD) is also well-established in South Asian populations. Insulin resistance, hypertension, and dyslipidemia are more common in South Asians and are key features of MetS that additionally promote atherosclerosis and increase the risk of CVD. South Asians with MetS have been found to have higher levels of circulating inflammatory markers and endothelial dysfunction, both of which are also associated with increased CVD risk [125].

Comparing South Asians to other Asian populations and non-Hispanic Whites in the USA, South Asians had higher proportional mortality rates from atherosclerotic cardiovascular disease (ASCVD), while Asian Americans – including Chinese, Filipinos, Japanese, Koreans, and Vietnamese – have a lower chance of developing ASCVD than the general population [6]. South Asians living in the USA and UK also have a higher prevalence of ASCVD, which begins at a younger age and is more aggressive than in people of other ethnicities [126, 127].

When compared to other ethnicities, South Asians have a higher prevalence of premature coronary heart disease [128]. Several traditional risk factors (diabetes, hypertension, dietary factors, obesity) and lipoprotein-associated risk factors (low HDL cholesterol levels, higher triglycerides, and elevated apolipoprotein B levels) likely contribute to premature coronary artery disease in South Asians [128]. A systematic review on the prevalence of MetS in South Asia reported that CVD occurs at a younger age in South Asians than in any other ethnic population [21].

CVD risk calculators are often used to estimate an individual's risk of developing CVD, accounting for factors such as age, sex, blood pressure, cholesterol levels, smoking status, and diabetes status to calculate an individual's risk score. Commonly used CVD risk calculators in the USA are the American Heart Association/American College of Cardiology (ACC/AHA) Pooled Cohort Equation and the Framingham Risk Score [129]. In the UK, QRISK® has been recommended by the National Institute for Health and Care Excellence (NICE 2014). South Asian ancestry is described as a "risk-enhancing factor" in the USA by the ACC/AHA guidelines [130]. Nonetheless, these calculators may not be as accurate for South Asians when compared to Caucasian cohorts, and studies have called for population-specific CVD risk models [127, 129, 131]. Within a large prospective study, South Asian individuals had a substantially higher risk of ASCVD as compared with individuals of European ancestry, but this risk was not captured by the Pooled Cohort Equations [127]. The study found that South Asians had over a twofold higher observed risk for CVD, while the predicted 10-year risk of CVD according to the AHA/ACC Pooled Cohort Equations and QRISK3 equations was nearly identical for South Asian and European ancestry individuals [127]. When using risk scores to determine the need for CVD preventive therapies, clinicians should be aware of risk model performance differences and potential limitations to accurately predict CVD risk across different race/ethnic groups such as South Asians [132].

Therapeutic Approaches for Metabolic Syndrome in South Asians

There are few studies investigating the differential response to medications or other therapeutic approaches used for MetS, CVD, or type 2 diabetes in South Asian populations compared to other ethnicities; the majority of recommendations and treatment goals are derived from studies performed in non-Hispanic, White populations [6]. There are also important differences between South Asians and Caucasians in the presentation of disease, diagnosis, awareness, behavior, and sociocultural factors, which can contribute to varied treatment and disease outcomes for South Asians [7]. This reflects a future need for interventions and therapies that are tailored to South Asian populations to ensure the success of treatment.

Culturally specific lifestyle interventions are likely the most effective way to prevent and manage MetS and its complications in different ethnic populations such as South Asians. These measures, in conjunction with community-based initiatives, could be effective in educating South Asians about the negative health effects of MetS and obesity in order to reduce the long-term complications of developing diabetes and/or CVD. Regarding lifestyle interventions, it has been suggested that South Asians need to participate in about 50% more minutes of physical activity than their White counterparts to glean the same metabolic health benefits [133]. Interactive group classes focused on increased physical activity and education have shown that both dietary and physical activity interventions can contribute to significant weight loss and a decrease in A1C among South Asian populations [6]. Lentils, whole grains, and vegetables are South Asian cooking staples that can be included in a healthy diet when considering dietary interventions. Incorporating micronutrient-dense but low-calorie fruits and vegetables into the diet is also one of the most cost-effective ways to combat micronutrient deficiency while decreasing excess calories in meals [41]. Furthermore, Ayurvedic medicine is a traditional medical system that has been practiced in South Asia for thousands of years. Turmeric, fenugreek, and cinnamon, among other Ayurvedic herbs and spices, have been traditionally used to improve blood glucose levels and insulin sensitivity [41]. However, many complementary and alternative medicines have not been rigorously scientifically studied for the treatment of MetS or diabetes. Traditional practices in South Asia such as religious fasting may impact metabolic health; thus, people with diabetes should be aware of the risks of hypoglycemia, dehydration, postural hypotension, and ketoacidosis when fasting and adjust their antihyperglycemic regimen under clinical supervision as appropriate [41].

Underrepresentation of South Asians in CVD outcome trials of recently approved glucose-lowering therapies is of particular concern given the large number of people with MetS, type 2 diabetes, CVD, and MetS who belong to this ethnic group. South Asians are likely to respond well to incretin-based therapies such as dipeptidyl peptidase-4 (DPP-4) inhibitors and glucagon-like peptide-1 (GLP-1) analogs [6]. DPP-4 inhibitors may be preferred for the treatment of South Asians with type 2 diabetes who are fasting given low risk of hypoglycemia [134]. Because of the significantly higher burden of CVD among South Asians, the South Asian Health Foundation suggests using GLP-1 receptor agonists be considered particularly to prevent CVD complications [134]. Moreover, GLP-1 receptor agonists have a favorable risk profile for hypoglycemia, making them potentially advantageous for use during fasting, and can reduce ectopic fat and lead to weight loss [134]. Of note, the MAGNA VICTORIA study investigated the efficacy of liraglutide in South Asian populations and found no difference in liraglutide efficacy between Western Europeans and South Asians [135]. SGLT2 inhibitors have been found to have a favorable safety profile in South Asians and can also be considered for CVD prevention in high-risk individuals [134].

Statins are recommended as first-line therapy for lowering low-density lipoprotein cholesterol (LDL-C) levels in patients with ASCVD and those at high risk of developing it. Statins such as rosuvastatin and atorvastatin are well-tolerated and effective in South Asian populations [136]. Besides statins, other lipid-lowering therapies such as ezetimibe and PCSK9 inhibitors may be considered for patients with ASCVD who cannot tolerate statins or who have persistently elevated LDL-C levels; these treatments appear safe and effective for South Asian populations [137, 138].

Another treatment option for metabolic syndrome is bariatric surgery. It has been demonstrated that gastric bypass surgery improves insulin sensitivity, lowers blood pressure and cholesterol levels, and leads to weight loss among obese Asian Indians in South India [139]. Clinical consideration of metabolic surgery in selected motivated individuals has been recommended for Asian Americans versus other ethnicities at lower BMI thresholds ($\geq 27.5 \text{ kg/m}^2$ vs. $\geq 30 \text{ kg/m}^2$, respectively) [6, 140]. Bariatric surgery has demonstrated efficacy in reducing total body fat, visceral fat area, and hepatic steatosis in South Asian populations [139, 141].

Conclusion

The term MetS refers to a collection of cardiometabolic conditions including abdominal (visceral) obesity, hypertension, hypertriglyceridemia, decreased HDL levels, and hyperglycemia. Though different organizations have established criteria for the diagnosis of MetS, NCEP ATP III or revised NCEP ATP III criteria are commonly used to identify the presence of MetS in the USA, while IDF and WHO criteria are also commonly used around the world. Nonetheless, there is consensus that ethnic-specific cutoffs for waist circumference should be used when diagnosing MetS in South Asians. Prevalence of MetS varies across different racial and ethnic populations; however, South Asians are at a higher risk of developing MetS and its components than Caucasians because of their unique genetic, lifestyle, and environmental risk factors. Excess total adipose tissue, visceral obesity, and fat accumulation at ectopic body sites are all associated with the increased risk of insulin resistance and MetS among South Asians. Furthermore, urbanization, acculturation, and migration all contribute to MetS prevalence among South Asians. Cardiovascular disease occurs at earlier ages and more aggressively in this population, and South Asians have among the highest prevalence rates of diabetes compared to other ethnicities. Lifestyle and behavioral modifications, community-based interventions, pharmacological interventions along with culturally specific tailored recommendations will be important to address the increasing prevalence of MetS and obesity in South Asians.

References

1. The World Fact Book: Central Intelligence Agency; 2017.
2. SAALT. (South Asians Learning Together). Demographic snapshot of South Asians in the United States. Retrieved from https://saalt.org/wp-content/uploads/2019/04/SAALT-Demographic-Snapshot-2019.pdf. 2019 April.
3. Rudra G. Here to stay: uncovering South Asian American history. Asian American/Asian Research Institute, The City University of New York. 2022 April 1.
4. Government of Canada SC. The Canadian census: a rich portrait of the country's religious and ethnocultural diversity. The Daily. 2022 October.
5. Peoples WDoMaI. South Asians Minority Rights Home 2022 September.
6. Volgman AS, Palaniappan LS, Aggarwal NT, Gupta M, Khandelwal A, Krishnan AV, et al. Atherosclerotic cardiovascular disease in South Asians in the United States: Epidemiology, risk factors, and treatments: a Scientific Statement from the American Heart Association. Circulation. 2018;138(1):e1–e34.
7. Pandit K, Goswami S, Ghosh S, Mukhopadhyay P, Chowdhury S. Metabolic syndrome in South Asians. Indian J Endocrinol Metab. 2012;16(1):44–55.
8. Han TS, Lean ME. A clinical perspective of obesity, metabolic syndrome and cardiovascular disease. JRSM Cardiovasc Dis. 2016;5:2048004016633371.
9. Silveira Rossi JL, Barbalho SM, Reverete de Araujo R, Bechara MD, Sloan KP, Sloan LA. Metabolic syndrome and cardiovascular diseases: going beyond traditional risk factors. Diabetes Metab Res Rev. 2022;38(3):e3502.
10. Noncommunicable diseases [Internet]. 2022 September.
11. Reaven GM. Banting lecture 1988. Role of insulin resistance in human disease. Diabetes. 1988;37(12): 1595–607.
12. Alberti KG, Eckel RH, Grundy SM, Zimmet PZ, Cleeman JI, Donato KA, et al. Harmonizing the metabolic syndrome: a joint interim statement of the International Diabetes Federation Task Force on Epidemiology and Prevention; National Heart, Lung, and Blood Institute; American Heart Association; World Heart Federation; International Atherosclerosis Society; and International Association for the Study of Obesity. Circulation. 2009;120(16):1640–5.
13. Tahapary DL, Harbuwono DS, Yunir E, Soewondo P. Diagnosing metabolic syndrome in a multi-ethnic country: is an ethnic-specific cut-off point of waist circumference needed? Nutr Diabetes. 2020;10(1):19.
14. Grundy SM, Cleeman JI, Daniels SR, Donato KA, Eckel RH, Franklin BA, et al. Diagnosis and management of the metabolic syndrome: an American Heart Association/National Heart, Lung, and Blood Institute Scientific Statement. Circulation. 2005;112(17): 2735–52.
15. Sperling LS, Mechanick JI, Neeland IJ, Herrick CJ, Després JP, Ndumele CE, et al. The cardiometabolic health alliance: working toward a new care model for the metabolic syndrome. J Am Coll Cardiol. 2015;66 (9):1050–67.
16. Misra A, Ramchandran A, Jayawardena R, Shrivastava U, Snehalatha C. Diabetes in South Asians. Diabet Med. 2014;31(10):1153–62.
17. WHO Expert Consultation. Appropriate body-mass index for Asian populations and its implications for policy and intervention strategies. Lancet. 2004:157–63.
18. Lear SA, Humphries KH, Kohli S, Chockalingam A, Frohlich JJ, Birmingham CL. Visceral adipose tissue accumulation differs according to ethnic background: results of the Multicultural Community Health Assessment Trial (M-CHAT). Am J Clin Nutr. 2007;86(2):353–9.
19. Lear SA, Humphries KH, Kohli S, Birmingham CL. The use of BMI and waist circumference as surrogates of body fat differs by ethnicity. Obesity (Silver Spring). 2007;15(11):2817–24.

20. Lear SA, James PT, Ko GT, Kumanyika S. Appropriateness of waist circumference and waist-to-hip ratio cutoffs for different ethnic groups. Eur J Clin Nutr. 2010;64(1):42–61.

21. Aryal N, Wasti SP. The prevalence of metabolic syndrome in South Asia: a systematic review. Int J Diabetes Dev Ctries. 2016;36(3):255–62.

22. Ranasinghe P, Mathangasinghe Y, Jayawardena R, Hills AP, Misra A. Prevalence and trends of metabolic syndrome among adults in the asia-pacific region: a systematic review. BMC Public Health. 2017;17(1): 101.

23. Hydrie MZ, Shera AS, Fawwad A, Basit A, Hussain A. Prevalence of metabolic syndrome in urban Pakistan (Karachi): comparison of newly proposed International Diabetes Federation and modified Adult Treatment Panel III criteria. Metab Syndr Relat Disord. 2009;7(2):119–24.

24. Ravikiran M, Bhansali A, Ravikumar P, Bhansali S, Dutta P, Thakur JS, et al. Prevalence and risk factors of metabolic syndrome among Asian Indians: a community survey. Diabetes Res Clin Pract. 2010;89(2): 181–8.

25. Zahid N, Claussen B, Hussain A. High prevalence of obesity, dyslipidemia and metabolic syndrome in a rural area in Pakistan. Diabetes Metab Syndr Clin Res Rev. 2008;2(1):13–9.

26. Chackrewarthy S, Gunasekera D, Pathmeswaren A, Wijekoon CN, Ranawaka UK, Kato N, et al. A Comparison between revised NCEP ATP III and IDF definitions in diagnosing metabolic syndrome in an urban Sri Lankan population: the Ragama Health Study. ISRN Endocrinol. 2013;2013:320176.

27. Chow CK, Naidu S, Raju K, Raju R, Joshi R, Sullivan D, et al. Significant lipid, adiposity and metabolic abnormalities amongst 4535 Indians from a developing region of rural Andhra Pradesh. Atherosclerosis. 2008;196(2):943–52.

28. Misra A, Khurana L. Obesity and the metabolic syndrome in developing countries. J Clin Endocrinol Metab. 2008;93(11 Suppl 1):S9–30.

29. Das M, Pal S, Ghosh A. Prevalence of cardiovascular disease risk factors by habitat: a study on adult Asian Indians in West Bengal. India Anthropol Anz. 2011;68(3):253–64.

30. Kanjilal S, Shanker J, Rao VS, Khadrinarasimhaih NB, Mukherjee M, Iyengar SS, et al. Prevalence and component analysis of metabolic syndrome: an Indian atherosclerosis research study perspective. Vasc Health Risk Manag. 2008;4(1):189–97.

31. Kamble P, Deshmukh PR, Garg N. Metabolic syndrome in adult population of rural Wardha, central India. Indian J Med Res. 2010;132(6):701–5.

32. Pemminati S, Prabha Adhikari MR, Pathak R, Pai MR. Prevalence of metabolic syndrome (METS) using IDF 2005 guidelines in a semi urban south Indian (Boloor Diabetes Study) population of Mangalore. J Assoc Physicians India. 2010;58:674–7.

33. Deepa M, Farooq S, Datta M, Deepa R, Mohan V. Prevalence of metabolic syndrome using WHO, ATPIII and IDF definitions in Asian Indians: the Chennai Urban Rural Epidemiology Study (CURES-34). Diabetes Metab Res Rev. 2007;23(2): 127–34.

34. Flowers E, Molina C, Mathur A, Prasad M, Abrams L, Sathe A, et al. Prevalence of metabolic syndrome in South Asians residing in the United States. Metab Syndr Relat Disord. 2010;8(5):417–23.

35. Rajpathak SN, Gupta LS, Waddell EN, Upadhyay UD, Wildman RP, Kaplan R, et al. Elevated risk of type 2 diabetes and metabolic syndrome among Asians and south Asians: results from the 2004 New York City HANES. Ethn Dis. 2010;20(3):225–30.

36. McKeigue PM, Marmot MG, Syndercombe Court YD, Cottier DE, Rahman S, Riemersma RA. Diabetes, hyperinsulinaemia, and coronary risk factors in Bangladeshis in east London. Br Heart J. 1988;60(5):390–6.

37. McKeigue PM, Shah B, Marmot MG. Relation of central obesity and insulin resistance with high diabetes prevalence and cardiovascular risk in South Asians. Lancet. 1991;337(8738):382–6.

38. McKeigue PM, Pierpoint T, Ferrie JE, Marmot MG. Relationship of glucose intolerance and hyperinsulinaemia to body fat pattern in south Asians and Europeans. Diabetologia. 1992;35(8):785–91.

39. McKeigue PM. Metabolic consequences of obesity and body fat pattern: lessons from migrant studies. Ciba Found Symp. 1996;201:54–64; discussion −7, 188–93

40. Tan CE, Ma S, Wai D, Chew SK, Tai ES. Can we apply the national cholesterol education program adult treatment panel definition of the metabolic syndrome to Asians? Diabetes Care. 2004;27(5):1182–6.

41. Jayawardena R, Sooriyaarachchi P, Misra A. Abdominal obesity and metabolic syndrome in South Asians: prevention and management. Expert Rev Endocrinol Metab. 2021;16(6):339–49.

42. Nestel P, Lyu R, Low LP, Sheu WH, Nitiyanant W, Saito I, et al. Metabolic syndrome: recent prevalence in East and Southeast Asian populations. Asia Pac J Clin Nutr. 2007;16(2):362–7.

43. Swarup S, Goyal A, Grigorova Y, Zeltser R. Metabolic syndrome. Treasure Island: StatPearls Publishing. Copyright © 2023, StatPearls Publishing LLC.: StatPearls; 2023.

44. Malandrino N, Bhat SZ, Alfaraidhy M, Grewal RS, Kalyani RR. Obesity and aging. Endocrinol Metab Clin N Am. 2023;52(2):317–39.

45. Gray LJ, Yates T, Davies MJ, Brady E, Webb DR, Sattar N, et al. Defining obesity cut-off points for migrant South Asians. PLoS One. 2011;6(10): e26464.

46. Rosenzweig JL, Bakris GL, Berglund LF, Hivert MF, Horton ES, Kalyani RR, et al. Primary prevention of ASCVD and T2DM in patients at metabolic risk: an

endocrine society* clinical practice guideline. J Clin Endocrinol Metab. 2019;104:3939–85.

47. Banerji MA, Faridi N, Atluri R, Chaiken RL, Lebovitz HE. Body composition, visceral fat, leptin, and insulin resistance in Asian Indian men. J Clin Endocrinol Metab. 1999;84(1):137–44.

48. Chandalia M, Abate N, Garg A, Stray-Gundersen J, Grundy SM. Relationship between generalized and upper body obesity to insulin resistance in Asian Indian men. J Clin Endocrinol Metab. 1999;84(7): 2329–35.

49. Chowdhury B, Lantz H, Sjostrom L. Computed tomography-determined body composition in relation to cardiovascular risk factors in Indian and matched Swedish males. Metabolism. 1996;45(5):634–44.

50. Shah NS, Luncheon C, Kandula NR, Khan SS, Pan L, Gillespie C, et al. Heterogeneity in obesity prevalence among Asian American adults. Ann Intern Med. 2022;175(11):1493–500.

51. Mohan V, Deepa M, Farooq S, Narayan KM, Datta M, Deepa R. Anthropometric cut points for identification of cardiometabolic risk factors in an urban Asian Indian population. Metabolism. 2007;56(7):961–8.

52. Razak F, Anand SS, Shannon H, Vuksan V, Davis B, Jacobs R, et al. Defining obesity cut points in a multiethnic population. Circulation. 2007;115(16):2111–8.

53. Misra A. Ethnic-specific criteria for classification of body mass index: a perspective for Asian Indians and American Diabetes Association Position Statement. Diabetes Technol Ther. 2015;17(9):667–71.

54. ElSayed NA, Aleppo G, Aroda VR, Bannuru RR, Brown FM, Bruemmer D, et al. 2. Classification and diagnosis of diabetes: standards of care in diabetes-2023. Diabetes Care. 2023;46(Suppl 1): S19–40.

55. Misra A, Khurana L, Isharwal S, Bhardwaj S. South Asian diets and insulin resistance. Br J Nutr. 2009;101 (4):465–73.

56. Aggarwal R, Bibbins-Domingo K, Yeh RW, Song Y, Chiu N, Wadhera RK, et al. Diabetes screening by race and ethnicity in the United States: equivalent body mass index and age thresholds. Ann Intern Med. 2022;175(6):765–73.

57. Sluyter JD, Plank LD, Rush EC. Identifying metabolic syndrome in migrant Asian Indian adults with anthropometric and visceral fat action points. Diabetol Metab Syndr. 2022;14(1):96.

58. Koh JH, Koh SB, Lee MY, Jung PM, Kim BH, Shin JY, et al. Optimal waist circumference cutoff values for metabolic syndrome diagnostic criteria in a Korean rural population. J Korean Med Sci. 2010;25 (5):734–7.

59. Eckel RH, Alberti KG, Grundy SM, Zimmet PZ. The metabolic syndrome. Lancet. 2010;375(9710):181–3.

60. Seo MH, Bae JC, Park SE, Rhee EJ, Park CY, Oh KW, et al. Association of lipid and lipoprotein profiles with future development of type 2 diabetes in nondiabetic Korean subjects: a 4-year retrospective, longitudinal study. J Clin Endocrinol Metab. 2011;96(12): E2050–4.

61. Kim SJ, Park YG, Kim JH, Han YK, Cho HK, Bang OY. Plasma fasting and nonfasting triglycerides and high-density lipoprotein cholesterol in atherosclerotic stroke: different profiles according to low-density lipoprotein cholesterol. Atherosclerosis. 2012;223 (2):463–7.

62. Ram CV, Farmer JA. Metabolic syndrome in South Asians. J Clin Hypertens (Greenwich). 2012;14(8): 561–5.

63. Arnett DK, Blumenthal RS, Albert MA, Buroker AB, Goldberger ZD, Hahn EJ, et al. 2019 ACC/AHA guideline on the primary prevention of cardiovascular disease: a report of the American College of Cardiology/American Heart Association Task Force on Clinical Practice Guidelines. Circulation. 2019;140(11): e596–646.

64. Bilen O, Kamal A, Virani SS. Lipoprotein abnormalities in South Asians and its association with cardiovascular disease: current state and future directions. World J Cardiol. 2016;8(3):247–57.

65. Fahed G, Aoun L, Bou Zerdan M, Allam S, Bou Zerdan M, Bouferraa Y, et al. Metabolic syndrome: updates on pathophysiology and management in 2021. Int J Mol Sci. 2022;23(2):786.

66. Joseph A, Kutty VR, Soman CR. High risk for coronary heart disease in Thiruvananthapuram city: a study of serum lipids and other risk factors. Indian Heart J. 2000;52(1):29–35.

67. Anand SS, Yusuf S, Vuksan V, Devanesen S, Teo KK, Montague PA, et al. Differences in risk factors, atherosclerosis and cardiovascular disease between ethnic groups in Canada: the study of health assessment and risk in ethnic groups (SHARE). Indian Heart J. 2000;52(7 Suppl):S35–43.

68. Gupta R, Gupta VP, Sarna M, Bhatnagar S, Thanvi J, Sharma V, et al. Prevalence of coronary heart disease and risk factors in an urban Indian population: Jaipur Heart Watch-2. Indian Heart J. 2002;54(1):59–66.

69. Sekhri T, Kanwar RS, Wilfred R, Chugh P, Chhillar M, Aggarwal R, et al. Prevalence of risk factors for coronary artery disease in an urban Indian population. BMJ Open. 2014;4(12):e005346.

70. Hughes LO, Wojciechowski AP, Raftery EB. Relationship between plasma cholesterol and coronary artery disease in Asians. Atherosclerosis. 1990;83(1):15–20.

71. Gopinath N, Chadha SL, Jain P, Shekhawat S, Tandon R. An epidemiological study of obesity in adults in the urban population of Delhi. J Assoc Physicians India. 1994;42(3):212–5.

72. Bhardwaj S, Misra A, Misra R, Goel K, Bhatt SP, Rastogi K, et al. High prevalence of abdominal, intra-abdominal and subcutaneous adiposity and clustering of risk factors among urban Asian Indians in North India. PLoS One. 2011;6(9):e24362.

73. Misra A, Pandey RM, Devi JR, Sharma R, Vikram NK, Khanna N. High prevalence of diabetes, obesity

and dyslipidaemia in urban slum population in northern India. Int J Obes Relat Metab Disord. 2001;25 (11):1722–9.

74. Ford ES, Li C, Zhao G, Pearson WS, Mokdad AH. Hypertriglyceridemia and its pharmacologic treatment among US adults. Arch Intern Med. 2009;169(6):572–8.

75. Basit A, Shera AS. Prevalence of metabolic syndrome in Pakistan. Metab Syndr Relat Disord. 2008;6(3): 171–5.

76. Rashid S, Sniderman A, Melone M, Brown PE, Otvos JD, Mente A, et al. Elevated cholesteryl ester transfer protein (CETP) activity, a major determinant of the atherogenic dyslipidemia, and atherosclerotic cardiovascular disease in South Asians. Eur J Prev Cardiol. 2015;22(4):468–77.

77. Yanai H, Tomono Y, Ito K, Furutani N, Yoshida H, Tada N. The underlying mechanisms for development of hypertension in the metabolic syndrome. Nutr J. 2008;7:10.

78. Cuspidi C, Meani S, Fusi V, Severgnini B, Valerio C, Catini E, et al. Metabolic syndrome and target organ damage in untreated essential hypertensives. J Hypertens. 2004;22(10):1991–8.

79. Schillaci G, Pirro M, Vaudo G, Gemelli F, Marchesi S, Porcellati C, et al. Prognostic value of the metabolic syndrome in essential hypertension. J Am Coll Cardiol. 2004;43(10):1817–22.

80. Gupta R. Meta-analysis of prevalence of hypertension in India. Indian Heart J. 1997;49(1):43–8.

81. Barnett AH, Dixon AN, Bellary S, Hanif MW, O'Hare JP, Raymond NT, et al. Type 2 diabetes and cardiovascular risk in the UK south Asian community. Diabetologia. 2006;49(10):2234–46.

82. Mohan B, Kumar N, Aslam N, Rangbulla A, Kumbkarni S, Sood NK, et al. Prevalence of sustained hypertension and obesity in urban and rural school going children in Ludhiana. Indian Heart J. 2004;56 (4):310–4.

83. Farrukh F, Abbasi A, Jawed M, Almas A, Jafar T, Virani SS, et al. Hypertension in women: a South-Asian Perspective. Front Cardiovasc Med. 2022;9: 880374.

84. Murphy C, Kanaganayagam GS, Jiang B, Chowienczyk PJ, Zbinden R, Saha M, et al. Vascular dysfunction and reduced circulating endothelial progenitor cells in young healthy UK South Asian men. Arterioscler Thromb Vasc Biol. 2007;27(4):936–42.

85. Chambers JC, McGregor A, Jean-Marie J, Kooner JS. Abnormalities of vascular endothelial function may contribute to increased coronary heart disease risk in UK Indian Asians. Heart. 1999;81(5):501–4.

86. Radhika G, Sathya RM, Sudha V, Ganesan A, Mohan V. Dietary salt intake and hypertension in an urban south Indian population – [CURES – 53]. J Assoc Physicians India. 2007;55:405–11.

87. Ferrannini E, Haffner S, Mitchell B, Stern M. Hyperinsulinaemia: the key feature of a cardiovascular and metabolic syndrome. Diabetologia. 1991;34:416–22.

88. Roberts CK, Hevener AL, Barnard RJ. Metabolic syndrome and insulin resistance: underlying causes and modification by exercise training. Compr Physiol. 2013;3(1):1–58.

89. Boden G, Shulman GI. Free fatty acids in obesity and type 2 diabetes: defining their role in the development of insulin resistance and beta-cell dysfunction. Eur J Clin Investig. 2002;32(Suppl 3):14–23.

90. Griffin ME, Marcucci MJ, Cline GW, Bell K, Barucci N, Lee D, et al. Free fatty acid-induced insulin resistance is associated with activation of protein kinase C theta and alterations in the insulin signaling cascade. Diabetes. 1999;48(6):1270–4.

91. Unger RH, Zhou YT. Lipotoxicity of beta-cells in obesity and in other causes of fatty acid spillover. Diabetes. 2001;50(Suppl 1):S118–21.

92. Patel P, Abate N. Body fat distribution and insulin resistance. Nutrients. 2013;5(6):2019–27.

93. Sharp PS, Mohan V, Levy JC, Mather HM, Kohner EM. Insulin resistance in patients of Asian Indian and European origin with non-insulin dependent diabetes. Horm Metab Res. 1987;19(2):84–5.

94. Raji A, Seely EW, Arky RA, Simonson DC. Body fat distribution and insulin resistance in healthy Asian Indians and Caucasians. J Clin Endocrinol Metab. 2001;86(11):5366–71.

95. Indulekha K, Anjana RM, Surendar J, Mohan V. Association of visceral and subcutaneous fat with glucose intolerance, insulin resistance, adipocytokines and inflammatory markers in Asian Indians (CURES-113). Clin Biochem. 2011;44(4): 281–7.

96. Unnikrishnan R, Gupta PK, Mohan V. Diabetes in South Asians: phenotype, clinical presentation, and natural history. Curr Diab Rep. 2018;18(6):30.

97. Gujral UP, Pradeepa R, Weber MB, Narayan KM, Mohan V. Type 2 diabetes in South Asians: similarities and differences with white Caucasian and other populations. Ann N Y Acad Sci. 2013;1281(1):51–63.

98. Petersen KF, Dufour S, Feng J, Befroy D, Dziura J, Dalla Man C, et al. Increased prevalence of insulin resistance and nonalcoholic fatty liver disease in Asian-Indian men. Proc Natl Acad Sci U S A. 2006;103(48):18273–7.

99. Shah A, Kanaya AM. Diabetes and associated complications in the South Asian population. Curr Cardiol Rep. 2014;16(5):476.

100. Mohan V, Sharp PS, Cloke HR, Burrin JM, Schumer B, Kohner EM. Serum immunoreactive insulin responses to a glucose load in Asian Indian and European type 2 (non-insulin-dependent) diabetic patients and control subjects. Diabetologia. 1986;29 (4):235–7.

101. Scholfield DJ, Behall KM, Bhathena SJ, Kelsay J, Reiser S, Revett KR. A study on Asian Indian and American vegetarians: indications of a racial

predisposition to glucose intolerance. Am J Clin Nutr. 1987;46(6):955–61.

102. Ramachandran A, Snehalatha C, Yamuna A, Murugesan N, Narayan KM. Insulin resistance and clustering of cardiometabolic risk factors in urban teenagers in southern India. Diabetes Care. 2007;30 (7):1828–33.

103. Hu FB. Globalization of diabetes: the role of diet, lifestyle, and genes. Diabetes Care. 2011;34(6): 1249–57.

104. Bavdekar A, Yajnik CS, Fall CH, Bapat S, Pandit AN, Deshpande V, et al. Insulin resistance syndrome in 8-year-old Indian children: small at birth, big at 8 years, or both? Diabetes. 1999;48(12):2422–9.

105. Ramachandran A, Mary S, Yamuna A, Murugesan N, Snehalatha C. High prevalence of diabetes and cardiovascular risk factors associated with urbanization in India. Diabetes Care. 2008;31(5):893–8.

106. Singh RB, Ghosh S, Niaz AM, Gupta S, Bishnoi I, Sharma JP, et al. Epidemiologic study of diet and coronary risk factors in relation to central obesity and insulin levels in rural and urban populations of north India. Int J Cardiol. 1995;47(3):245–55.

107. Abate N, Chandalia M. Ethnicity, type 2 diabetes & migrant Asian Indians. Indian J Med Res. 2007;125 (3):251–8.

108. Mohanty SA, Woolhandler S, Himmelstein DU, Bor DH. Diabetes and cardiovascular disease among Asian Indians in the United States. J Gen Intern Med. 2005;20(5):474–8.

109. Patel JV, Vyas A, Cruickshank JK, Prabhakaran D, Hughes E, Reddy KS, et al. Impact of migration on coronary heart disease risk factors: comparison of Gujaratis in Britain and their contemporaries in villages of origin in India. Atherosclerosis. 2006;185(2): 297–306.

110. Needham BL, Mukherjee B, Bagchi P, Kim C, Mukherjea A, Kandula NR, et al. Acculturation strategies among South Asian immigrants: the Mediators of Atherosclerosis in South Asians Living in America (MASALA) Study. J Immigr Minor Health. 2017;19 (2):373–80.

111. Khan SA, Jackson RT, Momen B. The relationship between diet quality and acculturation of immigrated South Asian American adults and their association with metabolic syndrome. PLoS One. 2016;11(6):e0156851.

112. Pilis W, Stec K, Zych M, Pilis A. Health benefits and risk associated with adopting a vegetarian diet. Rocz Panstw Zakl Hig. 2014;65(1):9–14.

113. Refsum H, Yajnik CS, Gadkari M, Schneede J, Vollset SE, Orning L, et al. Hyperhomocysteinemia and elevated methylmalonic acid indicate a high prevalence of cobalamin deficiency in Asian Indians. Am J Clin Nutr. 2001;74(2):233–41.

114. Lip GY, Luscombe C, McCarry M, Malik I, Beevers G. Ethnic differences in public health awareness, health perceptions and physical exercise: implications for heart disease prevention. Ethn Health. 1996;1(1):47–53.

115. Lauderdale DS, Rathouz PJ. Body mass index in a US national sample of Asian Americans: effects of nativity, years since immigration and socioeconomic status. Int J Obes Relat Metab Disord. 2000;24(9):1188–94.

116. Gadgil MD, Anderson CAM, Kandula NR, Kanaya AM. Dietary patterns in Asian Indians in the United States: an analysis of the metabolic syndrome and atherosclerosis in South Asians Living in America study. J Acad Nutr Diet. 2014;114(2):238–43.

117. Kesaniemi YK, Danforth E Jr, Jensen MD, Kopelman PG, Lefèbvre P, Reeder BA. Dose-response issues concerning physical activity and health: an evidence-based symposium. Med Sci Sports Exerc. 2001;33(6 Suppl):S351–8.

118. Daniel M, Wilbur J, Fogg LF, Miller AM. Correlates of lifestyle: physical activity among South Asian Indian immigrants. J Community Health Nurs. 2013;30(4):185–200.

119. UK Prospective Diabetes Study. XII: Differences between Asian, Afro-Caribbean and white Caucasian type 2 diabetic patients at diagnosis of diabetes. UK Prospective Diabetes Study Group. Diabet Med. 1994;11(7):670–7.

120. International Diabetes Federation (IDF). IDF diabetes Atlas 10th edition [Internet]. IDF diabetes Atlas 10th Ed. diabetesatlas.org; 2021. Available from: https:// diabetesatlas.org/data/en/.

121. Shaw JE, Sicree RA, Zimmet PZ. Global estimates of the prevalence of diabetes for 2010 and 2030. Diabetes Res Clin Pract. 2010;87(1):4–14.

122. Cheng YJ, Kanaya AM, Araneta MRG, Saydah SH, Kahn HS, Gregg EW, Fujimoto WY, Imperatore G. Prevalence of diabetes by race and ethnicity in the United States, 2011-2016.JAMA. 2019; 322: 2389–2398. https://doi.org/10.1001/jama.2019. 19365.

123. Chowdhury TA, Lasker SS. Complications and cardiovascular risk factors in South Asians and Europeans with early-onset type 2 diabetes. QJM. 2002;95(4):241–6.

124. Ogurtsova K, da Rocha Fernandes JD, Huang Y, Linnenkamp U, Guariguata L, Cho NH, et al. IDF Diabetes Atlas: global estimates for the prevalence of diabetes for 2015 and 2040. Diabetes Res Clin Pract. 2017;128:40–50.

125. Chait A, den Hartigh LJ. Adipose tissue distribution, inflammation and its metabolic consequences, including diabetes and cardiovascular disease. Front Cardiovasc Med. 2020;7:22.

126. Kalra D, Vijayaraghavan K, Sikand G, Desai NR, Joshi PH, Mehta A, et al. Prevention of atherosclerotic cardiovascular disease in South Asians in the US: A clinical perspective from the National Lipid Association. J Clin Lipidol. 2021;15(3):402–22.

127. Patel AP, Wang M, Kartoun U, Ng K, Khera AV. Quantifying and understanding the higher risk of atherosclerotic cardiovascular disease among South Asian individuals: results from the UK

Biobank prospective cohort study. Circulation. 2021;144(6):410–22.

128. Ahmed ST, Rehman H, Akeroyd JM, Alam M, Shah T, Kalra A, et al. Premature coronary heart disease in South Asians: burden and determinants. Curr Atheroscler Rep. 2018;20(1):6.

129. Badawy M, Naing L, Johar S, Ong S, Rahman HA, Tengah D, et al. Evaluation of cardiovascular diseases risk calculators for CVDs prevention and management: scoping review. BMC Public Health. 2022;22 (1):1742.

130. Grundy SM, Stone NJ, Bailey AL, Beam C, Birtcher KK, Blumenthal RS, et al. 2018 AHA/ACC/ AACVPR/AAPA/ABC/ACPM/ADA/AGS/APhA/ ASPC/NLA/PCNA guideline on the management of blood cholesterol: a report of the American College of Cardiology/American Heart Association Task Force on Clinical Practice Guidelines. Circulation. 2019;139(25):e1082–e143.

131. Findlay SG, Kasliwal RR, Bansal M, Tarique A, Zaman A. A comparison of cardiovascular risk scores in native and migrant South Asian populations. SSM Popul Health. 2020;11:100594.

132. Zinzuwadia A, Li C, Dashti H, Chen L, Cade B, Karlson E, et al. Abstract P021: performance of pooled cohort equations and MESA risk score across race/ethnicity and socioeconomic status to estimate 10-year cardiovascular risk in diverse New England cohort. Circulation. 2022;145:AP021–AP021.

133. Iliodromiti S, Ghouri N, Celis-Morales CA, Sattar N, Lumsden MA, Gill JM. Should physical activity recommendations for South Asian adults be ethnicity-specific? evidence from a cross-sectional study of south asian and white european men and women. PLoS One. 2016;11(8):e0160024.

134. Hanif W, Ali SN, Bellary S, Patel V, Farooqi A, Karamat MA, et al. Pharmacological management of South Asians with type 2 diabetes: consensus recommendations from the South Asian Health foundation. Diabet Med. 2021;38(4):e14497.

135. Bizino MB, Jazet IM, van Eyk HJ, Rensen PCN, Geelhoed-Duijvestijn PH, Kharagjitsingh AV, et al. Efficacy of liraglutide on glycemic endpoints in people of Western European and South Asian descent with T2DM using multiple daily insulin injections: results of the MAGNA VICTORIA studies. Acta Diabetol. 2021;58(4):485–93.

136. Deedwania PC, Gupta M, Stein M, Ycas J, Gold A. Comparison of rosuvastatin versus atorvastatin in South-Asian patients at risk of coronary heart disease (from the IRIS Trial). Am J Cardiol. 2007;99(11): 1538–43.

137. Hao Q, Aertgeerts B, Guyatt G, Bekkering GE, Vandvik PO, Khan SU, et al. PCSK9 inhibitors and ezetimibe for the reduction of cardiovascular events: a clinical practice guideline with risk-stratified recommendations. BMJ. 2022;377:e069066.

138. Choi JY, Na JO. Pharmacological Strategies beyond statins: ezetimibe and PCSK9 inhibitors. J Lipid Atheroscler. 2019;8(2):183–91.

139. Chandru S, Pramodkumar TA, Pradeepa R, Jebarani S, Prasad Y, Meher D, Praveen RP, et al. Impact of bariatric surgery on body composition and metabolism among obese Asian Indians with prediabetes and diabetes. J Diabet. 2021;12(2):208–17.

140. Committee ADAPP. 8. Obesity and weight management for the prevention and treatment of type 2 diabetes: standards of medical care in diabetes – 2022. Diabetes Care. 2021;45(Supplement_1):S113–S24.

141. Wijetunga U, Bulugahapitiya U, Wijeratne T, Jayasuriya A, Ratnayake G, Kaluarachchi V, et al. SAT-116 efficacy of bariatric surgery in improving obesity in South Asians. J Endocr Soc. 2019;3(Supplement_1) SAT–116. https://doi.org/10.1210/js. 2019-SAT-116

142. Health NIo. Clinical guidelines for the identification, evaluation, and treatment of overweight and obesity in adults-the evidence report. Obes Res. 1998;6(2): 51S–209S.

143. WHO Consultation on Obesity (1999: Geneva, Switzerland) & World Health Organization. (2000). Obesity: preventing and managing the global epidemic: report of a WHO consultation. World Health Organization. https://apps.who.int/iris/handle/10665/42330

144. Bhowmik B, Afsana F, Siddiquee T, Munir SB, Sheikh F, Wright E, et al. Comparison of the prevalence of metabolic syndrome and its association with diabetes and cardiovascular disease in the rural population of Bangladesh using the modified National Cholesterol Education Program Expert Panel Adult Treatment Panel III and International Diabetes Federation definitions. J Diabetes Investig. 2015;6(3):280–8.

145. Mehata S, Shrestha N, Mehta RK, Bista B, Pandey AR, Mishra SR. Prevalence of the metabolic syndrome and its determinants among Nepalese adults: findings from a nationally representative cross-sectional study. Sci Rep. 2018;8(1):14995.

146. Katulanda P, Ranasinghe P, Jayawardana R, Sheriff R, Matthews DR. Metabolic syndrome among Sri Lankan adults: prevalence, patterns and correlates. Diabetol Metab Syndr. 2012;4(1):24.

147. Lee WY, Park JS, Noh SY, Rhee EJ, Kim SW, Zimmet PZ. Prevalence of the metabolic syndrome among 40,698 Korean metropolitan subjects. Diabetes Res Clin Pract. 2004;65(2):143–9.

148. Dou XF, Zhang HY, Sun K, Wang DW, Liao YH, Ma AQ, et al. Metabolic syndrome strongly linked to stroke in Chinese. Zhonghua Yi Xue Za Zhi. 2004;84(7):539–42.

149. Chuang SY, Chen C, Tsai ST, Chou P. Clinical identification of the metabolic syndrome in Kinmen. Acta Cardiologica Sinica. 2002;18:16–23.

150. Thomas GN, Ho SY, Janus ED, Lam KS, Hedley AJ, Lam TH. The US National Cholesterol Education

Programme Adult Treatment Panel III (NCEP ATP III) prevalence of the metabolic syndrome in a Chinese population. Diabetes Res Clin Pract. 2005;67(3): 251–7.

151. FER P, Sy RG, Ty-Willing T, editors. Prevalence of metabolic syndrome among adult Filipinos, International Congress Series. Elsevier; 2004.

152. Executive Summary of The Third Report of The National Cholesterol Education Program (NCEP).

Expert Panel on Detection, Evaluation, And Treatment of High Blood Cholesterol In Adults (Adult Treatment Panel III). JAMA. 2001;285(19):2486–97.

153. Nakanishi N, Takatorige T, Fukuda H, Shirai K, Li W, Okamoto M, et al. Components of the metabolic syndrome as predictors of cardiovascular disease and type 2 diabetes in middle-aged Japanese men. Diabetes Res Clin Pract. 2004;64(1):59–70.

Obesity in East Asia

Yong-Moon Mark Park, Mee Kyoung Kim, and Junxiu Liu

Contents

Abstract

The worldwide prevalence of obesity has increased over the last several decades. Because of differences in the way obesity is defined, especially abdominal obesity, a direct comparison of obesity prevalence may not be appropriate between Asian countries and others. Despite the different definitions of obesity, the obesity epidemic is also observed in the countries in East Asia in parallel with marked environmental and lifestyle changes. This review focuses on the recent trends of general and abdominal obesity in East Asian countries – China, Japan, South Korea (Republic of Korea), and Taiwan. In addition to data on the obesity epidemic, a large body of evidence related to normal-weight individuals with "metabolic obesity" has been reported in East Asian countries. This phenotype is important from a public health perspective because Asian populations are more likely to develop increased visceral adiposity and insulin resistance compared with other populations with the same level of body mass index (BMI). Moreover, a "healthy obesity" state described in various populations may not be the case in East Asian populations. We will review the epidemiological and clinical implications of

Y.-M. M. Park (✉)
Department of Epidemiology, Fay W. Boozman College of Public Health, University of Arkansas for Medical Sciences, Little Rock, AR, USA
e-mail: ypark@uams.edu

M. K. Kim
Division of Endocrinology and Metabolism, Department of Internal Medicine, Yeouido St. Mary's Hospital, College of Medicine, The Catholic University of Korea, Seoul, South Korea
e-mail: makung@catholic.ac.kr

J. Liu
Department of Population Health Science and Policy, Icahn School of Medicine at Mount Sinai, New York, NY, USA
e-mail: Junxiu.Liu@Mountsinai.Org

© Springer Nature Switzerland AG 2023
R. S. Ahima (ed.), *Metabolic Syndrome*,
https://doi.org/10.1007/978-3-031-40116-9_8

these phenotypes in the populations of East Asian countries.

Keywords

Obesity · Body mass index · Waist circumference · Metabolic syndrome · Metabolic health · Metabolically obese normal weight · Metabolically healthy obese · East Asia

Introduction

The epidemic of obesity across the lifespan from childhood to adulthood has become a major public health concern in East Asian populations. This is mainly due to the adoption of Western diet and reduction in physical activity resulting from a rapid socioeconomic transition and urbanization over the last several decades [8, 37, 73]. Correspondingly, obesity prevalence increased dramatically in East Asian populations. Obesity in the pediatric population is also of particular concern due to the critical developmental periods predisposing individuals to adulthood obesity and other future health outcomes.

For epidemiological purposes, the body mass index (BMI) is a measure of general obesity and the waist circumference is a measure of central (abdominal) obesity. For Asians, general obesity has been defined as a BMI ≥ 25 kg/m^2 based on the recommendation from the International Obesity Task Force (IOTF) and the World Health Organization (WHO) Regional Office for the Western Pacific Region [68]. WHO expert consultation also proposed an alternative criterion of general obesity in Asians as BMI ≥ 27.5 kg/m^2 [18]. However, there is no consensus on a standard definition for abdominal obesity. Thus, several cutoffs have been proposed to determine abdominal obesity according to different countries or ethnicities. Each country in East Asia has its own recommended waist circumference threshold for abdominal obesity (Table 1).

In addition to these recommendations, a number of studies have identified the appropriate cutoff for abdominal obesity in East Asian countries in relation to metabolic syndrome or its components [2, 3, 26, 35, 47, 55, 67, 77, 82], multiple cardiovascular risk factors [34, 60, 62, 97], or insulin resistance [30, 43, 70]. However,

Table 1 Current recommended waist circumference thresholds for abdominal obesity

Population	Organization	Male, cm	Female, cm
Europid	IDF	≥ 94	≥ 80
Caucasian	WHO	≥ 94 (increased risk) ≥ 102 (higher risk)	≥ 80 (increased risk) ≥ 88 (higher risk)
US	AHA/NHLBI (ATP III)	≥ 102	≥ 88
Asian	IDF/WHO	≥ 90	≥ 80
Korea	KSSO	≥ 90	≥ 85
China	Cooperative Task Force	≥ 85	≥ 80
Japan	Japanese Obesity Society	≥ 85	≥ 90
Middle East, Mediterranean, and sub-Saharan African	IDF	≥ 94	≥ 80

IDF International Diabetes Federation, *WHO* World Health Organization, *AHA* American Heart Association, *NHLBI* National Heart, Lung, and Blood Institute, *ATP III* Adult Treatment Panel III, *KSSO* Korean Society for the Study of Obesity

Adapted from Yoon, Rev Endocrinol Metab 2014;29:418–426 with permission from Korean Endocrine Society [94]

most studies are limited to a cross-sectional design where inferences regarding causality and temporality could be precluded in the association between abdominal obesity and health outcomes. In this chapter, we focus on the prevalence and trends of general and central obesity in children and adults in East Asian countries – China, Japan, South Korea, and Taiwan.

The risk of developing obesity-related complications is well correlated with the degree of obesity. However, not all obese individuals are uniformly affected. Even in the same BMI category, a subgroup of individuals with obesity and normal cardiometabolic characteristics has been designated as "metabolically healthy obese (MHO)," compared with "metabolically unhealthy obese (MUO)" individuals who exhibit cardiometabolic characteristics that are not within normal ranges [33, 38, 75]. In the same context, some normal-weight individuals are prone to cardiometabolic abnormalities and have been described as "metabolically obese normal weight (MONW)" or "normal weight obesity (NWO)" compared to their metabolically normal counterparts in the same BMI category or individuals who are "metabolically healthy normal weight (MHNW)" [13, 39, 48, 76, 86]. Other researchers used the term "metabolically unhealthy non-obese (MUNO)," similar to the term "MONW," using the term "non-obese" instead of "normal weight."

Prevalence and Trends of Obesity in East Asia

General and Abdominal Obesity in Adults

Prevalence and trends of general and abdominal obesity in adults among East Asian countries are shown in Table 2.

China

The main source of data on the nationally representative estimate of obesity prevalence in China is the China Health and Nutrition Survey (CHNS), which is an ongoing open cohort and an international collaborative project between the Carolina Population Center at the University of North Carolina at Chapel Hill and the National Institute of Nutrition and Food Safety at the Chinese Center for Disease Control and Prevention [74]. The CHNS is a large-scale, nationwide cross-sectional survey designed to explore how the health and nutritional status of the Chinese population has been affected by social and economic changes [74]. Samples have been drawn from nine provinces (Liaoning, Heilongjiang, Jiangsu, Shandong, Henan, Hubei, Hunan, Guangxi, and Guizhou) using a multistage, random cluster process [74]. Based on CHNS data collected between 1993 and 2009, using the general obesity criteria proposed by WHO expert consultation for Chinese (BMI $\geq$ 27.5 kg/m^2), the overall prevalence of general obesity has gradually and significantly increased from 4% in 1993 to 10.7% in 2009 [85]. For males, the prevalence of general obesity increased from 2.9% in 1993 to 11.4% in 2009 [85]. Females have also experienced an increasing trend of general obesity from 5.0% in 1993 to 10.1% in 2009 [85]. A similar increasing trend in overweight has been observed for both males and females from 1993–2009. From 2014–2018, data from China Patient-Centered Evaluative Assessment of Cardiac Events (PEACE) Million Persons Project reported that the overall prevalence of obesity among adults aged 35–75 years were 16.0% for males and 14.4% for females. Data from China Chronic Disease and Risk Factors Surveillance reported that, in 2018, the prevalence of overweight and obesity was 45.0% and 9.0%, respectively.

From 1993–2009, the overall prevalence of abdominal obesity, defined by waist circumference $\geq$ 90 cm for males and $\geq$ 80 cm for females, increased significantly from 18.6% in 1993 to 37.4% in 2009 [85]. Females had a much higher prevalence of abdominal obesity than males across the same time period [85]. In 2009, almost half (45.9%) of the female population had abdominal obesity while nearly a third (27.8%) of the male had abdominal obesity. In 2014–2018, the prevalence of abdominal obesity was 32.7% for females and 36.6% for males among Chinese population aged 35–75 years.

Table 2 Prevalence and trend of general obesity and abdominal obesity for adults among East Asian countries

	Survey year	Sample	Age range	Definition criteria	Prevalence of overweight	Prevalence of obesity
General obesity						
China	1993 [74]	CHNS	≥18	OW: BMI 25–27.49; obese:≥27.5	Overall: 9.4%; 8% (M); 10.7% (F)	Overall: 4%; 2.9% (M); 5.0% (F)
	1997 [74]	CHNS	≥18	OW: BMI 25–27.49; obese:≥27.5	Overall:11.3%;10.4% (M); 12.1% (F)	Overall: 6.2%; 5.5% (M); 6.7% (F)
	2000 [74]	CHNS	≥18	OW: BMI 25–27.49; obese:≥27.5	Overall: 13.8%;13.7% (M); 13.9% (F)	Overall: 8.0%; 7.2% (M); 8.6% (F)
	2004 [74]	CHNS	≥18	OW: BMI 25–27.49; obese ≥27.5	Overall: 14.9%;15.0% (M); 14.9% (F)	Overall: 8.7%; 8.2% (M); 9.2% (F)
	2006 [74]	CHNS	≥18	OW: BMI 25–27.49; obese:≥27.5	Overall: 15.4; 16.5% (M); 14.4% (F)	Overall: 9.2%; 9.4% (M); 9.0% (F)
	2009 [74]	CHNS	≥18	OW: BMI 25–27.49; obese ≥27.5	Overall: 15.7%;17.1% (M); 14.4% (F)	Overall: 10.7%; 11.4% (M); 10.1% (F)
	2013 [55]	CHNS	≥18	OW: BMI 25–30; obese: BMI ≥ 30	28.3% (M); 27.4% (F)	3.8% (M) and 4.9% (F)
	2014–2018 [50]	PEACE	35–75	obese: ≥28.0	NA	16.0% (M); 14.4% (F)
	2018 [73]	CCDRFS	18–69	OW: BMI ≥ 25; obese ≥ 30	Overall: 45.0%; 40.9% (M); 36.7% (F)	Overall: 9.0%; 8.1% (M); 7.2% (F)
Japan	1976–80 [83]	NNS-J	≥20	Preobese: 25–29.9; obese: BMI ≥ 30	14.5% (M); 15.7% (F)	0.84% (M); 2.33% (F)
	1991–1995 [83]	NNS-J	≥20	Preobese: 25–29.9; obese: BMI ≥ 30	20.5% (M); 14.7% (F)	2.01% (M); 2.30% (F)
	2013 [55]	NNS-J	≥18	OW:BMI25–30; obese: BMI ≥ 30	28.9% (M); 17.6% (F)	4.5% (M); 3.3% (F)
South Korea	2001	KNHANES	≥20	BMI ≥ 25		Overall: 30.6%, 32.4% (M) and 29.4% (F)
	1998 [26]	KNHANES	≥20	OW: BMI ≥ 23; obese:BMI ≥ 25	50.8% (M); 47.3% (F)	26.0% (M); 26.5% (F)
	2001 [26]	KNHANES	≥20	OW: BMI ≥ 23; obese: BMI ≥ 25	57.4% (M); 51.9% (F)	32.4% (M); 29.3% (F)
	2005 [26]	KNHANES	≥20	OW: BMI ≥ 23; obese: BMI ≥ 25	62.5% (M); 50.0% (F)	35.1% (M); 28.0% (F)
	2007–2009 [26]	KNHANES	≥20	OW: BMI ≥ 23; obese:BMI ≥ 25	62.6% (M); 48.9% (F)	36.3% (M); 27.6% (F)
	2007 [8]	KNHANES	≥20	Obese: BMI ≥ 25		Overall: 32.1%, 36.7% (M) and 27.6% (F)
	2012 [8]	KNHANES	≥20	Obese: BMI ≥ 25		Overall: 32.8%, 36.8% (M) and 28.9% (F)

(continued)

Table 2 (continued)

	Survey year	Sample	Age range	Definition criteria	Prevalence of overweight	Prevalence of obesity
	2017 [8]	KNHANES	≥20	Obese: BMI ≥ 25		Overall: 34.4%, 42.3% (M) and 26.6% (F)
	2009 [78]	K-NHIS	≥20	Obese: BMI ≥ 25		Overall: 29.7%, 35.6% (M) and 23.9% (F)
	2014 [78]	K-NHIS	≥20	Obese: BMI ≥ 25		Overall: 31.1%, 38.8% (M) and 23.7% (F)
	2019 [78]	K-NHIS	≥20	Obese: BMI ≥ 25		Overall: 36.3%, 46.2% (M) and 27.3% (F)
	2013 [55]	K-NHIS	≥18	OW: BMI 25–30; obese: BMI ≥ 30	36.9% (M); 27.2% (F)	6.8% (M); 5.8% (F)
Taiwan	1993–1996 [48]	NAHSIT	≥20	OW: 25 < BMI < 30; obese: BMI > 30	21.10%	4.00%
	2000–2001 [14]	NHRIS	≥20	OW:BMI ≥ 24; obese: BMI ≥ 27	28.9% (M), 18.7% (F)	15.9% (M), 10.7% (F)
	2005–2008 [79]	NAHSIT	≥18	OW: BMI ≥ 24; obese: BMI ≥ 27	31.87% (M); 19.75% (F)	18.90% (M); 17.13% (F)
	2013 [55]		≥18	OW:BMI 25–30; obese: BMI ≥ 30	33.8% (M); 30.9% (F)	4.3% (M); 6.4% (F)
	2013–2014 [5]	NAHSIT	≥19	OW: BMI ≥ 24; obese: BMI ≥ 27	Overall: 43.4%	Overall: 22.0%
Abdominal obesity						
China					Prevalence of central obesity	
	1993 [74]	CHNS	≥18	WC ≥ 90 cm (M) and ≥ 80 cm (F)	Overall: 18.6%; 8.5% (M); 27.8% (F)	
	1997 [74]	CHNS	≥18	WC ≥ 90 cm (M) and ≥ 80 cm (F)	Overall:22.6%; 13.8% (M); 30.8% (F)	
	2000 [74]	CHNS	≥18	WC ≥ 90 cm (M) and ≥ 80 cm (F)	Overall: 28.8%; 19.5% (M); 37.1% (F)	
	2004 [74]	CHNS	≥18	WC ≥ 90 cm (M) and ≥ 80 cm (F)	Overall: 31.4%; 21.6% (M); 40.3% (F)	
	2006 [74]	CHNS	≥18	WC ≥ 90 cm (M) and ≥ 80 cm (F)	Overall: 32.8%; 23.2% (M); 41.4% (F)	
	2009 [74]	CHNS	≥18	WC ≥ 90 cm (M) and ≥ 80 cm (F)	Overall: 37.4%; 27.8 (M); 45.9% (F)	
	2014–2018 [50]	PEACE	35–75	WC ≥ 90 cm (M) and ≥ 85 cm (F)	36.6% (M); 32.7 (F)	

(continued)

Table 2 (continued)

	Survey year	Sample	Age range	Definition criteria	Prevalence of overweight	Prevalence of obesity
South Korea	1998 [57]	KNHANES	≥20	WC ≥ 90 cm (M) and ≥ 85 cm (F)	Overall: 22.4%, 20.6% (M); 24.1% (F)	
	2005 [57]	KNHANES	≥20	WC ≥ 90 cm (M) and ≥ 85 cm (F)	Overall: 23.9%, 24.0% (M); 23.8% (F)	
	2007–2009 [57]	KNHANES	≥20	WC ≥ 90 cm (M) and ≥ 85 cm (F)	Overall: 24.1%, 24.8% (M); 23.5% (F)	
	2009 [78]	KNHIS	≥20	WC ≥ 90 cm (M) and ≥ 85 cm (F)	Overall: 19.0%, 20.7% (M); 16.2% (F)	
	2014 [78]	KNHIS	≥20	WC ≥ 90 cm (M) and ≥ 85 cm (F)	Overall: 20.2%, 22.9% (M); 16.5% (F)	
	2019 [78]	KNHIS	≥20	WC ≥ 90 cm (M) and ≥ 85 cm (F)	Overall: 23.9%, 29.3% (M); 19.0% (F)	

NAHSIT Nutrition and Health Surveys in Taiwan, *NHRIS* National Health Research Institute Survey, *CHNS* China Health and Nutrition Surveys, *PEACE* China Patient-Centered Evaluative Assessment of Cardiac Events Million Persons Project, *CCDRFS* China Chronic Disease and Risk Factors Surveillance, *KNHANES* Korea National Health and Nutrition Examination Survey, *JNNS* Japan National Nutrition Survey, *OW* overweight, *WC* waist circumference, *KNHIS* Korea National Health Insurance Service, *M* male, *F* female

Japan

The National Nutrition Survey, Japan (NNS-J) is the main source of obesity prevalence estimates in Japan using a representative of the Japanese population. The NNS-J is a cross-sectional survey conducted annually since 1948 for large random samples of the Japanese population and covering around 5000 households in 300 randomly selected census units [95].

The prevalence of general obesity, defined by the NNS-J as BMI ≥ 30 kg/m^2, in men increased from 0.84% in 1976–1980 to 2.01% in 1991–1995, whereas the prevalence of general obesity in women did not materially change over this 20-year period (from 2.33% in 1976–80 to 2.30% in 1991–1995). In addition, in people aged 20–29 years, during the studied period, trends in overweight and obesity (BMI ≥ 25 kg/m^2) increased in young men and decreased in young women [96].

When analyzing NNS-J data during 1976–2005 for individuals aged 20–69 years, particularly for changes in the prevalence of overweight and obesity (BMI ≥ 25 kg/m^2) with age by birth cohort, the prevalence in men increased in cohorts born more recently, whereas the prevalence in women decreased in cohorts born more recently [20]. In an additional analysis of NNS-J data from 1973–2016 in individuals aged ≥65 years, the prevalence of overweight and obesity increased and nearly tripled in men (around 11% in 1973 to 30% in 2016), whereas the prevalence in women tended to increase until 2002 then decreased (around 22% in 1973 and 20% in 2016) [81].

South Korea

The Korea National Health and Nutrition Examination Survey (KNHANES) is the most important source of the nationally representative estimate of obesity prevalence in South Korea. First established in 1998, KNHANES has been conducted every year by the Ministry of Health and Welfare of Korea, targeting nationally representative noninstitutionalized civilians in South Korea [45].

General obesity, defined as a BMI ≥ 25 kg/m^2 based on the Asia-Pacific regional guidelines of

WHO, had a higher prevalence in males than in females. The prevalence of obesity for males increased from 26% in 1998 to 36.3% in 2007–2009 with an upward trend during the 12-year period, whereas the prevalence of obesity in females increased until 2001 and then exhibited a downward trend from 2005 to 2007–2009 [31]. Similar trends were observed for overweight (a BMI $\geq$ 23 kg/m^2) for both males and females [31].

Based on the KNHANES data collected between 2007 and 2017, the prevalence of obesity in South Korea increased along with significant secular changes in men but not in women. The overall prevalence of obesity was 32.1% in 2007, which increased to 34.4% in 2017 [9]. The prevalence of obesity in men significantly increased from 36.7% in 2007 to 42.3% in 2017. Conversely, the prevalence of obesity in women was 27.6% in 2007 and 26.6% in 2017, a nonsignificant change during the same period [9]. According to the 2020 Korean Society for the Study of Obesity (KSSO) Treatment Guideline, obesity classes were divided into three classes: class I obesity, BMI 25.0–29.9 kg/m^2; class II obesity, 30.0–34.9 kg/m^2; and class III obesity, $\geq$ 35.0 kg/m^2 [42].

The obesity prevalence in the overall South Korean population has steadily increased between 2009 and 2019, from 29.7% in 2009 to 36.3% in 2019 [61, 89]. Obesity prevalence increased significantly in men from 35.6% in 2009 to 46.2% in 2019 and from 23.9% in 2009 to 27.3% in 2019 in women [89]. The prevalence of obesity in all three classes increased for the total population over the past 11 years. The prevalence of class II obesity was 3.2% in the total population, 3.4% in men, and 3.1% in women in 2009; these prevalences increased to 5.4%, 6.3%, and 4.4% in 2019, respectively. The overall prevalence of class III obesity increased by nearly threefold over the past 11 years from 0.30% in 2009 to 0.89% in 2019: 3.7 times in men (0.26% in 2009 to 0.96% in 2019) and 2.3 times in women (0.35% in 2009 to 0.81% in 2019) [89].

In terms of abdominal obesity, defined as a waist circumference $\geq$ 90 cm for males and $\geq$ 85 cm for females, the prevalence slightly increased among men, whereas the prevalence slightly decreased among women over recent decades. Specifically, the overall prevalence of abdominal obesity increased from 22.4% in 1998 to 24.1% in 2007–2009. Males showed an upward trend from 20.6% in 1998 to 24.8% in 2007–2009, whereas the prevalence in females decreased from 24.1% in 1998 to 23.5% in 2007–2009 [65]. Between 2009 and 2019, the prevalence of abdominal obesity increased in both men and women, but most prominently in men [89], from 19.0% to 23.9% in the total population, 20.7% to 29.3% in men, and 16.2% to 19.0% in women. Abdominal obesity prevalence in men increased regardless of age over this 11-year period, and this trend was most evident among young men in their 20s and 30s. In 2019, the prevalence of abdominal obesity was 22.6% in men in their 20s and 32.4% in men in their 30s [89]. A steep increase in the prevalence of general obesity during the transition period from the 20s to the 30s was also observed. In 2019, the prevalence of general obesity (BMI $\geq$ 25) was 41% in men in their 20s and 52.2% in men in their 30s [89]. This phenomenon may be more strongly associated with environmental, social, and lifestyle changes in the transition period than other biological and genetic factors.

Taiwan

In Taiwan, the data source most commonly used for estimating the prevalence and trend of obesity in adults across the years are national surveys. We used the Nutrition and Health Surveys in Taiwan (NAHSIT) and National Health Research Institute Survey (NHRIS) to demonstrate the obesity prevalence and trend from 1993–1996 to 2005–2008 [57, 91]. In 1993–1996 of NAHSIT, the overall prevalence of obesity, defined as a BMI $\geq$ 30 kg/m^2 for adults aged $\geq$20 years, was 4%, while the prevalence of general obesity, defined as a BMI $\geq$ 27 kg/m^2 for those aged $\geq$18 years, was 18.9% for males and 17.13% for females [57]. The NHRIS prevalence of obesity for 2000–2001 was 15.9% for males and 10.7% for females [16]. However, because of different studied age ranges and obesity criteria, one needs to be cautious when comparing the prevalence of obesity across years directly. Data from 2013–2014 NAHSIT reported that the overall prevalence of overweight and obesity among participants aged 19 years and older was 43.4% and 22.0%, respectively. According to the Global Burden of Disease Study, South Korea has the highest prevalence of obesity in males, while Taiwan has a higher obesity prevalence in females [64].

General Obesity in Children

Like Western countries, childhood obesity is also on the rise in East Asian countries (Table 3). In China, examining the CHNS with IOTF criteria, the prevalence of childhood obesity significantly increased from 6.1% in 1993 to 13.1% in 2009 [54]. In 2010, based on the Chinese National Survey on Students' Constitution and Health, 10.9% of boys and 5.1% of girls had larger than 120% of the mean body weight based on height [79]. According to 2015–2019 China National Nutrition Surveys (CNNs), the prevalence of obesity was 3.6% for children aged less than 6 years and 7.9% for children aged 6 to 17 years [69].

In Japan, NNS-J data and IOTF criteria were used to estimate the prevalence and trend of childhood obesity (Table 3) [58]. The prevalence of childhood obesity increased from 1.8% in 1976 to 4.6% in 1980 among both boys and girls aged 6–8 years.

In South Korea, according to the National Growth Survey (NGS), the prevalence of obesity, defined as a BMI $\geq$ 95th percentile among children aged 2–18 years, increased from 5.8% in 1997 to 9.7% in 2005 [66]. According to KNHANES, from 2001–2007, the prevalence of obesity based on IOTF criteria among children aged 2–9 years decreased from 3.8% in 2001 to 1.0% in 2007 for girls, whereas the prevalence in boys increased from 5.5% in 2001 to 10.5% in 2007. Moreover, the prevalence of obesity among children aged 10–19 years demonstrates that, for boys, the prevalence decreased from 5.8% in 1998 to 5.6% in 2005 and then increased to 6.0% in 2007. In contrast, for girls, the prevalence of obesity increased from 1.6% in 1998 to 2.8% in 2005 and then decreased to 1.8% in 2007.

In Taiwan, the prevalence of obesity among children aged 12–15 years, defined as >120% of age and sex-specific mean body weight, increased from 12.4% in 1980–1982 to 14.8% in 1986–1988 for boys and 10.1% in 1980–1982 and 11.1% in 1986–1988 for girls [32, 64]. During 2001–2002, 12.0% of children aged 6–12 years had obesity, defined as a BMI $\geq$ 95th percentile according to NAHSIT [17].

Metabolic Health and Obesity in East Asia

Epidemiological and Clinical Implications of the MONW Phenotype

It is important to recognize MONW individuals in the East Asian populations, as they are more prone to develop increased visceral fat and insulin resistance than any other race or ethnicity with similar BMIs [63]. The prevalence of the MONW phenotype varies from 10–40% according to the definition of metabolic obesity and the populations used in each study (Table 4). Multiple studies have reported that the MONW phenotype is associated with an increased risk of cardiometabolic morbidity and mortality in the East Asian population. Lee et al. demonstrated that the MONW phenotype was independently associated with abnormal lipid profiles, such as elevated total cholesterol and triglycerides in both men and women [48]. Kim et al. evaluated 2078 normal-weight subjects ($18.5 \leq BMI < 25$ kg/m^2) and analyzed the data from atherosclerosis using coronary computed tomography, angiography, and pulse wave velocity [40]. They found that the NWO phenotype, defined by the highest tertile of gender-specific body fat percentage by sex (men $\geq 25.4\%$ and women $\geq 31.4\%$), was independently associated with the presence of soft plaques, meaning that NWO individuals may have a higher risk of subclinical atherosclerosis compared with MHNW individuals. Yoo et al. also demonstrated that the MONW phenotype, defined by the presence of metabolic syndrome and $18.5 \leq BMI < 25$ kg/m^2, was independently associated with carotid atherosclerosis compared to the MHNW phenotype among 1012 individuals

Table 3 Prevalence and trend of general obesity for children among East Asian countries

	Survey year	Sample	Age range	Overweight and obesity criteria	Prevalence of overweight	Prevalence of obesity
China						
	1993 [46]	CHNS	6–17	IOTF		6.10%
	1997 [46]	CHNS	6–17	IOTF		7.00%
	2000 [46]	CHNS	6–17	IOTF		7.40%
	2004 [46]	CHNS	6–17	IOTF		10.10%
	2006 [46]	CHNS	6–17	IOTF		10.30%
	2009 [46]	CHNS	6–17	IOTF		13.10%
	2010 [70]	CNSSCH	7–18	100–119.9% of standard weight for height by age and sex; ≥120% of standard weight for height	Overall: 19.2%; 23.4%(B); 14.5% (G)	Overall: 8.1%; 10.9% (B);5.1% (G)
	2015–2019	CNNs	<6, 6–17	IOTF	6.8% (<6 years); 11.1% (6–17 years)	3.6% (<6 years); 7.9% (6–17 years)
Japan	1976–1980 [49]	NNS-J	6–8	IOTF	7.9%(B); 8.7%(G)	1.8%(B); 1.8%(G)
			9–11	IOTF	10.7%(B); 9.3%(G)	1.6%(B); 1.3%(G)
			12–14	IOTF	9.2%(B); 8.6%(G)	1.0%(B); 0.5%(G)
	1981–1985 [49]	NNS-J	6–8	IOTF	9.1%(B); 10.8%(G)	2.1%(B); 1.9%(G)
			9–11	IOTF	11.9%(B); 10.3%(G)	2.1%(B); 0.9%(G)
			12–14	IOTF	12.6%(B); 9.6%(G)	2.1%(B); 0.5%(G)
	1986–1990 [49]	NNS-J	6–8	IOTF	12.5%(B); 13.2%(G)	3.8%(B); 2.8% (G)
			9–11	IOTF	15.4%(B); 12.8%(G)	3.3%(B); 1.2%(G)
			12–14	IOTF	12.2%(B); 10.0%(G)	2.1%(B); 1.2%(G)
	1991–1995 [49]	NNS-J	6–8	IOTF	13.9%(B); 14.7%(G)	3.7%(B); 3.1%(G)
			9–11	IOTF	19.1%(B); 14.8%(G)	4.1%(B); 2.0%(G)
			12–14	IOTF	14.6%(B); 9.0%(G)	2.5%(B); 1.6%(G)
	1996–2000 [49]	NNS-J	6–8	IOTF	15.3%(B); 14.6%(G)	4.6%(B); 4.6%(G)
			9–11	IOTF	18.4%(B); 17.2%(G)	4.0%(B); 3.0%(G)
			12–14	IOTF	14.9%(B); 11.2%(G)	2.7%(B); 1.0%(G)

(continued)

Table 3 (continued)

	Survey year	Sample	Age range	Overweight and obesity criteria	Prevalence of overweight	Prevalence of obesity
South Korea	1997 [58]	NGS	2–18	BMI ≥ 85th; BMI ≥ 95th	Overall: 13.0%; 12.4%(B); 13.8%(G)	Overall: 5.8%; 6.1% (B); 5.5%(G)
	2005 [58]	NGS	2–18	BMI ≥ 85th; BMI ≥ 95th	Overall: 19.0%; 19.7%(B); 18.2%(G)	Overall: 9.7%; 11.3%(B); 8.0%(G)
	2001 [36]	K-NHANES	2–9	IOTF	21.1%(B); 16.9%(G)	5.5%(B); 3.8%(G)
	2005 [36]	K-NHANES	2–9	IOTF	15.6%(B); 17.3%(G)	3.2%(B); 3.8%(G)
	2007 [36]	K-NHANES	2–9	IOTF	24.4%(B); 15.7%(G)	10.5%(B); 1.9%(G)
	1998 [36]	K-NHANES	10–19	IOTF	16.2%(B); 13.8%(G)	2.0%(B); 1.0%(G)
	2001 [36]	K-NHANES	10–19	IOTF	27.8%(B); 16.7%(G)	5.8%(B); 1.6%(G)
	2005 [36]	K-NHANES	10–19	IOTF	27.3% (B);16.9% (G)	5.6%(B); 2.8%(G)
	2007 [36]	K-NHANES	10–19	IOTF	29.4%(B); 16.4%(G)	6.0%(B); 1.0%(G)
Taiwan	1980–1982 [56]	NS	12–15	OW: 110 ± 120% of age and sex specific mean body weight; obese is >120% of mean body weight	13.0%(B); 11.3%(G)	12.4%(B); 10.1%(G)
	1986–1988 [27]	NS	12–15	OW: 110 ± 120% of age and sex specific mean body weight; obese is >120% of mean body weight	10.9%(B); 13.1%(G)	14.8%(B); 11.1%(G)
	1994–1996 [15]	TCHS	12–15	Overweight is defined as body weight at 110 ± 120% of mean body weight and obese is defined as >120% of mean body weight at same age and gender stratum	11.6%(B); 10.2%(G)	16.4%(B); 11.1%(G)
	2001–2002 [15]	NAHSIT	6–12	BMI ≥ 85th; BMI ≥ 95th	Overall: 15.0%; 15.5% (B) and 14.4% (G)	Overall: 12.0%; 14.7% (B) and 9.1% (G)

CNSSCH Chinese National Survey on Students' Constitution and Health, *CNNs* China National Nutrition Surveys, *IOTF* the International Obesity Task Force, BMI ≥ age-sex-specific BMI cutoff that corresponds to a BMI of 30 kg/m^2 at age 18, *NNS-J* Japan-National Nutrition Survey, *NGS* National Growth Survey, *NS* National Survey, *TCHS* Taipei Children Heart Study, *NHS* Nutrition and Health Survey, *CHNS* China Health and Nutrition Survey, *B* boys, *G* girls

(mean age 50.8 years) who received health exams [93]. Choi et al. conducted a prospective cohort study with a ten-year follow-up in 2317 elderly people aged >60 years in which MONW individuals were designated as BMI < 23 kg/m^2 with metabolic syndrome determined by modified

NCEP-ATP III criteria [14]. They found that all-cause and cardiovascular disease (CVD) mortality rates were significantly higher in MONW individuals compared to overweight or obese individuals. Analyzing the 2007–2014 KNHANES data, Seo et al. also demonstrated that individuals

Table 4 Prevalence of metabolically obese normal weight (MONW) phenotype in East Asia

Study	Country	Nationally representative sample	Population characteristic	Definition	Prevalence among normal weight population
[19]	China	Yes	3552 participants ($\geq$ 18 years)	$18.5 \leq$ BMI < 23 kg/m^2, Wildman criterion	47.9%
[24]	Japan	No	8090 nondiabetic subjects (5884 men and 2206 women) (aged 24–80 years)	BMI < 25 kg/m^2 with two or more of metabolic syndrome components defined by IDF	21.1% among total population
[23]	Japan	No	27,478 nondiabetic subjects (17,730 men and 9748 women)	BMI < 25 kg/m^2 with two or more of metabolic syndrome components defined by IDF	14.9% among total population
[40]	South Korea	Yes	5267 participants (2227 men, 3040 women) ($\geq$ 20 years)	BMI < 25 kg/m^2 with metabolic syndrome, defined by NCEP-ATP III guideline (2002)	12.7% (15.6% in men, 10.7% in women)
[49]	South Korea	No	8987 nondiabetic subjects (3632 men and 5355 women) ($\geq$ 40 years)	$18.5 \leq$ BMI < 23 kg/m^2 with a HOMA-IR in the highest quartile	Men (14.2%), women (12.9%)
[12]	South Korea	Yes	1736 nondiabetic women (1197 premenopausal women and 539 postmenopausal women) ($\geq$ 19 years)	$18.5 \leq$ BMI < 25 kg/m^2 with (HOMA-IR) in the highest quartile	18.7% for premenopausal women and 19.2% for postmenopausal women
[33]	South Korea	Yes	5313 men and 6904 women ($\geq$ 20 years)	$18.5 \leq$ BMI < 23 kg/m^2 greater than 26% body fat in men and greater than 36% body fat in women	36% for men, 29% for women
[53]	South Korea	Yes	17,029 nondiabetic subjects (7185 men and 9844 women) ($\geq$ 20 years)	$18.5 \leq$ BMI < 23 kg/m^2 with HOMA-IR in the highest quartile	10.54% for men and 13.26% for women
[77]	South Korea	Yes	323,175 subjects ($\geq$ 20 years)	$18.5 \leq$ BMI < 25 kg/m^2 with ≥ 1 metabolic disease component (hypertension, diabetes, and dyslipidemia)	17.3% among total population
[90]	Taiwan	Yes	2143 participants (1020 men and 1123 women) ($\geq$ 20 years)	BMI < 24 kg/m^2, high waist circumference (≥ 80 cm for women and ≥ 90 cm for men)	1.7% for men and 4.0% for women among total population
[80]	Taiwan	No	1180 participants ($\geq$ 65 years)	$18.5 \leq$ BMI < 24 kg/m^2 with metabolic syndrome defined by NCEP-ATP III guideline (2002) Wildman criterion	16.3%

HOMA-IR homeostasis model assessment of insulin resistance, *NCEP-ATP III (2002)* the National Cholesterol Education Program Adult Treatment Panel III (NCEP-ATPIII 2002), *IDF* International Diabetes Federation [1], Wildman criterion [84]

with the MONW phenotype, defined by the presence of metabolic syndrome and a BMI < 25 kg/m^2, had a higher prevalence of stroke than those with MHO in 25,744 subjects aged $\geq$40 years [78]. Yang et al. reported that the MONW group, defined by $18.5 \leq$ BMI < 25 kg/m^2 with $\geq$1 metabolic disease component (hypertension, diabetes, and dyslipidemia), had a significantly higher risk of all-cause and cardio-vascular mortality, whereas the MHO group had a lower mortality risk, compared to the MHNW group [88]. A similar pattern was noted for cancer and other-cause mortality. Metabolically unhealthy status was associated with a higher risk of all-cause and cardiovascular mortality regardless of BMI levels [88].

There is no consensus on the definition of the MONW or NWO phenotype. Thus, several studies have explored the criteria for identifying the MONW or NWO phenotype and related risk factors in East Asia. Kim et al. investigated the optimal cutoffs for percentage body fat (BF) to identify the NWO phenotype with the presence of at least one cardiovascular risk factor as the outcome, using data from KNHANES [39]. They suggested that 26% BF in men and 36% BF in women would be the best cutoff for defining NWO individuals. Lee et al. proposed a novel criterion for defining the MONW phenotype using the TyG index, calculated as: Ln[fasting triglycerides (mg/dL) × fasting plasma glucose (mg/dL)/2] [51, 52]. They determined the cutoff value of the TyG index using 7541 nondiabetic nationally representative normal weight subjects ($18.5 \leq BMI < 25$ kg/m^2) in South Korea and found that the TyG index predicted incident diabetes in a study of 3185 participants from a prospective community-based cohort study [52]. Du et al. used data from CHNS to assess the capability of lipid accumulation product (LAP) and visceral adiposity index (VAI) to determine the MONW phenotype and found that both LAP and VAI were highly associated with the MONW phenotype independent of the several different MONW criteria [19].

The major determinants of the MONW phenotype include genetics and lifestyle characteristics [21]. A number of studies have provided evidence of risk factors for the MONW phenotype in East Asia. In a study of a representative South Korean population, the MONW phenotype was associated with older age, lower education, moderate alcohol consumption, and moderate-intensity exercise [46]. In addition, Choi et al. found that the MONW characteristics vary before and after menopause, indicating that young age, rural residence, higher BMI, high systolic blood pressure, low HDL cholesterol, high white blood cell count, and lack of regular exercise were associated with the MONW phenotype in pre-menopausal women whereas only high alanine aminotransferase was associated in postmenopausal women [13]. For the association between the MONW phenotype and dietary patterns, Choi et al. showed that a reduced intake of carbohydrates and carbohydrate snacks is inversely associated with a MONW phenotype, especially in women, in whom a MONW phenotype was defined as $18.5 \leq BMI < 25$ kg/m^2 with metabolic syndrome based on the International Diabetes Federation consensus [12]. Yoo et al. demonstrated that higher serum ferritin levels are associated with the MONW phenotype, defined by modified NCEP-ATP III criteria, in a representative South Korean population of young adults aged 19–39 years with normal weight ($18.5 \leq BMI < 25$ kg/m^2) [92]. In another KNHANES study of 1813 normal weight adults ($18.5 \leq BMI < 25$ kg/m^2), the findings revealed that lower serum zinc levels are associated with the MONW phenotype defined by the highest quartile on the Homeostatic Model Assessment for Insulin Resistance (HOMA-IR) [87].

Epidemiological and Clinical Implications of the MHO Phenotype

Because there is no universal definition of metabolic health, large variations have been observed in the prevalence of the MHO phenotype ranging from 10–57%, depending on the definition of metabolic obesity and populations examined in each study (Table 5). In addition, much debate centers on whether the MHO phenotype is definitely healthy [44]. In one South Korean study, MHO was defined as a BMI ≥ 25 kg/m^2 with 1 or no metabolic syndrome components determined by modified NCEP-ATPIII, and MUO was defined as a BMI ≥ 25 kg/m^2 with two or more metabolic syndrome components [9]. From 2007–2017, the prevalence of MHO significantly increased only in women (women: 6.7–8.6%; men: 10.8–10.4%), while that of MUO significantly increased only in men (women: 18–20.8%; men: 25.8–31.8%) [9].

With an age- and gender-dependent prevalence between ~10% and 30%, MHO is not a rare condition.

Chen et al. studied the association between metabolic health and chronic kidney disease [7]. They demonstrated that the MUO, but not the MHO phenotype, was associated with an increased risk of chronic kidney disease compared to normal-weight individuals. However, a number of studies have shown that the MHO phenotype may be at increased risk of cardiovascular disease (CVD) in East Asia. Chang et al. assessed the coronary artery calcium (CAC) scores in MHO individuals in 14,828 apparently healthy adults in which metabolic health was determined as not having any metabolic syndrome component and having a HOMA-IR < 2.5. They found that MHO individuals had a higher prevalence of subclinical coronary atherosclerosis compared with MHNW individuals [5]. Jung et al. also found that the MHO phenotype is associated with the prevalence of subclinical coronary atherosclerotic burden defined by >50% stenosis, presence of plaque, and elevated CAC scores, compared with MHNW individuals in a study of 4009 health examinees in which MHO was defined as a BMI $\geq$ 25 kg/m^2 with Wildman criteria [29]. Lee et al. examined the association between the MHO phenotype and the risk of hypertension in a community-based prospective cohort study with an eight-year follow-up. They demonstrated that MHO individuals had a higher risk of incident hypertension compared with MHNW individuals [50]. Heianza et al. studied the risk of incident diabetes across various metabolic phenotypes and found that the MHO phenotype was associated with a higher risk of developing diabetes than the MHNW phenotype [25].

Transition from healthy to unhealthy metabolic phenotype contributes to adverse health outcomes. Heianza et al. evaluated stability and changes in metabolic health status in a prospective cohort study using a nondiabetic Japanese population [23]. They found that a persistent MUO status increased the risk of incident diabetes, and transition from MHO to MUO status was also associated with incident diabetes compared to individuals who maintained an MHNW phenotype.

However, there is mounting evidence that MHO is not a permanent state. Recent, large longitudinal studies have demonstrated that the MHO status represents a transient condition that involves a temporal expression of the dynamics in continuous variables. Cho et al. explored the influence of phenotypic transitions on the risk of developing CKD among individuals with MHO using a Korean National Health Screening Cohort [11]. In that study, MHO was defined as a BMI $\geq$ 25 kg/m^2 with 1 or no metabolic risk factor determined by modified NCEP-ATP III criteria. The prevalence of MHO was 9.2%, and the majority of MHO participants exhibited phenotypic shifts on the following biennial health examination: 47.6% remained in the MHO group at follow-up, 34.8% remained obese and transitioned to a metabolically unhealthy status (MHO to MUO), 12.1% lost weight and were metabolically healthy without obesity (MHO to MHNO) at follow-up, and 5.5% lost weight but transitioned to a metabolically unhealthy status (MHO to MUNO) [11]. They showed that people who remained obese or progressed to a metabolically unhealthy status (stable MHO, MHO to MUO, and MHO to MUNO groups) were all at elevated risk of CKD [11]. It is possible that MHO might not constitute a separate biologically defined subset of people with obesity. The MHO phenotype is regarded as an intermediate stage between a healthy, normal-weight and an unhealthy, obese status [10]. Kim et al. analyzed 3,479,514 metabolically healthy subjects ($\geq$ 20 years) from the Korean National Health Screening Program who underwent health examination between 2009 and 2010, with a follow-up after 4 years [41]. During the 4 years, 31.5% of the subjects in the MHO group and 11.1% in the MHNW group converted to a metabolically unhealthy phenotype [41]. The transition to a MUO phenotype was associated with an increased risk of type 2 diabetes. In contrast, the MHO individuals were characterized by preserved insulin sensitivity, low visceral fat accumulation, low inflammatory activity, and a lack of metabolic and cardiovascular complications.

Persistence of MHO was related to a younger age, sustained lower waist circumference, more peripheral fat distribution in women, and

Table 5 Prevalence of metabolically healthy obese (MHO) phenotype in East Asia

Study	Country	Nationally representative sample	Population characteristic	Definition	Prevalence among obese population
[6]	China	No	2324 subjects ($\geq$ 18 years)	BMI $\geq$ 24 kg/m² with no insulin resistance or any metabolic syndrome components except abdominal obesity	11.8% among total population
[19]	China	Yes	7765 participants ($\geq$ 18 years)	BMI $\geq$ 27.5 kg/m² with none or one of metabolic syndrome components defined by NCEP-ATP III guideline (2002)	10.7%
[24]	Japan	No	8090 nondiabetic subjects (5884 men and 2206 women) (aged 24–80 years)	BMI $\geq$ 25 kg/m² with none or one of metabolic syndrome components defined by IDF	44.1%
[23]	Japan	No	27,478 nondiabetic subjects (17,730 men and 9748 women)	BMI $\geq$ 25 kg/m² with none or one of metabolic syndrome components defined by IDF	11.0%
[40]	South Korea	Yes	5267 participants (2227 men, 3040 women) ($\geq$ 20 years)	BMI $\geq$ 25 kg/m² without metabolic syndrome defined by NCEP-ATP III guideline (2002)	47.9% (44.3% in men, 51.0% in women)
[49]	South Korea	No	8987 nondiabetic subjects (3632 men and 5355 women) ($\geq$ 40 years)	BMI $\geq$ 25 kg/m² with a HOMA-IR in the lowest quartile	Men (10.7%), women (14.5%)
[13]	South Korea	No	2317 participants (2227 men, 3040 women) ($\geq$60 years)	BMI $\geq$ 25 kg/m² without metabolic syndrome defined by NCEP-ATP III guideline (2002)	57.6%
[43]	South Korea	No	2352 participants (aged 40–69 years)	BMI $\geq$ 25 kg/m² with none of metabolic syndrome components defined by NCEP-ATP III guideline (2002)	18.1%
[77]	South Korea	Yes	323,175 subjects ($\geq$ 20 years)	BMI $\geq$ 25 kg/m² without metabolic disease component (hypertension, diabetes, and dyslipidemia)	16.5% among total population
[10]	South Korea	Yes	514,866 subjects	BMI $\geq$ 25 kg/m² with none or one of metabolic syndrome components determined by modified NCEP-ATP III guideline	9.2% among total population
[8]	South Korea	Yes	36.5 million ($\geq$ 20 years) in 2007 41.7 million ($\geq$ 20 years) in 2017	BMI $\geq$ 25 kg/m² with none or one of metabolic syndrome components determined by modified NCEP-ATP III guideline	8.7% (10.8% in men, 6.7% in women) in 2007 9.5% (10.4% in men, 8.6% in women) in 2017
[27]	Taiwan	Yes	1547 participants (629 men and 918 women) (aged 18–59 years)	BMI $\geq$ 25 kg/m² without metabolic syndrome defined by modified AHA guideline (2005)	28.5% (24.2% for men and 34.8% for women)

HOMA-IR Homeostasis model assessment of insulin resistance, *NCEP-ATP III (2002)*, the National Cholesterol Education Program Adult Treatment Panel III (2002), *IDF* International Diabetes Federation [1], AHA guideline (2005), [22]; Wildman criterion [84].

favorable diabetes and CVD outcomes [4]. However, there are individuals maintaining their MHO status over a long period, which did not translate into reduced CVD risk to the level of metabolically healthy lean subjects. Thus, MHO should not be considered as a safe condition, which does not require obesity treatment, but rather it should guide decision-making for personalized, risk-stratified obesity treatment [4]. It is possible the MHO phenotype may benefit from healthy diets to reduce mortality risk, which may be not the case in the MUO phenotype [72]. In contrast, the MONW phenotype would benefit from a high diet quality to lower mortality risk [71], although no specialized lifestyle intervention for MONW phenotype has been established yet [21].

Conclusions

The prevalence of obesity has increased continuously in East Asia for the past several decades, most prominently in men. However, the magnitude and trends of obesity in East Asia, which are comprised of high-income countries, are different from other Asian countries and populations undergoing a similar stage of obesity transition [28]. Obesity prevalence is relatively small in East Asian countries, but there still has been an enormous increase in obesity prevalence among adults, particularly in men, and a smaller increase among children.

Asian populations tend to have unfavorable metabolic risk profiles compared to any other race or ethnicity with the same level of BMI. MONW individuals at a higher metabolic risk include those with predominantly visceral and ectopic fat accumulation relative to BMI. Identifying modifiable risk factors in people with MONW who are seemingly healthy but at high risk for cardiometabolic disease could be beneficial to preventing cardiovascular morbidity and mortality in East Asian populations. In contrast, individuals with MHO phenotype, who are obese but maintain normal metabolic function, may not be a healthy status in East Asian populations. Metabolic health status may be a better predictor of CVD risk and mortality than a more visibly obese phenotype. Understanding the differences

and overlap of metabolic and obesity phenotypes are important for identifying high-risk groups prone to obesity-related complications such as type 2 diabetes and CVD, and for implementation of personalized treatment.

References

1. Alberti KG, Zimmet P, Shaw J. Metabolic syndrome – a new world-wide definition. A consensus statement from the International Diabetes Federation. Diabet Med. 2006;23(5):469–80. https://doi.org/10.1111/j.1464-5491.2006.01858.x.
2. Baik I. Optimal cutoff points of waist circumference for the criteria of abdominal obesity: comparison with the criteria of the International Diabetes Federation. Circ J. 2009;73(11):2068–75.
3. Bao Y, Lu J, Wang C, Yang M, Li H, Zhang X, Zhu J, Lu H, Jia W, Xiang K. Optimal waist circumference cutoffs for abdominal obesity in Chinese. Atherosclerosis. 2008;201(2):378–84. https://doi.org/10.1016/j.atherosclerosis.2008.03.001.
4. Blüher M. Metabolically healthy obesity. Endocr Rev. 2020;41(3) https://doi.org/10.1210/endrev/bnaa004.
5. Chang Y, Kim BK, Yun KE, Cho J, Zhang Y, Rampal S, Zhao D, Jung HS, Choi Y, Ahn J, Lima JA, Shin H, Guallar E, Ryu S. Metabolically-healthy obesity and coronary artery calcification. J Am Coll Cardiol. 2014;63(24):2679–86. https://doi.org/10.1016/j.jacc.2014.03.042.
6. Chang HC, Yang HC, Chang HY, Yeh CJ, Chen HH, Huang KC, Pan WH. Morbid obesity in Taiwan: prevalence, trends, associated social demographics, and lifestyle factors. PLoS One. 2017;12(2):e0169577. https://doi.org/10.1371/journal.pone.0169577.
7. Chen S, Zhou S, Wu B, Zhao Y, Liu X, Liang Y, Shao X, Holthofer H, Zou H. Association between metabolically unhealthy overweight/obesity and chronic kidney disease: the role of inflammation. Diabetes Metab. 2014;40(6):423–30. https://doi.org/10.1016/j.diabet.2014.08.005.
8. Cheng TO. The current state of cardiology in China. Int J Cardiol. 2004;96(3):425–39. https://doi.org/10.1016/j.ijcard.2003.10.011.
9. Chin SO, Hwang YC, Ahn HY, Jun JE, Jeong IK, Ahn KJ, Chung HY. Trends in the prevalence of obesity and its phenotypes based on the Korea National Health and nutrition examination survey from 2007 to 2017 in Korea. Diabetes Metab J. 2022;46(5):808–12. https://doi.org/10.4093/dmj.2021.0226.
10. Cho YK, Jung CH. Metabolically healthy obesity: epidemiology, criteria, and implications in chronic kidney disease. J Obes Metab Syndr. 2022;31(3):208–16. https://doi.org/10.7570/jomes22036.
11. Cho YK, Lee J, Kim HS, Park JY, Lee WJ, Kim YJ, Jung CH. Impact of transition in metabolic health and obesity on the incident chronic kidney disease: a

Nationwide Cohort Study. J Clin Endocrinol Metab. 2020;105(3) https://doi.org/10.1210/clinem/dgaa033.

12. Choi J, Se-Young O, Lee D, Tak S, Hong M, Park SM, Cho B, Park M. Characteristics of diet patterns in metabolically obese, normal weight adults (Korean National Health and Nutrition Examination Survey III, 2005). Nutr Metab Cardiovas Dis. 2012;22(7):567–74. https://doi.org/10.1016/j.numecd.2010.09.001.

13. Choi JY, Ha HS, Kwon HS, Lee SH, Cho HH, Yim HW, Lee WC, Park YM. Characteristics of metabolically obese, normal-weight women differ by menopause status: the Fourth Korea National Health and Nutrition Examination Survey. Menopause (New York, NY). 2013a;20(1):85–93. https://doi.org/10.1097/gme.0b013e31825d26b6.

14. Choi KM, Cho HJ, Choi HY, Yang SJ, Yoo HJ, Seo JA, Kim SG, Baik SH, Choi DS, Kim NH. Higher mortality in metabolically obese normal-weight people than in metabolically healthy obese subjects in elderly Koreans. Clin Endocrinol. 2013b;79(3):364–70. https://doi.org/10.1111/cen.12154.

15. Chu NF. Prevalence and trends of obesity among school children in Taiwan – the Taipei Children Heart Study. Int J Obes Relat Metab Disord. 2001;25(2):170–6. https://doi.org/10.1038/sj.ijo.0801486.

16. Chu NF. Prevalence of obesity in Taiwan. Obes Rev. 2005;6(4):271–4. https://doi.org/10.1111/j.1467-789X.2005.00175.x.

17. Chu N, Pan W. Prevalence of obesity and its comorbidities among schoolchildren in Taiwan. Asia Pac J Clin Nutr. 2007;16:601.

18. Consultation WE. Appropriate body-mass index for Asian populations and its implications for policy and intervention strategies. Lancet. 2004;363(9403):157–63. https://doi.org/10.1016/s0140-6736(03)15268-3.

19. Du T, Yu X, Zhang J, Sun X. Lipid accumulation product and visceral adiposity index are effective markers for identifying the metabolically obese normal-weight phenotype. Acta Diabetol. 2015; https://doi.org/10.1007/s00592-015-0715-2.

20. Funatogawa I, Funatogawa T, Nakao M, Karita K, Yano E. Changes in body mass index by birth cohort in Japanese adults: results from the National Nutrition Survey of Japan 1956–2005. Int J Epidemiol. 2009;38 (1):83–92. https://doi.org/10.1093/ije/dyn182.

21. Gómez-Zorita S, Queralt M, Vicente MA, González M, Portillo MP. Metabolically healthy obesity and metabolically obese normal weight: a review. J Physiol Biochem. 2021;77(1):175–89. https://doi.org/10.1007/s13105-020-00781-x.

22. Grundy SM, Cleeman JI, Daniels SR, Donato KA, Eckel RH, Franklin BA, Gordon DJ, Krauss RM, Savage PJ, Smith SC, Jr., Spertus JA, Costa F. Diagnosis and management of the metabolic syndrome: an American Heart Association/National Heart, Lung, and Blood Institute Scientific Statement. Circulation. 2005;112(17):2735–52. https://doi.org/10.1161/circulationaha.105.169404.

23. Heianza Y, Kato K, Kodama S, Suzuki A, Tanaka S, Hanyu O, Sato K, Sone H. Stability and changes in metabolically healthy overweight or obesity and risk of future diabetes: Niigata wellness study. Obesity (Silver Spring, Md). 2014;22(11):2420–5. https://doi.org/10.1002/oby.20855.

24. Heianza Y, Arase Y, Tsuji H, Fujihara K, Saito K, Hsieh SD, Tanaka S, Kodama S, Hara S, Sone H. Metabolically healthy obesity, presence or absence of fatty liver, and risk of type 2 diabetes in Japanese individuals: Toranomon Hospital Health Management Center Study 20 (TOPICS 20). J Clin Endocrinol Metab. 2014a;99(8):2952–60. https://doi.org/10.1210/jc.2013-4427.

25. Heianza Y, Kato K, Kodama S, Ohara N, Suzuki A, Tanaka S, Hanyu O, Sato K, Sone H. Risk of the development of type 2 diabetes in relation to overall obesity, abdominal obesity and the clustering of metabolic abnormalities in Japanese individuals: does metabolically healthy overweight really exist? The Niigata Wellness Study. Diabet Med. 2015;32(5):665–72. https://doi.org/10.1111/dme.12646.

26. Hou XG, Wang C, Ma ZQ, Yang WF, Wang JX, Li CQ, Wang YL, Liu SM, Hu XP, Zhang XP, Jiang M, Wang WQ, Ning G, Zheng HZ, Ma AX, Sun Y, Song J, Lin P, Liang K, Liu FQ, Li WJ, Xiao J, Gong L, Wang MJ, Liu JD, Yan F, Yang JP, Wang LS, Tian M, Zhao RX, Jiang L, Chen L. Optimal waist circumference cut-off values for identifying metabolic risk factors in middle-aged and elderly subjects in Shandong Province of China. Biomed Environmental Sci. 2014;27(5):353–9. https://doi.org/10.3967/bes2014.060.

27. Hwang LC, Bai CH, Sun CA, Chen CJ. Prevalence of metabolically healthy obesity and its impacts on incidences of hypertension, diabetes and the metabolic syndrome in Taiwan. Asia Pac J Clin Nutr. 2012;21 (2):227–33.

28. Jaacks LM, Vandevijvere S, Pan A, McGowan CJ, Wallace C, Imamura F, Mozaffarian D, Swinburn B, Ezzati M. The obesity transition: stages of the global epidemic. Lancet Diabetes Endocrinol. 2019;7(3): 231–40. https://doi.org/10.1016/s2213-8587(19)30026-9.

29. Jung CH, Lee MJ, Hwang JY, Jang JE, Leem J, Yang DH, Kang JW, Kim EH, Park JY, Kim HK, Lee WJ. Association of metabolically healthy obesity with subclinical coronary atherosclerosis in a Korean population. Obesity (Silver Spring, Md). 2014;22(12): 2613–20. https://doi.org/10.1002/oby.20883.

30. Kamezaki F, Sonoda S, Nakata S, Kashiyama K, Muraoka Y, Okazaki M, Tamura M, Abe H, Takeuchi M, Otsuji Y. Proposed cutoff level of waist circumference in Japanese men: evaluation by homeostasis model assessment of insulin resistance levels. Intern Med. 2012;51(16):2119–24.

31. Kang HT, Shim JY, Lee HR, Park BJ, Linton JA, Lee YJ. Trends in prevalence of overweight and obesity in Korean adults, 1998–2009: the Korean National Health and Nutrition Examination Survey. J Epidemiol. 2014;24(2):109–16.

32. Kao M, Huang H, Tzeng M, Lee N, Shieh M. The nutritional status in Taiwan – anthropometric'measurement 1986–1988 (Ì) body weight and body height. J Chin Nutr Soc. 1991;16:63–84.

33. Karelis AD, St-Pierre DH, Conus F, Rabasa-Lhoret R, Poehlman ET. Metabolic and body composition factors in subgroups of obesity: what do we know? J Clin Endocrinol Metab. 2004;89(6):2569–75. https://doi.org/10.1210/jc.2004-0165. 89/6/2569 [pii]

34. Kashihara H, Lee JS, Kawakubo K, Tamura M, Akabayashi A. Criteria of waist circumference according to computed tomography-measured visceral fat area and the clustering of cardiovascular risk factors. Circ J. 2009;73(10):1881–6.

35. Kawada T, Otsuka T, Inagaki H, Wakayama Y, Li Q, Li YJ, Katsumata M. Optimal cut-off levels of body mass index and waist circumference in relation to each component of metabolic syndrome (MetS) and the number of MetS component. Diabetes Metab Syndr. 2011;5(1):25–8. https://doi.org/10.1016/j.dsx.2010.05.012.

36. Khang YH, Park MJ. Trends in obesity among Korean children using four different criteria. Int J Pediatr Obes. 2011;6(3–4):206–14. https://doi.org/10.3109/17477166.2010.490270.

37. Kim S, Moon S, Popkin BM. The nutrition transition in South Korea. Am J Clin Nutr. 2000;71(1):44–53.

38. Kim HY, Kim CW, Lee CD, Choi JY, Park CH, Bae SH, Yoon SK, Han K, Park YM. Can "healthy" normal alanine aminotransferase levels identify the metabolically obese phenotype? Findings from the Korea national health and nutrition examination survey 2008–2010. Dig Dis Sci. 2014a;59(6):1330–7. https://doi.org/10.1007/s10620-013-2995-0.

39. Kim MK, Han K, Kwon HS, Song KH, Yim HW, Lee WC, Park YM. Normal weight obesity in Korean adults. Clin Endocrinol. 2014b;80(2):214–20. https://doi.org/10.1111/cen.12162.

40. Kim S, Kyung C, Park JS, Lee SP, Kim HK, Ahn CW, Kim KR, Kang S. Normal-weight obesity is associated with increased risk of subclinical atherosclerosis. Cardiovasc Diabetol. 2015;14:58. https://doi.org/10.1186/s12933-015-0220-5.

41. Kim JA, Kim DH, Kim SM, Park YG, Kim NH, Baik SH, Choi KM, Han K, Yoo HJ. Impact of the dynamic change of metabolic health status on the incident Type 2 diabetes: a Nationwide Population-Based Cohort Study. Endocrinol Metab (Seoul). 2019;34(4):406–14. https://doi.org/10.3803/EnM.2019.34.4.406.

42. Kim BY, Kang SM, Kang JH, Kang SY, Kim KK, Kim KB, Kim B, Kim SJ, Kim YH, Kim JH, Kim JH, Kim EM, Nam GE, Park JY, Son JW, Shin YA, Shin HJ, Oh TJ, Lee H, Jeon EJ, Chung S, Hong YH, Kim CH. 2020 Korean Society for the Study of obesity guidelines for the Management of Obesity in Korea. J Obes Metab Syndr. 2021;30(2):81–92. https://doi.org/10.7570/jomes21022.

43. Koh JH, Koh SB, Lee MY, Jung PM, Kim BH, Shin JY, Shin YG, Ryu SY, Lee TY, Park JK, Chung CH. Optimal waist circumference cutoff values for metabolic syndrome diagnostic criteria in a Korean rural population. J Korean Med Sci. 2010;25(5):734–7. https://doi.org/10.3346/jkms.2010.25.5.734.

44. Kramer CK, Zinman B, Retnakaran R. Are metabolically healthy overweight and obesity benign conditions? A systematic review and meta-analysis. Ann Intern Med. 2013;159(11):758–69. https://doi.org/10.7326/0003-4819-159-11-201312030-00008.

45. Kweon S, Kim Y, Jang MJ, Kim Y, Kim K, Choi S, Chun C, Khang YH, Oh K. Data resource profile: the Korea National Health and Nutrition Examination Survey (KNHANES). Int J Epidemiol. 2014;43(1):69–77. https://doi.org/10.1093/ije/dyt228.

46. Lee K. Metabolically obese but normal weight (MONW) and metabolically healthy but obese (MHO) phenotypes in Koreans: characteristics and health behaviors. Asia Pac J Clin Nutr. 2009;18(2):280–4.

47. Lee SY, Park HS, Kim DJ, Han JH, Kim SM, Cho GJ, Kim DY, Kwon HS, Kim SR, Lee CB, Oh SJ, Park CY, Yoo HJ. Appropriate waist circumference cutoff points for central obesity in Korean adults. Diabetes Res Clin Pract. 2007;75(1):72–80. https://doi.org/10.1016/j.diabres.2006.04.013.

48. Lee SH, Ha HS, Park YJ, Lee JH, Yim HW, Yoon KH, Kang MI, Lee WC, Son HY, Park YM, Kwon HS. Identifying metabolically obese but normal-weight (MONW) individuals in a nondiabetic Korean population: the Chungju Metabolic disease Cohort (CMC) study. Clin Endocrinol. 2011;75(4):475–81. https://doi.org/10.1111/j.1365-2265.2011.04085.x.

49. Lee S-H, Ha H-S, Park Y-J, Lee J-H, Yim H-W, Yoon K-H, Kang M-I, Lee W-C, Son H-Y, Park Y-M. Prevalence and characteristics of metabolically obese but normal weight and metabolically healthy but obese in middle-aged Koreans: the Chungju Metabolic Disease Cohort (CMC) Study. Endocrinol Metab. 2011;26(2):133–41.

50. Lee SK, Kim SH, Cho GY, Baik I, Lim HE, Park CG, Lee JB, Kim YH, Lim SY, Kim H, Shin C. Obesity phenotype and incident hypertension: a prospective community-based cohort study. J Hypertens. 2013;31(1):145–51. https://doi.org/10.1097/HJH.0b013e32835a3637.

51. Lee SH, Kwon HS, Park YM, Ha HS, Jeong SH, Yang HK, Lee JH, Yim HW, Kang MI, Lee WC, Son HY, Yoon KH. Predicting the development of diabetes using the product of triglycerides and glucose: the Chungju Metabolic Disease Cohort (CMC) study. PLoS One. 2014;9(2):e90430. https://doi.org/10.1371/journal.pone.0090430.

52. Lee SH, Han K, Yang HK, Kim HS, Cho JH, Kwon HS, Park YM, Cha BY, Yoon KH. A novel criterion for identifying metabolically obese but normal weight individuals using the product of triglycerides and glucose. Nutr Diabetes. 2015;5:e149. https://doi.org/10.1038/nutd.2014.46.

53. Lee SH, Han K, Yang HK, Kim MK, Yoon KH, Kwon HS, Park YM. Identifying subgroups of obesity using the product of triglycerides and glucose: the Korea National Health and Nutrition Examination Survey, 2008–2010. Clin Endocrinol. 2015;82(2):213–20. https://doi.org/10.1111/cen.12502.

54. Liang YJ, Xi B, Song AQ, Liu JX, Mi J. Trends in general and abdominal obesity among Chinese children and adolescents 1993–2009. Pediatr Obes. 2012;7(5):355–64. https://doi.org/10.1111/j.2047-6310.2012.00066.x.

55. Lim S, Kim JH, Yoon JW, Kang SM, Choi SH, Park YJ, Kim KW, Cho NH, Shin H, Park KS, Jang HC. Optimal cut points of waist circumference (WC) and visceral fat area (VFA) predicting for metabolic syndrome (MetS) in elderly population in the Korean Longitudinal Study on Health and Aging (KLoSHA). Arch Gerontol Geriatr. 2012;54(2): e29–34. https://doi.org/10.1016/j.archger.2011. 07.013.

56. Lin Y, Chu C, Hong C, Huang P. Assessment of nutritional status of the youth in Taiwan, I: body height and body weight. J Chin Nutr Soc. 1985;10:91–105.

57. Lin YC, Yen LL, Chen SY, Kao MD, Tzeng MS, Huang PC, Pan WH. Prevalence of overweight and obesity and its associated factors: findings from National Nutrition and Health Survey in Taiwan, 1993–1996. Prev Med. 2003;37(3):233–41.

58. Matsushita Y, Yoshiike N, Kaneda F, Yoshita K, Takimoto H. Trends in childhood obesity in Japan over the last 25 years from the national nutrition survey. Obes Res. 2004;12(2):205–14.

59. Mu L, Liu J, Zhou G, Wu C, Chen B, Lu Y, Lu J, Yan X, Zhu Z, Nasir K, Spatz ES, Krumholz HM, Zheng X. Obesity prevalence and risks among Chinese adults: findings from the China PEACE Million Persons Project, 2014–2018. Circ Cardiovasc Qual Outcomes. 2021;14(6):e007292. https://doi.org/10.1161/circoutcomes.120.007292.

60. Nakamura K, Nanri H, Hara M, Higaki Y, Imaizumi T, Taguchi N, Sakamoto T, Horita M, Shinchi K, Tanaka K. Optimal cutoff values of waist circumference and the discriminatory performance of other anthropometric indices to detect the clustering of cardiovascular risk factors for metabolic syndrome in Japanese men and women. Environ Health Prev Med. 2011;16(1):52–60. https://doi.org/10.1007/s12199-010-0165-y.

61. Nam GE, Kim YH, Han K, Jung JH, Rhee EJ, Lee SS, Kim DJ, Lee KW, Lee WY. Obesity fact sheet in Korea, 2019: prevalence of obesity and abdominal obesity from 2009 to 2018 and social factors. J Obes Metab Syndr. 2020;29(2):124–32. https://doi.org/10.7570/jomes20058.

62. Narisawa S, Nakamura K, Kato K, Yamada K, Sasaki J, Yamamoto M. Appropriate waist circumference cutoff values for persons with multiple cardiovascular risk factors in Japan: a large cross-sectional study. J Epidemiol. 2008;18(1):37–42.

63. Nazare JA, Smith JD, Borel AL, Haffner SM, Balkau B, Ross R, Massien C, Almeras N, Despres JP. Ethnic influences on the relations between abdominal subcutaneous and visceral adiposity, liver fat, and cardiometabolic risk profile: the international study of prediction of intra-abdominal adiposity and its relationship with Cardiometabolic risk/intra-abdominal adiposity. Am J Clin Nutr. 2012;96(4):714–26. https://doi.org/10.3945/ajcn.112.035758.

64. Ng M, Fleming T, Robinson M, Thomson B, Graetz N, Margono C, Mullany EC, Biryukov S, Abbafati C, Abera SF, et al. Global, regional, and national prevalence of overweight and obesity in children and adults during 1980–2013: a systematic analysis for the Global Burden of Disease Study 2013. Lancet. 2014;384 (9945):766–81. https://doi.org/10.1016/S0140-6736 (14)60460-8.

65. Oh SW. Obesity and metabolic syndrome in Korea. Diabetes Metab J. 2011;35(6):561–6. https://doi.org/10.4093/dmj.2011.35.6.561.

66. Oh K, Jang MJ, Lee NY, Moon JS, Lee CG, Yoo MH, Kim YT. Prevalence and trends in obesity among Korean children and adolescents in 1997 and 2005. Korean J Pediatr. 2008;51(9):950–5.

67. Oka R, Kobayashi J, Yagi K, Tanii H, Miyamoto S, Asano A, Hagishita T, Mori M, Moriuchi T, Kobayashi M, Katsuda S, Kawashiri M-a, Nohara A, Takeda Y, Mabuchi H, Yamagishi M. Reassessment of the cutoff values of waist circumference and visceral fat area for identifying Japanese subjects at risk for the metabolic syndrome. Diabetes Res Clin Pract. 2008;79 (3):474–81. https://doi.org/10.1016/j.diabres.2007. 10.016.

68. Organization WH (2000) International association for the study of obesity, International Obesity Taskforce. The Asia-Pacific perspective: redefining obesity and its treatment:15–21.

69. Pan XF, Wang L, Pan A. Epidemiology and determinants of obesity in China. Lancet Diabetes Endocrinol. 2021;9(6):373–92. https://doi.org/10.1016/s2213-8587(21)00045-0.

70. Park YM, Kwon HS, Lim SY, Lee JH, Yoon KH, Son HY, Yim HW, Lee WC. Optimal waist circumference cutoff value reflecting insulin resistance as a diagnostic criterion of metabolic syndrome in a nondiabetic Korean population aged 40 years and over: the Chungju Metabolic Disease Cohort (CMC) study. Yonsei Med J. 2010;51(4):511–8. https://doi.org/10.3349/ymj.2010.51.4.511.

71. Park YM, Fung TT, Steck SE, Zhang J, Hazlett LJ, Han K, Lee SH, Merchant AT. Diet quality and mortality risk in metabolically obese Normal-weight adults. Mayo Clin Proc. 2016a;91(10):1372–83. https://doi.org/10.1016/j.mayocp.2016.06.022.

72. Park YM, Steck SE, Fung TT, Zhang J, Hazlett LJ, Han K, Merchant AT. Mediterranean diet and mortality risk in metabolically healthy obese and metabolically unhealthy obese phenotypes. Int J Obes. 2016b;40(10): 1541–9. https://doi.org/10.1038/ijo.2016.114.

73. Popkin BM. The nutrition transition and obesity in the developing world. J Nutr. 2001;131(3):871S–3S.

74. Popkin BM, Du S, Zhai F, Zhang B. Cohort profile: the China Health and Nutrition Survey--monitoring and understanding socio-economic and health change in China, 1989–2011. Int J Epidemiol. 2010;39(6): 1435–40. https://doi.org/10.1093/ije/dyp322.

75. Primeau V, Coderre L, Karelis A, Brochu M, Lavoie M, Messier V, Sladek R, Rabasa-Lhoret R. Characterizing the profile of obese patients who are metabolically healthy. Int J Obes. 2010;35(7):971–81.

76. Ruderman NB, Schneider SH, Berchtold P. The "metabolically-obese," normal-weight individual. Am J Clin Nutr. 1981;34(8):1617–21.

77. Seo JA, Kim BG, Cho H, Kim HS, Park J, Baik SH, Choi DS, Park MH, Jo SA, Koh YH, Han C, Kim

NH. The cutoff values of visceral fat area and waist circumference for identifying subjects at risk for metabolic syndrome in elderly Korean: Ansan Geriatric (AGE) cohort study. BMC Public Health. 2009;9:443. https://doi.org/10.1186/1471-2458-9-443.

78. Seo YG, Choi HC, Cho B. The relationship between metabolically obese non-obese weight and stroke: the Korea National Health and Nutrition Examination Survey. PLoS One. 2016;11(8):e0160846. https://doi.org/10.1371/journal.pone.0160846.

79. Sun H, Ma Y, Han D, Pan CW, Xu Y. Prevalence and trends in obesity among China's children and adolescents, 1985–2010. PLoS One. 2014;9(8):e105469. https://doi.org/10.1371/journal.pone.0105469.

80. Tsou M. Metabolic syndrome in metabolic obese, non-obese elderly in northern Taiwan. Adv Aging Res. 2012;1:53–9. https://doi.org/10.4236/aar.2012.13007.

81. Tarui I, Okada E, Okada C, Saito A, Takimoto H. Trends in BMI among elderly Japanese population: findings from 1973 to 2016 Japan National Health and Nutrition Survey. Public Health Nutr. 2020;23(11):1907–15. https://doi.org/10.1017/s1368980019004828.

82. Wang W, Luo Y, Liu Y, Cui C, Wu L, Wang Y, Wang H, Zhang P, Guo X. Prevalence of metabolic syndrome and optimal waist circumference cut-off points for adults in Beijing. Diabetes Res Clin Pract. 2010;88 (2):209–16. https://doi.org/10.1016/j.diabres.2010.01.022.

83. Wang L, Zhou B, Zhao Z, Yang L, Zhang M, Jiang Y, Li Y, Zhou M, Wang L, Huang Z, Zhang X, Zhao L, Yu D, Li C, Ezzati M, Chen Z, Wu J, Ding G, Li X. Body-mass index and obesity in urban and rural China: findings from consecutive nationally representative surveys during 2004–18. Lancet. 2021;398 (10294):53–63. https://doi.org/10.1016/s0140-6736 (21)00798-4.

84. Wildman RP, Muntner P, Reynolds K, McGinn AP, Rajpathak S, Wylie-Rosett J, Sowers MR. The obese without cardiometabolic risk factor clustering and the normal weight with cardiometabolic risk factor clustering: prevalence and correlates of 2 phenotypes among the US population (NHANES 1999–2004). Arch Intern Med. 2008;168(15):1617–24.

85. Xi B, Liang Y, He T, Reilly KH, Hu Y, Wang Q, Yan Y, Mi J. Secular trends in the prevalence of general and abdominal obesity among Chinese adults, 1993–2009. Obes Rev. 2012;13(3):287–96. https://doi.org/10.1111/j.1467-789X.2011.00944.x.

86. Yajnik CS, Yudkin JS. The YY paradox. Lancet. 2004;363(9403):163.

87. Yang HK, Lee SH, Han K, Kang B, Lee SY, Yoon KH, Kwon HS, Park YM. Lower serum zinc levels are associated with unhealthy metabolic status in normal-weight adults: the 2010 Korea National Health and Nutrition Examination Survey. Diabetes Metab. 2015; https://doi.org/10.1016/j.diabet.2015.03.005.

88. Yang HK, Han K, Kwon HS, Park YM, Cho JH, Yoon KH, Kang MI, Cha BY, Lee SH. Obesity, metabolic health, and mortality in adults: a nationwide population-based study in Korea. Sci Rep. 2016;6: 30329. https://doi.org/10.1038/srep30329.

89. Yang YS, Han BD, Han K, Jung JH, Son JW. Obesity fact sheet in Korea, 2021: trends in obesity prevalence and obesity-related comorbidity incidence stratified by age from 2009 to 2019. J Obes Metab Syndr. 2022;31(2): 169–77. https://doi.org/10.7570/jomes22024.

90. Yeh WT, Chang HY, Yeh CJ, Tsai KS, Chen HJ, Pan WH. Do centrally obese Chinese with normal BMI have increased risk of metabolic disorders? Int J Obes. 2005;29(7):818–25. https://doi.org/10.1038/sj.ijo.0802975.

91. Yeh CJ, Chang HY, Pan WH. Time trend of obesity, the metabolic syndrome and related dietary pattern in Taiwan: from NAHSIT 1993–1996 to NAHSIT 2005–2008. Asia Pac J Clin Nutr. 2011;20(2):292–300.

92. Yoo KD, Ko SH, Park JE, Ahn YB, Yim HW, Lee WC, Park YM. High serum ferritin levels are associated with metabolic risk factors in non-obese Korean young adults: Korean National Health and Nutrition Examination Survey (KNHANES) IV. Clin Endocrinol. 2012;77(2):233–40. https://doi.org/10.1111/j.1365-2265.2011.04248.x.

93. Yoo HJ, Hwang SY, Hong HC, Choi HY, Seo JA, Kim SG, Kim NH, Choi DS, Baik SH, Choi KM. Association of metabolically abnormal but normal weight (MANW) and metabolically healthy but obese (MHO) individuals with arterial stiffness and carotid atherosclerosis. Atherosclerosis. 2014;234(1):218–23. https://doi.org/10.1016/j.atherosclerosis.2014.02.033.

94. Yoon YS, Oh SW. Optimal waist circumference cutoff values for the diagnosis of abdominal obesity in korean adults. Endocrinol Metab (Seoul). 2014;29(4):418–26. https://doi.org/10.3803/EnM.2014.29.4.418.

95. Yoshiike N, Matsumura Y, Iwaya M, Sugiyama M, Yamaguchi M. National Nutrition Survey in Japan. J Epidemiol. 1996;6(3 Suppl):S189–200. https://doi.org/10.2188/jea.6.3sup_189.

96. Yoshiike N, Seino F, Tajima S, Arai Y, Kawano M, Furuhata T, Inoue S. Twenty-year changes in the prevalence of overweight in Japanese adults: the National Nutrition Survey 1976–95. Obes Rev. 2002;3(3):183–90.

97. Zeng Q, He Y, Dong S, Zhao X, Chen Z, Song Z, Chang G, Yang F, Wang Y. Optimal cut-off values of BMI, waist circumference and waist:height ratio for defining obesity in Chinese adults. Br J Nutr. 2014;112 (10):1735–44. https://doi.org/10.1017/s0007114514 002657.

Part II

Genetic Factors

Evolution of Obesity

8

John R. Speakman

Contents

Abstract

Obesity is the result of a gene by environment interaction. A genetic legacy from our evolutionary past interacts with our modern environment to make some people obese. Why we have a genetic predisposition to obesity is problematical, because obesity has many negative consequences. How could natural selection favor the spread of such a disadvantageous

J. R. Speakman (✉)
State Key Laboratory of Molecular Developmental Biology, Institute of Genetics and Developmental Biology, Chinese Academy of Sciences, Beijing, People's Republic of China

Institute of Biological and Environmental Sciences, University of Aberdeen, Aberdeen, Scotland, UK
e-mail: J.speakman@abdn.ac.uk

trait? From an evolutionary perspective, three different types of explanation have been proposed to resolve this anomaly. The first is that obesity was once adaptive, in our evolutionary past. For example, it may have been necessary to support the development of large brains, or it may have enabled us to survive (or sustain fecundity) through periods of famine. People carrying so-called thrifty genes that enabled the efficient storage of energy as fat between famines would be at a selective advantage. In the modern world, however, people who have inherited these genes deposit fat in preparation for a famine that never comes, and the result is widespread obesity. The key problem with these adaptive scenarios is to understand why, if obesity was historically so advantageous, many people did not inherit these alleles and

© Springer Nature Switzerland AG 2023
R. S. Ahima (ed.), *Metabolic Syndrome*,
https://doi.org/10.1007/978-3-031-40116-9_9

in modern society remain slim. The second type of explanation is that most mutations in the genes that predispose us to obesity are neutral and have been drifting over evolutionary time – so-called drifty genes, leading some individuals to be obesity prone and others obesity resistant. The third type of explanation is that obesity is neither adaptive nor neutral and may never even have existed in our evolutionary past, but it is favored today as a maladaptive by-product of positive selection on some other trait. Examples of this type of explanation are the suggestion that obesity results from variation in brown adipose tissue thermogenesis, or the idea that we over consume energy to satisfy our needs for protein (the protein leverage hypothesis). This chapter reviews the evidence for and against these different scenarios, concluding that adaptive scenarios are unlikely, but the other ideas may provide possible evolutionary contexts in which to understand the modern obesity phenomenon.

Keywords

Obesity · Evolution · Adaptation · Natural selection · Thrifty genotype · Drifty genes · Genetic drift · Brown adipose tissue · Protein leverage hypothesis

Introduction

The obesity epidemic is a recent phenomenon (▶ Chap. 1, "Overview of Metabolic Syndrome" on "Epidemiology"). In as little as 50 years, there has been a progressive rise in the worldwide prevalence of obesity. A trend that started in the Western world [43] has rapidly spread to developing countries; until today, the only places yet to experience the epidemic are a few areas in sub-Saharan Africa. This change in the fatness of individuals over such a short timescale cannot reflect a change in the genetic makeup of the populations involved [106]. Most of the recent changes must therefore be driven by environmental factors (Chapter "Diet and Obesity (Macronutrients, Micronutrients, Nutritional Biochemistry)" on "Environmental

Factors"). Yet, even among the most obese countries, there remain large populations of individuals who remain lean (e.g., [44, 102]). These individual differences in obesity susceptibility mostly reflect genetic factors ([4, 49, 122]; Chapter "Genetics of Obesity" on "Genetic Factors"). The obesity epidemic is therefore a consequence of a gene by environment interaction [74, 128, 141]. Some people have a genetic predisposition to deposit fat, reflecting their evolutionary history, which results in obesity when exposed to the modern environment.

However, this interpretation of why we become obese has a major problem. We know that obesity is a predisposing factor for several serious noncommunicable diseases (Chapter "Metabolic Syndrome, GERD, Barrett's Esophagus" on "Diseases Associated with Obesity"). The fact that a large contribution to obesity is genetic yet obesity leads to an increase in the risk of developing these serious diseases is an issue, because the theory of evolution suggests that natural selection will only favor individuals that exhibit phenotypic traits that lead to increases in fitness (survival or fecundity). How is it possible for natural selection to have favored the spread of genes for obesity – a phenotype that has a negative impact on survival? This might be explained if obesity led to increases in fecundity that offset the survival disadvantage, but in fact obese people also have reduced fecundity ([170]; but see [116]), making the anomaly even worse. How did the predisposition to obesity evolve? What were the key events in our evolutionary history that led us to the current situation?

Why Do Animals and Humans Have Adipose Tissue?

The first law of thermodynamics states that energy can be neither created nor destroyed, but only transformed, and the second law states that there is an overall direction in the transformation, such that disorder (entropy) increases. Living organisms must obey these fundamental physical laws, and they have major consequences. Being low entropy systems, living things need to continuously fight against the impetus for entropy to increase. Complex organic molecules like proteins, lipids, DNA, and RNA become damaged and corrupted and must be continuously recycled and rebuilt to maintain their function. Doing this requires the continuous transformation of large amounts of energy. Hence, even when an organism is outwardly doing nothing, it still uses up large amounts of energy to maintain its low entropy state. However, living organisms must also grow, move around to find mates and food, defend themselves against attack by pathogens, and reproduce: processes which all require energy. The requirement for energy by living beings is continuous. Although energy sustains many different life processes, in animals, it can be obtained only by feeding, and feeding is discontinuous. Since energy cannot be created or destroyed, this means that animals need to have some mechanism(s) to store energy so that the episodic supply can be matched to the continuous requirement. The key storage mechanisms that allow us to get from one meal to the next are glucose and particularly glycogen in the liver and skeletal muscle. A useful analogy for this system is a regular bank account [135]. Money is periodically deposited into the account (similar to food intake) where it is stored temporarily (like glucose and glycogen stores) and is depleted by continuous spending (energy expenditure). The presence of the bank account acts as an essential buffer between discontinuous income and continuous spending.

There are, however, numerous situations where animals struggle to get enough food to meet the demands. In these instances, animals need a more long-term storage mechanism than glucose and glycogen stores, and this is generally provided by body fat. Returning to the analogy of a bank account – body fat is like a savings account. During periods when food is abundantly available, animals can deposit energy into their body fat (savings account), so that it is available for periods in the future when demand will exceed supply [64]. So adipose tissue exists primarily as a buffer that is used to supply energy during periods when food supply is insufficient to meet energy demands.

Why Do We Get Obese?

Given this background to why adipose tissue exists, there have been three different types of evolutionary explanation for why in modern society we fill up these fat stores to tremendous levels (Table 1: also reviewed in [133, 135]). First, there is the adaptive viewpoint. This suggests that obesity was adaptive in the past, but in the changed environment of the modern world, the positive consequences of being obese have been replaced by negative impacts. Second, there is the neutral viewpoint. This suggests that obesity has not been subject to strong selection in the past, but rather the genetic predisposition has arisen by neutral evolutionary processes like genetic drift. Finally there is the maladaptive viewpoint. This suggests that obesity has never been advantageous and that historically people were never obese (except some rare genetic mutations). However, the modern propensity to become obese is a by-product of positive selection on some other advantageous trait. Because evolution is by definition a genetic process, evolutionary explanations seek to explain where the genetic variation that causes a predisposition to obesity comes from. There is another set of ideas that are related to evolutionary explanations but do not concern genetic changes – for example, the "thrifty phenotype" hypothesis [52, 112, 163], the "thrifty epigenotype" hypothesis [147], and the oxymoronic "nongenetic evolution" hypothesis [5] (Table 1). This chapter does not concern these non-evolutionary ideas, but a treatment of some of them can be found elsewhere in this volume (Chapter "Fetal Metabolic Programming," Aitkin).

Adaptive Interpretations of Obesity

The primary adaptive viewpoint is that during our evolution accumulation of fat tissue provided a fitness advantage and was therefore positively selected by natural selection. This positive selection in the past is why some individuals have a predisposition to become obese today in spite of its negative effects. Humans are not the only animals to become obese [64]. There are several

Table 1 A summary of the main "evolutionary" and "quasi-evolutionary" ideas about the origins of obesity. Evolutionary ideas pertain to the genetic variation in susceptibility to obesity, while "quasi-evolutionary" arguments include trans-generational effects that are nongenetic. The "thrifty epigenome" model is a hybrid where genetic effects are fixed by epigenetic effects. The present chapter only concerns the evolutionary theories

Evolutionary theories

1 Adaptive scenarios

Hypothesis	Main feature	References
Thrifty gene hypothesis	Famine survival	[99] + many others
	Famine fecundity	[107, 112]
Loss of uricase	Efficiency of fructose use	[64]
Brain development	Fat required to support large brain	[106]
Fitness first	Obesity paradox	[116]

2. Neutral scenarios

Drifty gene hypothesis	Release from predation	[131, 132]

3. Maladaptive scenarios

Protein leverage hypothesis	Regulation of protein intake	[124]
Thermogenic variation	Variation in BAT activity	[119]
		[60]
		Selleyah et al. 2013

Quasi-evolutionary theories

Hypothesis	Main feature	References
Thrifty phenotype	Fetal programming	[52]
Thrifty epigenotype	Epigenetic consolidation of genotype	[147]
Nongenetic evolution	Trans-generational maternal effects	[5]

other groups of mammals and birds that deposit large amounts of body fat at levels equivalent to human obesity, for example, deposition of fat in some mammals prior to the hibernation (e.g., [13, 71, 73, 86, 138, 158]) and the deposition of fat in some birds prior to migration (e.g., [67, 95, 96, 118]). Several other animals show cycles in fat storage in relation to the annual cycle even though they do not engage in migration or hibernation – including voles [69, 70, 78] and hamsters

[9, 157] – mostly to facilitate breeding. These animal examples of obesity have in common the fact that deposition of fat is a preparatory response for a future shortfall in energy supply or an increase in demand [64]. For the hibernating animal, it will be unable to feed during winter, and for the migrating animal, it will also have no access to food when crossing barriers such as large deserts or oceans. Although humans neither seasonally hibernate nor migrate, a number of authors have made direct comparisons between these processes in wild animals and obesity in humans [64]. This is because humans must often deal with shortfalls of energy supply during periods of famine. Famine reports go back almost as long as people have been able to write [36, 54, 88]. The argument was therefore made that human obesity in our ancient past probably served the function of facilitating survival through famines [99], like fat storage in hibernators facilitates survival through hibernation. Famines would have provided a strong selection on genes that favored the deposition of fat during periods between famines. Individuals with alleles that favored efficient fat deposition would survive subsequent famines, while individuals with alleles that were inefficient at fat storage would not [99]. This idea, called the "thrifty gene hypothesis" was first published more than 50 years ago (more in the context of selection for genes predisposing to diabetes than obesity which was presumed to underpin the efficiency of fat storage) [99]. It has since been reiterated in various forms specifically with respect to obesity [17, 21, 34, 35, 76, 77, 101, 107–110, 113, 160, 162].

In detail, the hypothesis is as follows. When humans were experiencing periodic famines, thrifty alleles were advantageous because individuals carrying them would become fat between famines, and this fat would allow them to survive the next famine. They would pass their versions of the thrifty genes to their offspring, who would then also have a survival advantage in subsequent famines. In contrast, individuals not carrying such alleles would not prepare for the next famine by depositing as much fat, and would die, along with their unthrifty alleles. Because food supplies were presumed to be always low, even between famines, the levels of obesity attained, even in those individuals who carried the thrifty alleles, were probably quite modest, and so individuals never became fat enough to experience the detrimental impacts of obesity on health. What changed since the 1950s was that the food supply in Europe and North America increased dramatically due to enormous increases in agricultural production. This elevation in food supply has gradually spread through the rest of the world. The consequence is people in modern society who carry the thrifty alleles more efficiently eat the abundant food and deposit enormous amounts of fat. Obese people are like boy scouts: always prepared. In this way, the alleles that were once advantageous have been *rendered detrimental by progress* [99].

Advocates of the thrifty gene idea agree on some fundamental details. First, that famines are frequent. Estimates vary, but values of once every 10 years or so are often cited after [65]. Second, famines cause massive mortality (figures of 15–30% mortality are commonly quoted). However, they differ in some important aspects. One area of discrepancy is how far back in our history humans have been exposed to periodic famine. Some have suggested that famine has been an "ever present" feature of our history [21, 108]. There is a problem, however, with this suggestion. If the "thrifty alleles" provided a strong selective advantage to survive famines and famines have been with us for this period of time, then these alleles would have spread to fixation in the entire population [129–131]. We would all have the thrifty alleles, and in modern society we would all be obese. Yet, even in the most obese societies, there remains a population of lean people comprising about 20% of the population [44, 102]. If famine provided a strong selective force for the spread of thrifty alleles, it is relevant to ask how come so many people managed to avoid inheriting them [129–131].

We can illustrate this issue in a more quantitative manner. If a thrifty allele existed that promoted greater fat storage such that individuals carrying two versions of that allele survived 3% better and those who carry one version would survive 1.5% better, then a random mutation to create the thrifty allele would spread from being in just one individual to the entire population of the

ancient world in about 600 famine events. Using the most conservative estimate of famine frequency, of once per 150 years, this is about 90,000 years or about 1/500th the time since *Australopithecus*. Any mutation therefore that produced a thrifty allele within the first 99.8% of hominin history with this effect on mortality would therefore have gone to fixation. We would therefore all have inherited these alleles, and we would all be obese [129, 130].

This calculation reveals a large difference between the "obesity" phenomena observed in animals and the obesity epidemic in humans. In animals, when a species prepares for hibernation, migration, or breeding, the entire population becomes obese. The reasons are clear [137]. If a bird migrates across an area of ocean and does not deposit enough fat for the journey, it plunges into the ocean short of its destination and the genes that caused it to not deposit enough fat are purged from the population. Selection is intense, and consequently all the animals become obese. If the same intense selection processes had operated in humans, as suggested by advocates of adaptive interpretations of obesity like the thrifty gene hypothesis (Prentice 2001b, 2005), then we too would all become obese when the environmental conditions proved favorable for us to do so. We do not.

Another school of thought, however, is that famine has not been a feature of our entire history but is linked to the development of agriculture [113]. Benyshek and Watson [11] suggested that hunter-gatherer lifestyles are resilient to food shortages because individuals can be mobile, and when food becomes short in one area, they can seek food elsewhere or modify their diet to exploit whatever is abundant. In contrast, agricultural-based societies are dependent on fixed crops, and if these fail due, for example, to adverse weather conditions, food supply can immediately become a problem (see also [12]). Because mutations happening in the last 12,000 years would not have had chance to spread through the entire population, this shorter timescale for the process of selection might then explain why in modern society some of us become obese, but others remain lean.

The problem with this scenario, however, is opposite to the problem with the "ever present" idea. Humans developed agriculture only within the last 12,000 years [31], which would be only about 80 famine events with significant mortality. To be selected a mutation causing a thrifty allele would consequently have to provide an enormous survival advantage to generate the current prevalence of obesity. Calculations suggest the per-allele survival benefit would need to be around 10%. Although it is often suggested that mortality in famines is very high and therefore a per-allele mortality effect of this magnitude could be theoretically feasible, such large mortality effects of famines are generally confounded by the problem of emigration, and true mortality is probably considerably lower. An additional problem is that for a mutation to be selected, all of this mortality would need to depend on differences in fat content attributable to a single genetic mutation. This also makes the critical assumption that the reason people die in famines is because they starve to death, and thus individuals with greater fat reserves would on average be expected to survive longer than individuals with lower fat reserves. Although there are some famines where it is clear that starvation has been the major cause of death (e.g., [61]), for most famines this is not the case, and the major causes of death are generally disease related [1, 54, 92, 152]. This does not necessarily completely refute the idea that body fatness is a key factor influencing famine survival. The spread of disease among famine victims is probably contributed to by individuals having compromised immune systems. A key player in the relationship between energy status and immune status is leptin [39, 83, 87]. Low levels of leptin may underpin the immunodeficiency of malnutrition. Because circulating leptin levels are directly related to adipose tissue stores, it is conceivable that leaner people would have more compromised immune systems and hence be more susceptible to disease during famines.

One way to evaluate the role of body fatness in famine survival is to examine patterns of famine mortality with respect to major demographic variables such as age and sex and compare these to the expectation based on known effects of sex and age on body fat storage and utilization [134]. Females have greater body fat stores and lower metabolic rates compared with men of equivalent body weight and stature. In theory therefore, females should survive famines longer than males if body fatness plays a major role in survival [57, 84]. With respect to age, older individuals have declining metabolic rate, but they tend to preserve their fat stores until they are quite old [139]. Consequently, older individuals would be expected to survive famines longer than younger adults if body fatness was the overriding consideration. Patterns of mortality during actual famines suggest that males have higher mortality than females [84]. However, with respect to age, the highest mortality usually occurs among the very young (less than 5 years of age, including elevated fetal losses) and elderly (increasing probability of mortality with age from the age of about 40 onwards) [16, 54, 91, 121, 159]. The age-related pattern of mortality in adults is the opposite of that predicted if body fatness is the most important consideration. However, the impact of sex is in agreement with the theoretical expectation. Despite this apparent correspondence in many famines, the magnitude of the female mortality advantage massively exceeds the expectation from body fatness differences [134]. Yet in other famines, there is no female mortality advantage at all. This points to famine mortality being a far more complex phenomenon than simple reserve exhaustion. For instance, with respect to age, older individuals that have passed reproductive age may sacrifice themselves to provide food to enable survival of their offspring. Alternatively, they may succumb to diseases more rapidly because of an age-related decline in immune function. The exaggerated effect of sex may be similarly explained by social factors – females, for example, may exchange sex for extra food or may have more access to food because they do more of the family cooking – the "proximity to the pot" phenomenon [84]. Overall, the data on causes of mortality during famine points to an extremely complex picture, where differences in body fatness probably play a relatively minor role in defining who lives and who dies.

Recognizing the problem with the suggestion that selection for genes that cause obesity has only been in force for the past 12,000 years, Prentice et al. [113] suggested that the impact of body fatness during famines on fitness is not on survival probability but mostly on fertility. There is strong support for this suggestion (e.g., [117]). For many famines, we have considerable evidence that fertility is reduced. During the Dutch hunger winter, for example, when Nazi Germany imposed a blockade on some areas of the Netherlands, there was a clear reduction in the number of births from the affected regions that could be picked up in enrolments to the army 18 years later, while adjacent regions that were not blockaded and did not suffer famine show no such reduction. The effect is profound with a decline during the famine amounting to almost 50%. Tracing back the exact time that effects were manifest suggests that the major impact was on whether females became pregnant or not, rather than an impact on fetal or infant mortality rates [145, 146]. Unlike the effect of fatness on mortality, there is also good reason to anticipate that differences in fertility would be strongly linked to differences in body fatness. This is because we know from eating disorders such as anorexia nervosa that individuals with chronically low body fat stop menstruating and become functionally infertile. Leptin appears to be a key molecule involved in the association between body fatness and reproductive capability [3]. This effect is not just restricted to females. Both male and female ob/ob mice which cannot produce functional leptin are both sterile: a phenotype that can be reversed by administration of leptin in both sexes (females, [22]; males, [97]). Note however, that leptin is also responsive to chronic food shortage as well as body composition [161], and there is a school of thought that amenorrhea in anorexia nervosa is not due to low body fatness but low food intake. If this was the case, then lowered fertility need not necessarily be restricted to lean individuals. This argument may also apply to the link between fat stores and immune status elaborated above. Moreover, there is another argument why reduced fertility is unlikely to be a major selective force during famines and that is because following famines, there is usually a compensatory boom in fertility that offsets any reduction during the famine years. Individuals that fail to get pregnant

during famines tend to become immediately pregnant once the famine is over. Thus if one looks at the period including only the famine years, then fertility seems to have a major impact on demography (and hence selection), but expanding the period to include the famine and the post famine period revealing the net impact of altered fertility on demographics (and hence selection) is negligible and certainly insufficient to provide the selective advantage necessary to select genes for obesity over the period since humans invented agriculture.

These arguments about selection on genes favoring obesity were made before we had good information about the common polymorphisms that cause obesity or their effect sizes on fat storage. Without such information, it was plausible to suggest that genes might exist that have a large impact on fat storage and hence survival or fertility during famines. This view became untenable with the advent of genome-wide association studies (GWAS) which identified the main genes with common polymorphisms associated with increased obesity risk [29]. These GWAS studies revolutionized our view of the genetics of obesity since the majority of identified SNPs had nothing to do with the established hunger signaling pathway, and their effect sizes were all relatively small. At present, there are about 50 genes (SNPs) suggested to be associated with BMI that that have per-allele effect sizes between 1.5 kg and 100 g [103, 104, 142, 164, 166]. On this basis, it has been suggested that the genetic architecture of obesity may involve hundreds or even thousands of genes each with a very small effect [56]. This reality about the genetic architecture of obesity makes the proposed model by Prentice et al. [113] that selection on these genes has only occurred over the past 12,000 years completely untenable, because SNPs causing differences in fat storage of 100–1000 g could not possibly cause differential survival or fecundity during famines of 10%.

Setting aside the suggestion that famines are a phenomenon of the age of agriculture, if periodic food crises sufficient to cause significant mortality did affect us throughout our evolutionary history, it is possible to imagine a scenario where genes of small effect might have such a small impact on fat storage, and hence famine survival (or fecundity), that their spread in the population would be incredibly slow. Therefore, they might not progress to fixation over the duration of our evolutionary history, and we would be left today with the observed genetic architecture of many incompletely fixed genes of small effect. Speakman and Westerterp [140] evaluated this idea by first predicting the impact of such polymorphisms of small effect on famine survival and then modeling the spread of such genes over the four million years of hominin evolution (assuming a 150-year frequency of famines). Using a mathematical model of body fat utilization under total starvation, combined with estimates of energy demand across the lifespan, it was shown that genes that had a per-allele effect on fat storage of 80 g would cause a mortality difference of about 0.3%. That is 10x lower than the assumed effect that had been previously used to model the spread of thrifty genes [130]. Nevertheless, despite this very low impact on famine survival, a mutation causing such a difference in fat storage would move to fixation in about 6000 famine events (about 900,000 years). Thus the scenario of genetic polymorphisms moving slowly to fixation is correct, but it implies that all the mutations identified as important in GWAS studies had occurred in the last million years or so – which we know is not correct. In addition, if the selection model is correct, we would anticipate, all else being equal, that genes with greater effect size would have greater prevalence, but that is not observed in the known GWAS SNPs ([140] using data from [142]).

Overall, the idea that the genetic basis of obesity is adaptive, resulting from selection in our evolutionary history which favored "thrifty" alleles, because of elevated survival or fecundity of the obese during famines, is not supported by the available data. Other adaptive scenarios could be envisioned. For example, Power and Schulkin [106] argue that we are fat because of the need to support development of our large brains. Rakesh and Syam [116] point to the benefits of milder levels of obesity for disease survival and fecundity. An alternative idea is that fat storage in human ancestors was promoted by the loss of the uricase gene in the Miocene [64], which enabled more efficient utilization of fructose to deposit fat. This fat then enabled greater survival during periods of famine. A common problem faced by such scenarios is the fact that even in the most obesogenic modern environments, many individuals do not become fat. Any proposed adaptive scenario must explain this variation. Perhaps the closest any adaptive idea comes to explaining this variation is the suggestion of Johnson et al. [64] that we lost the uricase gene early in our evolution because of the advantages for conversion of fruit sugars to fat (i.e., everyone inherited this mutation), but this only leads to obesity in modern society in individuals with high intakes of fructose. This however does not explain the known genetic variation between individuals that predisposes to obesity [4].

The Neutral Viewpoint

Evolution is a complex process. We often regard natural selection as being the primary force generating genetic change. However, this is a naive viewpoint, and among evolutionary biologists, it is well recognized that natural selection is one of a number of processes including phyletic heritage, founder effects, neutral mutations, and genetic drift that underlie genetic variations between individuals in a population. We should be cautious not to interpret everything biological from the perspective of adaptation by natural selection. The emerging field of "evolutionary medicine" is rapidly learning to appreciate this fact, and there is an increasing recognition that other "nonadaptive" evolutionary processes may be important to understand the evolutionary background to many human diseases [33, 115, 154, 173]. The "drifty gene" hypothesis is a nonadaptive explanation for the evolutionary background of the risk of developing obesity [131, 132]. This hypothesis starts from the observation that many wild animals can accurately regulate their body fatness. Several models are available to understand this regulation [141], but a particularly useful idea is the suggestion that body weight is bounded by upper and lower limits or intervention points [58, 75, 131], called the dual intervention point model [141]. If an individual varies in weight between the two limits, then nothing happens, but if its body weight decreases below the lower limit or above the upper limit, it will intervene physiologically to control its weight. Body weight is kept relatively constant (between the two limits) in the face of environmental challenges. These upper and lower limits may be selected for by different evolutionary pressures: the lower limit by the risk of starvation and the upper limit by the risk of predation.

Considerable research suggests that this fundamental balance of risks of starvation keeping body masses up (i.e., setting the lower intervention point) and risks of predation keeping body masses down (i.e., setting the upper intervention point) is a key component of body mass regulation in birds [2, 15, 25–27, 46, 48, 51, 72, 155, 172], small mammals [8, 18, 19, 100, 148], and larger animals such as cetaceans [85]. The "starvation-predation" trade-off has become a generalized framework for understanding the regulation of adiposity between and within species [59, 62, 79, 167], and laboratory studies are now starting to probe the metabolic basis of the effects of stochastic food supply and predation risk on body weight regulation [93, 94, 151, 171].

The drifty gene hypothesis suggests that early hominins probably also had such a regulation system. During the early period of human evolution between 6 and 2 million years ago (Pliocene), large predatory animals were far more abundant [55]. Our ancestors (*Paranthropines* and *Australopithecines*) were also considerably smaller than modern humans, making them potential prey to a wide range of predators. At this stage of our evolution, it seems most likely that upper and lower intervention points evolved to be relatively close together, and the early hominids probably had close control over their body weights.

Several major events however happened in our evolutionary history around 2.5 million to 2.0 million years ago. The first was the evolution of social behavior. This would have allowed several individuals to band together to enhance their ability to detect predators and protect each other from their attacks. In a similar manner, some modern primates, for example, vervet monkeys, have

evolved complex signaling systems to warn other members of their social groups about the approach of potential predators [7, 23]. This alone may have been sufficient to dramatically reduce predation risk. A second change was the discovery of fire and weapons [105, 144], powerful means for early *Homo* to protect themselves against predation. Social structures would have greatly augmented these capacities. Modern non-hominid apes such as chimpanzees (*Pan troglodytes*) also use weapons such as sticks to protect themselves against predators such as large snakes, and it has been concluded that bands of early hominids with even quite primitive tools could easily succeed in defending themselves in confrontations with potential predators [153].

The consequence was that the predation pressure that maintained the upper intervention point effectively disappeared. It has been suggested that because there was no selective pressure causing this intervention point to change, the genes that defined it were then subject to mutation and random drift [131] – hence, the "drifty" gene hypothesis [132]. Genetic drift is a process that is favored by low effective population size. The suggestion that early *Homo* species had a small effective population size (around 10,000 despite a census population of around one million) [37, 53] would create a genetic environment where drift effects could be common. Mutations and drift for two million years would generate the necessary genetic architecture, but this is insufficient to cause an obesity epidemic. By this model virtually, the same genetic architecture would also have been present 20,000 years ago (after 1,980,000 years of mutation and drift compared to two million years today). Why did the obesity epidemic not happen then? There have been two separate factors of importance that restricted the potential for people to achieve their drifted upper intervention points – the level of food supply and the social distribution of it [106]. Before the Neolithic, the most important factor was probably the level of food supply. Paleolithic individuals probably could not increase their body masses sufficiently to reach their drifted upper intervention points because there was insufficient food available. At this stage, each individual or small group would be foraging entirely for their own needs.

Things changed in the Neolithic with the advent of agriculture. Subsistence agriculture is not much different from hunter-gathering – in that each individual grows and harvests food for themselves and/or a small group. As yields from agricultural practice improved, however, the numbers of people needed to grow and harvest food as a percentage of the total population declined. It is at this stage that more complex human societies emerged [31].

Human societies are only feasible because it is possible for a subset of individuals to grow and harvest food to sustain a larger number of individuals. This wider group of individuals is then able to perform activities that would be unfeasible if they had to spend all their time growing and harvesting food. Such activities include religion, sport, politics, the arts and war, as well as building projects with stone, making pottery, iron, and bronze-ware which all require high temperatures of a kiln and mining ores. These activities were only possible when yields from crops became high enough to allow some individuals to stop raising crops and do other things. However, a crucial additional element was the societal control of food supply, so that food produced by one section of society can be distributed to those that do not produce it. This effectively requires the development of monetary and class systems, most of which have their origins in the wake of Neolithic agriculture. This central control of food supply is important because people can only attain their drifted upper intervention points if there is an adequate supply of food for them to do so.

In the Paleolithic, most people could not get access to these resources because there were insufficient resources available. After the Neolithic, most people could also not get access to unlimited food supplies because of the central control of food supply. Because most people would normally have body weights in the region between their upper and lower intervention points, they would not experience a physiological drive forcing them to seek out such food. An exception might be during the rare periods of famine (see above). This pattern of food access led to the development of a class-related pattern of variation in body weight. In the lower classes, where food supply was restricted, people did not move to their upper intervention points, whereas in higher levels of society, where access to food was effectively unlimited, attainment of the drifted upper intervention point became possible. Consequently at this stage, obesity was restricted to the wealthy and powerful. Not all wealthy and powerful people became obese (only those with the genetic predisposition to do so – i.e., with high drifted upper intervention points), but none of the poorer classes did. Obesity became a status symbol [14, 106]. Reports of obese people date from at least early Greek times. In the fifth Century BC, Hippocrates suggested some potential cures for obesity [114]. This implies two things. There would be no need for a cure for obesity if nobody suffered from it, so it must have been common enough to warrant his attention. Second, Hippocrates did not regard obesity as advantageous or desirable – but something that needed to be "cured." This provides additional evidence against the famine-based "thrifty gene" hypothesis, since obesity 2500 years ago, when famines were still supposed to be a major selective pressure, should have been viewed as advantageous if that theory was correct.

Estimates by agricultural historians of the levels of food production support the idea that most people in the past were under socially restricted food supply. In the late 1700s, for example, it has been estimated that 70% of Britain and 90% of France were consuming less than 12 MJ/day. If only 10% of the population had free access to unlimited energy, then only people in this proportion of the population would be expected to reach their drifted upper intervention points. Obesity prevalence would be expected to be less than 3%. This was the actual prevalence of obesity in the USA in 1890. It seems that the social control of food supply only started to change in Western societies after the First World War. This period (1920s) saw a wave of obesity in Western societies [32], but this was reversed when the Western world went back to war in the 1940s, especially in countries where food rationing was introduced. The modern obesity epidemic reflects a second wave of obesity as easy access to nutritional resources became widespread across all social levels after World War II ended. Nowadays, anyone in the West can afford to overconsume energy [135]. For example, a person in the USA earning the minimum wage of 7.25$ per hour (2013) and working a standard 38 h week would have an annual income of about 14,300 US$. Assuming half of this was available to buy food, this person could buy annually 2865 McDonalds' happy meals (about eight per day), containing about 3700 cal, about 47% more energy than the daily intake requirement of a man and 84% more than the daily intake requirement of a woman. In 2013, it was estimated that earners of minimum wage had lower income than those on welfare in the majority of states in the USA. It has been frequently noted that obesity increases coincidental with the economic transition from being largely rural to largely urban. Explanations for this trend have largely concerned alterations in levels of physical activity and increased access to food resources. The current model is completely consistent with these interpretations because it suggests that only following such economic transitions are individuals able to achieve their drifted upper intervention points.

The GWAS provides some support for this model. SNPs predisposing to obesity have not been under strong positive selection [68, 127], and similar lack of strong positive selection is also observed in GWAS targets linked to type 2 diabetes [6]. This absence of selection is also supported by the absence of any link between prevalence and effect size among these SNPs [140]. Finally, the genes that have been identified appear to include a large proportion of centrally acting genes that are related to appetite and food intake (e.g., [47]). It is entirely conceivable that the centrally acting genes that have been identified to date somehow define the upper intervention point. Overall, this model provides a nonadaptive explanation for why some people get obese but others do not.

The Maladaptive Scenario

The maladaptive viewpoint is that obesity has never been advantageous. Historically, it may have never even existed, except in some rare individuals with unusual genetic abnormalities – perhaps represented in Paleolithic sculptures such as the "Venus of Willendorf." However, the idea is that genes that ultimately predispose us to obesity become selected as a by-product of selection on some other trait that was advantageous. The best example of a "maladaptive" interpretation of the evolution of obesity is the suggestion that it is caused by individual variability in the capacity of brown adipose tissue to burn off excess caloric intake [123].

Brown adipose tissue is found uniquely in mammals (▶ Chap. 17, "Adipose Structure (White, Brown, Beige)," Vidal-puig et al.). Contrasting white fat which contains a single large fat droplet, brown adipocytes typically contain large multilocular lipid droplets and abundant mitochondria. These mitochondria contain a unique protein called uncoupling protein 1 (UCP-1) which resides on the inner membrane. UCP-1 acts as a pore via which protons in the intermembrane space can return to the mitochondrial matrix. However, unlike protons traveling from the intermembrane space to the matrix via ATP synthase, the protons moving via UCP-1 are not coupled to the formation of ATP (hence, the name "uncoupling protein"). The chemiosmotic potential energy carried by the protons traveling via UCP-1 is therefore released directly as heat, which is the primary function of BAT – to generate heat for thermoregulation. Unsurprisingly, then BAT is found abundantly in small mammals and in the neonates of larger mammals (including humans), which have an unfavorable surface-to-volume ratio for heat loss. The weight of BAT, and hence its capacity to generate heat, varies in relation to thermoregulatory demands. During winter, the amount of BAT and UCP-1 increases [40, 41, 89]. During summer, BAT and UCP-1 are lower [40, 90, 168].

During the late 1970s, it was suggested that BAT might have an additional function: to "burn off" excess calorie intake [60, 119]. This idea fell out of favor because it was commonly believed that adult humans do not have significant deposits of BAT. However, active BAT was discovered in adult humans in 2007 [98], and since that time the idea that variability in BAT function might result in the variable susceptibility to obesity has reemerged [123]. This has been supported by observations that the amount and activity of BAT is inversely related to obesity [28, 156] and that there is an age-related reduction in BAT activity, correlated with the age-related increase in body fatness [28, 169]. Moreover, the seasonal changes and responses to cold exposure in animals are also observed in humans [120], suggesting important functional activity. Experimental studies in rodents have established that transplanting extra BAT tissue into an individual can protect both against diet-induced [81, 143] and genetic obesity [82].

The "maladaptive" scenario for the evolution of obesity is therefore as follows. Individuals are presumed to vary in their brown adipose tissue thermogenesis as a result of their variation in evolutionary exposure to cold [123], which necessitated the use of BAT for thermogenesis. Some individuals might have high levels of active BAT, while others might have lower levels, either because their exposure to cold was lower or because they avoided cold exposure by other mechanisms such as development of clothing and the use of fire. Consequently, high levels of BAT would be one of a number of alternative adaptive strategies for thermoregulation. Because of this diversity of potential strategies, a genetic predisposition to develop high and active levels of BAT would only be present in some individuals and populations. This would lead to individual and population variation in the ability to recruit BAT for its secondary function: burning off excess energy intake.

A key question, however, is why individuals might have excessive intake of energy in the first place. Especially since this notion appears diametrically opposed to the fundamental assumption underlying the thrifty gene hypothesis that energy supply is almost always limited, one potential explanation for this effect is that individuals may not only eat food for energy but also for some critical nutrient. When food is of high quality, it may be that by eating enough food to meet the daily energy demands is enough to also meet demands for the critical nutrient. Any excess nutrient intake could be excreted. Two scenarios

might alter this situation. Energy demands might decline. This could, for example, be precipitated by an increase in sedentary behavior in modern society [24, 111]. If individuals continued to eat food to meet their energy demands, then they would reduce their intake, but this might mean their intake of the critical nutrient was now below requirements, and they would be nutrient deficient. However, direct measurements of energy demand in humans in both Europe and North America since the 1980s do not support the idea that activity energy demands have declined [149, 165]. Nevertheless, another scenario is that the quality of the food might change and the ratio of energy to the critical nutrient might increase. Again, if individuals continued to eat to meet their energy requirements, then intake of the nutrient would become deficient. In both of these scenarios to avoid nutrient deficiency, individuals might consume more food to meet their demands for the nutrient. The result would be that their consumption of energy would then exceed their demands.

A strong candidate for the nutrient that may drive overconsumption of energy is protein. This idea is called the "protein leverage hypothesis" [124] and is elaborated in full detail in the book *The Nature of Nutrition* by Simpson and Raubenheimer [125]. By this hypothesis, the main driver of food intake is always the demand for protein. That is, people and animals primarily eat to satisfy their protein requirements, and energy balance comes along as a passenger. The idea has lots to commend it. Across human societies, the intake of protein, despite very diverse diets, is almost constant – consistent with this being the primary regulated nutrient. In contrast, energy intakes are widely divergent. Moreover, we know that diets which include a high ratio of protein to energy (e.g., the Atkins diet) are effective for weight loss. A review of 34 studies of dietary intake showed that dietary protein was negatively associated with energy intake [50]. Several experimental studies of diet choice in rodents also point to protein content as the factor regulating energy intake and hence body weight (e.g., [63, 126]). Hence, the protein leverage theory may provide a necessary backdrop to the brown adipose tissue idea. It has also been noted that the protein leverage hypothesis may also explain why in modern society individuals increase their body mass to their upper intervention points as part of the "drifty gene" idea detailed above [135]. Note however that other studies suggest little evidence in support of the protein leverage hypothesis in food intake records over time in the USA [10], but this may reflect the poverty of the food intake reports rather than the theory [30].

If humans do overconsume energy because of the requirement for protein, then the ability to burn off the excess energy might then depend on levels of brown adipose tissue. Individuals with large BAT depots might burn off the excess and remain lean, while those with lower levels of BAT might be unable to burn off the excess consumption and become obese. By this interpretation, obesity is a maladaptive consequence of variation in adaptive selection on brown adipose tissue capacity. The environmental trigger is the change in the energy to nutrient ratio in modern food that stimulates overconsumption of energy. There is no need by this viewpoint to infer that obesity has ever provided an advantage or even that we have in our history ever been fat.

If brown adipose tissue is a key factor that influences the propensity to become fat, then one would anticipate that knocking out the UCP-1 gene in mice would lead to obesity. Enerbäck et al. [38] knocked out UCP-1, but the result did not support the hypothesis, because the mice did not become any more obese than wild-type mice when exposed to a high-fat diet. One potential issue with this experiment was that the genetic background of these mice was a mix of two strains, one susceptible and the other not susceptible to weight gain on a high-fat diet. The experiment was repeated but with the mice now backcrossed onto a pure C57BL/6 background (a strain that is susceptible to high-fat diet-induced weight gain) [80]. However, now the mice lacking UCP-1 were actually more resistant to the high-fat diet-induced obesity than the wild-type mice, but the protective effect was abolished when the mice were raised at 27 °C. This confusion was further compounded when the same mice were studied at 30 °C, at which temperature the KO mice became

fat even on a chow diet, and this effect was multiplied with high-fat feeding [42]. This is very confusing because at 30 °C, one would anticipate that UCP-1 would not be active in the mice that had it, and hence they should not differ from the KO animals. So the impact of knocking out the UCP-1 gene ranges from being protective from obesity at 20 °C to neutral at 27 °C to highly susceptible at 30 °C. These data for the UCP-1 KO mouse raise some interesting questions about the hypothetical role of BAT in the development of obesity in humans. In particular in some circumstances, not having functional BAT is not an impediment to burning off excess intake (i.e., the UCP1 KO mice at 20 °C). It is unclear then why humans could not also burn off excess intake by other methods – for example, physical activity or shivering.

A second major problem with this BAT idea is that the obesity genes identified so far from the GWAS studies [142, 166] are not associated with brown adipose tissue function but instead appear mostly linked to development or expressed in the brain and linked to individual variation in food intake (e.g., the gene FTO: [20, 136]). This lack of a link to the genetics suggests that evolutionary variability in thermoregulatory requirements probably did not drive individual variations in BAT thermogenic capacity (but see Takenaka et al. [150] for a perspective on the evolution of human thermogenic capacity relative to the great apes). Finally, there are other potential explanations for why there might be an association between BAT depot size and obesity [28, 156]. Adipose tissue acts as an insulator, and thermoregulatory demands in the obese are reduced because of shift downwards in the thermoneutral zone [66]. Severely obese people may be under heat stress because of their reduced capacity to dissipate heat at ambient temperatures where lean people are in the thermoneutral zone. In these circumstances, the requirement for thermoregulatory heat production would be reduced, and hence it is potentially the case that the association between BAT activity and adiposity comes about because obesity reduces the need for BAT and not because variation in BAT causes variation in the capacity to burn off excess intake.

Conclusion

Many ideas have been presented that try to explain the evolutionary background of the genetic contribution to the obesity epidemic. These can be divided into three basic types of idea. Adaptive interpretations suggest that fat has been advantageous during our evolutionary history. Theories include the thrifty gene hypothesis and the idea that high body fat was necessary to support our brain development. These ideas generally struggle to explain the diverse in obesity levels observed in modern society. Neutral interpretations emphasize that the propensity to become obese does not have any advantage but is a by-product of mutation and genetic drift in some key control features. The dominant idea is the drifty gene hypothesis. Finally, obesity may be a maladaptive consequence of positive selection on some other systems. Examples of this type of explanation are the brown adipose tissue hypothesis and the protein leverage hypothesis.

Cross-References

▶ Adipose Structure (White, Brown, Beige)
▶ Body Composition Assessment
▶ Endocrine Disorders Associated With Obesity
▶ Genetics of Lipid Disorders
▶ Genetics of Type 2 Diabetes
▶ Linking Obesity, Metabolism, and Cancer
▶ Non-alcoholic Fatty Liver Disease
▶ Obesity and Cardiovascular Disease
▶ Obesity and Metabolic Syndrome in South Asians
▶ Obesity in Middle East
▶ Overview of Metabolic Syndrome
▶ Connecting Obesity and Reproductive Disorders
▶ Sarcopenic Obesity
▶ Type 2 Diabetes: Etiology, Epidemiology, Pathogenesis, and Treatment

References

1. Adamets S. Famine in nineteenth and twentieth century Russia: mortality by age, cause and gender. Chapter 8. In: Dyson T, O'Grada C, editors. Famine demography. Perspectives from the past and present. International studies in demography series. Oxford: Oxford University Press; 2002. p. 158–80.
2. Adriaensen F, et al. Stabilizing selection on blue tit fledgling mass in the presence of sparrowhawks. Proc R Soc Lond Ser B. 1998;265:1011–6.
3. Ahima RS, Dushay J, Flier SN, et al. Leptin accelerates the onset of puberty in normal female mice. J Clin Invest. 1997;99:391–5.
4. Allison DB, Kaprio J, Korkeila M, et al. The heritability of BMI among an international sample of monozygotic twins reared apart. Int J Obes. 1996;20:501–6.
5. Archer E. The childhood obesity epidemic as a result of nongenetic evolution: the maternal resources hypothesis. Mayo Clin Proc. 2015;90:77–92.
6. Ayub Q, et al. Revisiting the thrifty gene hypothesis via 65 loci associated with susceptibility to type 2 diabetes. Am J Hum Genet. 2014;94:176–85.
7. Baldellou M, Henzi SP. Vigilance, predator detection and the presence of supernumerary males in vervet monkey troops. Anim Behav. 1992;43:451–61.
8. Banks PB, Norrdahl K, Korpimaki E. Nonlinearity in the predation risk of prey mobility. Proc R Soc B. 2000;267:1621–5.
9. Bartness TJ, Wade GN. Photoperiodic control of seasonal body weight cycles in hamsters. Neurosci Biobehav Rev. 1984;9:599–612.
10. Bender RL, Dufour DL. Protein intake, energy intake, and BMI among USA adults from 1999–2000 to 2009–2010: little evidence for the protein leverage hypothesis. Am J Hum Biol. 2015;27:261–2.
11. Benyshek DC, Watson JT. Exploring the thrifty genotype's food-shortage assumptions, a cross-cultural comparison of ethnographic accounts of food security among foraging and agricultural societies. Am J Phys Anthropol. 2006;131:120–6.
12. Berbesque JC, et al. Hunter-gatherers have less famine than agriculturalists. Biol Lett. 2014;10:20130853.
13. Boswell T, Woods SC, Kenagy GJ. Seasonal changes in body mass, insulin and glucocorticoids of free-living golden mantled ground squirrels. Gen Comp Endocrinol. 1994;96:339–46.
14. Brewis AA. Obesity: cultural and biocultural perspectives. New York: Rutgers University Press; 2010.
15. Brodin A. Mass-dependent predation and metabolic expenditure in wintering birds: is there a trade-off between different forms of predation? Anim Behav. 2001;62:993–9.
16. Cai Y, Feng W. Famine, social disruption, and involuntary fetal loss: evidence from Chinese survey data. Demography. 2005;42:301–22.
17. Campbell BC, Cajigal A. Diabetes: energetics, development and human evolution. Med Hypotheses. 2001;57:64–7.
18. Carlsen M, Lodal J, Leirs H, et al. The effect of predation risk on body weight in the field vole, *Microtus agrestis*. Oikos. 1999;87:277–85.
19. Carlsen M, Lodal J, Leirs H, et al. Effects of predation on temporary autumn populations of subadult *Clethrionomys glareolus* in forest clearings. Int J Mamm Biol. 2000;65:100–9.

20. Cecil JE, Tavendale R, Watt P, et al. An obesity associated FTO gene variant and increased energy intake in children. N Engl J Med. 2008;359: 2558–66.

21. Chakravarthy MV, Booth FW. Eating, exercise, and "thrifty" genotypes: connecting the dots toward an evolutionary understanding of modern chronic diseases. J Appl Physiol. 2004;96:3–10.

22. Chehab FF, Lim ME, Lu RH. Correction of the sterility defect in homozygous obese female mice by treatment with human recombinant leptin. Nat Genet. 1996;12:318–20.

23. Cheney DL, Seyfarth RM. Vervet monkey alarm calls – manipulation through shared information. Behaviour. 1985;94:150–66.

24. Church TS, Thomas DM, Tudor-Loke C, et al. Trends over 5 decades in US occupation related physical activity and their associations with obesity. PLoS One. 2011;6:e19657.

25. Covas R, et al. Stabilizing selection on body mass in the sociable weaver *Philetairus socius*. Proc R Soc Lond Ser B. 2002;269:1905–9.

26. Cresswell W. Diurnal and seasonal mass variation in blackbirds *Turdus merula*: consequences for mass-dependent predation risk. J Anim Ecol. 1998;67: 78–90.

27. Cuthill IC, et al. Body mass regulation in response to changes in feeding predictability and overnight energy expenditure. Behav Ecol. 2000;11:189–95.

28. Cypress AM, Lehman S, Williams G, et al. Identification and importance of brown adipose tissue in adult humans. N Engl J Med. 2009;360:1509–17.

29. Day FR, Loos RJF. Developments in obesity genetics in the era of genome wide association studies. J Nutrigenet Nutrigenomics. 2011;4:222–38.

30. Dhurandhar NV, Schoeller DA, Brown AW, et al. Energy balance measurement: when something is *not* better than nothing. Int J Obes. 2015;39:1109–13.

31. Diamond J. Guns, germs and steel: the fates of human societies. New York: W.W. Norton; 1995.

32. DuBois E. Basal metabolism in health and disease. Philadelphia: Lea and Febiger; 1936.

33. Dudley JT, Kim Y, Liu L, et al. Human genomic disease variants: a neutral evolutionary explanation. Genome Res. 2012;22:1383–94.

34. Eaton SB, Konner M, Shostak M. Stone agers in the fast lane: chronic degenerative diseases in evolutionary perspective. Am J Med. 1988;84:739–49.

35. Eknoyan G. A history of obesity, or how what was good became ugly and then bad. Adv Chronic Kidney Dis. 2006;13:421–7.

36. Elia M. Hunger disease. Clin Nutr. 2000;19:379–86.

37. Eller E, Hawks J, Relethford JH. Local extinction and recolonisation, species effective population size and modern human origins. Hum Biol. 2009;81: 805–24.

38. Enerbäck S, Jacobsson A, Simpson EM, et al. Mice lacking mitochondrial uncoupling protein are cold-sensitive but not obese. Nature. 1997;387:90–4.

39. Faggioni R, Feingold KR, Grunfeld C. Leptin regulation of the immune response and the immunodeficiency of malnutrition. FASEB J. 2001;15: 2565–71.

40. Feist DD, Feist CF. Effects of cold, short day and melatonin on thermogenesis, body weight and reproductive organs in Alaskan red backed voles. J Comp Physiol B. 1986;156:741–6.

41. Feist DD, Rosenmann M. Norepinephrine thermogenesis in seasonally acclimatized and cold acclimated red-backed voles in Alaska. Can J Physiol Pharmacol. 1976;54:146–53.

42. Feldmann HM, Golozoubova V, Cannon B, et al. UCP1 ablation induces obesity and abolishes diet-induced thermogenesis in mice exempt from thermal stress by living at thermoneutrality. Cell Metab. 2009;9:203–9.

43. Flegal KM, Shepherd JA, Looker CA, et al. Overweight and obesity in the United States: prevalence and trends 1960–1994. Int J Obes. 1998;22:39–47.

44. Flegal KM, et al. Prevalence and trends in obesity among US adults, 1999–2008. JAMA. 2010;303: 235–41.

45. Franks PW. Gene by environment interactions in type 2 diabetes. Curr Diabetes Rep. 2011;11:552–61.

46. Fransson T, Weber TP. Migratory fuelling in blackcaps (*Sylvia atricapilla*) underperceived risk of predation. Behav Ecol Sociobiol. 1997;41:75–80.

47. Fredriksson R, Hagglund M, Olszewski PK, et al. The obesity gene, FTO, is of ancient origin, upregulated during food deprivation and expressed in neurons of feeding related nuclei of the brain. Endocrinology. 2008;149:2062–71.

48. Gentle LK, Gosler AG. Fat reserves and perceived predation risk in the great tit, Parus major. Proc R Soc Lond Ser B. 2001;268:487–91.

49. Ginsburg E, Livshits G, Yakovenko K, et al. Major gene control of human body height, weight and BMI in five ethnically different populations. Ann Hum Genet. 1998;62:307–22.

50. Gosby AK, Conigrave AD, Raubenheimer D, et al. Protein leverage and energy intake. Obes Rev. 2014;15:183–91.

51. Gosler AG, Greenwood JJD, Perrins C. Predation risk and the cost of being fat. Nature. 1995;377:621–3.

52. Hales CN, Barker DJ. Type 2 (non-insulin-dependent) diabetes mellitus: the thrifty phenotype hypothesis. Diabetologia. 1992;35:595–601.

53. Harding RM, Fullerton SM, Griffiths RC, et al. Archaic African and Asian lineages in the genetic ancestry of modern humans. Am J Hum Genet. 1997;60:772–89.

54. Harrison GA, editor. Famine. Oxford: Oxford University Press; 1988.

55. Hart D, Susman RW. Man the hunted. Primates, predators and human evolution. Boulder: Westview Press; 2005.

56. Hebebrand J, Volckmar AL, Knoll N, et al. Chipping away the 'missing heritability': GIANT steps forward

in the molecular elucidation of obesity – but still lots to go. Obes Facts. 2010;3:294–303.

57. Henry CJK. Body mass index and the limits to human survival. Eur J Clin Nutr. 1990;44:329–35.

58. Herman CP, Polivy J. A boundary model for the regulation of eating. In: Stunkard AJ, Stellar E, editors. Eating and its disorders. New York: Raven Press; 1984.

59. Higginson AD, McNamara JM, Houston AI. The starvation-predation trade-off predicts trends in body size, muscularity and adiposity between and within taxa. Am Nat. 2012;179:338–50.

60. Himms-Hagen J. Obesity may be due to malfunctioning brown fat. Can Med Assoc J. 1979;121:1361–4.

61. Hionidou V. Why do people die in famines? Evidence from three Island populations. Popul Stud A J Demogr. 2002;56:65–80.

62. Houston AI, McNamara JM, Hutchinson JMC. General results concerning the trade-off between gaining energy and avoiding predation. Philos Trans R Soc. 1993;341:375–97.

63. Huang X, Hancock DP, Gosby AK, et al. Effects of dietary protein to carbohydrate balance on energy intake, fat storage, and heat production in mice. Obesity. 2013;21:85–92.

64. Johnson RJ, Steinvinkel P, Martin SL, et al. Redefining metabolic syndrome as a fat storage condition based on studies of comparative physiology. Obesity. 2013;21:659–64.

65. Keys A, Brozek J, Henschel A, et al. The biology of starvation, vol. 2. Minneapolis: University of Minnesota Press; 1950.

66. Kingma B, Frijns A, van Marken LW. The thermoneutral zone: implications for metabolic studies. Front Biosci. 2012;E4:1975.

67. Klaasen M, Biebach H. Energetics of fattening and starvation in the long distance migratory garden warbler (*Sylvia borin*) during the migratory phase. J Comp Physiol. 1994;164:362–71.

68. Koh XH, Liu XY, Teo YY. Can evidence from genome-wide association studies and positive natural selection surveys be used to evaluate the thrifty gene hypothesis in East Asians? PLoS One. 2014;10: e10974.

69. Krol E, Speakman JR. Regulation of body mass and adiposity in the field vole, *Microtus agrestis*: a model of leptin resistance. J Endocrinol. 2007;192: 271–8.

70. Krol E, Redman P, Thomson PJ, et al. Effect of photoperiod on body mass, food intake and body composition in the field vole, *Microtus agrestis*. J Exp Biol. 2005;208:571–84.

71. Krulin G, Sealander JA. Annual lipid cycle of the gray bat *Myotis grisescens*. Comp Biochem Physiol. 1972;42A:537–49.

72. Kullberg C, Fransson T, Jakobsson S. Impaired predator evasion in fat blackcaps (*Sylvia atricapilla*). Proc R Soc Lond Ser B. 1996;263:1671–5.

73. Kunz TH, Wrazen JA, Burnet CD. Changes in body mass and fat reserves in pre-hibernating little brown bats (*Myotis lucifugus*). Ecoscience. 1998;5:8–17.

74. Levin BE. Developmental gene x environmental interactions affecting systems regulating energy homeostasis and obesity. Front Neuroendocrinol. 2010;31:270–83.

75. Levitsky DA. Putting behavior back into feeding behavior: a tribute to George Collier. Appetite. 2002;38:143–8.

76. Lev-Ran A. Thrifty genotype: how applicable is it to obesity and type 2 diabetes? Diabetes Rev. 1999;7: 1–22.

77. Lev-Ran A. Human obesity: an evolutionary approach to understanding our bulging waistline. Diabetes Metab Res Rev. 2001;17:347–62.

78. Li XS, Wang DH. Regulation of body weight and thermogenesis in seasonally acclimatized Brandt's voles (*Microtus brandtii*). Horm Behav. 2005;48: 321–8.

79. Lima SL. Predation risk and unpredictable feeding conditions – determinants of body mass in birds. Ecology. 1986;67:377–85.

80. Liu XT, Rossmeisl M, McClaine J, et al. Paradoxical resistance to diet-induced obesity in UCP-1 deficient mice. J Clin Investig. 2003;111:399–407.

81. Liu XM, et al. Brown adipose tissue directly regulates whole body energy metabolism and energy balance. Cell Res. 2013;23:851–4.

82. Liu XM, et al. Brown adipose tissue transplantation reverses obesity in the Ob/Ob mouse. Endocrinology. 2015;156:2461–9.

83. Lord GM, Matarese G, Howard LK, et al. Leptin modulates T-cell immune response and reverse starvation induced immunosuppression. Nature. 1998;394:897–901.

84. Macintyre K. Famine and the female mortality advantage. Chpt 12. In: Dyson T, O'Grada C, editors. Famine demography. Perspectives from the past and present. International studies in demography series. Oxford: Oxford University Press; 2002. p. 240–60.

85. MacLeod R, MacLeod CD, Learmouth JA, et al. Mass-dependent predation risk in lethal dolphin porpoise interactions. Proc R Soc B. 2007;274:2587–93.

86. Martin SL. Mammalian hibernation: a naturally reversible model for insulin resistance in man. Diab Vasc Dis Res. 2008;5:76–81.

87. Matarese G. Leptin and the immune system: how nutritional status influences the immune response. Eur Cytokine Netw. 2000;11:7–13.

88. McCance RA. Famines of history and of today. Proc Nutr Soc. 1975;34:161–6.

89. McDevitt RM, Speakman JR. Central limits to sustainable metabolic-rate have no role in cold-acclimation of the short-tailed field vole (*Microtus-agrestis*). Physiol Zool. 1994;67:1117–39.

90. McDevitt RM, Speakman JR. Summer acclimatization in the short-tailed field vole, *Microtus agrestis*. J Comp Physiol B. 1996;166:286–93.

91. Menken J, Campbell C. Forum: on the demography of South Asian famines. Health Transit Rev. 1992;2: 91–108.
92. Mokyr J, Grada CO. Famine disease and famine mortality: lessons from Ireland, 1845–1850. Centre for Economic Research working paper 99/12. Dublin: University College Dublin; 1999.
93. Monarca RI, da Luz MM, Wang DH, et al. Predation risk modulates diet induced obesity in male C57BL/6 mice. Obesity. 2015a; in press.
94. Monarca R, da Luz MM, Speakman JR. Behavioural and physiological responses of wood mice (*Apodemus sylvaticus*) to experimental manipulations of predation and starvation risk. Physiol Behav. 2015b;149:331–9.
95. Moore F, Kerlinger P. Stopover and fat deposition by North American wood warblers (*Parulinae*) following spring migration over the Gulf of Mexico. Oecologia. 1987;74:47–54.
96. Moriguchi S, Amano T, Ushiyama K, et al. Seasonal and sexual differences in migration timing and fat deposition in greater white-fronted goose. Ornithol Sci. 2010;9:75–82.
97. Mounzih K, Lu RH, Chehab FF. Leptin treatment rescues sterility of genetically obese Ob/Ob males. Endocrinology. 1997;138:1190–3.
98. Nedergaard J, Bengtsson T, Cannon B. Unexpected evidence for active brown adipose tissue in adult humans. Am J Phys. 2007;293:E444–52.
99. Neel JV. Diabetes mellitus a 'thrifty' genotype rendered detrimental by 'progress'? Am J Hum Genet. 1962;14:352–3.
100. Norrdahl K, Korpimaki E. Does mobility or sex of voles affect risk of predation by mammalian predators? Ecology. 1998;79:226–32.
101. O'Rourke RW. Metabolic thrift and the basis of human obesity. Ann Surg. 2014;259:642–8.
102. Ogden CL, Carroll MD, Curtin LR, et al. Prevalence of overweight and obesity in the United States, 1999–2004. JAMA. 2006;295:1549–55.
103. Okada Y, Kubo M, Ohmiya H, et al. Common variants at CDKAL1 and KLF9 are associated with body mass index in east Asian populations. Nat Genet. 2012;44:302–U105.
104. Paternoster L, Evans DM, Nohr EA, et al. Genome wide population based association study of extremely overweight a young adults – the GOYA study. PLoS One. 2012;6:e24303.
105. Platek SM, Gallup GG, Fryer BD. The fireside hypothesis: was there differential selection to tolerate air pollution during human evolution? Med Hypotheses. 2002;58:1–5.
106. Power ML, Schulkin J. The evolution of obesity. Baltimore: John Hopkins University Press; 2009. 408 p.
107. Prentice AM. Obesity and its potential mechanistic basis. Br Med Bull. 2001;60:51–67.
108. Prentice AM. Early influences on human energy regulation: thrifty genotypes and thrifty phenotypes. Physiol Behav. 2005a;86:640–5.
109. Prentice AM. Starvation in humans: evolutionary background and contemporary implications. Mech Ageing Dev. 2005b;126:976–81.
110. Prentice AM. The emerging epidemic of obesity in developing countries. Int J Epidemiol. 2006;35: 93–9.
111. Prentice AM, Jebb SA. Obesity in Britain – gluttony or sloth. Br Med J. 1995;311:437–9.
112. Prentice AM, Rayco-Solon P, Moore SE. Insights from the developing world: thrifty genotypes and thrifty phenotypes. Proc Nutr Soc. 2005;64:153–61.
113. Prentice AM, Hennig BJ, Fulford AJ. Evolutionary origins of the obesity epidemic: natural selection of thrifty genes or genetic drift following predation release? Int J Obes. 2008;32:1607–10.
114. Procope J. Hippocrates on diet and hygiene. London: Zeno; 1952.
115. Puzyrev VP, Kucher AN. Evolutionary ontogenetic aspects of pathogenetics of chronic human diseases. Russ J Genet. 2011;47:1395–405.
116. Rakesh TP, Syam TP. Milder forms of obesity may be a good evolutionary adaptation: 'fitness first' hypothesis. Hypothesis. 2015;13:e4.
117. Razzaque A. Effect of famine on fertility in a rural area of Bangladesh. J Biosoc Sci. 1988;20:287–94.
118. Repenning M, Fontana CS. Seasonality of breeding moult and fat deposition of birds in sub-tropical lowlands of southern Brazil. Emu. 2011;111:268–80.
119. Rothwell NJ, Stock MJ. Role for brown adipose tissue in diet induced thermogenesis. Nature. 1979;281:31–5.
120. Saito M, et al. High incidence of metabolically active brown adipose tissue in healthy adult humans effects of cold exposure and adiposity. Diabetes. 2009;58: 1526–31.
121. Scott S, Duncan SR, Duncan CJ. Infant mortality and famine – a study in historical epidemiology in northern England. J Epidemiol Community Health. 1995;49:245–52.
122. Segal N, Allison DB. Twins and virtual twins: bases of relative body weight revisited. Int J Obes. 2002;26: 437–41.
123. Sellayah D, Cagampang FR, Cox RD. On the evolutionary origins of obesity: a new hypothesis. Endocrinology. 2014;155:1573–88.
124. Simpson SJ, Raubenheimer D. Obesity: the protein leverage hypothesis. Obes Rev. 2005;6:133–42.
125. Simpson SJ, Raubenheimer D. The nature of nutrition: a unifying framework from animal adaptation to human obesity. Princeton: Princeton University Press; 2010. 248pp.
126. Sorensen A, Mayntz D, Raubenheimer D, et al. Protein-leverage in mice: the geometry of macronutrient balancing and consequences for fat deposition. Obesity. 2008;16:566–71.

127. Southam L, Soranzo N, Montgomery SB, et al. Is the thrifty genotype hypothesis supported by evidence based on confirmed type 2 diabetes and obesity susceptibility variants? Diabetologia. 2010;52:1846–51.

128. Speakman JR. Obesity – the integrated roles of environment and genetics. J Nutr. 2004;134:2090S–105S.

129. Speakman JR. Thrifty genes for obesity and the metabolic syndrome – time to call off the search? Diab Vasc Dis Res. 2006a;3:7–11.

130. Speakman JR. The genetics of obesity: five fundamental problems with the famine hypothesis. In: Fantuzzi G, Mazzone T, editors. Adipose tissue and Adipokines in health and disease. New York: Humana Press; 2006b.

131. Speakman JR. A nonadaptive scenario explaining the genetic predisposition to obesity: the "predation release" hypothesis. Cell Metab. 2007;6:5–12.

132. Speakman JR. Thrifty genes for obesity, an attractive but flawed idea, and an alternative perspective: the 'drifty gene' hypothesis. Int J Obes. 2008;32:1611–7.

133. Speakman JR. Evolutionary perspectives on the obesity epidemic: adaptive, maladaptive and neutral viewpoints. Annu Rev Nutr. 2013a;33:289–317.

134. Speakman JR. Sex and age-related mortality profiles during famine: testing the body fat hypothesis. J Biosoc Sci. 2013b;45:823–40.

135. Speakman JR. If body fatness is under physiological regulation, then how come we have an obesity epidemic? Physiology. 2014;29:88–98.

136. Speakman JR. The 'fat mass and obesity related' (FTO) gene: mechanisms of impact on obesity and energy balance. Curr Obes Rep. 2015;4:73–91.

137. Speakman JR, O'Rahilly S. Fat – an evolving issue. Dis Model Mech. 2012;5:569–73.

138. Speakman JR, Rowland A. Preparing for inactivity: how insectivorous bats deposit a fat store for hibernation. Proc Nutr Soc. 1999;58:123–31.

139. Speakman JR, Westerterp KR. Association between energy demands, physical activity and body composition in adult humans between 18 and 96 years of age. Am J Clin Nutr. 2010;92:826–34.

140. Speakman JR, Westerterp KR. A mathematical model of weight loss during total starvation: more evidence against the thrifty gene hypothesis. Dis Model Mech. 2013;6:236–51.

141. Speakman JR, Levitsky DA, Allison DB, et al. Set-points, settling points and some alternative models: theoretical options to understand how genes and environments combine to regulate body adiposity. Dis Model Mech. 2011;4:733–45.

142. Speliotes EK, Willer CJ, Berndt SI, et al. Association analyses of 249,796 individuals reveal 18 new loci associated with body mass index. Nat Genet. 2010;42:937–48.

143. Stanford KI, et al. Brown adipose tissue regulates glucose homeostasis and insulin sensitivity. J Clin Invest. 2013;123:215–23.

144. Stearns PN. The encyclopedia of world history. 6th ed. Boston: Houghton Mifflin; 2001.

145. Stein Z, Susser M. Fertility, fecundity, famine – food rations in Dutch famine 1944–45 have a causal relation to fertility and probably to fecundity. Hum Biol. 1975;47:131–54.

146. Stein ZA, Susser M, Saenger G, et al. Famine and human development: the Dutch hunger winter of 1944–1945. New York: Oxford University Press; 1975.

147. Stöger R. The thrifty epigenotype: an acquired and heritable predisposition for obesity and diabetes? BioEssays. 2008;30:156–66.

148. Sundell J, Norrdahl K. Body size-dependent refuges in voles: an alternative explanation of the chitty effect. Ann Zool Fenn. 2002;39:325–33.

149. Swinburn BA, et al. Estimating the changes in energy flux that characterize the rise in obesity prevalence. Am J Clin Nutr. 2009;89:1723–8.

150. Takenaka A, Nakamura S, Mitsunaga F, et al. Human specific SNP in obesity genes, adrenergic receptor beta 2(ADRB2), beta 3(ADRb3), and PPARgama 2 (PPARG) during primate evolution. PLoS One. 2012;7:e43461.

151. Tidhar WL, Bonnier F, Speakman JR. Sex- and concentration-dependent effects of predator feces on seasonal regulation of body mass in the bank vole Clethrionomys glareolus. Horm Behav. 2007;52:436–44.

152. Toole MJ, Waldman RJ. An analysis of mortality trends among refugee populations in Somalia, Sudan, and Thailand. Bull World Health Organ. 1988;66:237–47.

153. Treves A, Naughton-Treves L. Risk and opportunity for humans coexisting with large carnivores. J Hum Evol. 1999;36:275–82.

154. Valles SA. Evolutionary medicine at twenty: rethinking adaptationism and disease. Biol Philos. 2012;27:241–61.

155. van der Veen IT. Effects of predation risk on diurnal mass dynamics and foraging routines of yellowhammers (Emberiza citrinella). Behav Ecol. 1999;10:545–51.

156. Van Marken-Lichtenbelt W, Vanhommerig JW, Smulders NM, et al. Cold-activated brown adipose tissue in healthy men. N Engl J Med. 2009;360:1500–8.

157. Wade GN, Bartness TJ. Seasonal obesity in Syrian hamsters – effects of age, diet, photoperiod and melatonin. Am J Phys. 1984;247:R328–34.

158. Ward JM, Armitage KB. Circannual rhythms of food consumption, body mass and metabolism in yellowbellied marmots. Comp Biochem Physiol. 1981;69A:621–6.

159. Watkins SC, Menken J. Famines in historical perspective. Popul Dev Rev. 1985;11:647–75.

160. Watnick S. Obesity: a problem of Darwinian proportions? Adv Chronic Kidney Dis. 2006;13:428–32.

161. Weigle DS, Duell PB, Connor WE, et al. Effect of fasting, refeeding and dietary fat restriction on plasma leptin levels. J Clin Endocrinol Metab. 1997;82:561–5.

162. Wells JCK. The evolution of human fatness and susceptibility to obesity: an ethological approach. Biol Rev. 2006;81:183–205.

163. Wells JC. The thrifty phenotype as an adaptive maternal effect. Biol Rev Camb Philos Soc. 2007;82:143–72.

164. Wen WQ, Cho YS, Zheng W, et al. Meta-analysis identifies common variants associated with body mass index in east Asians. Nat Genet. 2012;44:307–U122.

165. Westerterp KR, Speakman JR. Physical activity energy expenditure has not declined since the 1980s and matches energy expenditures of wild mammals. Int J Obes. 2008;32:1256–63.

166. Willer CJ, Speliotes EK, Loos RJF, et al. Six new loci associated with body mass index highlight a neuronal influence on body weight regulation. Nat Genet. 2009;41:25–35.

167. Witter MS, Cuthill IC. The ecological costs of avian fat storage. Philos Trans R Soc Lond B. 1993;340: 73–92.

168. Wunder BA, Dobkin DS, Gettinger RD. Shifts in thermogenesis in prairie vole (*Microtus ochrogaster*)-strategies for survival in a seasonal environment. Oecologia. 1977;29:11–26.

169. Yoneshiro T, et al. Age-related decrease in cold-activated brown adipose tissue and accumulation of body fat in fealthy humans. Obesity. 2011;19: 1755–60.

170. Zaadstra BM, Siedell JC, Vannord PAH, et al. Fat and female fecundity – prospective study of effect of body fat distribution on conception rates. Br Med J. 1993;306:484–7.

171. Zhang LN, Mitchell SE, Hambly C, et al. Physiological and behavioral responses to intermittent starvation in C57BL/6J mice. Physiol Behav. 2012;105: 376–87.

172. Zimmer C, Boos M, Poulin N, et al. Evidence of the trade-off between starvation and predation risk in ducks. PLoS One. 2011;6:e22352.

173. Zinn AR. Unconventional wisdom about the obesity epidemic. Am J Med Sci. 2010;340:481–91.

Genetics of Type 2 Diabetes

9

Struan F. A. Grant

Contents

S. F. A. Grant (✉)
Center for Spatial and Functional Genomics, Divisions of
Human Genetics and Endocrinology & Diabetes,
Children's Hospital of Philadelphia; Department of
Genetics, Department of Pediatrics, Institute of Diabetes,
Obesity and Metabolism, Perelman School of Medicine,
University of Pennsylvania, Philadelphia, Pennsylvania,
USA
e-mail: grants@chop.edu

© Springer Nature Switzerland AG 2023
R. S. Ahima (ed.), *Metabolic Syndrome*,
https://doi.org/10.1007/978-3-031-40116-9_11

Abstract

The promise of high-throughput genomics has started to deliver novel insights in the genetic etiology of type 2 diabetes and its related traits. In particular, genome-wide association studies (GWAS) have revealed new biological underpinnings to metabolic traits, with particular focus being on the strongest loci *TCF7L2* and

FTO. However, many challenges still lie ahead as much of the "missing heritability" of such traits remains to be elucidated, with only a proportion of the genetic component to type 2 diabetes being characterized to date. Undeterred, investigators are aiming to use what has been found to already attempt risk prediction models, while laboratory-based researchers are trying to elucidate functional mechanisms. However, the latter have a number of challenges as these well-established signals still have to fully characterize the causal tissue, the causal variant, and often the actual causal gene. However, once advances are made of these fronts, the future looks bright with respect to the development of novel therapeutics and diagnostics for type 2 diabetes and its related traits.

Keywords

Heredity · Genome-wide association studies · Polygenic risk score

Introduction

Type 2 diabetes (T2D) is a member of the complex traits that are both common and known to have a genetic component. The reason T2D is considered complex is that there are two primary processes underpinning the disorder, i.e., insulin resistance and defects in insulin secretion. It is widely believed that discrete genetic factors play a role in these two mechanisms, which in turn influence T2D susceptibility. Insulin resistance is widely influenced by obesity, where a separate genetic etiology has also been implicated. However, teasing out the genetic factors contributing to the pathogenesis of T2D, where there is also such a marked environmental influence on risk, has proved challenging. So much so that before the era of GWAS, T2D was referred to as the "geneticist's nightmare," and the prospect of discovering the underlying genetic factors in this polygenic trait was equated to discovering the "Holy Grail."

Before one embarks on a genetic hunt for variants contributing to the pathogenesis of a disease, one has to convince oneself that there is indeed a genetic component to the trait. In the context of T2D, there is evidence from concordance observations when contrasting monozygotic twins with dizygotic twins, while segregation analyses in families have led to the conclusion that the sibling risk for T2D is approximately 3.5-fold [1]. As such, investigators have been motivated to seek out the genetic contributors to this common disease affecting many populations.

Candidate Gene and Family-Based Studies

In the relative dark ages before the advent of GWAS (i.e., prior to 2005), the only approach for assessing genes and their putative roles in complex traits was the *candidate gene approach*. Although a number of genes were robustly implicated in the pathogenesis of T2D during that period, the candidate gene approach was heavily biased by the "winner's curse" [2], where an investigator would select their favorite gene based on an already known role in the pathogenesis of the trait but would only formally report the finding if an association with a variant reached a significance level of $P = 0.05$. As such, there was an inherent bias in what result was reported, thus many of these loci were not replicated by peer investigative groups.

The handful of candidate genes for T2D that held up include peroxisome proliferator-activated receptor gamma (*PPARG*), calpain 10 (*CAPN10*), and "potassium inwardly rectifying channel, subfamily J, member 11" (*KCNJ11*) [3–5].

The first opportunity to carry out a hypothesis-free approach was with the advent of genome-wide linkage studies. These studies were enabled by panels of hundreds of microsatellites in complete linkage equilibrium, therefore, if a region of the genome was shared within and across families with a given trait, it could be detected by this approach. When it came to complex traits including T2D, regions of significant linkage were indeed detected [6] but the resolution of the approach was very crude, resulting in an average region of approximately 10–20 Mb, meaning that many hundreds of genes were harbored in such a wide location, i.e., the short list of genes was still very long. Trying to drill down on the linked region using follow-up association testing with additional microsatellites and/or with SNPs proved challenging. Although relatively successful for syndromic disorders, this approach did not yield many robust novel genes for complex diseases, largely due to the fact that the principle drivers of linkage signals are rare variants with high risk while it is now widely considered that the modest effect "common variant, common disease" hypothesis is more likely to underpin complex traits. As such if a variant is common it is unlikely that it will have very high impact as the selective pressure against it is so high. Thus the "age of enlightenment" came about in 2005, when the GWAS was able to detect such variants.

Genome-Wide Association Studies (GWAS)

In order to allow for genome-wide assessment of association, technological advances were required in order to move away from simple single gene assessments. The outcomes from the HapMap project [7, 8] proved feasible to leverage for this endeavor as it was observed that SNPs "travel" in blocks, i.e., regions of linkage disequilibrium (LD) occur in discrete "LD blocks." It became clear that a given LD block harbors a lot of redundancy with respect to information content, where there is a limited amount of haplotype diversity, and thus can be captured by small subset of the variants in the LD block and the rest can be subsequently inferred or "imputed" [9].

As such, rather than having to genotype the millions of common SNPs in the genome (minor allele frequency > 5%) in order to assess the genome for association with complex traits, one can leverage handpicked "tag-SNPs" that capture all common variation and can be boiled down to just hundreds of thousands of SNPs. As a consequence, this number of SNPs can be arrayed on a single chip, thus facilitating high-throughput genotyping in a cost-effect manner.

By genotyping thousands of patients and thousands of controls with such arrays the discovery of novel loci associated with common diseases has been facilitated, including for T2D (see below). Indeed, now many hundreds of variants have been reported for various common diseases, but unlike the candidate gene era, these variants are generally highly replicable and coincide with genes that suggest novel biology underpinning such traits. Indeed, for the first time in complex trait genetics research there is strong consensus among investigators on the robustness of a vast majority of these observations. The NHGRI and EBI maintain a queryable record of these reports and can be found at https://www.ebi.ac.uk/gwas.

The resulting data can be presented in a simple graph, where the x-axis represents the geographical order down each chromosome in turn while the y-axis reveals the strength of the association via a P value. One requires a large number of cases and controls in order to overcome the inevitable correction for multiple testing given the large number of SNPs being tested; after all, every 20th SNP will yield a P value of 0.05 by chance, so this cannot be considered the appropriate bar for significance in this setting; rather it has been calculated that there is a finite level of common diversity in the genome, so a specific bar for significance at the genome-wide level is $P = 5 \times 10^{-8}$. If that level of significance is achieved, there is a strong likelihood that this signal will replicate, a step which is indeed expected from a GWAS observation before it is considered publishable. These signals appear as spikes in graphs thus rendering them as plots resembling the New York City skyline; indeed, they are referred to as "Manhattan Plots" and what researchers are looking for are "Empire State Building"–type signals.

When one turns to the specific signals resulting from GWAS efforts of T2D, the first such report was in 2007 [10]. In that study, a number of loci achieved genome-wide significance, with the strongest "Empire State Building" signal being across the gene encoding transcription factor 7-like 2 (*TCF7L2*, formerly known as *TCF4*) [10]. Indeed, our group first published this association a year earlier through a rare success story of an association follow-up effort to a linkage signal [11] which has gone on to be replicated in diverse populations, in Europe, Asia, and Africa [12], and is now considered the strongest common genetic association with T2D in most ethnicities [13, 14]. Findings related to functional studies of *TCF7L2* and T2D are described below to exemplify the challenges with such follow-up efforts.

In addition to agreeing on the *TCF7L2* signal, the first T2D GWAS reports [10, 15–18] revealed signals within loci that harbored the following genes: "homeobox hematopoietically expressed" (*HHEX*), "solute carrier family 30 (zinc transporter), member 8" (*SLC30A8*), "CDK5 regulatory subunit associated protein 1-like 1" (*CDKAL1*), "insulin-like growth factor 2 mRNA-binding protein 2" (*IGF2BP2*), "cyclin-dependent kinase inhibitor 2A/B" (*CDKN2A/B*), and an intragenic region on 11p12. However, GWAS efforts in East Asians, where the haplotypic structure is substantially different from Europeans, revealed a different set of signals, with "KQT-like subfamily, member 1" (*KCNQ1*) being the gene harboring the strongest association [19, 20]. Furthermore, a strong association with common variants within the gene encoding "solute carrier family 16, member 11" (*SLC16A11*) has been shown to confer risk for T2D in Mexicans [21].

When one has exhausted the mining of the initial GWAS efforts in a given cohort, and in order to get the most of the large financial investment, investigators combine their datasets in order to find additional "Chrysler" and "Woolworth building"-type signals. The first such "meta-analysis" of T2D GWAS efforts in cohorts of European ancestry [22] revealed six additional loci corresponding to the following genes: "ADAM metallopeptidase with thrombospondin type 1 motif, 9" (*ADAMTS9*), "tetraspanin 8"/ "leucine-rich repeat-containing G protein-coupled receptor 5" (*TSPAN8-LGR5*), "cell division cycle 123 homolog"/"calcium/calmodulin-dependent protein kinase ID" (*CDC123-CAMK1D*), *NOTCH2*, "thyroid adenoma associated" (*THADA*), and "juxtaposed with another zinc finger gene 1" (*JAZF1*).

Larger and larger subsequent meta-analyses through the combination of more and more datasets revealed additional common variants but with diminishingly small effects [22–40], with the largest trans-ethnic meta-analysis derived from Europeans, African Americans, Hispanics, South Asians, and East Asians, made up of 228,499 cases and 1,178,783 controls, revealing genome-wide significant 568 signals [40].

Although in excess of 550 loci have now been established for T2D, it is clear that only a degree of the "missing heritability" [41] for the disease has been found, thus a substantial proportion of the genetic etiology of this disease still remains to be characterized.

T2D Risk Prediction

Undeterred by the fact that only a minority of the missing heritability has been predicted to be uncovered for T2D, investigators have already aimed to look at the predictive power of the robust variants established to date, especially if one is to consider the cumulative risk.

When the first "low-hanging fruit' variants had been uncovered, it was initially suggested that they did not add sufficient predictive power to other nongenetic predictors already known. For instance, a study of 18 variants did show that the risk of T2D was increased by 12% per risk allele [42], and that risk was increased by 2.6-fold when contrasting subjects who had the lowest genotype risk score with those who had the highest. However, this risk score model did not aid in prediction when one considered familial history of diabetes and/or other known risk factors. A parallel study published in the same issue of the *New England Journal of Medicine* made a similar conclusion, with only marginal improvement in predictive power when contrasted with clinical risk factors alone [43].

However, as more loci have been established to be associated with T2D over time, there is a general opinion that the risk predictive power is improving. A study of 40 SNPs suggested that the predicted risk of developing T2D was better in younger people [44]. Subsequent studies have suggested a degree of predictive power if harnessing in excess of 30 variants, particularly if combined with clinical risk factors [45–47]. But as long as a proportion of the missing heritability remains elusive, the predictive power of such collections of variants remains suboptimal and hinders diagnostic attempts, including direct to consumer testing efforts.

Sequencing Efforts: Missense Variants

The prevailing view is that much of the missing heritability is beyond the detection bandwidth of GWAS, where the still-to-be-characterized variants are not as common and do not confer very sizeable risk of T2D. In order to detect such variants one will need to collect larger and larger cohorts and carry out extensive sequencing efforts, of which the analytical challenges are very demanding. Indeed, more recent and larger scale sequencing efforts have accelerated the discovery of such variants [48, 49].

Some key success stories have been described, particularly when looking at specific geographic regions using sequencing technologies. The most obvious example is the common Arg684Ter missense variant within the "TBC1 domain family, member 4" (*TBC1D4*) gene uncovered in Greenland, which confers a staggering tenfold risk for homozygotes but its effects appear limited to that country. Although limited in its diagnostic applicability, this approach in an isolated population did uncover a bona fide novel possible therapeutic generalizable target for the disease.

Rare variants contributing to T2D have also been reported in other populations, with Iceland proving a rich source of such events, including uncovering variants in the genes encoding cyclin D2 (*CCND2*), peptidylglycine alpha-amidating monooxygenase (*PAM*), and pancreatic and duodenal homeobox 1 (*PDX1*) [50]. In addition, an investigative group uncovered rare loss-of-function variants in the "solute carrier family 30" (*SLC30A8*) gene that actually confers protection from T2D, suggesting a rich possibility for intervention opportunities [51]. Furthermore, a rare variant in the HNF1 homeobox A (*HNF1A*) gene has been found specifically in Latinos [52].

Collectively, these newly sequencing-identified variants do not explain much more of the missing heritability of T2D than what was found solely with GWAS, and the remaining such variants are going to be increasingly difficult to uncover. But as analytical and technical breakthroughs occur then the portfolio of rare, impactful, and not-so-impactful missense variants should be detected on a more regular basis. However, rare variants with modest effects in noncoding regions will prove far more challenging to fully elucidate.

GWAS Outcomes for Obesity

T2D and increased body mass index (BMI) are well known to be strongly correlated. As with other complex traits, many loci have been implicated in conferring risk for obesity. However, the first such locus suggested by this approach, insulin-induced gene 2 (*INSIG2*), failed to be widely replicated by others [53–57].

However, now 941 loci have been robustly established by GWAS as a consequence of larger and larger meta-analyses [58–66]. In fact, the "Empire State Building" signal on chromosome 16 for obesity/increased BMI was initially uncovered in a GWAS of T2D [67], but the authors of the study observed that the association was lost when corrected for BMI. Another study published around the same time also implicated the same locus as a consequence of a study of population markers [68]. This signal resides within the "fat mass and obesity associated" (*FTO*) gene and accounts for only approximately 1% of the predicted genetic component to obesity.

Indeed, subjects homozygous for the *FTO* BMI-increasing allele have been found to weigh on average 3 kg more than subjects carrying the other allele [69]. Interestingly, children homozygous for the BMI-decreasing allele of *FTO* eat significantly less than those carrying the BMI-increasing allele, pointing to a possible mechanism where the BMI-decreasing allele protects against overeating due to neuronal signaling for satiety [70, 71].

Functional Follow-Up of GWAS-Implicated Loci

The fact that the loci uncovered from GWAS do not explain the entire genetic architecture of complex traits has not deterred researchers from starting to look at the functional role of the signals already reported. After all, even though each locus does not explain a big proportion of the genetic component of common traits, these highly reproducible signals could represent generalizable targets for novel therapeutic intervention opportunities.

The loci that have received the most attention in this context have been the "Empire State Building" signals that have come up in T2D and obesity. As such, this section is going to highlight what has been found with efforts on *TCF7L2* and *FTO* loci to exemplify the sort of approaches that can be used to translate these findings.

The main challenge is that when a signal is observed in a given GWAS, all that one really is observing is a signal that is overrepresented in the DNA of a set of patients as compared to a set of controls, so one has very little clue on what the causal variant or causal tissue is with respect to where the site of action is. Furthermore, there is even doubt if the actual causal gene has been identified. These issues are tackled below as we go through the functional studies outlined.

Causal Variant

Before one can proceed to resolving the function of a GWAS-implicated locus, the best place to start is to determine what precisely the tag-SNPs are capturing. As mentioned above, it is unlikely the actual causal variant was physically present on the genotyping array, rather an SNP in LD with the causal variant has "traveled" through the generations with it. Elucidating the actual causal lesion at the multitude of GWAS loci has proved very challenging and to date only a handful of loci in the complex trait area have been resolved [72].

However, given that the *TCF7L2* locus for T2D was reported nearly a decade ago, it has received widespread attention and thus represents one of the few loci where the causal variant is presumed to have been identified. By leveraging the fact that different ethnic groups have different haplotypic structures, and assuming the same locus contributes to a trait across multiple races, one can fine map down the number of variants that the causal variant must be. These are known as "credible sets" and allow investigators to have a manageable shortlist of variants to work with [72].

Following on from refinement studies in Africans and resequencing efforts in African Americans [73, 74], Bayesian modeling strongly supported the previous reports by implicating rs7903146 within the third intron as being the causal variant at this locus [72]. Of particular note is that the risk T allele of rs7903146 is common in populations of European and African ancestry but not in East Asians, which is consistent with the fact that the association is present in that population but is often too difficult to detect as the variant is somewhat more rare in that ethnicity [75–80].

The same approach has now implicated shortlists of variants for other GWAS-implicated T2D and obesity loci [38, 65, 72].

Causal Tissue

TCF7L2

Although there is wide consensus that the causal susceptibility variant at the *TCF7L2* locus is the T allele of rs7903146, it is still very unclear in which tissue(s) it exerts its effect. But with the causal lesion now determined, that gives this locus a head start over its contemporary loci which have not received the same amount of attention. Given that the variant resides in an intronic region, many researchers have investigated it from a regulatory point of view by studying aspects of allele-specific expression, splicing, and chromatin state [81]. Many studies have been carried out to understand the mechanism by which TCF7L2 plays a regulatory role in T2D pathogenesis. With the fact that T2D is a metabolic disease, the primary tissues that have received most attention have been the pancreatic islet [82], liver [83], adipose tissue

[84], and the enteroendocrine L cell [85]. This work is outlined below.

Pancreatic Islet

As the *TCF7L2* locus association is stronger in cohorts with leaner T2D cases [64], the prevailing view is that the lesion is involved in insulin secretion as opposed to insulin resistance. It is therefore not surprising that the majority of studies published to date have focused on the pancreatic islet, with many key studies suggesting that the risk variant influences beta cell function and thus subsequent progression to diabetes [86, 87].

Leveraging small interfering RNA in human islets to deplete levels of TCF7L2 has led to an observation of reduced β-cell proliferation and elevated β cell apoptosis. In addition, glucose-stimulated insulin secretion has been shown to be impacted by the loss of TCF7L2 in islets derived from either mice or humans, while conversely overexpression of *TCF7L2* in islets resulted in resistance to glucose and cytokine-induced apoptosis [88]. Furthermore, using a dominant-negative *TCF7L2* model in rodent INS-1 cells led to the repression of proliferation, leading to the conclusion that TCF7L2 is involved in the maintenance of beta cell mass [89].

There have been some reports that *TCF7L2* mRNA levels in human pancreatic islets are elevated as the number of T2D risk alleles increases, and that the overexpression of *TCF7L2* in the same tissue leads to reduced insulin secretion [82, 90], but some other reports have not observed such an effect [91]. However, one key study did show that risk allele of rs7903146 was more abundant in the open chromatin fraction of pancreatic islets using formaldehyde-assisted isolation of DNA combined with sequencing (FAIRE-seq) suggesting that role of this variant is related to an allele-specific effect on transcriptional activity, promoter usage, and/or splicing [81].

Despite the abundance of interesting mRNA expression results, the main debate concerning TCF7L2 in pancreatic islet beta cells is the distinct paucity of TCF7L2 protein levels in the beta cell. Indeed, immunohistochemical staining in adult mouse pancreatic islets failed to detect the TCF7L2 protein [85], and similar results were seen in human beta cells [92]. Furthermore, the generation of a conditional *TCF7L2* knockout mouse model [93–95] revealed that deleting the gene from β cells had no impact on embryonic development of the endocrine pancreas, β cell proliferation, or expression of the key genes operating in that tissue. As such, there is a need to explore other tissues and mechanisms. For example, it has been suggested that TCF7L2 influences nicotine action in the brain, via a habenula-pancreas axis driving the pathogenesis of diabetes [96].

Liver

When one examines the liver-specific deletion in the *TCF7L2* knockout mouse model, hepatic lipid metabolism was not affected [93], suggesting that the gene's function impacts postnatal metabolic adaptation rather than during the development of the embryo. It became clear that key genes related to glycogen metabolism were significantly reduced in *TCF7L2* knockout rodent newborn liver in contrast with their wild-type littermates, including glycogen synthase 2 (*GYS2*). Genes related to gluconeogenesis were also impacted, such as phosphoenolpyruvate carboxykinase 1 (*PCK1*) and glucose-6-phosphate, catalytic subunit (*G6PC*) [93].

Gastrointestinal Tract

The gastrointestinal tract remains a popular area to investigate the role of *TCF7L2* function in the context of T2D. The full knockout mouse is embryonic lethal as a consequence of a defect in the proliferation of crypt stem cells in the small intestine [97]. Those studying the gastrointestinal tract are motivated by the hypothesis that *TCF7L2* plays a pivotal role in glucose homeostasis via the insulinotropic hormone glucagon-like peptide 1 (GLP-1), which is known to be produced in the enteroendocrine L cells of the small intestine [98]. It is also well known that *TCF7L2* occupies the promoter of the proglucagon gene, a crucial precursor to GLP-1, and is involved in its transcriptional control based on the work in intestinal GLUTag cells. In this setting, the dominant-negative mutant for *TCF7L2* depletes proglucagon mRNA levels [85], thus dramatically impacting GLP-1 levels in the intestinal tract [85].

Furthermore, immunohistochemistry with a TCF7L2-specific monoclonal antibody in human cells revealed a very restricted expression pattern that was limited to normal intestinal and mammary epithelium, together with the related carcinomas observed in the same tissues [99].

And finally, it has been known for over 15 years that missense mutations in *TCF7L2* (formerly TCF4) cause colorectal cancer [100], thus further implicating the role of this gene in the intestinal tract – see more details below.

Adipose Tissue

Despite there being less motivation to investigate a role for TCF7L2 in insulin resistance, there have been reports showing that *TCF7L2* expression levels are reduced in subcutaneous adipose tissue from patients with T2D [101]. In addition, tissue-specific alternative splicing of *TCF7L2* has been reported, in particular in the adipose setting [102–104], suggesting that the coordinated expression of this gene in this tissue is physiologically relevant and meaningful to metabolic control.

Connection to Cancer

As mentioned above, prior to its reported association with T2D, *TCF7L2* was already well established as a colorectal cancer susceptibility gene [105, 106]. This is partly due to the fact that TCF7L2 plays a role in regulating the expression of key genes involved in the control of the G1 to S phase transition in the cell cycle, including cyclin D1 and c-myc [107, 108]. Furthermore, extensive resequencing of genomic DNA from colorectal adenocarcinomas has revealed recurrent *TCF7L2* gene fusions with its neighboring gene, *VTI1A,* thus contributing to the pathogenesis of this cancer [109].

However, the role *TCF7L2* in cancer is complex. When one conducts a GWAS in most of the common cancers, the "Empire State Building" signal is located in a gene desert on chromosome 8q24 [110–123]. Subsequent follow-up of this multicancer locus revealed that the mechanism was through an extreme upstream TCF7L2 occupancy site that was involved in the transcriptional control of the *MYC* gene [124–126].

Going beyond *TCF7L2,* an interesting pattern is beginning to emerge, where many of the strongest associated GWAS-implicated T2D risk alleles protect against prostate cancer [127], including *THADA, JAZF1,* and *TCF2* (also known as *HNF1B*) [22, 128, 129].

As such, the link between T2D and cancer at the GWAS level is clear and is a potential clue on the functional mechanism of many of these key loci in metabolism. However, irrespective of the actual causal tissue (and indeed it may be all of the above as opposed to being restricted to just one), TCF7L2 is now extensively considered a "master regulator" of the canonical Wnt signaling pathway, where it plays a crucial role in multiple development processes [130–134]. Indeed, the mining of ChIP-seq data derived from multiple tissue-derived cell lines reveals that the list of genes bound by TCF7L2 are consistently and significantly enriched for both endocrine-related pathways and GWAS-implicated loci for various cardio-metabolic traits [92, 135, 136].

FTO

The *FTO* gene has received extensive attention, including being the subject of an article in *Science* characterizing FTO as encoding a "2-oxoglutarate-dependent nucleic acid demethylase" [137]. The areas of the body where it is most expressed, namely in key areas of the brain that influence appetite [137, 138], makes a lot of sense with respect to role in the pathogenesis of obesity from an increased energy intake perspective [70].

The mouse model lacking the *Fto* gene showed increased energy expenditure and was leaner, suggesting that targeting *FTO* could protect against obesity [69, 139, 140]. Conversely, the *Fto* ubiquitously overexpressing mouse reveals an increase in body and fat mass, primarily related to increased food intake [69].

The data suggest that FTO operates via CNS mechanisms, likely via the hypothalamus, to control feeding and metabolism. While there is excitement that FTO may be a therapeutic target for obesity, further investigation is necessary to discover the causal gene at this genomic region.

Causal Gene

GWAS has now delivered a large number of genomic signals that are associated with a myriad of common diseases and complex traits. Many of these loci have been widely validated and are thus considered robust observations by the community. However, these reports only represent a genomic signal and not necessarily, as often presumed, the localization of a culprit gene. This is due to the fact that gene expression can be controlled locally or via large genomic distances; indeed, most regulatory elements do not control the nearest genes and can reside tens or hundreds of kb away.

One clear example of this in highlighting how ignoring this basic concept in molecular biology can lead to misdirected research efforts is the strong associated signal with common obesity and *FTO*. Hundreds of scientific papers have been published studying the role of FTO in the context of obesity and/or BMI determination; however, two key papers revealed that this signal was actually an enhancer for at least the neighboring *IRX3* and *IRX5* genes [141, 142] leveraging chromatin conformation capture (3C)-based techniques. Such approaches can aid in the identification of causal genes at such loci by identifying genomic regions that are in physical contact with the locus of interest, although the search can be complicated by temporal effects [143]. Once the causal genes are actually identified with greater confidence, development can take place for therapeutic and diagnostic purposes.

Genetics of Early Life: Implications for T2D in Later Life

It is well established that many of the risk factors for common diseases of middle and old age often have their origins in childhood. If one can determine the genetic basis to these observations then possible early-stage interventions could be developed.

For instance, a link between low birth weight and the development of metabolic disease in adulthood has been established [144]. Genetic variation at the locus harboring the glucokinase (*GCK*) gene, which encodes a protein involved in pancreatic glucose-sensing and has been implicated by GWAS analyses of T2D related traits, has been shown to have differing effects on birth weight depending whether it is carried by the mother or the fetus [145]. This exemplifies the importance of endogenous fetal insulin-secreting capacity in order to determine antenatal growth, which is also known as the "fetal insulin hypothesis" [146].

Taking this concept one step further, a study consisting of >15,000 subjects and over 8000 mothers showed that for each maternal risk-conferring rs7903146 allele within *TCF7L2* increased birth weight while the combined effect of 3–4 maternal risk-conferring alleles of *TCF7L2* and *GCK* showed an even more marked impact [147]; however, the *TCF7L2* interaction with birth weight is not universally agreed upon [148, 149], possibly due to statistical power differences between study designs.

Such reports have led to subsequent studies looking at other T2D GWAS loci in the context of birth weight, with positive reports for loci including *CDKAL1*, *HHEX-IDE*, *CDKN2A/B*, *JAZF1, and IGFBP2* [149–153]. However, the full significance of these observations requires additional follow-up to fully understand the mechanism of action.

A meta-analysis of six European ancestry cohorts with GWAS data for birth weight identified variants associated with lower birth weight [154], with a subsequent larger meta-analysis from the same consortium revealing additional loci [155–157]. Of particular note were the adenylate cyclase 5 (*ADCY5*) and *CDKAL1* loci, as they are already established for T2D; however, it appears that their primary role is in much earlier life.

Another influence of childhood on adulthood is in the context of obesity. Indeed, approximately 70% of children who are obese during adolescence become obese adults [158–160] and are thus at much higher risk of disease in later life, including T2D. It has therefore been important to uncover the genetic determinants of childhood obesity as it would not only have implications for pediatric health but also for diseases of old age. Furthermore, it is also highly likely that it is easier to distill out genetic loci contributing to obesity in the pediatric setting where the influence of environmental confounders is lessened.

Cross-sectional cohort studies have consistently reported an age-dependent effect of high-risk *FTO* variants on BMI. The first reports revealed that there was no influence on fetal growth or birth weight, while the effect on BMI became most pronounced by the age of 7 years [67]. Indeed, a subsequent study found a negative association between the key *FTO* variant and BMI before the age of 2 years old and only took effect after that time point [161]. Furthermore, there is a growing picture that very few of the risk alleles first detected in the adult GWAS analyses of BMI have an influence on birth weight [162], which is in contrast to risk variants reported for T2D [163].

The Early Growth Genetics Consortium went on to conduct the largest GWAS for childhood obesity reported to date [164, 165] and observed many of the detected loci in adults but with a much lower sample number, supporting the notion that the pediatric setting is a more sensitive setting to uncover obesity genes.

LADA: A Major Confounder in Genetic Studies of T2D

With the search for more and more subtle effect size variants in T2D-related traits, there is an increasing risk that artifacts will be detected and inappropriate assignment of loci to the disease. After all, the *TCF7L2* locus confers a relative risk of 1.4 while the more recent loci are closer to 1.1. As sample sizes increase in ever bigger meta-analyses, the likelihood that comorbidities are driving some new signals is ever more likely, especially when hunting for loci that yield sub 1.1 odds ratios.

A clear example of this is the fact that among any given group of randomly selected T2D patients there will be in fact islet antibody–

positive subjects present at a frequency of 8–10% [166, 167]. There is good recent evidence to believe that subjects often referred to as "latent autoimmune diabetes in adults" (LADA) cases will be driving some of the more recent signals reported in massive meta-analyses of T2D GWAS. Indeed, the well-established autoimmune loci harboring the GLIS family zinc finger 3 (*GLIS3*) and "zinc finger, MIZ-type containing 1" (*ZMIZ1*) genes, respectively, have been reported to be associated with T2D [168]. Moreover, the most recent GWAS meta-analysis of T2D in African Americans reported two loci [34], *HLA-B and INS-IGF2*, both of which are well-known type 1 diabetes (T1D) loci.

Motivated by such observations we conducted the first GWAS of LADA, revealing that the lead signals were indeed established T1D loci. However, we also found that there were positive genome-wide genetic correlations with both T1D and T2D [169].

Conclusion

Although there have been huge advances in elucidating the genetics of T2D-related traits, much is still to be uncovered. Apart from the missing heritability that remains to be characterized, there remains challenges when it comes to determining the causal tissue, causal variant, and even the causal gene for many of the established GWAS loci. Once advances are made in these key areas, a better understanding of the genetic etiology of T2D will be in place and new therapeutic and diagnostic opportunities should present themselves.

References

1. Rich SS. Mapping genes in diabetes. Genetic epidemiological perspective. Diabetes. 1990;39(11):1315–9.
2. Lohmueller KE, Pearce CL, Pike M, Lander ES, Hirschhorn JN. Meta-analysis of genetic association studies supports a contribution of common variants to susceptibility to common disease. Nat Genet. 2003;33 (2):177–82.
3. Altshuler D, Hirschhorn JN, Klannemark M, Lindgren CM, Vohl MC, Nemesh J, et al. The common PPARgamma Pro12Ala polymorphism is

associated with decreased risk of type 2 diabetes. Nat Genet. 2000;26(1):76–80.
4. Gloyn AL, Weedon MN, Owen KR, Turner MJ, Knight BA, Hitman G, et al. Large-scale association studies of variants in genes encoding the pancreatic beta-cell KATP channel subunits Kir6.2 (KCNJ11) and SUR1 (ABCC8) confirm that the KCNJ11 E23K variant is associated with type 2 diabetes. Diabetes. 2003;52(2):568–72.
5. Horikawa Y, Oda N, Cox NJ, Li X, Orho-Melander M, Hara M, et al. Genetic variation in the gene encoding calpain-10 is associated with type 2 diabetes mellitus. Nat Genet. 2000;26(2):163–75.
6. Reynisdottir I, Thorleifsson G, Benediktsson R, Sigurdsson G, Emilsson V, Einarsdottir AS, et al. Localization of a susceptibility gene for type 2 diabetes to chromosome 5q34-q35.2. Am J Hum Genet. 2003;73(2):323–35.
7. The International HapMap Project. Nature. 2003;426 (6968):789–96.
8. A haplotype map of the human genome. Nature. 2005;437(7063):1299–320.
9. Stephens M, Smith NJ, Donnelly P. A new statistical method for haplotype reconstruction from population data. Am J Hum Genet. 2001;68(4):978–89.
10. Sladek R, Rocheleau G, Rung J, Dina C, Shen L, Serre D, et al. A genome-wide association study identifies novel risk loci for type 2 diabetes. Nature. 2007;445(7130):881–5.
11. Grant SF, Thorleifsson G, Reynisdottir I, Benediktsson R, Manolescu A, Sainz J, et al. Variant of transcription factor 7-like 2 (TCF7L2) gene confers risk of type 2 diabetes. Nat Genet. 2006;38(3):320–3.
12. Cauchi S, El Achhab Y, Choquet H, Dina C, Krempler F, Weitgasser R, et al. TCF7L2 is reproducibly associated with type 2 diabetes in various ethnic groups: a global meta-analysis. J Mol Med. 2007;85 (7):777–82.
13. Zeggini E, McCarthy MI. TCF7L2: the biggest story in diabetes genetics since HLA? Diabetologia. 2007;50(1):1–4.
14. Weedon MN. The importance of TCF7L2. Diabet Med. 2007;24(10):1062–6.
15. Wellcome Trust Case Control Consortium. Genome-wide association study of 14,000 cases of seven common diseases and 3000 shared controls. Nature. 2007;447(7145):661–78.
16. Saxena R, Voight BF, Lyssenko V, Burtt NP, de Bakker PI, Chen H, et al. Genome-wide association analysis identifies loci for type 2 diabetes and triglyceride levels. Science. 2007;316(5829):1331–6.
17. Zeggini E, Weedon MN, Lindgren CM, Frayling TM, Elliott KS, Lango H, et al. Replication of genome-wide association signals in UK samples reveals risk loci for type 2 diabetes. Science. 2007;316(5829):1336–41.
18. Scott LJ, Mohlke KL, Bonnycastle LL, Willer CJ, Li Y, Duren WL, et al. A genome-wide association study of type 2 diabetes in Finns detects multiple susceptibility variants. Science. 2007;316(5829):1341–5.
19. Unoki H, Takahashi A, Kawaguchi T, Hara K, Horikoshi M, Andersen G, et al. SNPs in KCNQ1 are associated with susceptibility to type 2 diabetes in East Asian and European populations. Nat Genet. 2008;40(9):1098–102.
20. Yasuda K, Miyake K, Horikawa Y, Hara K, Osawa H, Furuta H, et al. Variants in KCNQ1 are associated with susceptibility to type 2 diabetes mellitus. Nat Genet. 2008;40(9):1092–7.
21. Williams AL, Jacobs SB, Moreno-Macias H, Huerta-Chagoya A, Churchhouse C, Marquez-Luna C, et al. Sequence variants in SLC16A11 are a common risk factor for type 2 diabetes in Mexico. Nature. 2014;506 (7486):97–101. Epub 2014/01/07. https://doi.org/10.1038/nature12828.
22. Zeggini E, Scott LJ, Saxena R, Voight BF, Marchini JL, Hu T, et al. Meta-analysis of genome-wide association data and large-scale replication identifies additional susceptibility loci for type 2 diabetes. Nat Genet. 2008;40(5):638–45.
23. Morris AP, Voight BF, Teslovich TM, Ferreira T, Segre AV, Steinthorsdottir V, et al. Large-scale association analysis provides insights into the genetic architecture and pathophysiology of type 2 diabetes. Nat Genet. 2012;44(9):981–90. Epub 2012/08/14. https://doi.org/10.1038/ng.2383.
24. Steinthorsdottir V, Thorleifsson G, Reynisdottir I, Benediktsson R, Jonsdottir T, Walters GB, et al. A variant in CDKAL1 influences insulin response and risk of type 2 diabetes. Nat Genet. 2007;39(6):770–5.
25. Voight BF, Scott LJ, Steinthorsdottir V, Morris AP, Dina C, Welch RP, et al. Twelve type 2 diabetes susceptibility loci identified through large-scale association analysis. Nat Genet. 2010;42(7):579–89.
26. Rung J, Cauchi S, Albrechtsen A, Shen L, Rocheleau G, Cavalcanti-Proenca C, et al. Genetic variant near IRS1 is associated with type 2 diabetes, insulin resistance and hyperinsulinemia. Nat Genet. 2009;41(10):1110–5.
27. Gudmundsson J, Sulem P, Steinthorsdottir V, Bergthorsson JT, Thorleifsson G, Manolescu A, et al. Two variants on chromosome 17 confer prostate cancer risk, and the one in TCF2 protects against type 2 diabetes. Nat Genet. 2007;39(8):977–83.
28. Dupuis J, Langenberg C, Prokopenko I, Saxena R, Soranzo N, Jackson AU, et al. New genetic loci implicated in fasting glucose homeostasis and their impact on type 2 diabetes risk. Nat Genet. 2010;42(2):105–16.
29. DIAbetes Genetics Replication And Meta-analysis (DIAGRAM) Consortium. Genome-wide trans-ancestry meta-analysis provides insight into the genetic architecture of type 2 diabetes susceptibility. Nat Genet. 46(3):234–44. Epub 2014/02/11. https://doi.org/10.1038/ng.2897.
30. Cho YS, Chen CH, Hu C, Long J, Ong RT, Sim X, et al. Meta-analysis of genome-wide association

studies identifies eight new loci for type 2 diabetes in east Asians. Nat Genet. 2011;44(1):67–72. Epub 2011/12/14. https://doi.org/10.1038/ng.1019.

31. Kooner JS, Saleheen D, Sim X, Sehmi J, Zhang W, Frossard P, et al. Genome-wide association study in individuals of South Asian ancestry identifies six new type 2 diabetes susceptibility loci. Nat Genet. 2011;43 (10):984–9. Epub 2011/08/30. https://doi.org/10.1038/ng.921.

32. Bouatia-Naji N, Bonnefond A, Cavalcanti-Proenca C, Sparso T, Holmkvist J, Marchand M, et al. A variant near MTNR1B is associated with increased fasting plasma glucose levels and type 2 diabetes risk. Nat Genet. 2009;41(1):89–94.

33. Lyssenko V, Nagorny CL, Erdos MR, Wierup N, Jonsson A, Spegel P, et al. Common variant in MTNR1B associated with increased risk of type 2 diabetes and impaired early insulin secretion. Nat Genet. 2009;41(1):82–8.

34. Ng MC, Shriner D, Chen BH, Li J, Chen WM, Guo X, et al. Meta-analysis of genome-wide association studies in African Americans provides insights into the genetic architecture of type 2 diabetes. PLoS Genet. 2014;10(8):e1004517. https://doi.org/10.1371/journal.pgen.1004517.

35. Zhao W, Rasheed A, Tikkanen E, Lee JJ, Butterworth AS, Howson JMM, et al. Identification of new susceptibility loci for type 2 diabetes and shared etiological pathways with coronary heart disease. Nature genetics. 2017;49(10):1450–7. Epub 2017/09/05. https://doi.org/10.1038/ng.3943.

36. Suzuki K, Akiyama M, Ishigaki K, Kanai M, Hosoe J, Shojima N, et al. Identification of 28 new susceptibility loci for type 2 diabetes in the Japanese population. Nat Genet. 2019;51(3):379–86. Epub 2019/02/06. https://doi.org/10.1038/s41588-018-0332-4.

37. Spracklen CN, Horikoshi M, Kim YJ, Lin K, Bragg F, Moon S, et al. Identification of type 2 diabetes loci in 433,540 East Asian individuals. Nature. 2020;582 (7811):240–5. Epub 2020/06/06. https://doi.org/10.1038/s41586-020-2263-3.

38. Mahajan A, Taliun D, Thurner M, Robertson NR, Torres JM, Rayner NW, et al. Fine-mapping type 2 diabetes loci to single-variant resolution using high-density imputation and islet-specific epigenome maps. Nat Genet. 2018;50(11):1505–13. Epub 2018/10/10. https://doi.org/10.1038/s41588-018-0241-6.

39. Mahajan A, Spracklen CN, Zhang W, Ng MCY, Petty LE, Kitajima H, et al. Multi-ancestry genetic study of type 2 diabetes highlights the power of diverse populations for discovery and translation. Nat Genet. 2022;54(5):560–72. Epub 2022/05/14. https://doi.org/10.1038/s41588-022-01058-3.

40. Vujkovic M, Keaton JM, Lynch JA, Miller DR, Zhou J, Tcheandjieu C, et al. Discovery of 318 new risk loci for type 2 diabetes and related vascular outcomes among 1.4 million participants in a multi-ancestry meta-analysis. Nat Genet. 2020;52(7):680–

91. Epub 2020/06/17. https://doi.org/10.1038/s41588-020-0637-y.

41. Manolio TA, Collins FS, Cox NJ, Goldstein DB, Hindorff LA, Hunter DJ, et al. Finding the missing heritability of complex diseases. Nature. 2009;461 (7265):747–53.

42. Meigs JB, Shrader P, Sullivan LM, McAteer JB, Fox CS, Dupuis J, et al. Genotype score in addition to common risk factors for prediction of type 2 diabetes. N Engl J Med. 2008;359(21):2208–19.

43. Lyssenko V, Jonsson A, Almgren P, Pulizzi N, Isomaa B, Tuomi T, et al. Clinical risk factors, DNA variants, and the development of type 2 diabetes. N Engl J Med. 2008;359(21):2220–32. Epub 2008/11/21. https://doi.org/10.1056/NEJMoa0801869.

44. de Miguel-Yanes JM, Shrader P, Pencina MJ, Fox CS, Manning AK, Grant RW, et al. Genetic risk reclassification for type 2 diabetes by age below or above 50 years using 40 type 2 diabetes risk single nucleotide polymorphisms. Diabetes Care. 2011;34 (1):121–5.

45. Hivert MF, Jablonski KA, Perreault L, Saxena R, McAteer JB, Franks PW, et al. Updated genetic score based on 34 confirmed type 2 diabetes Loci is associated with diabetes incidence and regression to normoglycemia in the diabetes prevention program. Diabetes. 2011;60(4):1340–8.

46. Andersson EA, Allin KH, Sandholt CH, Borglykke A, Lau CJ, Ribel-Madsen R, et al. Genetic risk socre of 46 type 2 diabetes risk variants with changes in plasma glucose and estimates of pancreatic β-cell function over 5 years of follow-up. Diabetes. 2013;62(10):3610–7.

47. Talmud PJ, Cooper JA, Morris RW, Dudbridge F, Shah T, Engmann J, et al. Sixty-five common genetic variants and prediction of type 2 diabetes. Diabetes. 2015;64(5):1830–40. https://doi.org/10.2337/db14-1504.

48. Mahajan A, Wessel J, Willems SM, Zhao W, Robertson NR, Chu AY, et al. Refining the accuracy of validated target identification through coding variant fine-mapping in type 2 diabetes. Nat Genet. 2018;50 (4):559–71. Epub 2018/04/11. https://doi.org/10.1038/s41588-018-0084-1.

49. Fuchsberger C, Flannick J, Teslovich TM, Mahajan A, Agarwala V, Gaulton KJ, et al. The genetic architecture of type 2 diabetes. Nature. 2016;536(7614):41–7. Epub 2016/07/12. https://doi.org/10.1038/nature18642.

50. Steinthorsdottir V, Thorleifsson G, Sulem P, Helgason H, Grarup N, Sigurdsson A, et al. Identification of low-frequency and rare sequence variants associated with elevated or reduced risk of type 2 diabetes. Nat Genet. 2014;46(3):294–8. Epub 2014/01/28. https://doi.org/10.1038/ng.2882.

51. Flannick J, Thorleifsson G, Beer NL, Jacobs SB, Grarup N, Burtt NP, et al. Loss-of-function mutations in SLC30A8 protect against type 2 diabetes. Nat

Genet. 2014;46(4):357–63. Epub 2014/03/04. https://doi.org/10.1038/ng.2915.

52. Estrada K, Aukrust I, Bjorkhaug L, Burtt NP, Mercader JM, Garcia-Ortiz H, et al. Association of a low-frequency variant in HNF1A with type 2 diabetes in a Latino population. JAMA. 2014;311(22):2305–14. Epub 2014/06/11. https://doi.org/10.1001/jama.2014.6511.

53. Loos RJ, Barroso I, O'Rahilly S, Wareham NJ. Comment on "A common genetic variant is associated with adult and childhood obesity". Science. 2007;315(5809):187. author reply

54. Dina C, Meyre D, Samson C, Tichet J, Marre M, Jouret B, et al. Comment on "A common genetic variant is associated with adult and childhood obesity". Science. 2007;315(5809):187. author reply

55. Rosskopf D, Bornhorst A, Rimmbach C, Schwahn C, Kayser A, Kruger A, et al. Comment on "A common genetic variant is associated with adult and childhood obesity". Science. 2007;315, 187(5809) author reply

56. Lyon HN, Emilsson V, Hinney A, Heid IM, Lasky-Su J, Zhu X, et al. The association of a SNP upstream of INSIG2 with body mass index is reproduced in several but not all cohorts. PLoS Genet. 2007;3(4):e61.

57. Hotta K, Nakamura M, Nakata Y, Matsuo T, Kamohara S, Kotani K, et al. INSIG2 gene rs7566605 polymorphism is associated with severe obesity in Japanese. J Hum Genet. 2008;53(9):857–62.

58. Loos RJ, Lindgren CM, Li S, Wheeler E, Zhao JH, Prokopenko I, et al. Common variants near MC4R are associated with fat mass, weight and risk of obesity. Nat Genet. 2008;40(6):768–75.

59. Willer CJ, Speliotes EK, Loos RJ, Li S, Lindgren CM, Heid IM, et al. Six new loci associated with body mass index highlight a neuronal influence on body weight regulation. Nat Genet. 2009;41(1):25–34.

60. Thorleifsson G, Walters GB, Gudbjartsson DF, Steinthorsdottir V, Sulem P, Helgadottir A, et al. Genome-wide association yields new sequence variants at seven loci that associate with measures of obesity. Nat Genet. 2009;41(1):18–24.

61. Speliotes EK, Willer CJ, Berndt SI, Monda KL, Thorleifsson G, Jackson AU, et al. Association analyses of 249,796 individuals reveal 18 new loci associated with body mass index. Nat Genet. 2010;42(11):937–48.

62. Okada Y, Kubo M, Ohmiya H, Takahashi A, Kumasaka N, Hosono N, et al. Common variants at CDKAL1 and KLF9 are associated with body mass index in east Asian populations. Nat Genet. 2012;44(3):302–6. Epub 2012/02/22. https://doi.org/10.1038/ng.1086.

63. Monda KL, Chen GK, Taylor KC, Palmer C, Edwards TL, Lange LA, et al. A meta-analysis identifies new loci associated with body mass index in individuals of African ancestry. Nat Gen. 2013. Epub 2013/04/16. https://doi.org/10.1038/ng.2608.

64. Wen W, Cho YS, Zheng W, Dorajoo R, Kato N, Qi L, et al. Meta-analysis identifies common variants associated with body mass index in east Asians. Nat Genet. 2012;44(3):307–11. Epub 2012/02/22. https://doi.org/10.1038/ng.1087.

65. Locke AE, Kahali B, Berndt SI, Justice AE, Pers TH, Day FR, et al. Genetic studies of body mass index yield new insights for obesity biology. Nature. 2015;518(7538):197–206. https://doi.org/10.1038/nature14177.

66. Yengo L, Sidorenko J, Kemper KE, Zheng Z, Wood AR, Weedon MN, et al. Meta-analysis of genome-wide association studies for height and body mass index in approximately 700,000 individuals of European ancestry. Hum Mol Genet. 2018;27(20):3641–9. Epub 2018/08/21. https://doi.org/10.1093/hmg/ddy271.

67. Frayling TM, Timpson NJ, Weedon MN, Zeggini E, Freathy RM, Lindgren CM, et al. A common variant in the FTO gene is associated with body mass index and predisposes to childhood and adult obesity. Science. 2007;316(5826):889–94.

68. Dina C, Meyre D, Gallina S, Durand E, Korner A, Jacobson P, et al. Variation in FTO contributes to childhood obesity and severe adult obesity. Nat Genet. 2007;39(6):724–6.

69. Church C, Moir L, McMurray F, Girard C, Banks GT, Teboul L, et al. Overexpression of Fto leads to increased food intake and results in obesity. Nat Genet. 2010;42(12):1086–92.

70. Cecil JE, Tavendale R, Watt P, Hetherington MM, Palmer CN. An obesity-associated FTO gene variant and increased energy intake in children. N Engl J Med. 2008;359(24):2558–66.

71. Wardle J, Carnell S, Haworth CM, Farooqi IS, O'Rahilly S, Plomin R. Obesity associated genetic variation in FTO is associated with diminished satiety. J Clin Endocrinol Metab. 2008;93(9):3640–3.

72. Maller JB, McVean G, Byrnes J, Vukcevic D, Palin K, Su Z, et al. Bayesian refinement of association signals for 14 loci in 3 common diseases. Nat Genet. 2012. Epub 2012/10/30. https://doi.org/10.1038/ng.2435.

73. Helgason A, Palsson S, Thorleifsson G, Grant SF, Emilsson V, Gunnarsdottir S, et al. Refining the impact of TCF7L2 gene variants on type 2 diabetes and adaptive evolution. Nat Genet. 2007;39(2):218–25.

74. Palmer ND, Hester JM, An SS, Adeyemo A, Rotimi C, Langefeld CD, et al. Resequencing and analysis of variation in the TCF7L2 gene in African Americans suggests that SNP rs7903146 is the causal diabetes susceptibility variant. Diabetes. 2011;60(2):662–8. https://doi.org/10.2337/db10-0134.

75. Chang YC, Chang TJ, Jiang YD, Kuo SS, Lee KC, Chiu KC, et al. Association study of the genetic polymorphisms of the transcription factor 7-like 2 (TCF7L2) gene and type 2 diabetes in the Chinese population. Diabetes. 2007;56(10):2631–7.

76. Ng MC, Park KS, Oh B, Tam CH, Cho YM, Shin HD, et al. Implication of genetic variants near TCF7L2, SLC30A8, HHEX, CDKAL1, CDKN2A/B, IGF2BP2, and FTO in type 2 diabetes and obesity in 6719 Asians. Diabetes. 2008;57(8):2226–33.

77. Ng MC, Tam CH, Lam VK, So WY, Ma RC, Chan JC. Replication and identification of novel variants at TCF7L2 associated with type 2 diabetes in Hong Kong Chinese. J Clin Endocrinol Metab. 2007;92 (9):3733–7.

78. Ren Q, Han XY, Wang F, Zhang XY, Han LC, Luo YY, et al. Exon sequencing and association analysis of polymorphisms in TCF7L2 with type 2 diabetes in a Chinese population. Diabetologia. 2008;51(7): 1146–52.

79. Yu M, Xu XJ, Yin JY, Wu J, Chen X, Gong ZC, et al. KCNJ11 Lys23Glu and TCF7L2 rs290487(C/T) polymorphisms affect therapeutic efficacy of repaglinide in Chinese patients with type 2 diabetes. Clin Pharmacol Ther. 2010;87(3):330–5.

80. Zheng X, Ren W, Zhang S, Liu J, Li S, Li J, et al. Association of type 2 diabetes susceptibility genes (TCF7L2, SLC30A8, PCSK1 and PCSK2) and proinsulin conversion in a Chinese population. Mol Biol Rep. 2012;39(1):17–23.

81. Gaulton KJ, Nammo T, Pasquali L, Simon JM, Giresi PG, Fogarty MP, et al. A map of open chromatin in human pancreatic islets. Nat Genet. 2010;42(3): 255–9.

82. Lyssenko V, Lupi R, Marchetti P, Del Guerra S, Orho-Melander M, Almgren P, et al. Mechanisms by which common variants in the TCF7L2 gene increase risk of type 2 diabetes. J Clin Invest. 2007;117(8):2155–63.

83. Boj SF, van Es JH, Huch M, Li VS, Jose A, Hatzis P, et al. Diabetes risk gene and Wnt effector Tcf7l2/ TCF4 controls hepatic response to perinatal and adult metabolic demand. Cell. 2012;151(7):1595– 607. Epub 2012/12/25. https://doi.org/10.1016/j.cell. 2012.10.053.

84. Kaminska D, Kuulasmaa T, Venesmaa S, Kakela P, Vaittinen M, Pulkkinen L, et al. Adipose tissue TCF7L2 splicing is regulated by weight loss and associates with glucose and fatty acid metabolism. Diabetes. 2012;61(11):2807–13. Epub 2012/10/23. https://doi.org/10.2337/db12-0239.

85. Yi F, Brubaker PL, Jin T. TCF-4 mediates cell type-specific regulation of proglucagon gene expression by beta-catenin and glycogen synthase kinase-3beta. J Biol Chem. 2005;280(2):1457–64. https://doi.org/ 10.1074/jbc.M411487200.

86. Florez JC, Jablonski KA, Bayley N, Pollin TI, de Bakker PI, Shuldiner AR, et al. TCF7L2 polymorphisms and progression to diabetes in the Diabetes Prevention Program. N Engl J Med. 2006;355(3): 241–50. Epub 2006/07/21. https://doi.org/10.1056/ NEJMoa062418.

87. Le Bacquer O, Kerr-Conte J, Gargani S, Delalleau N, Huyvaert M, Gmyr V, et al. TCF7L2 rs7903146 impairs islet function and morphology in non-diabetic individuals. Diabetologia. 2012;55(10): 2677–81.

88. Shu L, Sauter NS, Schulthess FT, Matveyenko AV, Oberholzer J, Maedler K. Transcription factor 7-like 2 regulates beta-cell survival and function in human pancreatic islets. Diabetes. 2008;57(3):645–53.

89. Liu Z, Habener JF. Glucagon-like peptide-1 activation of TCF7L2-dependent Wnt signaling enhances pancreatic beta cell proliferation. J Biol Chem. 2008;283(13):8723–35.

90. Cauchi S, Froguel P. TCF7L2 genetic defect and type 2 diabetes. Curr Diab Rep. 2008;8(2):149–55.

91. Elbein SC, Chu WS, Das SK, Yao-Borengasser A, Hasstedt SJ, Wang H, et al. Transcription factor 7-like 2 polymorphisms and type 2 diabetes, glucose homeostasis traits and gene expression in US participants of European and African descent. Diabetologia. 2007;50(8):1621–30.

92. Zhao J, Schug J, Li M, Kaestner KH, Grant SF. Disease-associated loci are significantly over-represented among genes bound by transcription factor 7-like 2 (TCF7L2) in vivo. Diabetologia. 2010;53 (11):2340–6.

93. Boj SF, van Es JH, Huch M, Li VS, José A, Hatzis P, et al. Diabetes risk gene and Wnt effector Tcf7l2/ TCF4 controls hepatic response to perinatal and adult metabolic demand. Cell. 2012;151(7): 1595–607.

94. da Silva XG, Mondragon A, Sun G, Chen L, McGinty JA, French PM, et al. Abnormal glucose tolerance and insulin secretion in pancreas-specific Tcf7l2-null mice. Diabetologia. 2012;55(10):2667–76.

95. Savic D, Ye H, Aneas I, Park SY, Bell GI, Nobrega MA. Alterations in TCF7L2 expression define its role as a key regulator of glucose metabolism. Genome Res. 2011;21(9):1417–25.

96. Duncan A, Heyer MP, Ishikawa M, Caligiuri SPB, Liu XA, Chen Z, et al. Habenular TCF7L2 links nicotine addiction to diabetes. Nature. 2019;574 (7778):372–7. Epub 2019/10/18. https://doi.org/10. 1038/s41586-019-1653-x.

97. Korinek V, Barker N, Moerer P, van Donselaar E, Huls G, Peters PJ, et al. Depletion of epithelial stem-cell compartments in the small intestine of mice lacking Tcf-4. Nat Genet. 1998;19(4):379–83.

98. Hansson O, Zhou Y, Renström E, Osmark P. Molecular function of TCF7L2: Consequences of TCF7L2 splicing for molecular function and risk for type 2 diabetes. Curr Diab Rep. 2010;10(6):444–51.

99. Barker N, Huls G, Korinek V, Clevers H. Restricted high level expression of Tcf-4 protein in intestinal and mammary gland epithelium. Am J Pathol. 1999;154 (1):29–35. https://doi.org/10.1016/S0002-9440(10) 65247-9.

100. Duval A, Rolland S, Tubacher E, Bui H, Thomas G, Hamelin R. The human T-cell transcription factor-4 gene: structure, extensive characterization of alternative splicings, and mutational analysis in colorectal cancer cell lines. Cancer Res. 2000;60(14):3872–9.

101. Cauchi S, Meyre D, Dina C, Choquet H, Samson C, Gallina S, et al. Transcription factor TCF7L2 genetic study in the French population: expression in human beta-cells and adipose tissue and strong association with type 2 diabetes. Diabetes. 2006;55(10):2903–8.

102. Kaminska D, Kuulasmaa T, Venesmaa S, Käkelä P, Vaittinen M, Pulkkinen L, et al. Adipose tissue TCF7L2 splicing is regulated by weight loss and associates with glucose and fatty acid metabolism. Diabetes. 2012;61(11):2807–13.

103. Prokunina-Olsson L, Kaplan LM, Schadt EE, Collins FS. Alternative splicing of TCF7L2 gene in omental and subcutaneous adipose tissue and risk of type 2 diabetes. PLoS One. 2009;4(9):e7231.

104. Prokunina-Olsson L, Welch C, Hansson O, Adhikari N, Scott LJ, Usher N, et al. Tissue-specific alternative splicing of TCF7L2. Hum Mol Genet. 2009;18(20):3795–804.

105. Karsak M, Cohen-Solal M, Freudenberg J, Ostertag A, Morieux C, Kornak U, et al. Cannabinoid receptor type 2 gene is associated with human osteoporosis. Hum Mol Genet. 2005;14(22):3389–96.

106. Woods A, James CG, Wang G, Dupuis H, Beier F. Control of chondrocyte gene expression by actin dynamics: a novel role of cholesterol/Ror-alpha signalling in endochondral bone growth. J Cell Mol Med. 2009;13(9B):3497–516.

107. Baker N, Morin PJ, Clevers H. The Ying-Yang of TCF/beta-catenin signaling. Adv Cancer Res. 2000;77:1–24.

108. Tetsu O, McCormick F. Beta-catenin regulates expression of cyclin D1 in colon carcinoma cells. Nature. 1999;389(6726):422–6.

109. Idris AI, van't Hof RJ, Greig IR, Ridge SA, Baker D, Ross RA, et al. Regulation of bone mass, bone loss and osteoclast activity by cannabinoid receptors. Nat Med. 2005;11(7):774–9.

110. Amundadottir LT, Sulem P, Gudmundsson J, Helgason A, Baker A, Agnarsson BA, et al. A common variant associated with prostate cancer in European and African populations. Nat Genet. 2006;38(6):652–8.

111. Yeager M, Orr N, Hayes RB, Jacobs KB, Kraft P, Wacholder S, et al. Genome-wide association study of prostate cancer identifies a second risk locus at 8q24. Nat Genet. 2007;39(5):645–9.

112. Haiman CA, Patterson N, Freedman ML, Myers SR, Pike MC, Waliszewska A, et al. Multiple regions within 8q24 independently affect risk for prostate cancer. Nat Genet. 2007;39(5):638–44.

113. Gudmundsson J, Sulem P, Manolescu A, Amundadottir LT, Gudbjartsson D, Helgason A, et al. Genome-wide association study identifies a second prostate cancer susceptibility variant at 8q24. Nat Genet. 2007;39(5):631–7.

114. Witte JS. Multiple prostate cancer risk variants on 8q24. Nat Genet. 2007;39(5):579–80.

115. Haiman CA, Le Marchand L, Yamamato J, Stram DO, Sheng X, Kolonel LN, et al. A common genetic risk factor for colorectal and prostate cancer. Nat Genet. 2007;39(8):954–6.

116. Zanke BW, Greenwood CM, Rangrej J, Kustra R, Tenesa A, Farrington SM, et al. Genome-wide association scan identifies a colorectal cancer susceptibility locus on chromosome 8q24. Nat Genet. 2007;39 (8):989–94.

117. Tomlinson I, Webb E, Carvajal-Carmona L, Broderick P, Kemp Z, Spain S, et al. A genome-wide association scan of tag SNPs identifies a susceptibility variant for colorectal cancer at 8q24.21. Nat Genet. 2007;39(8):984–8.

118. Yang J, Weedon MN, Purcell S, Lettre G, Estrada K, Willer CJ, et al. Genomic inflation factors under polygenic inheritance. Eur J Hum Genet. 2011;19(7):807–12.

119. Golding J, Pembrey M, Jones R. ALSPAC—the Avon Longitudinal Study of Parents and Children. I. Study methodology. Paediatr Perinat Epidemiol. 2001;15 (1):74–87.

120. Leary SD, Smith GD, Rogers IS, Reilly JJ, Wells JC, Ness AR. Smoking during pregnancy and offspring fat and lean mass in childhood. Obesity (Silver Spring, Md). 2006;14(12):2284–93.

121. Jones RW, Ring S, Tyfield L, Hamvas R, Simmons H, Pembrey M, et al. A new human genetic resource: a DNA bank established as part of the Avon longitudinal study of pregnancy and childhood (ALSPAC). Eur J Hum Genet. 2000;8(9):653–60.

122. Rivas MA, Beaudoin M, Gardet A, Stevens C, Sharma Y, Zhang CK, et al. Deep resequencing of GWAS loci identifies independent rare variants associated with inflammatory bowel disease. Nat Genet. 2011;

123. Enciso-Mora V, Broderick P, Ma Y, Jarrett RF, Hjalgrim H, Hemminki K, et al. A genome-wide association study of Hodgkin's lymphoma identifies new susceptibility loci at 2p16.1 (REL), 8q24.21 and 10p14 (GATA3). Nat Genet. 2010;42(12):1126–30. Epub 2010/11/03. https://doi.org/10.1038/ng.696.

124. Pomerantz MM, Ahmadiyeh N, Jia L, Herman P, Verzi MP, Doddapaneni H, et al. The 8q24 cancer risk variant rs6983267 shows long-range interaction with MYC in colorectal cancer. Nat Genet. 2009;41 (8):882–4.

125. Tuupanen S, Turunen M, Lehtonen R, Hallikas O, Vanharanta S, Kivioja T, et al. The common colorectal cancer predisposition SNP rs6983267 at chromosome 8q24 confers potential to enhanced Wnt signaling. Nat Genet. 2009;41(8):885–90.

126. Ingalls AM, Dickie MM, Snell GD. Obese, a new mutation in the house mouse. Obes Res. 1996;4(1): 101. Epub 1996/01/01

127. Frayling TM, Colhoun H, Florez JC. A genetic link between type 2 diabetes and prostate cancer. Diabetologia. 2008;51(10):1757–60.

128. Houseknecht KL, Baile CA, Matteri RL, Spurlock ME. The biology of leptin: a review. J Anim Sci. 1998;76(5):1405–20. Epub 1998/06/11

129. Echwald SM, Rasmussen SB, Sorensen TI, Andersen T, Tybjaerg-Hansen A, Clausen JO, et al. Identification of two novel missense mutations in the human OB gene. Int J Obes Relat Metab Disord. 1997;21(4):321–6. Epub 1997/04/01

130. He X. A Wnt-Wnt situation. Dev Cell. 2003;4(6): 791–7.

131. van Es JH, Barker N, Clevers H. You Wnt some, you lose some: oncogenes in the Wnt signaling pathway. Curr Opin Genet Dev. 2003;13(1):28–33.

132. Helgadottir A, Manolescu A, Helgason A, Thorleifsson G, Thorsteinsdottir U, Gudbjartsson DF, et al. A variant of the gene encoding leukotriene A4 hydrolase confers ethnicity-specific risk of myocardial infarction. Nat Genet. 2006;38(1):68–74.

133. He TC, Sparks AB, Rago C, Hermeking H, Zawel L, da Costa LT, et al. Identification of c-MYC as a target of the APC pathway. Science. 1998;281(5382): 1509–12.

134. Kinzler KW, Vogelstein B. Lessons from hereditary colorectal cancer. Cell. 1996;87(2):159–70.

135. Johnson ME, Zhao J, Schug J, Deliard S, Xia Q, Guy VC, et al. Two novel type 2 diabetes loci revealed through integration of TCF7L2 DNA occupancy and SNP association data. BMJ Open Diabetes Res Care. 2014;2(1):e000052. Epub 2014/12/04. https://doi.org/10.1136/bmjdrc-2014-000052.

136. Norton L, Fourcaudot M, Abdul-Ghani MA, Winnier D, Mehta FF, Jenkinson CP, et al. Chromatin occupancy of transcription factor 7-like 2 (TCF7L2) and its role in hepatic glucose metabolism. Diabetologia. 2011;54(12):3132–42.

137. Gerken T, Girard CA, Tung YC, Webby CJ, Saudek V, Hewitson KS, et al. The obesity-associated FTO gene encodes a 2-oxoglutarate-dependent nucleic acid demethylase. Science. 2007;318(5855): 1469–72.

138. Lein ES, Hawrylycz MJ, Ao N, Ayres M, Bensinger A, Bernard A, et al. Genome-wide atlas of gene expression in the adult mouse brain. Nature. 2007;445(7124):168–76. Epub 2006/12/08. https://doi.org/10.1038/nature05453.

139. Church C, Lee S, Bagg EA, McTaggart JS, Deacon R, Gerken T, et al. A mouse model for the metabolic effects of the human fat mass and obesity associated FTO gene. PLoS Genet. 2009;5(8):e1000599.

140. Fischer J, Koch L, Emmerling C, Vierkotten J, Peters T, Bruning JC, et al. Inactivation of the Fto gene protects from obesity. Nature. 2009;458(7240): 894–8.

141. Smemo S, Tena JJ, Kim KH, Gamazon ER, Sakabe NJ, Gomez-Marin C, et al. Obesity-associated variants within FTO form long-range functional connections with IRX3. Nature. 2014;507(7492):371–5. Epub 2014/03/22. https://doi.org/10.1038/nature13138.

142. Claussnitzer M, Dankel SN, Kim KH, Quon G, Meuleman W, Haugen C, et al. FTO Obesity Variant Circuitry and Adipocyte Browning in Humans. N Engl J Med. 2015;373(10):895–907. https://doi.org/10.1056/NEJMoa1502214.

143. Sobreira DR, Joslin AC, Zhang Q, Williamson I, Hansen GT, Farris KM, et al. Extensive pleiotropism and allelic heterogeneity mediate metabolic effects of IRX3 and IRX5. Science. 2021;372(6546):1085–91. Epub 2021/06/05. https://doi.org/10.1126/science.abf1008.

144. Whincup PH, Kaye SJ, Owen CG, Huxley R, Cook DG, Anazawa S, et al. Birth weight and risk of type 2 diabetes: a systematic review. JAMA. 2008;300 (24):2886–97.

145. Hattersley AT, Beards F, Ballantyne E, Appleton M, Harvey R, Ellard S. Mutations in the glucokinase gene of the fetus result in reduced birth weight. Nat Genet. 1998;19(3):268–70. Epub 1998/07/14. https://doi.org/10.1038/953.

146. Hattersley AT, Tooke JE. The fetal insulin hypothesis: an alternative explanation of the association of low birthweight with diabetes and vascular disease. Lancet. 1999;353(9166):1789–92. Epub 1999/05/29. https://doi.org/10.1016/S0140-6736(98)07546-1.

147. Freathy RM, Weedon MN, Bennett A, Hypponen E, Relton CL, Knight B, et al. Type 2 diabetes TCF7L2 risk genotypes alter birth weight: a study of 24,053 individuals. Am J Hum Genet. 2007;80(6):1150–61.

148. Mook-Kanamori DO, de Kort SW, van Duijn CM, Uitterlinden AG, Hofman A, Moll HA, et al. Type 2 diabetes gene TCF7L2 polymorphism is not associated with fetal and postnatal growth in two birth cohort studies. BMC Med Genet. 2009;10:67. Epub 2009/07/21. https://doi.org/10.1186/1471-2350-10-67.

149. Pulizzi N, Lyssenko V, Jonsson A, Osmond C, Laakso M, Kajantie E, et al. Interaction between prenatal growth and high-risk genotypes in the development of type 2 diabetes. Diabetologia. 2009;52(5): 825–9.

150. van Hoek M, Langendonk JG, de Rooij SR, Sijbrands EJ, Roseboom TJ. Genetic variant in the IGF2BP2 gene may interact with fetal malnutrition to affect glucose metabolism. Diabetes. 2009;58(6):1440–4. Epub 2009/03/05. https://doi.org/10.2337/db08-1173.

151. Freathy RM, Bennett AJ, Ring SM, Shields B, Groves CJ, Timpson NJ, et al. Type 2 diabetes risk alleles are associated with reduced size at birth. Diabetes. 2009;58(6):1428–33.

152. Zhao J, Li M, Bradfield JP, Wang K, Zhang H, Sleiman P, et al. Examination of type 2 diabetes loci implicates CDKAL1 as a birth weight gene. Diabetes. 2009;58(10):2414–8.

153. Morgan AR, Thompson JM, Murphy R, Black PN, Lam WJ, Ferguson LR, et al. Obesity and diabetes genes are associated with being born small for gestational age: results from the Auckland Birthweight Collaborative study. BMC Med Genet. 2010;11:125. Epub 2010/08/18. https://doi.org/10.1186/1471-2350-11-125.

154. Freathy RM, Mook-Kanamori DO, Sovio U, Prokopenko I, Timpson NJ, Berry DJ, et al. Variants in ADCY5 and near CCNL1 are associated with fetal

growth and birth weight. Nat Genet. 2010;42(5): 430–5.

155. Horikoshi M, Yaghootkar H, Mook-Kanamori DO, Sovio U, Taal HR, Hennig BJ, et al. New loci associated with birth weight identify genetic links between intrauterine growth and adult height and metabolism. Nat Genet. 2013;45(1):76–82. Epub 2012/12/04. https://doi.org/10.1038/ng.2477.

156. Warrington NM, Beaumont RN, Horikoshi M, Day FR, Helgeland O, Laurin C, et al. Maternal and fetal genetic effects on birth weight and their relevance to cardio-metabolic risk factors. Nat Genet. 2019;51(5): 804–14. Epub 2019/05/03. https://doi.org/10.1038/ s41588-019-0403-1.

157. Horikoshi M, Beaumont RN, Day FR, Warrington NM, Kooijman MN, Fernandez-Tajes J, et al. Genome-wide associations for birth weight and correlations with adult disease. Nature. 2016;538(7624): 248–52. Epub 2016/09/30. https://doi.org/10.1038/ nature19806.

158. Nicklas TA, Baranowski T, Cullen KW, Berenson G. Eating patterns, dietary quality and obesity. J Am Coll Nutr. 2001;20(6):599–608.

159. Whitaker RC, Wright JA, Pepe MS, Seidel KD, Dietz WH. Predicting obesity in young adulthood from childhood and parental obesity. N Engl J Med. 1997;337(13):869–73.

160. Parsons TJ, Power C, Logan S, Summerbell CD. Childhood predictors of adult obesity: a systematic review. Int J Obes Relat Metab Disord. 1999;23 (Suppl 8):S1–107.

161. Hardy R, Wills AK, Wong A, Elks CE, Wareham NJ, Loos RJ, et al. Life course variations in the associations between FTO and MC4R gene variants and body size. Hum Mol Genet. 2010;19(3):545–52. Epub 2009/11/ 03. https://doi.org/10.1093/hmg/ddp504.

162. Andersson EA, Pilgaard K, Pisinger C, Harder MN, Grarup N, Faerch K, et al. Do gene variants influencing adult adiposity affect birth weight? A population-based study of 24 loci in 4744 Danish individuals. PLoS One. 2010;5(12):e14190. Epub 2010/12/15. https://doi.org/10.1371/journal.pone. 0014190.

163. Manco M, Dallapiccola B. Genetics of pediatric obesity. Pediatrics. 2012;130(1):123–33. Epub 2012/06/ 06. https://doi.org/10.1542/peds.2011-2717.

164. Bradfield JP, Taal HR, Timpson NJ, Scherag A, Lecoeur C, Warrington NM, et al. A genome-wide association meta-analysis identifies new childhood obesity loci. Nat Genet. 2012;44:526–31.

165. Bradfield JP, Vogelezang S, Felix JF, Chesi A, Helgeland O, Horikoshi M, et al. A trans-ancestral meta-analysis of genome-wide association studies reveals loci associated with childhood obesity. Hum Mol Genet. 2019;28(19):3327–38. Epub 2019/09/11. https://doi.org/10.1093/hmg/ddz161.

166. Grant SF, Hakonarson H, Schwartz S. Can the genetics of type 1 and type 2 diabetes shed light on the genetics of latent autoimmune diabetes in adults? Endocr Rev. 2010;31(2):183–93.

167. Basile KJ, Guy VC, Schwartz S, Grant SF. Overlap of genetic susceptibility to type 1 diabetes, type 2 diabetes, and latent autoimmune diabetes in adults. Curr Diab Rep. 2014;14(11):550. https://doi.org/10.1007/ s11892-014-0550-9.

168. Andersen MK, Sterner M, Forsen T, Karajamaki A, Rolandsson O, Forsblom C, et al. Type 2 diabetes susceptibility gene variants predispose to adult-onset autoimmune diabetes. Diabetologia. 2014. Epub 2014/ 06/08; https://doi.org/10.1007/s00125-014-3287-8.

169. Cousminer DL, Ahlqvist E, Mishra R, Andersen MK, Chesi A, Hawa MI, et al. First genome-wide association study of latent autoimmune diabetes in adults reveals novel insights linking immune and metabolic diabetes. Diabetes Care. 2018;41(11):2396–403. Epub 2018/09/27. https://doi.org/10.2337/dc18-1032.

Genetics of Lipid Disorders 10

Nora L. Nock

Contents

N. L. Nock (✉)
Department of Epidemiology and Biostatistics, Case
Western University School of Medicine, Cleveland, OH,
USA
e-mail: nln@case.edu

© Springer Nature Switzerland AG 2023
R. S. Ahima (ed.), *Metabolic Syndrome*,
https://doi.org/10.1007/978-3-031-40116-9_12

Abstract

This chapter focuses on the genetics of common lipid disorders, collectively referred to as "dyslipidemia," a component of the metabolic syndrome (MetSyn). We begin by providing a brief background on the lipids discussed in this chapter. Then, we discuss specific variants in key candidate genes and their role in related pathways that have been associated with individual lipid levels and dyslipidemia in larger-scale studies. In addition, we comment on associations observed in genome-wide association studies (GWAS) and sequencing studies. We also discuss how the use of more sophisticated statistical methods (e.g., genetic risk scores and pathway modeling) are helping to better understand the collective effects of multiple variants in multiple genes on these lipid traits. We conclude by providing perspectives for future directions.

Keywords

Obesity · Metabolic syndrome · Dyslipidemia · Genetics · Cholesterol · Triglycerides

Introduction

Dyslipidemia is characterized by an aggregation of lipoprotein abnormalities including high serum triglycerides (TG), low high-density lipoprotein cholesterol (HDL-C), and high or increased small low-density lipoprotein cholesterol (LDL-C). Lipoproteins, which contain lipids and apolipoproteins (APO), are responsible for transporting water-insoluble lipids (e.g., cholesterol and TG) in plasma from the intestines and liver, where they are absorbed and synthesized, respectively, to peripheral tissues (e.g., muscle, adipose) for utilization, processing, and/or storage [105].

There are several subtypes of lipoproteins that have specific functions including the following (from smallest to largest): (1) chylomicrons, which transport dietary TG from the intestines to the peripheral tissue and liver; (2) very LDL (VLDL) particles, which transport TG from the liver to peripheral tissues; (3) intermediate density lipoproteins (IDL), which are produced from VLDL particle metabolism and may be taken up by the liver or further hydrolyzed to LDL; and (4) HDL, which is key in "reverse cholesterol transport" or shuttling cholesterol from peripheral cells to the liver [105]. When LDL becomes lipid-depleted, small dense LDL (sdLDL) particles are formed that have a lower affinity for the LDL receptor (LDLR), more susceptibility to oxidation and a higher affinity for macrophages, and, thus, sdLDL particles can also contribute to the atherosclerotic process [13, 114]. Plasma triglycerides (TG) integrate multiple TG-rich lipoprotein particles, predominantly, intestinally synthesized chylomicrons in the postprandial state and hepatically synthesized VLDL in the fasted state.

Dyslipidemia is defined within the context of the metabolic syndrome (MetSyn), which is a clustering of metabolic traits including dyslipidemia as well as hypertension (raised systolic and/or diastolic blood pressure), dysglycemia (high fasting glucose), and obesity (high body mass index (BMI) and/or waist circumference). Multiple definitions for MetSyn have been proposed by organizations including the World Health Organization (WHO) [4], European Group Insulin Resistance (EGIR) [15], National Cholesterol Education Program Adult Treatment Panel III (NCEP ATP III) [47], International Diabetes Federation (IDF) [5], American Heart Association/National Heart, Lung, and Blood Institute (AHA/NHLBI) [64], and the joint interim statement proposed by the AHA/NHLBI, IDF, and others [6]. The dyslipidemia component of MetSyn has been fairly consistently defined as having TG $\geq$150 mg/l, HDL-C <40 mg/dl (1.03 mmol/l, in males) or <50 mg/dl (1.29 mmol/l in females) or drug treatment for elevated TG or low HDL-C (2001; [5, 6]). However, the World Health Organization (WHO) [4] proposed slightly lower limits for HDL-C (male: <0.9 mmol/l (35 mg/dl); female: <1.0 mmol/l (39 mg/dl)), and the EGIR [15] recommended that dyslipidemia be defined by HDL-C <1.0 mmol/l (39 mg/dl) or TG >2.0 mmol/l (177 mg/dl). Although the aforementioned guidelines exist, many authors have chosen to use cut points other than those specific in the context of MetSyn when defining dyslipidemia; therefore, in this chapter, we attempt to clarify the specific values and parameters used when referring to dyslipidemia. Furthermore, although LDL-C remains the primary target of therapy for the management of high blood cholesterol, there is currently no recommended value for LDL-C levels in the context of MetSyn. However, we note that the NCEP ATPIII guidelines for recommended drug therapy are based on LDL-C values ranging from ≥100 mg/dl to ≥190 mg/dl, depending on the presence/absence of other coronary heart disease (CHD) risk factors [63].

Dyslipidemia is quite common in developed nations, and its prevalence is rising worldwide, which may be attributed, in part, to the rising rates of overweight and obesity [69]. According to the National Health and Nutrition Examination Survey (NHANES) III, conducted in 1988–1994 in the USA, which used the NCEP ATP III criteria, the age-adjusted prevalence of dyslipidemia defined by high TG or low HDL-C was approximately 30.0% and 37.1%, respectively [50]. In a study using the Health Survey for England (HSE) (2003–2006) survey data and NHANES (1999–2006) data, the prevalence of low HDL-C (defined in both males and females as <40 mg/dl) was 10.0% in England and 19.2% in the USA [124]. Interestingly, trends in the USA and England have indicated that during the past two decades, there has been an increase in the proportion of individuals diagnosed with high cholesterol (≥240 mg/dl) that achieve therapeutic control [163]. In the USA, 54.0% of men (95% CI, 47.6–60.4) and 49.7% of women (95% CI, 44.3–55.0) in 2006 compared to 10.8% of men (95% CI, 8.0–13.6) and 8.6% (95% CI, 6.7–10.6) of women in 1993 had high total serum cholesterol and were on cholesterol-lowering medication [163]. In England, in 2006, 35.5% of men (95% CI, 32.8–38.3) and 25.7% of women (95% CI, 23.4–28.1) were on cholesterol-lowering medication as opposed to 0.6% of men (95% CI, 0.3–1.3) and 0.4% of women (95% CI, 0.1–0.7%) in 1993 [163]. Prevalence rates may also vary by whether or not relevant drug

treatments have been considered, which should include not only cholesterol-lowering therapies (e.g., statins) but other drugs (e.g., tamoxifen, glucocorticoids) that are known to alter TG and cholesterol levels [56].

Although the environment plays a substantive role in the manifestation of dyslipidemia, there is a strong genetic component. Heritability estimates reported for dyslipidemia typically range from 0.20 to 0.60 [42, 58, 74, 104, 193], and a recent review suggests HDL-C heritability may even extend up to 80% [154]. There have been many common genetic variants in the form of single nucleotide polymorphisms (SNPs) that have been associated with dyslipidemia. In this chapter, we update our previous summary of associations that have been reported between SNPs with a minor allele frequency (MAF) greater than 0.05 and HDL-C, LDL-C, and TG levels [137]. We note that, together, common variants have been estimated to explain less than 10% of HDL-C levels in the general population [104]; however, we purport that this is likely an underestimation of the genetic contribution and that more elegant statistical modeling methods that combine SNPs in a more biologically meaningful way will enable a better estimate and understanding of the collective role that genetic variants play in the manifestation of dyslipidemia and MetSyn. In the last section of this chapter, we review studies that have undertaken such more complex modeling strategies to better understand the aggregate effects of SNPs in dyslipidemia and MetSyn and provide insights to additional potential future directions.

Genetics of HDL-C

In Table 1, we list common SNPs associated with HDL-C that were initially tabulated in Boes et al. [23], which reviewed studies with sample sizes of 500 or greater, as well as other common SNPs in large studies that were identified in and since our previous review [137]. Variants in Table 1 are organized by gene acronyms which are listed in alphabetical order. Below, we describe variants in genes based on their involvement in relevant

Table 1 Genetic polymorphisms associated with HDL-C

Gene	Polym.	rs number	MAF	Ethn.	Sample size	Results (effect size, p-value)	Reference
ABCA1	C(−297)T	rs2246298	0.25 (T)	A	1625 (GP)	$p = 0.0455$	[175]
ABCA1	G(−273)C	rs1800976	0.40 (C)	A	1626 (GP); 735 (HBP)	+1.9/+2.7 mg/dl (1/2copies); $p = 0.03$ +1.9/+5.0 mg/dl (1/2 copies); $p = 0.03$	[175]
ABCA1	G(−273)C	rs1800976	0.38 (T)	Tu	2332 (GP)	+0.7/+1.9 mg/dl (1/2 copies); $p < 0.02$	[77]
ABCA1	G378C	rs1800978	0.13 (C)	W	5040 (GP)	−1.2/−2.7 mg/dl (1/2 copies); $p = 0.03$	[150]
ABCA1		rs3890182	0.13 (A)	W	5287 (GP)	−1/−3 mg/dl (1/2 copies); $p = 0.003$	[95]
ABCA1		rs2275542		A	<1880 (GP)	$p = 0.006$	[175]
ABCA1		rs2515602	0.27	B	1943 (P)	M; $p = 0.034$; F; $p < 0.001$	[101]
ABCA1	G596A	rs2853578	0.28 (A)	W	2468 (CVD) 834 (Co)	0.2/+2.8 mg/dl (1/2 copies); $p = 0.02$	[196]
ABCA1	G2310A	rs2066718	0.03 (A)	W	9123 (P)	F: higher levels in carriers; $p = 0.02$	[53]
ABCA1	G2706A	rs2066718	0.05 (A)	Tu	2458 (GP)	M: +2.0 mg/dl for heteroz.; $p < 0.01$	[77]
ABCA1	G2472A G2868A	rs2066718	0.06 (A)	Tu	2105 (GP)	F: +3.1 mg/dl for carriers; $p = 0.0005$	[77]
ABCA1	1883 M	rs4149313	0.12 (G)	W	9123 (P)	F: + heteroz.; $p = 0.05$	[53]
ABCA1	32b. + 30 ABC32			W	1543 (P)	−2.2 mg/dl for carriers; $p = 0.0040$	[35]
ABCA1	R1587K	rs2230808	0.24 (A)	W	9123 (P)	M: −1.5 mg/dl for heteroz.; $p = 0.008$	[53]
ABCA1	G4759A	rs2230808	0.26 (K)	W	779 (CVD)	−1.5 mg/dl for carriers; $p = 0.03$	[32]
ABCA1	50b.3038 ABC50	rs41474449		W	1543 (P)	+1.6 mg/dl for carriers; $p = 0.043$	[35]
ABCA1		rs3890182	0.12 (A)	EA	25,167	$p = 4.53E-07$	[41]
ADH5	A > G	rs2602836	0.44 (G)	EA AA, A	188,577 (Meta)	$p = 5 \times 10-9$	[198]
ANGPTL1	G > A	rs4650994	0.49 (A)	EA AA, A	188,577 (Meta)	$p = 7 \times 10-9$	[198]
ATG7	C > T	rs2606736	0.37(T)	EA AA, A	188,577 (Meta)	$p = 5 \times 10-8$	[198]
APOA1	T84C (HaeIII)	rs5070	0.23 (C)	A	1637 (GP)	+1.9/+5.4 mg/dl (1/2copies); $p = 0.0005$	[174]
APOA1	MspI RFLP	rs5069	0.31 (C)	B	3831 (P)	M/F; $p = $ n.s/0.022	[25]

(continued)

Table 1   (continued)

Gene	Polym.	rs number	MAF	Ethn.	Sample size	Results (effect size, p-value)	Reference
APOA1		rs28927680	0.93 (G)	EA	25,167	$p = 8.61E-09$	[41]
APOA1		rs964184	0.86 (C)	EA	25,167	$p = 6.08E-10$	[41]
APOA5-A4/A1		rs964184	0.14 (G)	C	5547	$-0.03(-0.04$ to $-0.01); p = 0.007$	[191]
APOA5	-1131 T > C	rs662799	0.06 (C)	UK	1696 (P)	-1.5 mg/dl/-5.4 mg/dl (1/2 copies); $p = 0.04$	[182]
APOA5	-1131 T > C	rs662799	0.07 (C)	W	1596 (SA PHIR)	-3.5 mg/dl per copy; $p = 0.00038$	[60]
APOA5	-1131 T > C	rs662799	0.23–0.30 (C)	C, Ma	2711 (C); 707 (M)	$-2.3/-5.4$ mg/dl 1/2 copies; $p < 0.0001$ $-1.2/-8.1$ mg/dl1/2 copies; $p < 0.0001$	[107]
APOA5	-1131 T > C	rs662799	0.34 (C)	A	521 Ho Co	-3.3 mg/dl per copy; $p < 0.001$	[204]
APOA5	$-3A > G$	rs651821	0.07	W	2056 (P)	M; $p = 0.30$; F; $p = 0.26$	[101]
APOA5	$-3A > G$	rs651821	0.18 (G)	C	2711 (GP)	$-2.3/-5.8$ mg/dl 1/2 copies; $p < 0.0001$	[107]
APOA5	$-3A > G$	rs651821	0.34 (C)	A	5207 (Ho Co, P)	-2.7 mg/dl per copy; $p < 0.001$	[204]
APOA5	$-3A > G$	rs651821	0.36 (G)	A	2417 (Ho Co)	$-3.9/-7.0$ mg/dl 1/2 copies; $p < 0.001$	[205]
APOA5	S19W	rs3135506	0.06 (W)	UK	1660 (P)	$-1.9/+1.2$ mg/dl (1/2 copies); $p = 0.02$	[182]
APOA5	56C > G	rs3135506	0.06 (G)	W	2347 (P)	-2.0 mg/dl for carriers; $p = 0.008$	[108]
APOA5		rs2072560	0.16 (A)	C	2711 (GP)	$-1.9/-3.9$ mg/dl (1/2 copies); $p = 0.003$	[107]
APOA5	IVS3 + 476 G > A	rs2072560		Ma	707 (P)	$-0.4/9.3$ mg/dl (1/2 copies); $p = 0.004$	[152]
APOA5	V153M	rs3135507		W	2557	F: -3.5 mg/dl for carriers; $p < 0.01$	[82]
APOA5	+553	rs2075291	0.07 (T)	A	5206 Ho Co	-4.6 mg/dl per copy; $p < 0.001$	[204]
APOA5	Gly185Cys	rs2075291	0.08 (T)	A	2417 Ho Co	$-5.0/-11.2$ mg/dl (1/2 copies); $p < 0.001$	[205]
APOA5	1259 T > C	rs2266788	0.18 (C)	C	2711 (GP)	$2.3/-3.1$ mg/dl 1/2 copies; $p < 0.0001$	[107]
APOB		rs11902417	0.78 (G)	E	17,723	$p = 3.7 \times 10-7$	[195]
APOC3	C455T	rs2854116	0.41 (C)	In	1308 (P)	$-3.1/-5.4$ mg/dl (1/2 copies); $p < 0.05$	[106]

(continued)

Table 1 (continued)

Gene	Polym.	rs number	MAF	Ethn.	Sample size	Results (effect size, p-value)	Reference
APOC3	PvuII	rs618354	0.49	A	F, 291 (GP)	F: +0.1/−4.2 mg/dl 1/2 copies; $p = 0.029$	[92]
APOC3	Sst1 RFLP	rs5128	0.09 (S2)	W	M, 1219 (P)	M: −1.8 mg/dl for carriers; $p = 0.04$.	[164]
APOC3	3′-utr/Sac I	rs5128	0.09 (+)	Hu	713 (P)	−5.0 mg/dl for heteroz.; $p = 0.0014$	[71]
APOC3	3238C > G	rs5128	0.07 (S2)	W	906 (GP)	+1.9 mg/dl for carriers; $p = 0.079$	[34]
APOE	Cys112Arg	rs429358	0.16 (A)	N	3575	$p = 0.001$	[151]
APOE	Cys112Arg	rs429358	0.12 (A) (E4)	L	1030	1.98 (1.05–3.74); men ($n = 425$); high versus low	[176]
BTN2A1	C > T	rs6929846		J; K	7471; 3529	CT or TT versus CC, $p = 0.005$; $p = 0.01$	[54]
C4orf52	G > A	rs10019888	0.18 (A)	EA AA, A	188,577 (Meta)	$p = 5 \times 10^{-8}$	[198]
CETP	G2708A	rs12149545	0.30 (A)	W	2683 GP 556 CVD	+1.9 mg/dl per copy; $p < 0.001$	[128]
CETP	G2708A	rs12149545	0.31 (A)	W	709 (CVD)	+1.5/+3.5 mg/dl (1/2 copies); $p = 0.0016$	[99]
CETP		rs3764261	0.14 (T)	C	4192	+0.07 mg/dl; $p = 4.3 \times 10^{-14}$	[115]
CETP	G971A	rs4783961	0.49 (A)	W	709 (CVD)	+1.2/+1.9 mg/dl (1/2 copies); $p = 0.09$	[99]
CETP	C629A	rs1800775	0.48 (A)	W	7083 (P)	+2.7/+5.4 mg/dl (1/2 copies); $p < 0.001$	[24]
CETP	C629A	rs1800775	0.51 (A)	W	847 M; 873 F (P)	+4.2 mg/dl for homoz.; $p < 0.002$	[17]
CETP	C629A	rs1800775	0.49 (A)	W	5287 (GP)	+3/+5 mg/dl (1/2 copies); $p = 2 \times 10^{-29}$	[95]
CETP	C629A	rs1800775	0.42 A	A	4050 (GP)	+2.2/+3.4 mg/dl 1/2 copies; $p = 3.28 \times 10^{-9}$	[181]
CETP	C629A	rs1800775	0.48 (A)	W	2683 GP; 556 CVD	+2.7 mg/dl per copy; $p < 0.001$	[128]
CETP	C629A	rs1800775	0.40 (A)	W	1214 (CVD); 574 (Co)	CVD: +2.0/3.5 mg/dl (1/2 copies) $p = 0.02$ Co: +3.3/6.1 mg/dl (1/2 copies); $p = 0.05$	[18]
CETP	C629A	rs1800775	0.44 (A)	W	709 (CVD)	+0.8/3.9 mg/dl (1/2 copies); $p < 0.0001$	[99]
CETP	C629A	rs1800775	0.50 (A)	W	309 (MI) 757 (Co)	+1.9/6.1 mg/dl (1/2 copies); $p < 0.0001$	[44]

(continued)

Table 1 (continued)

Gene	Polym.	rs number	MAF	Ethn.	Sample size	Results (effect size, p-value)	Reference
CETP	C629A	rs1800775	0.48 (A)	W	498 (CVD) 1107(Co)	+2.9/4.4 mg/dl (1/2 copies); $p < 0.001$	[51]
CETP	Taq1B	rs708272	0.40 (B2)		13,677 (Meta)	+1.2/+3.8 mg/dl (1/2 copies); $p < 0.0001$	[21]
CETP	Taq1B	rs708272			>10,000 (Meta)	+4.6 mg/dl for homoz.; $p < 0.00001$	[20]
CETP	Taq1B	rs708272	0.42 (B2)	W	7083 (P)	+2.7/5.0 mg/dl (1/2 copies); $p < 0.001$	[24]
CETP	Taq1B	rs708272	0.44 (B2)	W	2916 (P)	+2.5/4.7 mg/dl (1/2 copies); $p < 0.001$	[141]
CETP	Taq1B	rs708272	0.43 0.26 (A)	W B	2056 1943 (P)	$p < 0.01$; $p < 0.02$	[101]
CETP	Taq1B	rs708272	0.44 0.27 (A)	W B	8764 (P)	+2.3/5.8 mg/dl (1/2 copies); $p < 0.001$ +3.8/9.8 mg/dl (1/2 copies); $p < 0.001$	[136]
CETP	Taq1B	rs708272	0.41 (A)	W	1503 (P)	+2 /+5 mg/dl (1/2 copies); $p < 0.001$	[166]
CETP	Taq1B	rs708272	0.33 (A)	A	4207 (GP)	+2.5/4.4 mg/dl (1/2 copies); $p = 1.25 \times 10{-}10$	[181]
CETP	Taq1B	rs708272	0.40 (A)	A	1729 (GP)	M: +1.2/3.5 mg/dl (1/2 copies); $p = 0.096$ F: +1.9/6.2 mg/dl (1/2 copies); $p < 0.001$	[189]
CETP	Taq1B	rs708272	0.42 (A)	W	2683 GP; 556 CVD	+2.7 mg/dl per copy; $p < 0.001$	[128]
CETP	Taq1B	rs708272	0.42 (A)	W	2392 CVD; 827 Co	+1.7/3.6 mg/dl (1/2 copies); $p < 0.001$	[196]
CETP	Taq1B	rs708272	0.40 (A)	W	1464 CVD	+2.1/3.0 mg/dl (1/2 copies); $p = 0.003$	[27]
CETP	Taq1B	rs708272	0.41 (A)	W	1200 CV; 571 (Co)	+2.6/+4.3 mg/dl (1/2 copies); $p < 0.02$	[18]
CETP	Taq1B	rs708272	0.44 (A)	W	499 CVD; 1105 Co	+2.1/3.6 mg/dl (1/2 copies); $p < 0.001$	[51]
CETP	Taq1B	rs708272	0.45 (A)	WS	851,265 Co; 586 TC	$p = 0.014$ (2 copies)	[169]
CETP	+784CCC	rs34145065	0.39 (A)	W	709 (CVD)	+1.2/3.5 mg/dl (1/2 copies); $p = 0.0009$	[99]
CETP	A373P	rs5880	0.05 (A)	W	8467 P; 1636 CV	5.4 mg/dl for heteroz.; $p < 0.0001$	[2]
CETP	Ile405Val	rs5882			>10,000 (Meta)	+1.9 mg/dl for homoz.; $p < 0.00001$	[20]

(continued)

Table 1 (continued)

Gene	Polym.	rs number	MAF	Ethn.	Sample size	Results (effect size, p-value)	Reference
CETP	A +16G/ Ex.14	rs61212082	0.32 (A)	W	6421 (P)	M: +1.5/2.3 mg/dl (1/2 copies); $p = 0.002$ F: +0.0/+2.3 mg/dl (1/2 copies); $p = 0.007$	[86]
CETP		rs61212082	0.30 (A)	W	1208 (CVD) 572 (Co)	+1.4/+3.1 mg/dl (1/2 copies); $p = 0.08$ +0.3 /+8.4 mg/dl (1/2 copies); $p = 0.003$	[18]
CETP		rs61212082	0.30 (A)	W	498 (CVD); 1108 (Co)	+1.2/+3.5 mg/dl (1/2 copies); $p < 0.05$ +1.5 /+1.5 mg/dl (1/2 copies); $p < 0.05$	[51]
CETP	D442G	rs2303790b	0.03 (A)	A	3469 (He Ex)	+4.9 mg/dl for heteroz.; $p < 0.001$	[209]
CETP	R451Q	rs1800777	0.04 (A)	W	8467 (P); 1636 (CVD)	5.4 mg/dl for heteroz.; $p < 0.001$	[2]
CETP	G + 82A/Ex15	rs1800777	0.03 (A)	W	1071 CV; 532 Co	3.6/5.2 mg/dl for heteroz.; $p = 0.06/ 0.07$	[18]
CETP		rs12596776	0.90 (C)	EA	25,167	$p = 1.18E-05$	[41]
CETP		rs9989419	0.39 (A)	EA	25,167	$p = 1.71E-53$	[41]
CPS1	A > C	rs1047891	0.33 (C)	EA AA, A	188,577 (Meta)	$p = 5 \times 10{-8}$	[198]
DAGLB	G > A	rs702485	0.45 (A)	EA AA, A	188,577 (Meta)	$p = 7 \times 10{-12}$	[198]
FAM13A	A > G	rs3822072	0.46 (G)	EA AA, A	188,577 (Meta)	$p = 4 \times 10{-12}$	[198]
FTO	A > G	rs1121980	0.43 (G)	EA AA, A	188,577 (Meta)	$p = 7 \times 10{-9}$	[198]
GATA2	C > A	rs7431368		S	2386 CAD; 2171 C	B = 1.67; s.e. = 0.82; $p = 0.043$	[133]
GSK3B	T > C	rs6805251	0.39 (C)	EA AA, A	188,577 (Meta)	$p = 1 \times 10{-8}$	[198]
HAS1	A > G	rs17695224	0.26 (G)	EA AA, A	188,577 (Meta)	$p = 2 \times 10{-13}$	[198]
HDGF-PMVK	G > T	rs12145743	0.34 (T)	EA AA, A	188,577 (Meta)	$p = 2 \times 10{-8}$	[198]
IKZF1	G > T	rs17695224	0.32 (T)	EA AA, A	188,577 (Meta)	$p = 1 \times 10{-8}$	[198]
KAT5	A > G	rs12801636	0.23 (G)	EA AA, A	188,577 (Meta)	$p = 3 \times 10{-8}$	[198]
LCAT	Gly230Arg			W	156 low; 160 high	Variant sig. only in low-HDL group	[129]

(continued)

Table 1 (continued)

Gene	Polym.	rs number	MAF	Ethn.	Sample size	Results (effect size, p-value)	Reference
LCAT	608C/T	rs5922		A	203 (CVD)	Increase in HDL; $p = 0.015$	[207]
LCAT		rs5922		A	150 Str; 122 Co	Lower HDL-C in heteroz.; $p < 0.05$	[210]
LCAT	P143L +511C > T			A	190 CVD; 209 (Co)	Association with low HDL-C; $p < 0.01$	[208]
LCAT		rs2292318	0.12 (A)	W	1442 CVD, Co	Increases HDL-C; $p = 2 \times 10{-}5$	[146]
LDLR	Exon 2	rs2228671		W	1543 (P)	+3.8 mg/dl for carriers; $p = 0.0056$	[35]
LDLR	1866C > T Asn591Asn	rs688 = rs57911429	0.12 (T)	A	2417 (Ho Co)	+1.5/+8.5 mg/dl (1/2 copies); $p = 0.0155$	[205]
LDLR	Exon 12/HincII	rs688 = rs57911429	0.39 (+)	Hu	713 (P)	2.3/4.3 mg/dl (1/2 copies); $p = 0.047$	[71]
LDLR	2052 T > C	rs5925 = rs57369606	0.17 (C)	A	2417 Ho Co	+1.2/+5.4 (1/2 copies); $p = 0.043$	[205]
LIPC	T-710C	rs1077834	0.22 (C)	W	9121 (P)	+3–4% per copy; $p < 0.001$	[8]
LIPC	C-514Ta	rs1800588	0.25 (T)	Va	>24,000 (Meta)	+1.5/+3.5 mg/dl (1/2 copies); $p < 0.001$	[86]
LIPC	Pos.-480 T	rs1800588	0.21 (T) 0.53 (T)	W B	8897 (P) 2909 (P)	W: +2.2/+3.8 mg/dl (1/2 copies); $p < 0.001$ B: +1.6/+4.0 mg/dl (1/2 copies); $p < 0.001$	[136]
LIPC		rs1800588	0.21 (T)	W	6239 (P)	+1.3/+4.3 mg/dl (1/2 copies); $p < 0.001$	[86]
LIPC		rs1800588	0.38 (T)	A	2170 (P)	+2.3/+2.7 mg/dl (1/2 copies); $p = 0.001$	[180]
LIPC		rs1800588	0.21 (T)	W	5287 (GP)	+1/+4 mg/dl (1/2 copies); $p = 4 \times 10{-}10$	[95]
LIPC		rs1800588	0.25 (T)	W	2773 (GP)	+1.5 mg/dl per copy; $p = 0.04$	[183]
LIPC		rs1800588	0.24 (T)	W	3319 CV 1385 Co	+1.0/+3.8 mg/dl (1/2 copies); $p = 0.001$	[196]
LIPC		rs1800588	0.51 (T)	A	5207 Ho Co	+2.5 mg/dl per copy; $p < 0.001$	[204]
LIPC		rs1800588	0.21 (T)	W	6412 (CVD)	+2.0–2.5 mg/dl per copy; $p < 0.001$	[127]
LIPC	G -250A	rs2070895	0.22 (A)	W	9121 (P)	+3–4% per copy; $p < 0.001$	[8]
LIPC		rs2070895		W	1543 (P)	+1.5 mg/dl for carriers; $p = 0.020$	[35]

(continued)

Table 1 (continued)

Gene	Polym.	rs number	MAF	Ethn.	Sample size	Results (effect size, p-value)	Reference
LIPC		rs2070895	0.32 (A)	W	514 (P)	M; $p = 0.001$	[39]
LIPC		rs2070895	0.23 (A)	W	5585 (P)	+3.9/3.9 mg/dl (1/2 copies); $p = 8 \times 10{-}10$	[61]
LIPC		rs2070895	0.51 (A)	A	5213 Ho Co	+2.7 mg/dl per copy; $p < 0.001$	[204]
LIPC		rs2070895	0.39 (A)	A	716 He Ex	+2.1 mg/dl for carriers; $p = 0.026$	[102]
LIPC		rs12594375	0.37 (A)	A	2970 (GP)	$p = 0.00003$	[84]
LIPC		rs8023503	0.38 (T)	A	2970 (GP)	$p = 0.0001$	[84]
LIPC	+1075C	rs3829462	0.05 (C)	A	823	+8.0 mg/dl for heteroz.; $p < 0.05$	[48]
LIPC		rs4775041	0.29C	EA	25,167	$p = 1.03E{-}16$	[41]
LIPC		rs261332	0.20 (A)	EA	25,167	$p = 1.99E{-}13$	[41]
LPC		rs261334	0.20 (T)	E	17,723	$p = 4.9 \times 10{-}22$	[195]
LIPG	$-384A > C$	rs3813082	0.12 (C)	A	541 (Co)	+1.3/+10.2 mg/dl (1/2 copies); $p = 0.021$	[83]
LIPG		rs3813082	0.12 (C)	A	340 (kids)	+0.7/+9.8 (1/2 copies); $p = 0.0086$	[206]
LIPG	584 C/T T111I	rs2000813	0.32 (I)	W	495 (GP)	M: 1.2/+2.7 mg/dl (1/2 copies); $p = 0.82$ F: 0.4 /+1.9 mg/dl (1/2 copies); $p = 0.09$	[145]
LIPG		rs2000813	0.24 (T)	A	541 (Co)	+0.5/+6.1 mg/dl (1/2 copies); $p = 0.048$	[83]
LIPG		rs2000813	0.30 (T)	A	265 CVD 265 Co	+3.7 for carries; $p = <0.02$	[184]
LIPG		rs2000813	0.29 (T)	W 90%	372 (CVD)	+1.6/+6.0 mg/dl (1/2 copies); $p = 0.035$	[118]
LIPG	C + 42 T/ln 5	rs2276269	0.44 (T)	W	594 (HDL)	Decreases HDL-C; $p = 0.007$	[122]
LIPG	T + 2864C/l n8	rs6507931	0.42 (C)	W	594 (HDL)	Decreases HDL-C; $p = 0.004$	[122]
LIPG	2237G > A	rs3744841	0.36 (A)	A	340 (kids)	4.0 mg/dl/ -4.3 mg/dl (1/2 copies); $p = 0.011$	[206]
LPL	D9N; Asp9Asn	rs1801177		$-$	5067 (Meta)	-3.1 mg/dl for heteroz.; $p = 0.002$	[200]
LPL	Gly188Glu			$-$	10,434 (Meta)	-9.7 mg/dl for heteroz.; $p < 0.001$	[200]

(continued)

Table 1 (continued)

Gene	Polym.	rs number	MAF	Ethn.	Sample size	Results (effect size, p-value)	Reference
LPL	N291S	rs268		−	14,912 (Meta)	−4.6 mg/dl for heteroz.; $p < 0.001$	[200]
LPL	HindIll; Int8	rs320	0.30 (H)	W	520 (P)	+5.5 mg/dl in H − H − versus H + H +; $p = 0.025$	[167]
LPL	HindIll; Int8	rs320	0.26 (H1)	W	1361 (P)	M: +3.5 mg/dl for heteroz.; $p = 0.0018$ F:+4.2 mg/dl for heteroz.; $p = 0.0212$	[78]
LPL	HindIll; Int8	rs320	0.32 (H)	W	906 (GP)	+1.9 mg/dl; $p = 0.003$	[34]
LPL	HindIll; Int8	rs320		A	550 (NGT) 465 (DM)	NGT: +3.0 mg/dl for carriers; $p < 0.05$ DM: +1.0 mg/dl for carriers; $p < 0.05$	[153]
LPL	HindIll; Int8	rs320	0.27–0.31	NHW, H	615(W); 579(H)	$p = 0.005$	[3]
LPL		rs326	0.44	B	1943 (P)	M; $p = 0.013$; F; $p = 0.004$	[101]
LPL	S447X Ser447Ter	rs328			4388 (Meta)	+1.5 mg/dl for heteroz.; $p < 0.001$	[200]
LPL	S447X Ser447Ter	rs328	0.10 (G)	W	8968 (P)	+2.8/+4.0 mg/dl (1/2 copies); $p < 0.001$	[136]
LPL	S447X Ser447Ter	rs328	0.07 (G)	B	2677 (P)	+3.1/+12.6 mg/dl (1/2 copies); $p < 0.001$	
LPL	S447X	rs328	0.11 (X)	A	4058 (P)	+3.1 mg/dl; $p < 0.001$	[112]
LPL		rs328		W	1543 (P)	+2.7 mg/dl; $p = 0.0017$	[35]
LPL		rs328			25,167	$p = 5.6E-22$	[41]
LPL		rs328	0.09 (G)	W	5287 (GP)	+3/+5 mg/dl (1/2 copies); $p = 3 \times 10{-12}$	[95]
LPL		rs325	0.89 (T)	E	17,723	$p = 7.8 \times 10{-25}$	[195]
MARCH8	C > A	rs970548	0.26 (A)	EA AA, A	188,577 (Meta)	$p = 2 \times 10{-10}$	[198]
MLXIPL		rs17145738	0.12 (T)	EA	25,167	$p = 1.64E-05$	[41]
MOGAT2	A > C	rs499974	0.19 (C)	EA AA, A	188,577 (Meta)	$p = 1 \times 10{-8}$	[198]
M-RAS		rs6782181	0.39 (G)	S	2429 CAD 2221 C		[7]
M-RAS		rs253662	0.19 (G)	S	2429 CAD 2221 C		[7]

(continued)

Table 1 (continued)

Gene	Polym.	rs number	MAF	Ethn.	Sample size	Results (effect size, p-value)	Reference
OR4C46	C > T	rs11246602	0.15 (T)	EA AA, A	188,577 (Meta)	$p = 2 \times 10{-}10$	[198]
PIGV-NR0B2	T > C	rs12748152	0.09 (C)	EA AA, A	188,577 (Meta)	$p = 1 \times 10{-}15$	[198]
PON1	Q192R	rs662 = rs60480675	0.30 (G)	W	1232 (P)	W: +0.1/+2.3 mg/dl (1/2 copies); $p = 0.041$	[179]
PON1	Gln192Arg	rs662 = rs60480675	0.67	B	554	−5.4/−6.7 mg/dl (1/2 copies); $p = 0.008$	[179]
PON1		rs662 = rs60480675	0.29 (R)	Hu	738 (P)	−3.1 mg/dl/ −3.1 mg/dl (1/2 copies); $p = 0.001$	[71]
PON1		rs662 = rs60480675	0.36 (R)	W-Bra	261 CVD, Co	M: +1.5/+2.7 mg/dl (1/2 copies); $p = 0.035$	[157]
PON1	C-107 T	rs705379	0.48 (C)	W	710 (CVD)	−3.1/−2.3 mg/dl (1/2 copies); $p = 0.006$	[19]
PON1	Leu55M	rs85456	0.20 (T)	M-A	741	$p = 0.02$	[29]
PPAR γ	C1431T	rs3856806	0.15 (T)	C	820	$p < 0.01$	[65]
RSPO3	C > T	rs1936800	0.49 (T)	EA AA, A	188,577 (Meta)	$p = 3 \times 10{-}10$	[198]
SETD2	A > G	rs2290547	0.20 (G)	EA AA, A	188,577 (Meta)	$p = 4 \times 10{-}9$	[198]
SCARB 1	Exon 8 C > T	rs5888	0.44 (T)	W	865 (P)	+1.9/2.7 mg/dl (1/2 copies); $p = 0.006$	[132]
SCARB 1	C1050T	rs5888	0.49 (T)	W	546 (CVD)	+2.3/+1.9 mg/dl (1/2 copies); $p = 0.03$	[22]
SNX13	T > G	rs4142995	0.38 (G)	EA AA, A	188,577 (Meta)	$p = 9 \times 10{-}12$	[198]
STAB1	A > G	rs13326165	0.21 (G)	EA AA, A	188,577 (Meta)	$p = 9 \times 10{-}11$	[198]
TMEM176A	C > T	rs17173637	0.12 (T)	EA AA, A	188,577 (Meta)	$p = 2 \times 10{-}10$	[198]
ZBTB42-AKT1	G > A	rs4983559	0.40 (A)	EA AA, A	188,577 (Meta)	$p = 1 \times 10{-}8$	[198]

Adapted from Nock and Pillai [137] and Boes et al. [23] with permission from Elsevier

Abbreviations: *MAF* minor allele frequency, *A* Asians, *AA* African-Americans, *Am* Amish, *A-I* Asian Indian, *B* Blacks, *C* Chinese, *CH* Caribbean Hispanics, *E* European, *EA* European America, *I* Inuit, *Ma* Malays, *N* Netherlands, *NHW* non-Hispanic whites, *H* Hispanics, *Hu* Hutterites, *J* Japanese, *K* Korean, *L* Lithuanian, *S* Saudi Arabian, *Tu* Turks, *UK* United Kingdom, *W-Bra* Caucasian Brazilians, *W* Whites/Caucasians, *WS* Western Siberian Caucasians, *Va* various, *Non-DM C0* non diabetic control subjects, *MI* myocardial infarction, *NGT* normal glucose tolerance, *DM* Diabetes mellitus, *Ho Sta* hospital staff, *HBP* hypertensive patients, *He Ex* health examination, *Cor Ang* coronary angiography, *hyperCH* hypercholesterolemia patients, *CVD* cardiovascular disease, *C* controls, *Ho Co* hospital-based controls, *GP* general population, *Meta* meta-analysis, *P* population based, *M* males, *F* females, + increase, − decrease, *n.s.* not significant; see text for full gene names

biological pathways including HDL-C synthesis and metabolism as well as relevant transport, receptor, and ligand-binding (via apolipoproteins) mechanisms.

Variation in Genes Involved in HDL-C Synthesis and Metabolism

One of the most notable genes involved in HDL-C synthesis and metabolism is the cholesterol ester transfer protein (CETP) gene located on chromosome 16 (16q21) whose variants have been associated with HDL-C. CETP is a key plasma protein that mediates the transfer of esterified cholesterol from HDL to APOB (see section "Variation in Genes Involved in HDL-C Transport and Binding") containing particles in exchange for TG. Three common polymorphisms (Table 1: TaqIB (rs708272); −629C > A (rs1800775); Ile405Val (rs5882)) can all modestly inhibit CETP activity and have been consistently associated with higher HDL-C levels [17, 18, 20, 21, 24, 44, 51, 95, 99, 169, 181, 186].

Another key gene involved in HDL-C metabolism is lipoprotein lipase (LPL) located on chromosome 8 (8p22), which encodes an enzyme involved in lipolysis of TG-containing lipoproteins such as VLDL and chylomicrons [130] that generate free fatty acids (FFA) that can be taken up by the liver, muscle, and adipose tissues [105]. Thus, LPL may only affect HDL-C levels indirectly [113] but can affect LDL levels directly (see section "Genetics of LDL-C"). Several SNPs in LPL have been associated with HDL-C (Table 1) [3, 34, 78, 101, 103, 112, 136, 167, 200], and many of these SNPs are in strong linkage disequilibrium (LD) with each other (e.g., rs320, rs326, rs13702, rs10105606) [23, 73].

The hepatic lipase (HL; LIPC) gene located on chromosome 15 (15q21) encodes a glycoprotein that is synthesized by liver cells (hepatocytes) and catalyzes the hydrolysis of TG and phospholipids [131], and following hydrolysis of TG by LPL, VLDL particles are reduced to IDL particles that may be further hydrolyzed by HL/LIPC to LDL or taken up by the liver [105]. Several HL/LIPC SNPs have been associated with HDL-C with, perhaps, the most consistent associations with rs1800588 and rs2070895 (Table 1; [8, 35, 39, 48, 61, 84, 86, 95, 102, 127, 136, 180, 183, 196, 204]).

The endothelial lipase (EL; LIPG) gene, located on chromosome 18 (18q21.1), is an enzyme expressed in endothelial cells that, in the presence of HL/LIPC, metabolizes larger (HDL3) to smaller (HDL2) HDL-C particles and increases the catabolism of APOA-I (see section "Variation in Genes Involved in HDL-C Transport and Binding") [89]. Several EL/LPIG polymorphisms have been associated with HDL-C levels (Table 1; [83, 118, 122, 145, 184, 206]). Only the nonsynonymous SNP, rs2000813, has been consistently associated with HDL-C levels in African-Americans [83, 184, 206].

The lecithin-cholesterol acyltransferase (LCAT) gene, located on chromosome 16 (16q22.1), catalyzes the esterification of free cholesterol and metabolizes larger HDL-C particles to smaller HDL-C particles in the presence of cofactor APOA-I [100, 130]. However, polymorphisms in LCAT have only been inconsistently associated with changes in HDL-C levels (Table 1; [22, 129, 146, 208, 210]).

Paraoxonase 1 (PON1), which is located on chromosome 7 (7q21.3), inhibits the oxidation of LDL [119] and may, therefore, only indirectly affect antioxidant properties of HDL-C. Several SNPs in PON1 have been associated with HDL-C levels including two nonsynonymous SNPs, rs662 and rs3202100, which are in strong LD; however, results have been inconsistent across studies (Table 1; [19, 71, 123, 157, 190]).

Variation in Genes Involved in HDL-C Transport and Binding

Many common variants in genes involved in HDL-C transport and binding have been implicated. The scavenger receptor class B type 1 (SCARB1; SR-B1) gene located on chromosome 12 (12q24.31) is a key gene, which has been shown to participate in the uptake of HDL in animals by transferring cholesterol from the HDL-C particle and releasing the lipid-depleted

HDL particle into the circulation [1, 131]. Polymorphisms in SCARB1 have been associated with HDL-C levels with the most notable being rs5888 (Table 1; [22, 35, 80, 132, 142, 160, 176]).

The LDL receptor (LDLR) gene located on chromosome 19 (19p13.2) participates in the uptake of LDL and chylomicron remnants by hepatocytes [105] and may only indirectly affect HDL-C levels. However, a few polymorphisms in LDLR have been associated with HDL-C levels (Table 1; [35, 71, 205]), but their impact is greater on LDL-C levels.

The ATP-binding cassette transporter A1 (ABCA1), located on chromosome 9 (9q31.1), plays a key role in "reverse cholesterol transport" by mediating the efflux of cholesterol and phospholipids from macrophages to the nascent lipid-free, APOA-1 HDL particle [28, 131]. Several polymorphisms have been fairly consistently associated with HDL-C levels, but different variants appear to drive this association in different ethnic groups (Table 1; [32, 35, 53, 77, 95, 100, 150, 175, 196]).

The apolipoprotein A-1 (APOA1; APOA-I) gene, located on chromosome 11 (11q23-24), encodes a ligand required for HDL-C binding to its receptors including SCARB1 and ABCA1 and is an important cofactor in "reverse cholesterol transport" [131, 155, 156]. Polymorphisms in APOA-I have been associated with HDL-C levels, but results across studies have been inconsistent (Table 1; [25, 92, 111, 174]). Apolipoprotein A-4 (APOA4; APOA-IV) gene is part of the "APOA1/C3/A4/A5 gene cluster" and a potent activator of LCAT which modulates the activation of LPL and transfer of cholesteryl esters from HDL to LDL [105]. Polymorphisms in APOA4 have not been as well studied, but rs5110 (Gln360His) and rs675 have been associated with reduced HDL-C levels [143, 152].

Apolipoprotein A-5 (APOA5; APOA-V), located predominantly on TG-rich chylomicrons and VLDL, activates LPL [82]. A few APOA5 SNPs have been associated with HDL-C levels with rs651821 and rs662799 having the most consistent results across studies (Table 1; [60, 82, 101, 108, 152, 182, 204, 205]). Recently, rs964184 in the APOA5-A4-C3-A1 cluster was

associated with HDL-C in the SMART (Second Manifestations of ARTerial disease) cohort [191].

Apolipoprotein C-3 (APOC3; APOC-III), an inhibitor of LPL and transferred to HDL during the hydrolysis of TG-rich lipoproteins [105, 131], has several SNPs that have been identified, but associations with HDL-C levels have been inconsistent (Table 1; [11, 25, 34, 71, 92, 106, 144, 152, 164]). Apolipoprotein E (APOE), a critical ligand for binding to hepatic receptors that remove VLDL and LDL particles from the circulation, has several SNPs that have been fairly consistent associated with HDL-C levels [35, 52, 62, 94, 176, 178, 192, 199, 201].

Variation in Genes Involved in Cell Proliferation, Inflammation, and Related Pathways

The M-RAS gene located on chromosome 3 (3q22.2) encodes a member of the membrane-associated family of Ras small GTPase proteins engaged in tumor necrosis factor-alpha-stimulated lymphocyte function that appears to play a role in adhesion signaling, which is an important aspect of atherosclerotic pathways [55]. Interestingly, a few common variants in M-RAS, most notably, rs6782181, have recently been associated with low HDL-C levels in a large study involving CAD cases and "controls" with "no significant coronary stenosis by angiography" [7]; however, this finding does not appear to have been replicated yet in other populations.

GATA2, an endothelial transcription factor, located on chromosome 3 (3q21.3), is a multicatalytic transcription factor that plays a major role in controlling growth factor responsiveness and regulating inflammatory processes [188]. The rs7431368 SNP of the GATA2 gene has recently been associated with low HDL-C levels in a large Saudi case-control study involving 2386 CAD cases and 2171 angiographed controls [133].

Peroxisome proliferator-activated receptor gamma (PPARγ) may play a key role in lipid metabolism by inducing the transcription of related genes. Recently, the rs3856808 variant in PPARγ was associated with HDL-C levels in a random sample of 820 Chinese from the prevention of multiple metabolic disorders and metabolic syndrome in the Jiangsu province cohort [66].

The butyrophilin subfamily 2 member A1 (BTN2A1) gene, located on chromosome 6 (6p22.1), encodes proteins that help in the production of milk fat globules and regulating immune function [140]. The rs6929846 variant of BTN2A1 has been associated with HDL-C levels in large cohorts of Japanese and Korean individuals [54]. The combination of the rs6929846 T allele of BTN2A1 with the rs662799 C allele of APOA5 has also been associated with 35% lower HDL-C levels in Japanese individuals [75].

Genetic Variants Associated with HDL-C Identified Through GWAS

Results from genome-wide association studies (GWAS) have confirmed associations between polymorphisms in viable candidate genes including CETP, LPL, HL/LIPIC, EL/LIPG, ABCA1, LCAT, and the APOA1/C3/A4/A5 gene cluster and HDL-C levels [23]. GWAS have also identified two novel putative loci associated with HDL-C levels in a large Chinese pediatric population [172]. Twenty-four novel loci, all of which had MAF >0.05 (Table 1), were recently identified in a joint GWAS and Metabochip meta-analysis in 188,577 individuals of European East Asian, South Asian, and African ancestry [198]. Other novel and candidate loci from GWAS have been summarized nicely in other reviews [154, 185].

Genetics of LDL-C

Table 1 lists genetic variants associated with LDL-C in larger-scale studies. Below, we describe variants in genes based on their involvement in relevant biological pathways including LDL-C-related enzymes, receptors and transporters, lipoprotein, and protease mechanisms.

Genetic Variation in Enzymes, Receptors and Transporters, and LDL-C

The most marketed drugs for lowering LDL-C are statins, which inhibit hydroxy-3-methylglutaryl coenzyme A reductase (HMGCR), the rate-limiting enzyme in cholesterol synthesis that is normally suppressed [45]. The human HMGCR gene is located on chromosome 5 (5q13.3-14). Only a few common HMGCR polymorphisms have been associated with LDL-C levels including rs3846662 (Table 2) [26, 76, 149, 185].

As mentioned above, the LDL receptor (LDLR) gene, located on chromosome 19 (19p13.2), helps to regulate the uptake of LDL and chylomicron remnants by hepatocytes [105]. Although not the focus of this review, we note that familial (monogenic) hypercholesterolemia (FH: OMIM No. 143890) is one of the most common inherited metabolic diseases due to mutations in LDLR (a frequency of approximately 1 in 500 (heterozygotes) to 1 in 1,000,000 (homozygotes)) with heterozygotes having a decreased receptors and a two to three-fold increase in LDL-C levels and homozygotes having a complete loss of LDLR function and a greater than fivefold increase in LDL-C [56]. Several common polymorphisms in LDLR have also been identified and associated with more modest changes in LDL-C levels, including rs17248720, which was associated with LDL-C levels in Spanish "normolipemic" controls from the Aragon Workers Health Study (AWHS) [40], and rs6511720, which was associated with LDL-C in a meta-analysis [185, 197].

The ATP-binding cassette transporters G5 and G8 (ABCG5/8) gene cluster, located on chromosome 2 (2p21), regulates the efflux of cholesterol back into the intestinal lumen and, in hepatocytes, the efflux of cholesterol into bile [59]. A few common variants in ABCG5/8 have been associated with LDL-C levels (Table 2); however, a recent meta-analysis failed to find an association between the ABCG5/G8 polymorphism, rs6544718, and plasma lipid levels [88, 185].

Table 2 Genetic polymorphisms associated with LDL-C (see Table 1 legend for details)

Gene	Polym.	rs number	MAF	Ethn.	Sample size	Results (effect size, p-value)	Reference
ABCG8		rs4299376	0.30 (G)	E	95,454 (Meta)	+2.75 mg/dl; $p = 2 \times 10{-}8$	[185]
ABCG8	A632V	rs6544718		Va	982	$p = 0.02$	[88]
ACAD11	T > G	rs17404153	0.14 (G)	EA AA, A	188,577 (Meta)	$p = 2 \times 10{-}9$	[198]
APOB		rs562338	0.18 (A)	Va	10,849	+4.89 mg/dl; $p = 3.6 \times 10{-}12$	[197]
APOB		rs754523	0.28 (A)	Va	6542	+2.78 mg/dl; $p = 1.3 \times 10{-}6$	[197]
APOB		rs693	0.42 (G)	Va	3222	+2.44 mg/dl; $p = 0.0034$	[197]
APOB	Thr98Ile	rs1367117	0.30 (A)	E	95,454 (Meta)	+4.05 mg/dl; $p = 4 \times 10{-}114$	[185]
APOB		rs7575840	0.28 (T)	F	5054	0.131; $p = 3.88 \times 10{-}9$	[68]
APOB		rs515135	0.19 (A)	Va	982	$p = 2.4 \times 10{-}20$	[195]
APOE		rs4420638	0.17 (G)	E	95,454 (Meta)	+7.14 mg/dl; $p = 9 \times 10{-}147$	[185]
APOE	Arg176 Cys	rs7412	0.06 (T)	N-HB	683	−22.52 mg/dl; $p < 0.0001$	[29]
APOE	Cys130 Arg	rs429358	0.076 (T)	M-A	739	10.54 mg/dl; $p < 0.0001$	[29]
APOE	Cys130 Arg	rs429358	0.10 (E2)	L	1030; 605 W	E2 versus E3 (women); 0.35 (0.22–0.57)	[176]
APOE	Cys130 Arg	rs429358	0.09 (E4)	L	1030; 425 M	E4 versus E3 (men); $p < 0.05$	[176]
APOC1		rs4420638	0.82 (A)	Va	10,806	+6.61 mg/dl; $p = 4.9 \times 10{-}24$	[197]
APOE/ C1/C4		rs10402271	0.67 (T)	Va	6519	+2.62 mg/dl; $p = 1.5 \times 10{-}5$	[197]
ANXA9-CERS2	G > A	rs267733	0.16 (A)	EA AA, A	188,577 (Meta)	$p = 5 \times 10{-}9$	[198]
BTN2A1		rs6929846		J	5958	T allele; $p = 0.046$	[79]
BRCA2	T > C	rs4942486	0.48 (C)	EA AA, A	188,577 (Meta)	$p = 2 \times 10{-}11$	[198]
CMTM6	T > C	rs7640978	0.09 (C)	EA AA, A	188,577 (Meta)	$p = 1 \times 10{-}8$	[198]

(continued)

Table 2 (continued)

Gene	Polym.	rs number	MAF	Ethn.	Sample size	Results (effect size, p-value)	Reference
CSNK1G3	G > A	rs4520754	0.46 (A)	EA AA, A	188,577 (Meta)	$p = 4 \times 10{-}12$	[198]
EHBP1	G > A	rs2710642	0.45 (A)	EA AA, A	188,577 (Meta)	$p = 6 \times 10{-}9$	[198]
FN1	T > C	rs1250229	0.27 (C)	EA AA, A	188,577 (Meta)	$p = 3 \times 10{-}8$	[198]
LDLR		rs6511720	0.11 (T)	E	95,454 (Meta)	-6.99 mg/dl; $p = 4 \times 10{-}117$	[185]
INSIG2	A > G	rs12464355	0.10 (G)	W	561 (child)	B = -0.12 ± 0.03; $p = 2.7 \times 10{-}5$	[96]
INSIG2	C > T	rs2042492	0.27 (T)	B	497 (child)	B = 0.04 ± 0.02; $p = 0.04$	[96]
INSIG2	A > G	rs10490626	0.08 (G)	EA AA, A	188,577 (Meta)	$p = 2 \times 10{-}12$	[198]
LDLR		rs6511720	0.90 (T)	Va	7442	$+9.17$ mg/dl; $p = 3.3 \times 10{-}19$	[197]
LDLR	C3130T	rs17248720	0.16 (T)	S	525 C		[40]
MIR148A	C > T	rs4722551	0.20 (T)	EA AA, A	188,577 (Meta)	$p = 4 \times 10{-}14$	[198]
PCSK9		rs11206510	0.81 (C)	Va	10,805	$+3.04$ mg/dl; $p = 5.4 \times 10{-}7$	[197]
PCSK9		rs2479409	0.30 (G)	E	95,454 (Meta)	$+2.01$ mg/dl; $p = 2 \times 10{-}28$	[185]
PCSK9	A443T Ala443Thr	rs28362263	0.06 (A)	B	1750	95.5 versus 106.9 mg/dl; $p < 0.001$	[81]
PCSK9	C679X	rs28362286		B	1750	81.5 versus 106.9 mg/dl; $p < 0.001$	[81]
PCSK9	E670G	rs505151	0.11 (G)	W	691	$p = 0.001$	[31]
PCSK9		rs11206510	0.81 (T)	EA	21,986 (Meta)	$p = 1.44E{-}05$	[41]
SCARB 1 C1050T rs5888 0.41 (T) L 1030 TT versus CC (men only): $p < 0.05$ [176]	C1050T	rs5888	0.41 (T)	L	1030	TT versus CC (men); $p < 0.05$	[176]
SNX5	C > A	rs2328223	0.21 (A)	EA AA, A	188,577 (Meta)	$p = 4 \times 10{-}9$	[198]

(continued)

Table 2 (continued)

Gene	Polym.	rs number	MAF	Ethn.	Sample size	Results (effect size, p-value)	Reference
SORT1		rs629301	0.22 (G)	E	95,454 (Meta)	−5.65 mg/dl; $p = 1 \times 10-170$	[185]
SOX17	A > G	rs10102164	0.21 (A)	EA AA, A	188,577 (Meta)	$p = 4 \times 10-11$	[198]
SPTLC3	A > G	rs364585	0.38 (G)	EA AA, A	188,577 (Meta)	$p = 4 \times 10-10$	[198]

Genetic Variation in Lipoproteins and LDL-C

Apolipoprotein B (APOB; main isoform: ApoB-100), located on chromosome 2 (2p23-24), is responsible for the uptake of LDL by LDLR, which clears approximately 60–80% of the LDL in "normal" individuals with the remaining taken up by LRP or SCARB1 [105]. Common polymorphisms in APOB have been identified and associated with changes in LDL-C (Table 2; [68, 185, 195, 197]).

As mentioned above, APOE, located on chromosome 19 (19q13.2), is a critical ligand for binding chylomicron remnants, VLDL, and IDL particles to hepatic receptors to remove these particles from the circulation [105]. The structural APOE gene is polymorphic with three common alleles, designated as ε2, ε3, and ε4, which encode for E2, E3, and E4 proteins, respectively. Recently, the ε2 allele has been associated with high LDL-C levels in Lithuanian women [176]; however, the APOE ε4 allele has been the most consistently associated with LDL-C levels [10, 29, 43, 185, 197].

Genetic Variation in Proteases and LDL-C Levels

Proprotein convertase subtilisin-like kexin type 9 (PCSK9), located on chromosome 1 (1p32.3), is a serine protease that degrades hepatic LDLR in endosomes [126]. Over 50 variants in PCSK9 have been shown to affect circulating levels of cholesterol; however, most of these are relatively rare [38]. However, a few common polymorphisms in PCSK9 have been associated with LDL-C levels (Table 2) [31, 46, 81, 185, 197].

Genetic Variation in Inflammatory and Immune Systems and LDL-C

As mentioned above, the BTN2A1 gene, located on chromosome 6 (6p22.1), encodes proteins that help in the production of milk fat globules and regulating immune function [140]. The rs6929846 variant of BTN2A1 has been associated with HDL-C levels in a large community-dwelling cohort of Japanese individuals [79].

Insulin-induced gene 2 (INSIG2) located on chromosome 2 (2q14.2) plays a role in regulating lipid storage as well as blocking further cholesterol synthesis when sterols are present in the cell [203]. Recently, a common variant in INSIG2, rs12464355, has been associated with LDL-C levels in a random sample of non-Hispanic white children from the Princeton School District Study, a prospective cohort of fifth through 12th graders [96]. However, in this same study, rs1352083, rs13393332, and rs2042492, all in strong LD (but not rs12464355) in the INSIG2 gene, were associated with LDL-C levels in African-American children [96].

GWAS, Exome Sequencing, and LDL-C

GWAS have confirmed associations between polymorphisms in viable candidate genes including APOB, APOE, LDLR, and PCSK9 and have identified novel SNPs associated with LDL-C levels with strong biological plausibility including an inhibitor of lipase (ANGPTL3) and a transcription factor activating triglyceride synthesis (MLXIPL) [185]. GWAS have also identified four novel putative loci associated with LDL-C levels in a large Chinese pediatric population [172]. Fifteen novel loci, 13 of which had MAF >0.05 (and are listed in Table 2), were recently identified in a joint GWAS and Metabochip meta-analysis in 188,577 individuals of European East Asian, South Asian, and African ancestry [198].

Exome sequencing can help to identify rare, low-frequency variants and confirm known candidate loci. Recently, 2005 individuals (1854 African-American, 1153 European-American) from seven population-based cohorts were exome sequenced (with at least $20\times$ coverage over 70% of the exome target) and evaluated for associations with LDL-C levels [109]. Interestingly, single-variant (univariate/multivariable) analyses only identified one variant near APOE that was statistically significant (rs1160983, $p = 7.6 \times 10^{-14}$) [109]; however, more elegant statistical methods identified additional novel variants and confirmed associations with candidate loci.

Genetics of Triglycerides (TG)

Table 3 lists genetic variants associated with TG in larger-scale studies. Below, we describe variants in genes based on their involvement in relevant biological pathways including binding (via apolipoproteins) as well as relevant enzymes, receptors, and transporter mechanisms. Because plasma TG integrate multiple TG-rich lipoprotein particles, it is not surprising that there is considerable overlap between the genetic variants associated with TG levels and the genetic variants associated with HDL-C and LDL-C levels. The Global Lipids Genetics Consortium (GLGC) found that 15 of the 32 loci associated with TG levels were also jointly associated with HDL-C levels, explaining 9.6% of the total variation in plasma TG, which corresponded to 25–30% of the total genetic contribution to TG variability [185]. However, most loci appear to be more strongly associated with one lipid phenotype, while only a few loci have similar effect sizes across lipid phenotypes. Furthermore, there is substantial genetic heterogeneity between major ethnic groups (e.g., between Caucasians and African-Americans).

Genetic Variation in Apolipoproteins and TG

As mentioned above, APOB, located on chromosome 2 (2p23–24), is the backbone of atherogenic lipoproteins. APOB polymorphisms have been predominantly associated with LDL-C [16], but GWAS revealed that a common SNP in APOB, rs1042034, has been associated with TG [90, 185]. Further, polymorphisms in the APOA1/C3/A4/A5 gene cluster, located on chromosome 11 (11q23), have been associated with TG as well as HDL-C levels [185, 191, 197]. An SNP in the APOE gene, rs439401, has been shown to be strongly associated with TG levels [71, 90, 185]. The combination of the rs662799 C allele of APOA5 and the rs6929846 T allele of BTN2A1 has been associated with 41% higher TG levels in Japanese and 24% higher TG levels in Korean individuals [12, 75]. Furthermore, the BUD13/ZNF259 A-C – A-G-C-C haplotype (ZNF259 rs2075290, ZNF259 rs964184, BUD13 rs10790162, BUD13 rs17119975, BUD13 rs11556024, BUD13 rs35585096), near APOA5 on chromosome 11q23.3 and involved in cell proliferation and signal transduction, has been associated with high TG in a random sample of 1181 Chinese individuals [12].

Angiopoietin-like 3 protein (ANGPTL3) inhibits LPL catalytic activity, but this process is reversible [170, 173]. Polymorphisms in ANGPTL3, most notably, rs2131925, have been associated with TG levels [90, 97, 110, 185, 197]. In addition, several nonsynonymous ANGPTL3 variants have been associated with TG levels [135] in the Dallas Heart Study, but these SNPs have not been validated yet in other populations.

Table 3 Genetic polymorphisms associated with TG (see Table 1 legend for details)

	Polym.	rs number	MAF	Ethn.	Sample size	Results (effect size, p-value)	Reference
AKR1C4	G > A	rs1832007	0.10 (A)	EA AA, A	188,577 (Meta)	$p = 2 \times 10{-}12$	[198]
ANGPTL3		rs2131925	0.32 (G)	E	96,598 (Meta)	-4.94 mg/dl; $p = 9 \times 10{-}43$	[185]
ANGPTL3		rs1748195	0.70 (G)	Va	9559	7.12 mg/dl; $p = 5.4 \times 10{-}8$	[197]
APOA5		rs964184	0.13 (G)	E	96,598 (Meta)	$+16.95$ mg/dl; $p = 7 \times 10{-}240$	[185]
APOA5-A4/A1		rs964184	0.14 (G)	C	5547	0.12 (0.10–0.15); $p = 1.1 \times 10{-}19$	[191]
APOA5/A4/C3/A1		rs12286037	0.94 (C)	Va	9738	25.82 mg/dl; $p = 1.6 \times 10{-}22$	[197]
APOA5		rs662799	0.05 (A)	Va	3248	16.88 mg/dl; $p = 2.7 \times 10{-}10$	[197]
APOA5/A4/C3/A1		rs2000571	0.17 (G)	Va	3209	6.93 mg/dl; $p = 8.7 \times 10{-}5$	[197]
APOA5/A4/C3/A1		rs486394	0.28 (A)	Va	3597	1.50 mg/dl; $p = 0.0073$	[197]
APOE		rs439401	0.40 (C)	C	4.192	$p = 2.2 \times 10{-}5$	[115]
APOE		rs439401	0.64 (C)	Va	Meta	$p = 5.5 \times 10{-}30$	[91]
BTN2A1	C > T	rs6929846		J	5958	T allele; $p = 0.001$	[79]
GATA2	C > A	rs7431368		S	2386 CAD 2171 C	B $= -1.49$; s.e. $= 0.67$; $p = 0.03$; $p = 0.ppp$	[133]
INSIG2	G > A	rs889904	0.58 (A)	B	497 (child)	B $= -0.06 \pm 0.03$; $p = 0.01$	[96]
INSR	A > G	rs7248104	0.42 (G)	EA AA, A	188,577 (Meta)	$p = 5 \times 10{-}10$	[198]
LRPAP1	G > A	rs6831256	0.42 (A)	EA AA, A	188,577 (Meta)	$p = 2 \times 10{-}12$	[198]
LIPC/HL		rs4775041	0.67 (G)	Va	8462	3.62 mg/dl; $p = 2.9 \times 10{-}5$	[197]
LIPC/HL		rs261342	0.22 (G)	Va	Meta	$p = 2.0 \times 10{-}13$	[91]
LPL		rs12678919	0.12 (G)	E	96,598 (Meta)	-13.64 mg/dl; $p = 2 \times 10{-}115$	[185]
LPL		rs10503669	0.90 (A)	Va	9711	11.57 mg/dl; $p = 1.6 \times 10{-}14$	[197]
LPL		rs2197089	0.58 (A)	Va	3202	3.38 mg/dl; $p = 0.0029$	[197]
LPL		rs6586891	0.66 (A)	Va	3622	4.60 mg/dl; $p = 5 \times 10{-}4$	[197]
LPL	S447X	rs328	0.90 (C)	EA	24,258	$p = 4.16E{-}30$	[41]
LPL	S447X	rs328	0.10 (X)	Va	43,242	$-0.15(-0.12$ to $-0.19)$ mmol/l	[165]
LPL	D9N	rs1801177	0.03 (N)	Va	21,040	0.14 (0.08–0.20) mmol/l	[165]
LPL	N291S	rs368	0.03 (S)	Va	27,204	0.19 (0.12–0.26) mmol/l	[165]
LPL		rs326	0.18 (G)	C	4192	$p = 2.3 \times 10{-}6$	[115]
LRP1		rs11613352	0.23 (T)	E	96,598 (Meta)	-2.70 mg/dl; $p = 4 \times 10{-}10$	[185]

(continued)

Table 3 (continued)

	Polym.	rs number	MAF	Ethn.	Sample size	Results (effect size, p-value)	Reference
MET	G > A	rs38855	0.47 (A)	EA AA, A	188,577 (Meta)	$p = 1 \times 10{-}8$	[198]
MPP3	C > A	rs8077889	0.22 (A)	EA AA, A	188,577 (Meta)	$p = 1 \times 10{-}8$	[198]
MLXIPL		rs17145738	0.12 (T)	E	96,598 (Meta)	-9.32 mg/dl; $p = 6 \times 10{-}58$	[185]
MLXIPL		rs17145738	0.84 (T)	Va	9741	8.21 mg/dl; $p = 5 \times 10{-}8$	[197]
MLXIPL		rs7811265	0.81 (A)	Va	Meta	7.91 mg/dl $p = 9.0 \times 10{-}59$	[91]
PDXDC1	T > C	rs3198697	0.43 (C)	EA AA, A	188,577 (Meta)	$p = 2 \times 10{-}8$	[198]
PEPD	G > A	rs731839	0.35 (A)	EA AA, A	188,577 (Meta)	$p = 3 \times 10{-}9$	[198]
PPAR γ	Pro12 Ala	rs180592	0.26 (Ala)	C	820	$p < 0.01$	[66]
SULF2	A > G	rs2281279		C	1319	"G" allele; $p = 0.049$	[70]
VEGFA	A > C	rs998584	0.49 (C)	EA AA, A	188,577 (Meta)	$p = 3 \times 10{-}15$	[198]

Adapted from Nock and Pillai [137] and Boes et al. [23] with permission from Elsevier

Abbreviations: *MAF* minor allele frequency, *A* Asians, *AA* African-Americans, *Am* Amish, *A-I* Asian Indian, *B* Blacks, *C* Chinese, *CH* Caribbean Hispanics, *E* European, *EA* European America, *I* Inuit, *Ma* Malays, *N* Netherlands, *NHW* non-Hispanic whites, *H* Hispanics, *Hu* Hutterites, *J* Japanese, *K* Korean, *L* Lithuanian, *S* Saudi Arabian, *Tu* Turks, *UK* United Kingdom, *W-Bra* Caucasian Brazilians, *W* Whites/Caucasians, *WS* Western Siberian Caucasians, *Va* various, *Non-DM C0* non diabetic control subjects, *MI* myocardial infarction, *NGT* normal glucose tolerance, *DM* Diabetes mellitus, *Ho Sta* hospital staff, *HBP* hypertensive patients, *He Ex* health examination, *Cor Ang* coronary angiography, *hyperCH* hypercholesterolemia patients, *CVD* cardiovascular disease, *C* controls, *Ho Co* hospital-based controls, *GP* general population, *Meta* meta-analysis, *P* population based, *M* males, *F* females, + increase, − decrease, *n.s.* not significant; see text for full gene names

Genetic Variation in Enzymes and Transcription Factors and TG

As mentioned above, LPL is an enzyme that hydrolyzes TG-rich particles in peripheral tissues (muscle, macrophages, adipose) generating FFA and glycerol for energy metabolism and storage [57]. Although more than 100 mutations in LPL have been identified [134], only a few common nonsynonymous SNPs have been consistently associated with TG levels including rs1801177, rs328, and rs268 [121, 158, 165, 185, 197]. Two of these SNPs, rs1801177 and rs328, have been shown to be in strong LD in Caucasians [165].

The MLX interacting protein-like (MLXIPL) gene, located on located on chromosome 7 (7q11.23), encodes a transcription factor of the Myc/Max/Mad superfamily that activates, in a glucose-dependent manner, carbohydrate response element-binding protein (CREBP), which is expressed in lipogenic tissues coordinating the subsequent activation of lipogenic enzymes such as fatty acid synthase (FAS) to convert dietary carbohydrate to TG [85]. The rs1745738 polymorphism, initially identified via GWAS, has been associated with TG levels in several studies [90, 185, 194, 197].

As mentioned above, GATA2, an endothelial transcription factor, is a multi-catalytic transcription factor that plays a major role in controlling growth factor responsiveness and regulating inflammatory processes [188]. The rs7431368 SNP of the GATA2 gene has recently been associated with high TG levels in a large Saudi case-control study involving 2386 CAD cases and 2171 angiographed controls [133].

Peroxisome proliferator-activated receptor gamma (PPARγ) may play a key role in lipid metabolism by inducing the transcription of related genes that sense and regulate lipid metabolism, and, recently, the rs180592 variant in PPARγ was associated with TG levels in a random sample of 820 Chinese from the prevention of multiple metabolic disorders and metabolic syndrome in the Jiangsu province cohort [66]. In addition, the PPARα "V" allele of rs1800206 and the "G" allele of rs4253778 (haplotype) have been shown to be associated with high TG in a Chinese Han population [65].

Genetic Variation in Storage and Inflammatory and Immune Systems and TG

The INSIG2 gene, located on chromosome 2 (2q14.2), plays a role in regulating lipid storage as well as blocking further cholesterol synthesis when sterols are present in the cell [203]. Recently, a common variant in INSIG2, rs889904, was associated with TG levels in African-American children [96]. However, none of the 13 SNPs evaluated in the INSIG2 gene were associated with the non-Hispanic white children in this study [96].

The sulfatase-2 (SULF2) gene, located on chromosome 20 (20q13.12), encodes for the heparin sulfate glucosamine-6-O-ensosulfatase that removes 6-O sulfate groups [161] and is a hepatic heparan sulfate proteoglycan (HSPG) remodeling enzyme involved in TG-rich lipoprotein (TRL) remnant clearance [30, 49]. Recently, the "G" allele of rs2281279 in SULF2 has been found to lower SULF2 mRNA expression in liver biopsies of "healthy" subjects [125], and the "G" allele of rs2281279 has been associated with TG in the Diabetes Care System cohort [70].

Further, the BTN2A1 gene, mentioned above, located on chromosome 6 (6p22.1), encodes proteins that help in the production of milk fat globules and regulating immune function [140]. The rs6929846 variant of BTN2A1 has been associated with TG levels in a large community-dwelling cohort of Japanese individuals [79].

GWAS and TG

GWAS have identified novel mutations and confirmed associations between polymorphisms in viable candidate genes including APOB, APOE, LPL, and MLXIPL [185]. A recent GWAS in a large Chinese pediatric population has identified six additional novel loci associated with TG levels [172]. Furthermore, eight novel loci, all of which had MAF >0.05 (Table 3), were recently identified in a joint GWAS and Metabochip meta-analysis in 188,577 individuals of European East Asian, South Asian, and African ancestry [198].

Genetics of Dyslipidemia

Several investigators have also evaluated many of the aforementioned genetic variants on "dyslipidemia" in addition to individual lipid phenotypes. For example, the rs6929846 variant of BTN2A1 has been associated with dyslipidemia (defined as HDL-C <1.04 mmol/l, LDL-C ≥3.64 mmol/l, TG ≥1.65 mmol/l, or on anti-dyslipidemic drugs), as well as high LDL (section "Genetic Variation in Inflammatory and Immune Systems and LDL-C") and high TG (section "Genetic Variation in Enzymes and Transcription Factors and TG") levels in a large community-dwelling cohort of Japanese individuals [79]. The PPARγ rs3856806 "T" allele, the PPARγ rs1805192 "Ala" allele, and the PPARα rs1800206 "V" allele have all been associated with an increased risk of dyslipidemia (defined as HDL-C <1.04 mmol/l for men, HDL-C <1.30 mmol/l for women, LDL-C ≥4.14 mmol/l, TG ≥2.26 mmol/l, or total cholesterol (TC) ≥6.24 mmol/l) in a Chinese Han population

[65]. In addition, the PPARα "V" allele of rs1800206 and the "G" allele of rs4253778 (haplotype) have been shown to be associated with a fivefold increased risk of dyslipidemia in this Chinese Han population [65].

The Niemann-Pick C1-like 1 (NPC1L1) gene, located on chromosome 7 (7p13), plays a role in intestinal cholesterol absorption, and decreases in LDL-C levels in response to Ezetimibe, a pharmacologic inhibitor of NPC1L1, have been observed [33]. The rs2072183, rs217428, and rs217434 polymorphisms in NPC1L1 have been associated with dyslipidemia in several studies [72, 93, 120].

Genetics of Dyslipidemia Using More Complex Modeling Approaches

Given the polygenic nature and complexity of dyslipidemia, a better understanding of the collective integration of these genetic determinants is needed, which will undoubtedly require more elegant statistical modeling methods. As stated throughout this chapter, there is some overlap between genetic variants associated with HDL-C, LDL-C, and TG levels as well as MetSyn, since dyslipidemia is a component of MetSyn. As a result, we need to better understand the aggregate effects of multiple variants as well as how the effects of variation in one gene are modified in the presence of other genes and their variants. Below, we discuss some more advanced approaches which have attempted to better understand the effects of multiple variants on lipid levels and dyslipidemia.

Genetics of Dyslipidemia Using Genetic Risk Scores

Methods to evaluate the aggregate effects of multiple variants in genes affecting dyslipidemia and MetSyn traits have included calculation of genetic "risk scores," which add the number of "risk alleles" in a weighted or unweighted manner. For example, higher genotype risk scores (GRS),

constructed by simply summing risk alleles in nine common SNPs, have been associated with decreasing HDL-C levels [95]. In addition, unweighted risk scores have been constructed by summing the number of "TG-raising" alleles at 32 loci and then placed in "risk bins" (categories) to show that higher risk scores were significantly associated with patients with high TG (hypertriglyceridemia, HTG) compared to controls [90, 185].

GRS constructed using a weighted sum where the weight was based on the effect size and the number of SNPs (i.e., 47 SNPs for HDL-C, 37 SNPs for LDL-C, 32 SNPs for TG) were found to be strongly associated with HDL-C, LDL-C and TG in all age groups of children and adults, ages 3–45 years, in the Cardiovascular Risk in Young Finns Study; however, the total variance explained in these lipid levels decreased slightly with increasing age (3–6 years, 11.8–26.7%; 18 years, 11.3–18.4%; 33–45 years, 7.4–13.1%) [187]. Using the area under the (AUC) receiver operating curve (ROC) and the Venkatraman test for correlated ROCs (Venkatraman 1996) and integrated model discrimination improvement, which compares the mean differences between predicted probabilities [148], they concluded that the discrimination of high TG (HTG) in adulthood increased when the TG GRS were added to a model that also contained the childhood lipid measurement [187]. We note that the GRS in the Tikkanen et al. [187] study contained SNPs in many of the genes summarized in this chapter including ABCA1, ANGPTL3, APOA1-C3-A4-A5, APOB, APOE, CETP, GALNT2, LDLR, LIPC, LIPG, LPA, LPL, MLXIPL, NPC1L1, PCSK9, PLTP, and SCARB1.

Additional studies in adults have also not found improved discrimination with the addition of GRS. For example, quantiles of unweighted GRS have been evaluated in two large British cohorts (British Women's Heart and Health Study, BWHS: $n = 3414$; Whitehall II, WHII: $n = 5059$), and when comparing the highest to the lowest quintiles of LDL-C GRS (derived from 23 SNPs), they observed higher LDL-C levels (mean difference: BWHS, 0.63 (0.50–0.76); WHII, 0.85 (0.76–0.94)) and an increased odds of developing coronary heart disease (CHD) (BWHS, 1.43 (1.02–2.00); WHII, 1.31 (0.99–1.72)) [168]. However, the GRS did not improve discrimination over the Framingham Risk Score, which incorporates age, gender, smoking, diabetes status, SBP, TC, and HDL-C for assessing the 10-year risk of developing CVD [9] when using AUC ROC methods [168].

In addition, weighted GRS constructed using 13 SNPs and 30 SNPs identified through associations with CVD in GWAS were found to be associated with CVD mortality (13 SNPs, 1.35 (1.10–1.81); 30 SNPs, 1.46 (1.08–1.16)), but neither AUC ROC analyses nor the net classification index approach indicated the addition of the GRS (both 13 and 30 SNP versions) did not significantly improve prediction capacity of CVD mortality [36]. Therefore, other more elegant methods may be needed to better understand the aggregate effects of multiple SNPs and their potential ability to predict disease.

Genetics of Dyslipidemia Using Multi-Locus Burden and Dimension Reduction Methods

Using exome sequencing data from 2005 individuals from seven cohort studies, genetic burden tests, which evaluate aggregate effects of rare variants with low MAF, confirmed associations with APOE, LDLR, and PCSK9 genes and identified novel variants in PNPLA5 which were subsequently replicated in an independent study of 2084 individuals of European descent [109].

Multifactor dimensionality reduction (MDR) [159] and generalized multifactor dimensionality reduction (GMDR) methods [116] have been used to evaluate genetic interactions at multiple loci. Interestingly, when six SNPs in the ZNF259/BUD13 region were evaluated using single-locus analyses in a sample of 1181 Chinese individuals, only one SNP (BUD13 rs17119975) was found to be marginally associated with TG ($p = 0.064$),

but GMDR analyses revealed significant associations between two loci (BUD13 rs17119975, BUD13 rs10790162) and three loci (ZNF259 rs2075290, BUD13 rs17119975, BUD13 rs10790162) interaction models using cross-validation and permutation testing procedures [12], which suggests that GMDR may provide better insight to genetic interactions that may not be obviously revealed in single-locus analyses.

Genetics of Dyslipidemia and MetSyn Using Causal Modeling and Pathway Approaches

We have used the multivariate statistical framework of structural equation modeling (SEM) to evaluate multiple genetic determinants of MetSyn and aggregate effects of individual genes by modeling MetSyn as a second-order factor supported by lower-order factor traits (e.g., dyslipidemia) together with multiple latent candidate gene constructs, which we mathematically define by multiple SNPs in each respective gene [139]. Using this approach with the Framingham Heart Study (Offspring Cohort, Exam 7; Affymetrix 50k Human Gene Panel) data, we found that the CETP gene had a very strong association with the dyslipidemia factor but was not statistically significantly associated with MetSyn directly. Furthermore, we found that the association between the CSMD1 gene and MetSyn diminished when modeled simultaneously with six other candidate genes, most notably CETP and STARD13 [139]. Our approach might also help identify and explain novel signals (e.g., CSMD1) in GWAS studies [147]. Furthermore, we have evaluated the latent gene construct approach in the 1000 Genomes Project exon 5 sequencing data (24,497 SNPs in 697 unrelated individuals in seven populations), and we found that the approach provides a viable framework for modeling the aggregate effects of rare and common variants in multiple genes, but more elegant methods are needed to better identify the initial list of candidate loci [138].

The use of other forms of "causal modeling" (edge/node; integrative genetics) has been proposed to more fully address the complexity of MetSyn by integrating potential effects of maternal nutrition and epigenetics [117, 202]. Furthermore, using gene enrichment analysis and protein-protein interaction network approaches, the retinoid X receptor and farnesoid X receptor (FXR), which have multiple interactions in metabolism, cell proliferation, and oxidative stress pathways, have been identified as key players in MetSyn [177].

Various other types of pathway and network analyses have also been used to model multiple variants and identify candidate pleiotropic loci. In a secondary analysis of the GWAS data from 188,577 individuals from Willer et al. [198] where 62 SNPs were associated with HDL-C, 30 SNPs associated with LDL-C, and 32 SNPs associated with TG (157 unique loci), which were integrated with several other data sets of other components of MetSyn (BMI, SBP, DBP, BMI, CRP) and disease phenotypes (CAD, T2DM), 87 autosomal regions with 181 SNPs in 56 genes were found to be pleiotropic [154]. Further evaluation of these data using interactome analysis (via the Reactome FI plug-in [37, 171]) and functionally interacting networks (via the Disease Association Protein-Protein Link Evaluator software [162]) identified a network of 18 genes that showed statistically significant direct connectivity including direct connections with a cluster of genes consistently implicated in lipid disorders (APOA1, APOB, APOC1, APOE, ABCA1, CETP, LDLR, LIPC, LPL, PCSK9, PLTP), which contributed to the authors' conclusion that they found strong evidence for pleiotropy in CAD and lipid traits [154].

Pharmacogenomics for Dyslipidemia and MetSyn

However, more elegant kinetic models may be required to understand the true influence of genetic variants on dyslipidemia and MetSyn phenotypes given the presence of multiple feedback loops and reversible reactions [14, 67], and pharmacogenomics is likely to have the most impact on the future of personalized medicine for lipid disorders. For example, statins remain the cornerstone for lowering lipids; however, the individual response to statins is influenced by the patient's underling genetics. Decent progress has already been made in understanding how genetic variation in CETP, HMGRC, ABCB1, CYP3A4, PCSK9, LDLR, and solute carrier organic anion transporter family member 1B1 (SLCOB1), which transports statins from the blood to the liver, affects statin pharmacology and lipid response [98]. However, a better understanding of statin pharmacogenomics utilizing relevant pathway and network analysis will undoubtedly help to improve personalized response to statins and, in turn, help reduce the burden of CAD and CVD.

Cross-References

▷ Dyslipidemia in Metabolic Syndrome
▷ Genetics of Type 2 Diabetes
▷ Non-alcoholic Fatty Liver Disease
▷ Overview of Metabolic Syndrome

References

1. Acton S, Rigotti A, Landschulz KT, et al. Identification of scavenger receptor SR-BI as a high density lipoprotein receptor. Science. 1996;271: 518–20.
2. Agerholm-Larsen B, Tybjaerg-Hansen A, Schnohr P, et al. Common cholesteryl ester transfer protein mutations, decreased HDL cholesterol, and possible decreased risk of ischemic heart disease: the Copenhagen City Heart Study. Circulation. 2000;102: 2197–203.
3. Ahn YI, Kamboh MI, Hamman RF, et al. Two DNA polymorphisms in the lipoprotein lipase gene and their associations with factors related to cardiovascular disease. J Lipid Res. 1993;34:421–8.
4. Alberti KG, Zimmet PZ. Definition, diagnosis and classification of diabetes mellitus and its complications. Part 1: diagnosis and classification of diabetes mellitus provisional report of a WHO consultation. Diabet Med. 1998;15:539–53.
5. Alberti KG, Zimmet P, Shaw J. The metabolic syndrome – a new worldwide definition. Lancet. 2005;366:1059–62.
6. Alberti KG, Eckel RH, Grundy SM, et al. Harmonizing the metabolic syndrome: a joint interim statement

of the International Diabetes Federation Task Force on Epidemiology and Prevention; National Heart, Lung, and Blood Institute; American Heart Association; World Heart Federation; International Atherosclerosis Society; and International Association for the Study of Obesity. Circulation. 2009;120:1640–5.

7. Alshahid M, Wakil SM, Al-Najai M, et al. New susceptibility locus for obesity and dyslipidaemia on chromosome 3q22.3. Hum Genomics. 2013;7:15.

8. Andersen RV, Wittrup HH, Tybjaerg-Hansen A, et al. Hepatic lipase mutations, elevated high-density lipoprotein cholesterol, and increased risk of ischemic heart disease: the Copenhagen City Heart Study. J Am Coll Cardiol. 2003;41:1972–82.

9. Anderson KM, Odell PM, Wilson PW, et al. Cardiovascular disease risk profiles. Am Heart J. 1991;121: 293–8.

10. Anoop S, Misra A, Meena K, et al. Apolipoprotein E polymorphism in cerebrovascular & coronary heart diseases. Indian J Med Res. 2010;132:363–78.

11. Arai Y, Hirose N. Aging and HDL metabolism in elderly people more than 100 years old. J Atheroscler Thromb. 2004;11:246–52.

12. Aung LH, Yin RX, Wu DF, et al. Association of the variants in the BUD13-ZNF259 genes and the risk of hyperlipidaemia. J Cell Mol Med. 2014;18:1417–28.

13. Austin MA, King MC, Vranizan KM, et al. Atherogenic lipoprotein phenotype. A proposed genetic marker for coronary heart disease risk. Circulation. 1990;82:495–506.

14. Bakker BM, van Eunen K, Jeneson JA, et al. Systems biology from micro-organisms to human metabolic diseases: the role of detailed kinetic models. Biochem Soc Trans. 2010;38:1294–301.

15. Balkau B, Charles MA. Comment on the provisional report from the WHO consultation. European Group for the Study of Insulin Resistance (EGIR). Diabet Med. 1999;16:442–3.

16. Benn M. Apolipoprotein B, levels, APOB alleles, and risk of ischemic cardiovascular disease in the general population, a review. Atherosclerosis. 2009;206: 17–30.

17. Bernstein MS, Costanza MC, James RW, et al. No physical activity x CETP 1b.-629 interaction effects on lipid profile. Med Sci Sports Exerc. 2003;35: 1124–9.

18. Blankenberg S, Tiret L, Bickel C, et al. Genetic variation of the cholesterol ester transfer protein gene and the prevalence of coronary artery disease. The AtheroGene case control study. Z Kardiol. 2004;93 (Suppl 4):IV16–23.

19. Blatter Garin MC, Moren X, James RW. Paraoxonase-1 and serum concentrations of HDL-cholesterol and apoA-I. J Lipid Res. 2006;47:515–20.

20. Boekholdt SM, Thompson JF. Natural genetic variation as a tool in understanding the role of CETP in lipid levels and disease. J Lipid Res. 2003;44:1080–93.

21. Boekholdt SM, Sacks FM, Jukema JW, et al. Cholesteryl ester transfer protein TaqIB variant, high-density lipoprotein cholesterol levels, cardiovascular risk, and efficacy of pravastatin treatment: individual patient meta-analysis of 13,677 subjects. Circulation. 2005;111:278–87.

22. Boekholdt SM, Souverein OW, Tanck MW, et al. Common variants of multiple genes that control reverse cholesterol transport together explain only a minor part of the variation of HDL cholesterol levels. Clin Genet. 2006;69:263–70.

23. Boes E, Coassin S, Kollerits B, et al. Genetic-epidemiological evidence on genes associated with HDL cholesterol levels: a systematic in-depth review. Exp Gerontol. 2009;44:136–60.

24. Borggreve SE, Hillege HL, Wolffenbuttel BH, et al. PREVEND Study Group. The effect of cholesteryl ester transfer protein -629C->A promoter polymorphism on high-density lipoprotein cholesterol is dependent on serum triglycerides. J Clin Endocrinol Metab. 2005;90(7):4198–204. https://doi.org/10.1210/jc.2005-0182. Epub 2005 Apr 19. PMID: 15840744.

25. Brown CM, Rea TJ, Hamon SC, et al. The contribution of individual and pairwise combinations of SNPs in the APOA1 and APOC3 genes to interindividual HDL-C variability. J Mol Med (Berl). 2006;84:561–72.

26. Burkhardt R, Kenny EE, Lowe JK, et al. Common SNPs in HMGCR in micronesians and whites associated with LDL-cholesterol levels affect alternative splicing of exon13. Arterioscler Thromb Vasc Biol. 2008;28:2078–84.

27. Carlquist J, Anderson JL. Inconsistencies in the genetic prediction of HDL cholesterol versus atherosclerosis. Curr Opin Cardiol. 2007;22:352–8.

28. Cavelier C, Rohrer L, von Eckardstein A. ATP-binding cassette transporter A1 modulates apolipoprotein A-I transcytosis through aortic endothelial cells. Circ Res. 2006;99:1060–6.

29. Chang MH, Yesupriya A, Ned RM, et al. Genetic variants associated with fasting blood lipids in the U.S. population: third national health and nutrition examination survey. BMC Med Genet. 2010;11:62.

30. Chen K, Williams KJ. Molecular mediators for raft-dependent endocytosis of syndecan-1, a highly conserved, multifunctional receptor. J Biol Chem. 2013;288:13988–99.

31. Chen SN, Ballantyne CM, Gotto AM Jr, et al. A common PCSK9 haplotype, encompassing the E670G coding single nucleotide polymorphism, is a novel genetic marker for plasma low-density lipoprotein cholesterol levels and severity of coronary atherosclerosis. J Am Coll Cardiol. 2005;45:1611–9.

32. Clee SM, Zwinderman AH, Engert JC, et al. Common genetic variation in ABCA1 is associated with altered lipoprotein levels and a modified risk for coronary artery disease. Circulation. 2001;103:1198–205.

33. Cohen JC, Pertsemlidis A, Fahmi S, et al. Multiple rare variants in NPC1L1 associated with reduced sterol absorption and plasma low-density lipoprotein levels. Proc Natl Acad Sci U S A. 2006;103:1810–5.

34. Corella D, Guillen M, Saiz C, et al. Associations of LPL and APOC3 gene polymorphisms on plasma lipids in a Mediterranean population: interaction with tobacco smoking and the APOE locus. J Lipid Res. 2002;43:416–27.

35. Costanza MC, Cayanis E, Ross BM, et al. Relative contributions of genes, environment, and interactions to blood lipid concentrations in a general adult population. Am J Epidemiol. 2005;161:714–24.

36. Cox AJ, Hsu FC, Ng MC, et al. Genetic risk score associations with cardiovascular disease and mortality in the Diabetes Heart Study. Diabetes Care. 2014;37:1157–64.

37. Croft DP, Madden JR, Franks DW, et al. Hypothesis testing in animal social networks. Trends Ecol Evol. 2011;26:502–7.

38. Davignon J, Dubuc G, Seidah NG. The influence of PCSK9 polymorphisms on serum low-density lipoprotein cholesterol and risk of atherosclerosis. Curr Atheroscler Rep. 2010;12:308–15.

39. de Andrade FM, Silveira FR, Arsand M, et al. Association between −250G/A polymorphism of the hepatic lipase gene promoter and coronary artery disease and HDL-C levels in a Southern Brazilian population. Clin Genet. 2004;65:390–5.

40. De Castro-Oros I, Perez-Lopez J, Mateo-Gallego R, et al. A genetic variant in the LDLR promoter is responsible for part of the LDL-cholesterol variability in primary hypercholesterolemia. BMC Med Genet. 2014;7:17.

41. Dumitrescu L, Carty CL, Taylor K, et al. Genetic determinants of lipid traits in diverse populations from the population architecture using genomics and epidemiology (PAGE) study. PLoS Genet. 2011;7(6): e1002138. https://doi.org/10.1371/journal.pgen. 1002138. Epub 2011 Jun 30. PMID: 21738485.

42. Edwards KL, Newman B, Mayer E, et al. Heritability of factors of the insulin resistance syndrome in women twins. Genet Epidemiol. 1997;14:241–53.

43. Eichner JE, Dunn ST, Perveen G, et al. Apolipoprotein E polymorphism and cardiovascular disease: a HuGE review. Am J Epidemiol. 2002;155: 487–95.

44. Eiriksdottir G, Bolla MK, Thorsson B, et al. The −629C > A polymorphism in the CETP gene does not explain the association of TaqIB polymorphism with risk and age of myocardial infarction in Icelandic men. Atherosclerosis. 2001;159:187–92.

45. Endo A. The discovery and development of HMG-CoA reductase inhibitors. J Lipid Res. 1992;33:1569–82.

46. Evans D, Beil FU. The E670G SNP in the PCSK9 gene is associated with polygenic hypercholesterolemia in men but not in women. BMC Med Genet. 2006;7:66.

47. Expert Panel on Detection, Evaluation, and Treatment of High Blood Cholesterol in Adults. Executive summary of the third report of the National Cholesterol Education Program (NCEP) Expert Panel on

detection, evaluation, and treatment of high blood cholesterol in adults (Adult Treatment Panel III). JAMA. 2001;285:2486–97.

48. Fang DZ, Liu BW. Polymorphism of HL +1075C, but not −480 T, is associated with plasma high density lipoprotein cholesterol and apolipoprotein AI in men of a Chinese population. Atherosclerosis. 2002;161: 417–24.

49. Foley EM, Gordts PL, Stanford KI, et al. Hepatic remnant lipoprotein clearance by heparan sulfate proteoglycans and low-density lipoprotein receptors depend on dietary conditions in mice. Arterioscler Thromb Vasc Biol. 2013;33:2065–74.

50. Ford ES, Giles WH, Dietz WH. Prevalence of the metabolic syndrome among US adults: findings from the third National Health and Nutrition Examination Survey. JAMA. 2002;287:356–9.

51. Freeman DJ, Samani NJ, Wilson V, et al. A polymorphism of the cholesteryl ester transfer protein gene predicts cardiovascular events in non-smokers in the West of Scotland coronary Prevention Study. Eur Heart J. 2003;24:1833–42.

52. Frikke-Schmidt R, Tybjaerg-Hansen A, Steffensen R, et al. Apolipoprotein E genotype: epsilon32 women are protected while epsilon43 and epsilon44 men are susceptible to ischemic heart disease: the Copenhagen City Heart Study. J Am Coll Cardiol. 2000;35:1192–9.

53. Frikke-Schmidt R, Nordestgaard BG, Jensen GB, et al. Genetic variation in ABC transporter A1 contributes to HDL cholesterol in the general population. J Clin Invest. 2004;114:1343–53.

54. Fujimaki T, Kato K, Oguri M, et al. Association of a polymorphism of BTN2A1 with dyslipidemia in East Asian populations. Exp Ther Med. 2011;2:745–9.

55. Galkina E, Ley K. Vascular adhesion molecules in atherosclerosis. Arterioscler Thromb Vasc Biol. 2007;27:2292–301.

56. Garg A, Simha V. Update on dyslipidemia. J Clin Endocrinol Metab. 2007;92:1581–9.

57. Goldberg IJ. Lipoprotein lipase and lipolysis: central roles in lipoprotein metabolism and atherogenesis. J Lipid Res. 1996;37:693–707.

58. Goode EL, Cherny SS, Christian JC, et al. Heritability of longitudinal measures of body mass index and lipid and lipoprotein levels in aging twins. Twin Res Hum Genet. 2007;10:703–11.

59. Graf GA, Yu L, Li WP, et al. ABCG5 and ABCG8 are obligate heterodimers for protein trafficking and biliary cholesterol excretion. J Biol Chem. 2003;278: 48275–82.

60. Grallert H, Sedlmeier EM, Huth C, et al. APOA5 variants and metabolic syndrome in Caucasians. J Lipid Res. 2007;48:2614–21.

61. Grarup N, Andreasen CH, Andersen MK, et al. The −250G > A promoter variant in hepatic lipase associates with elevated fasting serum high-density lipoprotein cholesterol modulated by interaction with physical activity in a study of 16,156 Danish subjects. J Clin Endocrinol Metab. 2008;93:2294–9.

62. Gronroos P, Raitakari OT, Kahonen M, et al. Relation of apolipoprotein E polymorphism to markers of early atherosclerotic changes in young adults – the Cardiovascular Risk in Young Finns Study. Circ J. 2008;72:29–34.

63. Grundy SM, Cleeman JI, Merz CN, et al. Implications of recent clinical trials for the National Cholesterol Education Program Adult Treatment Panel III guidelines. J Am Coll Cardiol. 2004;44:720–32.

64. Grundy SM, Cleeman JI, Daniels SR, et al. Diagnosis and management of the metabolic syndrome: an American Heart Association/National Heart, Lung, and Blood Institute scientific statement. Curr Opin Cardiol. 2006;21:1–6.

65. Gu SJ, Guo ZR, Zhou ZY, et al. PPAR alpha and PPAR gamma polymorphisms as risk factors for dyslipidemia in a Chinese Han population. Lipids Health Dis. 2014a;13:23.

66. Gu SJ, Guo ZR, Zhou ZY, et al. Peroxisome proliferator-activated receptor γ polymorphisms as risk factors for dyslipidemia. Mol Med Rep. 2014b;10(5):2759–63. https://doi.org/10.3892/mmr.2014.2553. Epub 2014 Sep 10. PMID: 25216344.

67. Gutierrez-Cirlos C, Ordonez-Sanchez ML, Tusie-Luna MT, et al. Familial hypobetalipoproteinemia in a hospital survey: genetics, metabolism and non-alcoholic fatty liver disease. Ann Hepatol. 2011;10:155–64.

68. Haas BE, Weissglas-Volkov D, Aguilar-Salinas CA, et al. Evidence of how rs7575840 influences apolipoprotein B-containing lipid particles. Arterioscler Thromb Vasc Biol. 2011;31:1201–7.

69. Halpern A, Mancini MC, Magalhaes ME, et al. Metabolic syndrome, dyslipidemia, hypertension and type 2 diabetes in youth: from diagnosis to treatment. Diabetol Metab Syndr. 2010;2:55.

70. Hassing HC, Surendran RP, Derudas B, et al. SULF2 strongly prediposes to fasting and postprandial triglycerides in patients with obesity and type 2 diabetes mellitus. Obesity (Silver Spring). 2014;22:1309–16.

71. Hegele RA, Brunt JH, Connelly PW. Multiple genetic determinants of variation of plasma lipoproteins in Alberta Hutterites. Arterioscler Thromb Vasc Biol. 1995;15:861–71.

72. Hegele RA, Guy J, Ban MR, et al. NPC1L1 haplotype is associated with inter-individual variation in plasma low-density lipoprotein response to ezetimibe. Lipids Health Dis. 2005;4:16.

73. Heid IM, Boes E, Muller M, et al. Genome-wide association analysis of high-density lipoprotein cholesterol in the population-based KORA study sheds new light on intergenic regions. Circ Cardiovasc Genet. 2008;1:10–20.

74. Herbeth B, Samara A, Ndiaye C, et al. Metabolic syndrome-related composite factors over 5 years in the STANISLAS family study: genetic heritability and common environmental influences. Clin Chim Acta. 2010;411:833–9.

75. Hiramatsu M, Oguri M, Kato K, et al. Synergistic effects of genetic variants of APOA5 and BTN2A1 on dyslipidemia or metabolic syndrome. Int J Mol Med. 2012;30:185–92.

76. Hiura Y, Tabara Y, Kokubo Y, et al. Association of the functional variant in the 3-hydroxy-3-methylglutaryl-coenzyme a reductase gene with low-density lipoprotein-cholesterol in Japanese. Circ J. 2010;74:518–22.

77. Hodoglugil U, Williamson DW, Huang Y, et al. Common polymorphisms of ATP binding cassette transporter A1, including a functional promoter polymorphism, associated with plasma high density lipoprotein cholesterol levels in Turks. Atherosclerosis. 2005;183:199–212.

78. Holmer SR, Hengstenberg C, Mayer B, et al. Lipoprotein lipase gene polymorphism, cholesterol subfractions and myocardial infarction in large samples of the general population. Cardiovasc Res. 2000;47:806–12.

79. Horibe H, Ueyama C, Fujimaki T, et al. Association of a polymorphism of BTN2A1 with dyslipidemia in community-dwelling individuals. Mol Med Rep. 2014;9:808–12.

80. Hsu LA, Ko YL, Wu S, et al. Association between a novel 11-base pair deletion mutation in the promoter region of the scavenger receptor class B type I gene and plasma HDL cholesterol levels in Taiwanese Chinese. Arterioscler Thromb Vasc Biol. 2003;23:1869–74.

81. Huang CC, Fornage M, Lloyd-Jones DM, et al. Longitudinal association of PCSK9 sequence variations with low-density lipoprotein cholesterol levels: the Coronary Artery Risk Development in Young Adults Study. Circ Cardiovasc Genet. 2009;2:354–61.

82. Hubacek JA. Apolipoprotein A5 and triglyceridemia. Focus on the effects of the common variants. Clin Chem Lab Med. 2005;43:897–902.

83. Hutter CM, Austin MA, Farin FM, et al. Association of endothelial lipase gene (LIPG) haplotypes with high-density lipoprotein cholesterol subfractions and apolipoprotein AI plasma levels in Japanese Americans. Atherosclerosis. 2006;185:78–86.

84. Iijima H, Emi M, Wada M, et al. Association of an intronic haplotype of the LIPC gene with hyperalphalipoproteinemia in two independent populations. J Hum Genet. 2008;53:193–200.

85. Iizuka K, Horikawa Y. ChREBP: a glucose-activated transcription factor involved in the development of metabolic syndrome. Endocr J. 2008;55:617–24.

86. Isaacs A, Sayed-Tabatabaei FA, Njajou OT, et al. The −514 C- > T hepatic lipase promoter region polymorphism and plasma lipids: a meta-analysis. J Clin Endocrinol Metab. 2004;89:3858–63.

87. Isaacs A, Aulchenko YS, Hofman A, Maitland-van der Zee AH, Stricker BH, Oostra BA, Witteman JC, van Duijn CM, et al. Epistatic effect of cholesteryl ester transfer protein and hepatic lipase on serum high-density lipoprotein cholesterol levels. J Clin Endocrinol Metab. 2007;92:2680–7.

88. Jakulj L, Vissers MN, Tanck MW, et al. ABCG5/G8 polymorphisms and markers of cholesterol metabolism: systematic review and meta-analysis. J Lipid Res. 2010;51:3016–23.

89. Jaye M, Krawiec J. Endothelial lipase and HDL metabolism. Curr Opin Lipidol. 2004;15:183–9.

90. Johansen CT, Hegele RA. Genetic bases of hypertriglyceridemic phenotypes. Curr Opin Lipidol. 2011;22:247–53.

91. Johansen CT, Wang J, Lanktree MB, et al. An increased burden of common and rare lipid-associated risk alleles contributes to the phenotypic spectrum of hypertriglyceridemia. Arterioscler Thromb Vasc Biol. 2011;31(8):1916–26. https://doi.org/10.1161/ATVBAHA.111.226365. Epub 2011 May 19.PMID: 21597005.

92. Kamboh MI, Bunker CH, Aston CE, et al. Genetic association of five apolipoprotein polymorphisms with serum lipoprotein-lipid levels in African blacks. Genet Epidemiol. 1999;16:205–22.

93. Kashiwabara Y, Kobayashi Y, Koba S, et al. Gene polymorphism and frequencies of the NPC1L1 gene (rs2072183, rs217434 and rs217428) in Japanese patients with dyslipidemia. J Clin Pharm Ther. 2014;39:551–4.

94. Kataoka S, Robbins DC, Cowan LD, et al. Apolipoprotein E polymorphism in American Indians and its relation to plasma lipoproteins and diabetes. The Strong Heart Study. Arterioscler Thromb Vasc Biol. 1996;16:918–25.

95. Kathiresan S, Melander O, Guiducci C, et al. Six new loci associated with blood low-density lipoprotein cholesterol, high-density lipoprotein cholesterol or triglycerides in humans. Nat Genet. 2008;40: 189–97.

96. Kaulfers AM, Deka R, Dolan L, et al. Association of INSIG2 polymorphism with overweight and LDL in children. PLoS One. 2015;10:e0116340.

97. Keebler ME, Sanders CL, Surti A, et al. Association of blood lipids with common DNA sequence variants at 19 genetic loci in the multiethnic United States National Health and Nutrition Examination Survey III. Circ Cardiovasc Genet. 2009;2:238–43.

98. Kitzmiller JP, Binkley PF, Pandey SR, et al. Statin pharmacogenomics: pursuing biomarkers for predicting clinical outcomes. Discov Med. 2013;16: 45–51.

99. Klerkx AH, Tanck MW, Kastelein JJ, et al. Haplotype analysis of the CETP gene: not TaqIB, but the closely linked −629C → A polymorphism and a novel promoter variant are independently associated with CETP concentration. Hum Mol Genet. 2003;12: 111–23.

100. Klos KL, Kullo IJ. Genetic determinants of HDL: monogenic disorders and contributions to variation. Curr Opin Cardiol. 2007;22:344–51.

101. Klos KL, Sing CF, Boerwinkle E, et al. Consistent effects of genes involved in reverse cholesterol transport on plasma lipid and apolipoprotein levels in CARDIA participants. Arterioscler Thromb Vasc Biol. 2006;26(8):1828–36. https://doi.org/10.1161/01.ATV.0000231523.19199.45. Epub 2006 Jun 8. PMID: 16763159.

102. Ko YL, Hsu LA, Hsu KH, et al. The interactive effects of hepatic lipase gene promoter polymorphisms with sex and obesity on high-density-lipoprotein cholesterol levels in Taiwanese-Chinese. Atherosclerosis. 2004;172:135–42.

103. Komurcu-Bayrak E, Onat A, Poda M, et al. The S447X variant of lipoprotein lipase gene is associated with metabolic syndrome and lipid levels among Turks. Clin Chim Acta. 2007;383:110–5.

104. Kronenberg F, Coon H, Ellison RC, et al. Segregation analysis of HDL cholesterol in the NHLBI Family Heart Study and in Utah pedigrees. Eur J Hum Genet. 2002;10:367–74.

105. Kwan BC, Kronenberg F, Beddhu S, et al. Lipoprotein metabolism and lipid management in chronic kidney disease. J Am Soc Nephrol. 2007;18: 1246–61.

106. Lahiry P, Ban MR, Pollex RL, et al. Common variants APOC3, APOA5, APOE and PON1 are associated with variation in plasma lipoprotein traits in Greenlanders. Int J Circumpolar Health. 2007;66: 390–400.

107. Lai CQ, Tai ES, Tan CE, et al. The APOA5 locus is a strong determinant of plasma triglyceride concentrations across ethnic groups in Singapore. J Lipid Res. 2003;44:2365–73.

108. Lai CQ, Demissie S, Cupples LA, et al. Influence of the APOA5 locus on plasma triglyceride, lipoprotein subclasses, and CVD risk in the Framingham Heart Study. J Lipid Res. 2004;45:2096–105.

109. Lange LA, Hu Y, Zhang H, et al. Whole-exome sequencing identifies rare and low-frequency coding variants associated with LDL cholesterol. Am J Hum Genet. 2014;94:233–45.

110. Lanktree MB, Anand SS, Yusuf S, et al. Replication of genetic associations with plasma lipoprotein traits in a multiethnic sample. J Lipid Res. 2009;50:1487–96.

111. Larson IA, Ordovas JM, Barnard JR, et al. Effects of apolipoprotein A-I genetic variations on plasma apolipoprotein, serum lipoprotein and glucose levels. Clin Genet. 2002;61:176–84.

112. Lee J, Tan CS, Chia KS, et al. The lipoprotein lipase S447X polymorphism and plasma lipids: interactions with APOE polymorphisms, smoking, and alcohol consumption. J Lipid Res. 2004;45:1132–9.

113. Lewis GF, Rader DJ. New insights into the regulation of HDL metabolism and reverse cholesterol transport. Circ Res. 2005;96:1221–32.

114. Littlewood TD, Bennett MR. Apoptotic cell death in atherosclerosis. Curr Opin Lipidol. 2003;14:469–75.

115. Liu L, Aboud O, Jones RA, et al. Apolipoprotein E expression is elevated by interleukin 1 and other interleukin 1-induced factors. J Neuroinflammation. 2011;8:175. https://doi.org/10.1186/1742-2094-8-175. PMID: 22171672.

116. Lou XY, Chen GB, Yan L, et al. A generalized combinatorial approach for detecting gene-by-gene and gene-by-environment interactions with application to nicotine dependence. Am J Hum Genet. 2007;80: 1125–37.

117. Lusis AJ, Attie AD, Reue K. Metabolic syndrome: from epidemiology to systems biology. Nat Rev Genet. 2008;9:819–30.

118. Ma K, Cilingiroglu M, Otvos JD, et al. Endothelial lipase is a major genetic determinant for high-density lipoprotein concentration, structure, and metabolism. Proc Natl Acad Sci U S A. 2003;100:2748–53.

119. Mackness MI, Arrol S, Durrington PN. Paraoxonase prevents accumulation of lipoperoxides in low-density lipoprotein. FEBS Lett. 1991;286:152–4.

120. Maeda T, Honda A, Ishikawa T, et al. A SNP of NPC1L1 affects cholesterol absorption in Japanese. J Atheroscler Thromb. 2010;17:356–60.

121. Mailly F, Tugrul Y, Reymer PW, et al. A common variant in the gene for lipoprotein lipase (Asp9 → Asn). Functional implications and prevalence in normal and hyperlipidemic subjects. Arterioscler Thromb Vasc Biol. 1995;15:468–78.

122. Mank-Seymour AR, Durham KL, Thompson JF, et al. Association between single-nucleotide polymorphisms in the endothelial lipase (LIPG) gene and high-density lipoprotein cholesterol levels. Biochim Biophys Acta. 2004;1636:40–6.

123. Manresa JM, Zamora A, Tomas M, et al. Relationship of classical and non-classical risk factors with genetic variants relevant to coronary heart disease. Eur J Cardiovasc Prev Rehabil. 2006;13:738–44.

124. Martinson ML, Teitler JO, Reichman NE. Health across the life span in the United States and England. Am J Epidemiol. 2011;173:858–65.

125. Matikainen N, Burza MA, Romeo S, et al. Genetic variation in SULF2 is associated with postprandial clearance of triglyceride-rich remnant particles and triglyceride levels in healthy subjects. PLoS One. 2013;8:e79473.

126. Maxwell KN, Fisher EA, Breslow JL. Overexpression of PCSK9 accelerates the degradation of the LDLR in a post-endoplasmic reticulum compartment. Proc Natl Acad Sci U S A. 2005;102: 2069–74.

127. McCaskie PA, Cadby G, Hung J, et al. The C-480 T hepatic lipase polymorphism is associated with HDL-C but not with risk of coronary heart disease. Clin Genet. 2006;70:114–21.

128. McCaskie PA, Beilby JP, Chapman CM, et al. Cholesteryl ester transfer protein gene haplotypes, plasma high-density lipoprotein levels and the risk of coronary heart disease. Hum Genet. 2007;121: 401–11.

129. Miettinen HE, Gylling H, Tenhunen J, et al. Molecular genetic study of Finns with hypoalphalipoproteinemia and hyperalphalipoproteinemia: a novel Gly230 Arg mutation (LCAT[Fin]) of lecithin:cholesterol acyltransferase (LCAT) accounts for 5% of cases with very low serum HDL cholesterol levels. Arterioscler Thromb Vasc Biol. 1998;18:591–8.

130. Miller M, Zhan M. Genetic determinants of low high-density lipoprotein cholesterol. Curr Opin Cardiol. 2004;19:380–4.

131. Miller M, Rhyne J, Hamlette S, et al. Genetics of HDL regulation in humans. Curr Opin Lipidol. 2003;14: 273–9.

132. Morabia A, Ross BM, Costanza MC, et al. Population-based study of SR-BI genetic variation and lipid profile. Atherosclerosis. 2004;175:159–68.

133. Muiya NP, Wakil S, Al-Najai M, et al. A study of the role of GATA2 gene polymorphism in coronary artery disease risk traits. Gene. 2014;544:152–8.

134. Murthy V, Julien P, Gagne C. Molecular pathobiology of the human lipoprotein lipase gene. Pharmacol Ther. 1996;70:101–35.

135. Musunuru K, Pirruccello JP, Do R, et al. Exome sequencing, ANGPTL3 mutations, and familial combined hypolipidemia. N Engl J Med. 2010;363: 2220–7.

136. Nettleton JA, Steffen LM, Ballantyne CM, et al. Associations between HDL-cholesterol and polymorphisms in hepatic lipase and lipoprotein lipase genes are modified by dietary fat intake in African American and White adults. Atherosclerosis. 2007;194:e131–40.

137. Nock NL, Chandran Pillai APL. Dyslipidemia: genetics and role in the metabolic syndrome. In: Kelishadi R, editor. Dyslipidemia – from prevention to treatment. Rijeka: InTech; 2012.

138. Nock N, Zhang L. Evaluating aggregate effects of rare and common variants in the 1000 Genomes Project exon sequencing data using latent variable structural equation modeling. BMC Proc. 2011;5(Suppl 9):S47.

139. Nock NL, Wang X, Thompson CL, et al. Defining genetic determinants of the Metabolic Syndrome in the Framingham Heart Study using association and structural equation modeling methods. BMC Proc. 2009;3(Suppl 7):S50.

140. Ogg SL, Weldon AK, Dobbie L, et al. Expression of butyrophilin (Btn1a1) in lactating mammary gland is essential for the regulated secretion of milk-lipid droplets. Proc Natl Acad Sci U S A. 2004;101:10084–9.

141. Ordovas JM, Cupples LA, Corella D, et al. Association of cholesteryl ester transfer protein-TaqIB polymorphism with variations in lipoprotein subclasses and coronary heart disease risk: the Framingham study. Arterioscler Thromb Vasc Biol. 2000;20:1323–9.

142. Osgood D, Corella D, Demissie S, et al. Genetic variation at the scavenger receptor class B type I gene locus determines plasma lipoprotein concentrations and particle size and interacts with type 2 diabetes: the Framingham study. J Clin Endocrinol Metab. 2003;88:2869–79.

143. Ota VK, Chen ES, Ejchel TF, et al. APOA4 polymorphism as a risk factor for unfavorable lipid serum profile and depression: a cross-sectional study. J Investig Med. 2011;59:966–70.

144. Pallaud C, Sass C, Zannad F, et al. APOC3, CETP, fibrinogen, and MTHFR are genetic determinants of carotid intima-media thickness in healthy men (the Stanislas cohort). Clin Genet. 2001;59:316–24.

145. Paradis ME, Couture P, Bosse Y, et al. The T111I mutation in the EL gene modulates the impact of dietary fat on the HDL profile in women. J Lipid Res. 2003;44:1902–8.

146. Pare G, Serre D, Brisson D, et al. Genetic analysis of 103 candidate genes for coronary artery disease and associated phenotypes in a founder population reveals a new association between endothelin-1 and high-density lipoprotein cholesterol. Am J Hum Genet. 2007;80:673–82.

147. Parra EJ, Below JE, Krithika S, et al. Genome-wide association study of type 2 diabetes in a sample from Mexico City and a meta-analysis of a Mexican-American sample from Starr County. Texas Diabetol. 2011;54:2038–46.

148. Pencina MJ, D'Agostino RB. Evaluation of the Framingham risk score in the European Prospective Investigation of Cancer-Norfolk cohort-invited commentary. Arch Intern Med. 2008;168:1216–8.

149. Polisecki E, Muallem H, Maeda N, et al. Genetic variation at the LDL receptor and HMG-CoA reductase gene loci, lipid levels, statin response, and cardiovascular disease incidence in PROSPER. Atherosclerosis. 2008;200:109–14.

150. Porchay I, Pean F, Bellili N, et al. ABCA1 single nucleotide polymorphisms on high-density lipoprotein-cholesterol and overweight: the D.E.S.I.R. study. Obesity (Silver Spring). 2006;14:1874–9.

151. Povel CM, Boer JM, Imholz S, et al. Genetic variants in lipid metabolism are independently associated with multiple features of the metabolic syndrome. Lipids Health Dis. 2011;10:118. https://doi.org/10.1186/1476-511X-10-118. PMID: 21767357.

152. Qi L, Liu S, Rifai N, et al. Associations of the apolipoprotein A1/C3/A4/A5 gene cluster with triglyceride and HDL cholesterol levels in women with type 2 diabetes. Atherosclerosis. 2007;192:204–10.

153. Radha V, Mohan V, Vidya R, et al. Association of lipoprotein lipase Hind III and Ser 447 Ter polymorphisms with dyslipidemia in Asian Indians. Am J Cardiol. 2006;97:1337–42.

154. Rankinen T, Sarzynski MA, Ghosh S, et al. Are there genetic paths common to obesity, cardiovascular disease outcomes, and cardiovascular risk factors? Circ Res. 2015;116:909–22.

155. Remaley AT, Stonik JA, Demosky SJ, et al. Apolipoprotein specificity for lipid efflux by the human ABCA1 transporter. Biochem Biophys Res Commun. 2001;280:818–23.

156. Rigotti A, Trigatti B, Babitt J, et al. Scavenger receptor BI – a cell surface receptor for high density lipoprotein. Curr Opin Lipidol. 1997;8:181–8.

157. Rios DL, D'Onofrio LO, Cerqueira CC, et al. Paraoxonase 1 gene polymorphisms in angiographically assessed coronary artery disease: evidence for gender interaction among Brazilians. Clin Chem Lab Med. 2007;45:874–8.

158. Rip J, Nierman MC, Ross CJ, et al. Lipoprotein lipase S447X: a naturally occurring gain-of-function mutation. Arterioscler Thromb Vasc Biol. 2006;26:1236–45.

159. Ritchie MD, Hahn LW, Roodi N, et al. Multifactor-dimensionality reduction reveals high-order interactions among estrogen-metabolism genes in sporadic breast cancer. Am J Hum Genet. 2001;69:138–47.

160. Roberts CG, Shen H, Mitchell BD, et al. Variants in scavenger receptor class B type I gene are associated with HDL cholesterol levels in younger women. Hum Hered. 2007;64:107–13.

161. Rosen SD, Lemjabbar-Alaoui H. Sulf-2: an extracellular modulator of cell signaling and a cancer target candidate. Expert Opin Ther Targets. 2010;14:935–49.

162. Rosen EY, Wexler EM, Versano R, et al. Functional genomic analyses identify pathways dysregulated by progranulin deficiency, implicating Wnt signaling. Neuron. 2011;71:1030–42.

163. Roth GA, Fihn SD, Mokdad AH. High total serum cholesterol, medication coverage and therapeutic control: an analysis of national health examination survey data from eight countries. Bull World Health Organ. 2010;89:92–101.

164. Russo GT, Meigs JB, Cupples LA, et al. Association of the Sst-I polymorphism at the APOC3 gene locus with variations in lipid levels, lipoprotein subclass profiles and coronary heart disease risk: the Framingham offspring study. Atherosclerosis. 2001;158:173–81.

165. Sagoo GS, Tatt I, Salanti G, et al. Seven lipoprotein lipase gene polymorphisms, lipid fractions, and coronary disease: a HuGE association review and meta-analysis. Am J Epidemiol. 2008;168:1233–46.

166. Sandhofer A, Tatarczyk T, Laimer M, et al. The Taq1B-variant in the cholesteryl ester-transfer protein gene and the risk of metabolic syndrome. Obesity. 2008;16:919–22.

167. Senti M, Elosua R, Tomas M, et al. Physical activity modulates the combined effect of a common variant of the lipoprotein lipase gene and smoking on serum triglyceride levels and high-density lipoprotein cholesterol in men. Hum Genet. 2001;109:385–92.

168. Shah S, Casas JP, Gaunt TR, et al. Influence of common genetic variation on blood lipid levels, cardiovascular risk, and coronary events in two British prospective cohort studies. Eur Heart J. 2013;34:972–81.

169. Shakhtshneider EV, Kulikov IV, Maksimov VN, et al. CETP gene polymorphism in the caucasian population of West Siberia and in groups contrast by total serum cholesterol levels. Bull Exp Biol Med. 2014;157:364–7.

170. Shan L, Yu XC, Liu Z, et al. The angiopoietin-like proteins ANGPTL3 and ANGPTL4 inhibit

lipoprotein lipase activity through distinct mechanisms. J Biol Chem. 2009;284:1419–24.

171. Shannon P, Markiel A, Ozier O, et al. Cytoscape: a software environment for integrated models of biomolecular interaction networks. Genome Res. 2003;13:2498–504.

172. Shen Y, Xi B, Zhao X, et al. Common genetic variants associated with lipid profiles in a Chinese pediatric population. Hum Genet. 2013;132:1275–85.

173. Shimizugawa T, Ono M, Shimamura M, et al. ANGPTL3 decreases very low density lipoprotein triglyceride clearance by inhibition of lipoprotein lipase. J Biol Chem. 2002;277:33742–8.

174. Shioji K, Mannami T, Kokubo Y, et al. An association analysis between ApoA1 polymorphisms and the high-density lipoprotein (HDL) cholesterol level and myocardial infarction (MI) in Japanese. J Hum Genet. 2004a;49:433–9.

175. Shioji K, Nishioka J, Naraba H, et al. A promoter variant of the ATP-binding cassette transporter A1 gene alters the HDL cholesterol level in the general Japanese population. J Hum Genet. 2004b;49:141–7.

176. Smalinskiene A, Petkeviciene J, Luksiene D, et al. Association between APOE, SCARB1, PPARalpha polymorphisms and serum lipids in a population of Lithuanian adults. Lipids Health Dis. 2013;12:120.

177. Sookoian S, Pirola CJ. Metabolic syndrome: from the genetics to the pathophysiology. Curr Hypertens Rep. 2011;13:149–57.

178. Srinivasan SR, Ehnholm C, Elkasabany A, et al. Influence of apolipoprotein E polymorphism on serum lipids and lipoprotein changes from childhood to adulthood: the Bogalusa Heart Study. Atherosclerosis. 1999;143:435–43.

179. Srinivasan SR, Li S, Chen W, et al. Q192R polymorphism of the paraoxanase 1 gene and its association with serum lipoprotein variables and carotid artery intima-media thickness in young adults from a biracial community. The Bogalusa Heart Study. Atherosclerosis. 2004;177:167–74.

180. Tai ES, Corella D, Deurenberg-Yap M, et al. Dietary fat interacts with the -514C > T polymorphism in the hepatic lipase gene promoter on plasma lipid profiles in a multiethnic Asian population: the 1998 Singapore National Health Survey. J Nutr. 2003a;133:3399–408.

181. Tai ES, Ordovas JM, Corella D, et al. The TaqIB and -629C > A polymorphisms at the cholesteryl ester transfer protein locus: associations with lipid levels in a multiethnic population. The 1998 Singapore National Health Survey. Clin Genet. 2003b;63:19–30.

182. Talmud PJ, Hawe E, Martin S, et al. Relative contribution of variation within the APOC3/A4/A5 gene cluster in determining plasma triglycerides. Hum Mol Genet. 2002a;11:3039–46.

183. Talmud PJ, Hawe E, Robertson K, et al. Genetic and environmental determinants of plasma high density lipoprotein cholesterol and apolipoprotein AI concentrations in healthy middle-aged men. Ann Hum Genet. 2002b;66:111–24.

184. Tang NP, Wang LS, Yang L, et al. Protective effect of an endothelial lipase gene variant on coronary artery disease in a Chinese population. J Lipid Res. 2008;49:369–75.

185. Teslovich TM, Musunuru K, Smith AV, et al. Biological, clinical and population relevance of 95 loci for blood lipids. Nature. 2010;466:707–13.

186. Thompson A, Di AE, Sarwar N, et al. Association of cholesteryl ester transfer protein genotypes with CETP mass and activity, lipid levels, and coronary risk. JAMA. 2008;299:2777–88.

187. Tikkanen E, Tuovinen T, Widen E, et al. Association of known loci with lipid levels among children and prediction of dyslipidemia in adults. Circ Cardiovasc Genet. 2011;4:673–80.

188. Tsai FY, Keller G, Kuo FC, et al. An early haematopoietic defect in mice lacking the transcription factor GATA-2. Nature. 1994;371:221–6.

189. Tsujita Y, Nakamura Y, Zhang Q, et al. The association between high-density lipoprotein cholesterol level and cholesteryl ester transfer protein TaqIB gene polymorphism is influenced by alcohol drinking in a population-based sample. Atherosclerosis. 2007;191:199–205.

190. van Aalst-Cohen ES, Jansen AC, Boekholdt SM, et al. Genetic determinants of plasma HDL-cholesterol levels in familial hypercholesterolemia. Eur J Hum Genet. 2005;13:1137–42.

191. van de Woestijne AP, van der Graaf Y, de Bakker PI, et al. Rs964184 (APOA5-A4-C3-A1) is related to elevated plasma triglyceride levels, but not to an increased risk for vascular events in patients with clinically manifest vascular disease. PLoS One. 2014;9:e101082.

192. Volcik KA, Barkley RA, Hutchinson RG, et al. Apolipoprotein E polymorphisms predict low density lipoprotein cholesterol levels and carotid artery wall thickness but not incident coronary heart disease in 12,491 ARIC study participants. Am J Epidemiol. 2006;164:342–8.

193. Wang X, Paigen B. Genetics of variation in HDL cholesterol in humans and mice. Circ Res. 2005;96:27–42.

194. Wang J, Ban MR, Zou GY, et al. Polygenic determinants of severe hypertriglyceridemia. Hum Mol Genet. 2008;17:2894–9.

195. Waterworth DM, Ricketts SL, Song K, et al. Genetic variants influencing circulating lipid levels and risk of coronary artery disease. Arterioscler Thromb Vasc Biol. 2010;30:2264–76.

196. Whiting BM, Anderson JL, Muhlestein JB, et al. Candidate gene susceptibility variants predict intermediate end points but not angiographic coronary artery disease. Am Heart J. 2005;150:243–50.

197. Willer CJ, Sanna S, Jackson AU, et al. Newly identified loci that influence lipid concentrations and risk of coronary artery disease. Nat Genet. 2008;40:161–9.

198. Willer CJ, Schmidt EM, Sengupta S, et al. Discovery and refinement of loci associated with lipid levels. NatGenet. 2013;45:1274–83.

199. Wilson PW, Myers RH, Larson MG, et al. Apolipoprotein E alleles, dyslipidemia, and coronary heart disease. The Framingham Offspring Study. JAMA. 1994;272:1666–71.

200. Wittrup HH, Tybjaerg-Hansen A, Nordestgaard BG. Lipoprotein lipase mutations, plasma lipids and lipoproteins, and risk of ischemic heart disease. A meta-analysis. Circulation. 1999;99:2901–7.

201. Wu K, Bowman R, Welch AA, et al. Apolipoprotein E polymorphisms, dietary fat and fibre, and serum lipids: the EPIC Norfolk study. Eur Heart J. 2007;28:2930–6.

202. Wu S, Mar-Heyming R, Dugum EZ, et al. Upstream transcription factor 1 influences plasma lipid and metabolic traits in mice. Hum Mol Genet. 2010;19: 597–608.

203. Yabe D, Brown MS, Goldstein JL. Insig-2, a second endoplasmic reticulum protein that binds SCAP and blocks export of sterol regulatory element-binding proteins. Proc Natl Acad Sci U S A. 2002;99:12753–8.

204. Yamada Y, Matsuo H, Warita S, et al. Prediction of genetic risk for dyslipidemia. Genomics. 2007;90: 551–8.

205. Yamada Y, Ichihara S, Kato K, et al. Genetic risk for metabolic syndrome: examination of candidate gene polymorphisms related to lipid metabolism in Japanese people. J Med Genet. 2008;45:22–8.

206. Yamakawa-Kobayashi K, Yanagi H, Endo K, et al. Relationship between serum HDL-C levels and common genetic variants of the endothelial lipase gene in Japanese school-aged children. Hum Genet. 2003;113:311–5.

207. Zhang K, Zhang S, Zheng K, et al. Study on the association of lecithin cholesterol acyltransferase gene polymorphisms with the lipid metabolism in coronary atherosclerotic heart disease. Zhonghua Yi Xue Yi Chuan Xue Za Zhi. 2003;20:135–7.

208. Zhang K, Zhang S, Zheng K, et al. Novel P143L polymorphism of the LCAT gene is associated with dyslipidemia in Chinese patients who have coronary atherosclerotic heart disease. Biochem Biophys Res Commun. 2004;318:4–10.

209. Zhong S, Sharp DS, Grove JS, et al. Increased coronary heart disease in Japanese-American men with mutation in the cholesteryl ester transfer protein gene despite increased HDL levels. J Clin Invest. 1996;97:2917–23.

210. Zhu XY, Xu HW, Hou RY, et al. Lecithin-cholesterol acyltransferase gene 608C/T polymorphism associated with atherosclerotic cerebral infarction. Zhonghua Yi Xue Yi Chuan Xue Za Zhi. 2006;23: 419–22.

Part III

Environmental Factors

Diet and Obesity

11

Laura E. Matarese

Contents

L. E. Matarese (✉)
Department of Internal Medicine, Division of
Gastroenterology, Hepatology and Nutrition, Brody
School of Medicine, East Carolina University, Greenville,
NC, USA
e-mail: mataresel@ecu.edu

Abstract

The global prevalence of overweight and obesity as a public health concern is well established and reflects the overall worldwide lack of success in achieving and maintaining a healthy body weight. The major concern is that obesity is associated with numerous comorbidities and is a risk factor for several of the leading causes of death, including cardiovascular disease, diabetes mellitus, and many types of cancer. These are for the large part preventable diseases. The cornerstone of obesity therapy has been diet, exercise, and behavioral modification. Considering the plethora of existing diet programs and the global expansion of the obesity crisis, a conclusion can be drawn that no one diet has been universally successful at inducing and maintaining weight loss and improving metabolic parameters. This enigma provides some evidence as to the complexity of obesity and weight management. The achievement of a healthy body weight is far more complex than a simple reduction of caloric intake relative to energy expenditure. The factors affecting obesity are complicated, dynamic, and interrelated and involve numerous host factors as well as the environment. Thus, any nutrition intervention should be individualized. This chapter will review the physiological basis of scientifically validated weight loss diets, their effects on energy expenditure, body weight, body composition, and metabolic parameters.

Keywords

Obesity · Caloric restriction · Weight loss · Carbohydrate-restricted diet · Fat-restricted diet · Glycemic index · Mediterranean diet · Microbiome

Introduction

Obesity and its related comorbidities are no longer diseases of Western cultures and have become a global epidemic. According to the World Health Organization (WHO), more than 1 billion people worldwide are obese – 650 million adults, 340 million adolescents, and 39 million children [83]. Unfortunately, this number is still increasing. The WHO estimates that by 2025, approximately 167 million people – adults and children – will become less healthy because they are overweight or obese.

Obesity is a complex, chronic disease that contributes to the development of diabetes, cardiovascular disease, hypertension, cancers, and serious medical conditions, resulting in an adverse effect on quality of life and an estimated worldwide economic burden in the trillions of dollars annually in both direct and indirect costs [14, 73, 84]. The seriousness of obesity has led to the search for an effective and lasting treatment. Treatment often includes a multipronged approach. There are three main categories of interventions: (i) lifestyle modification including dietary changes, physical activity, and behavioral modification, (ii) pharmacotherapy, and (iii) surgery. Although the mechanisms differ, each of these interventions is designed to generate a negative energy balance and induce weight loss. Recently, the role of the microbiota and its effects on body weight has come to light as an important factor and possibly a potential interventional target. This chapter will focus on dietary interventions including macronutrients, micronutrients, and the nutritional biochemistry forming the basis for the design of the specific diet.

Popular Diets in the Lay Literature

There are well over 1000 weight loss diets that have been popularized in the lay literature and throughout the media with new diets appearing on a regular basis. The sheer number of available diets would suggest that as a global society, we have not been successful in managing this disease. Most of these weight loss plans have little to no scientific evidence behind them. They may recommend fasting, cleansing routines, and elimination of one or more food groups or suggest consumption of a particular type of food or a specific macronutrient. In the short term, these diets may produce weight loss simply because individuals have changed their usual eating habits. Although they may produce weight loss in the short term, the effects are generally not lasting. There are, however, some diets that are based on sound nutritional, physiological, and biochemical principles which have been studied under controlled conditions.

The Weight Loss Equation: Is Math Really That Simple?

The induction of weight loss has been traditionally thought of in terms of an equation: energy intake exceeding expenditure leads to weight gain, energy intake less than energy expenditure results in weight loss, and energy intake equivalent to expenditure result in weight maintenance. This concept is often attributed to the laws of thermodynamics that define the fundamentals of heat and work. But when these laws which govern the physical aspects of temperature, energy, and entropy are applied to living biological systems, the equation becomes far more complex. Biological systems are complicated and contain numerous variables beyond temperature, energy, and entropy. The second law of thermodynamics, the law of dissipation, states that the entropy increases during any spontaneous process and that for any irreversible reaction, there is a loss or dissipation of energy in that reaction. This is the law that describes the inefficiency in biological systems associated with metabolic processes. From a metabolic standpoint, it is impossible for a biological system to turn a given amount of energy into an equivalent amount of work. Thus, a "calorie" is not always a "calorie." Calories are not converted to energy on a one-to-one basis because of this loss of energy, this inefficiency, described by the second law of thermodynamics. Oxidation of carbohydrates is more thermodynamically efficient and requires less energy than oxidation of protein or fat which is why carbohydrate is the preferred fuel for the body. Inefficient protein and fat oxidation leads to extra energy loss, thus creating a metabolic advantage during weight loss interventions [24]. Whether or not this metabolic advantage is clinically relevant has been debated, and it is most likely only one of the factors affecting weight loss.

Factors Affecting Weight Loss

To consider weight loss as the mere application of an intervention designed to reduce intake and increase expenditure to mobilize adipose stores for fuel is an oversimplification. There are numerous biochemical, physiological, psychological, emotional, economic, and social factors associated with weight loss and gain (Table 1). These are multifaceted, interrelated, and dynamic such that a change in one factor will often affect others [52].

Genetic Factors

Genes influence every aspect of human physiology, development, adaptation, and disease progression. It is intriguing to think that there may be a genetic component to obesity and that alteration of the genetic expression could influence the progression to obesity or that some of these genes may influence the response to weight loss interventions [35]. The existence of one or more family members who are overweight or obese suggests that there may be a genetic component and that it may also be associated with specific socio-environmental factors [64]. Yet, it is not unusual to find both lean and obese members within the same family. The *LEP* gene that is located on chromosome 7 encodes for leptin

Table 1 Factors influencing weight loss

Individual host factors
Genetics
Body composition (lean muscle vs. adipose tissue)
Age
Insulin sensitivity and insulin resistance
Hormones (ghrelin and leptin)
Gut microbiota
Energy expenditure
Physical activity
Thermal effects of food
Resting energy expenditure
Diet composition
Satiety value
Macronutrient composition
Food supply (ultra-processed foods, refined sugar, high fructose corn syrup)
Psychosocial and economic
Behaviors
Religious and cultural practices
Poverty and food insecurity
Iatrogenic
Medications

which regulates energy intake and energy expenditure [33]. Leptin levels fall during fasting and mediate central adaptive responses by decreasing energy expenditure via suppression of sympathetic, thyroid, and reproductive functions and increasing during refeeding. Leptin signals through the leptin receptor (*LEPR*) [12]. The obesity-related effects of leptin are predominantly mediated by a long isoform that contains an intracellular domain (*LEPRb*), which is expressed in several regions of the central nervous system [25]. This shows that genes that are either enriched or exclusively expressed within the brain and CNS have a central role in obesity [47]. These interactions are complex and point to a key role for the brain in the control of body weight [48].

The percentage of persons affected by obesity that can be attributed to genetics varies widely, depending on the population examined, and ranges from 6% to 85% [86]. These estimated ranges vary depending on the individual and the degree of overweight. For some, genes may account for just 25% of the predisposition to be overweight, while for others, the genetic influence is as high as 70–80%.

At least 71 genes have been implicated in the development of obesity [18]. One of the genes known to contribute to polygenic obesity is the fat mass–obesity-associated (FTO) gene [7]. There are other gene mutations that have been associated with morbid obesity including Alstrom syndrome, Bardet–Biedl syndrome, Cohen syndrome, Ayazi syndrome, MOMO syndrome, and Prader–Willi syndrome. These observations provide a strong argument for a genetic component. Yet obesity cannot be attributed to genetics in all cases.

It is also possible that the development of obesity begins in utero during fetal development at which time nutritional, hormonal, physical, and psychological processes are preprogrammed to activate specific physiological functions at defined periods later in life [72]. It is not uncommon for women with gestational diabetes to give birth to large babies. The presence of obesity-promoting genes does not condemn an individual to a destiny of obesity and the related health concerns. Healthy environments and lifestyles can influence gene-related risks.

Physical Activity

One cannot overlook the contribution of physical activity to weight loss and maintenance. Engagement in physical activity, both aerobic exercise and strength training, will influence the metabolic rate and caloric expenditure. This is not only important for inducing weight loss but also for maintaining weight loss [69]. Physical activity also affects insulin sensitivity [70]. The positive changes on insulin sensitivity are sustained if exercise is sustained [37]. This in turn may affect the success of a planned dietary intervention. With aging, there is a reduction in the lean body mass, physical activity, and energy expenditure, all of which will result in increased weight gain if one continues to consume the same level of calories throughout the life span.

Insulin

There has been a renewed interest in action of insulin, particularly insulin sensitivity, in the lay literature with supplements and diets proposing to induce weight loss by affecting insulin sensitivity. If weight gain and loss are related to insulin, does it matter if someone is insulin-sensitive or insulin-resistant? The topic has been hotly debated. There have been numerous studies in the animal literature, genetic models, behavioral models, and human feeding studies [51]. The concept is that a high glycemic load diet stimulates insulin secretion, decreases fat oxidation, lowers energy expenditure, stimulates stress hormone secretion, limits the availability of metabolic fuels in the late postprandial period, and increases voluntary food intake [50, 66, 79]. These effects have been demonstrated in feeding studies. Cornier et al. conducted a small, controlled study on obese non-diabetic women over a 4-month feeding period [13]. The participants received a high-carbohydrate low-fat (60:20) or a low-carbohydrate high-fat (40:40) diet. Both diets were hypocaloric.

The high-carbohydrate low-fat diet was more effective in producing weight loss in the insulin-sensitive women, and the low-carbohydrate high-fat diet was more effective in the insulin-resistant women. The differences were not explained by caloric intake, physical activity, or resting metabolic rate. A similar study was conducted by Ebbeling et al. In this study, a low-glycemic diet resulted in greater weight loss in those individuals who were insulin-resistant [19]. Based on these results, it has been proposed that reducing the glycemic load may be important to achieve weight loss in those individuals with high insulin secretion.

However, the issue is complex and may involve more than insulin sensitivity or resistance. The Diet Intervention Examining The Factors Interacting with Treatment Success (DIETFITS) study was designed to test whether (i) a set of three single nucleotide polymorphism (SNP) genotype patterns or (ii) baseline differences in insulin secretion or both predisposed individuals to differences in weight loss while on a low-fat diet versus a low-carbohydrate diet [28]. The study included 609 overweight adults who were randomized to receive a healthy low-fat diet or a healthy low-carbohydrate diet over a 12-month period. Weight change was not significantly different between the two diet groups, and neither genotype pattern nor baseline insulin secretion was associated with the dietary effects on weight loss.

Hormones

In addition to insulin, there is also a role of hormones such as ghrelin and leptin in the development of obesity. Leptin is synthesized by adipocytes and secreted into the circulation at a level which is proportional to energy stores in adipose tissue. Leptin is a product of the *LEP* gene and stimulates the neural circuits that decrease food intake and increase energy expenditure [25]. In contrast, ghrelin is an orexigenic gut hormone which is decreased in obesity [74]. These hormones affect the appetite and satiety level, and the differences among individuals and

populations are still being elucidated. The effects of adipokines and gut hormones on weight loss may be related to the glycemic load or other nutrients in the diet or function independently. The ability to manipulate the secretion of these hormones may someday aid in the prevention and treatment of obesity.

Food Supply

Our food supply has changed dramatically over the years and has become far more ultra-processed and inclusive of highly refined sugars, chemicals, and preservatives. The overall refinement in the diet has also led to a reduction in fiber intake which in turn affects satiety and the health of the gut microbiota. Ultra-processed foods have been associated with metabolic syndrome and non-alcoholic fatty liver disease (NAFLD) [38]. The influence of the food supply on the development of obesity is also closely related to socioeconomic factors. When there are economic constraints, people will purchase low-cost foods, which tend to be processed, low in nutritional value and high in calories, fat, refined carbohydrates, and synthetic food additives.

Gut Microbiome

We are now beginning to appreciate the influence of the gut microbiota on health and disease. Intestinal dysbiosis has been linked to the metabolic syndrome [22, 75]. This dysbiosis influences the storage and release of energy from the adipocytes. Some of these components which affect the gut microbiota, in particular diet, are modifiable. Diets such as the Western diet have become a growing health concern, as they are strongly associated with obesity and related metabolic diseases, promoting inflammation and both structural and behavioral changes in gut microbiota [45]. The impact of single food components (macronutrients and micronutrients), salt, food additives, and different dietary habits (i.e., vegan and vegetarian, gluten-free, ketogenic, high-sugar, Western-type, and Mediterranean diets) on gut microbiota composition have been described [63]. The mechanisms behind these beneficial microbial metabolite effects are related to the ability of the gut microbiota to ferment complex dietary residues, generally fibers, that are resistant to digestion by enteric enzymes [57]. This process provides energy for the microbiota and culminates in the release of short-chain fatty acids (SCFAs) which are utilized for the metabolic needs of the colon and the host. It is the SCFAs that mediate the metabolic effects of the microbiota. Butyrate has a significant role in the colonic health-promoting and antineoplastic properties of the microbiota. Butyrate is the preferred energy source for colonocytes; it maintains mucosal integrity and suppresses inflammation and carcinogenesis through effects on immunity, gene expression, and epigenetic modulation. Undigested protein residues and fat-stimulated bile acids are also metabolized by the microbiota into inflammatory and/or carcinogenic metabolites, which increase the risk of neoplastic progression and metabolic disease [57]. Other components of the diet can affect the microbiome. For example, the use of artificial sweeteners was linked to the changes in the gut microbiota [67].

Most of the data surrounding the effects of the microbiota on weight loss have been extrapolated from epidemiological or animal studies. For example, dietary fiber has been shown to be protective and reduce body weight in several conditions [2]. Women who consume more refined grains tend to have greater weight gain than those who consume viscous or fermentable fibers [46]. In one study, the use of fiber supplements has been shown to result in greater weight loss [3].

It is tempting to think we can routinely and uniformly change the gut microbiota to achieve a specific and desired effect [10]. But the factors that influence these changes are multiple and complex. We know that diet can influence commensal microbiota. The overall composition of the diet also has a major impact on the gut microbiome [54, 85]. A diet high in fiber, fruits, and vegetables such as the Mediterranean diet can have beneficial effects on the microbiome.

There are numerous factors which affect the ecology of gut microbiota. Even the process of aging will influence the gut microbiota [9]. There are differences in individual characteristics such as lifestyle, antibiotic use, bile acids, country of residence, and, eventually, frailty. Individuals with obesity have a microbiome that is different from lean individuals. There are two phyla, mainly anaerobes, that appear to be linked to obesity, *Firmicutes* (positively) and *Bacteroidetes* (negatively). However, it is uncertain if these microorganisms cause obesity or are a result of obesity. For bifidobacteria, a consistent difference was found in the meta-analysis between obese subjects and 189 controls from six published studies showing that the digestive microbiota of the obese group was significantly depleted in bifidobacteria [4].

Prebiotics can modulate the gut microbiota. Prebiotics such as inulin, fructo-oligosaccharides, galacto-oligosaccharides, resistant starch, xylo-oligosaccharides, and arabinoxylan oligosaccharides support the growth of the beneficial bacteria and SCFA production in the gut. This results in improved barrier function and resistance to inflammatory stimuli, increased mineral absorption, and modulation of lipid metabolism, possibly by suppression of lipogenic enzymes and thus decreased synthesis of lipoproteins and triglycerides [39]. Prebiotics have been shown to improve glucose homeostasis via stimulation of glucagon-like peptide 1 secretion [17]. However, not all dietary fibers are prebiotics and not all prebiotics are fibers. Many fermentable dietary fibers are preferential fuels used by specific microbes or groups of microbes within the intestinal microbiota. Other less fermentable dietary fibers may influence the microbiota overall but do not have prebiotic activity. Although many prebiotics are considered fibers, dietary nutrients, including specific fatty acids within plants, may have prebiotic activity [71].

Probiotics also alter the microbiome. In general, the mechanisms that underlie beneficial effects of probiotics are attributed to exclusion of pathogenic microorganisms by production of bactericides and competition for nutrients, modulation of inflammatory responses through interaction with immune cells in the gut, and modulation of gene expression affecting host metabolism and gut barrier function [81]. The beneficial effects are strain-specific and dose dependent. Thus, there are no generic probiotic effects. The specific uses of probiotics to alter disease pathogenesis require further investigation.

The question becomes: can we modulate the gut microbiota to induce weight loss? At this point it is important to recognize that there is no substitute for a healthy lifestyle. Although promising, the gut microbiota and microbiota-derived metabolites may or may not have the therapeutic effect necessary to prevent or change the development or progression of the disease. What is more important is to fully understand how different dietary patterns modulate the composition of gut microbiota and whether these changes are long-term and lead to causal health effects.

Intermittent Fasting as a Tool to Change Metabolism

Intermittent fasting is an umbrella term used to describe various meal timing schedules that cycle between voluntary fasting (or reduced calorie intake) and non-fasting over a given period. It is also known as intermittent energy restriction and time-restricted eating. In general, only water, black coffee, and black tea are allowed during fasting. The idea of intermittent fasting is to induce a "metabolic switch." The circadian clock regulates eating, sleeping, hormones, physiologic, and metabolic processes. Eating throughout waking hours without exercise results in oxidation of calories consumed and not mobilization of adipose stores. During fasting, glycogen stores are depleted, and there is a "switch" to lipolysis after breakdown of the muscle. Regimens that exclude or restrict evening energy intake led to reduced postprandial insulin and glucose levels during the day [58]. There is increased fatty acid oxidation in the liver, increased production of the HDL precursor apolipoprotein A (apoA), and decreased production of the LDL precursor apolipoprotein B (apoB). Additionally, intermittent fasting, especially time-restricted feeding, is reported to restore key microbiota, reset the composition of the microbiome, and restore the cyclical fluctuations [58].

There are limited data on the effects of fasting on patients with metabolic syndrome (MetS) [68, 78, 80, 82]. Most of the studies evaluated changes in cardiovascular risk parameters but not necessarily MetS. A Cochrane review of intermittent fasting for the prevention of cardiovascular disease concluded that intermittent fasting may result in more weight loss than usual eating over 3 months but not when compared against energy-restricted diets for 3 months or longer. Intermittent fasting did not affect blood glucose levels when compared to usual eating over 3 months, energy restriction diets over 3 months, or energy restriction diets over 3–12 months. Overall weight loss and changes in blood glucose were small and not clinically significant [1].

The TREAT randomized clinical trial was a 12-week prospective study which compared consistent meal timing to time-restricted eating. There were no statistically significant changes in estimated energy intake or energy expenditure between groups. Time-restricted eating did not confer cardiometabolic benefits or change relevant metabolic markers. There were no significant within-group or between-group differences in fasting glucose, fasting insulin levels, and insulin resistance measured by HOMA-IR, HbA1c, triglycerides, or total cholesterol, LDL, or HDL cholesterol levels. There was no significant change in whole-body fat mass in the time-restricted eating or the consistent mealtime groups. However, appendicular lean mass was decreased significantly in the time-restricted eating group but not in the consistent meal timing group. The authors concluded that results of this study did not support the efficacy of time-restricted eating for weight loss, highlighted the importance of control interventions, and cautioned about the potential effects of time-restricted eating on appendicular muscle mass [49]. Although currently there is no compelling scientific evidence to support the use of intermittent fasting over consistent mealtime consumption, intermittent fasting may be of benefit in those individuals who cannot stop eating once they start. However, the loss of lean muscle mass is a concern since the muscle is a metabolically active tissue. The loss of lean body mass during time-restricted eating may be mitigated by increasing the number of meals within the eating window, increasing the protein content of the diet, or providing supplements such as whey protein or hydroxy-beta-methylbutyrate (HMB) to increase muscle mass and function as well as resistance training. However, these interventions have not been validated in clinical trials.

Somewhat related to the concept of intermittent fasting is the speed and frequency of eating. Garcidueñas-Fimbres et al. conducted a narrative review to summarize the evidence regarding the impact of eating speed and eating frequency on adiposity, MetS, or diet quality. The results of this review suggested that children and adults with a faster eating speed may be at higher risk of developing adiposity, MetS, or its components. A higher eating frequency may be associated with diet quality improvement, lower adiposity, and lower risk of developing MetS or its components. But the mechanisms by which these eating behaviors influence the development of MetS are yet to be determined.

Dietary Macronutrients

Most dietary interventions focus on modification of the macronutrient portion of the diet (i.e., carbohydrate, protein, and fat). When the percentage of one macronutrient is changed, there will be a corresponding increase or decrease in the other macronutrients. A diet may or may not define the characteristics of each of these macronutrients. For example, a carbohydrate is not a uniform organic compound and may be defined as simple or complex, by the glycemic index (GI), glycemic load (GL), or fiber content (viscous vs. fermentable). Proteins have varying amino acid profiles and may be derived from land animal, plant, or marine sources. In addition, these protein sources may contain varying amounts and types of fat. There are also some protein sources such as those derived from dairy sources which contain some carbohydrate. Fat sources include monosaturated, polyunsaturated, saturated, and trans fats. Depending on the composition included in the weight loss diet these will vary in the content of omega-3, omega-6, and omega-9 fatty acids. Foods are generally composites of each of these macronutrients. Therefore, the lack of precision in defining the dietary prescription makes comparisons of weight loss diets difficult.

Low-Carbohydrate and Ketogenic Diets: Metabolic Rationale

The use of low-carbohydrate and ketogenic diets has been extensively studied. The metabolic rationale for the restriction is that when the carbohydrate content of the diet is sufficiently reduced, especially simple and highly refined carbohydrates, there will be a decline in blood glucose and insulin levels, which in turn will shift metabolism from lipogenesis to lipolysis, resulting in weight loss. Accordingly, when the carbohydrate content of the diet is reduced, there is a corresponding increase in the protein and fat content. The oxidation of protein and fat for energy results in the production of ketones, which cause an increase in satiety and a voluntary caloric reduction. The oxidation of protein and fat is less efficient than the oxidation of carbohydrate. The extra energy required to oxidize protein and fat may be as high as 400–600 kcal/day [24]. Aside from the additional energy required to metabolize protein and fat, increasing the protein content of the diet has been shown to have a beneficial effect on the resting energy expenditure (REE) and total energy expenditure (TEE) during weight loss [20, 59]. Lipolysis is maintained even if there is an excess of calories because glycerol from fat is utilized as a gluconeogenic precursor. Thus, the rapid weight loss observed during the use of ketogenic diets is multifactorial and results from a combination of increased lipolysis, decreased de novo lipogenesis, increased energy expenditure from the conversion of glycerol and glycogenic amino acids to glucose, as well as the satiety value associated with ketones and higher protein intake.

The exact amount of carbohydrate required to produce these metabolic alterations has been debated and not clearly elucidated. It should also be noted that a low-carbohydrate diet is not necessarily a ketogenic diet. By far, the most highly studied ketogenic diet is the Atkins dietary approach. The diet has evolved since its initial introduction in 1972 and now offers different levels of carbohydrate restriction. The Atkins 40 diet prescribes 55–65% fat, 20–30% protein, and 10–15% carbohydrate. For more rapid weight loss, the Atkins 20 diet is suggested providing 60–70% fat, 20–30% protein, and 10–15% carbohydrate. The classic ketogenic diet recommends 75–90% fat, 5–20% protein, and less than 5% carbohydrate.

Considering the wide range of dietary carbohydrate levels used in studies, Feinman and colleagues proposed that a low-carbohydrate diet be defined as less than 130 g/day or less than 26% of total energy and a very low-carbohydrate ketogenic diet be defined as carbohydrate between 20 and 50 g/day or less than 10% of a 2000 kcal/day diet, whether or not ketosis occurs [23].

Another approach to controlling carbohydrate intake has been with the utilization of the glycemic index (GI) which measures the rate at which blood glucose levels rise when a particular food is ingested and how quickly the blood glucose levels drop. This ranking system was originally developed to aid those with diabetes and manage their carbohydrate intake relative to insulin requirements. Pure glucose has a rating of 100; thus, the closer a food is to glucose, GI of 100, the higher the GI rating. Foods with a low GI rating will be absorbed more slowly, keeping blood glucose levels lower and more sustained. The GI has inherent irregularities. For example, white bread and whole wheat bread have very similar GI rankings as do brown and white rice, yet clearly the whole grain choices are healthier. The glycemic load (GL) is the mathematical product of the GI and the amount of carbohydrate in the diet. Diets with a high GL result in higher postprandial insulin concentration than those with a low GL.

Low-Fat and Very Low-Fat Diets: Metabolic Rationale

Fat is the most calorically dense of all the macronutrients with 9 kcal/g. It was therefore logical to assume that reduction in dietary fat would result in a reduction of energy intake and body weight. As with the other macronutrients, the exact composition of a low-fat diet varies but is generally 20–30% of calories from fat, and a very low-fat diet is often as low as 10% of calories from fat. As the dietary fat content is reduced, the carbohydrate is increased, and, in some instances, there may be a slight increase in the protein content of the diet. These diets tended to be lower in calories when properly employed and resulted in weight loss when done correctly. However, in practice, the low-fat and very low-fat diets were low in satiety value and often lead to overconsumption. Some consumers believed that a low-fat diet meant they could eat as many calories as desired as long as these foods were low in fat. In this case, the dietary fat was replaced with carbohydrates, primarily in the form of simple sugars and refined carbohydrates, increasing caloric intake by 200 calories a day [23, 77]. Overall, the low-fat diet prescribed for the management of obesity and lowering of cardiovascular risk factors failed to produce the desired results [23]. The use of a low-fat diet without calorie restriction will not result in weight loss.

The Mediterranean Diet: Rationale and Effects

There is a wealth of information regarding the use of the Mediterranean Diet (Med Diet) and its effects on the microbiome. The Med Diet has been linked to many health benefits, including reduced mortality risk and the prevention of many diseases. The Med Diet centers around fruits, vegetables, olive oil, nuts, legumes, and whole grains. It is based on the regular consumption of mono-unsaturated fatty acids (MUFAs) and poly-unsaturated fatty acids (PUFAs), polyphenols, and other antioxidants. It also includes a high intake of prebiotic fiber and low-glycemic carbohydrates and greater consumption of plant proteins than animal proteins [15]. Consumption of Med Diet has been shown to alter the composition of the microbiota with higher levels of *Bacteroidetes* because of lower animal protein intake and higher bifidobacterial counts and higher total SCFAs because of greater consumption of plant-based nutrients, such as vegetable proteins and polysaccharides [26]. This has been confirmed by other reports that high-level consumption of plant-based foods and high-level adherence to a Med Diet beneficially impact the gut microbiota and metabolomic profile [16, 53]. These findings demonstrated a link between adherence to the Med Diet and improvements to the diversity and richness of gut microbiota.

Randomized Controlled Dietary Interventional Trials with Different Diets

Many of the diet studies have been based on observation or long-term epidemiological studies. Comparisons of controlled interventional trials of weight loss diets are difficult due to differences in study design and outcome parameters. There are numerous differences in the composition of the diets, the length of time of the intervention, the outcome parameters (i.e., weight loss, metabolic parameters, body composition), adherence, and setting (inpatient vs. outpatient). Additionally, some of the diet interventions employed an isocaloric prescription, while others allowed the patients to consume an unrestricted amount in order to evaluate the effects on appetite.

Owing to the difficulty that many individuals have following a diet plan for weight reduction, many turn to programs that offer partial meal replacements (MR) or total meal replacements (TMR). Meal replacements are typically formulated as prepackaged shakes, soups, and bars, which offer another option for reducing energy intake. The OPTIFAST program (OP) is one example of a TMR weight loss intervention. Originally developed in the 1970s as a very low-calorie diet (VLCD) providing 420 kcal/d, the OPTIFAST program has evolved to include comprehensive behavioral intervention and a higher calorie intake. The OPTIWIN multicenter clinical trial was designed to test the effectiveness of OP compared to a food-based dietary plan over a 26- and 52-week period. Both groups received comprehensive behavioral intervention for weight loss. The results demonstrated that a comprehensive behavioral weight loss intervention with TMR led to greater clinically significant weight loss at 26 and 52 weeks compared with a well-established food-based behavioral intervention. Fat mass loss was greater for OP; lean mass loss was proportional to total weight loss [5]. This study provided evidence of the safety and efficacy of the OP and provides an option for those individuals who have difficulty following a food-based program.

There have been several human trials (Table 2) which compared isocaloric diets containing a low versus high carbohydrate content [6, 30, 31, 34, 43, 44, 56, 60–62, 87]. The fact that these studies were isocaloric is an important point and permits the

Table 2 Isocaloric weight loss intervention trials with varying carbohydrate (CHO) contents

	% CHO		Weight loss (kg $\pm$ SEM)		
References	Low	High	Low CHO	High CHO	p
Young et al. [87]	7	23	16.2 $\pm$ 0.9	11.9 $\pm$ 0.8	<0.05
Rabast et al. [61]	10	68	14.0 $\pm$ 1.4	9.8 $\pm$ 1.0	0.10
Rabast et al. [62]	12	70	12.5 $\pm$ 0.9	9.5 $\pm$ 0.7	<0.01
Piatti et al. [60]	35	60	4.5 $\pm$ 0.4	6.4 $\pm$ 0.9	0.3
Golay et al. [31]	15	45	8.9 $\pm$ 0.6	7.5 $\pm$ 0.5	0.1
Golay et al. [30]	25	45	10.2 $\pm$ 0.7	8.6 $\pm$ 0.8	0.13
Lean et al. [44]	35	58	6.8 $\pm$ 0.8	5.6 $\pm$ 0.8	0.1
Baba et al. [6]	25	68	8.3 $\pm$ 0.7	6.0 $\pm$ 0.6	<0.05
Greene et al. [34]	5	55	10.4 $\pm$ 2.1	7.7 $\pm$ 1.1	0.25
Layman et al. [43]	44	59	7.5 $\pm$ 1.4	7.0 $\pm$ 1.4	0.8
Noakes et al. [56]	4	70	8.0 $\pm$ 0.6 kg	6.7 $\pm$ 0.7 kg	0.18

Adapted with permission from Fine and Feinman [24]

examination of effect based on the macronutrient percentages. Overall, greater weight loss was observed in the lower-carbohydrate diets in comparison with the higher-carbohydrate diets.

If diet is modified relative to the individual's usual intake, it is likely to produce weight loss regardless of the composition of the diet. To investigate the effects of altering the macronutrient content of weight loss diets, Shai et al. conducted a 2-year trial in which 322 moderately obese individuals were randomized to one of three diets: a calorie-restricted low-fat diet providing less than 30% fat, a calorie-restricted Mediterranean diet supplying less than 35% fat, or a very low-carbohydrate (less than 20 g initially up to 120 g carbohydrate) diet with no calorie restrictions [65]. Each of the diets resulted in weight loss. However, the low-carbohydrate diet produced the greatest weight loss followed by the Mediterranean diet and then low fat. Interestingly, the amount of weight loss was similar between the low-carbohydrate and Mediterranean diet at about the 1-year mark and continuing up to 2 years. The ratio of serum total cholesterol to HDL cholesterol decreased in all groups, with the low-carbohydrate group showing the greatest improvement with a relative decrease of 20% compared with the low-fat group with a decrease of 12%.

Gardner et al. evaluated the effects of four popular weight loss diets with varying levels of carbohydrate in a public health setting over the course of 1 year [27]. They randomized 311 overweight premenopausal women to the Atkins diet (<20 g carbohydrate/day, no calorie restriction), Zone (40% carbohydrate, calorie restricted), LEARN (55–60% carbohydrate, calorie restricted), and Ornish (<10% fat, no calorie restriction). The participants were provided with books explaining the diet and attended weekly instructions for 2 months. Subjects on the Atkins diet (low carbohydrate) had the greatest weight loss and had the highest retention in the study. The Atkins group also experienced the greatest improvement in metabolic effects, with significant changes in HDL cholesterol, triglycerides, and systolic blood pressure. These studies demonstrate that the low-carbohydrate diet, despite unrestricted caloric intake, is at least as effective if not more efficacious as other dietary plans with regard to weight loss and improvement in metabolic parameters.

The effects of the low-carbohydrate or a low-fat diet on weight loss and cardiovascular risk factors were evaluated over the course of 1 year in a randomized trial [8]. Participants without cardiovascular disease or diabetes (n = 148) were randomized to a low-carbohydrate or low-fat diet along with dietary counseling at regular intervals throughout the trial. The low-carbohydrate diet was more effective for weight loss and cardiovascular risk factor reduction than the low-fat diet.

There are some concerns regarding the inflammatory nature of high-fat ketogenic diets and the potential to increase LDL cholesterol. Gardner et al. conducted a randomized, crossover, interventional trial in individuals with prediabetes and type 2 diabetes mellitus (T2DM) comparing the ketogenic diet and the Med Diet [29]. The well-formulated ketogenic diet (WFKD) included non-starchy vegetables and excluded added sugars, refined grains, legumes, fruits, and whole, intact grains. The Med Diet also excluded added sugars and refined grains but included non-starchy vegetables, legumes, fruits, and whole, intact grains. The diets were switched at 12 weeks. The HbA1c values were not different between diet phases. The WFKD led to a greater decrease in triglycerides but also had potential untoward risks from elevated LDL cholesterol and lower nutrient intakes from after 12 weeks but improved from baseline on both diets avoiding legumes, fruits, and whole, intact grains, as well as being less sustainable. In contrast to these findings, Ebbeling et al. found that a low-carbohydrate diet, high in saturated fat, had benefits for insulin-resistant dyslipoproteinemia and lipoprotein(a), without adverse effects on LDL cholesterol or inflammation [21]. It is difficult to explain the differences between these two well-designed, well-controlled studies. It may be that the participants in each of these studies differed in genetic predisposition, some differences in the level of restriction in the test diets or perhaps transient hypercholesterolemia secondary to rapid weight loss. Nonetheless, the results reflect the complexities of diet interventions.

Systematic Reviews and Meta-analyses

The studies evaluating the role of diet on weight loss and metabolic parameters provide some insight into their effectiveness. However, many of the studies had small samples, were conducted over a short period of time, and may or may not have used appropriate controls. Because of the difficulties in evaluating the efficacy or these diets, several systematic reviews and meta-analyses have been conducted to try and discern whether there are advantages of one dietary approach over the other. Hession et al. conducted a systematic review of the effects of low-carbohydrate diets with low-fat diets on weight loss and coronary disease risk factors [36]. A total of 13 studies that lasted at least 6 months with a total of 1222 participants were included. The data demonstrate that low-carbohydrate, high-protein diets are more effective at 6 months and are as effective as low-fat diets in reducing weight and cardiovascular risk parameters for up to 1 year. In addition, higher retention rates were found in the low-carbohydrate group compared with the low-fat group.

Johnston et al. conducted a meta-analysis of popular weight loss diet programs [40]. The outcome parameters were weight loss at 6 and 12 months. There was no evaluation of other metabolic parameters. A total of 48 studies including 7268 participants were included in the analysis. Although not statistically significant, the largest weight loss was associated with low-carbohydrate diet both at 6 and 12 months. With a lack of statistical significance between the different weight loss interventions, it may be that the best practice should be to recommend a diet that a patient is likely to adhere to in order to lose weight.

The degree to which the carbohydrate content of a diet is considered "low" versus "high" makes comparison difficult. But what if the carbohydrate content of the diet is "balanced" or "moderate"? Low-carbohydrate versus balanced-carbohydrate diets for reducing weight and cardiovascular risk was evaluated in a Cochrane systematic review [55]. There were 61 parallel-arm randomized controlled trials in adults (18 years and older) who were overweight or living with obesity, without or

with type 2 diabetes, and with or without cardiovascular conditions or risk factors. Fifty-eight studies were included in the meta-analysis. Trials had to compare low-carbohydrate weight-reducing diets to balanced-carbohydrate (45–65% of total energy) weight-reducing diets, have a weight-reducing phase of 2 weeks or longer, and be explicitly implemented for the primary purpose of reducing weight, with or without advice to restrict energy intake. Most trials investigated low-carbohydrate diets (>50 g to 150 g per day or <45% of total energy expenditure), followed by very-low (≤50 g per day or <10% of total energy expenditure), and then incremental increases from very low to low. The most common diets compared were low-carbohydrate, balanced-fat (20–35% of total energy expenditure), and high-protein (>20% of total energy expenditure) treatment diets versus control diets balanced for the three macronutrients. In most trials the energy prescription or approach used to restrict energy intake was similar in both groups. The low-carbohydrate diets result in little to no difference in weight loss over the short term (3–8.5 months) and long term (1–2 years) compared to balanced-carbohydrate weight-reducing diets, in people with or without type 2 diabetes. In the short term, the average difference in weight loss was about 1 kg, and in the long term, the average difference was less than 1 kg. People lost weight on both diets in some trials, most likely reflecting a change in usual eating habits. The amount of weight lost on average varied greatly with both diets across the trials from less than 1 kg in some trials and up to about 12 kg in others in the short term and long term. Similarly, low-carbohydrate weight-reducing diets resulted in little to no difference in diastolic blood pressure, HbA1c, and LDL cholesterol for up to 2 years.

Kastorini et al. conducted a systematic review and random-effects meta-analysis of epidemiological studies and randomized controlled trials, to assess the effect of a Med Diet on MetS and its components [41]. Fifty original research studies (35 clinical, 2 prospective, and 13 cross-sectional trials), with 534,906 participants, were included in the analysis. The combined effect of prospective studies and clinical trials showed that adherence to the Med Diet was associated with reduced risk of MetS. Results from clinical studies revealed the protective role of the Med Diet on components of MetS, like waist circumference, high-density lipoprotein cholesterol, triglycerides, systolic and diastolic blood pressure, and glucose. The results from epidemiological studies also confirmed those of clinical trials.

Effects of Diet on Body Composition

There are limited data of the effect of the macronutrient composition of the diet on body composition beyond absolute weight loss. Brehm et al. [11] randomized healthy women to receive a low-fat or very low-carbohydrate diet. Weight loss and reduction of body fat as measured by DXA were greatest in the group receiving the very low-carbohydrate diet both at 3 and 6 months. Blood pressure, lipids, fasting glucose, and insulin were within normal limits for both groups at the beginning of the trial but continued to improve throughout the study period. The greatest weight loss occurred in the low-carbohydrate diet, and those individuals had the greatest reduction in body fat.

However, there are conflicting data. In a study to determine whether low-carbohydrate high-protein (LCHP) diets were more effective in promoting loss of weight, and body fat was conducted by Landers et al. [42]. Individuals were randomized to receive one of three diet plans: (i) a low-carbohydrate high-protein ketogenic diet, (ii) the Zone diet, and (iii) a conventional hypocaloric diabetic exchange diet that supplied less than 10%, 40%, and 50% of calories from carbohydrate, respectively. Body composition was measured before and after the intervention treatment period with DXA. The mean weight loss was 5.1 kg for those who completed the 12 week program. There were no significant differences in total weight, fat, or lean body mass loss when compared to diet group. Attrition was substantial for all plans at 43%, 60%, and 36% for LCHP, Zone, and conventional diets, respectively.

The effects of diet interventions on changes in fat location may be an important factor. One of the

key components of MetS is increased abdominal fat mass. Veum et al. randomly assigned abdominally obese men to a very high-fat, low-carbohydrate (VHFLC; 73% of energy fat and 10% of energy carbohydrate) or low-fat, high-carbohydrate (LFHC; 30% of energy fat and 53% of energy carbohydrate) diets to evaluate possible differential effects on visceral fat mass and body composition [76]. The diets were isocaloric and modestly energy-restrictive with an equal percentage total energy intake from protein (17% of energy). The diets also emphasized low-processed, lower-glycemic foods. Fat mass was quantified with computed tomography imaging. Total body weight decreased similarly on both diets, resulting in a 3.6–3.7 reduction in BMI points. Visceral fat and subcutaneous fat volume decreased on average by 21–27% and 21–25%, respectively, with no significant group differences in absolute or relative score changes from baseline to 12 weeks.

But the effects of diet on body composition may not be as simple as evaluating differences in the macronutrient content of the diet. Goni et al. noted that the adenylate cyclase 3 (ADCY3) gene is involved in the regulation of several metabolic processes including the development and function of the adipose tissue. They studied the effects of the ADCY3 rs10182181 genetic variant on changes in body composition in 147 overweight or obese subjects after 16 weeks of the dietary intervention of a moderately high-protein diet or a low-fat diet. In the moderately high-protein group, the G allele was associated with a lower decrease of fat mass, trunk, and android fat and a greater decrease in lean mass. Conversely, the low-fat group carrying the G allele was associated with a greater decrease in trunk, android, gynoid, and visceral fat. The authors concluded that individuals carrying the G allele of the rs10182181 polymorphism may benefit more in terms of weight loss and improvement of body composition measurements when undertaking a hypocaloric low-fat diet as compared to a moderately high-protein diet [32].

It also appears that the time frame of eating may affect body composition. The TREAT randomized clinical trial which compared consistent meal timing to time-restricted eating demonstrated a significant reduction in appendicular lean mass as compared to consistent meal timing [49]. The muscle is desirable from a functional standpoint. But it is also a metabolically active tissue which could influence the ability to maintain weight loss.

Conclusion

Obesity is a global problem and a major health concern due to the associated comorbidities. The foundation of obesity therapy has been diet, exercise, and behavioral modification. However, no one diet alone has been universally successful at inducing and maintaining weight loss and improving metabolic parameters, reflecting the complexity of the disease. Although many diets have shown weight loss in the short term, very few have demonstrated long-term success. Additionally, any potentially negative consequences of these diets, such as changes in the gut microbiota, need to be evaluated for their long-term effects. The factors affecting obesity are complex, dynamic, and interrelated and involve numerous host factors as well as the environment. Interventions to induce weight loss should have solid physiological and metabolic basis and be scientifically validated. Ultimately, the best diet is the one that patients can adhere to in order to achieve their health goals.

References

1. Allaf M, Elghazaly H, Mohamed OG, et al. Intermittent fasting for the prevention of cardiovascular disease. Cochrane Database Syst Rev. 2021; https://doi.org/10.1002/14651858.CD013496.pub2.

2. Anderson JW, Pasupuleti VK. Nutraceuticals and diabetes prevention and management. In: Pasupuleti VK, Anderson JW, editors. Nutraceuticals, glycemic health and Type 2 diabetes. Oxford, UK: Wiley-Blackwell; 2008. p. 1–9.

3. Anderson JW, Baird P, Davis RH, Ferreri S, Knudtson M, Koraym A, Waters V, Williams CL. Health benefits of dietary fiber. Nutr Rev. 2009;67:188–205.

4. Angelakis E, Armougom F, Million M, et al. The relationship between gut microbiota and weight gain in humans. Future Microbiol. 2012;7(1):91–109.

5. Ard JD, Lewis KH, Rothberg A, et al. Effectiveness of a Total Meal Replacement Program (OPTIFAST Program) on weight loss: results from the OPTIWIN Study. Obesity. 2019;27:22–9. https://doi.org/10.1002/oby.22303.

6. Baba NH, Sawaya S, Torbay N, et al. High protein vs high carbohydrate hypoenergetic diet for the treatment of obese hyperinsulinemic subjects. Int J Obes Relat Metab Disord. 1999;23:1202–6.

7. Baturin AK, Pogozheva AV, Sorokina E, et al. The study of polymorphism rs9939609 FTO gene in patients with overweight and obesity. Vopr Pitan. 2011;80(3):13–7.

8. Bazzano LA, Hu T, Reynolds K, et al. Effects of low-carbohydrate and low-fat diets: a randomized trial effects of low-carbohydrate and low-fat diets. Ann Intern Med. 2014;161:309–18.

9. Biagi E, Candela M, Fairweather-Tait S, et al. Ageing of the human metaorganism: the microbial counterpart. Age. 2012;34:247–67.

10. Brahe LK, Astrup A, Larsen LH. Can we prevent obesity-related metabolic diseases by dietary modulation of the gut microbiota? Adv Nutr. 2016;7:90–101. https://doi.org/10.3945/an.115.010587.

11. Brehm BJ, Seeley RJ, Daniels SR, et al. A randomized trial comparing a very low carbohydrate diet and a calorie-restricted low-fat diet on body weight and cardiovascular risk factors in healthy women. J Clin Endocrinol Metab. 2003;88:1617–23.

12. Chen H, et al. Evidence that the diabetes gene encodes the leptin receptor: identification of a mutation in the leptin receptor gene in db/db mice. Cell. 1996;84:491–5.

13. Cornier MA, Donahoo WT, Pereira R, et al. Insulin sensitivity determines the effectiveness of dietary macronutrient composition on weight loss in obese women. Obes Res. 2005;13(4):703–9.

14. d'Errico M, Pavlova M, Spandonaro F. The economic burden of obesity in Italy: a cost-of-illness study. Eur J Health Econ. 2022;23:177–92.

15. Davis C, Bryan J, Hodgson J, Murphy K. Definition of the Mediterranean diet: a literature review. Nutrients. 2015;7:9139–53. https://doi.org/10.3390/nu7115459.

16. De Filippis F, Pellegrini N, Vannini L, Jeffery IB, La Storia A, Laghi L, Serrazanetti DI, Di Cagno R, Ferrocino I, Lazzi C, et al. High-level adherence to a Mediterranean diet beneficially impacts the gut microbiota and associated metabolome. Gut. 2016;65:1812–21.

17. Delzenne NM, Cani PD, Neyrinck AM. Modulation of glucagon-like peptide 1 and energy metabolism by inulin and oligofructose: experimental data. J Nutr. 2007;137:2547S–51S.

18. Doo M, Kim Y. Association between ESR1 rs1884051 polymorphism and dietary total energy and plant

protein intake on obesity in Korean men. Nutr Res Pract. 2011;5(6):527–32.

19. Ebbeling CB, Leidig MM, Feldman HA, et al. Effects of a low–glycemic load vs low-fat diet in obese young adults: a randomized trial. JAMA. 2007;297:2092–102.

20. Ebbeling CB, Swain JF, Feldman HA, et al. Effects of dietary composition on energy expenditure during weight-loss maintenance. JAMA. 2012;307(24):2627–34.

21. Ebbeling CB, Knapp A, Johnson A, et al. Effects of a low-carbohydrate diet on insulin-resistant dyslipoproteinemia – a randomized controlled feeding trial. Am J Clin Nutr. 2022;115:154–62.

22. Everard A, Cani PD. Diabetes, obesity and gut microbiota. Best Pract Res Clin Gastroenterol. 2013;27:73–83.

23. Feinman RD, Pogozelski WK, Astrup A, et al. Dietary carbohydrate restriction as the first approach in diabetes management: critical review and evidence base. Nutrition. 2015;31(1):1–13.

24. Fine EJ, Feinman RD. Thermodynamics of weight loss diets. Nutr Metab. 2004;1(15):1–8.

25. Friedman JM, Halaas JL. Leptin and the regulation of body weight in mammals. Nature. 1998;395:763–70.

26. Garcia-Mantrana I, Selma-Royo M, Alcantara C, Collado MC. Shifts on gut microbiota associated to Mediterranean diet adherence and specific dietary intakes on general adult population. Front Microbiol. 2018;9:890.

27. Gardner CD, Kiazand A, Alhassan S, et al. Comparison of the Atkins, Zone, Ornish, and LEARN diets for change in weight and related risk factors among overweight premenopausal women: the ATO Z Weight Loss Study: a randomized trial. JAMA. 2007;297(9):969–77.

28. Gardner CD, Trepanowski JF, Del Gobbo LC, et al. Effect of low-fat vs low-carbohydrate diet on 12-month weight loss in overweight adults and the association with genotype pattern or insulin secretion the DIETFITS Randomized Clinical Trial. JAMA. 2018;319(7):667–79.

29. Gardner CD, Landry MJ, Perelman D, et al. Effect of a ketogenic diet versus Mediterranean diet on glycated hemoglobin in individuals with prediabetes and type 2 diabetes mellitus: the interventional Keto-Med randomized crossover trial. Am J Clin Nutr. 2022;116:640–52.

30. Golay A, Eigenheer C, Morel Y, et al. Weight-loss with low or high carbohydrate diet? Int J Obes Relat Metab Disord. 1996a;20:1067–72.

31. Golay A, Allaz AF, Morel Y, et al. Similar weight loss with low- or high-carbohydrate diets. Am J Clin Nutr. 1996b;63:174–8.

32. Goni L, Ignacio Riezu-Boj J, Milagro FI, et al. Interaction between an ADCY3 genetic variant and two weight-lowering diets affecting body fatness and body composition outcomes depending on macronutrient distribution: a randomized trial. Nutrients. 2018;10:789. https://doi.org/10.3390/nu10060789.

33. Green ED, Maffei M, Braden VV, et al. The human obese (OB) gene: RNA expression pattern and mapping on the physical, cytogenetic, and genetic maps of chromosome 7. Genome Res. 1995;5(1):5–12.

34. Greene P, Willett W, Devecis J, et al. Pilot 12-week feeding weight-loss comparison: low-fat vs low-carbohydrate (ketogenic) diets. Obes Res. 2003;11:A23.

35. Hainer V, Hermann T, Asimina M. Treatment modalities of obesity: what fits whom? Diabetes Care. 2008;31:269–77.

36. Hession M, Rolland C, Kulkarni U, et al. Systematic review of randomized controlled trials of low-carbohydrate vs. low-fat/low-calorie diets in the management of obesity and its comorbidities. Obes Rev. 2008;10:36–50.

37. Houmard JA, Tyndall GL, Midyette JB, et al. Effect of reduced training and training cessation on insulin sensitivity and muscle GLUT-4. J Appl Physiol. 1996;81:1162–8.

38. Ivancovsky-Wajcman D, Fliss-Isakov N, Webb M, Bentov I, et al. Ultra-processed food is associated with features of metabolic syndrome and non-alcoholic fatty liver disease. Liver Int. 2021;41:2635–45.

39. Jackson KG, Taylor GRJ, Clohessy AM, Williams CM. The effect of the daily intake of inulin on fasting lipid, insulin and glucose concentrations in middle-aged men and women. Br J Nutr. 1999;82:23–30.

40. Johnston BC, Kanters S, Bandayrel K, et al. Comparison of weight loss among named diet programs in overweight and obese adults. A meta-analysis. JAMA. 2014;312:923–33.

41. Kastorini CM, Milionis HJ, Esposito K, Giugliano D, Goudevenos JA, Panagiotakos DB. The effect of Mediterranean diet on metabolic syndrome and its components: a meta-analysis of 50 studies and 534,906 individuals. J Am Coll Cardiol. 2011;57:1299–313.

42. Landers P, Wolfe M, Glore S, et al. Effect of weight loss plans on body composition and diet duration. J Okla State Med Assoc. 2002;95(5):329–31.

43. Layman DK, Boileau RA, Erickson DJ, et al. A reduced ratio of dietary carbohydrate to protein improves body composition and blood lipid profiles during weight loss in adult women. J Nutr. 2003;133:411–7

44. Lean ME, Han TS, Prvan T, et al. Weight loss with high and low carbohydrate 1200 kcal diets in freeliving women. Eur J Clin Nutr. 1997;51:243–8.

45. Ley RE, Bäckhed F, Turnbaugh P, Lozupone CA, Knight RD, Gordon JI. Obesity alters gut microbial ecology. Proc Natl Acad Sci U S A. 2005;102:11070–5.

46. Liu S, Willett WC, Manson JE, et al. Relation between changes in intakes of dietary fiber and grain products and changes in weight and development of obesity

among middle-aged women. Am J Clin Nutr. 2003;78: 920–7.

47. Locke AE, et al. Genetic studies of body mass index yield new insights for obesity biology. Nature. 2015;518:197–206.

48. Loos RJF, Yeo GSH. The genetics of obesity: from discovery to biology. Nat Rev. 2022;23:120–33.

49. Lowe DA, Wu N, Rohdin-Bibby L, et al. Effects of time-restricted eating on weight loss and other metabolic parameters in women and men with overweight and obesity: the TREAT Randomized Clinical Trial. JAMA Intern Med. 2020;180:1491–9.

50. Ludwig DS. The glycemic index: physiological mechanisms relating to obesity, diabetes, and cardiovascular disease. JAMA. 2002;287(18):2414–23.

51. Ludwig DS, Ebbeling CB. The carbohydrate-insulin model of obesity beyond "calories in, calories out". JAMA Intern Med. 2018;178(8):1098–103.

52. Matarese LE, Pories WJ. Adult weight loss diets: metabolic effects and outcomes. Nutr Clin Pract. 2014;29 (6):759–67.

53. Mitsou EK, Kakali A, Antonopoulou S, Mountzouris KC, Yannakoulia M, Panagiotakos DB, Kyriacou A. Adherence to the Mediterranean diet is associated with the gut microbiota pattern and gastrointestinal characteristics in an adult population. Br J Nutr. 2017;117:1645–55.

54. Muegge BD, Kuczynski J, Knights D, Clemente JC, González A, Fontana L, Henrissat B, Knight R, Gordon JI. Diet drives convergence in gut microbiome functions across mammalian phylogeny and within humans. Science. 2011;332:970–4.

55. Naude CE, Brand A, Schoonees A, et al. Low-carbohydrate versus balanced-carbohydrate diets for reducing weight and cardiovascular risk. Cochrane Database Syst Rev. 2022;(1):CD013334. https://doi. org/10.1002/14651858.CD013334.pub2.

56. Noakes M, Foster PR, Keogh JB, et al. Comparison of isocaloric very low carbohydrate/high saturated fat and high carbohydrate/low saturated fat diets on body composition and cardiovascular risk. Nutr Metab. 2006;3: 7. https://doi.org/10.1186/1743-7075-3-7.

57. O'Keefe SJD. Diet, microorganisms and their metabolites, and colon cancer. Nat Rev Gastroenterol Hepatol. 2016;13(12):691–706.

58. Patterson RE, Laughlin GA, LaCroix AZ, et al. Intermittent fasting and human metabolic health. J Acad Nutr Diet. 2015 Aug;115(8):1203–12. https://doi.org/ 10.1016/j.jand.2015.02.018.

59. Pereira MA, Swain J, Goldfine AB, et al. Effects of a low–glycemic load diet on resting energy expenditure and heart disease risk factors during weight loss. JAMA. 2004;292:2482–90.

60. Piatti PM, Magni F, Fermo I, et al. Hypocaloric high-protein diet improves glucose oxidation and spares lean body mass: comparison to high-carbohydrate diet. Metabolism. 1994;43:1481–7.

61. Rabast U, Kasper H, Schonborn J. Comparative studies in obese subjects fed carbohydrate-restricted and high carbohydrate 1,000-calorie formula diets. Nutr Metab. 1978;22:269–77.

62. Rabast U, Hahn A, Reiners C, et al. Thyroid hormone changes in obese subjects during fasting and a very-low-calorie diet. Int J Obes. 1981;5:305–11.

63. Rinninella E, Cintoni M, Raoul P, et al. Food components and dietary habits: keys for a healthy gut microbiota composition. Nutrients. 2019;11:2393. https:// doi.org/10.3390/nu11102393.

64. Serene TE, Shamarina S, Mohd NM. Familial and socio-environmental predictors of overweight and obesity among primary school children in Selangor and Kuala Lumpur. Malays J Nutr. 2011;17(2):151–62.

65. Shai I, Schwarzfuchs D, Henkin Y, et al. Weight loss with a low-carbohydrate, Mediterranean or low-fat diet. N Engl J Med. 2008;359(3):229–41.

66. Solomon TP, Haus JM, Cook MA, et al. A low-glycemic diet lifestyle intervention improves fat utilization during exercise in older obese humans. Obesity (Silver Spring). 2013;21(11):2272–8.

67. Suez J, Korem T, Zeevi D, et al. Artificial sweeteners induce glucose intolerance by altering the gut microbiota. Nature. 2014;514(7521):181–6.

68. Swiatkiewicz I, Wozniak A, Taub PR. Time-restricted eating and metabolic syndrome: current status and future perspectives. Nutrients. 2021;13:221.

69. Swift DL, McGee JE, Earnest CP, Carlisle E, Nygard M, Johannsen NM. The effects of exercise and physical activity on weight loss and maintenance. Prog Cardiovasc Dis. 2018 Jul-Aug;61(2):206–13.

70. Swift DL, Houmard JA, Slentz CA, Kraus WE. Effects of aerobic training with and without weight loss on insulin sensitivity and lipids. PLoS One. 2018b;13(5): e0196637.

71. Tappenden KA. Prebiotics. In: Matarese LE, Mullin G, Tappenden KA, editors. The health professionals guide to gastrointestinal nutrition. 2nd ed. The Academy of Nutrition and Dietetics; 2023. p. 254–64.

72. Tounian P. Programming towards childhood obesity. Ann Nutr Metab. 2011;58(Suppl 2):30–41.

73. Tremmel M, Gerdtham U-G, Nilsson PM, Saha S. Economic burden of obesity: a systematic literature review. Int J Environ Res Public Health. 2017;14:435.

74. Tschöp M, Weyer C, Tataranni PA, Devanarayan V, Ravussin E, Heiman ML. Circulating ghrelin levels are decreased in human obesity. Diabetes. 2001;50 (4):707–9. https://doi.org/10.2337/diabetes.50.4.707.

75. Vallianou N, Stratigou T, Christodoulatos GS, Dalamaga M. Understanding the role of the gut microbiome and microbial metabolites in obesity and obesity-associated metabolic disorders: current evidence and perspectives. Curr Obes Rep. 2019;8:317–32.

76. Veum VL, Laupsa-Borge J, Eng O, et al. Visceral adiposity and metabolic syndrome after very high–fat and low-fat isocaloric diets: a randomized controlled trial. Am J Clin Nutr. 2017;105:85–99.

77. Volek JS, Phinney STD. A new look at carbohydrate-restricted diets: Separating fact from fiction. Nutr Today. 2013;48(2):E1–7.

78. Vrdoljak J, Kumric M, Vilovic M, et al. Can fasting curb the metabolic syndrome epidemic? Nutrients. 2022;14:456. https://doi.org/10.3390/nu14030456.

79. Walsh CO, Ebbeling CB, Swain JF, Markowitz RL, Feldman HA, Ludwig DS. Effects of diet composition on postprandial energy availability during weight loss maintenance. PLoS One. 2013;8(3):e58172.

80. Wang X, Li Q, Liu Y, et al. Intermittent fasting versus continuous energy-restricted diet for patients with type 2 diabetes mellitus and metabolic syndrome for glycemic control: A systematic review and meta-analysis of randomized controlled trials. Diabetes Res Clin Pract. 2021;179:109003.

81. Warren M, Martindale R. Probiotics. In: Matarese LE, Mullin G, Tappenden KA, editors. The health professionals guide to gastrointestinal nutrition. 2nd ed. The Academy of Nutrition and Dietetics; 2023. p. 265–79.

82. Wilkinson MJ, Manoogian ENC, Zadourian A, Lo H, Fakhouri S, Shoghi A, Wang X, Fleischer JG, Navlakha S, Panda S, et al. Ten-hour time-restricted eating reduces weight, blood pressure, and atherogenic lipids in patients with metabolic syndrome. Cell Metab. 2020;31:92–104.

83. World Health Organization. Global action plan on physical activity 2018–2030: more active people for a healthier world. World Health Organization; 2019.

84. World Health Organization. Obesity and overweight fact sheet. World Health Organizations Web site. 2022. https://www.who.int/news-room/fact-sheets/detail/obesity-and-overweight, Accessed Sept 2022.

85. Wu GD, Chen J, Hoffmann C, Bittinger K, Chen Y, Keilbaugh SA, Bewtra M, Knights D, Walters WA, Knight R, et al. Linking long-term dietary patterns with gut microbial enterotypes. Science. 2011;334:105–8.

86. Yang W, Kelly T, He J. Genetic epidemiology of obesity. Epidemiol Rev. 2007;29:49–61.

87. Young CM, Scanlan SS, Im HS, et al. Effect of body composition and other parameters in obese young men of carbohydrate level of reduction diet. Am J Clin Nutr. 1971;24:290–6.

The Built Environment and Metabolic Syndrome

12

Thao Minh Lam, Nicolette R. den Braver, and Jeroen Lakerveld

Contents

Abstract

The built environment encompasses important infrastructure and characteristics that drive health behaviors and health outcomes. In this chapter, we summarize and reflect upon epidemiological evidence of built environmental factors that have been studied in relation to cardiometabolic disease risk and outcomes.

Keywords

Exposome · Food environment · Dietary behavior · Walkability · Green space · Physical activity · Type 2 diabetes · Obesity · Cardiovascular diseases

T. M. Lam (✉) · N. R. den Braver · J. Lakerveld
Epidemiology and Data Science, Amsterdam University Medical Centers location Vrije Universiteit Amsterdam, Amsterdam, The Netherlands

Health Behaviours and Chronic Diseases Programme, Amsterdam Public Health Institute, Amsterdam, The Netherlands

Upstream Team, Amsterdam University Medical Centers location Vrije Universiteit Amsterdam, Amsterdam, The Netherlands
e-mail: t.m.lam@amsterdamumc.nl

Introduction

The built environment includes the human-made design and layout of the communities in which people live, work, and play. The built environment is visible and omnipresent; people spend most of their time operating, interacting, and changing the built environment. Overall, the combinations of exposures and lifestyle behaviors are referred to as the "exposome," a concept that captures the totality of non-genetic exposures over the life course [1]. The built environment, together with the social and physicochemical

© Springer Nature Switzerland AG 2023
R. S. Ahima (ed.), *Metabolic Syndrome*,
https://doi.org/10.1007/978-3-031-40116-9_59

environments, makes up the external exposome – the exposures that are measured outside of the body [2]. The impact of the exposome is major; it is estimated that our environment explains about 70% of the noncommunicable chronic disease burden [3]. Therefore, understanding the built environment could provide key entry points to reduce preventable chronic conditions.

Specifically, the built environment contains characteristics that increase or reduce the risk of cardiometabolic diseases including obesity, type 2 diabetes (T2D), and cardiovascular diseases (CVD). The built environment can have a direct influence on these diseases, for instance, via air pollutants that induce systemic inflammation of the body [4]. The built environment can also have an indirect impact, for instance, through an abundance of unhealthy food sources in the neighborhood which drives residents to have unhealthy diets or through poor walkability of neighborhoods that inhibits physical activity behaviors [5]. These unhealthy lifestyle behaviors are established behavioral risk factors for obesity – now considered a chronic relapsing disease which in turn acts as a gateway to a range of other noncommunicable diseases, such as T2D, CVDs, and cancer [6].

When researching built environmental exposures, especially their influence on cardiometabolic outcomes, the various environmental characteristics can be categorized into different domains. For instance, the exposure to fast-food restaurants, supermarkets, and greengrocers can be gathered under the domain "food environment." Likewise, characteristics such as walkability and the availability of sports facilities can be classified under the "physical activity environment" (Fig. 1). Here, it is important to note that such classifications are often arbitrary. In fact, components could potentially overlap across the environments. For example, population density could be an indicator for urbanization, for walkability, and for higher food outlet density. Moreover, in real life, exposures never present themselves in a structured, siloed way. Rather, they combine and interact in a dynamic, complex manner. A typical commuting trip to the office likely involves exposure to a mixture of environmental characteristics along the way, with

fast-food outlets, green space, various air pollutants, and other determinants of behaviors and health. At behavioral level, diet and physical activity have been shown to be complementary in causing physiological changes related to metabolic syndrome [7]. Therefore, it is important to consider this interdependence at both environmental and behavioral levels when studying the built environment's associations on health.

Early built environment studies often focused on urbanization, using proxies such as population density or migration patterns, and in particular urban sprawl as the main exposures of interest [8, 9], due to their relevance for cardiometabolic disease risks. However, the gap in the body mass index (BMI) between urban and rural residents is closing worldwide, with an unprecedented attributable increase in BMI in rural areas [10]. Therefore, instead of examining urbanization or the urban/rural disparity alone, more efforts are being made on identifying changes in underlying built environmental factors that drive cardiometabolic disease outcomes.

In this chapter, we outline conceptual framework encompassing built environmental factors at neighborhood level and cardiometabolic outcomes across two main domains: the food environment and the physical activity environment. We summarize the evidence across these domains and provide a reflection on methodological challenges in environmental epidemiology and discuss potential ways to further this research field. Environmental nuisance such as air, noise, and light pollution is a byproduct of human activities in the built environment and could arguably be considered as a component of the built environment, but these factors are not discussed here.

The Food Environment

Dietary behaviors or dietary patterns largely depend on habitual food choices and, to a certain extent, impulsive decisions. These are complex human behaviors, which may be partly driven by the exposure to food options in the environment [11]. Traditionally, the food environment encompasses the variety, availability, and density of food

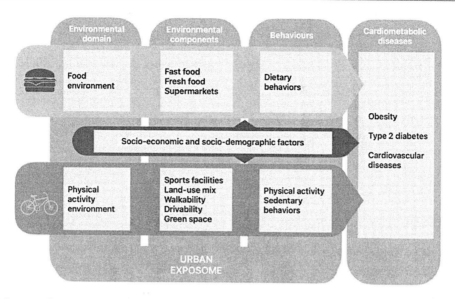

Fig. 1 Conceptual model of environmental domains relevant to lifestyle behaviors and cardiometabolic disease

outlets within a community or neighborhood available to its residents. With the increasing digitalization of every aspect of society, the food environment is also undergoing major changes [12]. Currently, some epidemiological evidence suggests that aspects of the neighborhood food environment, such as higher availability of fast-food and convenience stores, might be associated with increased intake of ultraprocessed meats, snacks, and sugar-sweetened beverages, while higher availability of healthy foods may promote better quality diets [13]. However, understanding the impact of the food environment on health outcomes is complex and has yielded mixed findings. Specifically for cardiometabolic disease outcome, epidemiological evidence is inconsistent, and the results are dominated by null findings [14–17]. Compared to research on the physical activity environment, food environments are much less consistent in the association with cardiometabolic diseases [14]. Studies have so far primarily examined the fast-food restaurant density, suggesting that higher density is associated with a higher cardiovascular disease (CVD) and total disease burden and mortality. However, data on other aspects of the food environment and health outcomes are scarce or lacking [17].

The majority of evidence in this field of research comes from the United States, with earlier studies focusing on socioeconomic inequality in terms of food access (food desert, food swamp, or fast food) and food security [18–20]. Luongo et al. (2020) reviewed food environmental studies in indigenous populations and found that traditional diets were healthier than retail food available to them, highlighting possible consequences of "food deserts" for vulnerable, remote populations [21]. Outcome-specific studies also indicated the role of deprivation in the association between food environments and health. Atanasova et al. (2022) reviewed causal studies with the retail food environment as exposure and found adverse BMI outcomes to be related especially for women and in Black and Hispanic populations [22]. Exposures to healthy food, on the other hand, were not associated with BMI; neither were changes in accessibility or availability of healthy food.

Across food outlet types, the most consistent evidence comes from studies on fast-food services, which were also predominantly conducted in the United States. In other countries, inconsistencies remain. For example, Mackenbach et al. (2019) and van Erpecum et al. (2022) both studied fast-food access and BMI in the

Dutch population [23, 24]. The former found that higher fast-food access was linked to lower BMI, the latter with higher BMI, while another Dutch study found no associations between fast-food exposures and BMI [25]. Another study suggested that the presence but not density of fast-food outlets, was relevant for T2D in The Netherlands [26]. Inconsistencies in such studies were the result of different definitions and operationalization of fast-food exposures, as well as chosen regions, choices of models, and consideration of potential confounders [27, 28].

In the recent years, some longitudinal studies were conducted that substantiated the evidence for the association between food environment and cardiometabolic outcomes. Three studies examined the changes in relative density of food outlets and observed associations with changes in T2D incidence in North and South America. In particular, reduced traditional fruits and vegetable stores and increased chain supermarkets in 53 cities in Mexico were associated with higher T2D incidence [29]. Increased fast-food outlets and reduced full-service restaurants in Utah, the United States, were also linked to higher T2D incidence [30]. Similarly, Polsky et al. (2016) found that increased proportion of fast food relative to all restaurants, but not absolute number of any particular outlet type was associated with increased incidence of T2D in Canada; which was significant especially in areas with more than three fast-food outlets [31]. These studies also highlight the need for relative food outlet measures either by expressing ratios between different outlet types or using combined measures including both healthy and unhealthy food outlets, since they performed better in associations with cardiometabolic disease outcomes [31, 32].

Natural experiments, where an accidental or planned change occurs completely out of the researchers' control, are a closer approximation of the causal effect and could be used to study health effect where controlled trials are infeasible (due to ethical concerns or costs). Natural experiments with the food environment are rare. However, one such study was conducted in Japan, where some residents of Iwanuma city were relocated to neighborhoods with lower distance to any food outlet types following a tsunami. Over the 2.5 years follow-up period, moving closer to any of food outlet type was shown to increase the risk of transition from normal weight to overweight/obesity and other cardiometabolic factors among the elderly residents [33].

In terms of existing research gaps, Den Braver et al. (2018) highlighted the inconsistent findings for T2D and emphasized the need to consider individual perceptions and their interactions with the food environment [16]. Additionally, Howell and Booth (2022) suggested that counterintuitive associations between food environment and health could potentially be explained by correlation between food outlets and neighborhood walkability [34]. Moreover, socioeconomic status remains a major confounder in these relationships [34]. Moreover, evidence from low-income countries where the incidence of metabolic syndrome is increasing the fastest is still missing.

Overall, the state of evidence on the relationship between the food environment and cardiometabolic health is characterized by inconsistencies and varied findings. Factors such as study design, measurement approaches, other contextual factors, and socioeconomic status have contributed to the mixed results found thus far. Further research – especially longitudinal and experimental – is necessary to enhance our understanding of the complex associations between the food environment, dietary behaviors, and cardiometabolic outcomes.

The Physical Activity Environment

The built environmental characteristics that are related to physical activity include the infrastructure of neighborhoods that might enforce or inhibit physical activity and sedentary behaviors (too much sitting). This includes aspects that are related to transportation, both active (cycling, walking, and use of public transport) or passive (car driving). Such infrastructural aspects are often classified according to the 6 Ds as first described by Ewing & Cervero [35]: density, diversity, design, destination accessibility, and distance to transit and demand management.

Later, even more Ds were added and researched (Table 1) [36]. Some of the Ds are more relevant at regional and national planning level, such as the jobs:housing ratio. Decision-making at this high level is difficult to evaluate, in terms of its effect on downstream outcome such as metabolic syndrome.

Within these Ds in particular and the physical activity environment in general, some factors are studied more extensively than others. Epidemiological studies in relation to obesity, T2D and CVD outcomes have been dominated by two main exposures, namely green space and walkability [14–16, 34, 37, 76]. On the other hand, relatively understudied aspects of the built environment are, for example, sports facilities, parking pressure, and safety. Safety could manifest as physical safety of urban infrastructure (think about lit pavements at night or safe road crossings) or in terms of crime rates (or "social" safety). Aesthetics of the neighborhood (including cleanliness and vandalism) could also contribute to or hinder more time spent outdoors, although it is highly subjective and contextual [38].

For green space, evidence suggests a potential protective effect against obesity and T2D [14, 16, 37, 39, 40]. Associations, however, vary based on the definition of green space used and the exact outcomes considered, as well as study design and population characteristics [34, 41, 42]. In terms of mechanism, De la Fuente et al.'s recent review postulated green space to function as a promoter of physical activity, which is the dominant theory, and specifically also as protector against air pollutants which may have obesogenic effects [43]. Similarly for T2D, recent literature reviews by Den Braver et al. (2018) and Ccami-Bernal et al. (2023) also suggested potential mediation of physical activity, such as walking [16, 44]. However, evidence of a formal mediation effect by physical activity is still inconclusive even though understanding such pathways provides useful insights for recommendations for practice [37, 39]. Depending on mechanism proposed, the operationalization of exposure to green space differs in research. It can be investigated as a percentage of green space in a certain area, the distance to nearest park/green space, or even

green space quality. Studies that looked at green space in combination with other neighborhood characteristics suggested that the protective effect of green space on T2D is stronger in areas with a higher availability of supermarkets [45]. However, also here, it is worth noting that most studies on green space and health outcomes have been conducted in North America and Australia, limiting the generalizability to other contexts [2, 34]. Ccami-Bernal et al.'s recent review on longitudinal evidence for green space and T2D incidence found that out of 13 studies included, 10 provided supportive evidence for an association between higher green space exposure (mainly density) and lower T2D incidence. Their review included evidence from various European, North American, Asian, and Australian studies. Further research is needed to fully elucidate the mechanistic pathways between green space, obesity to T2D [2, 14, 34]. In terms of CVD-related outcomes, Gascon et al. (2016) conducted a systematic review of primary studies and found an inverse association between residential greenness and CVD mortality [46]. However, evidence for specific sub-types of CVD such as ischemic heart diseases remain inconclusive [47, 48].

Studies on walkability and cardiometabolic risks have also shown varied results due to the diversity in study designs and measures used, although most studies suggest a protective effect of walkability. The number of components in a walkability index ranges anywhere from three (population density, land-use mix, intersection density) up to seven (retail and service density, block size, public transport density, green space), depending on the context [49, 50]. The most commonly used walkability index is Walk Score® whose associations with walking have been demonstrated across different geographic contexts [51 54]. Two recent longitudinal studies have examined the association between walkability and BMI, showing potential beneficial cardiometabolic effect. Lang et al. (2022) found higher Walk Score® to be associated with lower odds of overweight and moderate-to-high-risk waist circumference in a racially diverse cohort in the USA [55]. Creatore et al. (2016) found residents in highest quintile of walkability index

Table 1 Evolution of Ds of urban planning, adapted from Giles-Corti et al. [36]

D variable		Description	Example
6Ds	Density	Compactness of neighborhood, low distance to amenities and transport and high amenities densities	Population density, residential density
	Diversity	Land-use diversity, compactness, less travel time, lower dependence on car	Land-use mix
	Design	Urban designs to promote walking, public transport, and increased physical activity	Intersection density, parks and open space, blue space, transport hubs and schools, sports facilities
	Destination accessibility	Employment, facilities, and daily amenities accessible by foot or public transport	Retail and service density, job density, health facilities within 500 m or 1000 m of residential neighborhood
	Distance to transit	Frequency and connectedness of public transport options	Distance to nearest train/bus/tram/ferry station
	Demand management	Parking supply and pricing policies to reduce attractiveness of owning and driving cars	Parking demand: supply ratio (parking pressure), percentage free/paid parking in the neighborhood
8Ds	Distribution of employment	Jobs to housing ratio in a region	Job-housing ratio
	Desirability	Safety features, attractiveness, accessibility, affordability, convenience, and comfort	Crime prevention, streetlight, reduced vandalism, safety cycling measures, etc.
11Ds	Destination proximity	Local destinations for walkability	Distance to the nearest facility (school, healthcare, retail/ service)
	Disaster mitigation	Climate change mitigation strategies	Greening of neighborhoods for heat resilience, open soil for water absorption
	Distributed intervention	Embedding equity in decision-making/for whom is the intervention designed?	Reduced public transport costs for children and 65+

to also have lower incidences of overweight, obesity, and T2D in Canada [56]. For CVD outcomes, Makhlouf et al. (2023) conducted a cross-sectional, ecological analysis in the United States using nation-wide surveillance data and found walkability to be associated with coronary arterial disease prevalence, which was significantly mediated by obesity and T2D but also blood pressure and high cholesterol [57]. These findings were also confirmed in a longitudinal analysis by Makram et al. (2023) who used registry data between 2016 and 2022 and showed that residents of walkable neighborhoods had significantly lower CVD risk factors over the years, compared to those from car-dependent neighborhoods [58].

Car dependency of neighborhoods has also been quantified in a so-called drivability index and drivability studies are of growing interest due to a worldwide increase in urbanization and urban sprawl. New urbanized neighborhoods are

often sprawled and characterized by a relatively low residential density, limited mix of land use, and consequent high car dependency. Two studies by Den Braver et al. (2022, 2023) examined a novel drivability index composed of three components: urban sprawl, pedestrian facilities, and parking availability for Toronto, Canada [59]. Living in highly drivable neighborhoods was associated with an increased risk of diabetes in the whole population, even when neighborhood walkability was high. Especially young and middle-income residents showed to be a vulnerable subgroup, as they were at twofold risks of T2D when living in highly drivable neighborhoods [60].

In summary, green space has shown potential protective effects against obesity and T2D, with associations influenced by various factors such as measurement approaches and contextual characteristics. Walkability has also been associated with reduced obesity and T2D risk, with varying strengths of associations based on measures and methods employed, study design, population characteristics, and built environment context [14, 16, 34]. Associations with CVD incidence or mortality have been shown, but the evidence is much less clear. More research into the specific mechanisms and contextual factors underlying these relationships is warranted, but the current evidence base provides ample entry points for infrastructural public health interventions and urban planning strategies.

Combined Exposures

Due to the intertwining nature between physical activity and diet [7], environmental factors related to both should also be studied together, as suggested by primary studies discussed earlier in this chapter. From exposure science, there are multiple methods to account for this co-occurrence; for example, multiple regression allows mutual adjustments of more than one environmental exposure. However, depending on data structure and number of observations, the limit in the number of predictors could easily be reached. In this instance, shrinkage methods whereby a matrix of (correlated) environmental factors are reduced and only the most statistically relevant factors for outcome of interest are retained. The advance of machine learning also allows for modeling of multiple exposures and accounting for nonlinearity and interaction between exposures. Another method is the use of composite indicators, where environmental factors are combined into one overarching index.

Several such indices have been developed with specific cardiometabolic outcomes in mind. For example, Marek and colleagues (2021) developed the healthy location index (HLI) for high-resolution mesh block administrative units in New Zealand [61]. The index components were combined based on their "health-promoting" (supermarkets, fruits and vegetables, PA facilities, green space, and blue space) or "health-constraining" nature (fast food, takeaways, dairy, gaming locations and alcohol sales points) [61]. A recent association study by Hobbs et al. (2022) showed that either lower access to health-constraining outlets, higher access to health-promoting outlets, or higher overall HLI index score was consistently associated with lower BMI and lower odds of T2D [62]. Similarly, Cebrecos et al. (2019) created the Heart-Healthy Hoods (HHH) Index for the city of Madrid (Spain) with factors across the food environment (food outlet diversity), walkability (including residential density, population density, retail and service density and street connectivity), alcohol, and tobacco selling points. An ecological association study showed an increased CVD prevalence in less heart-healthy neighborhoods [63]. Lam et al. (2023) developed the Obesogenic Built environment CharacterisTics (OBCT) index with factors across the food environment (healthy and unhealthy) and PA environment (walkability, bikeability, drivability? and sports facilities) for all neighborhoods in The Netherlands [64]. Cross-sectional analysis with cardiometabolic outcomes in several Dutch cohorts showed that each increase in neighborhood obesogenicity was associated with higher BMI, blood pressure, and hypertension, but not blood lipids (unpublished observation). Both HLI and HHH index results could potentially extend our conceptual framework as other built environment factors related to health behaviors such as alcohol intake, smoking, and gaming could also be promoting metabolic syndrome. Furthermore, when weighted by their contribution to specific health outcomes (as in the case of HHH index), associations were demonstrated to be even stronger. Overall, the associations between indices and health outcomes remained relatively small but given their large reach (whole populations are exposed to the built environment) the public health impact could be large. Finally, composite indicators are useful tool to involve nontechnical stakeholders, since they could effectively rank and benchmark areas (blocks, regions, neighborhoods) and highlight areas in need of priority in case of limited resources.

Methodological Notes

Increasingly complex methods are being used to assess exposures to the built environment. Traditionally, most environmental exposures in epidemiological studies are modeled around residential addresses. However, people spend considerable amount of their time either in commute or at certain destinations (work, school, recreational facilities, etc.). Destination exposure, especially around work and along the commute pathway, is increasingly included in studies and shown to be of importance for behaviors and health [65–67]. Furthermore, some built environment exposures are consequent of behaviors which are restricted or facilitated by age, mobility, or socioeconomic status. To this end, innovative methods such as agent-based modeling or other machine learning approaches could be useful in modeling exposures based on predetermined conditions, by taking interactions and nonlinearity into account [68–70].

While most studies look for objective measures of the built environment modeled in geographic information systems, some studies argue for integration of subjective measures, since perceptions are sometimes more important for behaviors, as for the case of walkability or park access [71, 72]. Others advocate for the use of both, since perceptions and attitudes could potentially mediate the effect of objective environmental features on behaviors [67, 73]. However, a caution for reverse causation is warranted here, as self-reported exposures may be a reflection of health behaviors and outcomes, rather than a determinant.

Specifically for the food environment, online groceries, food shopping, and third-party delivery services increase accessibility and availability of food. As a consequence, people rely less on their immediate residential or work neighborhood for food. Moreover, food advertising and consumer engagement (surveys, advertisement-games, giveaways) are becoming increasingly pervasive on social media and research on their potential influence on food choice has only just begun. This poses challenges to understanding the food environment typology, our interactions therewith, and how these interactions lead to dietary choices and cardiometabolic health risks [12].

In terms of study design: Since the conceptual model in Fig. 1 postulates physical activity and diet as behaviors that could potentially modify disease risks, it is also useful to elucidate the literature on built environment and behaviors before linking it further to disease outcome. Wherever data are available, hypotheses on the role of environments on cardiometabolic risks through physical activity and diet should be tested, e.g., using formal mediation or other path analysis methods [67].

In terms of analysis, as argued earlier in this chapter, the relation between a built environment exposure and metabolic syndrome may interact or be confounded by other environmental factors. For example, Macdonald et al. (2018) suggested that fast-food exposure may co-locate with other "environmental bads," such as alcohol shops, tobacco, and gambling outlets, especially in more socially deprived areas [74]. Moreover, Lamichane et al. reported that areas with a higher socioeconomic status have more supermarkets present than areas with a low socioeconomic status [75]. This emphasizes the importance of adjusting for or stratifying by neighborhood characteristics including neighborhood socioeconomic status. Moreover, residential self-selection could play a crucial role on the causal pathway between built environment and health. This issue postulates that people do not randomly select their residence; instead, this decision is likely influenced by their preferences, attitudes, and socioeconomic situation. Any association found between built environment and dietary or travel behaviors and ultimately cardiometabolic health could therefore be biased if not adjusted for residential self-selection. However, the relative contribution between residential self-selection and built environment on health is still a topic of debate [73]. Ultimately, more longitudinal studies are desirable to ascertain causal effect between built environment and cardiometabolic health [14, 15, 17, 39].

Conclusion and Implications for Practice

The importance of the built environment for population health has been theorized and increasingly researched by academics. As a result, the current evidence has expanded over the past decade and points toward some environmental factors that are consistently associated with cardiometabolic risk. Especially, fast-food exposure, green space, and walkability have been consistently related to cardiometabolic health outcomes. However, for various domains, regions, and outcomes, evidence is less consistent or available. In regard to public health interventions, this may not necessarily be problematic. Is evidence required in order for policy makers and other interventionists to design and implement approaches? And if so, how much? It is likely that high scientific standards are not related to, nor required for more or less on-the-ground action. Rather, a better recognition and application of health policies is required, including that of policies related to urban design, public transportation, licensing of food outlets, and reduction of car use. Such policies for greener, safer, and more physically active societies go hand in hand with the goal of improving global health.

References

1. Wild CP. Complementing the genome with an "exposome": the outstanding challenge of environmental exposure measurement in molecular epidemiology. Cancer Epidemiol Biomark Prev. 2005;14(8):1847–50.
2. Beulens JWJ, Pinho MGM, Abreu TC, den Braver NR, Lam TM, Huss A, et al. Environmental risk factors of type 2 diabetes – an exposome approach. Diabetologia. 2022;65:263–74. https://link.springer.com/article/10.1007/s00125-021-05618-w
3. Forouzanfar MH, Afshin A, Alexander LT, Biryukov S, Brauer M, Cercy K, et al. Global, regional, and national comparative risk assessment of 79 behavioural, environmental and occupational, and metabolic risks or clusters of risks, 1990–2015: a systematic analysis for the Global Burden of Disease Study 2015. Lancet. 2016;388(10053).1659–724.
4. Poursafa P, Kamali Z, Fraszczyk E, Boezen HM, Vaez A, Snieder H. DNA methylation: a potential mediator between air pollution and metabolic syndrome. Clin Epigenet. 2022;14:1–13. https://doi.org/10.1186/s13148-022-01301-y.
5. Saelens BE, Sallis JF, Frank LD. Environmental correlates of walking and cycling: findings from the transportation, urban design, and planning literatures. Ann Behav Med. 2003;25:80–91. http://www.cnu.org

6. WHO Regional Office for Europe. WHO European Regional Obesity report 2022. 2022. 1–220 p. http://apps.who.int/bookorders
7. Baranowski T. Why combine diet and physical activity in the same international research society? Int J Behav Nutr Phys Act. 2004;1(1):1–10. https://ijbnpa.biomedcentral.com/articles/10.1186/1479-5868-1-2
8. Ewing R, Meakins G, Hamidi S, Nelson AC. Relationship between urban sprawl and physical activity, obesity, and morbidity – update and refinement. Heal Place. 2014;26:118–26. https://doi.org/10.1016/j.healthplace.2013.12.008.
9. Angkurawaranon C, Jiraporncharoen W, Chenthanakij B, Doyle P, Nitsch D. Urban environments and obesity in southeast Asia: a systematic review, meta-analysis and Meta-regression. PLoS One. 2014;9(11):1–19.
10. Bixby H, Bentham J, Zhou B, Di Cesare M, Paciorek CJ, Bennett JE, et al. Rising rural body-mass index is the main driver of the global obesity epidemic in adults. Nature. 2019;569(7755):260–4.
11. Lakerveld J, Mackenbach J. The upstream determinants of adult obesity. Obes Facts. 2017;10(3):216–22. http://www.karger.com/ofa
12. Granheim SI, Løvhaug AL, Terragni L, Torheim LE, Thurston M. Mapping the digital food environment: a systematic scoping review. Obes Rev. 2022;23(1):1–18.
13. Moore LV, Diez Roux AV, Nettleton JA, Jacobs DR. Associations of the local food environment with diet quality – a comparison of assessments based on surveys and geographic information systems. Am J Epidemiol. 2008;167(8):917–24.
14. Lam TM, Vaartjes I, Grobbee DE, Karssenberg D, Lakerveld J. Associations between the built environment and obesity: an umbrella review. Int J Health Geogr. 2021;20(1):1–24. https://doi.org/10.1186/s12942-021-00260-6.
15. Mackenbach JD, Rutter H, Compernolle S, Glonti K, Oppert J-MM, Charreire H, et al. Obesogenic environments: a systematic review of the association between the physical environment and adult weight status, the SPOTLIGHT project. BMC Public Health. 2014;14(1):233. http://www.embase.com/search/results?subaction=viewrecord&from=export&id=L605806669
16. Den Braver NR, Lakerveld J, Rutters F, Schoonmade LJ, Brug J, Beulens JWJ. Built environmental characteristics and diabetes: a systematic review and meta-analysis. BMC Med. 2018;16(1).12. https://pubmed.ncbi.nlm.nih.gov/29382337
17. Meijer P, Numans H, Lakerveld J. Associations between the neighbourhood food environment and cardiovascular disease: a systematic review. European Journal of Preventive Cardiology, zwad252, 2023. https://doi.org/10.1093/eurjpc/zwad252
18. Casagrande SS, Whitt-Glover MC, Lancaster KJ, Odoms-Young AM, Gary TL. Built environment and health behaviors among African Americans. A

systematic review. Am J Prev Med. 2009;36(2):174–81. https://doi.org/10.1016/j.amepre.2008.09.037.

19. Lovasi GS, Hutson MA, Guerra M, Neckerman KM. Built environments and obesity in disadvantaged populations. Epidemiol Rev. 2009;31(1):7–20.

20. Larson NI, Story MT, Nelson MC. Neighborhood environments: disparities in access to healthy foods in the U.S. Am J Prev Med. 2009 Jan;36(1):74–81.

21. Luongo G, Skinner K, Phillipps B, Yu Z, Martin D, Mah CL. The retail food environment, store foods, and diet and health among indigenous populations: a scoping review. Curr Obes Rep. 2020;9(3):288–306.

22. Atanasova P, Kusuma D, Pineda E, Frost G, Sassi F, Miraldo M. The impact of the consumer and neighbourhood food environment on dietary intake and obesity-related outcomes: a systematic review of causal impact studies. Soc Sci Med. 1982;2022(299): 1–25.

23. Mackenbach JD, Beenackers MA, Noordzij JM, Groeniger JO, Lakerveld J, van Lenthe FJ. The moderating role of self-control and financial strain in the relation between exposure to the food environment and obesity: the GLOBE study. Int J Environ Res Public Health. 2019;16(4):674. https://www.mdpi.com/1660-4601/16/4/674/htm

24. van Erpecum CPL, van Zon SKR, Bültmann U, Smidt N. The association between fast-food outlet proximity and density and body mass index: findings from 147,027 lifelines cohort study participants. Prev Med (Baltim). 2022;155:106915.

25. Harbers MC, Beulens JWJ, Boer JM, Karssenberg D, Mackenbach JD, Rutters F, et al. Residential exposure to fast-food restaurants and its association with diet quality, overweight and obesity in The Netherlands: a cross-sectional analysis in the EPIC-NL cohort. Nutr J. 2021;20(1):56. https://doi.org/10.1186/s12937-021-00713-5.

26. Ntarladima AM, Karssenberg D, Poelman M, Grobbee DE, Lu M, Schmitz O, et al. Associations between the fast-food environment and diabetes prevalence in The Netherlands: a cross-sectional study. Lancet Planet Health. 2022;6(1):e29–39. http://www.thelancet.com/article/S2542519621002989/fulltext

27. Wilkins E, Radley D, Morris M, Hobbs M, Christensen A, Marwa WL, et al. A systematic review employing the GeoFERN framework to examine methods, reporting quality and associations between the retail food environment and obesity. Health Place. 2019;57:186–99.

28. Wilkins E, Morris M, Radley D, Griffiths C. Methods of measuring associations between the retail food environment and weight status: importance of classifications and metrics. SSM – Popul Heal. 2019;8. https://www.scopus.com/inward/record.uri?eid=2-s2.0-85066995717&doi=10.1016%2Fj.ssmph.2019.100404&partnerID=40&md5=8d1b32e1e45515f0bc25577c59d89b21

29. Pérez-Ferrer C, Auchincloss AH, Barrientos-Gutierrez T, Colchero MA, de Oliveira CL, Carvalho de Menezes M, et al. Longitudinal changes in the retail food environment in Mexico and their association with diabetes. Health Place. 2020;66:102461.

30. Zick CD, Curtis DS, Meeks H, Smith KR, Brown BB, Kole K, et al. The changing food environment and neighborhood prevalence of type 2 diabetes. SSM Popul Health. 2023;21:101338. https://doi.org/10.1016/j.ssmph.2023.101338.

31. Polsky JY, Moineddin R, Glazier RH, Dunn JR, Booth GL. Relative and absolute availability of fast-food restaurants in relation to the development of diabetes: a population-based cohort study. Can J Public Health. 2016;107:eS27–33.

32. Cobb LK, Appel LJ, Manuel Franco M, Jones-Smith JC, Alana Nur A, Anderson CAM, et al. The relationship of the local food environment with obesity: a systematic review of methods, study quality, and results. Obesity (Silver Spring). 2015;23(7):1331–44.

33. Hikichi H, Aida J, Kondo K, Tsuboya T, Kawachi I. Residential relocation and obesity after a natural disaster: a natural experiment from the 2011 Japan earthquake and tsunami. Sci Rep. 2019;9(1):1–11. https://doi.org/10.1038/s41598-018-36906-y.

34. Howell NA, Booth GL. The weight of place: built environment correlates of obesity and diabetes. Endocr Rev. 2022;43:966–83.

35. Ewing R, Cervero R. Travel and the built environment. J Am Plan Assoc. 2010;76(3):265–94.

36. Giles-Corti B, Moudon AV, Lowe M, Cerin E, Boeing G, Frumkin H, et al. What next? Expanding our view of city planning and global health, and implementing and monitoring evidence-informed policy. Lancet Glob Health. 2022;10:e919–26.

37. Dendup T, Feng X, Clingan S, Astell-Burt T. Environmental risk factors for developing type 2 diabetes mellitus: a systematic review. Int J Environ Res Public Health. 2018;15(1):78.

38. Hoenink JC, Lakerveld J, Rutter H, Compernolle S, De Bourdeaudhuij I, Bárdos H, et al. The moderating role of social neighbourhood factors in the association between features of the physical neighbourhood environment and weight status. Obes Facts. 2019;12(1):14–24. http://www.karger.com/ofawww.karger.com/ofa

39. Chandrabose M, Rachele JN, Gunn L, Kavanagh A, Owen N, Turrell G, et al. Built environment and cardio-metabolic health: systematic review and meta-analysis of longitudinal studies. Obes Rev. 2019;20(1): 41–54. http://www.embase.com/search/results?subaction=viewrecord&from=export&id=L624078773

40. Doubleday A, Knott CJ, Hazlehurst MF, Bertoni AG, Kaufman JD, Hajat A. Neighborhood greenspace and risk of type 2 diabetes in a prospective cohort: the multi-ethnicity study of atherosclerosis. Environ Heal A Glob Access Sci Source. 2022;21(1):1–10. https://doi.org/10.1186/s12940-021-00824-w.

41. Lachowycz K, Jones AP. Greenspace and obesity: a systematic review of the evidence. Obes Rev. 2011;12 (501):183–9.

42. Klompmaker JO, Hoek G, Bloemsma LD, Gehring U, Strak M, Wijga AH, et al. Green space definition

affects associations of green space with overweight and physical activity. Environ Res. 2018;160:531–40.

43. De la Fuente F, Saldías MA, Cubillos C, Mery G, Carvajal D, Bowen M, et al. Green space exposure association with type 2 diabetes mellitus, physical activity, and obesity: a systematic review. Int J Environ Res Public Health. 2021;18:1–18.

44. Ccami-Bernal F, Soriano-Moreno DR, Fernandez-Guzman D, Tuco KG, Castro-Díaz SD, Esparza-Varas AL, et al. Green space exposure and type 2 diabetes mellitus incidence: a systematic review. Health Place. 2023;82:103045. https://doi.org/10.1016/j.healthplace.2023.103045.

45. India-Aldana S, Kanchi R, Adhikari S, Lopez P, Schwartz MD, Elbel BD, et al. Impact of land use and food environment on risk of type 2 diabetes: a national study of veterans, 2008–2018. Environ Res. 2022;212 (PA):113146. https://doi.org/10.1016/j.envres.2022.113146.

46. Gascon M, Triguero-Mas M, Martínez D, Dadvand P, Rojas-Rueda D, Plasència A, et al. Residential green spaces and mortality: a systematic review. Environ Int. 2016;86:60–7. https://doi.org/10.1016/j.envint.2015.10.013.

47. Yuan Y, Huang F, Lin F, Zhu P, Zhu P. Green space exposure on mortality and cardiovascular outcomes in older adults: a systematic review and meta-analysis of observational studies. Aging Clin Exp Res. 2021;33 (7):1783–97. https://doi.org/10.1007/s40520-020-01710-0.

48. Twohig-Bennett C, Jones A. The health benefits of the great outdoors: a systematic review and meta-analysis of greenspace exposure and health outcomes. Environ Res. 2018;166:628–37. https://doi.org/10.1016/j.envres.2018.06.030.

49. Liao B, van den Berg PEW, van Wesemael PJV, Arentze TA. Empirical analysis of walkability using data from The Netherlands. Transp Res Part D Transp Environ. 2020;85. https://doi.org/10.1016/j.trd.2020.102390.

50. Lam TM, Wang Z, Vaartjes I, Karssenberg D, Ettema D, Helbich M, et al. Development of an objectively measured walkability index for The Netherlands. Int J Behav Nutr Phys Act. 2022;19(1):50. https://pubmed.ncbi.nlm.nih.gov/35501815

51. Frank LD, Appleyard BS, Ulmer JM, Chapman JE, Fox EH. Comparing walkability methods: creation of street smart walk score and efficacy of a code-based 3D walkability index. J Transp Heal. 2021;21:101005.

52. Winters M, Teschke K, Brauer M, Fuller D. Bike score®: associations between urban bikeability and cycling behavior in 24 cities. Int J Behav Nutr Phys Act. 2016;13:18. https://pubmed.ncbi.nlm.nih.gov/26867585

53. Brown SC, Pantin H, Lombard J, Toro M, Huang S, Plater-Zyberk E, et al. Walk score®: associations with purposive walking in recent Cuban immigrants. Am J Prev Med. 2013;45(2):202–6.

54. Twardzik E, Judd S, Bennett A, Hooker S, Howard V, Hutto B, et al. Walk score and objectively measured physical activity within a national cohort. J Epidemiol Community Health. 2019;73(6):549–56. http://jech.bmj.com/

55. Lang IM, Antonakos CL, Judd SE, Colabianchi N. A longitudinal examination of objective neighborhood walkability, body mass index, and waist circumference: the REasons for geographic and racial differences in stroke study. Int J Behav Nutr Phys Act. 2022;19(1):1–15. https://doi.org/10.1186/s12966-022-01247-7.

56. Creatore MI, Glazier RH, Moineddin R, Fazli GS, Johns A, Gozdyra P, et al. Association of neighborhood walkability with change in overweight, obesity, and diabetes. JAMA. 2016;315(20):2211–20.

57. Makhlouf MHE, Motairek I, Chen Z, Nasir K, Deo SV, Rajagopalan S, et al. Neighborhood walkability and cardiovascular risk in the United States. Curr Probl Cardiol. 2023;48(3):1–13.

58. Makram OM, Nwana N, Nicolas JC, Gullapelli R, Pan A, Bose B, et al. Favorable neighborhood walkability is associated with lower burden of cardiovascular risk factors among patients within an integrated health system: the Houston Methodist learning health system outpatient registry. Curr Probl Cardiol. 2023;48(6):101642. https://doi.org/10.1016/j.cpcardiol.2023.101642.

59. den Braver NR, Lakerveld J, Gozdyra P, van de Brug T, Moin JS, Fazli GS, et al. Development of a neighborhood drivability index and its association with transportation behavior in Toronto. Environ Int. 2022;163:107182. https://doi.org/10.1016/j.envint.2022.107182.

60. Den Braver NR, Beulens JWJ, Wu CF, Fazli GS, Gozdyra P, Howell NA, et al. Higher neighborhood drivability is associated with a higher diabetes risk in younger adults : a population-based cohort study in Toronto, Canada. Diabetes Care. 2023;46:1177–84.

61. Marek L, Hobbs M, Wiki J, Kingham S, Campbell M. The good, the bad, and the environment: developing an area-based measure of access to health-promoting and health-constraining environments in New Zealand. Int J Health Geogr. 2021;20(1):16. https://doi.org/10.1186/s12942-021-00269-x.

62. Hobbs M, Milfont TL, Marek L, Yogeeswaran K, Sibley CG. The environment an adult resides within is associated with their health behaviours, and their mental and physical health outcomes: a nationwide geospatial study. Soc Sci Med. 2022;301:114801.

63. Cebrecos A, Escobar F, Borrell LN, Díez J, Gullón P, Sureda X, et al. A multicomponent method assessing healthy cardiovascular urban environments: the Heart Healthy Hoods Index. Health Place. 2019;55:111–9. https://doi.org/10.1016/j.healthplace.2018.11.010.

64. Lam TM, Wagtendonk AJ, den Braver NR, Karssenberg D, Vaartjes I, Timmermans EJ, et al. Development of a neighborhood obesogenic built environment characteristics index for The Netherlands. Obesity (Silver Spring). 2023;31(1):214–24.

65. Burgoine T, Forouhi NG, Griffin SJ. Associations between exposure to takeaway food outlets, takeaway food consumption, and body weight in Cambridgeshire, UK: population based, cross. BMJ. 2014;1464:1–10. https://doi.org/10.1136/bmj.g1464.

66. Sarkar C, Lai KY, Zhang R, Ni MY, Webster C. The association between workplace built environment and metabolic health: a systematic review and meta-analysis. Health Place. 2022;76:102829. https://doi.org/10.1016/j.healthplace.2022.102829.

67. Drewnowski A, Buszkiewicz J, Aggarwal A, Rose C, Gupta S, Bradshaw A. Obesity and the built environment: a reappraisal. Obesity (Silver Spring). 2019;28 (1):22–30. https://onlinelibrary.wiley.com/doi/abs/10.1002/oby.22672

68. Sonnenschein T, Scheider S, de Wit GA, Tonne CC, Vermeulen R. Agent-based modeling of urban exposome interventions: prospects, model architectures, and methodological challenges. Exposome. 2022;2(1). https://academic.oup.com/exposome/article/2/1/osac009/6754814

69. Ohanyan H, Portengen L, Huss A, Traini E, Beulens JWJ, Hoek G, et al. Machine learning approaches to characterize the obesogenic urban exposome. Environ Int. 2022;158:107015.

70. Ohanyan H, Portengen L, Kaplani O, Huss A, Hoek G, Beulens JWJ, et al. Associations between the urban exposome and type 2 diabetes: results from penalised regression by least absolute shrinkage and selection operator and random forest models. Environ Int. 2022;170:107592.

71. Den Braver NR, Rutters F, Wagtendonk AJ, Kok JG, Harms PP, Brug J, et al. Neighborhood walkability, physical activity and changes in glycemic markers in people with type 2 diabetes: the Hoorn diabetes care system cohort. Health Place. 2021;69:102560.

72. Petrunoff NA, Edney S, Yi NX, Dickens BL, Joel KR, Xin WN, et al. Associations of park features with park use and park-based physical activity in an urban environment in Asia: a cross-sectional study. Health Place. 2022;75:102790.

73. van Wee B, Cao J. Residential self-selection in the relationship between the built environment and travel behavior: a literature review and research agenda. In: Cao XJ, Ding C, Yang J, editors. Urban transport and land use planning. 1st ed. Amsterdam: Elsevier; 2020. p. 75–94. https://doi.org/10.1016/bs.atpp.2020.08.004.

74. Macdonald L, Olsen JR, Shortt NK, Ellaway A. Do 'environmental bads' such as alcohol, fast food, tobacco, and gambling outlets cluster and co-locate in more deprived areas in Glasgow City, Scotland? Health Place. 2018;51:224–31. https://doi.org/10.1016/j.healthplace.2018.04.008.

75. Lamichhanea AP, Warren J, Puett R, Porter DE, Bottai M, Mayer-Davis EJ, et al. Spatial patterning of supermarkets and fast food outlets with respect to neighborhood characteristics. Health Place. 2013;23 (1):1–7. https://www.ncbi.nlm.nih.gov/pmc/articles/PMC3624763/pdf/nihms412728.pdf

76. European Journal of Preventive Cardiology, zwad241, https://doi.org/10.1093/eurjpc/zwad241

Social and Community Networks and Obesity

13

Houssem Ben Khalfallah, Mariem Jelassi,
Narjes Bellamine Ben Saoud, and Jacques Demongeot

Contents

H. B. Khalfallah · M. Jelassi · N. B. B. Saoud
RIADI Laboratory, ENSI, Manouba University, La
Manouba, Tunisia
e-mail: houssembenkhalfallah@gmail.com;
mariem.jelassi@ensi-uma.tn;
narjes.bellamine@ensi.rnu.tn

J. Demongeot (✉)
AGEIS Laboratory, UGA, La Tronche, France
e-mail: jacques.demongeot@univ-grenoble-alpes.fr

© Springer Nature Switzerland AG 2023
R. S. Ahima (ed.), *Metabolic Syndrome*,
https://doi.org/10.1007/978-3-031-40116-9_19

Abstract

This chapter aims to apply a mathematical approach of the social and community networks in the discrete dynamic modeling context of a current pandemic, obesity, identified as a major worldwide risk for cardiometabolic disease by the World Health Organization (WHO). After providing an overview on the social and community networks and the main mathematical tools necessary to model an epidemic propagation in a discrete framework using the Hopfield-type propagation equation, we present the application of these tools to the obesity epidemic using real data observed in Tunisian and French high schools. After a discussion of the obtained results of model simulations, a medico-social explanation is proposed for the "contagion mechanism" and for prevention of the obesity spread in a dedicated community through adolescent social networks.

Keywords

Social networks · Obesity · Discrete dynamic · Epidemic modeling · Graph centrality

Introduction

Obesity was declared by the WHO in 1997 as a major public health problem and a global epidemic killing more individuals than many contagious infectious diseases [54]. Obesity can be considered as a social contagious disease because many of its determinants come from a sociocultural heritage transmitted through families [11, 35–38, 61]. To be able to act on the spread of obesity through prevention strategies, we need a mathematical model of transmission of the disease and a simulation tool for this model. Then, it will be possible to establish scenarios for combating the spread of obesity and develop effective prevention and treatment strategies. We will focus on the following topics: overview of social and community networks, mathematical aspects of the network modeling, application to the obesity

spread, interest of network simulations for public health policies of obesity factor prevention, conclusion, and perspectives of application to other contagious diseases.

Overview of Social and Community Networks

Social Network Modeling

Social network modeling is a technique used to represent interactions between individuals. Such networks are made up of a set of nodes (or vertices) representing individuals that are connected by edges (or links) representing the relations among them. These edges can be directed or not, depending on the network application. Directed networks are commonly used to model systems in which the direction of the relationships is important, such as in social networks where the edges represent friendships or connections and the direction of the edge represents the flow of information or influence from one person to another. Undirected networks are used in systems in which the direction of the relationships is not important, such as in social networks where the edges represent symmetric relationships, such as romantic partnerships or friendships between school pupils, with no direction of influence. In ecology, for example, network models are used to represent interactions among different species in a food web. In this case, the nodes in the network represent the species, and the edges represent the interactions (e.g., predator-prey, mutualism, etc.) [8]. By simulating the dynamics of the network, researchers can study how changes in one part of the food web, e.g., the introduction of a new species, may affect the entire ecosystem [57].

Social network analysis (SNA) and community analysis are both fields of network analysis (NA) that study the connections and interactions among individuals and groups. The goal of SNA is to understand the patterns and behaviors of individuals and groups in a network, as well as the effects of these patterns on the overall network. SNA and community analysis are widely used to identify key individuals or groups in a network, understand how information spreads through a network, and predict future behavior or outcomes in a network.

The data used in SNA and community analysis can come from a variety of sources, including surveys, social media, and online interactions. SNA is the study of the structure, dynamics, and functions of social networks. It focuses on the connections between individuals or groups in a network and the patterns and behaviors that emerge from these connections (Fig. 1). SNA involves the use of mathematical and computational methods, such as graph theory, centrality measures, and network visualization, to model and analyze these interactions.

Community analysis focuses on the groups or communities that form within a network and the dynamics and interactions among these groups.

This can include identifying of subgroups within a network, understanding how individuals form and maintain relationships within a group, and analyzing the role of groups in shaping individual behavior or outcomes. Community analysis may use a combination of quantitative and qualitative methods, including survey data, ethnographic observations, and interviews, to study the groups and communities within a network. The goal of community analysis is to identify and understand patterns of organization within a group or network of individuals or organizations, like groups of individuals or nodes that are more tightly connected to one another, or identifying key individuals or nodes that serve as hubs within the network. It can be used in a variety of fields, including sociology, anthropology, political science, and computer science, to gain insights into social networks, online communities, and other types of groups.

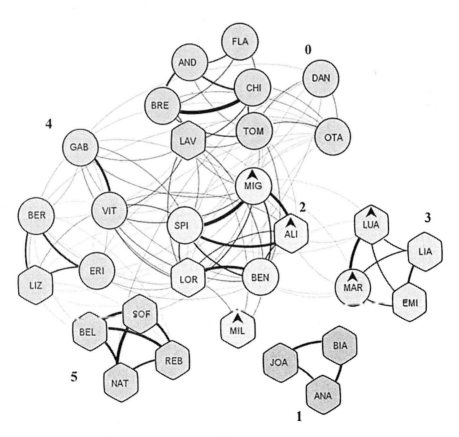

Fig. 1 A social network of children's free-play activity [67]

Network Analysis in Epidemiology

Network analysis (NA) in epidemiology is used, through SNA and community analysis, to study infectious diseases spread within a population by identifying patterns of social interactions and connections among individuals. In particular, these methods help understand the spread of diseases in complex populations with diverse social structures and behaviors. NA takes into account factors such as the age, sex, occupation, and other demographic characteristics of individuals, as well as their social networks and patterns of movement, which allow researchers to understand how a disease is transmitted, which individuals or groups are most at risk, and how to target interventions to slow or stop the spread of the disease [68]. One of the key applications of SNA in epidemiology is contact tracing, which involves identifying and tracking individuals who have been in close contact with an infected person (Figs. 2 and 3). SNA can be used to create a map of the social connections between individuals and identify individuals who are at high risk of infection based on their proximity to infected individuals in the network [18, 84]. It is used to identify key individuals or groups within a network who may be important in the transmission of a disease, such as individuals with many connections or who occupy central positions in the network. These individuals or groups, known as "bridge" or "super-spreader" individuals, may be particularly important to target with interventions, as their ability to spread the disease to many other individuals within the network [84].

Another application of SNA in epidemiology is understanding the role of different types of social connections in the spread of a disease. For example, researchers can use SNA to identify the different types of contacts (e.g., family, friends, work, etc.) that are most likely to transmit the disease and target interventions to those groups [87]. An example of using SNA in epidemiology is the study of the spread of influenza. Researchers used SNA to map the social network of individuals in a community and identified key individuals who played a significant role in the spread of the disease. This information can be used to target interventions, such as vaccination of these key individuals to reduce the spread of influenza in the community [43]. Another example of using SNA in epidemiology is the study of the spread of sexually transmitted

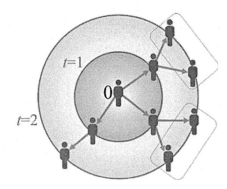

Fig. 3 Interaction graph in a contagious network representing the spread of the epidemic outbreak of a social contagious disease, from a first infectious "patient zero" (located at his "influence sphere" center), progressively infecting at $t = 1$ and $t = 2$ his neighbors in successive regions (rectangles) of the contagion network

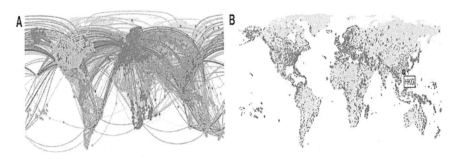

Fig. 2 Complexity in global, network-driven contagion phenomena. (**A**) The global mobility network. (**B**) Temporal snapshot of a simulated global pandemic with initial outbreak location in Hong Kong (HKG) [14]

infections (STIs) among adolescents. Researchers used SNA to map the sexual network of adolescents and identified high-risk individuals and groups who were more likely to spread STIs. This information can be used to target interventions and education efforts to reduce the spread of STIs [81].

Mathematical Aspects of the Network Modeling

The Obesity Transition Rule

Among the mathematical tools of network modeling applied to contagious diseases, we will choose an extension of the Boolean approach by Hopfield [2, 27–35, 55, 76], which consists in defining three states, 1 (or S) for normal weight, 2 (or W) for overweight, and 3 (or O) for obese, and a rule fixing the transition between these three states. The stochastic version of the Hopfield transition rule allows the calculation of the weight state

$O_i(t + 1)$ of an individual i at time $t + 1$ as a function of the state $O_k(t)$s of its neighbors ks belonging to its neighborhood $N(i)$, i.e., the set of the individuals linked to i (including himself) in the oriented interaction graph of a contagion network linking the individuals of the studied population (Fig. 3), by using a potential function denoted P_i and defined as follows:

$$P_i(t) = \sum_{k \in N(i)} w_{ik} O_k(t) \quad (1)$$

where w_{ik} is the interaction coefficient measuring the influence individual k has on individual i, its value being equal to 1, (respectively, 0 or -1) in the absence of precise estimation, if it is "obesogenic" (respectively, zero or normalizing). If T_i denotes a tolerance parameter, such as $1/T_i$ quantifies the global level of influence exerted on individual i by the individuals k belonging to its neighborhood $N(i)$, the stochastic transition rule is as follows:

$$\begin{cases} T_i = 0, O_i(t) = 1 \text{ or } 3: \text{if } P_i(t) > 0, \\ O_i(t + 1) = \inf(3, O_i(t) + 1); \text{if } P_i(t) \leq 0, O_i(t + 1) = \sup(1, O_i(t) - 1), \\ T_i = 0, O_i(t) = 2: \text{Proba}(O_i(t + 1) = 1) = \text{Proba}(O_i(t + 1) = 3) = \frac{1}{2}, \\ T_i > 0: \forall j, h \in \{1, 23\}, \text{Proba}(\{O_i(t + 1) = j | O_i(t) = h\}) = \frac{u(j, h)e^{v(j,h)P_i(t)/T_i}}{\sum_{l=0,1,2} u(j, l)e^{v(j,l)P_i(t)/T_i}} \end{cases} \quad (2)$$

where $u(j,h) = 1$, if $|j\text{-}h| \leq 1$, $u(j,h) = 0$, if $|j\text{-}h| > 1$, and $v(j,h) = 1$, if $j \geq \inf(3, h + 1)$, $v(j,h) = 0$, if $j < \inf(3, h + 1)$.

In Eq. (1), the function P_i is the analogue of the Hamiltonian function of the Hopfield model [55], and the tolerance parameter $1/T_i$ is the analogue of the temperature: higher is T_i, nearer the value $\frac{1}{2}$ (resp. $1/3$) is the probability to remain in same state j or change to its neighbor state, if $j = 1$ or 3 (resp. $j = 2$), which corresponds to an absence of influence of the previous state on the future state, regardless of the weight status.

The Notion of Centrality in the Contagion Network

The centrality for an individual in a contagious network quantifies the degree of influence that individual exerts on the weight state of his or her neighbors in the interaction graph of the network [13]. There are four classical types of centrality (Fig. 3). The first is the *betweenness centrality*, defined for *an individual k* [7]:

$$C^{betw}(k) = \sum_{i \neq j \neq k \in G} \frac{\beta_{ij}(k)}{\beta_k} \qquad (3)$$

where $\beta_{ij}(k)$ σ_{st} is the total number of the shortest paths from the individual i s to individual j t passing through the individual k, and $\beta_k = \sum_{i \neq j \in G} \beta_{ij}(k)$. The second type of centrality is the *degree centrality*, defined from the notions of out-, in-, or total-degree of an individual i, corresponding to the number of arrows of the interaction graph, respectively, exiting, entering, or both in the individual i. For example, the total-degree centrality is defined by:

$$C_i^{tot-deg} = \frac{\sum_{j=1,\ldots,n; j \neq i} |a_{ij}|}{n-1} \qquad (4)$$

where $a_{ij} = \text{sign}(w_{ij})$ denotes the general coefficient of the signed incidence matrix A of the graph G. The third type of centrality is the *closeness centrality*. The closeness is the inverse of the average farness, which is defined by averaging a distance between individuals i and $j \neq i$:

$$C_i^{clo} = \frac{n-1}{\sum_{j=1,\ldots,n; j \neq i} L(i,j)} \qquad (5)$$

where the distance can be $L(i,j)$, i.e., the length of the closest path between i and j.

The last type of classical centrality is the *spectral centrality* or *eigencentrality*, which takes into account the fact that the neighbors of an individual i in the interaction graph G can also be highly connected to other individuals of G, considering that connections to highly connected individuals contribute to the centrality of i more than connections to weakly connected individuals. Hence, the spectral centrality of the individual i better represents the global influence of i on the whole contagion network and is defined by [73]:

$$C_i^{spec} = \frac{\sum_{j \in N(i)} w_{ij} V_j}{\lambda} \qquad (6)$$

where λ is the dominant eigenvalue of the incidence matrix of the interaction graph G and V is its eigenvector. The four classical centralities

above can be very different, but they have each an intrinsic interest: (i) betweenness centrality relates to the global connectivity of an individual with all individuals of the network, (ii) degree centralities correspond to the local connectivity with only the nearest individuals, (iii) closeness centrality measures the relative proximity with other individuals for a given distance on the interaction graph, and (iv) spectral centrality corresponds to the ability to be connected to, possibly, a few numbers of individuals, but having a high connectivity, being important hub-relays for wide sub-networks [76]. Despite the complementary properties of the classical centralities, a new notion of centrality, called entropy centrality, has been introduced by Jelassi [61] to take into account not only the connectivity but also the heterogeneity of the distribution of states of the neighbors of an individual i:

$$C^{entropy}_i = -\sum_{k=1,\ldots,si} \nu_k \log_2 \nu_k \qquad (7)$$

where ν_k denotes the kth frequency among the s_i frequencies of the histogram of the state values observed in the neighborhood $N(i)$ of the individual i, i.e., the set of the individuals out- or in-linked to the individual i.

Application to the Spread of Obesity

Modeling the spread of obesity within social networks involves using data and statistical techniques to understand how obesity spreads among individuals who are connected in a social network, by analyzing factors such as the strength of social ties, demographic characteristics, and other variables that may influence the likelihood of obesity spreading from one person to another.

Recent research in this field has used advanced network analysis techniques, such as SNA and agent-based modeling (ABM), to study the spread of obesity in large-scale social networks by using data from social media platforms, electronic health records, and other sources to construct detailed representations of social networks and track the spread of obesity over time in order to understand how social networks can influence an individual's likelihood of becoming obese [20, 22, 36]. The Framingham Heart Study has examined the spread of obesity over 32 years in a large social network and showed that an individual's likelihood of becoming obese increased by 57% if he or she had a friend who became obese and by 40% if a sibling became obese. The study also found that the effect was stronger among close friends and siblings than distant connections and that the risk was greater for women than men [21].

Another example of a community analysis in epidemiology is the study of the distribution and determinants of obesity in a specific community [59, 60]. This type of study could involve collecting data on the body mass index (BMI) and other health-related measures from a representative sample of community members and analyzing the data to identify patterns and trends in obesity within the community. Other studies have been conducted in schools to examine the potential risk factors for obesity, such as diet, physical activity level, and access to healthy food options [71, 90].

In the present work, our study is based on a multi-level model, combining individual and social levels. We will use data collected from a survey targeting middle school students in Tunisia, North Africa. This survey includes questions on a student's eating habits, favorite activities, perception of surroundings, personality, parental and friendly relationships, etc. We will examine obesity spread through a middle school community of 274 students, aged between 13 and 15 years old, including 16 of them with obesity or who are overweight (Fig. 4). The individual level corresponds to individual parameters such as age, obesity state (S, normal weight; W, overweight; O, obese) and tolerance (trend of an individual to be connected with individuals having obesity).

The environment of an individual consists of social network, i.e., family member (parent, sibling), friend, colleague, etc. [59]. The obesity state transition of an individual is regulated by eating habits and physical activities, as well as by the influence by social network, which affects obesity state variations.

For example, an individual in the obesity state S (normal weight) and tolerance 0 can be influenced only by individuals connected to them with the same obesity state S, while an individual in the obesity state S with a tolerance value equal to 1 can be influenced by their neighbors having the obesity state S or W. Thus, the obesity values may change during the simulation. Each individual can thus change (increase or decrease) risk for obesity, according to their

Fig. 4 Student network. Red nodes represent overweight and obese, and node area size is proportional to out-degree (number of outgoing links)

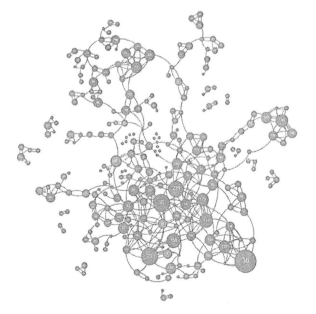

Table 1 Individual state transitions according to tolerance parameter

Tolerance/ initial state	S (normal weight)	W (overweight)	O (obese)
0	S → S	W → W	O → O
1	S → {S,W}	W → {S,W,O}	O → {W,O}
2	S → {S,W,O}	W → {S,W,O}	O → {S,W,O}

obesity state and the influence of their neighbors. Possible transitions between obesity states are summarized in Table 1.

Obesity Factors for Network Simulation for Public Health Policies and Prevention

The identification of obesity factors is essential to define an effective prevention policy. Figure 5 shows the obesity determinants of an individual over their lifetime classified into three categories. Most of these determinants exert their influence within the framework of family or social context and are related to the genetic and educational factors, which justifies the qualifier of social contagious disease. The first category describes environmental factors, including diet and physical factors, social structure, and social determinants. The second category characterizes psychological and behavioral factors. The third category represents biological factors [94]. All the determinants of obesity are based on the genetic, educational, social, and environmental background of an individual [10, 83].

Environmental Factors

The environment is defined as a set of complex factors, chemical, physical, and biotic. It is also an aggregation of social and cultural conditions, which act on an organism or ecological community and ultimately determine its form and survival. From this definition, some articles evoke the relationships between the environment and obesity. It turns out that the environment of an

individual plays a major role on eating behaviors. Some research has highlighted mechanisms favoring the increasing prevalence of overweight and obesity in a so-called "obesogenic" environment [52]. In a given population, each individual lives in certain conditions, interacts with other individuals, and has their own position. This means that at the population level, the environment of an individual is characterized by physical factors like food environment, physical environment, etc. and social factors such as social network, social status, etc.

Physical Factors

We consider only the purely physical factors (such as soil, climate, water supply) and all physical elements of the environment such as food environments and infrastructure that influence growth and development. This definition concurs with that of Rizzuto [79], which states that physical factors represent pollution and indoor environments, and that of Larson [65], which considers physical environment or settings referring to daycare, schools, workplaces, retail food stores, restaurants, and fast food outlets. For example, air pollution related to traffic is associated with the BMI [62] and can induce an endocrine disruption which could be obesogenic via the hypothalamic-pituitary-adrenal axis (HPS axis), CNS metabolic pathways, insulin resistance, etc.

Studies have also highlighted the contribution of the neighborhood and the place where an individual lives. It has been shown that the food environment (access to food stores, fast food, restaurants, etc.) and the physical activity environment influence the weight of individuals [12, 86, 99]. In addition, the presence of parks and green areas has been found to be related to obesity, e.g., the number of parks and their cleanliness are negatively correlated with the obesity rate [77, 89]. Physical environmental factors are also defined by the type of street where people live, the presence of sidewalks and bicycle paths, as well as access to recreational facilities (sports and recreation centers, gymnasia, golf courses, tennis courts, swimming pools, public open space, and

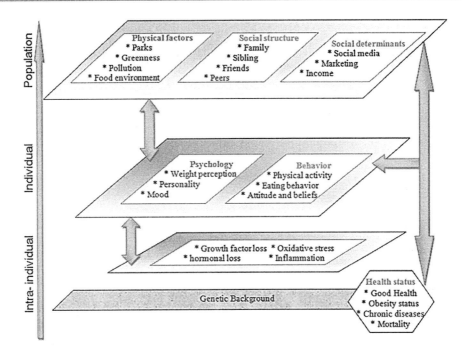

Fig. 5 Multi-level classification of obesity risk factors

beach or river foreshores) [50]. Excess weight gain is associated with the absence of sidewalks, absence of paths for walking, and the limitation of access to recreational facilities.

Social Factors

Social structure can be seen as a system organized by a characteristic pattern of relationships in which individuals form a social structure. This can be modeled as a social network made up of family, friends, colleagues, etc. [65]. The social structure was defined by Rizzuto as income distribution and gender equality [79]. Studies have focused on the relationship between the obesity status of an individual (normal weight, overweight, or obese) and their social network, demonstrating that it depends on the nature of the relationship and age of the individual [21, 46, 85]. It turns out that during childhood, an individual is much more influenced by their family's eating behavior and the individual's physical activity [51, 78]. Lazzeri studied a cohort of young people

between the ages of 11 and 15 and was able to demonstrate that the higher the education of one of the parents, the more unlikely it is that they are overweight [66].

In broader social groups, research has not been able to establish causality between an adolescent's body weight and that of their friends [5]. De La Haye [25] studied weight similarities in a group of teenage friends to determine whether these are due to contagion or friend selection based on homophily, and the conclusion, based on stochastic models, was that the similarity of weight in a network of friends was caused by a phenomenon of selection, i.e., adolescents have eating behaviors similar to those of their friends [46, 56]. This result agrees with that of Schaefer who used social network analysis based on the study of random graphs [85]. Fitzgerald proved the hypothesis that friends play an important role in adolescent physical activity levels [45], further supporting the hypothesis of a contagion phenomenon. On the other hand, Cohen-Cole found that obesity is due to environmental factors [23] rather than a contagion phenomenon as proposed by Christakis and Fowler [21, 47].

To determine the impact of collective behavior on the spread of the obesity epidemic, several mathematical tools have been used [69]. At the population level, the research carried out has been based on the study of dynamical systems [47], while at the individual level, ABM and SNA have been used [34, 93, 97]. Within this wide range of tools, it has been suggested that SNA is probably the best-known methodological approach in obesity that offers an illustrative example of more broadly applicable considerations in interpreting research results [65].

Social Network Analysis

Social determinants are defined as exogenous forces in society such as marketing and media or elements that define an individual's way of life such as income. These determinants, defined as the social macro-environment, include income and socioeconomic status, cultural norms and values, food marketing, and agricultural and food policy [65]. Wamala et al. studied these social determinants and more particularly socioeconomic status in relation to obesity. They found that low socioeconomic status is an important determinant of overweight and obesity in middle-aged Swedish women [97]. A study on obesogenic factors found that the number of fathers with obesity in low- and middle-income municipalities was higher than in high-income areas [51]. However, there was no association between income and maternal obesity status. The lower the parents' income, the more the children did sedentary activities and participated less in physical activities.

Another important aspect of social determinants is food marketing. Indeed, this aspect may seem trivial but contributes to the increase in the obesity. The influence of packaging on the food choices has been studied [16], showing that package design can alter the perception of quantity and increase preference for oversized portions. Food marketing can also be used as a prevention, as some community social marketing campaigns used this strategy to encourage low-income groups to take up sport [98].

Psychological and Behavioral Factors

At the individual level, psychological and behavioral factors are the direct consequence of the interaction of an individual with his physical and social environment. These factors can be divided into factors related to personality, lifestyle, or individual attitudes and beliefs. Indeed, Rizzuto demonstrated that many dietary factors such as diet, energy intake, physical activity, obesity, smoking, alcohol consumption, behavioral factors (e.g., sleep, stress), and cultural factors are important in the etiology of non-communicable diseases [79].

Behavioral factors, and more particularly lifestyle, studied in obesity research are generally dietary habits (such as the consumption of soft drinks [72] or alcohol [58]) and low level of physical activity [1]. Physical activities can be divided according to their influence on obesity rates. Indeed, physical activity – past or present sports activities [1, 58, 91], number of hours spent watching television [50], or video games [72] – all affect obesity. They may be an influence of sex on behaviors. For example, in men, having no leisure and consumption of sweets and smoking are associated with an increase in the BMI. In women, other factors seem more influential, such as lack of sleep and frequent consumption of soft drinks [58].

Other researchers have highlighted the relationship between behavior and environmental factors. A study showed that students changed eating behaviors from unhealthy to healthy due to positive social and environmental influences [24], which supports the hypothesis of the phenomenon of contagion. Students with similar eating behaviors tended to form distinct groups, supporting the selection hypothesis in the creation of social networks. There are strong associations between individuals and their friends in eating behaviors and physical activity in young adults [5]. The type of neighborhood restaurants may have different roles with respect to leisure time physical activity and overweight or obesity in individuals regardless of gender.

The psychological determinants include the mood, well-being [96], self-evaluation [4], anxiety [63], stress [70], impulsivity [17, 53, 96], and weight perception [1, 5, 22, 42, 58, 82]. Sutin et al. showed that personality traits are influenced by weight gain, and in turn, weight gain may be due to personality change [92]. They also found that significant weight gain is associated with increased impulsivity and possibly aggressivity [88], an observation that supported Hartmann's finding that children with compulsive eating, or hyperphagia, are significantly more impulsive [53]. Martyn-Nemeth et al. explained the relationship of low self-esteem and stress to the adoption of unhealthy eating behavior [70]. Other research has shown that obesity in women is associated with anxiety, depression, and well-being [58].

Another important psychological aspect is weight perception. It seems that women frequently overestimate their weight, while men often underestimate it [22]. A study has shown that overestimation of weight among normal weight adolescents and accurate perceptions of weight among overweight adolescents were associated with higher rates of disordered eating behaviors [42]. In another research, carried out on a cohort of never-married Indian women, it turned out that one in four overweight women and one in ten obese women considered themselves to be of normal weight [1]. Research has shown that the social structure to which an individual belongs can affect the perception of obesity. African-American women with obesity believe that people can be attractive and healthy at larger sizes [9], consistent with the view that the perception of body shapes and preferences for particular levels of fat are culturally determined of [3].

Biological Factors

Obesity is associated with excess adiposity; ectopic fat in the liver, muscle, and several organs; inflammation; oxidative stress; and hormone dysregulation [80]. These factors regulate eating, energy balance, and the pathogenesis of diabetes, cardiovascular disease, non-alcoholic fatty liver, dementia, and other diseases in individuals. However, the rising obesity trends globally are attributed mainly to environmental factors and influence of family, school, or social networks.

Network Simulations

After applying the obesity transition rule in a system with two states (normal weight S and overweight or obese O), we found that, in most cases, the ratio of overweight and obese remains limited or even becomes zero in some cases. However, in the case where the sample is half of tolerance equal to 1 and half of tolerance equal to 2, and by assigning the tolerance values by alternation between 1 and 2 starting with the first student, the obesity epidemic spreads rapidly in the studied sample (Fig. 6g and h). On the other hand, if we reverse the order used to assign tolerance values, the epidemic does not spread (Fig. 6i). This result shows that among people with a tolerance equal to 2 who find themselves in the scenario where obesity is spreading (Fig. 6g), some are not only influenceable by their homophilic character but also very influential in their social network, since they are the cause of the epidemic outbreak.

In the context of obesity contagion, high-degree centrality individuals are those who have many close connections to other individuals in the network and may therefore be more likely to influence the spread of obesity (Fig. 7a), while high-betweenness centrality individuals may be those who connect disconnected groups and facilitate the spread of obesity, since they act as bridges (Fig. 7b). Spectral centrality is also used to identify individuals or groups that are central to the network structure and may play a significant role in the spread of obesity (Fig. 7c). And high-closeness centrality individuals may be those who are well connected to other individuals in the network and have a significant impact on the spread of obesity due to their central location (Fig. 7d), since this centrality compute the average distance between a node and all other nodes in a network.

According to the collected data and the network topology, some network centrality measures

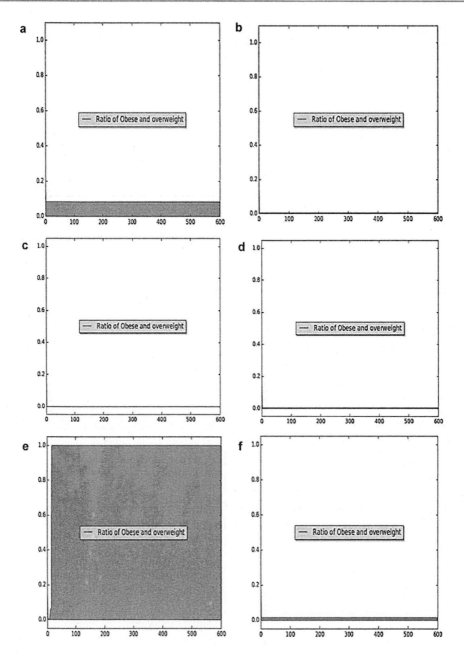

Fig. 6 Ratio of overweight and obese students with (**a**) tolerance equal to 0, (**b**) tolerance equal to 1, (**c**) tolerance equal to 2, (**d**) half of the students with tolerance equal to 0 and half to 1, (**e**) half of the students with tolerance equal to 0 and half to 2, (**f**) half of the students with tolerance equal to 1 and half to 0, (**g**) half of the students with tolerance equal to 1 and half to 2, (**h**) half of the students with tolerance equal to 2 and half to 0, (**i**) half of the students with tolerance equal to 2 and half to 1, the opposite of (**g**). In each case where half of the students have tolerance i and half tolerance j, we have assigned the tolerance values by alternation between i and j starting with the same student and then, following the same order

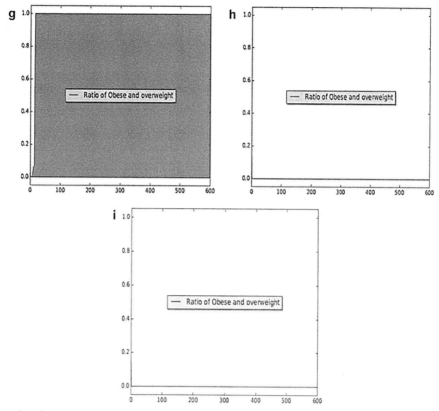

Fig. 6 (continued)

could be more suitable than others. In social sciences, spectral centrality could be interesting in many cases, since this measure evaluates the importance of an individual by the importance of the individuals with whom he maintains links. In other words, the basic question that makes an individual influential is not the number of his connections, but rather the influence of those he knows. If the aim of the public health policy is to diminish the number of obese individuals, the identification of the obese hubs is important: a nutritional rehabilitation on a part of these obese or overweight hubs can reduce drastically the number of obese or overweight individuals in their neighborhood.

For example, if we diminish their influence by increasing their tolerance parameter T_i, we can suppress their influence and then reduce the risk to become obese at their contact. Suppose that we start with an interaction network of 100 individuals including 100 obese or overweight and zero normal weight, with interaction weights w_{ij} chosen at random either 0 or 1.

The simulations have been done by using only two states, normal weight (S) and overweight or obese (W). Figure 8 shows that, by increasing the value of the tolerance parameter T_i for the eight most influential overweight or obese individuals in the sense of the spectral centrality (Fig. 7c), the mean percentage of normal weight individuals increases until the value ½, corresponding to a random choice equilibrated between the normality on the one hand and overweight or obesity on the other hand. That shows that the states of the nodes of the network can be regularized to the normality after a campaign targeted at the most influential obese or overweight individuals (in the sense of the spectral centrality) of the interaction network [59, 60].

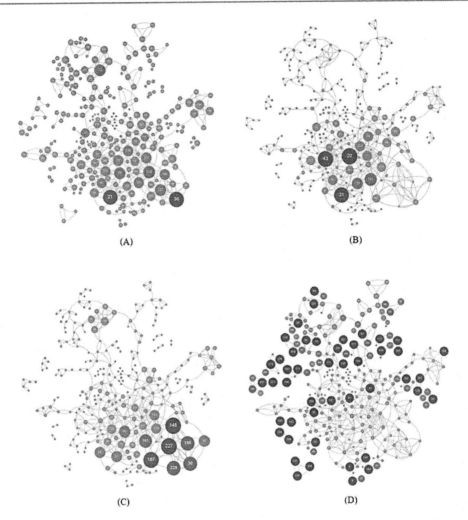

Fig. 7 Students' network centrality analysis. (**A**) Degree centrality. (**B**) Betweenness centrality. (**C**) Spectral centrality. (**D**) Closeness centrality

Conclusion

We have shown that a discrete modeling approach using an automata network makes it possible to account for the dissemination of a contagious disease such as the obesity and also to simulate the impact of public health measures, such as a therapeutic education of the individuals most involved in the dissemination of the disease. This approach has only concerned studies on well-identified school communities, but it provides a methodology that could be used in the general population, to simulate and evaluate the effect of preventive measures, based essentially, in the case of obesity, on learning lifestyle and dietary measures to regress the disease in patients in whom obesity is still reversible, and to reduce the impact of the transmission of bad eating habits by individuals with the most contact and influence in family, educational, and social networks. Many contagious diseases have an infectious origin, and the modeling of their dissemination requires a network approach similar to those used for the social contagious diseases. Their spread involves infectious agents. The elucidation of COVID-19 pathogenesis and spread provided a recent opportunity for modeling [6, 15, 19, 26, 27, 41, 44, 48, 49, 64, 100, 101], taking into account determinants like age, vaccination, and environmental factors [39, 40, 74, 75].

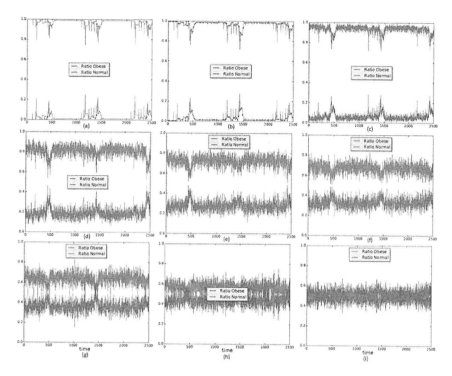

Fig. 8 Percentages of obese or overweight (red) and normal weight (green) individuals evolving from an initial population with 100 obese or overweight and zero normal weight, with increasing values of T_i for the eight individuals who are the most influential (in the sense of the spectral centrality): (**a**) $T_i = 0.1$, (**b**) $T_i = 0.5$, (**c**) $T_i = 1$, (**d**) $T_i = 2$, (**e**) $T_i = 3$, (**f**) $T_i = 4$, (**g**) $T_i = 5$, (**h**) $T_i = 10$, and (**i**) $T_i = 100$

References

1. Agrawal P, Gupta K, Mishra V, et al. Effects of sedentary lifestyle and dietary habits on body mass index change among adult women in India: findings from a follow-up study. Ecol Food Nutr. 2013;52: 387–406.
2. Albert R, Thakar J. Boolean modeling: a logic-based dynamic approach for understanding signaling and regulatory networks and for making useful predictions. WIREs Syst Biol Med. 2014;6:353–69.
3. Allon N. The stigma of overweight in everyday life. Psychological aspects of obesity: a handbook. New York: Van Nostrand Reinhold; 1982. p. 130–74.
4. Annesi JJ. Effects of improved self-appraisal and mood factors on weight loss in obese women initiating supported exercise. J Complement Integr Med. 2011;8:1378.
5. Barclay KJ, Edling C, Rydgren J. Peer clustering of exercise and eating behaviours among young adults in Sweden: a cross-sectional study of ego-centric network data. BMC Public Health. 2013;13:784.
6. Barrat A, Barthélémy M, Vespignani A. Dynamical processes on complex networks. Cambridge: Cambridge University Press; 2008.
7. Barthélémy M. Betweenness centrality in large complex networks. Eur Phys J B. 2004;38:163–8.
8. Bascompte J. Mutualistic networks. Front Ecol Environ. 2009;7:429–36.
9. Befort CA, Thomas JL, Daley CM, et al. Perceptions and beliefs about body size, weight and weight loss among obese African American women: a qualitative inquiry. Health Educ Behav. 2008;35:410–26.
10. Belsky DW, Mott TE, Sugden K, et al. Development and evaluation of a genetic risk score for obesity. Biodemography Soc Biol. 2013;59(85):100.
11. Ben Khalfallah H, Jelassi M, Demongeot J, et al. Decision support systems in Healthcare: systematic review, meta-analysis and prediction, with example of COVID-19. AIMS Bioeng. 2023;10:27–52.
12. Boone-Heinonen J, Diez-Roux AV, Go DC, et al. The neighborhood energy balance equation: does neighborhood food retail environment + physical activity environment = obesity? The CARDIAstudy. PLoS One. 2013;8:e85141.

13. Böttcher L, Woolley-Meza O, Goles E, et al. Connectivity disruption sparks explosive epidemic spreading. Phys Rev E. 2016;93:042315S.

14. Brockmann D, Helbing D. The hidden geometry of complex, network-driven contagion phenomena. Science. 2013;342:1337–42.

15. Buscarino A, Fortuna L, Frasca M, et al. Disease spreading in populations of moving agents. Europhys Lett. 2008;82:38002.

16. Chandon P, Wansink B. Does food marketing need to make us fat? A review and solutions. Nutr Rev. 2012;70:571–93.

17. Chapman BP, Fiscella K, Duberstein P, et al. Can the influence of childhood socioeconomic status on men's and women's adult bodymass be explained by adult socioeconomic status or personality? Findings from a national sample. Health Psychol. 2009;28:419.

18. Chen YD, Tseng C, King CC, et al. Incorporating geographical contacts into social network analysis for contact tracing in epidemiology: a study on Taiwan SARS data. Intell Security Informatics: Biosurveillance. 2007;4506:23–36.

19. Cheng HY, Jian SW, Liu DP, et al. Contact tracing assessment of COVID-19 transmission dynamics in Taiwan and risk at different exposure periods before and after symptom onset. JAMA Intern Med. 2020;180:1156–63.

20. Chomutare T, Xu A, Iyengar MS. Social network analysis to delineate interaction patterns that predict weight loss performance. In: IEEE 27th international symposium on computer-based medical systems. New York: IEEE; 2014. p. 271–6.

21. Christakis NA, Fowler JH. The spread of obesity in a large social network over 32 years. N Engl J Med. 2007;357(4):370–9.

22. Christensen VT. My sibling, my weight. How gender, sibling gender, sibling weight and sibling weight level perception influence weight perception accuracy. Nutr Diabetes. 2014;4:e103.

23. Cohen-Cole E, Fletcher JM. Is obesity contagious? Social networks vs. environmental factors in the obesity epidemic. J Health Econ. 2008;27:1382–7.

24. Dabbaghian V, Mago VK, Wu T, et al. Social interactions of eating behavior among high school students: a cellular automata approach. BMC Med Res Methodol. 2012;12:155.

25. De La Haye K, Robins G, Mohr P, et al. Homophily and contagion as explanations for weight similarities among adolescent friends. J Adolesc Health. 2011;49(4):421–7.

26. Demongeot J, Magal P. Spectral method in epidemic time series. Biology. 2022;11:1825.

27. Demongeot J, Sené S. Asymptotic behavior and phase transition in regulatory networks. II Simulations. Neural Netw. 2008;21:971–9.

28. Demongeot J, Sené S. Phase transitions in stochastic non-linear threshold Boolean automata networks on Z^2: the boundary impact. Adv Appl Math. 2018;98: 77–99.

29. Demongeot J, Sené S. About block-parallel Boolean networks: a position paper. Nat Comput. 2020;19: 5–13.

30. Demongeot J, Elena A, Sené S. Robustness in neural and genetic networks. Acta Biotheor. 2008a;56: 27–49.

31. Demongeot J, Jezequel C, Sené S. Asymptotic behavior and phase transition in regulatory networks. I Theoretical results. Neural Netw. 2008b;21:962–70.

32. Demongeot J, Ben Amor H, Gillois P, et al. Robustness of regulatory networks. A generic approach with applications at different levels: physiologic, metabolic and genetic. Int J Mol Sci. 2009;10:4437–73.

33. Demongeot J, Elena A, Noual M, et al. "Immunetworks", attractors and intersecting circuits. J Theor Biol. 2011;280:19–33.

34. Demongeot J, Hansen O, Hessami H, Jannot AS, Mintsa J, Rachdi M, Taramasco C. Random modelling of contagious diseases. Acta Biotheoretica. 2013; 61:141–72.

35. Demongeot J, Elena A, Jelassi M, et al. Smart homes and sensors for surveillance and preventive education at home: example of obesity. Information. 2016;7:50.

36. Demongeot J, Jelassi M, Taramasco C. From susceptibility to Frailty in social networks: the case of obesity. Math Pop Stud. 2017;24:219–45.

37. Demongeot J, Jelassi M, Hazgui H, et al. Biological networks entropies: examples in neural memory networks, genetic regulation networks and social epidemic networks. Entropy. 2018;20:36.

38. Demongeot J, Jelassi M, Taramasco C. Big data approach for managing the information from genomics, proteomics, and wireless sensing in e-Health. In: Dey N, Bhatt C, Ashour A, editors. Big Data and remote sensing: acquisition, visualisation and interpretation. New York: Springer; 2019. p. 1–37.

39. Demongeot J, Oshinubi K, Rachdi M, et al. Estimation of daily reproduction rates in COVID-19 outbreak. Computation. 2021;9:109.

40. Demongeot J, Griette Q, Magal P, et al. Modelling vaccine efficacy for COVID-19 outbreak in New York City. Biology. 2022;11:345.

41. Demongeot J, Griette Q, Maday Y, et al. A Kermack-McKendrick model with age of infection starting from a single or multiple cohorts of infected patients. Proc R Soc A. 2023;479:0381.

42. Eichen DM, Conner BT, Daly BP, et al. Weight perception, substance use, and disordered eating behaviors: comparing normal weight and overweight high-school students. J Youth Adolescence. 2012;41:1–13.

43. Ferguson NM, Cummings DA, Cauchemez S, et al. Strategies for containing an emerging influenza pandemic in Southeast Asia. Nature. 2005;437:209–14.

44. Ferretti L, Wymant C, Kendall M, et al. Quantifying SARS-CoV-2 transmission suggests epidemic control with digital contact tracing. Science. 2020;368: eabb6936.

45. Fitzgerald A, Fitzgerald N, Aherne C. Do peers matter? A review of peer and/or friends' influence on

physical activity among American adolescents. J Adolesc. 2012;35:941–58.

46. Fletcher A, Bonell C, Sorhaindo A. You are what your friends eat: systematic review of social network analyses of young people's eating behaviours and body weight. J Epidemiol Community Health. 2011;65:548–55.

47. Fowler JH, Christakis NA. Estimating peer effects on health in social networks: a response to Cohen-Cole and Fletcher; trogdon, nonnemaker, pais. J Health Econ. 2008;27:1400.

48. Funk S, Gilad E, Watkins C, et al. The spread of awareness and its impact on epidemic outbreaks. Proc Natl Acad Sci U S A. 2009;106:6872–7.

49. Gaudart J, Landier J, Huiart L, et al. Factors associated with spatial heterogeneity of Covid-19 in France: a nationwide ecological study. Lancet Public Health. 2021;6:e222–31.

50. Giles-Corti B, Macintyre S, Clarkson JP, et al. Environmental and lifestyle factors associated with overweight and obesity in Perth, Australia. Am J Health Promot. 2003;18:93–102.

51. Gregori D, Foltran F, Ghidina M, et al. Familial environment in high- and middle low-income municipalities: a survey in Italy to understand the distribution of potentially obesogenic factors. Public Health. 2012;126:731–9.

52. Harrington DW, Elliott SJ. Weighing the importance of neighbourhood: a multilevel exploration of the determinants of overweight and obesity. Soc Sci Med 2009;68:593–600.

53. Hartmann AS, Czaja J, Rief W, et al. Personality and psychopathology in children with and without loss of control over eating. Compr Psychiatry. 2010;51:572–8.

54. Haththotuwa RN, Wijeyaratne CN, Senarath U. Worldwide epidemic of obesity. In: Mahmood TA, Arulkumaran S, Chervenak FA, editors. Obesity and obstetrics. 2nd ed. Amsterdam: Elsevier; 2020. p. 3–8.

55. Hopfield JJ. Neural networks and physical systems with emergent collective computational abilities. Proc Natl Acad Sci U S A. 1982;79:2554–8.

56. Houldcroft L, Haycraft E, Farrow C. Peer and friend influences on children's eating. Soc Dev. 2014;23:19–40.

57. Ings TC, Montoya JM, Bascompte J, et al. Ecological networks–beyond food webs. J Anim Ecol. 2009;78:253–69.

58. Inoue M, Toyokawa S, Inoue K, et al. Lifestyle, weight perception and change in body mass index of Japanese workers: My health up study. Public Health. 2010;124:530–7.

59. Jelassi M. Modélisation, simulation et analyse multi-échelle de réseaux sociaux complexes: Application à l'aide à la prévention des maladies contagieuses (PhD Thesis). Université Grenoble Alpes; 2017.

60. Jelassi M, Ben Miled S, Bellamine Ben Saoud N, Demongeot J. Obesity determinants: a systematic review. In: 2015 third World Conference on Complex Systems (WCCS). New York: IEEE; 2015. p. 1–6.

61. Jelassi M, Oshinubi K, Rachdi M, et al. Epidemic dynamics on social interaction networks. AIMS Bioeng. 2022;9:348–61.

62. Jerrett M, McConnell R, Wolch J, et al. Traffic-related air pollution and obesity formation in children: a longitudinal, multilevel analysis. Environ Health. 2014;13:49.

63. Jorm AF, Korten AE, Christensen H, et al. Association of obesity with anxiety, depression and emotional well-being: a community survey. Aust N Z J Public Health. 2003;27:434–40.

64. Kammegne B, Oshinubi K, Babasola T, et al. Mathematical modelling of spatial distribution of COVID-19 outbreak using diffusion equation. Pathogens. 2023;12:88.

65. Larson N, Story M. A review of environmental influences on food choices. Ann Behav Med. 2009;38:56–73.

66. Lazzeri G, Giacchi MV, Spinelli A, et al. Overweight among students aged 11-15 years and its relationship with breakfast, area of residence and parents' education: results from the Italian HBSC 2010 cross-sectional study. Nutr J. 2014;13:69.

67. Lira P, Moretti C, Guimarães D, et al. Group cohesiveness in children free-play activity: a social network analysis. Int J Psychol. 2021;56:941–50.

68. Lloyd AL, Valeika S. Network models in epidemiology: an overview. In: Blasius B, Jürgen Kurths J, Stone L, editors. Complex population dynamics: nonlinear modeling in ecology, epidemiology and genetics, vol. 7. Singapore: World Scientific; 2007. p. 189–214.

69. Luke DA, Stamatakis KA. Systems science methods in public health: dynamics, networks, and agents. Annu Rev Public Health. 2012;33:357–76.

70. Martyn-Nemeth P, Penckofer S, Gulanick M, et al. The relationships among self-esteem, stress, coping, eating behavior, and depressive mood in adolescents. Res Nurs Health. 2009;32:96–109.

71. McConnell P, Wendel J. Solving the child obesity problem: how schools can be part of the solution. ICAN: Infant, Child Adolescent Nutr. 2010;2:232–6.

72. Nagel G, Wabitsch M, Galm C, et al. Determinants of obesity in the Ulm research on metabolism, exercise and lifestyle in children. Eur J Pediatr. 2009;168:1259–67.

73. Negre CFA, Morzan UN, Hendrickson HP, et al. Eigenvector centrality for characterization of protein allosteric pathways. Proc Natl Acad Sci U S A. 2021;115:12201–8.

74. Oshinubi K, BuHamra S, Alkandari N, et al. Age dependent epidemic modelling of COVID-19 outbreak in Kuwait, France and Cameroon. Healthcare. 2022a;10:482.

75. Oshinubi K, Fougère C, Demongeot J. A model for the lifespan loss due to a viral disease: example of the COVID-19 outbreak. Infect Dis Rep. 2022b;14:321–40.

76. Parmer T, Rocha LM, Radicchi F. Influence maximization in Boolean networks. Nat Commun. 2022;13: 3457.

77. Pereira G, Christian H, Foster S, et al. The association between neighborhood greenness and weight status: an observational study in Perth Western Australia. Environ Health. 2013;12:49.

78. Po'e EK, Heerman WJ, Mistry RS, et al. Growing right onto wellness (grow): a family-centered, community-based obesity prevention randomized controlled trial for preschool child parent pairs. Contemp Clin Trials. 2013;36:436–49.

79. Rizzuto D, Fratiglioni L. Lifestyle factors related to mortality and survival: amini-review. Gerontology. 2014;60:327–35.

80. Rohrmann S, Shiels MS, Lopez DS, et al. Body fatness and sex steroid hormone concentrations in US men: results from NHANES III. Cancer Causes Control. 2011;22:1141–51.

81. Salganik MJ, Heckathorn DD. Sampling and estimation in hidden populations using respondent-driven sampling. Sociol Methodol. 2004;34:193–240.

82. Sánchez-Villegas A, Madrigal H, Martínez-González M, et al. Perception of body image as indicator of weight status in the European Union. J Hum Nutr Diet. 2001;14:93–102.

83. Sanderson SC, Diefenbach MA, Streicher SA, et al. Genetic and lifestyle causal beliefs about obesity and associated diseases among ethnically diverse patients: a structured interview study. Public Health Genomics. 2013;16:83–93.

84. Saraswathi S, Mukhopadhyay A, Shah H, et al. Social network analysis of COVID-19 transmission in Karnataka. India Epidemiol Infect. 2020;148:e320.

85. Schaefer DR, Simpkins SD. Using social network analysis to clarify the role of obesity in selection of adolescent friends. Am J Public Health. 2014;104: 1223–9.

86. Seliske L, Pickett W, Rosu A, et al. The number and type of food retailers surrounding schools and their association with lunchtime eating behaviors in students. Int J Behav Nutr Phys Activity. 2013;10:19.

87. Shoham DA, Messer LC. Social network analysis for epidemiology. In: Oakes JM, Kaufman JS, editors. Methods in social epidemiology. 2nd ed. San Francisco: Jossey Bass; 2017. p. 212–38.

88. Simon GE, Von Kor M, Saunders K, et al. Association between obesity and psychiatric disorders in the US adult population. Arch Gen Psychiatry. 2006;63: 824–30.

89. Stark JH, Neckerman K, Lovasi GS. The impact of neighborhood park access and quality on body mass index among adults in New York city. Prev Med. 2014;64:63–8.

90. Story M, Nanney MS, Schwartz MB. Schools and obesity prevention: creating school environments and policies to promote healthy eating and physical activity. Milbank Q. 2009;87:71–100.

91. Suder A. Body fatness and its social and lifestyle determinants in young working males from Kracow, Poland. J Biosoc Sci. 2009;41:139–54.

92. Sutin AR, Costa PT Jr, Chan W, et al. I know not to, but I can't help it: weight gain and changes in impulsivity-related personality traits. Psychol Sci. 2013;24:1323–8.

93. Taramasco C, Demongeot J. Collective intelligence, social networks and propagation of a social disease, the obesity. In: EIDWT'11, IEEE Proceedings, Piscataway. 2011;86–90.

94. Tzanetakou IP, Katsilambros NL, Benetos A, et al. Is obesity linked to aging? Adipose tissue and the role of telomeres. Ageing Res Rev. 2012;11:220–9.

95. Valente TW, Fujimoto K, Chou CP, Spruijt-Metz D. Adolescent affiliations and adiposity: asocial network analysis of friendships and obesity. J Adolesc Health. 2009;45:202–4.

96. Viner R, Haines MM, Taylor SJ, et al. Bodymass, weight control behaviors, weight perception and emotional wellbeing in a multiethnic sample of early adolescents. Int J Obes. 2006;30:1514.

97. Wamala SP, Wolk A, Orth-Gomér K. Determinants of obesity in relation to socio-economic status among middle-aged Swedish women. Prev Med. 1997;26: 734–44.

98. Withall R, Jago R, Fox KR. The effect a of community-based social marketing campaign on recruitment and retention of low-income groups into physical activity programmes – a controlled before-and-after study. BMC Public Health. 2012;12:836.

99. Xu X, Short SE, Liu T. Dynamic relations between fast-food restaurant and body weight status: longitudinal and multilevel analysis of Chinese adults. J Epidemiol Community Health. 2013;67:271–9.

100. Xu Z, Yang D, Wang L, et al. Statistical analysis supports UTR (untranslated region) deletion theory in SARS-CoV-2. Virulence. 2022;13:1772–89.

101. Xu Z, Wei D, Zeng Q, et al. More or less deadly? A mathematical model that predicts 1 SARS-CoV-2 evolutionary direction. Comput Biol Med. 2023;153:106510.

Part IV

Pathophysiology

Principles of Energy Homeostasis

14

Rexford S. Ahima

Contents

Abstract

Mammals have evolved complex mechanisms to obtain energy from food; store excess energy in the forms of glycogen, fat, and protein; and utilize energy efficiently for vital functions. Obesity develops when energy intake exceeds energy expenditure. While obesity treatment is mostly focused on reducing food intake, studies suggest that increasing energy expenditure through physical activity and adaptive thermogenesis is an important strategy for sustaining weight loss and improving health. This chapter will describe fundamental concepts of bioenergetics and provide a framework for understanding the pathogenesis and treatment of metabolic syndrome.

Keywords

Obesity · Diet · Energy intake · Energy expenditure · ATP · Thermogenesis · Physical activity

R. S. Ahima (✉)
Department of Medicine, Division of Endocrinology, Diabetes and Metabolism, Johns Hopkins University School of Medicine, Baltimore, MD, USA
e-mail: ahima@jhmi.edu

© Springer Nature Switzerland AG 2023
R. S. Ahima (ed.), *Metabolic Syndrome*,
https://doi.org/10.1007/978-3-031-40116-9_48

Introduction

Energy metabolism is controlled by genetic and environmental factors which affect energy intake and energy expenditure (Fig. 1a). Energy balance is attained when energy intake is equal to energy expenditure. When energy intake exceeds energy expenditure, a state of positive energy balance occurs, and this leads to obesity, a condition characterized by increased body weight, especially fat, in adipose tissue and other organs. A state of negative energy balance ensues when energy intake in markedly reduced in relation to energy expenditure. There is profound individual variability in the time to attain energy balance and the patterns of weight gain and weight loss. Over the past three decades, we have gained substantial insights into the genetic, epigenetic, and environmental factors favoring overeating, obesity, and metabolic syndrome [45, 62]. It is difficult to lose weight and maintain weight loss over long periods due to metabolic, behavioral, neuroendocrine, and autonomic responses that promote weight regain and maintain energy stores in adipose tissue [1, 28, 45, 62]. Multiple neuronal and hormonal signals oppose the state of weight reduction and predispose toward positive energy storage. For example, the fall in leptin counteracts weight loss by stimulating appetite and decreasing energy expenditure [1]. Hyperinsulinemia promotes energy storage in the forms of glycogen, fat, and protein [45, 62]. Important inferences about the pathogenesis and treatment of obesity and metabolic syndrome can be drawn from fundamental concepts of energy metabolism.

Energy Intake

Energy needed for metabolic and physiological functions is derived from the chemical energy bound in macronutrient components of food, i.e., carbohydrates, fats, proteins, and ethanol. Food digestion is facilitated by cooking, chewing, mixing with saliva, gastric movements, and enzymes which blend the food into chyme [20, 77]. In the upper intestine, the chyme is digested further to produce glucose, fatty acids, and amino acids which are absorbed [20, 77]. The chemical energy in nutrients is released and converted into heat, mechanical, and other forms of energy. Fats and carbohydrates are the main sources of dietary energy [33, 37]. Proteins are also an important source of energy, especially when total dietary energy intake is limited [33, 37]. Ethanol is often overlooked as a source of energy in food, but its contribution to total energy intake is significant in people who regularly consume alcoholic beverages [33].

The unit of energy in the International System of Units is the joule (J), which is the energy expended when 1 kg is moved 1 meter by a force of 1 Newton [37]. The conversion factors for joules and calories are 1 kJ = 0.239 kcal and 1 kcal = 4.184 kJ. The *ingested energy* (IE) or gross energy (GE) is the maximum amount of energy measured after complete combustion to carbon dioxide and water in a bomb calorimeter. Incomplete digestion of food in the small intestine, and fermentation of unabsorbed carbohydrate in the colon, results in the loss of *fecal energy* (FE) and *gaseous energy* (GaE). Short-chain fatty acids are formed in the intestine, some of which are absorbed and available as energy. Some energy is lost as *urinary energy* (UE) in the form of urea and other nitrogenous waste compounds derived from incomplete catabolism of protein. Food energy remaining after accounting for these losses is known as *metabolizable energy* (ME), most of which is available for ATP production. Some of the ME is utilized during metabolic processes associated with digestion, absorption, and intermediary metabolism of food and can be measured as heat production referred to as *diet-induced thermogenesis* (DIT) or *thermic effect of food* (TEF). The *net metabolizable energy* (NME) is obtained by subtracting the energy lost to microbial fermentation and DIT from the ME.

The ME was classically defined as the food energy available for heat production and later defined as the amount of energy available for whole body (total) heat production in a state of nitrogen and energy balance [37]. The NME is defined on the basis of the ATP-producing capacity of food instead of the total heat-producing

Fig. 1 (**a**) Energy homeostasis. Genetic and environmental factors affect food intake and energy expenditure. Energy balance is achieved when energy intake is equal to expenditure. Obesity is a state of positive energy balance in which the excess energy is stored mainly as fat. (**b**) Body energy stores of a lean 70 kg man

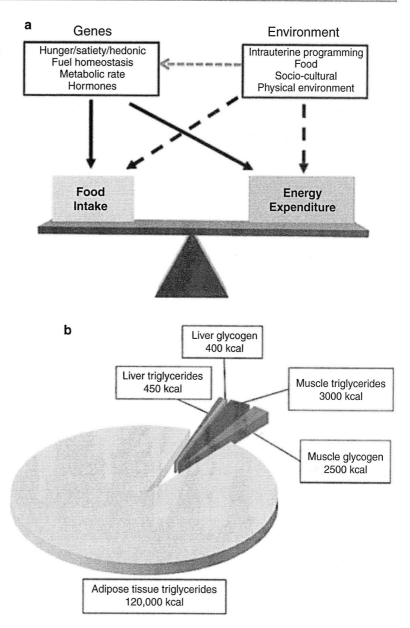

capacity. Strictly, the NME refers to the food energy available for body functions requiring ATP. The measurement of *food energy content* is by chemical analysis or estimated from food composition tables. The Atwater general factor system of food energy is based on the heat of combustion of protein, fat, and carbohydrate, corrected for energy losses via digestion, absorption, and urinary excretion. The ME values are 17 kJ/g (4.0 kcal/g) for protein, 37 kJ/g (9.0 kcal/g) for fat, 17 kJ/g (4.0 kcal/g) for carbohydrates, and 29 kJ/g (7.0 kcal/g) for ethanol [33, 37].

Dietary recommendations must meet energy requirements in addition to providing all essential nutrients necessary for attainment and maintenance of optimal health and physiological functions. The daily human energy requirement is estimated from the measurement of energy expenditure plus the extra energy needed for growth, pregnancy, and lactation. A state of *energy balance* is attained when the dietary energy intake is equal to total energy expenditure. A person is considered to be in a *steady state* when the energy balance is maintained over a long period. Recommended food intake, referred to as *daily requirement* or *recommended daily intake*, represents an average of energy needs over a certain number of days and does not indicate exactly how much energy should be consumed daily. Energy requirements are estimated from data from group of individuals of the same gender, age, BMI, and *physical activity level* (PAL) [33, 37]. However, there are individual variations due to differences in lifestyle and other factors that alter energy requirements within a population [33, 37].

The *food energy density* is defined as the amount of energy contained in a gram of food. *Very low energy density foods* contain less than 0.6 calories/gram, e.g., lettuce, apple, tomato, strawberry, broccoli, grapefruit, nonfat milk, carrot, and vegetable soup. *Low energy density foods* contain 0.6–1.5 calories/gram, e.g., oatmeal, whole milk, beans, banana, broiled fish, fat-free yogurt, baked potato, and cooked whole grain rice. *Medium energy density foods* contain 1.5–4 calories/gram, e.g., egg, roast chicken, bagel, white bread, ham, cream cheese, raisin, pretzel, cake with frosting, and cheddar cheese. *High energy density foods* contain more than 4 calories/gram, e.g., mayonnaise dressing, chocolate chip cookies, potato chips, bacon, butter, and peanut butter. Low energy density foods have a high content of water, complex carbohydrate, and fiber content, while the high energy density foods have a low content of water and fiber content and a content of high sugar and fat.

Energy Expenditure

The daily energy expenditure consists of the sleeping metabolic rate and energy used during arousal. Energy expenditure decreases to a minimum during sleep and increases during arousal as a result of activity-induced energy expenditure and diet-induced energy expenditure (thermic effect of food). The daily energy expenditure varies as a function of body size and body composition (determinants of resting energy expenditure), food intake, and physical activity.

Basal metabolism. This refers to the energy required to maintain the functions essential for life, such as the maintenance of cellular structure, metabolic pathways, temperature, cardiorespiratory, and brain functions [11, 13, 36, 63, 64]. The basal metabolic rate (BMR), also known as the standard metabolic rate (SMR), is the rate of energy expenditure measured under standard conditions that include being awake in the supine position after 10–12 h of overnight fasting, 8 h of physical rest, a state of mental relaxation, and thermoneutral conditions, i.e., an environmental temperature that does not elicit heat generation or dissipation. The BMR is the largest component of energy expenditure and represents 45–70% of the daily total energy expenditure (TEE). The BMR is heritable, correlated with body size, body composition, sex, age, and sympathetic nervous system (SNS) activity [11, 14, 36, 63, 68, 78]. The fat-free mass (FFM) accounts for two-thirds of the BMR variance between individuals [12, 38]. Men have higher BMR compared to women, and aging is associated with a decline in BMR, and these differences are attributable to FFM [12, 38]. The BMR can be estimated based on age, sex, and weight (Table 1).

In contrast to the BMR, the resting metabolic rate (RMR) or resting energy expenditure (REE) measures the amount of energy used in a relaxed but not postabsorptive state and requires the subject to be in a thermoneutral environment [92]. The less stringent criteria make the RMR or REE more practical than BMR for clinical and research studies.

Energy expenditure related to feeding. Eating requires energy for ingestion and digestion of food and for absorption, transport, interconversion, oxidation, and storage of nutrients. The amount and content of food are determinants of *diet-induced energy expenditure (DEE)*, also known by various terms such as *thermic effect of food* (TEF), *diet-induced thermogenesis (DIT)*, and *specific dynamic action (SDA)* [16, 81]. The DEE is measured as the difference between energy expenditure after food consumption and resting energy expenditure (REE), divided by the

Table 1 Estimates of basal metabolic rate from body weight

Age (*years*)	BMR: MJ/day	BMR: kcal/day
Males		
<3	0.249 kg − 0.127	59.512 kg − 30.4
3–10	0.095 kg + 2.110	22.706 kg + 504.3
10–18	0.074 kg + 2.754	17.686 kg + 658.2
18–30	0.063 kg + 2.896	15.057 kg + 692.2
30–60	0.048 kg + 3.653	11.472 kg + 873.1
>60	0.049 kg + 2.459	11.711 kg + 587.7
Females		
<3	0.244 kg − 0.130	58.317 kg − 31.1
3–10	0.085 kg + 2.033	20.315 kg + 485.9
10–18	0.056 kg + 2.898	13.384 kg + 692.6
18–30	0.062 kg + 2.036	14.818 kg + 486.6
30–60	0.034 kg + 3.538	8.126 kg + 845.6
>60	0.038 kg + 2.755	9.082 kg + 658.5

rate of nutrient energy intake. The DEE is different for various ingested nutrients, 0–3% for fat, 5–10% for carbohydrate, and 20–30% for protein. In normal weight healthy subjects on a mixed diet and in energy balance, the DEE is estimated as 10% of the total amount of energy ingested over 24 hours.

Adaptive thermogenesis. This refers to heat production in response to ambient temperature. Cold exposure induces non-shivering thermogenesis in brown adipose tissue and shivering thermogenesis in skeletal muscle. Non-shivering thermogenesis is a major thermoregulatory mechanism against cold exposure in rodents, and it is mediated through activation of SNS activity and generation of heat by uncoupling protein (UCP)-1 [25]. As discussed later, browning of adipose tissue occurs in humans and plays an important role in adaptive thermogenesis and the pathogenesis of obesity.

Physical activity. Activity-induced energy expenditure (ΛEE), the most variable component of the total daily energy expenditure (TEE), is derived from total energy expenditure (TEE) minus resting energy expenditure (REE) and diet-induced energy expenditure (DEE). Physical activity may be divided into *obligatory* and *discretionary* activities. Obligatory activities include work, other daily activities such as self-care, caring for the family and other home activities, going to school, and other demands imposed by the economic, social, and cultural environment. Discretionary activities include exercise for fitness and health and other optional but desirable activities for social interaction. The physical activity level (PAL) can be estimated from the 24-h TEE and REE ratio (PAL = TEE/REE) [37]. A sedentary or light activity person has a PAL of 1.40–1.69, a moderately active or active person has a PAL of 1.70–1.99, and a very active person has a PAL of 2.0–2.4.

Growth, pregnancy, and lactation. The energy required for growth comprises of energy needed for the synthesis of growing tissues and energy deposited in growth tissues. The energy cost of growth is about 35% of TEE in the first 3 months of age, falls to 5% at 12 months and 3% in the second year, remains at 1–2% until mid-adolescence, and is minimal in the late teenage years [37]. During pregnancy, energy is needed for growth of the fetus, placenta, and maternal tissues, such as the uterus, breasts, and fat stores, as well as meeting the demands of maternal metabolism at rest and during physical activity. The energy cost of lactation comprises of energy required to produce and secrete breast milk. In addition to increasing their food intake, lactating women derive part of the higher energy requirement from fat stores accumulated during pregnancy.

Measurement of Energy Expenditure

The concept that energy expenditure is related to chemical combustion was proposed by Lavoisier [26]. Energy expenditure can be measured by *direct calorimetry*. The subject is housed in a testing chamber, the non-evaporative heat loss is measured from the temperature gradient across the walls of an insulated chamber, and evaporative heat loss is measured in the water vapor in the test chamber. The total heat loss is measured as the sum of evaporative and non-evaporative loss. *Direct calorimetry* is accurate, but it requires a specialized testing facility [34].

Indirect calorimetry is based on the principle that the combustion of food to generate energy requires oxygen consumption. *Indirect calorimetry* estimates energy expenditure from the rates of respiratory gas exchange and nitrogen excretion [48, 59]. The heat produced by the utilization of oxygen varies according to the contents of carbohydrate, fat, and protein. Indirect calorimetry is often used to measure BMR or RMR for hours using a ventilation hood or for days in a respiratory chamber. A constant supply of fresh air is provided to the subject, and the respiratory gas exchange is measured by analyzing the air inflow and outflow and the flow rate. Oxygen consumption, carbon dioxide production, and urinary nitrogen excretion are measured. Energy expenditure = MR (kcal/day) = 3.941 VO_2 (L/day) + 1.106 VCO_2 (L/day) − 2.17 N Urine (g/day), where MR = metabolic rate, VO_2 = oxygen consumption, VCO_2 = carbon dioxide production, and N Urine = nitrogen excreted in urine. The urinary nitrogen derived from incomplete combustion of protein is small, and it is estimated to be 12 g/day (0.5 g/h). The ratio of VCO_2 and VO_2 is known as the respiratory quotient (RQ) or respiratory exchange ratio (RER) and ranges from 0.7 to1.0. The RQ is 1 when carbohydrate is the sole fuel being oxidized and 0.7 when fat is the sole fuel being oxidized. The proportion of energy utilized from carbohydrate or fat can be estimated using standard equations [48, 59].

Indirect calorimetry techniques for the measurement of energy expenditure in humans utilize a facemask, ventilated hood, or respiration chamber (whole room calorimeter). A facemask is used to measure REE and physical activity (treadmill exercise) (AEE), and a ventilated hood encloses the head only and is used to measure REE and energy expenditure during nutrient digestion, absorption, and storage (DEE). A room calorimeter is an airtight room ventilated with fresh air. The subject is fully enclosed in the chamber which allows physical activity, and air is pumped in and blown out into a mixing chamber where samples are collected for measurements of oxygen and carbon dioxide.

The *doubly labeled water* technique is based on the principle that oxygen in the respiratory carbon dioxide is in equilibrium with the oxygen in the body water. The doubly labeled water technique involves enriching the body water with an isotope of oxygen and an isotope of hydrogen and then determining the washout kinetics. It allows the TEE to be measured in subjects under free-living conditions over a period of 1–4 weeks [61, 70, 76]. A single oral dose of water enriched in deuterium (^2H) and ^{18}oxygen (^{18}O) is given orally to label the body water. After equilibrium is reached in 3–6 h, ^{18}O is lost as $CO^{18}O$ and H_2 ^{18}O, and deuterium is lost in water. ^{18}O and ^2H enrichment is measured by isotope ratio mass spectrometry in the urine or saliva. Carbon dioxide production rate is based on the difference in turnover rates between the oxygen and hydrogen labels. The difference between the slopes for the log-transformed disappearance rates of ^2H and ^{18}O is proportional to the amount of carbon dioxide produced. Based on a 24-h respiratory quotient value of 0.85, the oxygen consumption and TEE values are calculated [61, 70, 76].

Assessment of body movement using *accelerometry* is a popular method for measuring physical activity [57]. Accelerometers can measure body movement and provide information about physical activity patterns over long periods. Recent advancements in sensor technologies have enabled the development of accelerometers with different capabilities. Piezo-resistive or piezo-capacitive sensors differentiate between physical activity intensity and postures. In order to capture physical activity patterns, the monitoring needs to be done over several days and weeks. Detection of specific types of activities may require a multiple sensor system [57]. It is noteworthy that accelerometers do not measure energy expenditure; therefore, the data may need to be compared to energy expenditure measured by the doubly labeled water method.

The TEE can be estimated by *factorial calculations* based on the time and energy cost of habitual activities [37] (Table 2). Factorial calculations combine the energy spent while sleeping, resting, working, and doing social or discretionary household and leisure activities, and the energy expenditure estimate is based on the time allocated to each activity and the corresponding energy cost.

Table 2 Factorial calculations of total energy expenditure

Main daily activities	Time allocation (h)	Energy cost[a] (PAR)	Time × energy cost	Mean PAL[b] (multiple of 24-h BMR)
Sedentary or light activity lifestyle				
Sleeping	8	1	8.0	
Personal care (dressing, bathing)	1	2.3	2.3	
Eating	1	1.5	1.5	
Cooking	1	2.1	2.1	
Sitting (e.g., office work, selling produce, tending shop)	8	1.5	12.0	
General household work	1	2.8	2.8	
Driving car to and from work	1	2.0	2.0	
Walking at varying paces without a load	1	3.2	3.2	
Light leisure activities (e.g., watching TV, chatting)	2	1.4	2.8	
Total	**24**		**36.7**	**36.7/24 = 1.53**
Active or moderately active lifestyle				
Sleeping	8	1	8.0	
Personal care (dressing, bathing)	1	2.3	2.3	
Eating	1	1.5	1.5	
Standing, carrying light loads (e.g., waiting on tables, arranging merchandise)[b]	8	2.2	17.6	
Commuting to and from work on the bus	1	1.2	1.2	
Walking at varying paces without a load	1	3.2	3.2	
Low intensity aerobic exercise	1	4.2	4.2	
Light leisure activities (e.g., watching TV, chatting)	3	1.4	4.2	
Total	**24**		**42.2**	**42.2/24 = 1.76**
Vigorous or vigorously active lifestyle				
Sleeping	8	1	8.0	
Personal care (dressing, bathing)	1	2.3	2.3	
Eating	1	1.4	1.4	
Cooking	1	2.1	2.1	
Non-mechanized strenuous work (e.g., agricultural work-planting, weeding, gathering)	6	4.1	24.6	
Collecting water and wood	1	4.4	4.4	
Non-mechanized domestic chores (sweeping, washing clothes and dishes by hand)	1	2.3	2.3	
Walking at varying paces without a load	1	3.2	3.2	
Miscellaneous light leisure activities	4	1.4	5.6	
Total	**24**		**53.9**	**53.9/24 = 2.25**

[a]Energy costs of activities expressed as multiples of the BMR or PAR
[b]Composite of the energy cost of standing, walking slowly, and serving meals or carrying a light load
[c]PAL = physical activity level or energy requirement expressed as a multiple of 24-h BMR

Energy Partitioning

Most of the energy in the body is stored as fat in adipose tissue (Fig. 1b). Figure 2 shows the weights and energy expenditure of key metabolic organs that contribute to the total energy expenditure. Various organs are involved in the production, storage, and utilization of energy [23, 24, 31, 62, 65, 71, 74] (Fig. 3). The liver is the main distributor of energy to other organs and maintains blood glucose levels within a narrow range

Fig. 2 (a) Organ weight (% body weight) and (b) organ energy expenditure (% whole body energy expenditure) in a healthy adult (Adapted from Ref. [42]. This is an open access article under the terms of the Creative Commons Attribution License, which permits use, distribution, and reproduction in any medium, provided the original work is properly cited)

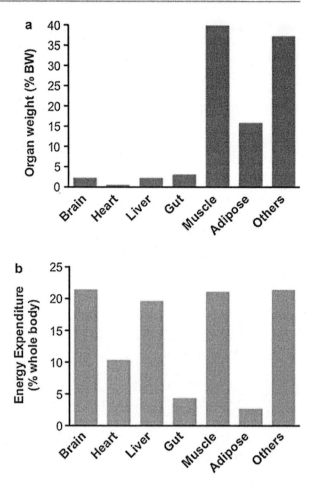

in response to intermittent food intake. The liver also produces urea and other nitrogenous waste products. After a carbohydrate-rich meal, glucose enters hepatocytes via GLUT2, and the glucose is phosphorylated by glucokinase to form glucose 6-phosphate (G6-P). Glucokinase has a higher Km for glucose, 10 mM, than other hexokinase isozymes, which allows hepatocytes to continue phosphorylating glucose when the blood glucose concentration is very high after eating. Conversely, the high Km of glucokinase limits glucose phosphorylation when the blood glucose concentration is low during fasting, thereby preventing the liver from consuming glucose. During fasting, G6-P is dephosphorylated by G6-Pase to supply blood glucose to the brain and other tissues. Some of the G6-P undergoes glycolysis to form pyruvate, decarboxylated to form acetyl-CoA, which is then oxidized by the citric acid

cycle to produce ATP. Acetyl-CoA also serves as a precursor of fatty acids, used for triglyceride, phospholipid, and cholesterol synthesis. G6-P can also enter the pentose phosphate pathway, producing NADPH for the synthesis of fatty acids and cholesterol and D-ribose 5-phosphate, a precursor for nucleotides.

Amino acids entering hepatocytes are used as precursors for protein synthesis or exported to other organs. Amino acids are transaminated, deaminated, and degraded in hepatocytes to produce pyruvate and other intermediates in the citric acid cycle. Ammonia released from amino acid catabolism is excreted as urea. Pyruvate generated from amino acids is converted to glucose and glycogen via gluconeogenesis, or to acetyl-CoA to be oxidized via the citric acid cycle and oxidative phosphorylation to produce ATP or converted to lipids. During the period between meals, a

a

Metabolic Pathways	Brain	Heart	Skeletal Muscle	GI Tract	Liver	Adipose Tissue
Gluconeogenesis I, II, III (PYR→GAP,GAP →G6P, G6P →GLC)					▓	
Glycogen synthesis (GLY →G6P)	▓				▓	
Glycogenolysis (G6P→GLY)	▓				▓	
Fatty acid synthesis (ACoA→FFA)						▓
Fatty acid oxidation (FFA →ACoA)		▓	▓		▓	
Lipolysis (TG→FFA+GLR)			▓			▓
TG synthesis (FFA+GRP→TG)			▓	▓		▓
Glycerol phosphorylation (GLR→GRP)			▓		▓	
GAP reduction (GAP→GRP)						▓
GRP oxidation (GRP→GAP)					▓	
Alanine breakdown (ALA→PYR)					▓	
Alanine synthesis (PYR→ALA)			▓			
Protein breakdown (Protein→ALA)			▓			

b

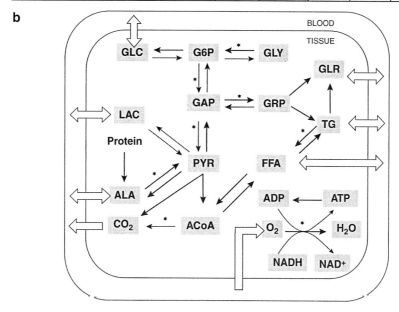

Fig. 3 (**a**) Organ-specific pathways for energy metabolism. Gray panels indicate the existence of a particular metabolic pathway. (**b**) Cellular metabolism of carbohydrate, fat, and amino acid. Abbreviations: *ADP* adenosine diphosphate, *ATP* adenosine triphosphate, *ACoA* acetyl-CoA, *AA* amino acids, *GLC* glucose, *G6P* glucose-6-phosphate, *GAP* glyceraldehyde-3-phosphate, *GLR* glycerol, *GRP* glycerol-3-phosphate, *GLY* glycogen, *FFA* free fatty acid, *LAC* lactate, *PYR* pyruvate, *TG* triglycerides (Adapted from Ref. [42]. This is an open access article under the terms of the Creative Commons Attribution License, which permits use, distribution, and reproduction in any medium, provided the original work is properly cited)

small amount of muscle protein is degraded to amino acids, which donate their amino groups via transamination to pyruvate, producing alanine, which is transported to the liver and deaminated into pyruvate, which is then converted to glucose via gluconeogenesis.

The liver plays an important role in lipid metabolism. Triglycerides are synthesized de novo or from the esterification of glycerol and fatty acyl-CoA. Fatty acids are the primary fuel for oxidative metabolism in hepatocytes, generating acetyl-CoA and NADH. Acetyl-CoA is oxidized via the citric acid cycle to produce ATP, and the excess acetyl-CoA is converted to acetoacetate and beta-hydroxybutyrate. These ketones are important fuels for the heart and brain during prolonged fasting. Acetyl-CoA derived from fatty acids is used for the synthesis of cholesterol, needed for membrane assembly, and for the synthesis of steroid hormones and bile salts. Fatty acids are also converted to phospholipids and triglycerides, which are exported via lipoproteins to adipose tissue for storage. Nonesterified fatty acids are bound to serum albumin and transported to the heart and skeletal muscles to be used as fuel.

White adipose tissue (WAT) is the main energy storage organ and comprises 15–20% of the mass of a normal adult (Fig. 1b). Adipocytes interact with the brain, liver, skeletal muscles, heart, and other organs. During periods of high carbohydrate intake, adipocytes are capable of converting glucose into fatty acids and fatty acids to triglycerides. However, most of the triglycerides stored in human adipocytes are derived from the VLDL exported from liver and chylomicrons from the intestinal tract. When energy demand rises, adipocyte lipases release free fatty acids from triglycerides which are transported to skeletal muscles and heart. Epinephrine stimulates adipocyte lipolysis via hormone-sensitive lipase (HSL), while insulin inhibits lipolysis. Most of the fatty acids generated by triacylglycerol lipase in adipocytes are re-esterified to triglycerides by glycerol kinase which uses glycerol phosphate derived mainly from pyruvate via glyceroneogenesis.

Skeletal muscle performs mechanical work necessary for maintaining body posture, breathing, and locomotion. Type I (slow-twitch; red) myofiber has low tension, is highly resistant to fatigue, and produces ATP via oxidative phosphorylation. Red muscle fiber is very rich in mitochondria and blood supply. Type II (fast-twitch; white) myofiber has fewer mitochondria than red muscle, is less vascular, generates greater tension and faster contraction, and is quicker to fatigue. Resting muscle uses mostly free fatty acids from adipose tissue and ketone bodies from the liver. These fuels are oxidized and degraded into acetyl-CoA, which enters the citric acid cycle for oxidative phosphorylation and ATP production. Moderately active muscle uses glucose in addition to fatty acids and ketones. The glucose is converted to pyruvate via glycolysis and then to acetyl-CoA and oxidized via the citric acid cycle. Maximum contraction of fast-twitch muscle rapidly depletes ATP, and this cannot be replenished by aerobic respiration. Glycogen stored in muscle is broken down to produce lactate, but the amount of glycogen in skeletal muscle is small and cannot sustain glycolysis during prolonged exercise. Thus, skeletal muscle also generates phosphocreatine to provide energy. After exercise, the lactate is transported from muscle to liver, and glucose is produced via gluconeogenesis and transported back to muscle to replenish the glycogen stores.

The brain has a very active oxidative metabolism, accounting for about 20% of oxygen consumption. The brain uses glucose as its main fuel, but it can also use fatty acids and ketones during starvation. The liver is the main source of glucose for the brain. Neurons metabolize glucose via glycolysis and the citric acid cycle, and this provides most of the ATP needed to establish and maintain the membrane electrical potential and also generate action potentials during neurotransmission.

Hormones Mediating Energy Homeostasis

The effects of gut hormones, adipokines, and other circulating factors involved in energy metabolism are described in other chapters. The blood glucose concentration is maintained within a narrow range around 4.5 mM. During feeding, insulin stimulates glucose uptake by muscle and adipose tissue and stimulates the synthesis of glycogen and triglycerides from glucose. Excess triglycerides are exported from the liver as VLDL. Insulin stimulates triglyceride synthesis in adipocytes from fatty acids released from the VLDL. During fasting, glucagon and epinephrine levels are increased and stimulate glycogenolysis by activating glycogen phosphorylase and inactivating glycogen synthase. As fasting is prolonged, glucagon inhibits glucose breakdown via glycolysis in the liver and stimulates glucose synthesis by gluconeogenesis by reducing the concentration of fructose 2,6-bisphosphate, an allosteric inhibitor of fructose 1,6-bisphosphatase and an activator of phosphofructokinase. Glucagon inhibits pyruvate kinase, leading to accumulation of phosphoenolpyruvate, which drives gluconeogenesis. Glucagon also stimulates the synthesis of phosphoenolpyruvate carboxykinase (PEPCK) which promotes gluconeogenesis. Ultimately, these effects of glucagon culminate in an increase in hepatic glucose output to supply glucose to the brain and other vital organs. During prolonged fasting, the fall in insulin and rise in glucagon and epinephrine levels trigger a switch from carbohydrate-based to fat-based metabolism. Epinephrine stimulates acetyl-CoA production via fatty acid oxidation and promotes the formation of ketones which are exported from the liver to heart, skeletal muscle, and brain to be used as energy substrates.

The conversion of cortisol to active or inactive metabolites has profound effects on carbohydrate, fat, and protein metabolism. Plasma cortisol is increased during starvation, acute infection, and in response to other stressors and stimulates glucose production, lipolysis, and proteolysis. In contrast to glucagon and epinephrine, cortisol acts relatively slowly through nuclear transcriptional mechanisms to control energy metabolism.

Brown Adipose Thermogenesis

Oxidative metabolism occurs within mitochondria through the citric acid cycle and electron transport chain [26]. Oxygen is consumed, water and carbon dioxide are produced, and the ATP generated is used for various cellular functions, including the maintenance of Na^+/K^+ and Ca^{2+} pumps. H^+, Na^+, K^+, and Ca^{2+} leak across membrane channels along electrochemical gradients, and the H^+ leak dissipates free energy in the form of heat and decreases the amount of ATP generated per molecule of oxygen split by the electron transport chain [30]. The *uncoupling* of oxidative phosphorylation is very prominent in brown adipose tissue (BAT) and is mediated by UCP1, a 32 kDa protein located in the inner mitochondrial transmembrane of brown adipocytes, which allows protons to reenter the mitochondrial matrix from the inner membrane space. BAT uses glucose and fatty acids as fuel, and the heat is liberated by H^+ rushing down its electrochemical gradient. BAT plays a critical role in thermogenesis in rodents [21, 22, 25, 40]. UCP1-deficient mice are hypersensitive to cold temperature and prone to obesity, whereas UCP1 expression in WAT results prevents obesity [21, 22, 40, 41].

BAT is located in the interscapular region of neonates, and it has been detected in the cervical and supraclavicular regions of adults, using ^{18}F-FDG-PET-CT scans and histological analysis of fat biopsies [18, 69, 85, 89, 96]. BAT activity is increased in response to cold exposure, β_3-adrenergic agonist, and ephedrine and results in weight loss [5, 6, 8, 72, 93]. Other factors implicated in the browning of adipose tissue include thyroid hormone, bile acids, leptin, melanocortin-4-receptor agonists, and FGF-21 [29].

Muscle Thermogenesis

Skeletal muscle makes up 45–55% body mass in mammals, is the major determinant of the basal metabolic rate, and increases energy expenditure through exercise and non-exercise physical activity. Skeletal muscle is the main site of insulin-stimulated and non-insulin dependent glucose uptake, thus serving a major role in glucose homeostasis and pathophysiology of type 2 diabetes. During acute exercise, skeletal muscle utilizes locally stored glycogen, and during prolonged physical activity, skeletal muscle switches from carbohydrate to fatty acid oxidation.

Skeletal muscle plays an important role in thermogenesis [65, 86, 90, 95]. Fidgeting and other non-exercise activities dissipate heat and prevent obesity [35, 46, 97]. Shivering thermogenesis occurs in skeletal muscle in response to cold exposure [86, 95]. Chronic exercise increases the expression of genes involved in mitochondrial respiration and fatty acid oxidation, which protect against obesity, diabetes, and hyperlipidemia [90]. Cold exposure also promotes a switch from white (glycolytic) to red (oxidative) myofibers by inducing the expression of nuclear coactivator PGC1α, which is also induced in brown fat in response to cold [47, 58].

Another mechanism for skeletal muscle thermogenesis is linked to the control of ATP turnover and Ca^{2+} gradient by the sarcoplasmic reticulum Ca^{2+} ATPase (SERCA) [9, 55]. Ca^{2+} promotes heat production from ATP hydrolysis during muscle relaxation or sustained contraction. The heat energy is released when the Ca^{2+} is pumped back into the sarcoplasmic reticulum by SERCA. Cold exposure induces the expression and activity of SERCA1 in skeletal muscle to increase muscle oxidative metabolism and heat production. Normally, the opening of sodium channels leads to the release of Ca^{2+} into the cytoplasm from sources outside the cell and the sarcoplasmic reticulum through ryanodine receptor (RyR). The RyR-mediated Ca^{2+} leak is an important mechanism for SERCA-activated heat production [9, 55]. Sarcolipin interacts with SERCA in the presence of Ca^{2+}, leading to uncoupling of the SERCA pump [9]. Mice lacking sarcolipin develop diet-induced obesity, confirming an important role of this pathway in muscle thermogenesis and energy homeostasis [9].

Energy Dysregulation in Obesity

The worldwide increase in obesity and metabolic syndrome is attributed to overconsumption of food, especially energy-dense foods rich in fat and sugar. The excess energy is deposited mainly as fat in adipose tissue, as well as in the liver, muscle, pancreatic beta-cells, and other tissues. Ectopic fat deposition (steatosis) leads to insulin resistance, oxidative injury, inflammation, and other changes that predispose to type 2 diabetes and greater cardiovascular risk. Food restriction is the main strategy for obesity treatment, but this alone is often unsuccessful due to an adaptive reduction in energy expenditure, increased hunger, and other physiological and behavioral responses that oppose weight loss [4, 44, 73, 75, 82, 94]. Discoveries in molecular genetics, in addition to population and laboratory studies, have enriched our knowledge of mechanisms underlying obesity and related diseases. Pathway analyses provide strong support for genetic loci related to CNS circuits and molecules related to energy metabolism and glucose homeostasis [49, 51, 52].

Some studies have demonstrated associations of RMR, TEF, RQ, or SNS activity with weight gain or weight loss [2, 7, 23, 31, 60, 68, 74, 78, 82]. A seminal experiment by Bouchard et al. [15] showed that monozygotic twins who were overfed displayed similar gains in body weight and fat between each twin pair, indicating a strong genetic influence on energy metabolism. It is possible that genetic factors predispose toward obesity by affecting multiple factors, such as food digestion, absorption, availability of metabolizable energy (ME), TEF, and mitochondrial energy metabolism. Reduced physical activity is often cited as a cause of obesity, but the evidence is debatable. Some studies have suggested that the increasing obesity trend parallels the sedentary lifestyle in various populations [17, 80]. Non-exercise physical activity may prevent the development of obesity [87]. Reduced physical activity may predispose to sarcopenia, insulin resistance, and metabolic syndrome, especially among older people [10, 39]. However, other researchers have found no major changes in physical activity to explain the increasing trend of obesity [91]. It has been proposed that energy balance may be easier to achieve at a higher level of energy expenditure [32]. Above a threshold physical activity level, the energy intake and energy expenditure are very sensitive to changes in each other within the "regulated zone" of energy balance [32]. In contrast, the energy intake and expenditure are weakly sensitive to changes in each other in the "unregulated zone" below the physical activity threshold, and this promotes overeating and weight regain following caloric restriction [32].

Attempts at weight loss are popular worldwide, and the initial weight loss through dieting is often successful, but the long-term maintenance of lost weight is challenging [4, 75]. Typically, dietary interventions result in early rapid weight loss, followed by weight plateau, and then progressive regain [4, 75]. A meta-analysis of weight loss studies involving hypocaloric diets showed that more than 50% of the initial lost weight was regained after 2 years, and more than 75% was regained after 5 years [4]. In the Look AHEAD study, patients with overweight and type 2 diabetes lost significant weight from intensive lifestyle intervention, structured meal plans and meal replacements during the first year; however, 50% of the initial weight lost was regained and persisted until 8 years [50]. Even bariatric surgery, which produces sustained weight loss, may be followed by weight regain [54].

Health care providers often advise patients that a modest caloric restriction will result in weight loss, one pound for 3500 kcal of calorie deficit, and this weight loss is progressive. For example, eliminating one can of soda, 300 kcal per day, is predicted to decrease body weight by 30 pounds in a year [28]. When patients fail to achieve and maintain this weight loss target, they are blamed for lacking in willpower. This weight loss dogma is based on the assumption that energy is stored in body fat. Weight reduction from the loss of body water, and the profound and sustained fall in energy expenditure resulting from caloric restriction are not considered [28, 66]. Endocrine and metabolic adaptations during weight loss trigger feedback regulation of food intake, and these mechanisms oppose continued weight loss and long-term weight maintenance.

Weight loss and weight regain are both influenced by biological, environmental, and social factors [3] (Fig. 4). Altering the macronutrient composition of diets has been proposed as a means of regulating hunger, satiety, and energy storage in adipose tissue. For example, low-carbohydrate/high-fat diets have been claimed to provide evidence for the "carbohydrate-insulin model of obesity," which posits that diets high in carbohydrates stimulate insulin secretion, which blunts fat oxidation and promotes fat accumulation, resulting in cellular energy starvation, which then drives hunger and overeating suppresses energy expenditure, and increases energy storage in adipose tissue [53]. However, contrary to the expectation of the carbohydrate-insulin model, eating a low-carbohydrate diet does not produce long-term weight loss [83]. Diets with higher protein content may increase satiety and energy expenditure but have no long-term benefit on weight loss [43]. Overall, long-term diet trials have not shown superiority of one diet over another with respect to weight loss.

Various mechanisms have been proposed to explain individual variability in obesity, weight loss, and weight regain. When a person gains weight, the excess energy is stored as triglycerides predominantly in existing adipocytes, leading to the formation of large hypertrophic adipocytes [84]. In the YoYo study, the adipocyte size decreased during weight loss on a 12-week low-calorie diet or a 5-week very-low-calorie diet, and similar to animal studies, there was an increase in the number of small adipocytes, a reduction in large adipocytes, and gradual restoration of adipocytes to their original size during weight regain [67, 88]. Studies have also shown changes in adipose stress markers, extracellular matrix remodeling, inflammatory cells, and insulin sensitivity during weight loss and weight regain [84]. Blood markers include lipid metabolites, adipokines, and inflammatory and oxidative stress markers [27, 56, 79]. Leptin is decreased and ghrelin is increased during weight loss, but these changes are not reliable predictors of weight regain [79].

Conclusions

The mechanisms of energy metabolism respond more robustly to negative energy balance than to positive energy balance. The energy balance

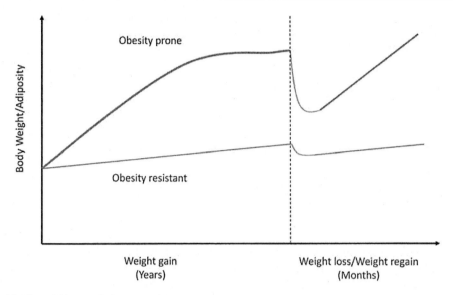

Fig. 4 (a) Natural history of obesity, weight loss, and weight regain in obesity-prone versus obesity-resistant individuals. Biological, environmental, and social factors affect the development of obesity. Typically, dietary interventions result in weight loss followed by weight regain

concept predicts that it would be easier to prevent the transition from a normal to obese weight than to produce a sustained weight loss in an obese person [19]. This concept offers a rational biological basis for the implementation of obesity prevention programs, aimed at promoting healthier food choices, increasing energy expenditure through physical activity in individuals and among the wider population, and developing cognitive skills and behaviors to sustain long-term healthy weight [19]. Obesity prevention demands changes in the "built environment" and a transformation of societal perceptions and practices regarding the causes and treatment of obesity and related diseases.

A better understanding of the principles of bioenergetics will facilitate new preventive and treatment approaches for obesity and metabolic diseases. Novel technologies to precisely measure energy intake, expenditure, and storage under free-living conditions will help in the development of accurate diagnostic tools and a better stratification of metabolic syndrome risk. Bioenergetic pathways of the gastrointestinal tract, liver, brown fat, white fat, skeletal muscle, and other tissues need to be thoroughly investigated to determine their contributions to whole body metabolism and how these pathways can be targeted specifically and safely for therapeutic purposes.

Cross-References

▷ Body Composition Assessment
▷ Carbohydrate, Protein, and Fat Metabolism in Obesity
▷ Diet and Obesity
▷ Overview of Metabolic Syndrome
▷ Sarcopenic Obesity
▷ The Built Environment and Metabolic Syndrome

Acknowledgments This work was supported by grants R01DK135751 and RF1 AG059621 from the US National Institutes of Health, and American Heart Association Obesity Research Network, and Cardiometabolic Health and Type 2 Diabetes Research Network.

References

1. Ahima RS. Digging deeper into obesity. J Clin Invest. 2011;121(6):2076–9. https://doi.org/10.1172/JCI58719.
2. Amatruda JM, Statt MC, Welle SL. Total and resting energy expenditure in obese women reduced to ideal body weight. J Clin Invest. 1993;92(3):1236–42. https://doi.org/10.1172/JCI116695.

3. Anastasiou CA, Karfopoulou E, Yannakoulia M. Weight regaining: from statistics and behaviors to physiology and metabolism. Metabolism. 2015;64(11):1395–407. https://doi.org/10.1016/j.metabol.2015.08.006. Epub 2015 Aug 15.

4. Anderson JW, Konz EC, Frederich RC, Wood CL. Long-term weight-loss maintenance: a meta-analysis of US studies. Am J Clin Nutr. 2001;74(5):579–84.

5. Astrup A. Thermogenesis in human brown adipose tissue and skeletal muscle induced by sympathomimetic stimulation. Acta Endocrinol Suppl (Copenh). 1986;278:1–32.

6. Astrup A, Bulow J, Madsen J, Christensen NJ. Contribution of BAT and skeletal muscle to thermogenesis induced by ephedrine in man. Am J Phys. 1985;248(5 Pt 1):E507–15.

7. Astrup A, Gotzsche PC, van de Werken K, Ranneries C, Toubro S, Raben A, Buemann B. Meta-analysis of resting metabolic rate in formerly obese subjects. Am J Clin Nutr. 1999;69(6):1117–22.

8. Baba S, Tatsumi M, Ishimori T, Lilien DL, Engles JM, Wahl RL. Effect of nicotine and ephedrine on the accumulation of 18F-FDG in brown adipose tissue. J Nucl Med. 2007;48(6):981–6. https://doi.org/10.2967/jnumed.106.039065.

9. Bal NC, Maurya SK, Sopariwala DH, Sahoo SK, Gupta SC, Shaikh SA, Pant M, Rowland LA, Bombardier E, Goonasekera SA, Tupling AR, Molkentin JD, Periasamy M. Sarcolipin is a newly identified regulator of muscle-based thermogenesis in mammals. Nat Med. 2012;18(10):1575–9. https://doi.org/10.1038/nm.2897.

10. Batsis JA, Mackenzie TA, Barre LK, Lopez-Jimenez F, Bartels SJ. Sarcopenia, sarcopenic obesity and mortality in older adults: results from the National Health and Nutrition Examination Survey III. Eur J Clin Nutr. 2014;68(9):1001–7. https://doi.org/10.1038/ejcn.2014.117.

11. Bogardus C, Lillioja S, Ravussin E, Abbott W, Zawadzki JK, Young A, Knowler WC, Jacobowitz R, Moll PP. Familial dependence of the resting metabolic rate. N Engl J Med. 1986;315(2):96–100. https://doi.org/10.1056/NEJM198607103150205.

12. Bosy-Westphal A, Eichhorn C, Kutzner D, Illner K, Heller M, Muller MJ. The age-related decline in resting energy expenditure in humans is due to the loss of fat-free mass and to alterations in its metabolically active components. J Nutr. 2003;133(7):2356–62.

13. Bosy-Westphal A, Reinecke U, Schlorke T, Illner K, Kutzner D, Heller M, Muller MJ. Effect of organ and tissue masses on resting energy expenditure in underweight, normal weight and obese adults. Int J Obes Relat Metab Disord. 2004;28(1):72–9. https://doi.org/10.1038/sj.ijo.0802526.

14. Bouchard C, Tremblay A, Nadeau A, Despres JP, Theriault G, Boulay MR, Lortie G, Leblanc C, Fournier G. Genetic effect in resting and exercise metabolic rates. Metab Clin Exp. 1989;38(4):364–70.

15. Bouchard C, Tremblay A, Despres JP, Nadeau A, Lupien PJ, Theriault G, Dussault J, Moorjani S, Pinault S, Fournier G. The response to long-term overfeeding in identical twins. N Engl J Med. 1990;322(21):1477–82. https://doi.org/10.1056/NEJM199005243222101.

16. Brundin T, Thorne A, Wahren J. Heat leakage across the abdominal wall and meal-induced thermogenesis in normal-weight and obese subjects. Metab Clin Exp. 1992;41(1):49–55.

17. Caleyachetty R, Echouffo-Tcheugui JB, Tait CA, Schilsky S, Forrester T, Kengne AP. Prevalence of behavioural risk factors for cardiovascular disease in adolescents in low-income and middle-income countries: an individual participant data meta-analysis. Lancet Diabetes Endocrinol. 2015;3:535. https://doi.org/10.1016/S2213-8587(15)00076-5.

18. Cypess AM, Lehman S, Williams G, Tal I, Rodman D, Goldfine AB, Kuo FC, Palmer EL, Tseng YH, Doria A, Kolodny GM, Kahn CR. Identification and importance of brown adipose tissue in adult humans. N Engl J Med. 2009;360(15):1509–17. https://doi.org/10.1056/NEJMoa0810780.

19. Eckel RH, Kahn SE, Ferrannini E, Goldfine AB, Nathan DM, Schwartz MW, Smith RJ, Smith SR. Obesity and type 2 diabetes: what can be unified and what needs to be individualized? J Clin Endocrinol Metab. 2011;96(6):1654–63. https://doi.org/10.1210/jc.2011-0585.

20. Elia M, Cummings JH. Physiological aspects of energy metabolism and gastrointestinal effects of carbohydrates. Eur J Clin Nutr. 2007;61(Suppl 1):S40–74. https://doi.org/10.1038/sj.ejcn.1602938.

21. Enerback S, Jacobsson A, Simpson EM, Guerra C, Yamashita H, Harper ME, Kozak LP. Mice lacking mitochondrial uncoupling protein are cold-sensitive but not obese. Nature. 1997;387(6628):90–4. https://doi.org/10.1038/387090a0.

22. Feldmann HM, Golozoubova V, Cannon B, Nedergaard J. UCP1 ablation induces obesity and abolishes diet-induced thermogenesis in mice exempt from thermal stress by living at thermoneutrality. Cell Metab. 2009;9(2):203–9. https://doi.org/10.1016/j.cmet.2008.12.014.

23. Flatt JP, Ravussin E, Acheson KJ, Jequier E. Effects of dietary fat on postprandial substrate oxidation and on carbohydrate and fat balances. J Clin Invest. 1985;76(3):1019–24. https://doi.org/10.1172/JCI112054.

24. Frayn KN. Adipose tissue as a buffer for daily lipid flux. Diabetologia. 2002;45(9):1201–10. https://doi.org/10.1007/s00125-002-0873-y.

25. Golozoubova V, Hohtola E, Matthias A, Jacobsson A, Cannon B, Nedergaard J. Only UCP1 can mediate adaptive nonshivering thermogenesis in the cold. FASEB J. 2001;15(11):2048–50. https://doi.org/10.1096/fj.00-0536fje.

26. Green DE, Zande HD. Universal energy principle of biological systems and the unity of bioenergetics. Proc Natl Acad Sci U S A. 1981;78(9):5344–7.

27. Greenway FL. Physiological adaptations to weight loss and factors favouring weight regain. Int J Obes. 2015;39(8):1188–96.

28. Hall KD, Sacks G, Chandramohan D, et al. Quantification of the effect of energy imbalance on bodyweight. Lancet. 2011;378(9793):826–37.

29. Harms M, Seale P. Brown and beige fat: development, function and therapeutic potential. Nat Med. 2013;19(10):1252–63. https://doi.org/10.1038/nm.3361.

30. Harper ME, Green K, Brand MD. The efficiency of cellular energy transduction and its implications for obesity. Annu Rev Nutr. 2008;28:13–33. https://doi.org/10.1146/annurev.nutr.28.061807.155357.

31. Hill JO, Peters JC, Reed GW, Schlundt DG, Sharp T, Greene HL. Nutrient balance in humans: effects of diet composition. Am J Clin Nutr. 1991;54(1):10–7.

32. Hill JO, Wyatt HR, Peters JC. Energy balance and obesity. Circulation. 2012;126(1):126–32. https://doi.org/10.1161/CIRCULATIONAHA.111.087213.

33. Human energy requirements: report of a joint FAO/WHO/UNU Expert Consultation. Food Nutr Bull. 2005;26(1):166.

34. Jequier E, Acheson K, Schutz Y. Assessment of energy expenditure and fuel utilization in man. Annu Rev Nutr. 1987;7:187–208. https://doi.org/10.1146/annurev.nu.07.070187.001155.

35. Johannsen DL, Ravussin E. Spontaneous physical activity: relationship between fidgeting and body weight control. Curr Opin Endocrinol Diabetes Obes. 2008;15(5):409–15. https://doi.org/10.1097/MED.0b013e32830b10bb.

36. Johnstone AM, Murison SD, Duncan JS, Rance KA, Speakman JR. Factors influencing variation in basal metabolic rate include fat-free mass, fat mass, age, and circulating thyroxine but not sex, circulating leptin, or triiodothyronine. Am J Clin Nutr. 2005;82(5):941–8.

37. Joint WHOFAOUNUEC. Protein and amino acid requirements in human nutrition. World Health Organ Tech Rep Ser. 2007;935:1–265.

38. Keys A, Taylor HL, Grande F. Basal metabolism and age of adult man. Metab Clin Exp. 1973;22(4):579–87.

39. Kim TN, Choi KM. The implications of sarcopenia and sarcopenic obesity on cardiometabolic disease. J Cell Biochem. 2015;116(7):1171–8. https://doi.org/10.1002/jcb.25077.

40. Kontani Y, Wang Y, Kimura K, Inokuma KI, Saito M, Suzuki-Miura T, Wang Z, Sato Y, Mori N, Yamashita H. UCP1 deficiency increases susceptibility to diet-induced obesity with age. Aging Cell. 2005;4(3):147–55. https://doi.org/10.1111/j.1474-9726.2005.00157.x.

41. Kopecky J, Clarke G, Enerback S, Spiegelman B, Kozak LP. Expression of the mitochondrial uncoupling protein gene from the aP2 gene promoter prevents genetic obesity. J Clin Invest. 1995;96(6):2914–23. https://doi.org/10.1172/JCI118363.

42. Kummitha CM, Kalhan SC, Saidel GM, Lai N. Physiol Rep. 2014;2(9), pii: e121590.

43. Larsen TM, Dalskov SM, van Baak M, et al. Diets with high or low protein content and glycemic index for weight-loss maintenance. N Engl J Med. 2010;363(22):2102–13.

44. Larson DE, Ferraro RT, Robertson DS, Ravussin E. Energy metabolism in weight-stable postobese individuals. Am J Clin Nutr. 1995;62(4):735–9.

45. Leibel RL, Rosenbaum M, Hirsch J. Changes in energy expenditure resulting from altered body weight. N Engl J Med. 1995;332(10):621–8. https://doi.org/10.1056/NEJM199503093321001.

46. Levine JA, Eberhardt NL, Jensen MD. Role of non-exercise activity thermogenesis in resistance to fat gain in humans. Science. 1999;283(5399):212–4.

47. Lin J, Wu H, Tarr PT, Zhang CY, Wu Z, Boss O, Michael LF, Puigserver P, Isotani E, Olson EN, Lowell BB, Bassel-Duby R, Spiegelman BM. Transcriptional co-activator PGC-1 alpha drives the formation of slow-twitch muscle fibres. Nature. 2002;418(6899):797–801. https://doi.org/10.1038/nature00904.

48. Livesey G, Elia M. Estimation of energy expenditure, net carbohydrate utilization, and net fat oxidation and synthesis by indirect calorimetry: evaluation of errors with special reference to the detailed composition of fuels. Am J Clin Nutr. 1988;47(4):608–28.

49. Locke AE, et al. Genetic studies of body mass index yield new insights for obesity biology. Nature. 2015;518(7538):197–206. https://doi.org/10.1038/nature14177.

50. Look AHEAD Research Group. Eight-year weight losses with an intensive lifestyle intervention: the look AHEAD study. Obesity (Silver Spring). 2014;22:5–13.

51. Loos RJ, Bouchard C. FTO: the first gene contributing to common forms of human obesity. Obes Rev. 2008;9(3):246–50. https://doi.org/10.1111/j.1467-789X.2008.00481.x.

52. Loos RJ, et al. Common variants near MC4R are associated with fat mass, weight and risk of obesity. Nat Genet. 2008;40(6):768–75. https://doi.org/10.1038/ng.140.

53. Ludwig DS, Friedman MI. Increasing adiposity: consequence or cause of overeating? JAMA. 2014;311(21):2167–8.

54. Magro DO, et al. Long-term weight regain after gastric bypass: a 5-year prospective study. Obes Surg. 2008;18:648–51.

55. Maurya SK, Bal NC, Sopariwala DH, Pant M, Rowland LA, Shaikh SA, Periasamy M. Sarcolipin is a key determinant of the basal metabolic rate, and its overexpression enhances energy expenditure and resistance against diet-induced obesity. J Biol Chem. 2015;290(17):10840–9. https://doi.org/10.1074/jbc.M115.636878.

56. Ochner CN, Barrios DM, Lee CD, Pi-Sunyer FX. Biological mechanisms that promote weight regain following weight loss in obese humans. Physiol Behav. 2013;120:106–13.

57. Plasqui G, Bonomi AG, Westerterp KR. Daily physical activity assessment with accelerometers: new insights and validation studies. Obes Rev. 2013;14(6):451–62. https://doi.org/10.1111/obr.12021.

58. Puigserver P, Wu Z, Park CW, Graves R, Wright M, Spiegelman BM. A cold-inducible coactivator of nuclear receptors linked to adaptive thermogenesis. Cell. 1998;92(6):829–39.

59. Ravussin E, Lillioja S, Anderson TE, Christin L, Bogardus C. Determinants of 24-hour energy expenditure in man. Methods and results using a respiratory chamber. J Clin Invest. 1986;78(6):1568–78. https://doi.org/10.1172/JCI112749.

60. Ravussin E, Lillioja S, Knowler WC, Christin L, Freymond D, Abbott WG, Boyce V, Howard BV, Bogardus C. Reduced rate of energy expenditure as a risk factor for body-weight gain. N Engl J Med. 1988;318(8):467–72. https://doi.org/10.1056/NEJM198802253180802.

61. Ravussin E, Harper IT, Rising R, Bogardus C. Energy expenditure by doubly labeled water: validation in lean and obese subjects. Am J Phys. 1991;261(3 Pt 1):E402–9.

62. Redman LM, Heilbronn LK, Martin CK, de Jonge L, Williamson DA, Delany JP, Ravussin E, Pennington CT. Metabolic and behavioral compensations in response to caloric restriction: implications for the maintenance of weight loss. PLoS One. 2009;4(2):e4377. https://doi.org/10.1371/journal.pone.0004377.

63. Rising R, Keys A, Ravussin E, Bogardus C. Concomitant interindividual variation in body temperature and metabolic rate. Am J Phys. 1992;263(4 Pt 1):E730–4.

64. Rolfe DF, Brown GC. Cellular energy utilization and molecular origin of standard metabolic rate in mammals. Physiol Rev. 1997;77(3):731–58.

65. Rosenbaum M, Goldsmith R, Bloomfield D, Magnano A, Weimer L, Heymsfield S, Gallagher D, Mayer L, Murphy E, Leibel RL. Low-dose leptin reverses skeletal muscle, autonomic, and neuroendocrine adaptations to maintenance of reduced weight. J Clin Invest. 2005;115(12):3579–86. https://doi.org/10.1172/JCI25977.

66. Rosenbaum M, Hirsch J, Gallagher DA, Leibel RL. Long-term persistence of adaptive thermogenesis in subjects who have maintained a reduced body weight. Am J Clin Nutr. 2008;88(4):906–12.

67. Rossmeislova L, et al. Weight loss improves the adipogenic capacity of human preadipocytes and modulates their secretory profile. Diabetes. 2013;62:1990–5.

68. Saad MF, Alger SA, Zurlo F, Young JB, Bogardus C, Ravussin E. Ethnic differences in sympathetic nervous system-mediated energy expenditure. Am J Phys. 1991;261(6 Pt 1):E789–94.

69. Saito M, Okamatsu-Ogura Y, Matsushita M, Watanabe K, Yoneshiro T, Nio-Kobayashi J, Iwanaga T, Miyagawa M, Kameya T, Nakada K, Kawai Y, Tsujisaki M. High incidence of metabolically active brown adipose tissue in healthy adult humans: effects of cold exposure and adiposity. Diabetes. 2009;58(7):1526–31. https://doi.org/10.2337/db09-0530.

70. Schoeller DA. Recent advances from application of doubly labeled water to measurement of human energy expenditure. J Nutr. 1999;129(10):1765–8.

71. Schulz LO, Schoeller DA. A compilation of total daily energy expenditures and body weights in healthy adults. Am J Clin Nutr. 1994;60(5):676–81.

72. Shekelle PG, Hardy ML, Morton SC, Maglione M, Mojica WA, Suttorp MJ, Rhodes SL, Jungvig L, Gagne J. Efficacy and safety of ephedra and ephedrine for weight loss and athletic performance: a meta-analysis. JAMA. 2003;289(12):1537–45. https://doi.org/10.1001/jama.289.12.1537.

73. Sims EA, Danforth E Jr, Horton ES, Bray GA, Glennon JA, Salans LB. Endocrine and metabolic effects of experimental obesity in man. Recent Prog Horm Res. 1973;29:457–96.

74. Smith SR, de Jonge L, Zachwieja JJ, Roy H, Nguyen T, Rood JC, Windhauser MM, Bray GA. Fat and carbohydrate balances during adaptation to a high-fat. Am J Clin Nutr. 2000;71(2):450–7.

75. Snook KR, Hansen AR, Duke CH, Finch KC, Hackney AA, Zhang J. (2017). Change in percentages of adults with overweight or obesity trying to lose weight, 1988–2014. JAMA. 2017;317(9):971–3.

76. Speakman JR. The history and theory of the doubly labeled water technique. Am J Clin Nutr. 1998;68(4):932S–8S.

77. Spiller RC. Intestinal absorptive function. Gut. 1994;35(1 Suppl):S5–9.

78. Spraul M, Ravussin E, Fontvieille AM, Rising R, Larson DE, Anderson EA. Reduced sympathetic nervous activity. A potential mechanism predisposing to body weight gain. J Clin Invest. 1993;92(4):1730–5. https://doi.org/10.1172/JCI116760.

79. Strohacker K, McCaffery JM, MacLean PS, Wing RR. Adaptations of leptin, ghrelin or insulin during weight loss as predictors of weight regain. Int J Obes (Lond). 2014;38(3):388–96. https://doi.org/10.1038/ijo.2013.118. Epub 2013 Jun 26

80. Swinburn BA, Sacks G, Hall KD, McPherson K, Finegood DT, Moodie ML, Gortmaker SL. The global obesity pandemic: shaped by global drivers and local environments. Lancet. 2011;378(9793):804–14. https://doi.org/10.1016/S0140-6736(11)60813-1.

81. Tataranni PA, Larson DE, Snitker S, Ravussin E. Thermic effect of food in humans: methods and results from use of a respiratory chamber. Am J Clin Nutr. 1995;61(5):1013–9.

82. Tataranni PA, Young JB, Bogardus C, Ravussin E. A low sympathoadrenal activity is associated with body weight gain and development of central adiposity in Pima Indian men. Obes Res. 1997;5(4):341–7.

83. Tobias DK, Chen M, Manson JE, Ludwig DS, Willett W, Hu FB. Effect of low-fat vs. other diet interventions on long-term weight change in adults: a

systematic review and meta-analysis. Lancet Diabetes Endocrinol. 2015;3(12):968–79.

84. van Baak MA, Mariman ECM. Nature reviews. Endocrinology. 2019;15:274–87.

85. van Marken Lichtenbelt WD, Vanhommerig JW, Smulders NM, Drossaerts JM, Kemerink GJ, Bouvy ND, Schrauwen P, Teule GJ. Cold-activated brown adipose tissue in healthy men. N Engl J Med. 2009;360(15):1500–8. https://doi.org/10.1056/NEJMoa0808718.

86. van Ooijen AM, van Marken Lichtenbelt WD, van Steenhoven AA, Westerterp KR. Cold-induced heat production preceding shivering. Br J Nutr. 2005;93(3):387–91.

87. Villablanca PA, Alegria JR, Mookadam F, Holmes DR Jr, Wright RS, Levine JA. Nonexercise activity thermogenesis in obesity management. Mayo Clin Proc. 2015;90(4):509–19. https://doi.org/10.1016/j.mayocp.2015.02.001.

88. Vink RG, Roumans NJ, Mariman EC, van Baak MA. Dietary weight loss-induced changes in RBP4, FFA, and ACE predict weight regain in people with overweight and obesity. Physiol Rep. 2017;5:e13450.

89. Virtanen KA, Lidell ME, Orava J, Heglind M, Westergren R, Niemi T, Taittonen M, Laine J, Savisto NJ, Enerback S, Nuutila P. Functional brown adipose tissue in healthy adults. N Engl J Med. 2009;360(15):1518–25. https://doi.org/10.1056/NEJMoa0808949.

90. Vybiral S, Lesna I, Jansky L, Zeman V. Thermoregulation in winter swimmers and physiological significance of human catecholamine thermogenesis. Exp Physiol. 2000;85(3):321–6.

91. Westerterp KR, Speakman JR. Physical activity energy expenditure has not declined since the 1980s and matches energy expenditures of wild mammals. Int J Obes. 2008;32(8):1256–63. https://doi.org/10.1038/ijo.2008.74.

92. Weststrate JA. Resting metabolic rate and diet-induced thermogenesis: a methodological reappraisal. Am J Clin Nutr. 1993;58(5):592–601.

93. Weyer C, Tataranni PA, Snitker S, Danforth E Jr, Ravussin E. Increase in insulin action and fat oxidation after treatment with CL 316,243, a highly selective beta3-adrenoceptor agonist in humans. Diabetes. 1998;47(10):1555–61.

94. Weyer C, Pratley RE, Salbe AD, Bogardus C, Ravussin E, Tataranni PA. Energy expenditure, fat oxidation, and body weight regulation: a study of metabolic adaptation to long-term weight change. J Clin Endocrinol Metab. 2000;85(3):1087–94. https://doi.org/10.1210/jcem.85.3.6447.

95. Wijers SL, Schrauwen P, Saris WH, van Marken Lichtenbelt WD. Human skeletal muscle mitochondrial uncoupling is associated with cold induced adaptive thermogenesis. PLoS One. 2008;3(3):e1777. https://doi.org/10.1371/journal.pone.0001777.

96. Zingaretti MC, Crosta F, Vitali A, Guerrieri M, Frontini A, Cannon B, Nedergaard J, Cinti S. The presence of UCP1 demonstrates that metabolically active adipose tissue in the neck of adult humans truly represents brown adipose tissue. FASEB J. 2009;23(9):3113–20. https://doi.org/10.1096/fj.09-133542.

97. Zurlo F, Ferraro RT, Fontvielle AM, Rising R, Bogardus C, Ravussin E. Spontaneous physical activity and obesity: cross-sectional and longitudinal studies in Pima Indians. Am J Phys. 1992;263(2 Pt 1):E296–300.

Carbohydrate, Protein, and Fat Metabolism in Obesity

15

Jose E. Galgani, Víctor Cortés, and Fernando Carrasco

Contents

J. E. Galgani (✉)
Departamento Ciencias de la Salud, Carrera de Nutrición y
Dietética, Facultad de Medicina, Pontificia Universidad
Católica de Chile, Santiago, Chile

Departamento de Nutrición, Diabetes y Metabolismo,
Escuela de Medicina, Pontificia Universidad Católica de
Chile, Santiago, Chile

Pennington Biomedical Research Center, Baton Rouge,
LA, USA
e-mail: jgalgani@uc.cl

V. Cortés
Departamento de Nutrición, Diabetes y Metabolismo,
Escuela de Medicina, Pontificia Universidad Católica de
Chile, Santiago, Chile
e-mail: vcortesm@uc.cl

F. Carrasco
Departamento de Nutrición. Facultad de Medicina,
Universidad de Chile, Santiago, Chile

Department of Nutrition, Clínica Las Condes, Santiago,
Chile
e-mail: fernandocarrasco@u.uchile.cl

© Springer Nature Switzerland AG 2023
R. S. Ahima (ed.), *Metabolic Syndrome*,
https://doi.org/10.1007/978-3-031-40116-9_21

Abstract

Macronutrient metabolism is essential for transferring energy contained in food to usable forms of cellular energy. The balance between energy from fuels flowing to cells and then expended during cellular work will determine body size. In the last decades, energy homeostasis has been challenged by an overwhelming dietary macronutrient availability that imposes a need for expanding adipose mass. The capacity to handle such higher energy and macronutrient fluxes impacts metabolic processes at the cellular and whole organism levels. Herein, we reviewed carbohydrate, fat, and protein metabolism, particularly comparing individuals with and without obesity.

Keywords

Fuel oxidation · Energy balance · Fuel partitioning · Cellular metabolism · Energy transfer

Introduction

All life forms require an exogenous energy supply and the biochemical machinery for transforming fuels into usable forms of cellular energy. This energy sustains processes for survival, including the maintenance of electrochemical gradients, macromolecule synthesis and breakdown, and thermogenesis, among others [1]. Energy resides in the carbon-hydrogen bonds of carbohydrates, lipids, and proteins. Such energy is transferred to energy carriers such as NADH and $FADH_2$. In the mitochondria, a sequence of reactions remove hydrogen atoms (i.e., dehydrogenation) from NADH and $FADH_2$ to generate a transmembrane proton (H^+) gradient that allows phosphorylation of ADP to ATP. There is a tight balance between ATP demand and synthesis, so carbohydrates, lipids, and proteins are oxidized depending on ATP demand. Because macronutrient excess does not increase ATP demand, excess energy is stored mainly as triglycerides (TAG) in white adipose tissue (WAT). If energy surplus persists over time, body mass increases, leading to obesity when a threshold of 30 kg of body weight per square meter is reached. Thus, the most notorious biological consequence of this energy imbalance is the expansion of WAT. The body weight will stabilize whenever the initial energy surplus matches the new energy demand imposed for the weight gained. Excessive fat accumulation is responsible for shortening life expectancy and multiple comorbidities [2, 3]. Insulin plays a pivotal role in regulating macronutrient metabolism; therefore, insulin resistance may alter carbohydrate, lipid, and protein metabolism in obesity. In turn, altered macronutrient metabolism leading to generation of metabolites that disrupt insulin signaling could contribute to perpetuating insulin resistance. Herein, we compare macronutrient metabolism in individuals with and without obesity and its potential relevance for understanding obesity-related metabolic disorders.

Macronutrient Intake Versus Oxidation in Obesity

Maintaining a stable body mass and composition implies that energy intake over time matches energy demand, resulting in a null energy balance.

In this condition, the net macronutrient storage is also null; thus, whole-body mass and composition remain constant. Therefore, null energy balance will necessarily occur when the average proportion of macronutrients oxidized (represented by the VCO_2:VO_2 ratio, so-called respiratory quotient (RQ) equals the proportion of dietary macronutrients available for oxidation (represented by the dietary VCO_2:VO_2 ratio, i.e., food quotient (FQ) over a given period [4, 5]. Individuals with obesity are not exempt from that principle. Lean and individuals with obesity displayed similar 24-h RQ when fed a weight-maintaining diet of similar macronutrient composition [6].

Whether lean and individuals with obesity differ in their ability to overcome energy deficit and excess has also been a matter of study. In particular, it has been hypothesized that obesity is associated with an abnormal response to energy deficit and excess, which can perpetuate the obesity phenotype. This hypothesis has been repeatedly refuted. For instance, both 24-h energy expenditure and 24-h RQ in response to an acute energy deficit or excess changed similarly in individuals with and without obesity [6, 7]. Of particular, relevance is a 96-h whole-body metabolic chamber study [8], where normal-weight volunteers and volunteers with obesity fed a hypercaloric diet (50% excess energy) showed a similar macronutrient oxidative disposal. Thus, no evidence currently supports an altered whole-body metabolic response in obesity under negative, neutral, or positive energy balance conditions. Yet, it is possible that organ and tissue-specific differences in macronutrient metabolism occur in obesity due to WAT expansion. Further analysis is presented below.

Carbohydrate Metabolism in Obesity

Overview of Glucose Metabolism

Carbohydrate is usually the primary source of dietary energy for humans, with glucose as the main energy substrate for cells. Red blood cells lack mitochondria and thus depend exclusively on glucose for energy provision. The brain and renal medulla also rely primarily on glucose as their energy source. Indeed, due to its high metabolic rate [~20% of whole-body basal metabolic rate [1]], the brain requires ~100 g of glucose per day. Such cellular glucose requirement is constant while dietary carbohydrate intake fluctuates over 24 h, being null during the sleeping time and episodic over the waking period. A complex neuroendocrine regulatory system provides a constant glucose supply to organs, tissues, and cells while preventing hypoglycemia during fasting and hyperglycemia after meals [9].

Cellular glucose uptake is one of the regulatory mechanisms of extracellular glucose concentration. Thus, after ingestion of a glucose load in healthy humans, 45–55% of dietary glucose is taken up by peripheral organs and the liver, respectively [9]. This efficient glucose uptake buffers the elevation in glycemia imposed by dietary carbohydrates. Glucose uptake proceeds through insulin-independent and insulin-dependent mechanisms [10]. High-blood glucose concentration represents an insulin-independent mechanism driving hepatic glucose uptake [11]. In turn, insulin promotes glucose uptake in skeletal muscle and adipose tissue by triggering GLUT4 translocation to the cell surface [10, 11]. Once glucose is taken up, it is oxidized or directed toward glycogen synthesis to prevent postprandial hyperglycemia. Postprandial suppression of hepatic glucose production is another mechanism to prevent hyperglycemia and maintain glycemia within a physiological range [11, 12].

Under conditions of null exogenous glucose supply, the glucose concentration gradient between the extracellular and intracellular compartments is sustained by the ability of the liver to release glucose into the circulation. This process is accomplished through the hydrolysis of hepatic glycogen and conversion of specific metabolites (lactate, pyruvate, glycerol, and some amino acids) to glucose (i.e., neoglucogenesis). Concomitantly, other tissues (e.g., skeletal muscle) adapt their energy supply and metabolism to alternative energy substrates (e.g., fatty acids) in order to spare glucose [13]. Finally, energy sufficiency at the cellular, organ, and whole-body levels is achieved after adapting fuel oxidation to fuel availability, a process known as metabolic flexibility [14]. In this metabolic scenario, insulin plays a pivotal role in determining fuel partitioning, so dietary macronutrient availability matches the oxidation rate.

Glucose Uptake and Phosphorylation

Cellular glucose uptake is a process that involves facilitated transport by members of a family of glucose transporter (GLUT) isoforms [15]. GLUT1 is expressed ubiquitously and is constitutively located in the plasma membrane. GLUT2 is present in pancreatic beta cells, hepatocytes, and the basolateral membrane of intestinal and kidney epithelial cells. GLUT2 has a high capacity but low affinity for glucose transport that allows the internalization of large amounts of glucose under hyperglycemic conditions. GLUT2 also mediates glucose efflux from the liver into the circulation under fasting conditions to prevent hypoglycemia. GLUT3 is expressed in the brain and has a high affinity for glucose. This feature allows it to provide a relatively constant glucose supply to the neurons, even when extracellular glucose concentration is low. GLUT4 is found in striated myocytes and adipocytes and is responsible for insulin-stimulated glucose uptake. GLUT4 translocation from the cytosol to the sarcolemma and transverse tubule membranes is stimulated by muscle contraction [16].

Glucose is rapidly phosphorylated through an ATP-dependent reaction catalyzed by hexokinases that prevent the outflow of newly incorporated glucose. The hexokinase isoform found in the liver (type 4 hexokinase or glucokinase) has a relatively low affinity for glucose, with a K_m double fasting glycemia (~5 mM). This feature allows hepatocytes to phosphorylate high glucose levels that reach the liver from the intestine after meals via the portal vein. Once glucose is converted to glucose-6-phosphate (G6P), it has two major metabolic fates: (i) glycolytic metabolism to pyruvate, which can then be converted to lactate (anaerobic condition) or oxidized to acetyl-coenzyme A (CoA) (aerobic condition) and (ii) conversion to glucose-1-phosphate (G1P), the precursor of glycogen synthesis. G6P can also enter the pentose phosphate pathway generating NADPH to fuel de novo lipogenesis (DNL) and sugar precursors for nucleoside synthesis.

Under noninsulin-stimulated conditions (e.g., overnight fasting), the circulating glucose is mostly taken up by nonskeletal muscle tissues (e.g., central nervous system) [10]. Individuals without or with obesity have similar blood glucose clearance rates [17], consistent with the observation that glucose uptake in fasting conditions relies on insulin-independent mechanisms. Indeed, the transport of 3-O-methylglucose (a nonmetabolizable glucose analog) [18] and the content of G6P [19] were similar in muscle biopsies from donors without or with obesity.

In contrast, upon insulin stimulation, the classical sigmoidal insulin dose-response curve for glucose uptake is right-shifted in obesity [20]. The most critical contributor to the lower whole-body glucose uptake in individuals with obesity is the diminished insulin-stimulated glucose clearance by skeletal muscle [21, 22]. Such impairment is noted across all major muscle groups [23]. At the molecular level, insulin-stimulated GLUT4 translocation is reduced in individuals with insulin resistance and obesity compared to normal-weight individuals. This finding is consistent with the impaired insulin-stimulated glucose transport detected in muscle biopsies of subjects with obesity versus lean individuals [18, 24]. These alterations have been described during the euglycemic-hyperinsulinemic glucose clamp procedure, a nonphysiological condition where a constant and continuous insulin dose is infused while glucose is co-infused at a variable rate, so euglycemia is maintained constant [25]. Under normal feeding conditions, for example, in response to a meal, the whole-body glucose uptake depends on the capacity of pancreatic beta cells to release as much insulin as required to compensate for defective insulin action. Obesity is associated with higher basal and postprandial insulin secretion [26]. Thus, hyperinsulinemia can partially or fully restore tissue glucose uptake and glycemic control in individuals with obesity when compared with lean individuals [26, 27] (Fig. 1).

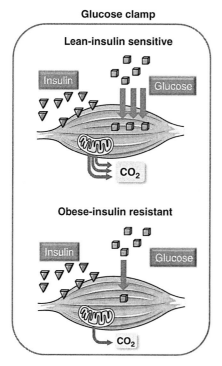
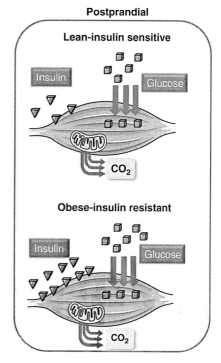

Fig. 1 The figure represents glucose uptake in individuals without obesity and high insulin sensitivity and individuals with obesity and low insulin sensitivity under two insulin-stimulated conditions: glucose clamp (supraphysiological) and postprandial (physiological). In the glucose clamp, insulin-stimulated glucose uptake is impaired in insulin-resistant versus insulin-sensitive subjects, which reduces intracellular glucose utilization and oxidation (CO_2 production). In the postprandial condition, hyperinsulinemia compensates for defective tissue insulin action, which partially or fully prevents the decrease in glucose uptake and glucose oxidation. Thus, during the glucose clamp condition, insulin resistance is manifested by decreased glucose uptake and oxidation at a similar circulating glucose and insulin concentration. In turn, insulin resistance is mainly characterized by hyperinsulinemia and normal glucose utilization in the postprandial condition

Glycolysis and Oxidation

The glycolytic processing of one mole of G6P yields two moles of pyruvate and a net production of two moles of ATP. Pyruvate can be converted to lactate through lactate dehydrogenase or oxidized to acetyl-CoA through the mitochondrial pyruvate dehydrogenase complex (PDH). In the mitochondria, acetyl-CoA enters the tricarboxylic acid (TCA) cycle, which undergoes oxidation to CO_2 to generate NADH and $FADH_2$. Obesity is associated with the differential partitioning of pyruvate to lactate and CO_2, resulting in elevated blood lactate concentration [28]. Indeed, lactate-to-glucose cycling is increased in children with versus without obesity [29]. The pathophysiological

relevance of this finding and its mechanistic basis remains unclear. At the molecular level, the conversion of pyruvate to lactate or acetyl-CoA is pivotal for cellular metabolic flexibility. In this regard, an animal model having defective PDH activity (by hyperacetylation of PDH Eα subunit) has impaired metabolic flexibility, enhanced lactate production, and higher fatty acid oxidation even in the fed state [30]. Such differential lactate metabolism in obesity appears not to influence oxidative glucose disposal. Concordantly, Owen et al. [31] observed similar oxidative disposal of glucose and other macronutrients in subjects with obesity compared to lean subjects over an 8-h feeding protocol. A complementary analysis detected similar whole-body glycolytic and oxidative disposal of a 75-g oral glucose load in insulin-sensitive and -resistant individuals, defined by the glucose clamp technique [32].

Glucose oxidation has also been assessed during euglycemic-hyperinsulinemic clamp conditions. The extent to which the RQ increases upon insulin stimulation is a marker of metabolic flexibility, which indicates the ability to increase glucose over fatty acid oxidation [14]. Individuals with obesity and insulin resistance show a lower increase in the skeletal muscle RQ than lean/insulin-sensitive individuals, indicating metabolic inflexibility [17] (Fig. 1). In turn, improvement of insulin sensitivity through weight loss enhanced skeletal muscle metabolic flexibility [17]. These findings have been considered a feature of an intrinsic cellular defect, mostly at the mitochondrial level, where the ability to switch lipid oxidation off is impaired in the transition from fasting to fed conditions. An alternative explanation for the impaired increase in glucose oxidation over lipid oxidation can be simply due to the lower cellular entry rate determined by the glucose clamping [14] (Fig. 1). Indeed, when taking into account the insulin-stimulated glucose disposal rate, the increase in the RQ parallels relates to insulin sensitivity [14, 33]. Likewise, patients with obesity and type 2 diabetes displayed similar metabolic flexibility before and after a one-year weight loss intervention when controlling for insulin-stimulated glucose disposal rate [33]. These findings suggest that metabolic inflexibility results from lower intracellular glucose availability rather than intrinsic cellular disparities between individuals with contrasting insulin sensitivity.

Glucose Storage

Conversion of G6P to G1P is mediated through phosphoglucomutase. G1P is then converted to uridine diphosphate (UDP) glucose and bound to a growing glycogen polymer. Insulin stimulates glycogen synthesis by relieving the glycogen synthase kinase 3-dependent inhibition on glycogen synthase. Also, insulin-mediated GLUT4 translocation to the plasma membrane increases glucose flux and availability of the substrates of glycogen

synthase [34]. Glycogen is synthesized by both the liver and skeletal muscle. The former has a higher glycogen content per gram of wet tissue, while skeletal muscle accounts for a higher proportion of the total body glycogen pool due to its higher contribution to the fat-free mass in adults.

Hepatic glycogen has a systemic role due to its contribution to glucose production for maintaining glycemia during fasting. In contrast, skeletal muscle glycogen mostly sustains local ATP production during contraction. Under limited exogenous glucose supply, glycogen hydrolysis increases G6P supply, which is then converted to glucose by the hepatic glucose-6-phosphatase. G6P cannot be converted to glucose in skeletal muscle because it lacks glucose-6-phosphatase. Individuals with obesity relative to their lean counterparts show lower glycogen synthase activity in fasting, while muscle glycogen content remains unaltered [19]. Under glucose clamp conditions, nonoxidative glucose disposal, primarily dependent on glycogen synthesis, is lower in individuals with obesity relative to lean individuals [35], possibly owing to decreased intracellular glucose availability and lower insulin-dependent glycogen synthase activity [36, 37]. In turn, in feeding conditions, whole-body nonoxidative glucose disposal was similar in women without and with obesity studied for 96 h in a whole-body metabolic chamber [8].

Hepatic Glucose Production

Hepatocytes can produce glucose via two mechanisms: (i) glycogenolysis, i.e., hydrolysis of stored glycogen, and (ii) gluconeogenesis, i.e., *de novo* glucose production from nonglucose precursors. Conditions of limited exogenous glucose supply are characterized by low-blood insulin: glucagon ratio. This hormonal milieu promotes glycogenolysis and gluconeogenesis. Biochemically, gluconeogenesis follows the reverse glycolytic flux, although some reactions are exclusive for glycolysis (i.e., glucose phosphorylation and the synthesis of fructose-6-phosphate and phosphoenolpyruvate). Thus, gluconeogenesis requires ATP to convert pyruvate, alanine, lactate, and glycerol to glucose.

Individuals with obesity show elevated basal (fasting) hepatic glucose production and impaired ability of insulin to suppress this process [20]. Epidemiological studies have consistently found a direct correlation between central obesity and insulin resistance and its systemic consequences, the so-called metabolic syndrome. Intrahepatic rather than visceral fat at the tissue level is associated with impaired hepatic glucose control [38]. These findings suggest that hepatic metabolic dysfunction, more than any other intra-abdominal organ, is central to the pathogenesis of insulin resistance. In concordance with this hypothesis, the surgical removal of visceral adipose tissue had little impact on insulin sensitivity in humans [39, 40]. The fact that less than 20% of portal vein free-fatty acids (FFA) come from visceral fat in individuals with or without obesity while 10% of the total FFA found in peripheral blood circulation comes from visceral fat challenges any causative role of visceral fat on metabolic disturbances [41].

De Novo Lipogenesis

The main metabolic fates of glucose are oxidation or glycogen synthesis. In circumstances of glucose excess and high-cellular energy status, glucose can also convert into palmitate (i.e., DNL), the main product of the endogenous fatty acid synthesis pathway. Oxidation of acetyl-CoA in the mitochondria originates citrate, a TCA intermediary. Under conditions of excess glucose supply, citrate leaves the mitochondria to be converted into acetyl-CoA and oxaloacetate by the action of citrate lyase in the cytosol. Acetyl-CoA is then carboxylated to malonyl-CoA in a reaction stimulated by insulin and catalyzed by acetyl-CoA carboxylase. Malonyl-CoA is the substrate of fatty acid synthase that generates palmitate in a multistep sequence of NADPH-dependent reactions.

DNL was postulated as partially responsible for the increased adiposity of subjects with obesity, particularly in individuals eating high-carbohydrate diets, where carbohydrate excess was converted into fat. Acheson et al. [42] measured the RQ of lean individuals consuming large amounts of glucose (500 g/day), and observed the expected increase in RQ. However, the RQ transiently reached values above 1.00, indicating that whole-body net DNL was minimal after short-term carbohydrate overfeeding. A subsequent calorimetric study compared lean and individuals with obesity after a 4-day isoenergetic diet (50% energy from carbohydrates) and a 4-day carbohydrate overfeeding (1.75-fold energy excess, 75% energy from carbohydrates) [43]. After carbohydrate overfeeding, both groups increased the whole-body net DNL over 5 h after glucose ingestion (3.25 g/kg fat-free mass). However, both after the isoenergetic diet and carbohydrate-enriched diet, individuals with obesity showed lower whole-body net DNL than lean individuals.

Later studies quantified in vivo hepatic DNL by incorporating newly synthesized fatty acids into circulating triglyceride-rich lipoproteins by stable isotopic labeling. Individuals with obesity showed higher hepatic DNL than lean individuals [44–46], a metabolic process strongly associated with hepatic and systemic insulin resistance [44, 46] and carbohydrate intake [47]. The effect of glucose and sucrose overfeeding on hepatic DNL was studied in women with and without obesity [45]. After a 4-day 50% surplus of energy as glucose or sucrose, hepatic DNL increased two- to threefold regardless of the obesity status and carbohydrate type [45].

Lipid Metabolism in Obesity

Overview of Lipid Metabolism

Lipids are key components of cells, fulfilling energetic, structural, and regulatory roles. Fatty acids and cholesterol are the most abundant dietary lipids. Dietary fatty acids are mainly stored as TAG in WAT, ~7600 kcal/kg. Cholesterol is mostly present in cellular membranes and is neither physiologically stored nor used as an energy substrate [48]. Because of its ability to buffer fluctuations in calorie intake, WAT is a major evolutionary adaptation against starvation. WAT secretes endocrine factors called adipokines, which integrate whole-body energy balance, feeding behavior, insulin sensitivity, and vascular function. WAT also regulates fertility, mating selection, offspring growth, immune function, and bone accrual [49]. Fatty acid oxidation fulfills 25–45% of daily energy needs in humans, which in an average healthy adult represents about 70–130 g of fat per day. Cholesterol is converted to sterols, steroids, and biliary acids, which have multiple biological functions.

Dietary TAG are hydrolyzed in the lumen of the small intestine by pancreatic lipase, and the released FFA and monoacylglycerol are then incorporated into bile acid micellae and absorbed by enterocytes. In the small intestine, fatty acids are esterified into TAG and, along with other lipids and fat-soluble vitamins, incorporated into chylomicrons. Then, chylomicrons reach the systemic circulation after being secreted into the splanchnic lymphatic circulation. On the endothelial cell surface, chylomicron's TAG are subjected to extracellular hydrolysis by lipoprotein lipase to release fatty acids to the WAT, skeletal muscle, and heart. The liver then clears chylomicron remnants through endocytic uptake mediated by the LDL receptor-related protein 1. In hepatocytes, the lipoprotein lipids are processed by the endolysosomal pathway to release fatty acids and cholesterol, which are then incorporated into very low-density lipoproteins (VLDL). Circulating VLDL's TAG are also a substrate for lipoprotein lipase.

Extracellular FFA are internalized by the cells through scavenger receptor FAT/CD36 and members of the fatty acid transport protein (FATP) family [50]. FAT/CD36 is highly expressed in the WAT and skeletal muscle, while its expression in the adult liver is low. Inside the cell, fatty acids bind to cytosolic fatty acid-binding proteins for intracellular transport and utilization, which are rapidly esterified with CoA by the members of the acyl-CoA synthetase family. Acyl-CoAs are then esterified to glycerol-3-phosphate for TAG and phospholipid synthesis in a series of reactions catalyzed by acyltransferases and phosphatases. In the muscle and liver, acyl-CoAs are mainly directed toward mitochondrial beta-oxidation for ATP synthesis. Fatty acids can also be esterified to sphingosine to form ceramide and other sphingolipids. Importantly, diacylglycerol (DAG) and ceramides are well-characterized intracellular messengers involved in signaling pathways that have been implicated in the pathogenesis of obesity-related insulin resistance [2].

Low insulin and increased glucagon levels during fasting promote intracellular TAG hydrolysis, releasing fatty acids and glycerol toward the extracellular medium. Because adipocytes lack glycerol kinase activity [51], glycerol cannot be transformed into glycerol-3-phosphate for the esterification of fatty acids to TAG. Thus, glycerol reaches the circulation for hepatic neoglucogenesis. In turn, FFA released to the extracellular space bind to plasma proteins, mostly albumin. Then, FFA are taken up in nonadipose tissues for reesterification, oxidation, or hepatic conversion to ketone bodies. In the liver, circulating FFA are the primary source for hepatic TAG synthesis and constitute the bulk of fatty acids incorporated in VLDL particles [52].

Lipid metabolism, including TAG synthesis and DNL, is regulated at the transcriptional level by the sterol regulatory element-binding protein (SREBP) 1c, carbohydrate-responsive element-binding protein (ChREBP), peroxisomal proliferator-activated receptor (PPAR)γ, and liver X receptor (LXR). These transcription factors belong to different molecular families. Furthermore, diverse signals regulate their activity. However, they extensively overlap in their repertory of target genes. Hence, whereas SREBP1c is regulated by insulin, ChREBP by glucose, PPARγ by fatty acids, and oxysterols activate LXR, all of them regulate the abundance of the enzymes involved in lipogenesis.

PPARγ is a lipogenic transcriptional regulator that has been targeted by drugs approved for clinical use (thiazolidinediones). Although endogenous PPARγ ligand remains unknown, pioglitazone and rosiglitazone (two types of thiazolidinediones) are effective insulin-sensitizers used in patients with type 2 diabetes. Some proposed lipids identified in vitro (polyunsaturated fatty acids and prostanoids) may be physiological agonists/antagonists of PPARγ; the evidence is tenuous. In contrast, there is strong evidence showing that 1-palmitoyl-2-oleoyl-sn-glycerol-3-phosphocholine is an endogenous ligand of PPARα in mouse liver [53].

Fatty Acid Uptake

The independent effect of overexpression of skeletal muscle- and liver-specific lipoprotein lipase on insulin resistance has been studied. In both cases, lipoprotein lipase overexpression (fourfold) elevated intrahepatic or intramuscular TAG content. Skeletal muscle showed higher contents of long-chain acyl-CoAs, DAG, and ceramides, whereas the liver showed higher content of long-chain acyl-CoAs. This intracellular lipid buildup was accompanied by tissue-specific insulin resistance [54], suggesting a pathogenic role of these particular lipid species in insulin resistance.

The plasma membrane fatty acid transporter FAT/CD36 also determines tissue lipid load, as shown in knockout mouse studies. This animal model shows reduced VLDL clearance, muscle fatty acid uptake, and high-plasma TAG concentration. Furthermore, mice lacking FAT/CD36 have low-muscle TAG content and a high DAG-to-TAG ratio [55]. These changes were associated with improved skeletal muscle insulin sensitivity but, unexpectedly, impaired hepatic insulin sensitivity [56]. Conversely, skeletal muscle-specific FAT/CD36 overexpression elevated plasma glucose and insulin concentrations, suggesting impaired insulin sensitivity and defective glucose homeostasis [57].

In humans, fatty acid uptake has been studied using giant sarcolemmal vesicles from donors with or without obesity. Vesicles from donors with obesity show elevated palmitate transport, membrane-associated FAT/CD36 content, and intramuscular TAG accumulation. Myotubes from donors with obesity also showed higher content of FAT/CD36 and oleic acid uptake [58]. At the whole-body level, individuals with obesity have increased rates of plasma palmitate clearance at any palmitate concentration, both in basal and insulin-stimulated conditions, compared to lean

participants [59]. Noteworthy, the clearance rates of plasma palmitate were inversely related to muscle insulin sensitivity, without differences between individuals with or without obesity [59]. In vivo assessment using the leg balance technique showed similar fasted and insulin-stimulated skeletal muscle fatty acid uptake rates in individuals with or without obesity [17]. Under exercise conditions, the plasma fatty acid tissue uptake is also similar in individuals with or without obesity [60].

Fatty Acid Oxidation

Fatty acids are the primary metabolic fuel for oxidation from fed to fasted conditions. Oxidation of saturated and unsaturated fatty acids can occur by alpha-, beta-, or omega-oxidation. Alpha-oxidation is essential for the catabolism of molecules that cannot be metabolized by beta-oxidation. Also, in the synthesis of alpha-hydroxy fatty acids, which are then incorporated into sphingolipids. Beta-oxidation is the primary catabolic pathway for fatty acids, which occurs mainly in the mitochondria and to a lower extent in peroxisomes. The metabolization of very long-chain fatty acids requires chain shortening by peroxisomal beta-oxidation to medium long-chain products, which are then transported to the mitochondria for complete beta-oxidation. Omega-oxidation of fatty acids proceeds in the endoplasmic reticulum and yields dicarboxylic acid products. Mitochondrial beta-oxidation is regulated at three enzyme-mediated steps: (i) fatty acid activation to acyl-CoA in the cytosol, (ii) acyl-carnitine translocation to the mitochondrial matrix (catalyzed by carnitine palmitoyltransferase [CPT] 1), and (iii) mitochondrial beta-oxidation through four sequential enzymatic reactions.

Impaired fatty acid oxidation due to mitochondrial abnormalities has been postulated as a driver of ectopic fat accumulation leading to obesity-related insulin resistance [17, 61]. In line with this hypothesis, Kim et al. observed reduced palmitate (CPT1-dependent) and palmitoylcarnitine (CPT1-independent) oxidation along with lower

CPT1 activity in muscle biopsies from donors with obesity versus lean individuals [61]. Similarly, skeletal muscle cells from donors with obesity showed lower oleic acid oxidation compared with normal weight individuals [58]. Concordantly, the skeletal muscle of individuals with obesity is characterized by lower lipid oxidation during fasting conditions but higher lipid oxidation during insulin-stimulated conditions [17]. Such alteration is a characteristic feature of metabolic inflexibility, where insulin-dependent suppression of lipid oxidation is lower in obesity [62]. Alteration in skeletal muscle lipid oxidation capacity is evident during moderate-intensity endurance exercise in individuals with obesity. It has consistently been observed that individuals with obesity have a higher reliance on fat oxidation due to enhanced nonplasma fatty acid oxidation [60, 63]. Thus, high skeletal muscle lipid accumulation often noted in obesity [64] promotes fat oxidation, decreasing the use of plasma fatty acids and carbohydrates as energy fuels [60, 62].

Fatty Acid Turnover

Whole-body FFA flux from WAT to blood and blood to tissues (e.g., liver, skeletal muscle) is called FFA turnover and determines blood FFA concentration. In obesity, due to WAT expansion, blood FFA concentration should increase even if the WAT lipolytic rate per tissue unit stays unaltered [65]. However, plasma FFA concentration is weakly associated with body fat mass or body mass index (r values <0.10) [66]. On the one hand, this pattern is due to a strong suppression of FFA release from WAT [62, 66], which contributes to lower FFA overflux to tissues. On the other hand, in obesity, there is a higher systemic FFA clearance rate, both in fasting and insulin-stimulated conditions [59]. Such adaptations maintain the blood FFA concentration at levels similar to lean individuals. However, it cannot entirely prevent FFA overflow into tissues, impacting intracellular FFA turnover and insulin sensitivity.

Increased fatty acid supply to tissues can increase TAG accumulation in lipid droplets, which are dynamic structures regulating intracellular fatty acid turnover. The balance between glycerolipid synthesis and intracellular lipolysis ultimately determines tissue lipid balance and the synthesis of lipid intermediates. It has been shown that increased lipolytic rates led to higher fatty acid availability and de novo ceramide synthesis in a muscle cell line overexpressing ATGL [67]. Incomplete TAG hydrolysis might also favor DAG accumulation [68].

The relevance of fatty acid turnover is highlighted by studies showing that individuals with versus without obesity have higher intramyocellular TAG, DAG, and ceramides contents [64, 69]. However, only body fatness relates directly to intramyocellular TAG content, whereas it does not associate with the muscle content of DAG or ceramides [69]. In turn, the DAG:TAG hydrolase activity ratio (an index of incomplete TAG hydrolysis), which is lower in obesity, determines the muscle DAG and ceramide contents [69].

Consequences of Altered Tissue Lipid Balance in Obesity

Obesity is characterized by increased WAT mass in subcutaneous and intra-abdominal depots. Obesity determines pathologic changes in the WAT, including hypertrophy of adipocytes, activated immune cell infiltration, abnormal vascular supply, and fibrotic extracellular matrix [2, 70]. This pathologically remodeled WAT cannot fully expand and thus leaks fatty acids toward tissues and cells that are not adapted to store massive amounts of these molecules [2, 70]. This phenomenon may explain why individuals with obesity commonly have augmented lipid accumulation in the liver, skeletal muscle, and heart. It also explains why patients with lipodystrophy (a severe paucity of WAT) show ectopic fat accumulation and severe insulin resistance. Remarkably, leptin, the most potent insulin sensitizer for patients with generalized lipodystrophy, decreases ectopic lipid overload and insulin resistance [71].

Excessive fat accumulation in nonadipose tissues, particularly at the intrahepatic level, is directly associated with impaired glucose tolerance, systemic insulin resistance, and increased circulating levels of enlarged VLDL particles [38, 72–74]. Interventions to decrease ectopic tissue lipid load are usually associated with improved insulin sensitivity, further supporting the role of excessive lipid levels in insulin resistance pathogenesis. For instance, thiazolidinediones reduce plasma FFA concentration and liver TAG content while enhancing insulin-stimulated glucose disposal rate in subjects with type 2 diabetes [75]. Notably, the role of exercise, a well-established insulin-sensitizing tool, on intramuscular TAG remains controversial. Some studies have shown that physical training decreases intramyocellular TAG [76], whereas others found the opposite result [77]. Nutritional interventions with or without exercise have also shown a correlation between liver and skeletal muscle ectopic reduction and improved insulin sensitivity. Thus, a Mediterranean diet with low carbohydrate content showed superior effects in reducing intrahepatic, pericardial, and pancreatic fat than a low-fat isocaloric diet in volunteers with obesity. The Mediterranean diet combined with moderate physical activity further decreased the visceral fat volume and improved insulin sensitivity and blood lipid profile [78].

Similarly, an alternate-day fasting scheme (600 kcal/d alternated with ad libitum every other day) for 3 months in individuals with obesity decreased intrahepatic fat content and body weight while improving insulin sensitivity [79]. These results suggest that decreasing intrahepatic and intramyocellular fat content improves insulin sensitivity. Noteworthy, the increased intramyocellular lipid content commonly observed in endurance-trained athletes does not associate with impaired muscle insulin sensitivity, a phenomenon known as the athlete's paradox [80]. Thus, qualitative differences in the accumulated lipids or the cellular adaptative mechanism overcoming intracellular lipid overload are critical determinants of insulin resistance rather than the total ectopic TAG load.

Protein Metabolism in Obesity

Overview of Protein Metabolism

Proteins are heterogeneous macromolecules with a broad range of molecular mass, structure, and functions. The biological properties of proteins are determined by their unique sequence of amino acids. These are organic structures containing at least one atom of nitrogen. Humans cannot synthesize some amino acids encoded in the genetic code (i.e., essential amino acids). These amino acids must be obtained from diet to match amino acid requirements for protein synthesis. Dietary amino acids and those derived from endogenous protein hydrolysis are energy substrates for humans, typically corresponding to 10–20% (60–120 g/day) of total energy needs. As a by-product of amino acid oxidation, nitrogen is lost in the urine, mainly as urea, implying that dietary amino acids must replace amino acids undergoing oxidation. Thus, the balance between protein oxidation (mainly assessed by nitrogen loss in the urine), synthesis, and intake is critical for preserving whole-body lean mass.

Dietary amino acids reach the liver via the portal vein, and a significant proportion is retained by hepatic tissue. Branched-chain amino acids (BCAA), i.e., valine, leucine, and isoleucine, are poorly metabolized by hepatocytes and are preferentially channeled to skeletal muscle for energy production and conversion into alanine and glutamine. These two latter amino acids are then released from muscle and taken up by the liver and other tissues for further utilization.

Amino acids turnover depends on the level of energy sufficiency that determines the extent to which amino acids are spared as an energy source, including the balance between protein synthesis and degradation [81]. Insulin is a key regulator of this balance, although its effectiveness depends on circulating insulin concentration. Thus, low circulating insulin concentration (similar to that observed in insulin-sensitive fasted individuals) in the presence of a high amino acid supply stimulates muscle protein synthesis without affecting skeletal muscle protein breakdown

[82]. However, increasing blood insulin concentration does not enhance protein synthesis but suppresses protein degradation [82]. At the molecular level, insulin increases Akt/PKB activity, stimulating the mammalian target of rapamycin complex 1 (mTORC1), a critical regulator of protein synthesis. Insulin also decreases protein degradation by inhibiting proteasome activity [83]. Similarly, IGF-1, another critical mediator activating PI3K/Akt pathway, can also inhibit the ubiquitin-proteasome system and protein degradation [84].

Protein Turnover in Obesity

Obesity-related hyperinsulinemia could promote protein accretion unless defective insulin action also extends to amino acid metabolism. Insulin regulation of glucose and amino acid metabolism may also differ in the molecular pathways involved. Several studies have compared whole-body amino acid metabolism in individuals with and without obesity. Some studies detected higher fasting proteolysis in obesity [85, 86], which becomes normalized after weight loss [87]. Other studies, however, observed a similar pattern in individuals with and without obesity [88, 89]. Upon insulin stimulation, proteolysis suppression appears preserved in obesity [86–89]. In turn, insulin-stimulated protein synthesis appears impaired [86] or preserved [88, 89] in obesity. Differences in study design (e.g., the method to correct for body size, comparison based on relative or absolute values, and insulin dose) can partly explain the lack of consistency across studies. Subject characteristics may also play a role, including body fat distribution and the degree of insulin resistance, which are heterogeneous among individuals with obesity. Taken together, an obesity-related pattern regarding whole-body protein metabolism is unclear.

At the organ level, skeletal muscle represents a target of interest. Obesity shows to impair protein synthesis in response to insulin or protein ingestion. This phenomenon, coined as "anabolic resistance," is associated with insulin resistance and low-grade inflammation [90]. Such anabolic resistance has been noted in individuals with obesity after ingestion of isolated milk protein [91] and co-infusion of insulin plus amino acids [92]. The pathophysiological relevance of this phenomenon is elusive because it does not seem to affect leg muscle mass or strength [92]. In addition, similar to the whole-body level, muscle resistance to the anabolic stimuli of food protein [93, 94] or insulin [88] is not consistently reported.

Branched-Chain Amino Acids (BCAA) and Obesity

For over 50 years, it has been known that circulating BCAA concentration is elevated in human obesity. Even more, there is evidence suggesting that high-blood BCAA is an independent risk factor for insulin resistance and type 2 diabetes [95]. Why blood BCAA is high in obesity, besides its pathophysiological relevance, remains unsolved. One possible explanation is that most dietary BCAA reach peripheral circulation, which prompts the idea that increased protein intake in individuals with obesity may lead to higher circulating BCAA. Indeed, there is a tight direct correlation between BCAA intake and blood BCAA concentration [96].

Impaired tissue clearance of circulating BCAA might also play a role. Isolated adipocytes from subcutaneous WAT of individuals with obesity showed lower expression of mitochondrial BCAA catabolic enzymes than adipocytes from lean donors [97]. Furthermore, the content of mitochondrial BCAA aminotransferase and branched-chain keto acid dehydrogenase subunit E1 (two catabolic enzymes of BCAA) in WAT increased after gastric bypass-induced weight loss, which mirrored the reduction in circulating BCAA concentration [98]. Although the contribution of WAT to whole-body BCAA metabolism appears minor [97], these studies suggest that high-blood BCAA concentration in obesity may not just be a consequence of higher food/protein intake.

Concluding Remarks

Obesity is the result of a chronic mismatch between energy intake and expenditure. This energy imbalance challenges the capacity of the body to handle and dispose of glucose and lipid macronutrients properly. Over time, positive energy balance leads to a new steady state, set at higher energy flux levels, in which macronutrient overflow matches macronutrient oxidation. Why, when individuals reach this new steady state, they cannot resolve the metabolic disturbance associated with excessive adiposity remains unknown.

It is possible that abnormally high steady-state energy flux, attributed to increased body size rather than elevated physical activity, might determine metabolic stress. On the other hand, tissue-specific metabolic disturbances may be undetectable when a whole-body approach is utilized. The fact that whole-body macronutrient oxidative and nonoxidative disposal under physiological conditions (e.g., in the transition from fasting to feeding conditions or over a 24-h period) is similar in individuals without and with obesity may underestimate subtle tissue-specific macronutrient unbalances.

The notion of obesity as a simple metabolic entity is unrealistic. Indeed, there are different subtypes of obesity, e.g., metabolically healthy and unhealthy obese [99]. Identifying tissue, cellular, and molecular determinants of metabolic adaptation to high-energy fluxes will require expanding our capabilities to study in vivo tissue metabolic dynamics. Furthermore, molecular insight to interindividual variation in the adaptation to overfeeding and weight gain would enhance our understanding of obesity-related metabolic disorders.

References

1. Rolfe DF, Brown GC. Cellular energy utilization and molecular origin of standard metabolic rate in mammals. Physiol Rev. 1997;77(3):731–58.
2. Klein S, Gastaldelli A, Yki-Jarvinen H, Scherer PE. Why does obesity cause diabetes? Cell Metab. 2022;34(1):11–20.
3. Fontaine KR, Redden DT, Wang C, Westfall AO, Allison DB. Years of life lost due to obesity. JAMA. 2003;289(2):187–93.
4. Hill JO, Peters JC, Reed GW, Schlundt DG, Sharp T, Greene HL. Nutrient balance in humans: effects of diet composition. Am J Clin Nutr. 1991;54(1):10–7.
5. Westerterp KR. Food quotient, respiratory quotient, and energy balance. Am J Clin Nutr. 1993;57 (5 Suppl):759S–64S; discussion 64S–65S.
6. Weyer C, Vozarova B, Ravussin E, Tataranni PA. Changes in energy metabolism in response to 48 h of overfeeding and fasting in Caucasians and Pima Indians. Int J Obes Relat Metab Disord. 2001;25(5):593–600.
7. Webb P, Annis JF. Adaptation to overeating in lean and overweight men and women. Hum Nutr Clin Nutr. 1983;37(2):117–31.
8. McDevitt RM, Poppitt SD, Murgatroyd PR, Prentice AM. Macronutrient disposal during controlled overfeeding with glucose, fructose, sucrose, or fat in lean and obese women. Am J Clin Nutr. 2000;72(2): 369–77.
9. Gerich JE. Physiology of glucose homeostasis. Diabetes Obes Metab. 2000;2(6):345–50.
10. Baron AD, Brechtel G, Wallace P, Edelman SV. Rates and tissue sites of non-insulin- and insulin-mediated glucose uptake in humans. Am J Physiol. 1988;255 (6 Pt 1):E769–74.
11. Ferrannini E, Bjorkman O, Reichard GA Jr, Pilo A, Olsson M, Wahren J, et al. The disposal of an oral glucose load in healthy subjects. A quantitative study. Diabetes. 1985;34(6):580–8.
12. Bonuccelli S, Muscelli E, Gastaldelli A, Barsotti E, Astiarraga BD, Holst JJ, et al. Improved tolerance to sequential glucose loading (Staub-Traugott effect): size and mechanisms. Am J Physiol Endocrinol Metab. 2009;297(2):E532–7.
13. Cahill GF Jr. Fuel metabolism in starvation. Annu Rev Nutr. 2006;26:1–22.
14. Galgani JE, Fernandez-Verdejo R. Pathophysiological role of metabolic flexibility on metabolic health. Obes Rev. 2021;22(2):e13131.
15. Holman GD. Structure, function and regulation of mammalian glucose transporters of the SLC2 family. Pflugers Arch. 2020;472(9):1155–75.
16. Klip A, McGraw TE, James DE. Thirty sweet years of GLUT4. J Biol Chem. 2019;294(30):11369–81.
17. Kelley DE, Goodpaster B, Wing RR, Simoneau JA. Skeletal muscle fatty acid metabolism in association with insulin resistance, obesity, and weight loss. Am J Physiol. 1999;277(6 Pt 1):E1130–41.
18. Dohm GL, Tapscott EB, Pories WJ, Dabbs DJ, Flickinger EG, Meelheim D, et al. An in vitro human muscle preparation suitable for metabolic studies. Decreased insulin stimulation of glucose transport in muscle from morbidly obese and diabetic subjects. J Clin Invest. 1988;82(2):486–94.
19. Allenberg K, Nilsson M, Landin K, Lindgarde F. Glycogen and lactate synthetic pathways in human skeletal muscle in relation to obesity, weight reduction and physical training. Eur J Clin Investig. 1988;18(3): 250–5.
20. Bonadonna RC, Groop L, Kraemer N, Ferrannini E, Del Prato S, DeFronzo RA. Obesity and insulin

resistance in humans: a dose-response study. Metabolism. 1990;39(5):452–9.

21. Laakso M, Edelman SV, Olefsky JM, Brechtel G, Wallace P, Baron AD. Kinetics of in vivo muscle insulin-mediated glucose uptake in human obesity. Diabetes. 1990;39(8):965–74.

22. Ramos PA, Lytle KA, Delivanis D, Nielsen S, LeBrasseur NK, Jensen MD. Insulin-stimulated muscle glucose uptake and insulin signaling in lean and obese humans. J Clin Endocrinol Metab. 2021;106(4): e1631–e46.

23. Koh HE, van Vliet S, Meyer GA, Laforest R, Gropler RJ, Klein S, et al. Heterogeneity in insulin-stimulated glucose uptake among different muscle groups in healthy lean people and people with obesity. Diabetologia. 2021;64(5):1158–68.

24. Goodyear LJ, Giorgino F, Sherman LA, Carey J, Smith RJ, Dohm GL. Insulin receptor phosphorylation, insulin receptor substrate-1 phosphorylation, and phosphatidylinositol 3-kinase activity are decreased in intact skeletal muscle strips from obese subjects. J Clin Invest. 1995;95(5):2195–204.

25. Gastaldelli A. Measuring and estimating insulin resistance in clinical and research settings. Obesity (Silver Spring). 2022;30(8):1549–63.

26. van Vliet S, Koh HE, Patterson BW, Yoshino M, LaForest R, Gropler RJ, et al. Obesity is associated with increased basal and postprandial beta-cell insulin secretion even in the absence of insulin resistance. Diabetes. 2020;69(10):2112–9.

27. Baron AD, Laakso M, Brechtel G, Hoit B, Watt C, Edelman SV. Reduced postprandial skeletal muscle blood flow contributes to glucose intolerance in human obesity. J Clin Endocrinol Metab. 1990;70(6): 1525–33.

28. Chondronikola M, Magkos F, Yoshino J, Okunade AL, Patterson BW, Muehlbauer MJ, et al. Effect of progressive weight loss on lactate metabolism: a randomized controlled trial. Obesity (Silver Spring). 2018;26(4): 683–8.

29. Stunff CL, Bougneres PF. Alterations of plasma lactate and glucose metabolism in obese children. Am J Physiol. 1996;271(5 Pt 1):E814–20.

30. Jing E, O'Neill BT, Rardin MJ, Kleinridders A, Ilkeyeva OR, Ussar S, et al. Sirt3 regulates metabolic flexibility of skeletal muscle through reversible enzymatic deacetylation. Diabetes. 2013;62(10):3404–17.

31. Owen OE, Mozzoli MA, Smalley KJ, Kavle EC, D'Alessio DA. Oxidative and nonoxidative macronutrient disposal in lean and obese men after mixed meals. Am J Clin Nutr. 1992;55(3):630–6.

32. Galgani JE, Ravussin E. Postprandial whole-body glycolysis is similar in insulin-resistant and insulin-sensitive non-diabetic humans. Diabetologia. 2012;55(3):737–42.

33. Galgani JE, Heilbronn LK, Azuma K, Kelley DE, Albu JB, Pi-Sunyer X, et al. Metabolic flexibility in response to glucose is not impaired in people with type 2 diabetes after controlling for glucose disposal rate. Diabetes. 2008;57(4):841–5.

34. Yki-Jarvinen H, Mott D, Young AA, Stone K, Bogardus C. Regulation of glycogen synthase and phosphorylase activities by glucose and insulin in human skeletal muscle. J Clin Invest. 1987;80(1): 95–100.

35. Young AA, Bogardus C, Wolfe-Lopez D, Mott DM. Muscle glycogen synthesis and disposition of infused glucose in humans with reduced rates of insulin-mediated carbohydrate storage. Diabetes. 1988;37(3):303–8.

36. Cline GW, Petersen KF, Krssak M, Shen J, Hundal RS, Trajanoski Z, et al. Impaired glucose transport as a cause of decreased insulin-stimulated muscle glycogen synthesis in type 2 diabetes. N Engl J Med. 1999;341(4):240–6.

37. Hojlund K, Birk JB, Klein DK, Levin K, Rose AJ, Hansen BF, et al. Dysregulation of glycogen synthase COOH- and NH2-terminal phosphorylation by insulin in obesity and type 2 diabetes mellitus. J Clin Endocrinol Metab. 2009;94(11):4547–56.

38. Fabbrini E, Magkos F, Mohammed BS, Pietka T, Abumrad NA, Patterson BW, et al. Intrahepatic fat, not visceral fat, is linked with metabolic complications of obesity. Proc Natl Acad Sci U S A. 2009;106(36): 15430–5.

39. Fabbrini E, Tamboli RA, Magkos F, Marks-Shulman PA, Eckhauser AW, Richards WO, et al. Surgical removal of omental fat does not improve insulin sensitivity and cardiovascular risk factors in obese adults. Gastroenterology. 2010;139(2):448–55.

40. Lima MM, Pareja JC, Alegre SM, Geloneze SR, Kahn SE, Astiarraga BD, et al. Visceral fat resection in humans: effect on insulin sensitivity, beta-cell function, adipokines, and inflammatory markers. Obesity (Silver Spring). 2013;21(3):E182–9.

41. Nielsen S, Guo Z, Johnson CM, Hensrud DD, Jensen MD. Splanchnic lipolysis in human obesity. J Clin Invest. 2004;113(11):1582–8.

42. Acheson KJ, Schutz Y, Bessard T, Anantharaman K, Flatt JP, Jequier E. Glycogen storage capacity and de novo lipogenesis during massive carbohydrate overfeeding in man. Am J Clin Nutr. 1988;48(2):240–7.

43. Minehira K, Vega N, Vidal H, Acheson K, Tappy L. Effect of carbohydrate overfeeding on whole body macronutrient metabolism and expression of lipogenic enzymes in adipose tissue of lean and overweight humans. Int J Obes Relat Metab Disord. 2004;28(10): 1291–8.

44. Marques-Lopes I, Ansorena D, Astiasaran I, Forga L, Martinez JA. Postprandial de novo lipogenesis and metabolic changes induced by a high-carbohydrate, low-fat meal in lean and overweight men. Am J Clin Nutr. 2001;73(2):253–61.

45. McDevitt RM, Bott SJ, Harding M, Coward WA, Bluck LJ, Prentice AM. De novo lipogenesis during controlled overfeeding with sucrose or glucose in lean and obese women. Am J Clin Nutr. 2001;74(6): 737–46.

46. Smith GI, Shankaran M, Yoshino M, Schweitzer GG, Chondronikola M, Beals JW, et al. Insulin resistance

drives hepatic de novo lipogenesis in nonalcoholic fatty liver disease. J Clin Invest. 2020;130(3):1453–60.

47. Schwarz JM, Neese RA, Turner S, Dare D, Hellerstein MK. Short-term alterations in carbohydrate energy intake in humans. Striking effects on hepatic glucose production, de novo lipogenesis, lipolysis, and whole-body fuel selection. J Clin Invest. 1995;96(6):2735–43.

48. Cortes VA, Busso D, Maiz A, Arteaga A, Nervi F, Rigotti A. Physiological and pathological implications of cholesterol. Front Biosci (Landmark Ed). 2014;19(3):416–28.

49. Trujillo ME, Scherer PE. Adipose tissue-derived factors: impact on health and disease. Endocr Rev. 2006;27(7):762–78.

50. Hajri T, Abumrad NA. Fatty acid transport across membranes: relevance to nutrition and metabolic pathology. Annu Rev Nutr. 2002;22:383–415.

51. Tan GD, Debard C, Tiraby C, Humphreys SM, Frayn KN, Langin D, et al. A "futile cycle" induced by thiazolidinediones in human adipose tissue? Nat Med. 2003;9(7):811–2; author reply 2.

52. Donnelly KL, Smith CI, Schwarzenberg SJ, Jessurun J, Boldt MD, Parks EJ. Sources of fatty acids stored in liver and secreted via lipoproteins in patients with nonalcoholic fatty liver disease. J Clin Invest. 2005;115(5):1343–51.

53. Chakravarthy MV, Lodhi IJ, Yin L, Malapaka RR, Xu HE, Turk J, et al. Identification of a physiologically relevant endogenous ligand for PPARalpha in liver. Cell. 2009;138(3):476–88.

54. Kim JK, Fillmore JJ, Chen Y, Yu C, Moore IK, Pypaert M, et al. Tissue-specific overexpression of lipoprotein lipase causes tissue-specific insulin resistance. Proc Natl Acad Sci U S A. 2001;98(13):7522–7.

55. Goudriaan JR, den Boer MA, Rensen PC, Febbraio M, Kuipers F, Romijn JA, et al. CD36 deficiency in mice impairs lipoprotein lipase-mediated triglyceride clearance. J Lipid Res. 2005;46(10):2175–81.

56. Goudriaan JR, Dahlmans VE, Teusink B, Ouwens DM, Febbraio M, Maassen JA, et al. CD36 deficiency increases insulin sensitivity in muscle, but induces insulin resistance in the liver in mice. J Lipid Res. 2003;44(12):2270–7.

57. Ibrahimi A, Bonen A, Blinn WD, Hajri T, Li X, Zhong K, et al. Muscle-specific overexpression of FAT/CD36 enhances fatty acid oxidation by contracting muscle, reduces plasma triglycerides and fatty acids, and increases plasma glucose and insulin. J Biol Chem. 1999;274(38):26761–6.

58. Katare PB, Dalmao-Fernandez A, Mengeste AM, Hamarsland H, Ellefsen S, Bakke HG, et al. Energy metabolism in skeletal muscle cells from donors with different body mass index. Front Physiol. 2022;13: 982842.

59. Cao C, Koh HE, Van Vliet S, Patterson BW, Reeds DN, Laforest R, et al. Increased plasma fatty acid clearance, not fatty acid concentration, is associated with muscle insulin resistance in people with obesity. Metabolism. 2022;132:155216.

60. Horowitz JF, Klein S. Oxidation of nonplasma fatty acids during exercise is increased in women with abdominal obesity. J Appl Physiol (1985). 2000;89(6):2276–82.

61. Kim JY, Hickner RC, Cortright RL, Dohm GL, Houmard JA. Lipid oxidation is reduced in obese human skeletal muscle. Am J Physiol Endocrinol Metab. 2000;279(5):E1039–44.

62. Groop LC, Bonadonna RC, Simonson DC, Petrides AS, Shank M, DeFronzo RA. Effect of insulin on oxidative and nonoxidative pathways of free fatty acid metabolism in human obesity. Am J Physiol. 1992;263(1 Pt 1):E79–84.

63. Goodpaster BH, Wolfe RR, Kelley DE. Effects of obesity on substrate utilization during exercise. Obes Res. 2002;10(7):575–84.

64. Kiefer LS, Fabian J, Rospleszcz S, Lorbeer R, Machann J, Kraus MS, et al. Distribution patterns of intramyocellular and extramyocellular fat by magnetic resonance imaging in subjects with diabetes, prediabetes and normoglycaemic controls. Diabetes Obes Metab. 2021;23(8):1868–78.

65. Frayn KN. Adipose tissue as a buffer for daily lipid flux. Diabetologia. 2002;45(9):1201–10.

66. Karpe F, Dickmann JR, Frayn KN. Fatty acids, obesity, and insulin resistance: time for a reevaluation. Diabetes. 2011;60(10):2441–9.

67. Liu L, Zhang Y, Chen N, Shi X, Tsang B, Yu YH. Upregulation of myocellular DGAT1 augments triglyceride synthesis in skeletal muscle and protects against fat-induced insulin resistance. J Clin Invest. 2007;117(6):1679–89.

68. Badin PM, Louche K, Mairal A, Liebisch G, Schmitz G, Rustan AC, et al. Altered skeletal muscle lipase expression and activity contribute to insulin resistance in humans. Diabetes. 2011;60(6):1734–42.

69. Moro C, Galgani JE, Luu L, Pasarica M, Mairal A, Bajpeyi S, et al. Influence of gender, obesity, and muscle lipase activity on intramyocellular lipids in sedentary individuals. J Clin Endocrinol Metab. 2009;94(9):3440–7.

70. Rutkowski JM, Stern JH, Scherer PE. The cell biology of fat expansion. J Cell Biol. 2015;208(5):501–12.

71. Oral EA, Simha V, Ruiz E, Andewelt A, Premkumar A, Snell P, et al. Leptin-replacement therapy for lipodystrophy. N Engl J Med. 2002;346(8):570–8.

72. Adiels M, Taskinen MR, Packard C, Caslake MJ, Soro-Paavonen A, Westerbacka J, et al. Overproduction of large VLDL particles is driven by increased liver fat content in man. Diabetologia. 2006;49(4):755–65.

73. Gastaldelli A, Cusi K, Pettiti M, Hardies J, Miyazaki Y, Berria R, et al. Relationship between hepatic/visceral fat and hepatic insulin resistance in nondiabetic and type 2 diabetic subjects. Gastroenterology. 2007;133(2):496–506.

74. Saponaro C, Sabatini S, Gaggini M, Carli F, Rosso C, Positano V, et al. Adipose tissue dysfunction and visceral fat are associated with hepatic insulin resistance

and severity of NASH even in lean individuals. Liver Int. 2022;42(11):2418–27.

75. Mayerson AB, Hundal RS, Dufour S, Lebon V, Befroy D, Cline GW, et al. The effects of rosiglitazone on insulin sensitivity, lipolysis, and hepatic and skeletal muscle triglyceride content in patients with type 2 diabetes. Diabetes. 2002;51(3):797–802.

76. Bergman BC, Butterfield GE, Wolfel EE, Casazza GA, Lopaschuk GD, Brooks GA. Evaluation of exercise and training on muscle lipid metabolism. Am J Physiol. 1999;276(1 Pt 1):E106–17.

77. Hoppeler H, Howald H, Conley K, Lindstedt SL, Claassen H, Vock P, et al. Endurance training in humans: aerobic capacity and structure of skeletal muscle. J Appl Physiol (1985). 1985;59(2):320–7.

78. Gepner Y, Shelef I, Schwarzfuchs D, Zelicha H, Tene L, Yaskolka Meir A, et al. Effect of distinct lifestyle interventions on mobilization of fat storage pools: CENTRAL magnetic resonance imaging randomized controlled trial. Circulation. 2018;137(11): 1143–57.

79. Ezpeleta M, Gabel K, Cienfuegos S, Kalam F, Lin S, Pavlou V, et al. Effect of alternate day fasting combined with aerobic exercise on non-alcoholic fatty liver disease: a randomized controlled trial. Cell Metab. 2023;35(1):56–70 e3.

80. Goodpaster BH, He J, Watkins S, Kelley DE. Skeletal muscle lipid content and insulin resistance: evidence for a paradox in endurance-trained athletes. J Clin Endocrinol Metab. 2001;86(12):5755–61.

81. Pellett PL, Young VR. The effects of different levels of energy intake on protein metabolism and of different levels of protein intake on energy metabolism: a statistical evaluation from the published literature. In: Scrimshaw NS, Schürch B, editors. Protein energy interactions. Lausanne: International Dietary Energy Consultancy Group Switzerland; 1992. p. 81–136.

82. Greenhaff PL, Karagounis LG, Peirce N, Simpson EJ, Hazell M, Layfield R, et al. Disassociation between the effects of amino acids and insulin on signaling, ubiquitin ligases, and protein turnover in human muscle. Am J Physiol Endocrinol Metab. 2008;295(3): E595–604.

83. James HA, O'Neill BT, Nair KS. Insulin regulation of proteostasis and clinical implications. Cell Metab. 2017;26(2):310–23.

84. Yoshida T, Delafontaine P. Mechanisms of IGF-1-mediated regulation of skeletal muscle hypertrophy and atrophy. Cells. 2020;9(9):1970.

85. Welle S, Barnard RR, Statt M, Amatruda JM. Increased protein turnover in obese women. Metabolism. 1992;41(9):1028–34.

86. Chevalier S, Marliss EB, Morais JA, Lamarche M, Gougeon R. Whole-body protein anabolic response is resistant to the action of insulin in obese women. Am J Clin Nutr. 2005;82(2):355–65.

87. Welle S, Statt M, Barnard R, Amatruda J. Differential effect of insulin on whole-body proteolysis and glucose

metabolism in normal-weight, obese, and reduced-obese women. Metabolism. 1994;43(4):441–5.

88. Guillet C, Delcourt I, Rance M, Giraudet C, Walrand S, Bedu M, et al. Changes in basal and insulin and amino acid response of whole body and skeletal muscle proteins in obese men. J Clin Endocrinol Metab. 2009;94(8):3044–50.

89. Solini A, Bonora E, Bonadonna R, Castellino P, DeFronzo RA. Protein metabolism in human obesity: relationship with glucose and lipid metabolism and with visceral adipose tissue. J Clin Endocrinol Metab. 1997;82(8):2552–8.

90. Paulussen KJM, McKenna CF, Beals JW, Wilund KR, Salvador AF, Burd NA. Anabolic resistance of muscle protein turnover comes in various shapes and sizes. Front Nutr. 2021;8:615849.

91. Smeuninx B, McKendry J, Wilson D, Martin U, Breen L. Age-related anabolic resistance of myofibrillar protein synthesis is exacerbated in obese inactive individuals. J Clin Endocrinol Metab. 2017;102(9):3535–45.

92. Murton AJ, Marimuthu K, Mallinson JE, Selby AL, Smith K, Rennie MJ, et al. Obesity appears to be associated with altered muscle protein synthetic and breakdown responses to increased nutrient delivery in older men, but not reduced muscle mass or contractile function. Diabetes. 2015;64(9):3160–71.

93. Kouw IWK, van Dijk JW, Horstman AMH, Kramer IF, Goessens JPB, van Dielen FMH, et al. Basal and postprandial myofibrillar protein synthesis rates do not differ between lean and obese middle-aged men. J Nutr. 2019;149(9):1533–42.

94. Beals JW, Skinner SK, McKenna CF, Poozhikunnel EG, Farooqi SA, van Vliet S, et al. Altered anabolic signalling and reduced stimulation of myofibrillar protein synthesis after feeding and resistance exercise in people with obesity. J Physiol. 2018;596(21):5119–33.

95. White PJ, McGarrah RW, Herman MA, Bain JR, Shah SH, Newgard CB. Insulin action, type 2 diabetes, and branched-chain amino acids: a two-way street. Mol Metab. 2021;52:101261.

96. Meguid MM, Matthews DE, Bier DM, Meredith CN, Soeldner JS, Young VR. Leucine kinetics at graded leucine intakes in young men. Am J Clin Nutr. 1986;43(5):770–80.

97. Lackey DE, Lynch CJ, Olson KC, Mostaedi R, Ali M, Smith WH, et al. Regulation of adipose branched-chain amino acid catabolism enzyme expression and cross-adipose amino acid flux in human obesity. Am J Physiol Endocrinol Metab. 2013;304(11):E1175–87.

98. She P, Van Horn C, Reid T, Hutson SM, Cooney RN, Lynch CJ. Obesity-related elevations in plasma leucine are associated with alterations in enzymes involved in branched-chain amino acid metabolism. Am J Physiol Endocrinol Metab. 2007;293(6):E1552–63.

99. Bluher M. Metabolically healthy obesity. Endocr Rev. 2020;41(3):bnaa004.

Brain Regulation of Feeding and Energy Homeostasis

16

Alison H. Affinati, Carol F. Elias, David P. Olson, and Martin G. Myers Jr

Contents

A. H. Affinati (✉)
Department of Internal Medicine, University of Michigan, Ann Arbor, MI, USA
e-mail: aaffinat@med.umich.edu; aaffinat@umich.edu

C. F. Elias
Department of Molecular and Integrative Physiology, University of Michigan, Ann Arbor, MI, USA

Department of Obstetrics and Gynecology, University of Michigan, Ann Arbor, MI, USA
e-mail: cfelias@umich.edu; cfelias@med.umich.edu

D. P. Olson
Department of Molecular and Integrative Physiology, University of Michigan, Ann Arbor, MI, USA

Department of Pediatrics, University of Michigan, Ann Arbor, MI, USA
e-mail: dpolson@med.umich.edu; dpolson@umich.edu

M. G. Myers Jr
Department of Internal Medicine, University of Michigan, Ann Arbor, MI, USA

Department of Molecular and Integrative Physiology, University of Michigan, Ann Arbor, MI, USA
e-mail: mgmyers@med.umich.edu; mgmyers@umich.edu

© Springer Nature Switzerland AG 2023
R. S. Ahima (ed.), *Metabolic Syndrome*,
https://doi.org/10.1007/978-3-031-40116-9_22

Abstract

In the past decades, it has become clear that homeostatic systems in the brain play a key role in the control of feeding and energy homeostasis. These neuronal circuits require the integration of diverse physiological components, from sensing energy demands and storage to behavioral responses, motor function, and reflex adjustments. Studies in various organisms including worms, flies, rodents, and humans have identified key molecular pathways, conserved genes, and neural circuits crucial for the control of individual components of energy homeostasis. Among them, the brain plays the fundamental role in feeding behavior, satiety, reward or hedonic consumption, energy expenditure, body weight and body composition, and glucose homeostasis. Although the role of the brain in the control of metabolism has been studied for over a century, the discovery of leptin and its cognate receptor in the mid-1990s and recent advances in molecular and genetic tools to study neural circuits and their function have accelerated the advancement of the field. In this chapter, we will highlight the main findings in recent years using these scientific tools with emphasis on the brain pathways and circuitry associated with the control of food intake and metabolism.

Keywords

Hypothalamus · Neuroendocrinology · Autonomic nervous system · Melanocortin · Lateral parabrachial nucleus · Paraventricular nucleus of the hypothalamus · Arcuate nucleus · Mesolimbic dopaminergic system

Introduction

The fundamental role of the central nervous system (CNS) in the regulation of feeding and energy homeostasis has been known for over a century. Clinical observations in patients with Fröhlich's syndrome (adiposogenital dystrophy) who display excessive subcutaneous fat due to adenopituitary tumors gave rise to an important debate on the relative contributions of the pituitary gland versus the overlying hypothalamus in the genesis of obesity in this syndrome. While Fröhlich, Crowe, and Cushing supported the importance of the pituitary gland in the control of adiposity, Aschner subsequently demonstrated that removal of the pituitary gland alone did not affect adiposity in dogs, suggesting that hypothalamic damage was the main cause of the obesity seen in Fröhlich's syndrome [1]. With the development of experimental techniques to lesion specific areas of the brain, Hetherington and Ranson reinforced Aschner's findings and proposed a crucial role for the hypothalamus in regulation of feeding and body weight. They observed that bilateral lesions of the medial hypothalamus of rats (without disturbing the pituitary gland) produced a profound increase in body weight and fat. On the other hand, lesions of the lateral hypothalamic area resulted in profound hypophagia, often leading to death by starvation. Together, these observations gave rise to the classic "dual center" model proposed by Stellar in 1954, which posited that the hypothalamus contains a "satiety center" (i.e., the ventromedial nucleus of the hypothalamus, the VMH) and a "feeding center" (i.e., the lateral hypothalamic area, the LHA) [2].

These ideas were later revised with the development of more refined and precise techniques.

For example, small electrolytic or excitotoxic lesions of the VMH and adjacent areas or knife cuts of projecting fibers failed to recapitulate hyperphagic obesity, challenging the concept of the VMH as the satiety center [3]. Concurrently, others questioned the interpretation of data from lesions of the LHA due to the potential interruption of the medial forebrain bundle (which contains the ascending fibers of the mesolimbic dopaminergic system), which might cause movement disorders or other behavioral changes [4].

The discovery of the leptin and its cognate receptor (LepRb) in the mid-1990s, together with the development of new molecular and genetic tools, has enabled targeted analysis of neural circuits and the identification of genetically defined neuronal populations associated with specific physiological components of energy homeostasis [5–7].

As a starting point, the neural control of metabolic function recapitulates the basic organizational principles of the CNS in general. The sensory (*input*) arm perceives and conveys information on nutritional state and energy stores to specific brain nuclei (*integrative centers*) that integrate multiple physiological signals and orchestrate a coordinated response via the motor (*output*) arm. The sensory arm relies on hormones, peptides, and other signals from peripheral organs and tissues that function as "metabolic cues." In this chapter, we will summarize what we have learned over the past three decades, primarily by using animal models and genetic tools. We will give special emphasis to the brain circuitry unraveled by studies performed in rodents, the preclinical animal model of choice in the field. Much of the information gleaned in rodents has been confirmed subsequently in humans.

Sensing Metabolic Cues: Humoral and Neural Components

The sensory (input) arm of the neural control of the metabolic function may be subdivided into humoral and neural components, according to the route used by the metabolic cues to access the CNS. Most of these signals enter the CNS via the hypothalamus (largely humoral signals) and brain stem (both humoral and neural signals).

Humoral Components

Metabolic signals derived from peripheral tissues are released into the circulation and directly act in specific hypothalamic and brain stem nuclei to control food intake, energy expenditure, and glucose homeostasis. Among them, hormones secreted by adipocytes (e.g., leptin), endocrine pancreas (e.g., insulin), and gastrointestinal tract (e.g., ghrelin) have been widely investigated in the context of the neural control of metabolic function.

Leptin, encoded by *Lep/LEP* (previously called *ob* for *obese*), is primarily synthesized and secreted by white adipose tissue [5]. During fasting, the fall in leptin levels represents a key signal for the neuroendocrine adaptations prompted by states of energy deficiency [8, 9]. These adaptive responses include decreased locomotor activity and thermogenesis, increased appetite and motivation for food, inhibition of the thyroid and reproductive axes, and activation of the adrenal axis. Leptin acts via its receptor, LepRb (encoded by *Lepr/LEPR*), which is highly expressed in several regions of the hypothalamus, including the arcuate nucleus (ARH), the VMH, the dorsomedial nucleus (DMH), and the LHA. In the brain stem, the ventral tegmental area (VTA), the periaqueductal gray matter (PAG), the lateral parabrachial nucleus (lPBN), and the nucleus of the solitary tract (NTS) also express LepRb [6, 7, 10, 11].

Insulin, produced by the pancreatic β cells, is crucial for the control of blood glucose; it stimulates glucose uptake by peripheral organs including the liver, muscle, and adipose tissue. Glucose uptake by neurons and glia is mediated by insulin-insensitive glucose transporters; hence, the acquisition and use of glucose by the brain are independent of insulin action. Insulin receptors are widespread in the CNS, however, and a host of evidence supports a role for brain insulin action in the control of energy balance (along with peripheral glucose homeostasis). For example, mice with brain deletion of insulin receptor display increased adiposity and higher susceptibility to obesogenic diet [12, 13], whereas selection of ablation insulin receptor from astrocytes dysregulates glucose homeostasis [14].

Ghrelin is primarily produced and released by endocrine cells of the stomach and small intestine. It was initially described as a potent growth hormone (GH) secretagogue, acting via the GH secretagogue receptor (GHSR). Soon after its discovery, several laboratories reported that peripheral or central injections of ghrelin potently stimulate food intake and decrease energy expenditure, leading to weight gain [15]. Ghrelin is also an important modulator of glucose homeostasis. Loss-of-function mutations in the ghrelin gene (*Ghrl*) increase glucose-stimulated insulin secretion, as well as insulin sensitivity [16]. Similarly, ghrelin infusion reduces insulin sensitivity and increases glucose levels. Some of ghrelin's actions may be mediated by direct effects on pancreatic islets, but many lines of evidence demonstrate major roles of ghrelin through GHSR in the brain. GHSR is abundant in the ARH and VMH, as well as several relevant brain stem sites, including the VTA, lPBN, and NTS [15].

To exert their effects, circulating hormones must cross the blood–brain barrier (BBB) to reach their receptors in the brain parenchyma. The BBB is composed of closely apposing endothelial cells, glia, and (in some areas) tanycytes. It is present in the entire brain with the exception of small areas located adjacent to the cerebral ventricles, called circumventricular organs (CVOs). The CVOs contain fenestrated blood vessels that allow diffusion and interchange of bigger molecules (peptides and hormones) between the brain parenchyma and the bloodstream, presumably without the need for active transport across the BBB [17]. Among the well-described CVOs, the median eminence and the area postrema (AP) are of particular interest here, given their proximity to metabolic sensing neurons in the ARH and the NTS, respectively. Circulating hormones may cross the BBB to access other brain regions via two mechanisms: (a) via lipid-mediated free diffusion and (b) via carrier- or receptor-mediated active transport. Most of the metabolic hormones

(e.g., leptin, insulin, and ghrelin) have BBB transporters that permit access to deep structures in the brain [18–20].

Neural Components: Visceral Inputs

The CNS control of energy homeostasis also relies on information conveyed by neuronal inputs. Sensory information is generated in each segment of the alimentary tract, from food taste, temperature, and texture in the mouth to mechanical and chemical signals in the stomach and intestine. These signals are conveyed by several cranial nerves carrying different modalities of sensory inputs. The upper segments of the alimentary tract (mouth and tongue) convey gustatory inputs (taste signals) to the rostral NTS via the facial (VII) and glossopharyngeal (IX) cranial nerves; the mid- and lower segments (pharynx, larynx, esophagus, stomach, and intestine, as well as the liver and the portal vein) transmit mechanical and chemical inputs to the medial and caudal NTS via the vagus (cranial nerve X). The different modalities of sensory inputs convey distinct information to the brain. For example, while gustatory inputs are associated with food selection and hedonic responses, mechano- and chemoreceptors signal nutritional content. In this regard, the vagus nerve represents the primary neural conduit for information from the viscera to the CNS [21].

The vagus nerve is composed of afferent (sensory) and efferent (motor) fibers. The afferent vagal branch is organized as a typical sensory nerve, i.e., pseudo-unipolar neurons with cell bodies located in a ganglion outside the CNS, the nodose ganglion (a.k.a. inferior ganglion of the vagus nerve (Fig. 1)). Vagal dendrites, which contain specialized receptors, are distributed in a topographic manner along the mid- and lower segments of the alimentary tract. The mechanoreceptors are concentrated in the pharynx, esophagus, and stomach, and the chemoreceptors are more abundant in the stomach, liver, and intestine [22]. The mechanoreceptors are found throughout the myenteric plexus and external smooth muscle layers. In the stomach, they sense gastric

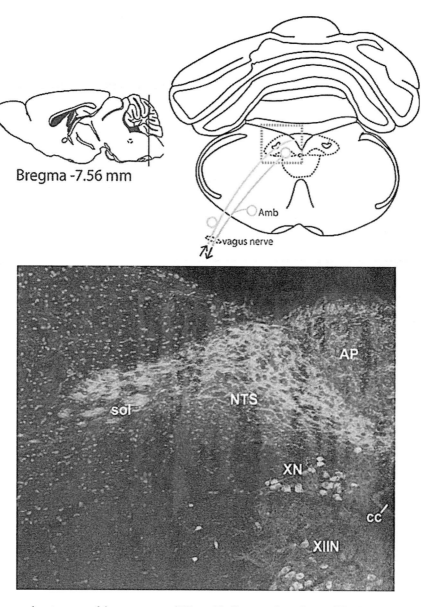

Fig. 1 Sensory and motor arms of the vagus nerve (*XN*). Sensory terminals innervate the area postrema (*AP*) and the nucleus of the solitary tract (*NTS*, pseudocolor *yellow*, using Nav1.8 reporter mice). Motor neurons in the motor nucleus of the vagus nerve (*DMV*) are represented in *blue* (choline acetyltransferase (ChAT) reporter mice). This image was kindly provided by Dr. Laurent Gautron, working in the University of Texas Southwestern Medical Center, Dallas

distension and provide signals that promote satiation. The chemoreceptors are distributed in the mucosal and submucosal layers of the gastrointestinal (GI) tract and in the liver and portal vein; these may sense changes in glucose, amino acids, and fatty acids. The chemoreceptor cells are also responsive to peptides produced in the GI mucosa in response to food intake, including (among others) ghrelin, cholecystokinin (CCK), amylin, peptide YY, and glucagon-like peptide-1 (GLP-1) [22, 23].

Measuring Ca^{+2}_i fluxes in nodose ganglion cells in vivo reveals that distinct subsets of vagal sensory neurons respond to gut stretch versus nutrient ingestion [24]. *Glp1r* expression marks stretch-responsive cells that receive information from mechanosensory terminals in the wall of the stomach (and in the intestine, to a lesser extent). Expression of the orphan GPCR *Gpr65* marks distinct nutrient-sensitive nodose cells, which innervate the intestinal villi. In addition to identifying additional markers for distinct vagal sensory cell types, single-cell RNA-sequencing and subsequent functional analysis of gut-innervating nodose neurons also revealed that stretch-sensitive (*Glp1r/Oxtr*) nodose cells decrease food intake, while nutrient-sensitive (*Gpr65/Vip/Sst*) nodose cells do not alter feeding, but rather modulate gastric pressure [25].

Brain Stem Pathways: Transducing Visceral and Humoral Inputs to Control Food Intake and Body Weight

Many humoral and neural signals of energy balance, including a variety of gut-derived signals, converge on the NTS (Fig. 2, [26, 27]). In addition to receiving vagally encoded information from the gut, many humorally conveyed signals (including gut peptides, such as amylin and CCK) activate AP cells that project onto an overlapping set of neurons in the medial NTS; medial NTS responses contribute to satiation.

The NTS receives and responds to many types of stimuli (not just feeding-related gut signals) and thus contains many different types of neurons that mediate distinct functions, including those that control respiration and cardiovascular function [28]. Groups of NTS neurons whose activation suppresses food intake include (among others) those that express cholecystokinin (*Cck*), *Lepr* (along with preproglucagon (*Gcg*), the processing of which in NTS neurons produces GLP-1), and calcitonin receptor (*Calcr*).

While most rodents are unable to vomit, stimuli associated with gut malaise in these animals promote a conditioned taste avoidance (CTA, in which the pairing of a novel flavor with an aversive stimulus prevents the subsequent ingestion of the flavor). Many stimuli that strongly activate NTS neurons as well as the artificial activation

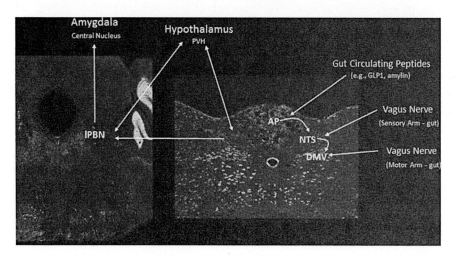

Fig. 2 Flow of information in the hindbrain. The area postrema (AP), a circumventricular organ that has direct access to the circulation, receives information about feeding status by sensing gut peptides (e.g., GLP1 and amylin). These cells project to the nucleus of the solitary tract (*NTS*), where the area postrema-derived information is integrated with information conveyed by vagal sensory afferents from the gut. This integrated information is not only passed to the dorsal motor nucleus of the vagus nerve (*DMV*) to stimulate vagal motor neurons efferent to the gut (controlling peristalsis, etc.) but is also passed forward to the lateral parabrachial nucleus (*lPBN*), an important center for anorexia, and to a variety of hypothalamic sites, including the paraventricular nucleus (*PVH*). Hypothalamic sites also project to the lPBN and NTS. The output of these nuclei promotes satiety. A subset of lPBN neurons projects to the central nucleus of the amygdala (CeA) to mediate a powerful anorectic signal

of several sets of NTS neurons (e.g., those that express *Cck*) promote CTA formation in addition to suppressing food intake. Hence, one model for the control of food intake by the NTS theorized the existence of a single type of appetite-suppressing NTS circuit by which moderate circuit activation promotes satiation, while stronger activation causes aversive responses.

This single circuit model does not fit well with the observation that consuming nutritious foods promotes a positively reinforcing response while suppressing feeding, however, since this would require the same circuit to mediate both positively and negatively reinforcing responses. Indeed, recent evidence suggests that some NTS circuits mediate satiation with neutral or positive valence, while distinct circuits promote aversive anorexia. For example, the activation of NTS *Calcr* neurons fails to promote a CTA (and may mediate positive reinforcement), despite suppressing food intake more strongly than does the activation of CTA-promoting NTS *Cck* cells [29]. The activation of *Lepr/Gcg*-expressing NTS neurons also strongly suppresses food intake but fails to promote a CTA [30, 31]. Hence, distinct NTS neuron types mediate the aversive versus non-aversive suppression of food intake.

The distinct gut-sensing nodose cell types innervate different regions of the NTS (nutrient-sensing *Gpr65* cells innervate a region proximal to the AP, while mechanosensing *Glp1r* cells innervate the lateral NTS) [24], consistent with the distinct downstream functions for each of these gut-innervating nodose cell types. Importantly, vagal sensory signaling from the gut transmits a positive valence/reinforcing signal in response to food ingestion [32]. Hence, vagal sensory signals from the gut appear to convey non-aversive and/or rewarding information while suppressing food intake and modulating gut motility. These findings suggest that aversive signals may travel to the brain by mechanisms other than the vagus – perhaps via the dorsal root ganglion (spinal sensory neurons) and/or by humoral signaling (including via the AP).

The AP, commonly referred to as the "vomiting center," plays important roles in aversive responses; indeed, inflammation of the AP in neuromyelitis optica spectrum disorders often presents with unremitting vomiting [27]. AP neurons mainly project locally and within the brain stem – primarily targeting the NTS and lPBN. Several recent studies have used single-cell sequencing methods to catalog AP neuron populations, revealing two overarching sets of glutamatergic (excitatory) neurons and one set of GABAergic (inhibitory) cells [33, 34]. One set of glutamatergic neurons, marked by the expression of *Calcr*, mediates non-aversive responses; the other (marked by *Glp1r*, *Gfral*, and *Casr*, among others) promotes strong CTA responses (consistent with the strong aversive responses provoked by ligands for these receptors – GLP-1R agonists, GDF-15, and vomitoxin, respectively) [27]. Many GABAergic AP neurons express *Gipr* [33, 34]; these project locally and may attenuate the function of glutamatergic AP neuron populations. The roles for AP neurons in the long-term control of feeding and in overall energy balance remain to be determined.

Activating projections from aversive NTS *Cck* neurons to the lPBN activates a set of lPBN calcitonin gene-related peptide (CGRP)-containing neurons and promotes the aversive suppression of food intake [35]. Furthermore, activating lPBN CGRP neurons suppresses food intake and promotes a CTA, while silencing lPBN CGRP cells blocks the CTA associated with a variety of gut malaise-promoting agents. Thus, lPBN CGRP cells mediate the suppression of food intake along with a variety of aversive affects associated with gut malaise and systemic illness. In contrast, stimulating non-aversive NTS *Calcr* cells does not activate lPBN CGRP cells, but rather activates a distinct (but as yet molecularly uncharacterized) set of lPBN cells [29]. Hence, the lPBN must contain multiple types of food intake-suppressing neuron types, some of which remain to be described. A distinct subset of lPBN neurons that express *Pdyn* monitors feeding and suppresses food intake, although less is understood about their potential role(s) in behavioral responses to other aversive signals [36].

While many early studies aimed at determining the function of NTS circuits in food intake identified roles for the NTS in the control of meal size, compensatory alterations in meal frequency during these studies generally resulted in unchanged long-term energy balance [27]. In contrast, silencing NTS *Calcr* neurons in mice increases food intake and body weight, especially in animals fed a palatable diet [29]. Hence, the endogenous activity of at least some NTS neurons plays a crucial role in the long-term restraint of food intake and adiposity, especially during exposure to palatable diets.

While silencing non-aversive NTS *Calcr* neurons promotes increased feeding and body weight, silencing aversive lPBN CGRP cells modestly increases meal size but not overall food intake and does not alter long-term parameters of energy balance [37]. Hence, non-aversive brain stem pathways housed in the NTS and/or lPBN might play a larger role in overall energy balance than aversive pathways (the latter of which would presumably be activated mainly during emergencies, such as toxin ingestion, rather than as part of a homeostatic feeding control system).

Importantly, in addition to roles played by brain stem nuclei in conveying gut- and nutrient-derived information rostrally, the NTS and lPBN receive information from hypothalamic structures and play an important role in mediating the control of food intake by these sites [26]. Both the NTS and lPBN receive direct inputs from the hypothalamus – especially from the PVH and the ARH nuclei; the lPBN plays prominent roles in the control of food intake by cells in both of these areas [37, 38].

Hypothalamic Systems That Control Energy Balance

Overall Organization

Many of the neural systems that control energy balance lie in the hypothalamus. Like the brain stem (and unlike more recently developed brain areas such as the cerebral cortex), the hypothalamus is not organized in a laminar manner but rather consists of clusters of neuronal soma called nuclei. The connections among these nuclei generate an integrated circuitry that collates relevant signals to produce a final output to motor neurons that control autonomic and endocrine systems or influence feeding behavior. Each of these nuclei contains many different (and even oppositely acting) types of neurons with distinct roles.

Within the medial region, the ARH, which lies immediately above the median eminence, has rapid access to circulating factors (see section "Humoral Components" discussed above) that signal energy balance [39]. The ARH makes strong reciprocal connections with the DMH, which integrates the ARH-derived signals with information from other hypothalamic sites (e.g., circadian cues, body temperature) (Fig. 3). The ARH and DMH each also make strong reciprocal connections with the PVH. The PVH and the DMH also receive direct input from the brain stem. The PVH represents a crucial hypothalamic output: PVH efferents to the brain stem and spinal cord control autonomic function, projections to the median eminence and posterior pituitary control endocrine function, and projections to the brain stem regulate feeding.

The VMH, especially the dorsomedial VMH, which lies between the anterior portions of the ARH and DMH, makes relatively few connections with these two nuclei but rather projects to rostral (e.g., preoptic area (POA) and bed nucleus of the stria terminalis (BST)) and brain stem regions (e.g., the periaqueductal gray matter (PAG)) associated with autonomic function [40]. Lateral to the ARH, VMH and DMH, lies the more loosely defined LHA, through which course projections among several limbic regions rostral and caudal to the hypothalamus. The LHA contains heterogeneous populations of neurons, many of which receive metabolic signals and project to the midbrain (including the dopaminergic VTA) and to rostral limbic regions such as the nucleus accumbens (NAc). The LHA represents a major conduit linking the hypothalamus to the mesolimbic dopaminergic system and other circuits that control motivation [41].

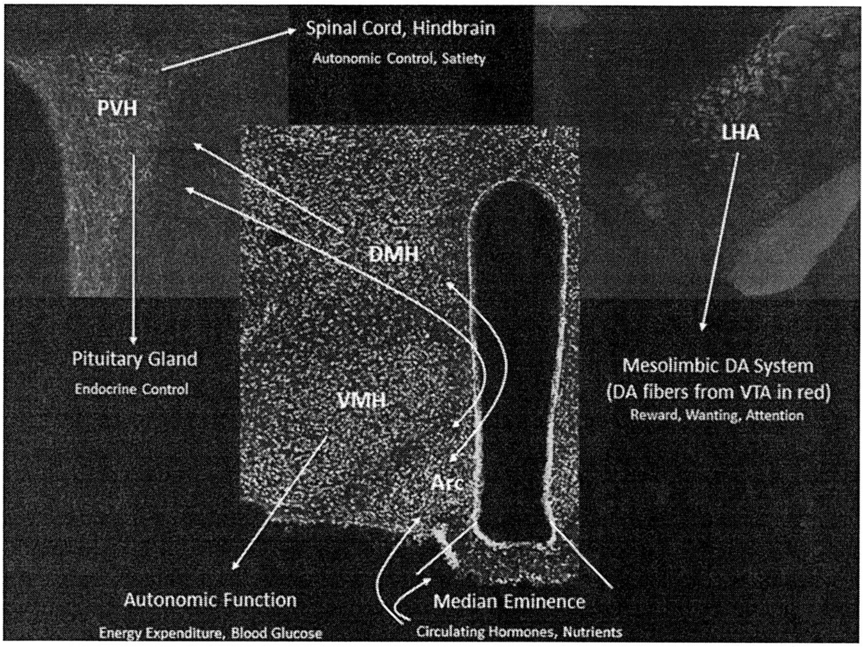

Fig. 3 Flow of information in the hypothalamus and roles of hypothalamic nuclei. The arcuate nucleus (*ARH*), which is located directly above the median eminence, has the most direct exposure to circulating hormones and nutrients and is enriched in receptors for these substances. ARH neurons, including the important POMC and AgRP neurons that comprise the inception site of the hypothalamic melanocortin system, project densely to the dorsomedial hypothalamic nucleus (DMH, where information is integrated with circadian, temperature, and other inputs) and to the paraventricular nucleus of the hypothalamus (PVH, the major output nucleus for the medial hypothalamus). The DMH makes reciprocal connections with the ARH and PVH. Projections from the PVH target the median eminence and pituitary gland for the regulation of endocrine function, the spinal cord to control sympathetic nervous system (*SNS*) function, and the hindbrain to modulate satiety. The ventromedial hypothalamic nucleus (*VMH*) senses glucose, along with some hormones that are sensed by the ARH, and projects to forebrain and hindbrain regions that control autonomic function, thereby controlling energy expenditure and blood glucose levels. The lateral hypothalamic area (*LHA*) contains many types of neurons that project into areas associated with attention, reward, and wanting, such as the mesolimbic dopamine system. The LHA represents a major conduit from hypothalamic homeostatic circuits into the brain's motivational circuitry

In the next sections, we describe in more detail the circuitry and function of each of these hypothalamic components.

Arcuate Nucleus

The ARH in rodents (tuberal nucleus in humans) resides in the medioventral portion of the hypothalamus surrounding the base of the third ventricle; it is intimately connected to the median eminence and hypophyseal portal vascular system by the infundibular stalk. The ARH contains several different groups of projection neurons, including those that produce pro-opiomelanocortin (POMC), agouti-related peptide (AgRP), or kisspeptin; the ARH also contains hypophysiotropic neurons, including distinct sets of neurons that produce growth hormone-releasing hormone (GHRH), somatostatin (SST), or dopamine.

The ARH contains tanycytes, in addition to the astrocytes, oligodendrocytes, and microglia that are found throughout the brain. The tanycyte cell bodies reside in the ventral ependymal lining of the third ventricle and elaborate characteristic arching lateral and ventral projections through the adjacent brain parenchyma. As a circumventricular organ with fenestrated capillaries, the median eminence provides neurons in the most medioventral portion of the ARH with relatively unfettered access to circulating hormones, cytokines, nutrients, and metabolites. Modulation of tanycytes by fasting and some peripheral signals appears to be able to expand this unfettered access of circulating factors deeper into the ARH parenchyma.

Neuropeptidergic neurons of the ARH, including cells that contain POMC, are among the earliest differentiated neurons of the CNS, at E10.5 in the mouse. A postnatal surge in adipocyte leptin secretion stimulates the formation of neural projections from ARH POMC and AgRP neurons to other hypothalamic nuclei, including the PVH and DMH [42].

Abundant genetic evidence from the clinic, together with animal studies, has identified the CNS melanocortin system (which includes POMC and AgRP neurons and their downstream targets that express the CNS melanocortin receptors (MC3R and MC4R)) as a critical component of the homeostatic neural circuitry regulating energy balance. Melanocortin peptides (α-, β-, and γ-MSH in humans; α- and γ-MSH in rodents) produced by POMC neurons are endogenous agonists of the two CNS melanocortin receptors, while AgRP is a competitive antagonist/inverse agonist at both receptors [43].

POMC and AgRP neurons are differentially regulated: leptin and signals of energy surfeit increase *Pomc* expression, while fasting activates (and feeding/leptin inhibit) AgRP neurons [43]. Activation of GHSR-containing AgRP neurons mediates a substantial portion of ghrelin-mediated hyperphagia. A study by Cowley et al. [44] first proposed a model to explain the homeostatic basis of body weight control, whereby these two neuron populations largely project to similar sites in the CNS but have opposing actions: α-MSH ultimately leading to decreased food intake and increased energy expenditure and AgRP increasing food intake and decreasing energy expenditure.

More recently studies have generally upheld this model but have shown that AgRP neurons mediate melanocortin-independent effects, as well. In addition to AgRP, AgRP neurons produce neuropeptide Y (NPY) and the fast inhibitory neurotransmitter GABA. AgRP and NPY both stimulate food intake following injection into the cerebrospinal fluid or specific hypothalamic nuclei, but mutant mice engineered to lack AgRP and/or NPY do not exhibit the predicted phenotype of decreased body weight, adiposity, and food intake [45]. These paradoxical findings have at least been partially explained by the primary role of GABA signaling from AgRP neurons in their acute actions to stimulate feeding, with the neuropeptides playing accessory or modulatory roles [46]. Additionally, ablation of AgRP neurons in the adult, but not in neonatal mouse, causes starvation and death, and this phenotype is independent of melanocortin signaling [47]. These findings suggest that developmental compensation during the early neonatal period can mitigate the effects of disturbances in the AgRP neuron.

Stimulation of AgRP neurons by either optogenetic or chemogenetic technology leads to the rapid onset of feeding, even in sated mice. There are apparently at least two parallel neural pathways mediating these effects, one a direct projection of AgRP neurons to the lPBN and a second polysynaptic circuit involving an inhibitory AgRP projection to MC4R-expressing glutamatergic neurons within the PVH that in turn project by a descending pathway to the lPBN [48].

Unlike the rapid stimulatory effects on food intake produced by the remote activation of AgRP neurons, activation of ARH POMC neurons only produces delayed inhibitory effects on food intake [49, 50]. Similarly, only long-term inhibition of POMC neurons was capable of increasing food intake [50]. Because the feeding inhibitory effects from optogenetic activation of POMC neurons were blocked by a melanocortin antagonist and POMC neuron activation could overcome coincident inhibition from AgRP neurons, the most parsimonious explanation for the delayed response is that melanocortin peptide release, and not other putative peptide and amino acid transmitters produced in POMC neurons, is of principal importance to POMC neuron function in the control of energy homeostasis.

Dorsomedial Nucleus

Even among the complex nuclei of the hypothalamus, the size and functional diversity of the DMH are substantial. While there are many recognized subdivisions of the DMH, it is probably most useful to distinguish among the dorsal component (DMHd, which borders the dorsal hypothalamic area or DHA), the compact central zone, and the ventral region (DMHv). The DMH plays a role in the control of many autonomic functions, including thermogenesis, heart rate, and blood pressure. Like the ARH, the DMH contains a substantial number of *Lepr*-expressing cells [51]. Dorsal DMH/DHA *Lepr* neurons interact with the thermal control systems of the medial preoptic area and PVH and play an important role in the control of body temperature by leptin. Consistently, deletion of LepRb in the prolactin-releasing hormone-expressing neurons of this region decreases body temperature and energy expenditure, promoting obesity in high-fat-fed animals [52].

Other data also suggest a role for the DMH in the control of food intake, including the inhibition of AgRP neurons. Correlative evidence suggests the potential for DMH leptin action (presumably the ventral DMH) in the control of feeding: the deletion of *Lepr* from distributed populations of hypothalamic cells that express the vesicular GABA transporter (vGat, *Slc32a1* gene) or neuronal nitric oxide synthase (nNOS, *Nos1* gene) each produces dramatic hyperphagia and obesity [53]. The distributions of these cells overlap mainly in the DMH, suggesting a potential role for DMH LepRb neurons in the suppression of feeding. Indeed, ablation of *Lepr* throughout the DMH promotes obesity in part by promoting hyperphagia [54]. Presumably, the variable effects on feeding that result from the various DMH perturbations reflect differences in the subregions of the DMH targeted in each study.

Paraventricular Nucleus: Hypothalamic Output

The PVH is a critical hypothalamic center that receives and integrates energy balance signals from a variety of brain regions and coordinates physiologic responses to maintain energy homeostasis predominantly through the autonomic nervous system. The PVH is a complex structure composed of a heterogeneous group of mostly glutamatergic neurons that have been classically described as parvocellular or magnocellular based on cell size and axonal projection patterns. The magnocellular neurons in the PVH, including those that express oxytocin (OXT) or vasopressin (AVP), project primarily to the posterior pituitary and release their contents directly into the systemic circulation to regulate peripheral tissue function. Importantly, however, dendritic release of these neuropeptides has been implicated in the overall control and coordination of PVH function [55].

The PVH parvocellular cells are more diverse and send projections within the central nervous system to three main areas: [1] the median eminence where secreted factors (e.g., corticotropin-releasing hormone or CRH) enter the portal hypophyseal circulation and regulate pituitary function; [2] the brain stem, including the dorsal vagal complex (composed of the NTS and DMV) and the parabrachial nucleus (PBN) – both of which have been implicated in feeding [56]; and [3] the preganglionic, sympathetic output centers such as the intermediolateral cell column of the spinal cord [57]. Parvocellular PVH neurons that respond to satiety signals, such as leptin, have been proposed to regulate feeding by modulating hindbrain responses to ascending feeding signals from the gut and periphery [50, 58]. It is important to note that hypothalamic factors secreted into the portal hypophyseal circulation at the median eminence undoubtedly contribute to both energy and metabolic homeostasis via regulation of pituitary hormone release.

The overall importance of the PVH in the regulation of energy balance is underscored by the massive obesity and metabolic abnormalities associated with alterations in PVH development or function. Rodents and humans harboring deleterious mutations in the hypothalamic transcription factor *single minded-1* (Sim1) develop a hypocellular PVH and hyperphagic obesity. Moreover, lesions of the PVH also result in hyperphagic obesity and glucose dysregulation. Neither the neural architecture nor the molecular mechanisms used by the PVH to maintain energy and metabolic homeostasis are well understood. This is in large part due to the cellular heterogeneity of the PVH, the density of its projection targets, and the vast array of afferent inputs that the PVH receives from many different brain regions [59].

The PVH serves as an important output center for peptide signals and conditions known to modulate food intake, including leptin, melanocortins (from the ARH), GLP-1 (presumably from the NTS), GLP-1R agonists, and dehydration [60]. The melanocortin system is perhaps the best studied of these pathways, as it is essential for energy balance in rodents and humans and is directly linked to PVH function [43, 61, 62]. POMC and AgRP neurons in the ARH produce melanocortin agonists and antagonists, respectively, and project to PVH neurons that express melanocortin receptors [63]. Endogenous and pharmacologic melanocortin agonists stimulate melanocortin receptor-bearing neurons to activate effector pathways that inhibit food intake and stimulate energy expenditure. Melanocortin action in PVH Sim1 neurons suppresses food intake [38], and ablation of most Sim1 neurons in adult mice results in profound hyperphagic obesity with decreased energy expenditure and altered locomotor activity [64]. In addition, selective deletion of MC4R from Sim1 cells leads to hyperphagic obesity [38].

Subsets of PVH neurons contain a variety of neuropeptides implicated in neuroendocrine and energy balance control, including OXT, CRH, AVP, thyrotropin-releasing hormone, and SST. The anorectic effects of pharmacologic doses of OXT and CRH agonists generated a great deal of interest in PVH OXT and CRH neurons as potential regulators of energy balance. At odds with this formulation are the findings that rodents lacking OXT or OXT neurons (or CRH/CRH receptors) demonstrate minimal energy balance phenotypes; neither does the activation of PVH OXT nor CRH neurons alter feeding [65]. In this regard it is important to note that OXT and CRH receptors are widely distributed in the CNS and that extra-PVH sources of these peptides may make important contributions to energy balance control. Whether the contradiction between pharmacologic studies and genetic approaches reflects developmental compensation to the systemic inactivation of these neuropeptides is not clear, but the profound effects of Sim1 neuron (pan-PVH) manipulation suggest that yet-to-be-defined PVH neurons distinct from OXT and CRH cells represent crucial mediators of energy balance.

With an array of genetic tools, cell-specific genetic changes in PVH cells have confirmed the critical role of the PVH in feeding regulation and have extended our understanding of the molecular components and neural circuitry of PVH function/action. MC4R action on Sim1 cells in the PVH is sufficient to normalize feeding in animals that lack MC4Rs elsewhere, and this is not attributable to direct MC4R action on OXT, CRH, or AVP neurons. Moreover, MC4R expression in Sim1 PVH neurons is required for body weight maintenance, indicating that PVH MC4R action is both necessary and sufficient for normal energy homeostasis [38, 66]. Remote activation of Sim1 PVH neurons using chemogenetic approaches suppresses feeding and increases energy utilization [61]. The effects of pan-PVH activation on parameters of energy balance are not assignable to PVH OXT, CRH, or AVP neurons, since chemogenetic manipulation of these populations had minor (if any) effects on energy balance. In contrast, cell-specific activation of neuronal nitric oxidase synthase (NOS1), brain-derived neurotrophic factor (BDNF), GLP-1R, calcitonin receptor (CALCR), or *Irs4*-expressing neurons (all subset of Sim1 PVH cells) significantly alter feeding indicating that multiple genetically defined PVH subsets play important roles in feeding and energy expenditure control [65, 67, 68]. Whether the modulation of feeding and energy expenditure can be mapped on to discrete neural circuits that emanate from the PVH requires additional investigation.

The PVH sends projections to a variety of brain regions within the central nervous system.

For the purposes of this discussion, we will high-light the functional roles of PVH projections to brain areas known to be important for food intake/energy expenditure, including the lPBN (feeding), NTS, and spinal cord (autonomic control). The importance of these specific PVH projections has been inferred based on published data demonstrating the importance of these target regions in energy balance. The combination of stereotaxic delivery of cell-specific viral tools into transgenic animals with technologies such as light-dependent neural activation (optogenetics) has made it possible to interrogate the physiologic function of specific PVH neuronal projections. Indeed, studies using these technologies have revealed a PVH → ARH orexigenic circuit and established the importance of PVH → lPBN projections for melanocortin action in the CNS [61, 69]. Similar approaches targeting other PVH projections will undoubtedly uncover additional important biological mechanisms underpinning energy balance regulation.

Ventromedial Nucleus

For several decades following the seminal studies of Hetherington and Ranson, in which the bilateral medial hypothalamic lesions (that included the VMH) produced hyperphagic obesity, the VMH was the main focus of attention regarding the neural control of energy homeostasis [70]. Following intense debate, these studies were supplanted by findings suggesting that the electrolytic lesions likely disrupted the neural connections of the medial hypothalamus, including projections from the ARH to and from the PVH [1, 3]. While still not completely resolved, the role of the VMH in energy balance has been clarified by recent studies using more specific molecular and cellular methods.

The VMH contains glucose-sensing neurons that sense changes in glucose levels, as well as those that express receptors for metabolic hormones (e.g., leptin and insulin) or for neuropeptides associated with energy balance [51, 71, 72]. To better understand the regulation and function of VMH circuits, several groups have examined the temporal and anatomic distribution of gene expression in the VMH. Of the identified genes, steroidogenic factor 1 (SF1, encoded by *Nr5a1/ NR5A1*) received a great deal of attention due to its VMH-specific expression within the CNS [73]. The restricted expression of SF1 has allowed the development of a series of genetically modified mouse models to interrogate VMH function. Mice with global loss-of-function mutations in SF1 show disrupted VMH development and neuron-specific ablation of SF1 or silencing of SF1 neurons results in morbid obesity – primarily due to decreased energy expenditure [74–76].

However, the VMH, like most hypothalamic nuclei, is not a homogeneous structure, but is composed of neurons with distinct transcriptional and neurochemical identities and characteristic projection patterns. Anatomically, the VMH consists of a dorsomedial component (VMHdm) and a ventrolateral component (VMHvl) with clearly demarcated functions. Not surprisingly, then, advances in single-cell genomics have revealed distinct transcriptional profiles for VMHdm neurons compared to VMHvl neurons. Remarkably, each of these anatomically defined regions is composed of over a dozen different transcriptionally defined cell types that respond to different stimuli and have distinct projection patterns [77, 78].

As our understanding of the heterogeneity of the VMH increases, many groups have sought to establish the roles for specific cell types within the VMH on energy homeostasis. For example, several groups have demonstrated that leptin signaling in VMH SF1 neurons is required for energy expenditure, glucose homeostasis, and adaptive thermogenesis and hence for the control of body weight [79, 80]. Indeed, activating only those neurons within the VMH that express *Lepr* results in decreased energy expenditure and thermogenesis, with only small changes in food intake [81]. Consistent with these finding, ablating neurons that express pituitary adenylate cyclase-activating polypeptide (PACAP), which partially colocalizes with *Lepr* and is regulated by leptin in the VMH, rapidly causes increased body weight due to decreased energy expenditure and reduced BAT thermogenesis but without changes in activity or food intake [82].

While the vlVMH has traditionally been studied for its role in aggression and sexual behavior, recently several groups have demonstrated that this area of the VMH may have a broad role in energy and glucose homeostasis as well [83, 84]. VMH neurons that express estrogen receptor (*Esr1*), which are located primarily in the vlVMH, are involved in brown adipose tissue thermogenesis and activity, while other vlVMH neurons that express relaxin/insulin-like family peptide receptor 4 (*Rxfp4*) regulate food intake [85]. Ablating these neurons results in decreased body weight due to a decrease in food intake on both normal chow and HFD.

In addition to identifying the function of specific, genetically defined neural populations within the VMH, other investigators have shown that VMH projections to specific locations have distinct functions in metabolism. For example, dmVMH neurons that project to the paraventricular thalamus (PVT) are involved in the inhibition of food intake, while those that project to the anterior BST (aBST) regulate glucose mobilization [86–88].

The VMH also plays a prominent role in the control of glucose homeostasis [72]. VMH neuron responses to glucose are heterogeneous: glucose-excited (GE) VMH neurons increase, and glucose-inhibited (GI) VMH neurons decrease their firing rate when glucose rises. Intra-VMH 2-deoxyglucose (a non-metabolizable glucose analog that mimics low glucose) injection increases plasma glucose, glucagon, noradrenaline, and adrenaline, suggesting a role in the counter-regulatory response to hypoglycemia, presumably by activating GI neurons. Activation of VMH neurons that project to the aBST mobilizes glucose and increases counter-regulatory hormones [86, 87], while VMH neurons that express the cholecystokinin b receptor (CCKBR) mobilize glucose and induce the counter-regulatory response without altering energy expenditure or body weight [76]. Conversely, leptin or melanocortin action in the VMH increases glucose uptake into tissues and/or decreases blood glucose (presumably via GE neurons). These findings support the notion that the VMH is a key component in the control of glucose homeostasis

via sensing changes in glucose levels and modulation of autonomic responses [72, 89, 90].

The VMH coordinates energy expenditure, physical activity, thermogenesis, and food intake in response to environmental, metabolic, and hormonal cues to mediate whole-body energy and glucose homeostasis. While recent studies have begun to illuminate the specific neural populations, circuits, and signaling molecules involved, the upstream regulatory inputs and the neural pathways that lie downstream of distinct VMH neurons to control each aspect of energy homeostasis remain poorly understood.

Lateral Hypothalamic Area and Mesolimbic Dopaminergic System

Unlike the control of autonomic and endocrine function, foraging for and eating food require the initiation and coordination of complex behaviors. While the neural circuits that generate motor patterns represent the ultimate outputs for these behaviors, these circuits also serve the brain's motivational systems [91]. The central control of motivation is mediated by the mesolimbic dopamine (DA) system, at the core of which lie DA neurons of the midbrain ventral tegmental area (VTA) [92]. The VTA DA neurons project to many places, including the nucleus accumbens, where DA release modulates motivation.

Several decades-old observations also suggested a role for the LHA in motivation. Not only does lesioning the LHA promote anhedonia and abrogate the motivation to feed in experimental animals, but also animals will self-administer activating current to the LHA, suggesting that LHA activation is rewarding/motivating [93]. Since the medial forebrain bundle, which carries axons from (among others) the VTA to the NAc, courses through the LHA, it was not initially clear whether the perturbation of the medial forebrain bundle or rather LHA neurons mediates these effects, however.

With the discovery and functional characterization of several discrete sets of LHA neurons, it became clear that LHA neurons themselves play an important role in the control of motivation, including the mesolimbic DA system. Indeed, the LHA integrates metabolic (e.g., leptin and melanocortins) and other homeostatic signals from the hypothalamus to modulate mesolimbic DA-dependent activity, attention, and motivation [11, 91]. Like the ARH, VMH, and DMH, the LHA contains many groups of neurons, some of which function antagonistically. Important LHA neurons include orexin (a.k.a. hypocretin)-containing cells, which project to a variety of midbrain and hindbrain sites. Orexin neurons are activated by signals of energy deficit (fasting, ghrelin, etc.) to promote arousal and food seeking; conversely, leptin inhibits orexin neurons [11, 91, 94]. Melanin-concentrating hormone (MCH)-expressing neurons in the LHA project widely through the forebrain, including to the NAc, and stimulate feeding [95]. Overexpression of MCH promotes increased feeding and weight gain, while the ablation of MCH or MCH neurons decreases feeding and promotes leanness.

In addition to the glutamatergic orexin and MCH neurons, the LHA also contains a substantial population of GABAergic neurons, many of which contain neuropeptides, including neurotensin and galanin. Optogenetic activation of GABAergic LHA neurons stimulates feeding, and this activation is associated with positive valence. Interestingly, these appetitive and consummatory responses are not encoded by the same neuron underscoring the complexity of LHA neurocircuitry [96]. While orexin neurons contain GHSR (the receptor for orexigenic ghrelin), neither orexin nor MCH cells contain LepRb [97]. Rather, a substantial subset of LHA GABA neurons coexpresses LepRb. Like the larger population of LHA GABA neurons, many LHA LepRb neurons also contain neurotensin and/or galanin. Both neurotensin- and galanin-expressing neurons in the LHA have been shown to modulate feeding behaviors [94, 98].

LHA LepRb neurons contribute to the control of feeding, energy expenditure, and energy balance by leptin, since intra-LHA leptin suppresses feeding in leptin-deficient animals, and deletion of LepRb in LHA neurotensin neurons decreases activity and energy expenditure while increasing adiposity [99]. LHA LepRb neurons project locally onto orexin (but not MCH) neurons, in addition to innervating the VTA and other midbrain sites [100]. While the action of ARH-derived melanocortins apparently drives the control of MCH neurons by leptin and energy balance, leptin action via LHA LepRb neurons inhibits the activity of orexin neurons, at least in part via galanin [41, 101]. LHA leptin action also promotes the expression of orexin; this somewhat counterintuitive bidirectional regulation of orexin neurons presumably reflects the need for leptin to reduce acute foraging activity while supporting the normal function of orexin to permit alertness and attention [100].

Leptin action via LHA neurotensin neurons also modulates the mesolimbic DA function, decreasing nucleus accumbens DA transport activity (hence increasing synaptic DA transmission) [99]. Since the chemogenetic activation of LHA neurotensin neurons increases nucleus accumbens DA concentration via the release of neurotensin in the VTA, intra-VTA neurotensin release by LHA LepRb neurons presumably represents a mechanism by which LHA LepRb neurons control mesolimbic DA function. While LHA LepRb neurons represent a major mechanism by which leptin and energy status control the mesolimbic DA system, some VTA cells also contain LepRb [102]. VTA LepRb neurons mainly project locally and to the central nucleus of the amygdala (rather than the nucleus accumbens), and the ablation of LepRb from DA neurons fails to alter energy balance or tested parameters of mesolimbic DA function. Thus, LHA LepRb neurons represent the primary link between leptin and the control of mesolimbic DA function and motivation.

Conclusions

The physiological regulation of varied components of the metabolic function relies on a coordinated action of humoral and neural signals, integrated brain circuits and orchestrated motor, and behavioral and reflex responses. With the use of molecular and genetic tools and new technology, we have a much clear picture of the role of specific neuronal populations and brain pathways associated with the control of many aspects of energy homeostasis. The "dual center" hypothesis has its heuristic value, but recent evidence using more precise tools has demonstrated the complexity of the system with the action of a series of hypothalamic and brain stem nuclei. We have also gained knowledge on the relevance of selective neurotransmitters/peptides and neural pathways in several aspects of the metabolic regulation. The next challenge will be to determine how each of these components is interconnected and integrated to generate a highly coordinated physiological system.

Cross-References

▶ Adipokines and Metabolism
▶ Adipose Structure (White, Brown, Beige)
▶ Bariatric Surgery
▶ Circadian Rhythms and Metabolism
▶ Gut Hormones and Metabolic Syndrome
▶ Insulin Resistance in Obesity
▶ Overview of Metabolic Syndrome
▶ Pancreatic Islet Adaptation and Failure in Obesity
▶ Pharmacotherapy of Obesity and Metabolic Syndrome

Acknowledgments The authors are supported by the National Institutes of Health grants (DK129722 to AHA, DK20572 (the Michigan Diabetes Research Center), DK056731, and DK132008 to MGM; DK104999 to DPO; DK117821 to DPO and MGM; HD61539, HD69702 to CFE), the Warren Alpert Foundation to AHA, the Marilyn H. Vincent Foundation to MGM, and the Whitehall Foundation to DPO.

References

1. Elmquist JK, Elias CF, Saper CB. From lesions to leptin. Neuron. 1999;22(2):221–32.
2. Stellar E. The physiology of motivation. Psychol Rev. 1954;61(1):5–22.
3. King BM. The rise, fall, and resurrection of the ventromedial hypothalamus in the regulation of feeding behavior and body weight. Physiol Behav. 2006;87(2):221–44.
4. Bernardis LL, Bellinger LL. The lateral hypothalamic area revisited: ingestive behavior. Neurosci Biobehav Rev. 1996;20(2):189–287.
5. Zhang Y, Proenca R, Maffei M, Barone M, Leopold L, Friedman JM. Positional cloning of the mouse obese gene and its human homologue. Nature. 1994;372(6505):425–32.
6. Tartaglia LA, Dembski M, Weng X, Deng N, Culpepper J, Devos R, et al. Identification and expression cloning of a leptin receptor. OB-R Cell. 1995;83(7):1263–71.
7. Chua SC, Chung WK, Wu-Peng XS, Zhang Y, Liu SM, Tartaglia L, et al. Phenotypes of mouse diabetes and rat fatty due to mutations in the OB (leptin) receptor. Science. 1996;271(5251):994–6.
8. Ahima RS, Saper CB, Flier JS, Elmquist JK. Leptin regulation of neuroendocrine systems. Front Neuroendocrinol. 2000;21(3):263–307.
9. Casanueva FF, Dieguez C. Neuroendocrine regulation and actions of leptin. Front Neuroendocrinol. 1999;20(4):317–63.
10. Elmquist JK, Bjørbaek C, Ahima RS, Flier JS, Saper CB. Distributions of leptin receptor mRNA isoforms in the rat brain. J Comp Neurol. 1998;395(4):535–47.
11. Myers MG, Münzberg H, Leinninger GM, Leshan RL. The geometry of leptin action in the brain: more complicated than a simple ARC. Cell Metab. 2009;9(2):117–23.
12. Brüning JC, Gautam D, Burks DJ, Gillette J, Schubert M, Orban PC, et al. Role of brain insulin receptor in control of body weight and reproduction. Science. 2000;289(5487):2122–5.
13. Kleinridders A, Ferris HA, Cai W, Kahn CR. Insulin action in brain regulates systemic metabolism and brain function. Diabetes. 2014;63(7):2232–43.
14. García-Cáceres C, Quarta C, Varela L, Gao Y, Gruber T, Legutko B, et al. Astrocytic insulin signaling couples brain glucose uptake with nutrient availability. Cell. 2016;166(4):867–80.
15. Nakazato M, Murakami N, Date Y, Kojima M, Matsuo H, Kangawa K, et al. A role for ghrelin in the central regulation of feeding. Nature. 2001;409(6817):194–8.
16. Sun Y, Asnicar M, Saha PK, Chan L, Smith RG. Ablation of ghrelin improves the diabetic but not obese phenotype of ob/ob mice. Cell Metab. 2006;3(5):379–86.
17. Johnson AK, Gross PM. Sensory circumventricular organs and brain homeostatic pathways. FASEB J. 1993;7(8):678–86.
18. Banks WA, Owen JB, Erickson MA. Insulin in the brain: there and Back again. Pharmacol Ther. 2012;136(1):82–93.
19. Banks WA. The blood-brain barrier: connecting the gut and the brain. Regul Pept. 2008;149(1–3):11–4.
20. Duquenne M, Folgueira C, Bourouh C, Millet M, Silva A, Clasadonte J, et al. Leptin brain entry via a tanycytic LepR–EGFR shuttle controls lipid metabolism and pancreas function. Nat Metab [Internet]. 2021; [cited 2021 Aug 8]; https://www.nature.com/articles/s42255-021-00432-5

21. Pavlov VA, Tracey KJ. The vagus nerve and the inflammatory reflex – linking immunity and metabolism. Nat Rev Endocrinol. 2012;8(12):743–54.

22. Berthoud HR. Multiple neural systems controlling food intake and body weight. Neurosci Biobehav Rev. 2002;26(4):393–428.

23. Chaudhri OB, Salem V, Murphy KG, Bloom SR. Gastrointestinal satiety signals. Annu Rev Physiol. 2008;70:239–55.

24. Williams EK, Chang RB, Strochlic DE, Umans BD, Lowell BB, Liberles SD. Sensory neurons that detect stretch and nutrients in the digestive system. Cell. 2016;166(1):209–21.

25. Bai L, Mesgarzadeh S, Ramesh KS, Huey EL, Liu Y, Gray LA, et al. Genetic identification of vagal sensory neurons that control feeding. Cell. 2019;179(5): 1129–1143.e23.

26. Grill HJ, Hayes MR. Hindbrain neurons as an essential hub in the neuroanatomically distributed control of energy balance. Cell Metab. 2012;16(3):296–309.

27. Cheng W, Gordian D, Ludwig MQ, Pers TH, Seeley RJ, Myers MG. Hindbrain circuits in the control of eating behaviour and energy balance. Nat Metab. 2022;4(7):826–35.

28. Do J, Chang Z, Sekerková G, McCrimmon DR, Martina M. A leptin-mediated neural mechanism linking breathing to metabolism. Cell Rep. 2020;33(6):108358.

29. Cheng W, Gonzalez I, Pan W, Tsang AH, Adams J, Ndoka E, et al. Calcitonin receptor neurons in the mouse nucleus tractus solitarius control energy balance via the non-aversive suppression of feeding. Cell Metab. 2020;31(2):301–312.e5.

30. Cheng W, Ndoka E, Hutch C, Roelofs K, MacKinnon A, Khoury B, et al. Leptin receptor-expressing nucleus tractus solitarius neurons suppress food intake independently of GLP1 in mice. JCI Insight. 2020;5(7):e134359.

31. Gaykema RP, Newmyer BA, Ottolini M, Raje V, Warthen DM, Lambeth PS, et al. Activation of murine pre-proglucagon-producing neurons reduces food intake and body weight. J Clin Invest. 2017;127(3): 1031–45.

32. Han W, Tellez LA, Perkins MH, Perez IO, Qu T, Ferreira J, et al. A neural circuit for gut-induced reward. Cell. 2018;175(3):665–678.e23.

33. Zhang C, Kaye JA, Cai Z, Wang Y, Prescott SL, Liberles SD. Area postrema cell types that mediate nausea-associated behaviors. Neuron. 2020;109:461. S0896627320308886

34. Ludwig MQ, Cheng W, Gordian D, Lee J, Paulsen SJ, Hansen SN, et al. A genetic map of the mouse dorsal vagal complex and its role in obesity. Nat Metab. 2021;3:530.

35. Roman CW, Sloat SR, Palmiter RD. A tale of two circuits: CCKNTS neuron stimulation controls appetite and induces opposing motivational states by projections to distinct brain regions. Neuroscience. 2017;358:316–24.

36. Chen J, Zhan C. Gut–vagus–NTS neural pathway in controlling feeding behaviors. Stress and Brain [Internet]. 2023; [cited 2023 Jun 13]; https://www.sciopen.com/article/10.26599/SAB.2023.9060033

37. Campos CA, Bowen AJ, Schwartz MW, Palmiter RD. Parabrachial CGRP neurons control meal termination. Cell Metab. 2016;23(5):811–20.

38. Shah BP, Vong L, Olson DP, Koda S, Krashes MJ, Ye C, et al. MC4R-expressing glutamatergic neurons in the paraventricular hypothalamus regulate feeding and are synaptically connected to the parabrachial nucleus. Proc Natl Acad Sci U S A. 2014;111(36): 13193–8.

39. Myers MG, Olson DP. SnapShot: neural pathways that control feeding. Cell Metab. 2014;19(4): 732–732.e1.

40. Canteras NS, Simerly RB, Swanson LW. Organization of projections from the ventromedial nucleus of the hypothalamus: APhaseolus vulgaris-Leucoagglutinin study in the rat. J Comp Neurol. 1994;348(1):41–79.

41. Opland DM, Leininger GM, Myers MG. Modulation of the mesolimbic dopamine system by leptin. Brain Res. 2010;1350:65–70.

42. Bouret SG. Trophic action of leptin on hypothalamic neurons that regulate feeding. Science. 2004;304(5667):108–10.

43. Cone RD. Anatomy and regulation of the central melanocortin system. Nat Neurosci. 2005;8(5): 571–8.

44. Cowley MA, Smart JL, Rubinstein M, Cerdán MG, Diano S, Horvath TL, et al. Leptin activates anorexigenic POMC neurons through a neural network in the arcuate nucleus. Nature. 2001;411(6836):480–4.

45. Qian S, Chen H, Weingarth D, Trumbauer ME, Novi DE, Guan X, et al. Neither agouti-related protein nor neuropeptide Y is critically required for the regulation of energy homeostasis in mice. Mol Cell Biol. 2002;22(14):5027–35.

46. Tong Q, Ye CP, Jones JE, Elmquist JK, Lowell BB. Synaptic release of GABA by AgRP neurons is required for normal regulation of energy balance. Nat Neurosci. 2008;11(9):998–1000.

47. Luquet S. NPY/AgRP neurons are essential for feeding in adult mice but can be ablated in neonates. Science. 2005;310(5748):683–5.

48. Deem JD, Faber CL, Morton GJ. AgRP neurons: regulators of feeding, energy expenditure, and behavior. FEBS J. 2022;289(8):2362–81.

49. Aponte Y, Atasoy D, Sternson SM. AGRP neurons are sufficient to orchestrate feeding behavior rapidly and without training. Nat Neurosci. 2011;14(3): 351–5.

50. Atasoy D, Betley JN, Su HH, Sternson SM. Deconstruction of a neural circuit for hunger. Nature. 2012;488(7410):172–7.

51. Scott MM, Lachey JL, Sternson SM, Lee CE, Elias CF, Friedman JM, et al. Leptin targets in the mouse brain. J Comp Neurol. 2009;514(5):518–32.

52. Dodd GT, Worth AA, Nunn N, Korpal AK, Bechtold DA, Allison MB, et al. The thermogenic effect of leptin is dependent on a distinct population of prolactin-releasing peptide neurons in the dorsomedial hypothalamus. Cell Metab. 2014;20(4): 639–49.

53. Leshan RL, Greenwald-Yarnell M, Patterson CM, Gonzalez IE, Myers MG. Leptin action through hypothalamic nitric oxide synthase-1-expressing neurons controls energy balance. Nat Med. 2012;18(5):820–3.

54. Rezai-Zadeh K, Yu S, Jiang Y, Laque A, Schwartzenburg C, Morrison CD, et al. Leptin receptor neurons in the dorsomedial hypothalamus are key regulators of energy expenditure and body weight, but not food intake. Mol Metab. 2014;3(7):681–93.

55. Brown CH, Ludwig M, Tasker JG, Stern JE. Somatodendritic vasopressin and oxytocin secretion in endocrine and autonomic regulation. J Neuroendocrinol. 2020;32(6):e12856.

56. Berthoud HR, Sutton GM, Townsend RL, Patterson LM, Zheng H. Brainstem mechanisms integrating gut-derived satiety signals and descending forebrain information in the control of meal size. Physiol Behav. 2006;89(4):517–24.

57. Biag J, Huang Y, Gou L, Hintiryan H, Askarinam A, Hahn JD, et al. Cyto- and chemoarchitecture of the hypothalamic paraventricular nucleus in the C57BL/6J male mouse: a study of immunostaining and multiple fluorescent tract tracing. J Comp Neurol. 2012;520(1):6–33.

58. Blevins JE, Schwartz MW, Baskin DG. Evidence that paraventricular nucleus oxytocin neurons link hypothalamic leptin action to caudal brain stem nuclei controlling meal size. Am J Phys Regul Integr Comp Phys. 2004;287(1):R87–96.

59. Ferguson AV, Latchford KJ, Samson WK. The paraventricular nucleus of the hypothalamus a potential target for integrative treatment of autonomic dysfunction. Expert Opin Ther Targets. 2008;12(6): 717–27.

60. Dalvi PS, Nazarians-Armavil A, Purser MJ, Belsham DD. Glucagon-like peptide-1 receptor agonist, exendin-4, regulates feeding-associated neuropeptides in hypothalamic neurons in vivo and in vitro. Endocrinology. 2012;153(5):2208–22.

61. Garfield AS, Li C, Madara JC, Shah BP, Webber E, Steger JS, et al. A neural basis for melanocortin-4 receptor-regulated appetite. Nat Neurosci. 2015;18(6):863–71.

62. Farooqi IS, Keogh JM, Yeo GSH, Lank EJ, Cheetham T, O'Rahilly S. Clinical spectrum of obesity and mutations in the melanocortin 4 receptor gene. N Engl J Med. 2003;348(12):1085–95.

63. Ellacott KLJ, Cone RD. The central melanocortin system and the integration of short- and long-term regulators of energy homeostasis. Recent Prog Horm Res. 2004;59:395–408.

64. Xi D, Gandhi N, Lai M, Kublaoui BM. Ablation of Sim1 neurons causes obesity through hyperphagia and reduced energy expenditure. PLoS One. 2012;7(4):e36453.

65. Li C, Navarrete J, Liang-Guallpa J, Lu C, Funderburk SC, Chang RB, et al. Defined paraventricular hypothalamic populations exhibit differential responses to food contingent on caloric state. Cell Metab. 2019;29(3):681–694.e5.

66. Balthasar N, Dalgaard LT, Lee CE, Yu J, Funahashi H, Williams T, et al. Divergence of Melanocortin pathways in the control of food intake and energy expenditure. Cell. 2005;123(3):493–505.

67. An JJ, Liao GY, Kinney CE, Sahibzada N, Xu B. Discrete BDNF neurons in the paraventricular hypothalamus control feeding and energy expenditure. Cell Metab. 2015;22(1):175–88.

68. Gonzalez IE, Ramirez-Matias J, Lu C, Pan W, Zhu A, Myers MG Jr, et al. Paraventricular calcitonin receptor–expressing neurons modulate energy homeostasis in male mice. Endocrinology. 2021;162(6):bqab072.

69. Krashes MJ, Shah BP, Madara JC, Olson DP, Strochlic DE, Garfield AS, et al. An excitatory paraventricular nucleus to AgRP neuron circuit that drives hunger. Nature. 2014;507(7491):238–42.

70. Hetherington AW, Ranson SW. Hypothalamic lesions and adiposity in the rat. Anat Rec. 1940;78(2): 149–72.

71. Elmquist JK, Ahima RS, Maratos-Flier E, Flier JS, Saper CB. Leptin activates neurons in ventrobasal hypothalamus and brainstem. Endocrinology. 1997;138(2):839–42.

72. Routh VH. Glucosensing neurons in the ventromedial hypothalamic nucleus (VMN) and hypoglycemia-associated autonomic failure (HAAF). Diabetes Metab Res Rev. 2003;19(5):348–56.

73. Ikeda Y, Luo X, Abbud R, Nilson JH, Parker KL. The nuclear receptor steroidogenic factor 1 is essential for the formation of the ventromedial hypothalamic nucleus. Mol Endocrinol. 1995;9(4):478–86.

74. Kim KW, Sohn JW, Kohno D, Xu Y, Williams K, Elmquist JK. SF-1 in the ventral medial hypothalamic nucleus: a key regulator of homeostasis. Mol Cell Endocrinol. 2011;336(1–2):219–23.

75. Majdic G, Young M, Gomez-Sanchez E, Anderson P, Szczepaniak LS, Dobbins RL, et al. Knockout mice lacking steroidogenic factor 1 are a novel genetic model of hypothalamic obesity. Endocrinology. 2002;143(2):607–14.

76. Flak JN, Goforth PB, Dell'Orco J, Sabatini PV, Li C, Bozadjieva N, et al. Ventromedial hypothalamic nucleus neuronal subset regulates blood glucose independently of insulin. J Clin Investig. 2020;130(6): 2943–52.

77. Kim DW, Yao Z, Graybuck LT, Kim TK, Nguyen TN, Smith KA, et al. Multimodal analysis of cell types in a hypothalamic node controlling social behavior. Cell. 2019;179(3):713–728.e17.

78. Affinati AH, Sabatini PV, True C, Tomlinson AJ, Kirigiti M, Lindsley SR, et al. Cross-species analysis

defines the conservation of anatomically segregated VMH neuron populations. elife. 2021;10:e69065.

79. Bingham NC, Anderson KK, Reuter AL, Stallings NR, Parker KL. Selective loss of leptin receptors in the ventromedial hypothalamic nucleus results in increased adiposity and a metabolic syndrome. Endocrinology. 2008;149(5):2138–48.

80. Dhillon H, Zigman JM, Ye C, Lee CE, McGovern RA, Tang V, et al. Leptin directly activates SF1 neurons in the VMH, and this action by leptin is required for normal body-weight homeostasis. Neuron. 2006;49(2):191–203.

81. Sabatini PV, Wang J, Rupp AC, Affinati AH, Flak JN, Li C, et al. tTARGIT AAVs mediate the sensitive and flexible manipulation of intersectional neuronal populations in mice. elife. 2021;10:e66835.

82. Hurley MM, Anderson EM, Chen C, Maunze B, Hess EM, Block ME, et al. Acute blockade of PACAP-dependent activity in the ventromedial nucleus of the hypothalamus disrupts leptin-induced behavioral and molecular changes in rats. Neuroendocrinology. 2020;110(3–4):271–81.

83. Musatov S, Chen W, Pfaff DW, Mobbs CV, Yang XJ, Clegg DJ, et al. Silencing of estrogen receptor alpha in the ventromedial nucleus of hypothalamus leads to metabolic syndrome. Proc Natl Acad Sci U S A. 2007;104(7):2501–6.

84. Xu Y, Nedungadi TP, Zhu L, Sobhani N, Irani BG, Davis KE, et al. Distinct hypothalamic neurons mediate estrogenic effects on energy homeostasis and reproduction. Cell Metab. 2011;14(4):453–65.

85. Lewis JE, Woodward OR, Nuzzaci D, Smith CA, Adriaenssens AE, Billing L, et al. Relaxin/insulin-like family peptide receptor 4 (Rxfp4) expressing hypothalamic neurons modulate food intake and preference in mice. Mol Metab. 2022;66:101604.

86. Meek TH, Nelson JT, Matsen ME, Dorfman MD, Guyenet SJ, Damian V, et al. Functional identification of a neurocircuit regulating blood glucose. Proc Natl Acad Sci U S A. 2016;113(14):E2073–82.

87. Faber CL, Matsen ME, Velasco KR, Damian V, Phan BA, Adam D, et al. Distinct neuronal projections from the hypothalamic ventromedial nucleus mediate glycemic and behavioral effects. Diabetes. 2018;67(12):2518–29.

88. Zhang J, Chen D, Sweeney P, Yang Y. An excitatory ventromedial hypothalamus to paraventricular thalamus circuit that suppresses food intake. Nat Commun. 2020;11(1):6326.

89. Sutton AK, Goforth PB, Gonzalez IE, Dell'Orco J, Pei H, Myers MG, et al. Melanocortin 3 receptor expressing neurons in the ventromedial hypothalamus promote glucose disposal. Proc Natl Acad Sci. 2021;118(15):e2103090118.

90. Minokoshi Y, Haque MS, Shimazu T. Microinjection of leptin into the ventromedial hypothalamus increases glucose uptake in peripheral tissues in rats. Diabetes. 1999;48(2):287–91.

91. Berthoud HR. Interactions between the "cognitive" and "metabolic" brain in the control of food intake. Physiol Behav. 2007;91(5):486–98.

92. Berridge KC. Motivation concepts in behavioral neuroscience. Physiol Behav. 2004;81(2):179–209.

93. Fulton S, Woodside B, Shizgal P. Modulation of brain reward circuitry by leptin. Science. 2000;287(5450):125–8.

94. Brown JA, Bugescu R, Mayer TA, Gata-Garcia A, Kurt G, Woodworth HL, et al. Loss of action via neurotensin-leptin receptor neurons disrupts leptin and ghrelin-mediated control of energy balance. Endocrinology. 2017;158(5):1271–88.

95. Georgescu D, Sears RM, Hommel JD, Barrot M, Bolaños CA, Marsh DJ, et al. The hypothalamic neuropeptide melanin-concentrating hormone acts in the nucleus accumbens to modulate feeding behavior and forced-swim performance. J Neurosci. 2005;25(11):2933–40.

96. Jennings JH, Ung RL, Resendez SL, Stamatakis AM, Taylor JG, Huang J, et al. Visualizing hypothalamic network dynamics for appetitive and consummatory behaviors. Cell. 2015;160(3):516–27.

97. Leininger GM, Jo YH, Leshan RL, Louis GW, Yang H, Barrera JG, et al. Leptin acts via leptin receptor-expressing lateral hypothalamic neurons to modulate the mesolimbic dopamine system and suppress feeding. Cell Metab. 2009;10(2):89–98.

98. Qualls-Creekmore E, Yu S, Francois M, Hoang J, Huesing C, Bruce-Keller A, et al. Galanin-expressing GABA neurons in the lateral hypothalamus modulate food reward and noncompulsive locomotion. J Neurosci. 2017;37(25):6053–65.

99. Leininger GM, Opland DM, Jo YH, Faouzi M, Christensen L, Cappellucci LA, et al. Leptin action via neurotensin neurons controls orexin, the mesolimbic dopamine system and energy balance. Cell Metab. 2011;14(3):313–23.

100. Louis GW, Leininger GM, Rhodes CJ, Myers MG. Direct innervation and modulation of orexin neurons by lateral hypothalamic LepRb neurons. J Neurosci. 2010;30(34):11278–87.

101. Goforth PB, Leininger GM, Patterson CM, Satin LS, Myers MG. Leptin acts via lateral hypothalamic area neurotensin neurons to inhibit orexin neurons by multiple GABA-independent mechanisms. J Neurosci. 2014;34(34):11405–15.

102. Fulton S, Pissios P, Manchon RP, Stiles L, Frank L, Pothos EN, et al. Leptin regulation of the mesoaccumbens dopamine pathway. Neuron. 2006;51(6):811–22.

Adipose Structure (White, Brown, Beige)

17

Vanessa Pellegrinelli, Antonio Vidal-Puig, and Stefania Carobbio

Contents

V. Pellegrinelli
Wellcome-MRC Institute of Metabolic Science and
Medical Research Council Metabolic Diseases Unit,
University of Cambridge, Cambridge, UK
e-mail: vp332@medschl.cam.ac.uk

A. Vidal-Puig
Wellcome-MRC Institute of Metabolic Science and
Medical Research Council Metabolic Diseases Unit,
University of Cambridge, Cambridge, UK

Centro de Investigacion Principe Felipe, Valencia, Spain
e-mail: ajv22@medschl.cam.ac.uk

S. Carobbio (✉)
Centro de Investigacion Principe Felipe, Valencia, Spain
e-mail: scarobbio@cipf.es

© Springer Nature Switzerland AG 2023
R. S. Ahima (ed.), *Metabolic Syndrome*,
https://doi.org/10.1007/978-3-031-40116-9_23

Abstract

Our understanding of adipose tissue physiology and pathophysiology has substantially increased during the last decade. Notably, white adipose tissue (WAT) dysfunction has been proposed as a critical determinant of obesity-associated metabolic complications. WAT is a complex metabolic organ composed of many cell types, including adipocytes, the primary cell type involved in energy storage. Adipocytes also synthesize numerous molecules that regulate energy balance, vascular homeostasis, and insulin sensitivity. In obesity, WAT expansion is associated with intensified structural remodeling that compromises the tissue's metabolic and secretory functions. Failure to efficiently store lipids in WAT results in a "*spillover*" of the excess lipids into non-adipose tissues, which further disrupts metabolic homeostasis and contributes to the development of obesity-related pathologies, known collectively as metabolic syndrome.

In contrast, brown adipose tissue (BAT) is an energy-dissipating thermogenic organ that produces heat by uncoupling mitochondrial fatty acid oxidation. Activation of BAT thermogenesis can ameliorate the effects of WAT dysfunction in metabolically compromised mouse models. The rediscovery of BAT in humans has raised the possibility that BAT could be a therapeutic target for metabolic syndrome. This chapter will discuss important structural and cellular features of the WAT and BAT and how obesity alters WAT and BAT structure, intercellular crosstalk, and function.

Keywords

White adipocyte · Brown adipose tissue · Beige adipocyte · Angiogenesis · Immune cells · Extracellular matrix

Introduction

Obesity is caused by sustained positive energy balance. Adipose tissue (AT) is the principal organ for energy storage in mammals, and excessive expansion of AT plays a central role in the pathology of obesity. AT is also a vital endocrine organ, regulating several aspects of metabolism, from appetite to nutrient partitioning and uptake by other tissues. Therefore, it is essential to understand the consequences of obesity on AT biology and function.

AT is a connective tissue composed predominantly of adipocytes, whose primary functions are the storage of energy as triglycerides (TGs) in lipid droplets and the coordinated mobilization of these lipids to fuel other organs. The AT also secretes hormones termed "*adipokines*" that help coordinate these functions and inform the central nervous system of energy supplies as a permissive level of control for costly physiological processes such as pregnancy. AT is distributed throughout the body in various depots with location-specific differences in structure, composition, and functions. For example, white AT (WAT) can be found subcutaneously (subcutaneous WAT, scWAT) and in the intra-abdominal cavity (visceral WAT, visWAT). WAT is characterized by its ability to expand to meet the storage demands determined by nutrient excess in positive energy balance. These lipids should be efficiently stored and released when energy supply to peripheral tissues is required.

The primary function of brown adipose tissue (BAT) is heat generation (thermogenesis) to maintain body temperature. Until the last decade, BAT was not much more than a *"rodent curiosity."* However, in the last 10–15 years, the realization that human infants and lean adults have BAT has massively reinvigorated the research in this area. Brown adipocytes are uniquely adapted for thermogenesis by uncoupling protein 1 (UCP1) expression in their mitochondria. UCP1 uncouples substrate oxidation from ATP synthesis, a process known as thermogenesis, primarily serves to defend the core body temperature in the face of heat loss to the environment.

WAT structure and function are maladapted in human obesity, particularly associated with metabolic complications. We have proposed the *AT expandability hypothesis* that suggests that WAT dysfunction is a crucial determinant of obesity-associated metabolic complications. Healthy WAT maintains metabolic homeostasis by locking excess nutrients and being able to expand and retract dynamically as energy availability fluctuates between surplus and shortfall. In contrast, in a chronic state of positive energy balance, WAT – especially visWAT – is constantly compelled to expand. Besides, the perception of the large amount of fat in severely obese individuals might suggest that WAT expansion capacity is not infinite and beyond a genetically/epigenetically determined limit; in the context of obesity, WAT becomes functionally impaired both as a storage and as endocrine organ. The excess lipid species then accumulate in vital metabolic organs such as skeletal muscle, liver, or kidney (referred to as ectopic lipid accumulation), which negatively affects their function known as "lipotoxicity," one of the fundamental pathogenic mechanisms associated with the development of the metabolic syndrome.

Conversely, from experiments with obese rodents, it is known that BAT activation removes nutrient excess by oxidizing lipids and glucose; this can limit weight gain and mitigate the negative impact of obesity on WAT and other organs. Therefore, promoting BAT thermogenesis has recently been considered a potential therapeutic approach to treating human obesity and its associated complications. However, the success of this strategy requires a better understanding of BAT structure and function in humans, areas that have only been rigorously investigated since 2009.

This chapter outlines the cellular and structural features and the biological functions of WAT and BAT; their anatomical distribution, plasticity, and development; and the roles of immune cells, the vascular network, the extracellular matrix, and the nervous system in regulating AT function. The impact of obesity on each of these aspects will also be described.

White and Brown Adipose Tissue: Cellular and Structural Features

Adipose Tissue Cellular and Structural Components

Adipocytes are the main cellular components of AT. In WAT, adipocytes are spherical cells that store fat in the form of TGs in a unilocular lipid droplet. Adipocyte diameter varies from 30 to 180 μm, depending on the anatomical location and lipid content. The lipid droplet is a dynamic structure, growing, and shrinking as lipids are added or removed, a process enabled by enzymes, lipid droplet proteins, and the cytoskeleton.

In contrast, BAT adipocytes store lipids in multiple, smaller lipid droplets. Multilocularity increases lipid droplet surface area and is more suited for the quick and titrated release of stored lipids for oxidation. Brown adipocytes also have more specialized mitochondria, which express UCP1, the mitochondrial inner membrane protein that enables heat production by uncoupling substrate oxidation from adenosine triphosphate (ATP) production. In rodents, UCP1-expressing multilocular adipocytes can also be dispersed in scWAT under conditions requiring increased heat production (e.g., chronic cold exposure). These UCP1-positive cells are termed "*beige*" or "*brite*" (brown-in-white) adipocytes. Whereas brown adipocytes are a homogenous population demarcated by connective tissue, beige adipocytes exist interspersed among white adipocytes within scWAT.

Adipocytes interact with other cellular components in AT, including the nonmyelinated nerve endings of noradrenergic sympathetic fibers, resident immune cells, and vascular cells, such as endothelial cells and pericytes. In addition, specific AT cellular components can be replenished by progenitor populations of preadipocytes and mesenchymal stem cells. Cells in AT also interact with the extracellular matrix (ECM), which is composed mainly of collagens and provides structural support and regulation of critical cellular functions such as survival and differentiation. The cellular composition of BAT and WAT is distinct and reflects their different functions. For example, there are more sympathetic nerve endings and capillaries per adipocyte in BAT compared to WAT. This difference is partly due to smaller adipocyte size and serves the increased requirements in BAT for gas exchange and the supply of oxidative substrates. Furthermore, in rodents, the developmental origins of BAT and WAT adipocytes are different, and even different WAT depots derive from distinct lineages [18]. Though this is impossible to interrogate in humans, the selective loss of particular WAT depots in different types of partial lipodystrophies suggests distinct origins for adipocytes of different WAT depots.

Adipose Tissue Cellular Subpopulation Heterogeneity

Until recently, the adipose tissue was considered as being formed of homogenous populations of different cell types. However, in the last few years, technological advancements, such as single-cell or single nuclei RNAseq, have been developed, which allow dissecting tissue subpopulation heterogeneity at the individual cell level and a high resolution. This transcriptional characterization of individual cells facilitates the progress in understanding the adipose tissue composition and functional compartmentalization specialization in physiological and pathophysiological conditions [27]. These approaches have been applied both for the study of the heterogeneity of the stromal vascular fraction as well as of the mature cells of different AT depots in murine and human models as well as other large animals [31]. Applying single-cell profiling methodologies to adipose tissue research has produced large complex datasets. Notably, many genes that discriminate different cell subpopulations are not associated with known cellular mechanisms, pointing to the many gaps in our knowledge of adipocyte and adipose tissue functions. Nevertheless, this work has produced consistent new findings. For instance, cells that can inhibit adipose differentiation, adipocyte subpopulations with higher lipolytic, hypertrophic or fibro-inflammatory potential, and adipocytes primed for thermogenic activity, all of which are characterized by specific markers, many newly identified thanks to this technology. The adipocyte subpopulations also differ between various adipose depots [125] and present gender dysmorphism affecting mechanisms related to preadipocyte activation and pathways controlling the adipogenic and pro-inflammatory properties of distinct progenitor subpopulations [109]. Single-cell RNA profiling also revealed that murine alternatively activated macrophage signaling is sufficient to induce browning in this depot in an SNS-independent manner [43]. Moreover, Jumabay et al. have reported a subpopulation of BAT progenitors that can undergo neurogenic differentiation [57]. Other single-cell -omics technology has been applied to study AT cell heterogeneity. For example, single-cell proteomic performed on WAT of lean and diet-induced obesity mice identified different subpopulations of tissue-resident macrophages characterized by different origins, i.e., embryonic versus bone marrow-derived, different proliferation capability as well as more or less active in phagocytosis, endocytosis, and antigen processing in vitro [33]. The future challenge is to understand the specific function of all these newly identified cellular subpopulations within the AT.

Anatomical Distribution of WAT

WAT is anatomically distributed into two main depots: **subcutaneous** (scWAT) and **visceral** (visWAT) (Fig. 1a). ScWAT is found below the skin, and depending on their anatomical location, different scWAT depots have different structural and ultrastructural features. For example, the scWAT depots localized to the abdominal area are characterized by large, tightly packed adipocytes, relatively poor vascularization, and a weak ECM. The structural scWAT is more fibrous and vascularized and is located in the limbs and hips. Finally, the fibrous scWAT is composed of smaller adipocytes and is particularly suited to tolerate mechanical stress in areas such as the heel by its enrichment with ECM components. Visceral WAT (visWAT) comprises intraperitoneal/intraabdominal depots, including omental, mesenteric, and gonadal depots (epididymal and paratesticular in males, periovarial and periuterine in females). Discrete visWAT depots are found in contact with organs such as the heart (pericardial), arteries (perivascular), and kidneys (retroperitoneal). Other AT depots include mammary AT, bone marrow AT, facial AT, and dermal AT [22]. Morphologically, adipocytes in visWAT are smaller than those in scWAT.

The amount and distribution of lipids between visWAT and scWAT depots differ depending on gender and age. For example, in females, scWAT is preferentially located in the gluteofemoral area, whereas in males, it is predominantly located in the abdominal area [119]. In males, abdominal WAT mass increases with age independently of adiposity, and in females, the postmenopausal period is associated with an increase in visWAT, potentially due to a relative increase in testosterone levels [55].

Anatomical Redistribution of WAT in Obesity

Obesity is characterized by an excessive increase in fat mass that predisposes to the development of metabolic complications such as cardiovascular diseases and type 2 diabetes. Existing adipocytes become enlarged (hypertrophy), and new adipocytes are recruited (hyperplasia) to accommodate the excess nutrients. Furthermore, in obesity, there is an anatomical repartitioning of WAT mass from scWAT to visWAT. Compared to scWAT, visWAT is more metabolically active and releases more pro-inflammatory cytokines and free fatty acids (FFAs) into circulation [38]. Therefore, the accumulation of intra-abdominal fat may negatively affect the function of other metabolic organs such as liver by increasing systemic inflammation and elevating FFA levels in the blood.

VisWAT dysfunction is associated with ectopic lipid accumulation in vital metabolic organs such as the liver, heart, pancreas, and skeletal muscle (Fig. 1b). Ectopic lipids can accumulate as intracellular lipids (e.g., within hepatocytes in the liver or within myocytes in muscle), form a new fat depot (e.g., intermuscular AT), or accumulate in other preexisting visWAT depots (e.g., pericardial and perivascular depots). Ectopic lipid accumulation causes a lipotoxic effect impairing insulin sensitivity, especially in myocytes and hepatocytes [10].

Men and women are equally susceptible to obesity but differ in the health consequences mainly due to their different body fat distribution. The incidence of CVD associated with an obese phenotype usually is higher in males than females. That is because men develop a larger visWAT around the visceral organs. In contrast, women exhibit a more abundant scWAT in the lower hip region, which protects them from the premature development of atherosclerosis and acute coronary syndromes by activating pro-inflammatory factors. In women, the cardiometabolic risk increases after menopause due to their increased visceral adiposity [70].

Anatomical Distribution of BAT

BAT has long been known to exist in infants. Infants are at a higher risk of losing core body temperature when exposed to a cold environment than adults due to their larger surface-area-to-volume ratio. Although newborns are born with scWAT for insulation, they still require BAT

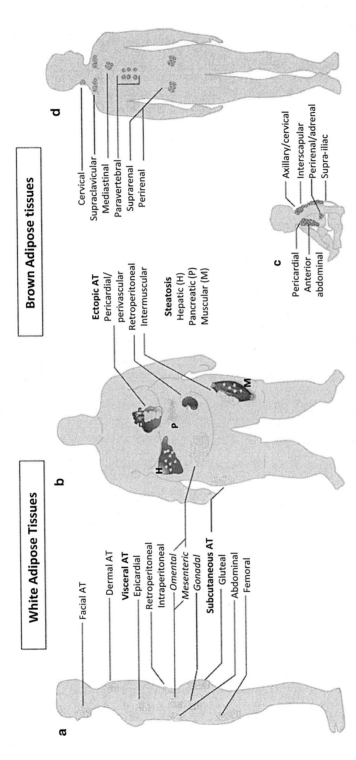

Fig. 1 Anatomical distribution of adipose tissue depots. (**a**) White adipose tissue (*AT*) depots in a lean adult [7]. Subcutaneous AT (*scWAT*) depots include gluteal, abdominal, and femoral depots. Visceral AT (*visWAT*) depots include epicardial, retroperitoneal, and intraperitoneal depots. Intraperitoneal depots can be further subdivided into omental, mesenteric, and gonadal depots (epididymal and paratesticular in males, periovarial and periuterine in females). Other depots are the facial and dermal AT. (**b**) Ectopic lipid accumulation in obesity. Lipids can accumulate in preexisting or new fat depots (visceral, pericardial, perivascular, retroperitoneal, and intermuscular AT) or within cells leading to steatosis in the liver, pancreas, and muscle. (**c**) Brown adipose tissue depots in infants [65]. These depots are strategically placed to protect and warm the blood flow of critical organs and areas of the body (in brackets as follows): supra-axillary/cervical (head), perirenal/adrenal (kidneys), interscapular (spinal cord), supra-iliac (lumbar and azygos veins), pericardial (heart), anterior abdominal (liver). (**d**) Brown adipose tissue depots persist in adults. Some brown adipose tissue depots persist in adults, including cervical, supraclavicular, mediastinal, paravertebral, suprarenal, and perirenal depots

thermogenesis to counteract excessive heat loss. BAT represents 1% of body weight in newborns and is topographically distributed in multiple depots protecting critical organs by warming their blood flow to these areas (Fig. 1c) [65].

Many infant BAT depots, such as the interscapular depot, postnatally lose their "brown" phenotype, including loss of UCP1 expression and increased adipocyte size [65]. However, some deeper BAT depots in infants (e.g., the perirenal depot) persist into adulthood (Fig. 1d). The use of metabolic image technology in the form of 2-[^{18}F]fluoro-2-deoxyglucose positron emission tomography coupled with computed tomography (FDG-PET/CT) demonstrates the presence of BAT in adult humans. FDG-PET measures the uptake and accumulation of FDG, a radioactive analog of glucose that cannot be metabolized. FDG-accumulating tissues are visualized using PET and identified as AT using CT. Biopsies have demonstrated the presence of UCP1 in several FDG-accumulating adipose tissue depots (Fig. 1d) [124].

As a percentage of body weight, adults have much less BAT compared to infants. Also, the likelihood of BAT detection is higher in females [88]. An exception to the gradual loss of BAT from birth through adulthood is the increased prevalence of BAT during puberty compared to childhood. Notably, BAT activity decreases with age, whereas the incidence of metabolic diseases increases with age. Moreover, decreased BAT activity is associated with surrogate parameters of metabolic dysfunction, such as increasing BMI, percent body fat, and plasma glucose levels [88].

Considering beige cells, data from rodents indicate that cold exposure preferentially recruits beige cells in scWAT compared to visWAT. However, it is still unclear whether UCP1-expressing adipocytes can be recruited in WAT depots of healthy humans. UCP1-expressing multilocular adipocytes have been reported in WAT of patients with pheochromocytomas and paragangliomas. These catecholamine-secreting cancers may mimic the effects of chronically increased sympathetic nervous tone to WAT in response to long-term cold exposure, stimulating beige cell recruitment in rodents. However, the recruitment of UCP1-expressing adipocytes has not been demonstrated in the WAT of healthy humans under physiological conditions, and unfortunately, FDG-PET/CT is not sensitive enough to distinguish clusters of thermogenic adipocytes in WAT [83].

In addition to whether beige adipocyte recruitment is a physiological phenomenon in humans, the question of whether the brown adipocytes in human BAT depots are more similar to rodent beige adipocytes or rodent brown adipocytes is also unresolved. For example, the UCP1-expressing adipocytes in adult human supraclavicular BAT occur in clusters interspersed among white adipocytes, a pattern reminiscent of the beige cells in rodent scWAT. In contrast, the human infant interscapular BAT depot is dominated by multilocular UCP1-expressing adipocytes separated from surrounding WAT by connective tissue. This structural arrangement is reminiscent of the rodent interscapular BAT depot [71].

In the last few years, new BAT and beige fat depots have been identified in murine models. Mesa et al. describe new pelvic and lower abdominal BAT depots located around the urethra, internal reproductive and urinary tract organs, and significant lower pelvic blood vessels, as well as between adjacent muscles where the upper hind leg meets the abdominal cavity. Whether the thermogenic activity of these BAT depots associated has any specific function has yet to be determined [78]. Similarly, Chan et al. identified and characterized a novel, naturally existing beige fat depot, thigh adipose tissue (tAT). Unlike classic WATs, tAT maintains beige fat morphology at room temperature, whereas high-fat diet (HFD) feeding or aging promotes the development of typical WAT features, namely unilocular adipocytes. tAT is covered by a muscular septum that separates it from scWAT, which raises the possibility that it may be intramuscular AT depot. Its actual function is still unclear, but a possibility is that tAT functions as a cushion surrounding the synovial joint between the femur and pelvis, perhaps maintaining a homeostatic temperature of the joint for movement or blood flow [21].

Metabolic Functions of Brown and White Adipose Tissue

Metabolic Function of WAT

Classically described as an organ for energy storage, WAT is also a metabolic, endocrine organ. WAT releases circulating factors central to the coordinated regulation of energy metabolism. Here, we will consider the mechanisms regulating WAT energy storage and mobilization, as this is most directly related to WAT structure. We point the readers to the chapter on adipokines (▶ Chap. 18, "Adipokines and Metabolism") for further information on the endocrine function of WAT.

Triglyceride Storage and Mobilization of Energy Reserves

In the postprandial state, nutrients are absorbed by the intestinal tract and enter the bloodstream. Most absorbed nutrients are stored in the liver, and WAT as glycogen and triglycerides, respectively. Insulin is the primary anabolic hormone orchestrating this process. To be stored in WAT, triglycerides (TGs) from blood are hydrolyzed into FFAs, taken up by the adipocyte, and re-esterified subsequently into TGs incorporated into the lipid droplet (Fig. 2a).

In the postabsorptive state, energy reserves are mobilized in response to catecholamines such as epinephrine, released by the adrenal medulla, and norepinephrine, by nerve endings of the sympathetic nervous system (SNS) within WAT. In a process termed lipolysis, catecholamines bind to β-adrenergic receptors (ARs) (primarily β3 subtype in mice and β1/2 in humans), activating protein kinase A (PKA) to initiate the breakdown of intracellular TGs into FFAs and glycerol, which are released into the circulation (Fig. 2a). These substrates are taken up by the liver and muscle (sites of FFA oxidation), and glycerol is used as a substrate for hepatic gluconeogenesis. Glucagon, secreted by endocrine pancreatic α-cells in response to catecholamines, plays a complementary role by promoting gluconeogenesis by the liver and, in rodents, lipolysis by WAT as well. Significantly, cold exposure also increases WAT lipolysis via the SNS; in this context, FFAs released by WAT are taken up by BAT and used as substrates for thermogenesis.

In the absence of a lipolytic stimulus, lipolysis is repressed by basal levels of catecholamines engaging α 2-ARs; these inhibitory receptors have a higher affinity for catecholamines compared to β-ARs. α 2-AR-mediated suppression of lipolysis is overwhelmed when the local concentration of catecholamines increases, activating pro-lipolytic β-ARs. Postprandially, lipolysis is also repressed by insulin.

Energy storage and mobilization show depot-specific differences. In particular, higher lipolytic rates are observed in visceral adipocytes compared to subcutaneous adipocytes due to increased lipolytic responsiveness to adrenergic stimulation and reduced sensitivity to the anti-lipolytic effects of insulin and α 2-AR signaling [38]. Because the blood supply of visWAT drains into the portal vein, in obesity, hepatic metabolism may be particularly impaired by the redistribution of fat mass to the more metabolically active visWAT and the consequently increased load of FFAs into the blood.

Altered Metabolic Function During Obesity

Obese WAT is characterized by an altered secretion profile of adipokines, discussed in ▶ Chap. 18, "Adipokines and Metabolism," and functionally altered energy storage and mobilization. Firstly, FFA uptake and triglyceride storage are facilitated by the upregulation of FFA uptake mechanisms. For instance, LPL expression and activity increase in obese scWAT and visWAT, and LPL expression positively correlates with BMI. Additionally, CD36 expression is induced during obesity and positively correlates with increased visWAT mass [74]. These processes promote WAT expansion. Secondly, the regulation of lipolysis is impaired due to reduced lipase activity and decreased responsiveness to catecholamines. In rats, it has been reported that obesity-induced inflammation and cytokine signaling activate ERK MAP kinase, which subsequently phosphorylates the β3AR on S247, causing an enhancement of adipocyte basal lipolysis, which is a hallmark of obesity states [48].

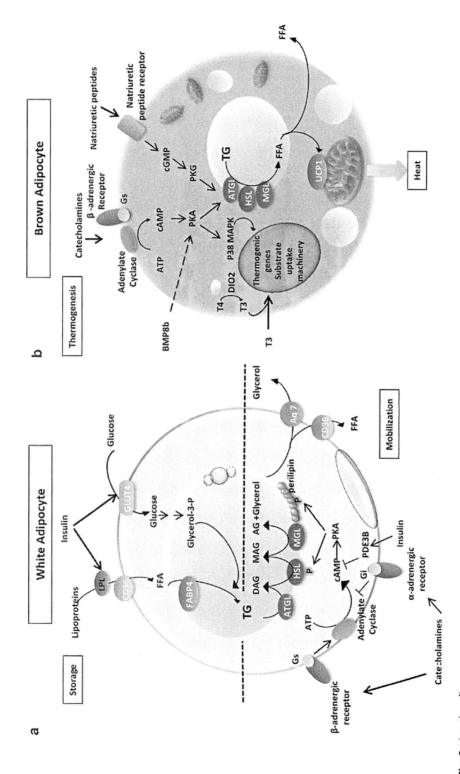

Fig. 2 (continued)

Metabolic Function of BAT

The metabolic function of BAT has been primarily studied in rodents. Their small body size and relatively increased surface-area-to-volume ratio mean that adult rodents depend on BAT thermogenesis to maintain their core body temperature. Heat production is an energy-expensive process that negatively affects energy balance and whole-body substrate utilization in rodents and humans.

Thermogenesis

Brown adipocytes are uniquely optimized for thermogenic function by UCP1. UCP1 resides in and regulates the proton permeability of the inner mitochondrial membrane (IMM). In mitochondria, substrate oxidation is coupled to electron transport to generate a proton gradient and a potential difference across the IMM. ATP is made using the energy released when protons flow down their electrochemical gradient across the IMM through ATP synthases. When activated by FFAs, UCP1 increases IMM proton permeability and thereby "uncouples" substrate oxidation from ATP synthesis, producing heat instead.

The metabolic rate of activated BAT is so elevated that intracellular lipid stores are quickly depleted, so the uptake of lipids and glucose from the blood must replenish oxidative substrates. The substrate uptake machinery of brown adipocytes is similar to that of white adipocytes. Like in WAT, insulin increases BAT's substrate uptake, coordinating BAT's metabolism with the fasted or fed state. However, the SNS is the primary regulator of BAT activation. In response to a thermogenic stimulus – a signal indicating an increased demand for heat production such as a decrease in environmental temperature – norepinephrine is released by sympathetic nerve endings in BAT and binds to β ARs on brown adipocytes. Of interest is that this is true for mice, but for humans, this is controversial. So far, different groups have come to different conclusions [20]. Whether human BAT thermogenesis is regulated by β1, β2, or β3 adrenergic receptors is debatable. The downstream signaling pathways have been

---

Fig. 2 (continued) Signaling pathways regulating adipocyte function. The molecular details of these pathways derive primarily from studies using rodent models. (a) The intracellular signaling pathways mediate the response of white adipocytes to extracellular signals (insulin, catecholamines, and glycerol) that promote energy storage and mobilization. Insulin promotes energy storage by adipocytes. Insulin stimulates the translocation of lipoprotein lipase (*LPL*) to the vascular walls of capillaries, where it hydrolyzes triglycerides, which are carried in the blood by lipoproteins. The resulting free fatty acids (*FFAs*) are taken up by adipocytes through membrane receptors, such as fatty acid translocase (CD36), and are rapidly sequestered by lipid-binding proteins, for example, fatty acid-binding protein 4 (*FABP4*). Insulin also regulates the translocation of GLUT4 glucose transporters to the plasma membrane, allowing glucose to enter the adipocyte by facilitated diffusion. Glucose uptake is essential for adipocyte lipid storage because FFAs must be reincorporated into triglyceride molecules so they can be stored in the lipid droplet, and this process requires glycerol-3-phosphate produced by glycolysis. Catecholamines drive energy mobilization. Catecholamines bind to β-adrenergic receptors to initiate the breakdown of intracellular TGs into FFAs released into the circulation. β-Adrenergic receptors (*ARs*) interact with the Gs subunits of heterotrimeric G proteins; Gs subunits activate adenylate cyclase, leading to increased production of cyclic AMP and subsequent protein kinase A (PKA) activation. PKA phosphorylates lipid droplet membrane proteins and lipases to stimulate lipolysis, releasing FFAs and glycerol that leave the adipocyte. In the absence of a lipolytic stimulus, lipolysis is repressed by basal catecholamines engaging α 2-ARs, coupled to Gi subunits that inhibit adenylate cyclase. Postprandially, insulin represses lipolysis through activation of the phosphodiesterase (PDE3B), which limits PKA activation by degrading cyclic AMP. (b) The intracellular signaling pathways that mediate the response of brown adipocytes to extracellular signals (catecholamines, natriuretic peptides, triiodothyronine, BMP8b) that mediate thermogenesis. Abbreviations: acylglycerol (*AG*), adenosine triphosphate (*ATP*), adipose triglyceride lipase (*ATGL*), cyclic AMP (*cAMP*), cyclic GMP (*cGMP*), diacylglycerol (*DAG*), fatty acid-binding protein 4 (*FABP4*), fatty acid translocase (*CD36*), free fatty acid (*FFA*), glucose transporter 4 (*GLUT4*), glycerol-3-phosphate (*glycerol-3-P*), lipoprotein lipase (*LPL*), monoacylglycerol (*MAG*), phosphodiesterase 3 B (*PDE3B*), protein kinase A (*PKA*), triglyceride (*TG*), triiodothyronine (*T3*), uncoupling protein 1 (*UCP1*)

studied primarily in rodent models. Lipolysis is activated similarly to white adipocytes except for a few key differences (Fig. 2b). Firstly, the FFAs freed from intracellular triglycerides are used for oxidation and UCP1 activation. Secondly, lipolysis in BAT is coordinated with a non-insulin-dependent upregulation of the substrate uptake machinery to increase the uptake of oxidative substrates, such as FFAs released into the blood by WAT lipolysis. Finally, sympathetic stimulation increases the transcription of critical thermogenic genes such as UCP1. In addition to cold exposure, BAT is also activated in rodents in response to excess nutrient consumption, for example, due to high-fat diet (HFD) feeding, a process known as diet-induced thermogenesis. Recently, UCP1-independent non-canonical mechanisms promoting thermogenesis in brown and beige adipocytes have been reported involving creatine substrate cycling and calcium cycling pathways [52].

Independently from the SNS, brown and beige adipocytes are regulated by several endocrine factors in rodents (Fig. 2b). Thyroid hormone is a key endocrine regulator of BAT thermogenesis. Though triiodothyronine (T3) has central effects that can regulate sympathetic tone to BAT, T3 is also generated locally by brown adipocytes [73].

T3 regulates the transcription of the UCP1 gene via thyroid hormone response elements in its promoter. The unliganded thyroid hormone receptor acts as a transcriptional repressor, and the binding of T3 to its receptor relieves this repression [96].

Other endocrine factors regulate the responsiveness of brown adipocytes to adrenergic stimulation by interacting with the cAMP/PKA pathway and its effectors. For example, BMP8b increases the maximal thermogenic response of brown adipocytes to adrenergic stimulation by potentiating PKA activity [132]. In addition, PKA shares many intracellular targets with protein kinase G (PKG). As a result, cardiac natriuretic peptides (CNPs), which act via PKG, can induce lipolysis and the expression of thermogenic genes in brown and white adipocytes, a response which is additive to that of norepinephrine [9]. Endocrine factors that bypass the sympathetic nervous pathways to regulate brown and beige adipocyte activity have also been identified (Table 1).

The relevance of endocrine activators to human BAT is under investigation. For example, in an isolated case, levothyroxine treatment for thyroid cancer also increased BAT mass and activity as a side effect, and upon withdrawal of levothyroxine treatment, BAT activity and mass decreased [112].

Table 1 Endocrine factors bypassing the sympathetic nervous pathways to regulate brown and beige adipocyte activity

Molecules	Mechanism of action	References
FGF21	Release of FGF21 by the liver within hours of birth is an important signal promoting thermogenesis in neonatal mice. FGF21 is also released by brown adipocytes themselves, acting locally to further increase BAT thermogenesis and systemically to induce beige adipocyte recruitment in WAT	[46]
Irisin, cardiotrophin-1	Recruit beige adipocytes in white adipose tissue by acting on white adipocytes and their precursors.	[11]
Lactate, nitrate, β-aminoisobutyric acid, adenosine	Activate brown adipocytes and recruit beige adipocytes	[99]
Meteorin	Induces M2 polarization of macrophages to recruit beige adipocytes in WAT	[98]
ANP/BNP	Induce WAT browning by promoting triglyceride lipolysis as well as uncoupling of mitochondrial respiration	[58]
Bile acids	Promote BAT thermogenic activity through activation of intracellular thyroid hormone signals by binding to their receptor TGR5	[131]
IL-27	Promotes adipocyte thermogenesis by activating p38 MAPK–PGC-1α signaling and stimulating the production of UCP1.	[129]
FGF15/19	Enhance BAT activity and metabolic rate.	[35]

Moreover, circulating levels of FGF21 and irisin are increased with cold exposure in humans, suggesting that these factors may be involved in cold-induced thermogenesis [68]. Other factors, such as bile acids secreted by the liver by binding to their receptor TGR5 in the adipocytes, promote BAT activation through the induction of intracellular thyroid hormone signaling [131]. A- type and B-type natriuretic peptides can induce WAT browning by promoting TG lipolysis and increasing UCP1 expression and function [58]. Finally, more recently, Wang et al. demonstrated that IL27Rα ko mouse developed obesity and showed decreased oxygen consumption, indicating that its ligand IL-27 through the p38 MAPK-PGC1α signaling pathway plays a role in promoting adipocyte thermogenesis and energy expenditure [129].

Regulation of Whole-Body Energy Metabolism

BAT activity can promote a negative energy balance and weight loss. In rodents, BAT thermogenesis is responsible for the ~60% increase in metabolic rate caused by decreasing housing temperature from 30 °C to 23 °C [16]. Indeed, BAT ablation or dysfunction in rodents decreases energy expenditure, causing an obese phenotype [32]. Conversely, BAT simulation by cold exposure or β 3-AR agonism increases energy expenditure, attenuates weight gain, and decreases adiposity in rodent models of obesity [44]. The full impact of BAT activation on human energy expenditure has not been fully clarified, but it is likely less than in rodents due to reduced dependence on BAT thermogenesis and lower BAT mass as percent of body weight. However, a direct link between increased BAT activity and adiposity

is suggested by the evidence that 2-h bouts of exposure to 17 °C for 6 weeks increased BAT activity and decreased adiposity in healthy volunteers [135].

In terms of whole-body metabolism, increased energy expenditure by BAT requires increased substrate uptake and utilization. Increased glucose and lipid disposal by activated BAT are sufficient to normalize hyperglycemia and hyperlipidemia in mouse models of diabetes [6]. The fact that sustained BAT activation introduces a negative energy balance may indicate that the main beneficial effects of BAT activation on diabetes and dyslipidemia are secondary to its effects on body weight. However, in some experiments, activation of BAT by chronic treatment with a β 3-AR agonist did not decrease body weight but decreased serum levels of glucose and FFAs and increased peripheral insulin sensitivity [72]. This change indicates that BAT activation directly improves glucose homeostasis, so the fact that BAT activation can also protect against obesity is an added advantage. BAT endocrine activity may also regulate whole-body energy metabolism. Some of the molecules described previously as thermogenic activators are also factors secreted by BAT itself. In particular, BAT production of certain factors known to regulate metabolism is sufficient to have a systemic impact (Table 2), suggesting that BAT may be an important node for regulating energy and glucose homeostasis.

In humans, the glucose uptake rate of cold-stimulated BAT per gram of tissue exceeds that of insulin-stimulated skeletal muscle, and evidence suggests that activated BAT may regulate glycemia. Indeed, fasting glucose levels are lower in individuals with detectable BAT than in those

Table 2 Factors with Endocrine Functions that Are Released by Brown Adipocytes

Molecules	Importance	References
T3	Regulates whole-body energy expenditure	[46]
FGF21, IL-6	Regulate glucose homeostasis	[46]
Leptin, adiponectin	Regulate appetite, and glucose and lipid metabolism. Expression is downregulated with increased BAT activity and therefore may be of lesser importance	[15]
CXCL14	Regulates the alternative activation and recruitment of macrophages	[19]
GDF15	Exerts anti-inflammatory effects on M1 macrophages	[14]
BMP8b/NRG4 axis	BMP8b induces the endogenous production of NRG4, which promotes the outgrowth and branching of sympathetic nerve axons	[128]

without detectable BAT, though a causal link has not been established [67]. Regarding endocrine function for human BAT, FGF21 expression has been detected in neonatal BAT and adult BAT induced by pheochromocytoma [47]. However, the secretion profile of physiological adult BAT has not been analyzed in healthy conditions or the context of obesity and metabolic disease. Other factors released from BAT, known as Batokines, such as CXCL14, GDF15, and BMP8b together with NRG4, have an impact on the recruitment and function of other cell types, such as macrophages and neurons [14, 19, 128].

Effect of Obesity on Thermogenesis and Regulation of Energy Metabolism

Though increasing BAT activity in rodent models of obesity has beneficial effects on energy balance and metabolism, BAT does become dysfunctional in the context of obesity in rodents. For example, in *ob/ob* mice, BAT is insulin-resistant, suggesting that, like other insulin-sensitive tissues, BAT is also negatively affected by hyperinsulinemia and hyperglycemia in the context of obesity. In line with this, a study investigating BAT activation by cold and insulin stimulation in humans measured reduced responsiveness to both of these stimuli in obese patients regarding glucose uptake and blood flow [86]. Similarly, basal and cold-induced FFA uptake is impaired in obese BAT, which reduces access to essential substrates for its metabolism [105]. Moreover, BAT mass and activity are minimized in obese patients due to reduced cell proliferation, preadipocyte differentiation, and increased apoptosis caused by catecholamine resistance, inflammation, ER, and oxidative stress [1]. On a positive note, a recent study measuring BAT activity in lean versus obese individuals after exposure to a standardized cooling protocol using a water-perfused vest showed that despite a significantly lower prevalence of BAT, the metabolic activity and thermogenic capacity of BAT appears to be still intact in obesity [63]. These findings support current efforts to harness BAT activity and/or to recruit new BAT as a therapeutic strategy to counteract obesity and its metabolic complications.

Adipose Tissue Plasticity

Adipogenesis

Both BAT and WAT are established in utero. In animal models, WAT depots have been found to derive from both the mesoderm and the neural crest so that distinct developmental origins may underlie the different gene expression patterns found in different WAT depots in humans. Rodent studies have shown that brown adipocytes derive from the paraxial mesoderm and interestingly share a Myf5$^+$ lineage origin with myocytes, whereas most white adipocytes have a Myf5$^-$ lineage origin (Fig. 3) [18]. In recent years, a more complex picture regarding the adipocytes' developmental origins and identity of the adipocytes, even within a same AT depot, has emerged. Lee et al. demonstrated that WAT is composed of at least three distinct adipocyte subpopulations that arise from different populations of adipocyte precursor cells and have distinct molecular markers (i.e., Wt1, Tagln, and Mx1). Moreover, they present differences in metabolism and differential responses to exogenous stimuli. These different types of adipocytes are found in each adipose depot in different proportions, contributing to the differing biology of individual adipose depots [69].

AT expansion in the adult is fundamental to the functional roles of WAT and BAT. As we have seen, WAT must expand if excessive calorie consumption and conversely contract by releasing FFAs in fasting conditions to act as an efficient storage organ. BAT is equally plastic and can expand or contract to match its thermogenic capacity to the thermogenic needs of the organism. In both cases, AT expansion requires the production of new adipocytes. Adipocytes are nondividing cells, so new adipocytes are made from undifferentiated precursor cells with proliferative capacity that persist in adult AT: mesenchymal stem cells and preadipocytes. Adipocyte differentiation encompasses the production of preadipocytes – which are committed to producing adipocytes – from mesenchymal stem cells and the terminal differentiation of preadipocytes into mature adipocytes.

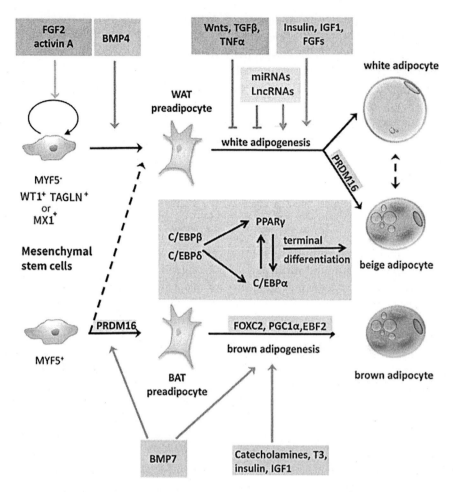

Fig. 3 Origins of adipocytes and transcriptional regulation of adipocyte differentiation. Mesenchymal stem cells and preadipocytes with proliferative and adipogenic capacity persist in adult AT. Rodent brown adipocytes derive from an MYF5[+] lineage, unlike most white adipocytes [18]. White adipocytes can originate also from Wt1[+], Tagln[+], or Mxt1[+] lineage precursors [69]. Beige adipocytes may derive from precursors or directly from white adipocytes [101] MiRNAs, and LncRNAs can exert both an inhibitory or an activator effect (*light yellow box*) [136]. C/EBPs and PPARγ transcription factors regulate adipogenesis, which is biased toward a thermogenic brown or beige phenotype by factors such as FOXC2, PGC1α, EBF2, and PRDM16 (transcriptional control in *blue boxes*) [107]. Extracellular signals can maintain the undifferentiated, proliferating state of mesenchymal stem cells (*purple box*) and promote (*green boxes*) or inhibit (*red boxes*) adipocyte differentiation [100, 118, 122])

White Adipocyte Differentiation

The first step of white adipocyte differentiation is the generation of preadipocytes from mesenchymal precursors. In vitro, mesenchymal precursors can be maintained in an undifferentiated, proliferating state by factors such as FGF2 and activin A and committed to the adipocyte cell lineage by BMP4 [118]. Adipogenesis is the production of adipocytes from preadipocytes, and extensive studies of this process in vitro have highlighted a cascade of transcription factors that regulates adipocyte differentiation (Fig. 3). C/EBPβ and C/EBPδ are induced first during mitotic clonal expansion of preadipocytes and subsequently induce C/EBPα (alpha) and PPARγ 2, which maintain the terminal differentiation of the adipocyte. This process is characterized by cell cycle arrest and the induction of mature white adipocyte machinery, such as the de novo lipogenic program, which is regulated by the transcription factor SREBP1c. More recently described new players in the regulations of adipocyte differentiation are miRNAs and LncRNA, which can both play as activators and inhibitors of this process [136].

In vitro, the white adipogenic transcriptional cascade can be initiated or suppressed by extracellular signals (Fig. 3) [100]. For example, insulin-like growth factor 1 (IGF-1) and glucocorticoids induce adipogenesis. Although FGF2 stimulates mesenchymal stem cell proliferation, this factor and other FGF family members (FGF1, FGF10) have also been shown to promote adipogenesis. In contrast, Wnt family members (such as WNT10b), TGF-β, and inflammatory cytokines (such as TNFα inhibit adipogenesis).

The identification of adipocyte precursors in the vasculature of murine and human scWAT (and rodent BAT) suggests that angiogenesis (the generation of new capillaries, discussed later) and adipogenesis are spatially and temporally coupled, linking the production of new adipocytes to the expansion of critical ancillary components such as capillary networks [118].

Brown and Beige Adipocyte Differentiation

Like in WAT, mesenchymal stem cells and pre-adipocytes with proliferative and adipogenic capacity persist in adult BAT. Because, at least in rodents, brown adipocytes share a Myf5$^+$ lineage origin with myocytes, a unique component of brown adipocyte differentiation is the repression of myogenic genes, a role ascribed to co-activator PRDM16 [106]. The source of beige adipocytes in rodent WAT is debated. These cells may arise by transdifferentiation of white adipocytes or adipogenesis from beige-specific precursors [101]. Recently, it has been reported that, upon cold exposure, another source of thermogenic adipocyte precursors is the vascular smooth muscle-derived Trpv1+ progenitors [108]. In line with this single-cell transcriptome of human and murine PVAT, the analysis identified a smooth muscle cell Myh-11$^+$ subpopulation that gives rise to this depot's thermogenic adipocytes [3].

In vitro studies using rodent cells suggest that the transcriptional cascade that controls terminal differentiation into mature brown, and presumably beige, adipocytes shares many similarities to that of white adipocytes, including transcriptional control by C/EBPs and PPARγ 2. However, specific transcription factors direct this process toward a brown versus white adipocyte cell fate. For example, FOXC2 modulates the expression and activity of adrenergic signaling molecules, PGC1α regulates both mitochondrial and thermogenic gene expressions, and PRDM16 represses white adipocyte genes during beige adipocyte recruitment (Fig. 3) [107]. More recently, EBF2 has been identified as a regulator of thermogenic adipocytes by recruiting the histone reader DPF3/BAF complex to the chromatin to allow its opening and transcription of BAT-specific genes [110].

Similar to brown adipocyte activation, brown adipogenesis is regulated by the SNS and endocrine mechanisms. For example, brown pre-adipocyte proliferation can be stimulated by insulin, IGF-1, and catecholamines (via the β 1-AR) [81]. Adrenergic signaling via the β 3-AR induces differentiation by promoting the transcription of thermogenic genes via transcriptional machineries such as PGC1α, CREB, and ATFII. Relief of thyroid hormone receptor repression of UCP1 transcription by T3 is essential for terminal brown adipocyte differentiation, as is insulin's induction of lipogenic genes during adipogenesis [81]. Interestingly, BMP7 alone can stimulate the differentiation of brown preadipocytes and commit mesenchymal precursors to a brown adipocyte cell fate [122].

Adipose Tissue Expansion

WAT expansion can be achieved by increasing adipocyte number (hyperplasia) and increasing the size of the preexisting adipocytes (hypertrophy). In the early stages of obesity, adipocyte size can increase up to 20-fold. More adipocytes are made to increase the storage capacity of AT. In order to maintain proper WAT function despite an increased caloric burden, hyperplasia rather than hypertrophy is the preferable adaptation because hypertrophy negatively affects adipocyte function, as suggested by the positive correlation between adipocyte size, insulin resistance, and increased risk of type 2 diabetes [76]. Adipocyte hypertrophy is also associated with inflammatory gene expression and an altered secretory profile. Unfortunately, hypertrophic AT displays a decreased adipogenic capacity, which aggravates hypertrophy by limiting the production of new adipocytes that could increase the tissue's storage capacity [53]. The overall failure of WAT as a storage organ of lipids occurs when its maximum storage capacity is reached, leading to lipotoxicity in non-adipose tissues. Of interest, some individuals, despite becoming obese, do not develop comorbidities. They represent 15–45% of obese individuals and are indicated as metabolically healthy obese (MHO). The reverse is also true. There are lean individuals (6–30%) who are excessively insulin-resistant, diabetic and with accelerated cardiovascular abnormalities similar if not worst to those of obese patients (metabolically obese normal weight individuals, MONW). Investigating these paradoxical phenotypes that uncouple adiposity from comorbidities can give important insights regarding the mechanisms causing these metabolic dysfunctions [50].

The body's demand for heat production by BAT also regulates BAT expansion. The maximal heat BAT can generate depending on the number of brown adipocytes. In rodents, when BAT thermogenesis is insufficient to maintain core body temperature, for example, in response to an acute reduction in environmental temperature, thermogenesis by muscle shivering makes up the difference. Over 4 weeks at the cooler temperature, BAT thermogenesis is "*adapted*" to fully meet the thermogenic requirement of the organism. This is achieved by increasing BAT mass ("recruitment") and its thermogenic capacity. A sustained increase in sympathetic tone to BAT stimulates BAT recruitment. Incidentally, chronic sympathetic stimulation of WAT also recruits beige cells. The term "acclimation" refers to the physiological regulation of BAT mass, so that

BAT thermogenesis balances heat loss to the environment at a new environmental temperature. BAT can expand or atrophy depending on the changing thermogenic demands of the organism.

Recent studies have demonstrated that chronic cold exposure can activate and recruit BAT in humans [135]. This observation is promising evidence that human BAT is an active, highly plastic "trainable" tissue responsive to physiological stimuli and that lessons learned from BAT recruitment in rodents have translational value. In humans, in the context of obesity, BAT is insulin-resistant, and the likelihood of BAT detection decreases as BMI and adiposity increase [88]. Moreover, given the evidence from rodent models, it is reasonable to hypothesize that insulin resistance in BAT may contribute to its reduced mass in obesity since insulin plays a crucial role in brown preadipocyte proliferation and differentiation. However, what represents good news is that a significant amount of BAT can be recruited in obese subjects using intermittent exposure to mild cold [40], indicating that the function of obese BAT can be rescued to a certain extent. In line with this, Jespersen et al. identified dormant brown adipocyte precursors in the perirenal region of lean human healthy individuals, which have the potential to be recruited and activated to restore dysfunctional metabolism and counteract obesity [56]. The effect of obesity on beige adipocyte recruitment is even less well understood.

Immunity in WAT and BAT

Macrophages

Macrophages are found in WAT, even in lean individuals; in rodents, resident macrophages may maintain WAT metabolic homeostasis. These macrophages have been identified as having a predominantly anti-inflammatory alternatively activated "M2" phenotype, expressing markers such as CD206 and CD163 [75]. The recent use of methodologies that allow investigation at a single-cell level further subdivides the lean ATMs based on TIM4, CD163, and MHCII. $CD163^+$ $TIM4^-$ macrophages originate from bone marrow monocytes. TIM4$^+$ macrophages seem instead to be of embryonic origin [33].

Obesity is characterized by increased local inflammation in WAT, especially visWAT, associated with a general increase in systemic inflammation levels. Local inflammation is promoted by adipocyte hypertrophy and hypoxia, which causes increased expression by adipocytes of inflammatory cytokines (e.g., TNFα, IL-6, and IL-1β) and chemokines (e.g., CCL2, CCL5, CXCL1, CXCL2, CXCL8).

Chemokines are chemoattractant cytokines that recruit and activate various immune cells, most importantly macrophages. Macrophages bind to and migrate through the endothelium (the single layer of endothelial cells of a capillary) by binding to adhesion molecules that are expressed by endothelial cells and induced by inflammatory cytokines (Fig. 4) [113]. In human obesity, macrophage infiltration is more pronounced in visWAT compared to scWAT. The classical paradigm that inflammatory cytokines

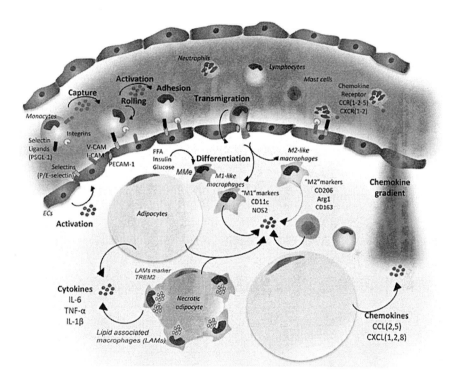

Fig. 4 Immune cell infiltration into obese adipose tissue and macrophage polarization. In obese WAT, hypertrophic and necrotic adipocytes secrete cytokines and chemokines that result in the accumulation of immune cells and tissue inflammation. Cytokines (TNFα, IL-6, and IL-1β) activate endothelial cells (*ECs*) to express various cellular adhesion molecules, including selectins, I-CAM, V-CAM, and PECAM-1 (intracellular, vascular, and platelet-endothelial cell adhesion molecule, respectively) [113]. Immune cells (monocytes, mast cells, neutrophils, and lymphocytes) are recruited to the endothelium by chemokines (CCL2, CCL5, CXCL1, CXCL2, CXCL8) binding to chemokine receptors. In a diapedesis process, the immune cells bind to the endothelium, become activated by cytokines, roll along the endothelium, and finally adhere, enabling their transmigration through the endothelium. Except for neutrophils, which remain adherent to the endothelium, most immune cells infiltrate AT through para- or transcellular mechanisms [113]. Monocytes differentiate within WAT into M1 (CD11c and NOS2 expressing) or M2 (CD206, Arg1, and CD163 expressing) macrophages according to their initial circulating phenotype and/or response to the local microenvironment. Another class of M1-like macrophages are the metabolically activated macrophages (MMe) that respond to nutrient stimuli such as insulin, FFAs, and glucose [62]. Macrophages expressing M1 and/or M2 markers are organized in crown-like structures around dead adipocytes and participate (lipid-associated macrophages or LAMs [54]), along with hypertrophic adipocytes and other infiltrating immune cells, to the maintenance of AT inflammation

and FFAs released by adipocytes contribute to polarizing infiltrating macrophages (and potentially resident "M2-like" macrophages) to an "M1-like" phenotype, which is characterized by the production of inflammatory cytokines, has been challenged in more recent years since a new population of pro-inflammatory ATMs has been identified, the so-called metabolically activated macrophages (MMe). These macrophages are activated by nutritional signals including glucose, insulin, and fatty acids and express surface receptors such as CD36, ABCA1, and PLIN2 that differ from the ones expressed by M1- and M2-like macrophages [62]. Within obese WAT, macrophages accumulate around the dead adipocytes forming the so-called crown-like structures, taking up cellular debris, and accumulating lipids [23]. Thanks to single-cell transcriptomic analyses, this subtype of ATMs has been identified as lipid-associated macrophages (LAM), characterized by the expression of the TREM2 surface marker [54]. Overall, this leads to a positive feedback loop that reinforces local inflammation and WAT dysfunction (Fig. 4): inflammatory cytokines released by macrophages and adipocytes alike further promote adipocyte inflammation, insulin resistance, altered production of adipokines, impaired adipogenesis, and vascular remodeling.

Other Immune Cells in Obese WAT

Immune cell infiltration into obese WAT is not limited to macrophages. In fact, in HFD-induced obese mice, the accumulation of T lymphocytes precedes macrophage infiltration into visWAT [59]. In the same model, early infiltration of B lymphocytes was also described in visWAT before any changes in body weight and insulin sensitivity [29]. Furthermore, neutrophil accumulation in the lumen of the vasculature of scWAT and visWAT positively correlates with BMI [85]. The accumulation of activated neutrophils in AT vessels may promote endothelial cell senescence and chemokine production, which could increase the infiltration of immune cells and further aggravate AT inflammation [103]. Finally, though the absolute

number of mast cells remains unchanged, mast cell degranulation activity is increased in the AT of obese patients, further contributing to inflammatory cytokine release [28]. Taken together, these alterations highlight how profoundly obesity induces inflammation in WAT. Of interest, single-cell sequencing and multi-omics analysis have contributed to the identification of new subpopulations of immune cells in obese WAT, which in the future will allow to precisely define the changes in immune composition and signaling networks that are associated with human obesity [25].

The Lymphatic System in WAT

There is a greater density of lymphoid structures in visWAT compared to scWAT, which may be significant in the context of inflammation in obesity. Apart from its roles in lipid absorption and immunity, the lymphatic system may also be a conduit for adipokines, which have been found in higher concentrations in lymph compared to the blood in humans [79]. Adipocyte-derived pro-inflammatory cytokines, including IL-6 and TNFα, were also found in lymph in lean subjects [79]. Obesity can significantly affect structural and functional changes in the lymphatic system. Pathological lesions in the lymphatic system caused by obesity are partly a result of the accumulation of inflammatory cells around the lymphatic vessels. The opposite is also true. Dysfunction in the lymphatic system may also be involved in the pathogenesis of obesity. Mouse models initially provided data linking lymphatic dysfunction with obesity with lymphatic defects [4].

Role of Macrophages in BAT

Macrophages seem to have an essential physiological role in controlling BAT activation in rodents. As well as regulating sympathetic tone to BAT, cold exposure also affects the phenotype of resident macrophages in rodent BAT, polarizing them to an M2 phenotype. It has been described by Nguyen et al. that these M2 macrophages then release norepinephrine, contributing to the adrenergic activation of brown adipocytes [84]. Furthermore, M2 polarization of WAT macrophages also has been shown in rodents to contribute to beige cell recruitment via norepinephrine secretion [95]. However, another group published data contradicting this finding. They showed that M2 macrophages do not express enough TH to produce norepinephrine in BAT and WAT [34]. Nowadays, it is still controversial whether M2 macrophages synthesize NE during thermogenesis. More recently, a part of M2 and other distinct subpopulations of macrophages have been identified in BAT and scWAT: the cholinergic ATMs (ChAMs) that activate thermogenic responses in brown or beige adipocytes through paracrine mechanisms upon cold exposure. On the other hand, thermogenic inhibitory ATM subsets, i.e., sympathetic innervation-regulatory- macrophages and catecholamines scavenging macrophages (SAMs) that block sympathetic innervation or import/degrade catecholamine respectively, have been identified in thermogenic adipose niches [97]. Adipose SAMs are recruited in obese conditions, suggesting their possible role in promoting inflammation. Moreover, BAT resident macrophages, by uptaking and eliminating the oxidatively damaged mitochondria released by the brown adipocytes, contribute to maintaining BAT thermogenic function. These findings reveal a homeostatic role of tissue-resident macrophages in the mitochondrial quality control of BAT [102]. Brown adipocytes, like white adipocytes, become hypertrophic in rodent models of obesity. This *"whitening"* of the BAT is also induced by other factors than obesity, including high ambient temperature, leptin receptor deficiency, β-adrenergic signaling impairment, and lipase deficiency, each of which is capable of inducing macrophage infiltration, brown adipocyte death, and crown-like structure (CLS) formation [61].

Vascularization of Adipose Tissue

Mechanisms of Angiogenesis in WAT

Blood is supplied to adipose tissues via arterioles that branch into capillary beds. Arterioles are composed of a layer of smooth muscle cells surrounding a layer of endothelial cells (the endothelium). Capillaries are smaller in diameter and lack a smooth muscle cell layer. The vasculature is a crucial structure contributing to WAT function, transporting lipids intended for storage in WAT and adipokines and FFAs released by WAT. AT perfusion can be regulated by vasodilatation or vasoconstriction mediated by factors secreted by endothelial cells and by the SNS via ARs expressed on smooth muscle cells.

The vascular network must be remodeled during AT expansion. Angiogenesis is the development of a vascular network from a preexisting one and requires the proliferation and migration of endothelial cells to form a new capillary (Fig. 5). The new vessel is stabilized upon maturation by the production of ECM components, which form the basement membrane, and the recruitment of pericytes, which are mural cells of blood vessels. Microvascular pericytes stabilize new vessels by producing factors such as angiopoietins that promote endothelial survival and represent a pool of adipocyte progenitors [121]. Angiogenesis is regulated by angiogenic factors produced by adipocytes, adipocyte precursors, vascular cells, and even macrophages (Fig. 5).

Vascular Dysfunction in Obese WAT

Obese WAT is characterized by increased angiogenic activity due to inflammation and hypoxia. For example, many inflammatory factors that are increased in obese WAT also have angiogenic properties, including cytokines (TNFα, IL-6, IL-1β) and some chemokines (CXCL2, CXCL8) [24]. Additionally, the expression of hypoxia-responsive angiogenic factors, such as VEGF, is upregulated in obese WAT and more so in visWAT compared to scWAT [126]. However, angiogenesis is insufficient to prevent the development of hypoxia, particularly in visWAT [126]. This defective angiogenesis may be caused by an impairment in vascular function, mainly due to dysfunctional endothelial cells.

As well as playing a pivotal role in angiogenesis, endothelial cells are essential regulators of vascular integrity. Firstly, they control the passage

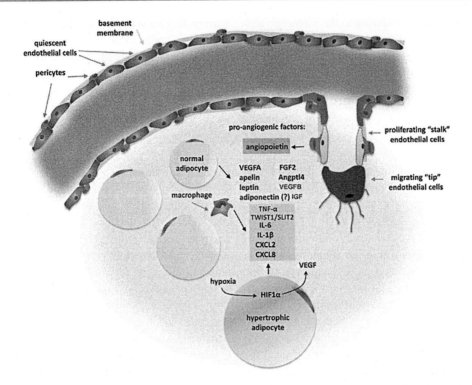

Fig. 5 Mechanisms of angiogenesis in obese adipose tissue. The primary structural cells of blood vessels are endothelial cells and pericytes. Angiogenesis is driven by pro-angiogenic factors released by pericytes (angiopoietins) and adipocytes (VEGF-A, VEGF-B, FGF2, apelin, Angptl4, leptin, IGF, potentially adiponectin) [12, 17, 36, 50, 64, 87, 117]. Macrophages and hypertrophic adipocytes in obese WAT secrete inflammatory factors with angiogenic properties, including cytokines (TNFα, IL-6, IL-1β), some chemokines (CXCL2, CXCL8) [24] and other signaling factors such as TWIST1 and SLIT2 [51]. Hypoxia also drives VEGF expression [30]. A new vessel is formed by the migration of endothelial "**tip cells**" at the tip of the new capillary and proliferating endothelial "stalk" cells that drive elongation. Endothelial cells produce ECM components to generate a new basement membrane, and pericytes stabilize the new vessel [117]

of materials from the tissue to the blood and vice versa. On top of acting as a semipermeable barrier, endothelial cells also respond to various stimuli by releasing factors that regulate vasodilation and vasoconstriction, such as nitric oxide (NO) and endothelin-1 (ET-1), respectively. Importantly, insulin is one such stimulus, so it is not surprising that endothelial cell dysfunction is linked to insulin resistance. Insulin resistance decreases NO production and increases endothelial cell expression of immune cell adhesion molecules, facilitating monocyte infiltration [93].

Furthermore, inflammatory factors such as IL-6 and TNFα inhibit insulin-induced NO production and vasodilatation while increasing the secretion of the vasoconstrictor ET-1 [2]. Overall, endothelial cell insulin resistance favors inflammation and vasoconstriction. Furthermore, endothelial cells from the visWAT of obese patients show increased expression of inflammatory markers, which may contribute to premature endothelial cell senescence, thereby further impairing vascular integrity [126].

Endothelial cell senescence could also be promoted by the angiogenic environment of obese WAT, given that adipocyte-derived VEGF-A causes endothelial cell senescence in vitro [126]. Indeed, the altered secretion profile of hypertrophic adipocytes may directly contribute to endothelial cell dysfunction. For example, adiponectin and leptin positively regulate endothelial cell function: both promote NO production, and adiponectin has anti-inflammatory and anti-apoptotic effects [60]. Thus, leptin resistance and reduced adiponectin expression in obesity may limit the beneficial actions of these adipokines on endothelial cells. Recently, Emont et al. confirmed, by single-cell RNAseq, that obesity causes a decrease in the expression of eight genes involved in promoting angiogenesis in both visWAT and scWAT. These genes are the "usual suspects," i.e., ADIPOQ, VEGF-A, IGF1, but new ones were also identified, FGFR1, MET, NAMPT, SCTR, and PRLR [31].

Finally, in vitro experiments suggest that endothelial cell dysfunction has a direct negative impact on adipocyte function. Cocultures of visWAT endothelial cells and adipocytes from obese subjects showed reduced lipolytic and insulin responses and increased inflammatory secretion profiles compared to cocultures of cells from lean subjects [91]. Treatment with angiopoietin-1, a pericyte-derived factor, reduced the inflammatory profile endothelial cells from obese visWAT, and coculture of these treated cells with adipocytes from obese visWAT reduced cytokine secretion by the adipocytes [91].

In summary, the combination of inflammation, altered adipokine secretion, and endothelial cell dysfunction undermines vascular integrity in obese WAT. Therefore, despite an adaptive increase in angiogenic activity in obese WAT, hypoxic areas still develop.

Angiogenesis in BAT

BAT is more vascularized than WAT. The vasculature plays a fundamental role in BAT thermogenesis as it is required to conduct BAT-generated heat throughout the body. In line with this, BAT activation is coupled to SNS-mediated vasodilatation and increased blood flow, ensuring adequate gas exchange [86]. Furthermore, angiogenesis accompanies BAT expansion in rodents in response to chronic cold exposure, ensuring the vascularization of newly formed brown adipocytes, which can derive from precursors residing in the vasculature. Mature brown adipocytes stimulate vascular remodeling by secreting angiogenic factors, including VEGF, FGF2, NO, and BMP8b. This response is not triggered by hypoxia; rather, it

may be a direct effect of adrenergic stimulation of brown adipocytes [133]. A reduction in capillary density accompanied by hypoxia is found in the BAT of diet-induced obese mice in association with "whitening" of brown adipocytes (accumulation of lipids, loss of mitochondria, and reduced adrenergic signaling) [111]. Interestingly, in this model, BAT functionality was rescued by delivery to VEGF-A to BAT, highlighting the dependence of thermogenesis on adequate vascularization.

Finally, beige cell recruitment in WAT is also coupled to increased vascular density, and experimentally increasing vascularization in adipose tissue by overexpression of VEGF is sufficient to recruit beige cells in WAT [133].

Adipose Tissue Extracellular Matrix

Structure, Composition, and Physiological Role of the Extracellular Matrix in WAT

The extracellular matrix (ECM) is a complex network of macromolecules that are produced by and surrounds the component cells of AT (Fig. 6a1). Collagen and elastin fibers are the major structural proteins of the ECM, and other components, such as fibronectin, laminins, and proteoglycans, bind them. The ECM provides structural support for the cells in AT and can also directly regulate AT function. For example, proteoglycans can regulate the release of secreted factors such as chemokines and growth factors. Additionally, the ECM communicates bidirectionally with cells via cellular binding integrins to ECM components such as fibronectin. Integrins are plasma membrane transmembrane proteins that are involved in both "outside-in" (ECM binding activates downstream signaling in cells) and "inside-out" signals (intracellular regulation of integrin/ECM binding activity) [49]. An important example of "outside-in" signaling is the interaction of ECM components with adipocyte cytoskeletal structures at focal adhesion complexes via integrins, thereby regulating cell shape (Fig. 6a2). This is relevant for adipogenesis, a process requiring drastic cellular morphology changes as spindle-shaped preadipocytes grow larger and rounder as they differentiate into mature adipocytes.

The ECM of adipocytes, known as the basement membrane (BM), is particularly enriched with collagen types IV and XVIII, laminin, and glycoprotein entactin [77]. In contrast, the ECM of preadipocytes is composed primarily of collagen types I and II and fibronectin [77]. Therefore, the preadipocyte ECM must be degraded during adipogenesis, and the mature adipocyte BM must be synthesized (Fig. 6a3). ECM turnover is mediated by enzymes that degrade existing ECM structures, such as fibrinolytic plasmin and matrix metalloproteinases (MMPs), and by enzymes involved in the modification and cross-linking of newly synthesized components, such as ADAM proteases and lysyl oxidase (LOX), respectively [77]. These processes are especially relevant to WAT expansion when existing ECM components must be degraded to create room for new and larger adipocytes, and the ECM must be restructured around the expanded tissue. Interestingly, ECM composition and evolution during adipogenesis differ between WAT depots. For example, collagen IV and fibronectin expressions are higher in visWAT, whereas collagen I expression is higher in scWAT [80].

WAT Fibrosis in Obesity

Fibrosis, the excessive deposition of ECM proteins, is induced in obese scWAT and visWAT around adipocytes and blood vessels [28]. Transcriptomic analyses of scWAT from obese subjects show induction of ECM components such as integrins, collagens, proteoglycans, laminins, proteases, and LOX [42]. In this line, matrisome analysis of monozygotic weight-discordant twins adipose tissue revealed a profound ECM remodeling and hypertrophic inflammatory phenotype. In context, the vital role of PEPD in collagen turnover has recently been described. Its depletion causes the accumulation of proline-containing dipeptide and, consequently, the development of AT fibrosis. That reflects the impact of decreased PEPD expression in obesity [92]. Indeed, it is likely that chronic low-grade

inflammation in obese WAT contributes to the development of fibrosis. In a time-course microarray study of the WAT of diet-induced obese mice, inflammatory-related genes were induced in visWAT prior to genes involved in fibrosis. Furthermore, macrophage accumulation into visWAT preceded the appearance of fibrosis in the same model [115]. Immune cells may promote fibrosis by promoting TGF-β signaling, either by secreting TGF-β and its family member activin A or by releasing MMP9, a protease that can activate TGF-β [120]. Activin A and TGF-β (beta) induce preadipocytes, endothelial cells, and mature adipocytes to synthesize ECM components; in particular, preadipocytes from obese scWAT adopt a fibroblast-like phenotype (Fig. 6b [28]. The resulting fibrosis can impose mechanical constraints that may negatively impact adipocyte function and limit adipose tissue expansion, exacerbating metabolic dysfunction. The ECM has also been reported to reprogram adipocyte metabolism and contribute to the phenotypic differences between visWAT and scWAT depots. Culturing visceral adipocytes in subcutaneous ECM rescues HFD-induced IR and promotes adipogenesis, whereas visceral ECM dampens glucose uptake and expression of adipogenic genes in subcutaneous adipocytes [114].

Structure, Composition, and Physiological Role of the Extracellular Matrix in BAT

Although the ECM is a well-described WAT, few studies focus on the BAT ECM and its remodeling in pathophysiological conditions. The BM of rodent brown adipocytes is known to contain collagen IV, laminin, and fibronectin and may be more enriched with heparin sulfate proteoglycan compared to the white adipocyte BM [41]. It would be expected that brown adipocytes in BAT might interact with their ECM similarly to white adipocytes in WAT.

Recent studies have highlighted how the BAT ECM may regulate BAT function. For example, MAGP-1 (microfibril-associated glycoprotein 1) stabilizes microfibril networks to confer tissue elasticity and also regulates cellular signaling by interacting with cell-surface receptors and modulating the bioavailability of growth factors such as TGF-β. MAGP-1-deficient mice displayed increased TGF-β activity in BAT and reduced thermogenesis and UCP1 gene expression, a phenotype rescued by TGF-β neutralization [26]. More recently, Gonzalez-Porras et al. showed that alterations in integrins and ECM proteins composition in AT could modulate its thermogenic capacity. Absence of laminin 4 and, as a consequence of their direct interaction, a decrease in integrin ITA7 expression promotes beiging [39]. Fibrosis in BAT may also impair thermogenesis. In one study, BAT inflammation and fibrosis were genetically induced in rodents by overexpression of endotrophin (a C-terminal cleavage product of the COL6α 3 chain), accompanied by reduced energy expenditure [116]. VEGF neutralization induced fibrosis in another rodent model; this led to capillary dropout in BAT, local hypoxia, immune cell infiltration, fibrosis, and ultimately brown adipocyte apoptosis [5]. It remains to be seen whether obesity is associated with BAT fibrosis and whether fibrosis negatively affects BAT activity in humans.

Innervation of Adipose Tissue

Nervous Networks in Adipose Tissue

Efferent sensory and afferent sympathetic nerves have been identified in rodent WAT and BAT [37]. In rodents, sympathetic innervation is greater in BAT compared to WAT and greater in scWAT compared to visWAT [82]. Nerve endings are in contact with adipocytes and blood vessels. As we have seen, the norepinephrine released from sympathetic nerves regulates AT perfusion and several components of AT function, from WAT lipolysis to BAT thermogenesis. In rodents, sympathetic stimulation of WAT also suppresses the release of leptin and adiponectin from WAT and can induce the secretion of autocrine and endocrine factors including BMP8b, FGF21, and T3 [46, 132].

Sympathetic activity is regulated by the hypothalamus, which receives information related to energy availability to regulate lipolysis and environmental and core body temperature to regulate thermogenesis. When a sympathetic response is required, this information is transmitted to sympathetic premotor neurons located in the rostral raphe pallidus and parapyramidal areas of the hindbrain, as determined by neuronal viral tracer studies in rodents [123]. These premotor neurons synapse with preganglionic neurons whose cell bodies reside in the spinal intermediolateral nucleus. Finally, these preganglionic neurons regulate the activity of the norepinephrine-releasing postganglionic neurons with nerve endings in AT [123]. Distinct regulation of sympathetic tone to different WAT and BAT depots has been observed in animal models because different depots are innervated by distinct populations of postganglionic neurons [13]. Along with norepinephrine, sympathetic nerves in rodent WAT and BAT also release neuropeptide Y (NPY), which has been shown to inhibit lipolysis and promote leptin release by human white adipocytes in vitro [37]. Interestingly, feedback loops between the sympathetic and sensory nervous systems in both WAT and BAT have been identified [104]. There is also evidence of WAT and BAT crosstalk via afferent sensory feedback to maintain thermoregulation. Interestingly, the activation of the parasympathetic nervous system (PSNS) may play an opposing role to that of the SNS. Reduced melanocortin signaling due to increased vagal activity within the splanchnic compartment actively facilitates adipose tissue expansion. Importantly, a lack of parasympathetic innervation in the WAT has been reported and therefore further research is needed to determine how the brain–melanocortin–vagus efferent axis regulates fat mass gain [45].

Nervous Remodeling in AT

In rodents, cold exposure increases the density of sympathetic innervation in BAT and WAT depots [127]. Indeed, during BAT recruitment in rodents, the nervous network is remodeled to innervate

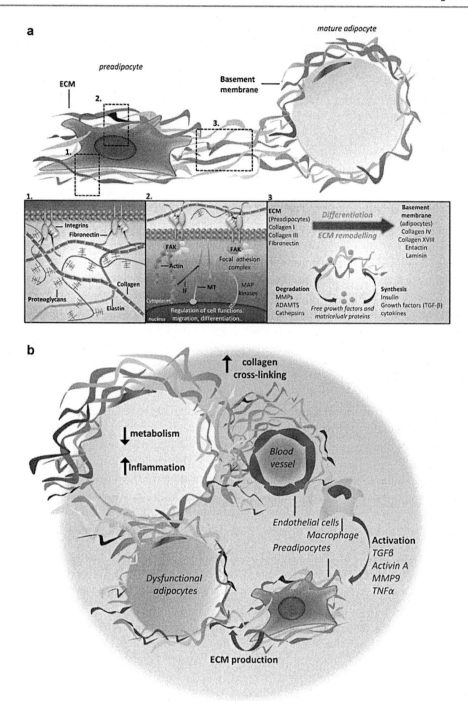

Fig. 6 The extracellular matrix of adipose tissue. (**a**) ECM composition, signaling, and remodeling in adipocytes. (*1*) The ECM is a network of macromolecules composed of structural proteins (collagens and elastin), adhesion proteins (fibronectin), and proteoglycans. (*2*) The ECM regulates cell functions such as migration and differentiation through interactions with extracellular receptors such as integrins [49]. This can occur via the activation of FAK (focal adhesion kinase) in focal adhesion complexes and downstream MAP kinase/actin-dependent signaling or directly through mechanical cues transmitted into cells via the cytoskeleton of microtubules (*MT*) and intermediary filaments. (*3*) ECM remodeling is a critical component of adipogenesis. The preadipocyte ECM primarily

new brown adipocytes [127]. The expression of several neurotrophins that regulate neuron survival and plasticity has been detected in human or rodent WAT and BAT and may underlie these observations. For example, nerve growth factor (NGF) is required for sympathetic neuron survival and is secreted by white and brown adipocytes [89]. Neurotrophins with chemoattractant (neuregulin 4) and chemorepellent (semaphorins) properties have also been detected [128]. Through the secretion of the cytokine Slit3 upon cold exposure, ATMs exert a modulatory function in the sympathetic innervation of adipose tissue by promoting sympathetic nerve growth and stimulating the synthesis and release of NE, which in turn stimulate thermogenesis [130]. A subset of macrophages, i.e., the cold-induced neuroimmune cells (CINCs), are recruited to the AT in response to cold and have been shown to coordinate the expression of genes involved in nerve survival and plasticity. These CINCs secrete neurotrophic factors such as BDNF, which have been reported to exert an essential role in WAT innervation [8].

Obesity is associated with reduced adrenergic responsiveness of BAT and WAT, a phenomenon attributed to adipocyte dysfunction. Additionally, changes at a central level, such as hypothalamic insulin resistance and neuroinflammation, have downstream effects on the nervous regulation of AT [94]. As inflammatory mediators have been shown to trigger neuritis and disrupt sensory neuron activity, it is conceivable that the increased production of cytokines in adipose tissue due to obesity-induced chronic inflammation may impair the ability of local sensory nerves to convey information from the adipose tissue to the brain. Indeed, sensory nerve dysfunctions in the initial stages of glucose intolerance in obese subjects have been reported [134].

Conclusions

In conclusion, proper AT function depends on the coordinated interaction of adipocytes, precursor cells, immune cells, blood vessels, nerves, and the ECM. Obesity is characterized by an absolute increase in and an anatomical redistribution of WAT mass, which leads to chronic inflammation, insulin resistance, and other metabolic complications. Obesity also alters the ultrastructure and cellular composition of WAT, negatively affecting WAT function and ultimately impairing its ability to buffer excess nutrients. This can lead to ectopic lipid accumulation in non-adipose tissues, further exacerbating metabolic dysfunction.

The rediscovery of BAT, a type of AT uniquely specialized for calorie burning, in adult humans has created the opportunity for novel therapeutic strategies to treat obesity and metabolic syndrome. Although WAT far outstrips BAT in terms of percent of body mass, in rodents, the high activity of BAT is an essential contributor to nutrient partitioning and utilization and body weight regulation. Therapeutically increasing BAT activity could theoretically eliminate excess nutrients, improving WAT function with knock-on effects on whole-body metabolism. The success of this approach will depend on a better understanding of BAT structure and function in

---

Fig. 6 (continued) comprises collagen I, III, and fibronectin [77]. The basement membrane (*BM*) is a specialized ECM surrounding mature adipocytes composed of collagen IV, XVIII, entactin, and laminin [66]. During differentiation, the preadipocyte ECM is degraded by proteases (MMPs, ADAMT, and cathepsins) [77]. This releases growth factors and matricellular proteins important for synthesizing the new mature adipocyte BM, stimulated by insulin, TGF-β, and cytokine signaling [77]. The ECM is also involved in the changes to cellular morphology associated with adipogenesis [77]. (**b**) Cellular and physiological contributors to fibrosis in WAT.

Preadipocytes, immune cells, endothelial cells, and mature adipocytes contribute to WAT fibrosis. Inflammation likely precedes fibrosis, as macrophages accumulate in obese WAT prior to fibrosis, where they promote inflammation (TNFα) as well as ECM synthesis via TGF-β and activin A signaling [120]. Preadipocytes are proposed as the major effectors of AT fibrosis. Fibrosis negatively impacts adipocyte metabolism by decreasing metabolic functions such as lipolysis and adipokine secretion and by inducing an inflammatory response [90]

healthy adult humans and whether potential BAT-based therapeutic strategies can overcome any limitations caused by the negative impact of obesity on BAT function.

Cross-References

▷ Adipokines and Metabolism
▷ Brain Regulation of Feeding and Energy Homeostasis
▷ Carbohydrate, Protein, and Fat Metabolism in Obesity
▷ Dyslipidemia in Metabolic Syndrome
▷ Linking Inflammation, Obesity, and Diabetes
▷ Principles of Energy Homeostasis

References

1. Alcala M, Calderon-Dominguez M, Serra D, Herrero L, Viana M. Mechanisms of impaired brown adipose tissue recruitment in obesity. Front Physiol. 2019;10:94. https://doi.org/10.3389/fphys.2019.00094.
2. Andreozzi F, Laratta E, Procopio C, Hribal ML, Sciacqua A, Perticone M, ... Sesti G. Interleukin-6 impairs the insulin signaling pathway, promoting production of nitric oxide in human umbilical vein endothelial cells. Mol Cell Biol. 2007;27(6):2372–83. https://doi.org/10.1128/MCB.01340-06.
3. Angueira AR, Sakers AP, Holman CD, Cheng L, Arbocco MN, Shamsi F, ... Seale P. Defining the lineage of thermogenic perivascular adipose tissue. Nat Metab. 2021;3(4):469–84. https://doi.org/10.1038/s42255-021-00380-0.
4. Antoniak K, Hansdorfer-Korzon R, Mrugacz M, Zorena K. Adipose tissue and biological factors. Possible link between lymphatic system dysfunction and obesity. Metabolites. 2021;11(9):617. https://doi.org/10.3390/metabo11090617.
5. Bagchi M, Kim LA, Boucher J, Walshe TE, Kahn CR, D'Amore PA. Vascular endothelial growth factor is important for brown adipose tissue development and maintenance. FASEB J. 2013;27(8):3257–71. https://doi.org/10.1096/fj.12-221812.
6. Bartelt A, Bruns OT, Reimer R, Hohenberg H, Ittrich H, Peldschus K, ... Heeren J. Brown adipose tissue activity controls triglyceride clearance. Nat Med. 2011;17(2):200–5. https://doi.org/10.1038/nm.2297.
7. Bjorndal B, Burri L, Staalesen V, Skorve J, Berge RK. Different adipose depots: their role in the development of metabolic syndrome and mitochondrial response to hypolipidemic agents. J Obes. 2011;2011:490650. https://doi.org/10.1155/2011/490650.
8. Blaszkiewicz M, Wood E, Koizar S, Willows J, Anderson R, Tseng YH, ... Townsend KL. The involvement of neuroimmune cells in adipose innervation. Mol Med. 2020;26(1):126. https://doi.org/10.1186/s10020-020-00254-3.
9. Bordicchia M, Liu D, Amri EZ, Ailhaud G, Dessi-Fulgheri P, Zhang C, ... Collins S. Cardiac natriuretic peptides act via p38 MAPK to induce the brown fat thermogenic program in mouse and human adipocytes. J Clin Invest. 2012;122(3):1022–36. https://doi.org/10.1172/JCI59701.
10. Boren J, Taskinen MR, Olofsson SO, Levin M. Ectopic lipid storage and insulin resistance: a harmful relationship. J Intern Med. 2013;274(1):25–40. https://doi.org/10.1111/joim.12071.
11. Bostrom P, Wu J, Jedrychowski MP, Korde A, Ye L, Lo JC, ... Spiegelman BM. A PGC1-alpha-dependent myokine that drives brown-fat-like development of white fat and thermogenesis. Nature. 2012;481(7382):463–8. https://doi.org/10.1038/nature10777.
12. Brakenhielm E, Veitonmaki N, Cao R, Kihara S, Matsuzawa Y, Zhivotovsky B, ... Cao Y. Adiponectin-induced antiangiogenesis and antitumor activity involve caspase-mediated endothelial cell apoptosis. Proc Natl Acad Sci U S A. 2004;101(8):2476–81. https://doi.org/10.1073/pnas.0308671100.
13. Brito NA, Brito MN, Bartness TJ. Differential sympathetic drive to adipose tissues after food deprivation, cold exposure or glucoprivation. Am J Physiol Regul Integr Comp Physiol. 2008;294(5):R1445–52. https://doi.org/10.1152/ajpregu.00068.2008.
14. Campderros L, Moure R, Cairo M, Gavalda-Navarro-A, Quesada-Lopez T, Cereijo R, ... Villarroya F. Brown adipocytes secrete GDF15 in response to thermogenic activation. Obesity (Silver Spring). 2019;27(10):1606–16. https://doi.org/10.1002/oby.22584.
15. Cannon B, Nedergaard J. Brown adipose tissue: function and physiological significance. Physiol Rev. 2004;84(1):277–359. https://doi.org/10.1152/physrev.00015.2003.
16. Cannon B, Nedergaard J. Nonshivering thermogenesis and its adequate measurement in metabolic studies. J Exp Biol. 2011;214(Pt 2):242–53. https://doi.org/10.1242/jeb.050989.
17. Cao R, Brakenhielm E, Wahlestedt C, Thyberg J, Cao Y. Leptin induces vascular permeability and synergistically stimulates angiogenesis with FGF-2 and VEGF. Proc Natl Acad Sci U S A. 2001;98(11):6390–5. https://doi.org/10.1073/pnas.101564798.
18. Carobbio S, Rosen B, Vidal-Puig A. Adipogenesis: new insights into brown adipose tissue differentiation. J Mol Endocrinol. 2013;51(3):T75–85. https://doi.org/10.1530/JME-13-0158.
19. Cereijo R, Gavalda-Navarro A, Cairo M, Quesada-Lopez T, Villarroya J, Moron-Ros S, ... Villarroya F. CXCL14, a brown adipokine that mediates brown-

fat-to-macrophage communication in thermogenic adaptation. Cell Metab. 2018;28(5):750–763.e6. https://doi.org/10.1016/j.cmet.2018.07.015.

20. Cero C, Lea HJ, Zhu KY, Shamsi F, Tseng YH, Cypess AM. beta3-adrenergic receptors regulate human brown/beige adipocyte lipolysis and thermogenesis. Insight. 2021;6(11):e139160. https://doi.org/10.1172/jci.insight.139160.

21. Chan M, Lim YC, Yang J, Namwanje M, Liu L, Qiang L. Identification of a natural beige adipose depot in mice. J Biol Chem. 2019;294(17):6751–61. https://doi.org/10.1074/jbc.RA118.006838.

22. Chen SX, Zhang LJ, Gallo RL. Dermal white adipose tissue: a newly recognized layer of skin innate defense. J Invest Dermatol. 2019;139(5):1002–9. https://doi.org/10.1016/j.jid.2018.12.031.

23. Cinti S, Mitchell G, Barbatelli G, Murano I, Ceresi E, Faloia E, . . . Obin MS. Adipocyte death defines macrophage localization and function in adipose tissue of obese mice and humans. J Lipid Res. 2005;46(11): 2347–55. https://doi.org/10.1194/jlr.M500294-JLR200.

24. Coppack SW. Pro-inflammatory cytokines and adipose tissue. Proc Nutr Soc. 2001;60(3):349–56. https://doi.org/10.1079/pns2001110.

25. Cottam MA, Caslin HL, Winn NC, Hasty AH. Multiomics reveals persistence of obesity-associated immune cell phenotypes in adipose tissue during weight loss and weight regain in mice. Nat Commun. 2022;13(1):2950. https://doi.org/10.1038/s41467-022-30646-4.

26. Craft CS, Pietka TA, Schappe T, Coleman T, Combs MD, Klein S, . . . Mecham RP. The extracellular matrix protein MAGP1 supports thermogenesis and protects against obesity and diabetes through regulation of TGF-beta. Diabetes. 2014;63(6):1920–32. https://doi.org/10.2337/db13-1604.

27. Deutsch A, Feng D, Pessin JE, Shinoda K. The impact of single-cell genomics on adipose tissue research. Int J Mol Sci. 2020;21(13):4773. https://doi.org/10.3390/ijms21134773.

28. Divoux A, Tordjman J, Lacasa D, Veyrie N, Hugol D, Aissat A, . . . Clement K. Fibrosis in human adipose tissue: composition, distribution, and link with lipid metabolism and fat mass loss. Diabetes. 2010;59(11): 2817–25. https://doi.org/10.2337/db10-0585.

29. Duffaut C, Galitzky J, Lafontan M, Bouloumie A. Unexpected trafficking of immune cells within the adipose tissue during the onset of obesity. Biochem Biophys Res Commun. 2009;384(4): 482–5. https://doi.org/10.1016/j.bbrc.2009.05.002.

30. Elias I, Franckhauser S, Bosch F. New insights into adipose tissue VEGF-A actions in the control of obesity and insulin resistance. Adipocytes. 2013;2(2): 109–12. https://doi.org/10.4161/adip.22880.

31. Emont MP, Jacobs C, Essene AL, Pant D, Tenen D, Colleluori G, . . . Rosen ED. A single-cell atlas of human and mouse white adipose tissue. Nature. 2022;603(7903):926–33. https://doi.org/10.1038/s41586-022-04518-2.

32. Feldmann HM, Golozoubova V, Cannon B, Nedergaard J. UCP1 ablation induces obesity and abolishes diet-induced thermogenesis in mice exempt from thermal stress by living at thermoneutrality. Cell Metab. 2009;9(2):203–9. https://doi.org/10.1016/j.cmet.2008.12.014.

33. Felix I, Jokela H, Karhula J, Kotaja N, Savontaus E, Salmi M, Rantakari P. Single-cell proteomics reveals the defined heterogeneity of resident macrophages in white adipose tissue. Front Immunol. 2021;12: 719979. https://doi.org/10.3389/fimmu.2021.719979.

34. Fischer K, Ruiz HH, Jhun K, Finan B, Oberlin DJ, van der Heide V, . . . Buettner C. Alternatively activated macrophages do not synthesize catecholamines or contribute to adipose tissue adaptive thermogenesis. Nat Med. 2017;23(5):623–30. https://doi.org/10.1038/nm.4316.

35. Fu L, John LM, Adams SH, Yu XX, Tomlinson E, Renz M, . . . Stewart TA. Fibroblast growth factor 19 increases metabolic rate and reverses dietary and leptin-deficient diabetes. Endocrinology. 2004;145(6):2594–603. https://doi.org/10.1210/en.2003-1671.

36. Gealekman O, Guseva N, Hartigan C, Apotheker S, Gorgoglione M, Gurav K, . . . Corvera S. Depot-specific differences and insufficient subcutaneous adipose tissue angiogenesis in human obesity. Circulation. 2011;123(2):186–94. https://doi.org/10.1161/CIRCULATIONAHA.110.970145.

37. Giordano A, Morroni M, Santone G, Marchesi GF, Cinti S. Tyrosine hydroxylase, neuropeptide Y, substance P, calcitonin gene-related peptide and vasoactive intestinal peptide in nerves of rat periovarian adipose tissue: an immunohistochemical and ultrastructural investigation. J Neurocytol. 1996;25(2): 125–36. https://doi.org/10.1007/BF02284791.

38. Giorgino F, Laviola L, Eriksson JW. Regional differences of insulin action in adipose tissue: insights from in vivo and in vitro studies. Acta Physiol Scand. 2005;183(1):13–30. https://doi.org/10.1111/j.1365-201X.2004.01385.x.

39. Gonzalez Porras MA, Stojkova K, Vaicik MK, Pelowe A, Goddi A, Carmona A, . . . Brey EM. Integrins and extracellular matrix proteins modulate adipocyte thermogenic capacity. Sci Rep. 2021;11(1):5442. https://doi.org/10.1038/s41598-021-84828-z.

40. Hanssen MJ, van der Lans AA, Brans B, Hoeks J, Jardon KM, Schaart G, . . . van Marken Lichtenbelt WD. Short-term cold acclimation recruits brown adipose tissue in obese humans. Diabetes. 2016;65(5): 1179–89. https://doi.org/10.2337/db15-1372.

41. Haraida S, Nerlich AG, Wiest I, Schleicher E, Lohrs U. Distribution of basement membrane components in normal adipose tissue and in benign and malignant

tumors of lipomatous origin. Mod Pathol. 1996;9(2): 137–44.

42. Henegar C, Tordjman J, Achard V, Lacasa D, Cremer I, Guerre-Millo M, . . . Clement, K. Adipose tissue transcriptomic signature highlights the pathological relevance of extracellular matrix in human obesity. Genome Biol. 2008;9(1):R14. https://doi.org/10.1186/gb-2008-9-1-r14.

43. Henriques F, Bedard AH, Guilherme A, Kelly M, Chi J, Zhang P, . . . Czech MP. Single-cell RNA profiling reveals adipocyte to macrophage signaling sufficient to enhance thermogenesis. Cell Rep. 2020;32(5):107998. https://doi.org/10.1016/j.celrep.2020.107998.

44. Himms-Hagen J, Cui J, Danforth E Jr, Taatjes DJ, Lang SS, Waters BL, Claus TH. Effect of CL-316,243, a thermogenic beta 3-agonist, on energy balance and brown and white adipose tissues in rats. Am J Phys. 1994;266(4 Pt 2):R1371–82. https://doi.org/10.1152/ajpregu.1994.266.4.R1371.

45. Holland J, Sorrell J, Yates E, Smith K, Arbabi S, Arnold M, . . . Perez-Tilve D. A brain-melanocortin-vagus axis mediates adipose tissue expansion independently of energy intake. Cell Rep. 2019;27(8): 2399–410. e2396. https://doi.org/10.1016/j.celrep.2019.04.089.

46. Hondares E, Iglesias R, Giralt A, Gonzalez FJ, Giralt M, Mampel T, Villarroya F. Thermogenic activation induces FGF21 expression and release in brown adipose tissue. J Biol Chem. 2011;286(15): 12983–90. https://doi.org/10.1074/jbc.M110.215889.

47. Hondares E, Gallego-Escuredo JM, Flachs P, Frontini A, Cereijo R, Goday A, . . . Villarroya F. Fibroblast growth factor-21 is expressed in neonatal and pheochromocytoma-induced adult human brown adipose tissue. Metabolism. 2014;63(3): 312–7. https://doi.org/10.1016/j.metabol.2013.11.014.

48. Hong S, Song W, Zushin PH, Liu B, Jedrychowski MP, Mina AI, . . . Banks AS. Phosphorylation of Beta-3 adrenergic receptor at serine 247 by ERK MAP kinase drives lipolysis in obese adipocytes. Mol Metab. 2018;12:25–38. https://doi.org/10.1016/j.molmet.2018.03.012.

49. Hu P, Luo BH. Integrin bi-directional signaling across the plasma membrane. J Cell Physiol. 2013;228(2): 306–12. https://doi.org/10.1002/jcp.24154.

50. Huang LO, Rauch A, Mazzaferro E, Preuss M, Carobbio S, Bayrak CS, . . . Loos RJF. Genome-wide discovery of genetic loci that uncouple excess adiposity from its comorbidities. Nat Metab. 2021;3(2):228–43. https://doi.org/10.1038/s42255-021-00346-2.

51. Hunyenyiwa T, Hendee K, Matus K, Kyi P, Mammoto T, Mammoto A. Obesity inhibits angiogenesis through TWIST1-SLIT2 signaling. Front Cell Dev Biol. 2021;9:693410. https://doi.org/10.3389/fcell.2021.693410.

52. Ikeda K, Yamada T. UCP1 dependent and independent thermogenesis in Brown and Beige adipocytes. Front Endocrinol (Lausanne). 2020;11:498. https://doi.org/10.3389/fendo.2020.00498.

53. Isakson P, Hammarstedt A, Gustafson B, Smith U. Impaired preadipocyte differentiation in human abdominal obesity: role of Wnt, tumor necrosis factor-alpha, and inflammation. Diabetes. 2009;58(7): 1550–7. https://doi.org/10.2337/db08-1770.

54. Jaitin DA, Adlung L, Thaiss CA, Weiner A, Li B, Descamps H, . . . Amit, I.. Lipid-associated macrophages control metabolic homeostasis in a Trem2-dependent manner. Cell. 2019;178(3):686–698.e14. https://doi.org/10.1016/j.cell.2019.05.054.

55. Janssen I, Powell LH, Kazlauskaite R, Dugan SA. Testosterone and visceral fat in midlife women: the Study of Women's Health Across the Nation (SWAN) fat patterning study. Obesity (Silver Spring). 2010;18(3):604–10. https://doi.org/10.1038/oby.2009.251.

56. Jespersen NZ, Feizi A, Andersen ES, Heywood S, Hattel HB, Daugaard S, . . . Scheele C. Heterogeneity in the perirenal region of humans suggests presence of dormant brown adipose tissue that contains brown fat precursor cells. Mol Metab. 2019;24:30–43. https://doi.org/10.1016/j.molmet.2019.03.005.

57. Jumabay M, Zhang L, Yao J, Bostrom KI. Progenitor cells from brown adipose tissue undergo neurogenic differentiation. Sci Rep. 2022;12(1):5614. https://doi.org/10.1038/s41598-022-09382-8.

58. Kimura H, Nagoshi T, Oi Y, Yoshii A, Tanaka Y, Takahashi H, . . . Yoshimura M. Treatment with atrial natriuretic peptide induces adipose tissue browning and exerts thermogenic actions in vivo. Sci Rep. 2021;11(1):17466. https://doi.org/10.1038/s41598-021-96970-9.

59. Kintscher U, Hartge M, Hess K, Foryst-Ludwig A, Clemenz M, Wabitsch M, . . . Marx, N.. T-lymphocyte infiltration in visceral adipose tissue: a primary event in adipose tissue inflammation and the development of obesity-mediated insulin resistance. Arterioscler Thromb Vasc Biol. 2008;28(7):1304–10. https://doi.org/10.1161/ATVBAHA.108.165100.

60. Kobashi C, Urakaze M, Kishida M, Kibayashi E, Kobayashi H, Kihara S, . . . Kobayashi M. Adiponectin inhibits endothelial synthesis of interleukin-8. Circ Res. 2005;97(12):1245–52. https://doi.org/10.1161/01.RES.0000194328.57164.36.

61. Kotzbeck P, Giordano A, Mondini E, Murano I, Severi I, Venema W, . . . Cinti S. Brown adipose tissue whitening leads to brown adipocyte death and adipose tissue inflammation. J Lipid Res. 2018;59(5):784–94. https://doi.org/10.1194/jlr.M079665.

62. Kratz M, Coats BR, Hisert KB, Hagman D, Mutskov V, Peris E, . . . Becker L. Metabolic dysfunction drives a mechanistically distinct proinflammatory phenotype in adipose tissue macrophages. Cell Metab. 2014;20(4):614–25. https://doi.org/10.1016/j.cmet.2014.08.010.

63. Kulterer OC, Herz CT, Prager M, Schmoltzer C, Langer FB, Prager G, ... Kiefer FW. Brown adipose tissue prevalence is lower in obesity but its metabolic activity is intact. Front Endocrinol (Lausanne). 2022;13:858417. https://doi.org/10.3389/fendo.2022.858417.

64. Kunduzova O, Alet N, Delesque-Touchard N, Millet L, Castan-Laurell I, Muller C, ... Valet P. Apelin/APJ signaling system: a potential link between adipose tissue and endothelial angiogenic processes. FASEB J. 2008;22(12):4146–53. https://doi.org/10.1096/fj.07-104018.

65. Lean ME. Brown adipose tissue in humans. Proc Nutr Soc. 1989;48(2):243–56. https://doi.org/10.1079/pns19890036.

66. LeBleu VS, Macdonald B, Kalluri R. Structure and function of basement membranes. Exp Biol Med (Maywood). 2007;232(9):1121–9. https://doi.org/10.3181/0703-MR-72.

67. Lee P, Greenfield JR, Ho KK, Fulham MJ. A critical appraisal of the prevalence and metabolic significance of brown adipose tissue in adult humans. Am J Physiol Endocrinol Metab. 2010;299(4):E601–6. https://doi.org/10.1152/ajpendo.00298.2010.

68. Lee P, Linderman JD, Smith S, Brychta RJ, Wang J, Idelson C, ... Celi FS. Irisin and FGF21 are cold-induced endocrine activators of brown fat function in humans. Cell Metab. 2014;19(2):302–9. https://doi.org/10.1016/j.cmet.2013.12.017.

69. Lee KY, Luong Q, Sharma R, Dreyfuss JM, Ussar S, Kahn CR. Developmental and functional heterogeneity of white adipocytes within a single fat depot. EMBO J. 2019;38(3):e99291. https://doi.org/10.15252/embj.201899291.

70. Li H, Konja D, Wang L, Wang Y. Sex differences in adiposity and cardiovascular diseases. Int J Mol Sci. 2022;23(16):9338. https://doi.org/10.3390/ijms23169338.

71. Lidell ME, Betz MJ, Dahlqvist Leinhard O, Heglind M, Elander L, Slawik M, ... Enerback S. Evidence for two types of brown adipose tissue in humans. Nat Med. 2013;19(5):631–4. https://doi.org/10.1038/nm.3017.

72. Liu X, Perusse F, Bukowiecki LJ. Mechanisms of the antidiabetic effects of the beta 3-adrenergic agonist CL-316243 in obese Zucker-ZDF rats. Am J Phys. 1998;274(5):R1212–9. https://doi.org/10.1152/ajpregu.1998.274.5.R1212.

73. Lopez M, Alvarez CV, Nogueiras R, Dieguez C. Energy balance regulation by thyroid hormones at central level. Trends Mol Med. 2013;19(7):418–27. https://doi.org/10.1016/j.molmed.2013.04.004.

74. Love-Gregory L, Abumrad NA. CD36 genetics and the metabolic complications of obesity. Curr Opin Clin Nutr Metab Care. 2011;14(6):527–34. https://doi.org/10.1097/MCO.0b013e32834bbac9.

75. Lumeng CN, Bodzin JL, Saltiel AR. Obesity induces a phenotypic switch in adipose tissue macrophage polarization. J Clin Invest. 2007;117(1):175–84. https://doi.org/10.1172/JCI29881.

76. Lundgren M, Svensson M, Lindmark S, Renstrom F, Ruge T, Eriksson JW. Fat cell enlargement is an independent marker of insulin resistance and 'hyperleptinaemia'. Diabetologia. 2007;50(3):625–33. https://doi.org/10.1007/s00125-006-0572-1.

77. Mariman EC, Wang P. Adipocyte extracellular matrix composition, dynamics and role in obesity. Cell Mol Life Sci. 2010;67(8):1277–92. https://doi.org/10.1007/s00018-010-0263-4.

78. Mesa AM, Medrano TI, Sirohi VK, Walker WH, Johnson RD, Tevosian SG, ... Cooke PS. Identification and characterization of novel abdominal and pelvic brown adipose depots in mice. Adipocytes. 2022;11(1):616–29. https://doi.org/10.1080/21623945.2022.2133415.

79. Miller NE, Michel CC, Nanjee MN, Olszewski WL, Miller IP, Hazell M, ... Frayn KN. Secretion of adipokines by human adipose tissue in vivo: partitioning between capillary and lymphatic transport. Am J Physiol Endocrinol Metab. 2011;301(4):E659–67. https://doi.org/10.1152/ajpendo.00058.2011.

80. Mori S, Kiuchi S, Ouchi A, Hase T, Murase T. Characteristic expression of extracellular matrix in subcutaneous adipose tissue development and adipogenesis; comparison with visceral adipose tissue. Int J Biol Sci. 2014;10(8):825–33. https://doi.org/10.7150/ijbs.8672.

81. Mur C, Valverde AM, Kahn CR, Benito M. Increased insulin sensitivity in IGF-I receptor – deficient brown adipocytes. Diabetes. 2002;51(3):743–54. https://doi.org/10.2337/diabetes.51.3.743.

82. Murano I, Barbatelli G, Giordano A, Cinti S. Noradrenergic parenchymal nerve fiber branching after cold acclimatisation correlates with brown adipocyte density in mouse adipose organ. J Anat. 2009;214(1):171–8. https://doi.org/10.1111/j.1469-7580.2008.01001.x.

83. Muzik O, Mangner TJ, Leonard WR, Kumar A, Janisse J, Granneman JG. 15O PET measurement of blood flow and oxygen consumption in cold-activated human brown fat. J Nucl Med. 2013;54(4):523–31. https://doi.org/10.2967/jnumed.112.111336.

84. Nguyen KD, Qiu Y, Cui X, Goh YP, Mwangi J, David T, ... Chawla A. Alternatively activated macrophages produce catecholamines to sustain adaptive thermogenesis. Nature. 2011;480(7375):104–8. https://doi.org/10.1038/nature10653.

85. Nijhuis J, Rensen SS, Slaats Y, van Dielen FM, Buurman WA, Greve JW. Neutrophil activation in morbid obesity, chronic activation of acute inflammation. Obesity (Silver Spring). 2009;17(11):2014–8. https://doi.org/10.1038/oby.2009.113.

86. Orava J, Nuutila P, Noponen T, Parkkola R, Viljanen T, Enerback S, ... Virtanen KA. Blunted metabolic responses to cold and insulin stimulation in brown adipose tissue of obese humans. Obesity (Silver Spring). 2013;21(11):2279–87. https://doi.org/10.1002/oby.20456.

87. Ouchi N, Kobayashi H, Kihara S, Kumada M, Sato K, Inoue T, ... Walsh K. Adiponectin stimulates angiogenesis by promoting cross-talk between AMP-activated protein kinase and Akt signaling in endothelial cells. J Biol Chem. 2004;279(2):1304–9. https://doi.org/10.1074/jbc.M310389200.

88. Ouellet V, Routhier-Labadie A, Bellemare W, Lakhal-Chaieb L, Turcotte E, Carpentier AC, Richard D. Outdoor temperature, age, sex, body mass index, and diabetic status determine the prevalence, mass, and glucose-uptake activity of 18F-FDG-detected BAT in humans. J Clin Endocrinol Metab. 2011;96(1):192–9. https://doi.org/10.1210/jc.2010-0989.

89. Peeraully MR, Jenkins JR, Trayhurn P. NGF gene expression and secretion in white adipose tissue: regulation in 3T3-L1 adipocytes by hormones and inflammatory cytokines. Am J Physiol Endocrinol Metab. 2004;287(2):E331–9. https://doi.org/10.1152/ajpendo.00076.2004.

90. Pellegrinelli V, Heuvingh J, du Route O, Rouault C, Devulder A, Klein C, ... Clement K. Human adipocyte function is impacted by mechanical cues. J Pathol. 2014;233(2):183–95. https://doi.org/10.1002/path.4347.

91. Pellegrinelli V, Rouault C, Veyrie N, Clement K, Lacasa D. Endothelial cells from visceral adipose tissue disrupt adipocyte functions in a three-dimensional setting: partial rescue by angiopoietin-1. Diabetes. 2014;63(2):535–49. https://doi.org/10.2337/db13-0537.

92. Pellegrinelli V, Rodriguez-Cuenca S, Rouault C, Figueroa-Juarez E, Schilbert H, Virtue S, ... Vidal-Puig A. Dysregulation of macrophage PEPD in obesity determines adipose tissue fibro-inflammation and insulin resistance. Nat Metab. 2022;4(4):476–94. https://doi.org/10.1038/s42255-022-00561-5.

93. Potenza MA, Addabbo F, Montagnani M. Vascular actions of insulin with implications for endothelial dysfunction. Am J Physiol Endocrinol Metab. 2009;297(3):E568–77. https://doi.org/10.1152/ajpendo.00297.2009.

94. Purkayastha S, Cai D. Neuroinflammatory basis of metabolic syndrome. Mol Metab. 2013;2(4):356–63. https://doi.org/10.1016/j.molmet.2013.09.005.

95. Qiu Y, Nguyen KD, Odegaard JI, Cui X, Tian X, Locksley RM, ... Chawla, A.. Eosinophils and type 2 cytokine signaling in macrophages orchestrate development of functional beige fat. Cell. 2014;157(6):1292–308. https://doi.org/10.1016/j.cell.2014.03.066.

96. Rabelo R, Reyes C, Schifman A, Silva JE. Interactions among receptors, thyroid hormone response elements, and ligands in the regulation of the rat uncoupling protein gene expression by thyroid hormone. Endocrinology. 1996;137(8):3478–87. https://doi.org/10.1210/endo.137.8.8754777.

97. Rahman MS, Jun H. The adipose tissue macrophages central to adaptive thermoregulation. Front Immunol. 2022;13:884126. https://doi.org/10.3389/fimmu.2022.884126.

98. Rao RR, Long JZ, White JP, Svensson KJ, Lou J, Lokurkar I, ... Spiegelman BM. Meteorin-like is a hormone that regulates immune-adipose interactions to increase beige fat thermogenesis. Cell. 2014;157(6):1279–91. https://doi.org/10.1016/j.cell.2014.03.065.

99. Roberts LD, Ashmore T, Kotwica AO, Murfitt SA, Fernandez BO, Feelisch M, ... Griffin JL. Inorganic nitrate promotes the browning of white adipose tissue through the nitrate-nitrite-nitric oxide pathway. Diabetes. 2015;64(2):471–84. https://doi.org/10.2337/db14-0496.

100. Rosen ED, MacDougald OA. Adipocyte differentiation from the inside out. Nat Rev Mol Cell Biol. 2006;7(12):885–96. https://doi.org/10.1038/nrm2066.

101. Rosenwald M, Perdikari A, Rulicke T, Wolfrum C. Bi-directional interconversion of brite and white adipocytes. Nat Cell Biol. 2013;15(6):659–67. https://doi.org/10.1038/ncb2740.

102. Rosina M, Ceci V, Turchi R, Chuan L, Borcherding N, Sciarretta F, ... Lettieri-Barbato D. Ejection of damaged mitochondria and their removal by macrophages ensure efficient thermogenesis in brown adipose tissue. Cell Metab. 2022;34(4):533–548.e12. https://doi.org/10.1016/j.cmet.2022.02.016.

103. Rouault C, Pellegrinelli V, Schilch R, Cotillard A, Poitou C, Tordjman J, ... Lacasa D. Roles of chemokine ligand-2 (CXCL2) and neutrophils in influencing endothelial cell function and inflammation of human adipose tissue. Endocrinology. 2013;154(3):1069–79. https://doi.org/10.1210/en.2012-1415.

104. Ryu V, Garretson JT, Liu Y, Vaughan CH, Bartness TJ. Brown adipose tissue has sympathetic-sensory feedback circuits. J Neurosci. 2015;35(5):2181–90. https://doi.org/10.1523/JNEUROSCI.3306-14.2015.

105. Saari TJ, Raiko J, U-Din M, Niemi T, Taittonen M, Laine J, ... Virtanen KA. Basal and cold-induced fatty acid uptake of human brown adipose tissue is impaired in obesity. Sci Rep. 2020;10(1):14373. https://doi.org/10.1038/s41598-020-71197-2.

106. Seale P, Bjork B, Yang W, Kajimura S, Chin S, Kuang S, ... Spiegelman BM. PRDM16 controls a brown fat/skeletal muscle switch. Nature. 2008;454(7207):961–7. https://doi.org/10.1038/nature07182.

107. Seale P, Conroe HM, Estall J, Kajimura S, Frontini A, Ishibashi J, ... Spiegelman BM. Prdm16 determines the thermogenic program of subcutaneous white adipose tissue in mice. J Clin Invest. 2011;121(1):96–105. https://doi.org/10.1172/JCI44271.

108. Shamsi F, Piper M, Ho LL, Huang TL, Gupta A, Streets A, ... Tseng YH. Vascular smooth muscle-derived Trpv1(+) progenitors are a source of cold-induced thermogenic adipocytes. Nat Metab. 2021;3(4):485–95. https://doi.org/10.1038/s42255-021-00373-z.

109. Shan B, Barker CS, Shao M, Zhang Q, Gupta RK, Wu Y. Multilayered omics reveal sex- and depot-dependent adipose progenitor cell heterogeneity. Cell Metab. 2022;34(5):783–799.e87. https://doi.org/10.1016/j.cmet.2022.03.012.

110. Shapira SN, Lim HW, Rajakumari S, Sakers AP, Ishibashi J, Harms MJ, ... Seale, P.. EBF2 transcriptionally regulates brown adipogenesis via the histone reader DPF3 and the BAF chromatin remodeling complex. Genes Dev. 2017;31(7):660–73. https://doi.org/10.1101/gad.294405.116.

111. Shimizu I, Aprahamian T, Kikuchi R, Shimizu A, Papanicolaou KN, MacLauchlan S, ... Walsh K. Vascular rarefaction mediates whitening of brown fat in obesity. J Clin Invest. 2014;124(5):2099–112. https://doi.org/10.1172/JCI71643.

112. Skarulis MC, Celi FS, Mueller E, Zemskova M, Malek R, Hugendubler L, ... Gorden P. Thyroid hormone induced brown adipose tissue and amelioration of diabetes in a patient with extreme insulin resistance. J Clin Endocrinol Metab. 2010;95(1):256–62. https://doi.org/10.1210/jc.2009-0543.

113. Springer TA. Adhesion receptors of the immune system. Nature. 1990;346(6283):425–34. https://doi.org/10.1038/346425a0.

114. Strieder-Barboza C, Baker NA, Flesher CG, Karmakar M, Patel A, Lumeng CN, O'Rourke RW. Depot-specific adipocyte-extracellular matrix metabolic crosstalk in murine obesity. Adipocytes. 2020;9(1):189–96. https://doi.org/10.1080/21623945.2020.1749500.

115. Strissel KJ, Stancheva Z, Miyoshi H, Perfield JW 2nd, DeFuria J, Jick Z, ... Obin MS. Adipocyte death, adipose tissue remodeling, and obesity complications. Diabetes. 2007;56(12):2910–8. https://doi.org/10.2337/db07-0767.

116. Sun K, Park J, Gupta OT, Holland WL, Auerbach P, Zhang N, ... Scherer PE. Endotrophin triggers adipose tissue fibrosis and metabolic dysfunction. Nat Commun. 2014;5:3485. https://doi.org/10.1038/ncomms4485.

117. Sundberg C, Kowanetz M, Brown LF, Detmar M, Dvorak HF. Stable expression of angiopoietin-1 and other markers by cultured pericytes: phenotypic similarities to a subpopulation of cells in maturing vessels during later stages of angiogenesis in vivo. Lab Investig. 2002;82(4):387–401. https://doi.org/10.1038/labinvest.3780433.

118. Tang QQ, Otto TC, Lane MD. Commitment of C3H10T1/2 pluripotent stem cells to the adipocyte lineage. Proc Natl Acad Sci USA. 2004;101(26):9607 11. https://doi.org/10.1073/pnas.0403100101.

119. Tchernof A, Belanger C, Morisset AS, Richard C, Mailloux J, Laberge P, Dupont P. Regional differences in adipose tissue metabolism in women: minor effect of obesity and body fat distribution. Diabetes. 2006;55(5):1353–60. https://doi.org/10.2337/db05-1439.

120. Tracy TF Jr. Editorial: acute pancreatitis and neutrophil gelatinase MMP9: don't get me started! J Leukoc

Biol. 2012;91(5):682–4. https://doi.org/10.1189/jlb.1111535.

121. Traktuev DO, Merfeld-Clauss S, Li J, Kolonin M, Arap W, Pasqualini R, ... March KL. A population of multipotent CD34-positive adipose stromal cells share pericyte and mesenchymal surface markers, reside in a periendothelial location, and stabilize endothelial networks. Circ Res. 2008;102(1):77–85. https://doi.org/10.1161/CIRCRESAHA.107.159475.

122. Tseng YH, Kokkotou E, Schulz TJ, Huang TL, Winnay JN, Taniguchi CM, ... Kahn CR. New role of bone morphogenetic protein 7 in brown adipogenesis and energy expenditure. Nature. 2008;454(7207):1000–4. https://doi.org/10.1038/nature07221.

123. Tupone D, Madden CJ, Morrison SF. Autonomic regulation of brown adipose tissue thermogenesis in health and disease: potential clinical applications for altering BAT thermogenesis. Front Neurosci. 2014;8:14. https://doi.org/10.3389/fnins.2014.00014.

124. van Marken Lichtenbelt WD, Vanhommerig JW, Smulders NM, Drossaerts JM, Kemerink GJ, Bouvy ND, ... Teule GJ. Cold-activated brown adipose tissue in healthy men. N Engl J Med. 2009;360(15):1500–8. https://doi.org/10.1056/NEJMoa0808718.

125. Vijay J, Gauthier MF, Biswell RL, Louiselle DA, Johnston JJ, Cheung WA, ... Grundberg E. Single-cell analysis of human adipose tissue identifies depot and disease specific cell types. Nat Metab. 2020;2(1):97–109. https://doi.org/10.1038/s42255-019-0152-6.

126. Villaret A, Galitzky J, Decaunes P, Esteve D, Marques MA, Sengenes C, ... Bouloumie A. Adipose tissue endothelial cells from obese human subjects: differences among depots in angiogenic, metabolic, and inflammatory gene expression and cellular senescence. Diabetes. 2010;59(11):2755–63. https://doi.org/10.2337/db10-0398.

127. Vitali A, Murano I, Zingaretti MC, Frontini A, Ricquier D, Cinti S. The adipose organ of obesity-prone C57BL/6J mice is composed of mixed white and brown adipocytes. J Lipid Res. 2012;53(4):619–29. https://doi.org/10.1194/jlr.M018846.

128. Wang GX, Zhao XY, Meng ZX, Kern M, Dietrich A, Chen Z, ... Lin JD. The brown fat-enriched secreted factor Nrg4 preserves metabolic homeostasis through attenuation of hepatic lipogenesis. Nat Med. 2014;20(12):1436–43. https://doi.org/10.1038/nm.3713.

129. Wang Q, Li D, Cao G, Shi Q, Zhu J, Zhang M, ... Yin Z. IL-27 signalling promotes adipocyte thermogenesis and energy expenditure. Nature. 2021;600(7888):314–8. https://doi.org/10.1038/s41586-021-04127-5.

130. Wang YN, Tang Y, He Z, Ma H, Wang L, Liu Y, ... Tang QQ. Slit3 secreted from M2-like macrophages increases sympathetic activity and thermogenesis in adipose tissue. Nat Metab. 2021;3(11):1536–51. https://doi.org/10.1038/s42255-021-00482-9.

131. Watanabe M, Houten SM, Mataki C, Christoffolete MA, Kim BW, Sato H, ... Auwerx J. Bile acids

induce energy expenditure by promoting intracellular thyroid hormone activation. Nature. 2006;439(7075): 484–9. https://doi.org/10.1038/nature04330.

132. Whittle AJ, Carobbio S, Martins L, Slawik M, Hondares E, Vazquez MJ, . . . Vidal-Puig A. BMP8B increases brown adipose tissue thermogenesis through both central and peripheral actions. Cell. 2012;149(4):871–85. https://doi.org/10.1016/j.cell. 2012.02.066.

133. Xue Y, Petrovic N, Cao R, Larsson O, Lim S, Chen S, . . . Cao Y. Hypoxia-independent angiogenesis in adipose tissues during cold acclimation. Cell Metab. 2009;9(1):99–109. https://doi.org/10.1016/j.cmet. 2008.11.009.

134. Yadav RL, Sharma D, Yadav PK, Shah DK, Agrawal K, Khadka R, Islam MN. Somatic neural alterations in non-diabetic obesity: a cross-sectional study. BMC Obes. 2016;3:50. https://doi.org/10. 1186/s40608-016-0131-3.

135. Yoneshiro T, Aita S, Matsushita M, Kayahara T, Kameya T, Kawai Y, . . . Saito M. Recruited brown adipose tissue as an antiobesity agent in humans. J Clin Invest. 2013;123(8):3404–8. https://doi.org/ 10.1172/JCI67803.

136. Zhang P, Wu S, He Y, Li X, Zhu Y, Lin X, . . . Shen L. LncRNA-mediated adipogenesis in different adipocytes. Int J Mol Sci. 2022;23(13). https://doi.org/ 10.3390/ijms23137488.

Adipokines and Metabolism

18

Rexford S. Ahima and Hyeong-Kyu Park

Contents

R. S. Ahima (✉)
Department of Medicine, Division of Endocrinology, Diabetes and Metabolism, Johns Hopkins University School of Medicine, Baltimore, MD, USA
e-mail: ahima@jhmi.edu

H.-K. Park
Department of Internal Medicine, Soonchunhyang University College of Medicine, Seoul, South Korea

Abstract

Adipose tissue is the main site of energy storage in the form of triglycerides. Mature adipocytes also produce enzymes, growth factors, cytokines, chemokines, and hormones (adipokines) implicated in the modulation of feeding, energy homeostasis, lipid and glucose metabolism, inflammation, coagulation, and cardiovascular system. Obesity alters the

© Springer Nature Switzerland AG 2023
R. S. Ahima (ed.), *Metabolic Syndrome*,
https://doi.org/10.1007/978-3-031-40116-9_24

expression, circulating levels, and signaling mechanisms of adipose-secreted factors, and these changes have been linked to the development of insulin resistance, type 2 diabetes, dyslipidemia, atherosclerosis, cancer, and other diseases.

Keywords

Adipose tissue · Adipokine · Leptin · Adiponectin · Resistin · Batokine · Obesity

Introduction

White adipose tissue (WAT), the main type of adipose tissue in mammals, is composed of specialized cells for lipid storage (adipocytes) embedded in a highly vascularized and innervated loose connective tissue. Mature white adipocytes contain a single large fat droplet occupying >90% of the cell volume, and the nucleus and cytoplasm are squeezed into the remaining cell volume, creating a signet ring appearance. In addition to adipocytes, WAT contains adipocyte progenitor cells, macrophages, leukocytes, fibroblasts, and endothelial cells. The highest amounts of WAT are found in the subcutaneous regions and surrounding abdominal and thoracic organs.

Triglycerides stored in white adipocytes represent the major energy reserves of the body and are in a constant state of flux in relation to feeding and fasting. Insulin is increased in response to meals, binds to the insulin receptor, and suppresses lipolysis via activation of phosphodiesterase 3B which hydrolyzes cAMP and inactivates protein kinase A (PKA). Insulin also suppresses lipolysis through a cAMP-independent pathway mediated by stimulation of protein phosphatase-1 which inactivates hormone-sensitive lipase (HSL). Epinephrine and norepinephrine levels increase during fasting and bind to their cognate receptors on adipocytes triggering activation of adenylate cyclase, increasing cAMP which activates PKA leading to phosphorylation and activation of HSL. In addition to HSL, adipocytes express other triglyceride hydrolases including desnutrin/ATGL, triacylglycerol hydrolase, and adiponutrin. Other proteins implicated in triglyceride metabolism in adipose tissue include perilipins, adipose fatty acid-binding protein (aP2), caveolin-1, aquaporin 7, and lipotransin. Perilipin-1 coats lipid droplets and prevents access of triglyceride lipases, thus limiting basal lipolysis. aP2 transports fatty acids to the plasma membrane to be released into plasma. Glycerol released from triglyceride hydrolysis is exported via aquaporin 7. Lipotransin may be involved in shuttling HSL from the cytosol to the lipid droplet during adipocyte stimulation.

In addition to enzymes and transporters involved in fuel homeostasis, adipose tissue produces and secretes several proteins including adhesion molecules, growth factors, adipokines, cytokines, chemokines, and complement and coagulation factors (Table 1). This chapter focuses on the biology of leptin, adiponectin, and resistin.

Brown adipose tissue (BAT) is composed of adipocytes rich in mitochondria and multiloculated lipid droplets, and localized mostly in the interscapular region of rodents and neonatal humans where it serves as thermogenic function. BAT regresses after infancy in humans but remains active in the cervical, mediastinal, paravertebral, and perirenal areas, oxidizing glucose and fatty acids and releasing energy in the form of heat in response to cold exposure, beta-adrenergic agonists, and thyroid hormone. In addition to thermoregulation, BAT synthesizes and secretes signaling molecules, known as batokines, which act via autocrine, paracrine, and endocrine mechanisms (Table 2). This chapter discusses the functions of fibroblast growth factor (FGF)-21, interleukin-6, and other batokines.

Leptin

Leptin is a 167-amino-acid peptide which is mainly produced and secreted by WAT and to a lesser extent by placenta, mammary gland, ovary, skeletal muscle, stomach, pituitary gland, and lymphoid tissue. Plasma leptin concentrations are proportional to the amount of body fat. In addition, leptin levels increase in response to overfeeding and

Table 1 Proteins produced by white adipose tissue

Enzymes and transporters	Receptors	Secreted proteins
Lipid metabolism	*Peptide and*	*Adipokines*
LPL	*glycoprotein*	Leptin
HSL	Insulin	Adiponectin
ATGL	Glucagon	Resistin (rodents)
Triacylglycerol	FSH	Angiotensinogen
hydrolase	GH	Fasting-induced adipose factor (angiopoietin-like protein-4)
Adiponutrin	Ang-II	Apelin
CETP	CCK-B/gastrin	Omentin
aP2	Adiponectin	Retinol-binding protein (RBP4)
CD36	*Nuclear*	Visfatin
ApoE	PPARγ	Vaspin
Perilipins	Glucocorticoid	*Cytokines*
Caveolin-1	Estrogen	TNF-α
Aquaporin 7	Progesterone	MIF
Lipotransin	Androgen	IL-1β, IL-4, IL-6, IL-8, IL-10, and IL-18
Glucose metabolism	Thyroid	*Chemokines*
IRS-1, IRS-2	Vitamin D	Chemerin
PI3K	NF-κB	MCP-1
Akt		MIP-1α
Protein kinase λ/ζ		*Complement factors*
GSK-3α		Adipsin
GLUT4		Acylation-stimulating protein
Steroid metabolism		*Acute phase proteins*
Aromatase		CRP
11β-HSD-1		Serum amyloid A3 (SAA3)
17β-HSD		Haptoglobin
Estrogen		*Growth/angiogenic/coagulation factors*
sulfotransferase		FGF-1, FGF-2, FGF-7, FGF-9, FGF-10, and FGF-18
		IGF-1
		HGF
		NGF
		VEGF
		TGF-β
		Angiopoietin-1 and angiopoietin-2
		Tissue factor
		PAI-1
		Extracellular matrix
		α2-Macroglobulin
		VCAM-1
		ICAM-1
		Collagen I, III, IV, and VI
		Fibronectin
		MMP1, MMP7, MMP9, MMP10, MMP11, MMP14, and MMP15
		Lysyl oxidase

during starvation [15, 19]. Leptin is secreted in a pulsatile manner and displays a circadian rhythm with a nadir at midafternoon and peak levels at midnight. The pulsatile leptin secretion is similar in obese and lean people, but the pulse amplitude is higher in obesity [56]. Leptin levels exhibit a sexual dimorphism, being higher in premenopausal women than men and declining in postmenopausal women. Subcutaneous fat produces more leptin than visceral fat, and this may in part contribute to higher leptin levels in women compared to men [68]. Besides sex steroids, leptin is increased by insulin and glucocorticoids and reduced by catecholamines and inflammatory cytokines [1].

Table 2 Metabolic mediators produced and secreted by brown adipose tissue

BMP-8b	Promotes sympathetic nerve activity via NRG-4 and enhances lipolysis via HSL in response to adrenergic stimulation
CXCL-14	Recruits alternatively activated M2 macrophages and promotes browning of WAT
Endothelin 1	Inhibits brown and beige adipogenesis and reduces energy expenditure
FGF-21	Enhances browning of WAT and BAT-mediated thermogenesis
GDF-15	Suppresses proinflammatory gene expression
IGF-1	Regulates glucose metabolism through BAT and systemic mechanisms
IGFBP-2	Enhances the differentiation of osteoclasts and increases bone remodeling
IL-6	Enhances browning of WAT, insulin sensitivity, and glucose homeostasis
Myostatin	Inhibits muscle growth and brown adipogenesis and impairs insulin sensitivity and glucose uptake
NRG-4	Enhances browning of WAT, reduces hepatic steatosis and hyperlipidemia, and improves glucose homeostasis
NGF	Promotes neurite outgrowth and sympathetic innervation
SLIT2-C	Enhances browning of WAT and glucose homeostasis
Triiodothyronine (T3)	Produced from type 2 deiodinase (Dio2) conversion of thyroxine (T4) and regulates development and metabolism
VEGF-A	Promotes angiogenesis and vascularization of BAT

Leptin Signaling

Leptin exerts its effects via leptin receptors (LepRs) located throughout the central nervous system (CNS). Four alternatively spliced isoforms of LepR have been identified in humans. The long isoform of leptin receptor (LepRb) is abundantly expressed in the hypothalamus and other brain regions, where it regulates energy homeostasis and neuroendocrine function, and considered as the main leptin receptor. LepRb is mainly responsible for inhibition of food intake and stimulation of energy expenditure, while the short isoforms of LepR are thought to mediate the transport of leptin across the blood–brain barrier. Evidence suggests that leptin transport into the hypothalamus is mediated by tanycytes through LepR [9].

Leptin binds to LepRb leading to activation of Janus kinase 2 (JAK2)–signal transducer and activator of transcription 3 (STAT3) (Fig. 1). Leptin signaling also interacts with insulin receptor substrate (IRS)–phosphatidylinositol 3-kinase (PI3K), SH2-containing protein tyrosine phosphatase 2 (SHP2)–mitogen-activated protein kinase (MAPK), $5'$ adenosine monophosphate-activated protein kinase (AMPK)/acetyl-CoA carboxylase (ACC), and other signaling pathways. Activation of JAK2–STAT3 signaling plays a crucial role in leptin's ability to regulate energy homeostasis. Leptin signaling is terminated by suppressor of cytokine signaling 3 (SOCS3) which inhibits JAK2–STAT3. Induction of protein tyrosine phosphatase 1B (PTP1B) also inhibits leptin signaling [21, 71].

Leptin acts directly on anorexigenic neurons that synthesize pro-opiomelanocortin (POMC) and cocaine- and amphetamine-regulated transcript (CART) and orexigenic neurons that synthesize Agouti-related peptide (AgRP) and neuropeptide Y (NPY). During fasting, plasma leptin levels decline rapidly leading to stimulation of AgRP and NPY and suppression of POMC and CART, thereby increasing food intake and decreasing energy expenditure [3]. The lateral hypothalamus contains neurons that express melanin-concentrating hormone (MCH) and orexins. These neuropeptides are decreased by leptin resulting in suppression of feeding [21]. Other leptin targets in the lateral hypothalamus innervate the ventral tegmental area (VTA), linking leptin to the hedonic control of feeding mediated by the mesolimbic dopaminergic system. Leptin also acts on ventromedial hypothalamic neurons that express the transcription factor steroidogenic factor 1 (SF-1). Mice with SF-1 deletion in the Ventromedial Hypothalamus are susceptible to obesity associated with impaired thermogenesis. Brain-derived neurotrophic factor

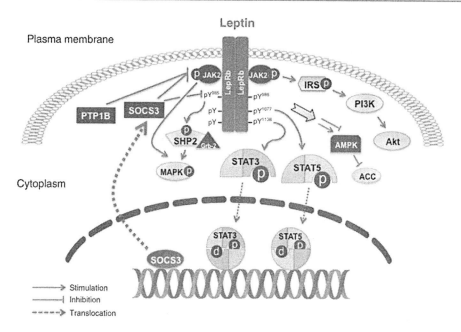

Fig. 1 Leptin signaling. Leptin binds to LepRb resulting in its dimerization and formation of LepRb/JAK2 complex. Activated JAK2 autophosphorylates and also phosphorylates Tyr^{985}, Tyr^{1077}, and Tyr^{1138} in LepRb. STAT3 and STAT5 bind to phospho-Tyr^{1138} and phospho-Tyr^{1077} in LepRb and are subsequently phosphorylated. The active STAT3 and STAT5 dimers translocate to the nucleus and activate the transcription of neuropeptides and other target genes. SOCS3, a target gene of STAT3, inhibits JAK2/STAT3 by interacting with phospho-Tyr^{985} or JAK2 and acting as a feedback inhibitor of leptin signaling. PTP1B inhibits leptin signaling through dephosphorylation of JAK2. After JAK2 activation, SH2-containing protein tyrosine phosphatase 2 (SHP2) binds to phospho-Tyr^{985} in LepRb and recruits the adaptor protein growth factor receptor-bound protein 2 (Grb2), leading to activation of the mitogen-activated protein kinase (MAPK) signaling pathway. Leptin activates MAPK independently of SHP2 and also regulates PI3K signaling through IRS phosphorylation. Forkhead box O1 (FoxO1), mammalian target of rapamycin (mTOR), and phosphodiesterase 3B (PDE3B) are important downstream targets of PI3K in the leptin signaling pathway. Leptin also regulates feeding and metabolism through 5′ adenosine monophosphate-activated protein kinase (AMPK) and acetyl-CoA carboxylase (ACC) in the brain and peripheral organs. (From [87]. Used with permission under the Creative Commons License)

in the Ventromedial Hypothalamus has been linked to leptin's effects on feeding and energy balance. Subpopulations of neurons in the nucleus tractus solitarius (NTS) express LepRb, glucagon-like peptide 1 (GLP-1), and cholecystokinin (CCK), and leptin acts synergistically with GLP-1 and CCK in the NTS to increase satiety.

In addition to regulating food intake, leptin stimulates sympathetic nervous activity and brown adipose tissue (BAT) thermogenesis [109]. The thermogenic effect of leptin is mediated partly via suppression of MCH and Forkhead box O1 (FoxO1). Mice lacking leptin and MCH are less obese than leptin-deficient *ob/ob* mice and display greater energy expenditure and locomotor activity compared to *ob/ob* mice. Leptin has neurotrophic effects on hypothalamic neurons implicated in feeding and energy homeostasis. Neural projections from the arcuate to paraventricular nucleus (PVN) are reduced in *ob/ob* mice and restored by leptin treatment in neonatal mice. Leptin administration in *ob/ob* mice rapidly normalizes synaptic inputs to POMC and AgRP neurons to levels seen in wild-type mice. Leptin's actions in neurodevelopment have been demonstrated as well in murine cerebral cortex and hippocampus. Brain imaging studies have also revealed structural and functional deficits reversible by leptin treatment in congenital leptin deficiency [62].

The role of leptin in energy homeostasis is most evident in leptin deficiency. *ob/ob* mice develop hyperphagia, low metabolic rate, and early onset obesity, associated with high expression of NPY and MCH and low expression of POMC in the hypothalamus [1]. Congenital leptin deficiency in humans also leads to hyperphagia and morbid obesity reversible by leptin treatment [29, 30]. In contrast, most obese people have high levels of leptin expression in adipose tissue and plasma leptin levels, and they respond poorly to leptin treatment (Fig. 2). This suggests "leptin resistance" in common forms of obesity arising from overnutrition and sedentary lifestyle [41, 67, 70]. Specific mechanisms underlying leptin resistance in "common obesity" are unknown

and may include impaired leptin transport across blood–brain barrier and disruption of leptin signaling via hypothalamic inflammation, endoplasmic reticulum stress, and unknown factors [77].

Effects of Leptin on Neuroendocrine System

Reduced leptin levels during fasting trigger various hormonal responses [1], including hypogonadotropic hypogonadism, suppression of thyroid and growth hormone (GH) levels, and activation of the hypothalamic–pituitary–adrenal axis in mice, which are prevented by leptin treatment [2, 15] (Fig. 2). Leptin replacement restores thyroid hormone, testosterone, and luteinizing hormone (LH) levels in fasted mice [2] and LH pulsatility and testosterone levels in starved human volunteers [2, 15]. Leptin replacement

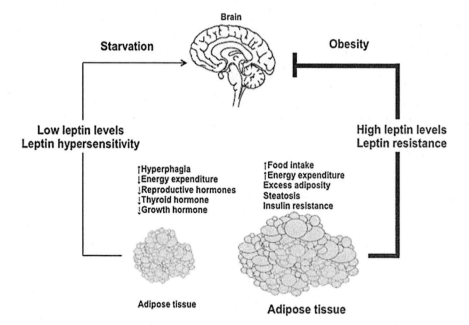

Fig. 2 Physiology of leptin in starvation and obesity. Leptin levels fall during starvation and stimulate food intake by increasing expression of orexigenic neuropeptides and decreasing expression of anorexigenic neuropeptides. In addition, the decline of leptin level modulates mesolimbic dopamine system and hindbrain circuits to increase food intake and also has effects on sympathetic nervous system to decrease energy expenditure. Low leptin levels trigger neuroendocrine adaptations resulting in suppression of thyroid hormone, reproductive hormone, and growth hormone. Leptin levels are increased in obesity, but the feedback response in the brain is blunted due to leptin resistance. (From [88]. License number 3674271217804, Elsevier Publishers)

facilitates pubertal development in *ob/ob* mice and leptin-deficient humans, establishing a crucial role of leptin in reproduction [30]. Leptin also prevents the pubertal delay associated with starvation and exerts a permissive effect on puberty in normal mice. Low leptin levels are also linked to impaired leptin pulsatility and hypogonadism in hypothalamic amenorrhea and lipoatrophy [14, 66]. Leptin treatment increases LH levels, LH pulse frequency, and estradiol levels and corrects abnormal thyroid and cortisol levels in hypothalamic amenorrhea [138]. Similarly, leptin replacement normalizes LH and sex steroid levels in individuals with generalized lipoatrophy [76].

These findings suggest that leptin is an important signal linking energy stores to the neuroendocrine axis. However, the underlying mechanisms are still unclear. Gonadotropin-releasing hormone (GnRH) neurons lack LepR; thus, it is likely that leptin acts indirectly to regulate the reproductive axis [35]. Although kisspeptin may mediate the effects of leptin, mice with selective deletion of LepR from hypothalamic Kiss1 neurons show normal pubertal development and fertility, indicating that leptin action in Kiss1 neurons is not essential for puberty and reproduction. Kiss1 neurons in the arcuate nucleus express LepR, but leptin signaling in these neurons occurs after completion of sexual maturation and is not crucial for leptin action during puberty.

Leptin regulates thyroid hormone by stimulating thyrotropin-releasing hormone (TRH) via upregulation of proTRH gene expression and increasing the processing of proTRH. Healthy humans have circadian and pulsatile levels of leptin and TSH, while congenital leptin deficiency results in a highly disorganized secretion of TSH. After leptin replacement, leptin-deficient individuals exhibit an increase in thyroid hormone levels but no change in TSH [30]. Leptin administration prevents the fasting-induced suppression of TSH pulses but does not reverse the fall in tri-iodothyronine (T3) levels [15]. In women with hypothalamic amenorrhea, leptin administration increases free T3 and T4 levels [138]. Leptin treatment also reverses the declines in T3 and T4 levels during weight loss [49, 103].

Metabolic Effects of Leptin

Leptin treatment decreases glucose, insulin, and lipids before weight loss is achieved in *ob/ob* mice. In individuals with congenital leptin deficiency, leptin replacement rapidly decreases insulin resistance, steatosis, and plasma lipids and glucose [30]. Similarly, leptin treatment decreases insulin resistance, steatosis, and glucose in generalized lipoatrophy ([7, 74, 76, 81, 117]; Petersen et al. 2002). Leptin decreases visceral fat in normal rats and in patients with lipoatrophy [55, 74]. CNS leptin administration inhibits de novo lipogenesis and enhances lipolysis in the adipose and liver. Leptin also stimulates fatty acid oxidation by activating AMPK in skeletal muscle and preventing the accumulation of lipid metabolites associated with lipotoxicity.

Studies in diabetic mice suggest that leptin administration normalizes glucose levels by suppressing glucagon and hepatic intermediary metabolites. CNS leptin treatment decreases glucose and glucagon through insulin-independent mechanisms. Leptin suppresses hepatic glucose production by ameliorating hyperglucagonemia and increasing peripheral glucose uptake, partly by targeting POMC- and AgRP-expressing neurons in the arcuate nucleus. Restoration of LepR expression in the arcuate nucleus decreases insulin and glucose in LepR-null mice. Moreover, a selective expression of LepRb in hypothalamic POMC neurons prevents diabetes in LepR-deficient *db/db* mice, independently of changes in feeding and weight. Deletion of leptin targets, SOCS3 or PTP1B, in POMC neurons also improves glucose metabolism. Furthermore, genetically mediated alteration of PI3K activity in POMC neurons affects hepatic insulin sensitivity. A selective reexpression of LepRb in AgRP neurons mediates antidiabetic actions of leptin in *db/db* mice by suppressing glucagon. Leptin inhibits insulin gene expression and glucose-stimulated insulin secretion, and insulin stimulates both leptin synthesis and secretion, thus establishing an adipose tissue–islet axis. Leptin also protects pancreatic β-cells from lipotoxicity.

Leptin has been linked to bone metabolism. In rodents, leptin alters cortical bone formation via β-adrenergic stimulation or GH/insulin-like growth factor (IGF)-1 effects on trabecular bone remodeling. Leptin may influence cortical bone metabolism through hypothalamic neuropeptides, e.g., NPY, which inhibits cortical bone formation. Leptin acts directly on marrow stromal cells to increase osteoblast differentiation and inhibit adipocyte differentiation. Leptin stimulates osteoblast proliferation and mineralization. Leptin's effect on bone biology is evident in leptin-deficient states in humans. Leptin treatment stimulates bone formation, bone mineral density, and content in the lumbar spine of patients with hypothalamic amenorrhea [118, 138]. Potential actions of leptin on bone may involve increased IGF-1 and estrogen and reduction of cortisol. Furthermore, leptin may inhibit bone formation via sympathetic nervous activation [126].

Effects of Leptin on Immunity

Leptin has important roles in modulating innate and adaptive immunity. Leptin stimulates neutrophil chemotaxis and macrophage phagocytosis, and production of proinflammatory cytokines, e.g., IL-6, IL-12, and TNF-α [13]. Leptin inhibits the proliferation of regulatory T cells, stimulates T helper 1 cells, and may contribute to protection from infections and the development of autoimmunity [58, 71]. Leptin treatment in *ob/ob* mice and short-term fasted wild-type mice reverses immune dysfunction associated with hypoleptinemia. Congenital leptin deficiency is associated with a higher incidence of infection, likely due to a reduction of circulating CD4+ T cells and impaired T cell proliferation and cytokine release [30]. In women with hypothalamic amenorrhea and chronic leptin deficiency, leptin replacement increases soluble TNF-α receptor and restores CD4+ T cell counts and proliferative responses, suggesting that leptin promotes immune reconstitution in chronic hypoleptinemia (Chan et al. 2005; [61]). Leptin treatment exacerbates experimental autoimmune encephalomyelitis, while leptin deficiency in *ob/ob* mice is protective against encephalomyelitis. Patients with multiple sclerosis have increased leptin levels in blood and cerebrospinal fluid and reduced peripheral regulatory T cells. These findings suggest potential roles of leptin in the pathogenesis of autoimmune diseases.

Clinical Uses of Leptin

Leptin has potent effects in states of leptin deficiency [133]. Leptin replacement reduces body weight and fat and reverses neuroendocrine and metabolic abnormalities in congenital leptin deficiency [30]. Leptin treatment restores menstrual cycles, normalizes the gonadal, thyroid, and adrenal axes, and improves bone mineral density and bone formation in women with hypothalamic amenorrhea and hypoleptinemia [118]. Leptin treatment also improves insulin sensitivity, dyslipidemia, and hepatic steatosis in patients with lipoatrophy [16, 74, 81].

In contrast to leptin deficiency, most forms of obesity are associated with leptin resistance [67, 70]. Clinical trials investigating the use of recombinant leptin or leptin sensitizers in people with obesity have produced minimal or no effect. The first clinical study involving administration of recombinant methionyl human leptin (r-metHuLeptin) in subjects with common (polygenic) obesity demonstrated no significant difference in body weight between the leptin-treated group and placebo group [36]. Similarly, weekly Fc-leptin administration did not produce a significant weight loss in obese subjects [42]. A combination of a very low-calorie diet and pegylated leptin treatment resulted in significant additional weight loss in overweight men. However, severe caloric restriction to 500 kcal/day combined with leptin treatment did not produce significant weight loss compared to placebo [43].

In patients with obesity and diabetes, leptin treatment did not reduce weight or affect glucose and insulin sensitivity [67]. Recombinant leptin treatment slightly reduced HbA1c but did not alter body weight or inflammatory markers in obese patients with type 2 diabetes [67]. Leptin treatment increased the total plasma leptin, leptin-binding protein, and antileptin antibody levels, likely limiting free leptin availability at the target tissues [70]. Leptin treatment in gastric bypass patients did not produce additional weight loss, and there were no changes in fat mass, resting energy expenditure, thyroid hormone, or cortisol [50].

A combination of leptin and amylin resulted in weight loss and prevented the reduction in energy expenditure associated with weight loss [105]. A combined therapy of leptin and pramlintide (an amylin analog) also resulted in more weight loss in subjects with obesity compared to leptin or pramlintide alone [101]. In a longer study, administration of metreleptin and pramlintide to obese subjects resulted in a significant weight loss, but some subjects developed antileptin antibodies which led to suspension of the study [23].

The varied responses to leptin treatment in obese subjects may be explained by differences in leptin formulation, endogenous leptin levels, and unknown factors mediating leptin resistance. Studies of rodent models suggest leptin sensitizers may offer therapeutic value. Amylin acts synergistically with leptin to reduce adiposity in obese rodents, while preventing the compensatory reduction in energy expenditure associated with weight loss [105, 132]. Metformin, exendin-4, and fibroblast growth factor (FGF)-21 have been shown to increase leptin sensitivity in rodents [48, 73]. Exercise also increases leptin sensitivity in human skeletal muscle.

Leptin replacement overcomes hunger, reduced energy expenditure, and neuroendocrine adaptation which drives weight regain in response to weight loss. In clinical studies, leptin replacement therapy restored thyroid hormone levels, sympathetic nervous activity, and energy expenditure and reversed declines in satiation in weight-reduced individuals [49, 103]. Brain imaging studies have shown that leptin prevents alterations in neuronal activity associated with weight loss-induced homeostatic, emotional, and cognitive control of food intake [104]. These findings raise the possibility that leptin treatment may promote weight loss maintenance.

Another potential clinical use of leptin is in the area of neurodegenerative disorders such as Alzheimer's disease. Some studies indicate that leptin promotes neurogenesis, axonal growth, synaptogenesis, and neuroprotection. Prospective studies have shown that low leptin levels are associated with higher risk of dementia and Alzheimer's disease [22, 57]. Impairments in leptin signaling have been detected in Alzheimer's disease [34, 64]. Neuroprotective actions of leptin and improvement in cognition in mouse models are seen in leptin treatment as well as a bioactive leptin fragment (leptin$_{116-130}$) [25]. Hexamers derived from leptin$_{116-130}$, i.e., leptin$_{116-121}$, $_{117-122}$, $_{118-123}$, $_{120-125}$, mimic the ability of full length leptin to increase AMPA receptor trafficking and hippocampal synaptic plasticity [25]. Leptin hexamers enhanced performance in episodic memory tasks and ameliorated the synapto-toxic effects of Aβ, indicating that leptin and leptin-derived peptides are potential therapeutics for Alzheimer's disease [25].

Adiponectin

Adipose Complement Related Protein of 30 kDa (Acrp30) was identified using a subtractive cloning strategy in 3T3-L1 adipocytes [111]. Shortly thereafter, other groups working independently cloned the same gene using other methods and named it as AdipoQ [39], apM1 [59], or GBP28 [78]. The consensus name, adiponectin, was proposed in 1999 [5]. Adiponectin is expressed mainly in adipose tissue and circulates in different multimeric forms [112] (Fig. 3).

The adiponectin promoter contains binding elements for C/EBPα, PPARγ, Sterol Regulatory Element-Binding Proteins, and LRH-1 (liver receptor homolog-1) (Liu and Liu 2010). FoxO1-C/EBPα complex activates adiponectin gene transcription, and this process is facilitated by SIRT1. In contrast, FoxO1 binds to PPARγ and blocks its target genes. Although the transcriptional regulation of adiponectin is important, studies indicate that the levels of adiponectin are mainly regulated through posttranslational modification, involving folding and processing in the endoplasmic reticulum and trafficking through the Golgi apparatus.

The structure of adiponectin consists of a signal sequence at the N-terminus, followed by a variable region, a collagenous domain, and a C-terminal globular domain. The N-terminal

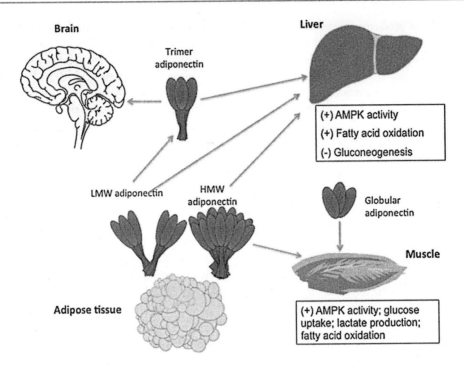

Fig. 3 Adiponectin proteins and target organs. The globular form of adiponectin, expressed in *E. coli*, stimulates fatty acid oxidation when it is administered in mice. The globular form of adiponectin is not detectable in mammalian tissues and unlikely to have a physiological function

region is important for the formation of multimers, intermolecular disulfide bond and secretion of adiponectin. In serum, adiponectin exists as globular, trimeric, hexameric, and high molecular weight (HMW) multimer. The globular adiponectin is produced by proteolytic cleavage of adiponectin. Adiponectin multimerization is regulated via hydroxylation and glycosylation. A disulfide bond between two trimers leads to the formation of a hexamer, and multimeric HMW adiponectin is formed by 12–18 monomeric adiponectin. The synthesis of adiponectin occurs in the endoplasmic reticulum of adipocytes and is regulated by endoplasmic reticulum resident protein 44 (ERp44), ER oxidoreductase1-Lα (Ero1-Lα), and disulfide-bond A oxidoreductase-like protein (DsbA-La). ERp44 retains adiponectin in the endoplasmic reticulum and inhibits secretion, and Ero1-Lα increases adiponectin secretion. After synthesis and assembly, adiponectin is exported to the Golgi network, packaged and released from adipocytes via constitutive and regulated secretion.

The trimeric adiponectin is the main form in human cerebrospinal fluid [53]. The high molecular weight (HMW, 18–36) multimer of adiponectin is abundant in plasma in females, and the trimeric and hexameric forms are abundant in plasma in males [33, 85, 90]. Unlike leptin, plasma adiponectin levels are reduced in obesity, increased following fasting, and decreased by refeeding [5]. The levels of HMW adiponectin are highly predictive of insulin sensitivity [86]. Insulin-sensitizing thiazolidinediones increase the levels of HMW adiponectin in human and mice [79]. Mice lacking adiponectin do not respond to thiazolidinedione treatment confirming that adiponectin plays an essential role in mediating the antidiabetic effect of thiazolidinediones [79].

Adiponectin Signaling

The functions of adiponectin are mediated via AdipoR1, AdipoR2, and T-cadherin. AdipoR1 and AdipoR2 contain seven-transmembrane domains that exhibit high sequence homology particularly in the membrane-spanning regions. These receptors have a unique feature that is opposite to the transmembrane topology of G-protein-coupled receptors. AdipoR1 and AdipoR2 have differences in binding affinities to adiponectin, tissue-specific expression, and signaling function. AdipoR1 mRNA is abundant in the skeletal muscle, spleen, lung, heart, kidney, and liver. AdipoR1 stimulates AMPK activation and inhibits gluconeogenesis and lipogenesis. AdipoR2 is highly expressed in the liver, induces PPARα, increases glucose uptake and fatty acid oxidation, and reduces oxidative injury and inflammation.

APPL1 and APPL2, adaptor proteins containing pleckstrin homology, phosphotyrosine binding domain, and leucine zipper motif, act downstream of AdipoR1 and AdipoR2. Adiponectin stimulation induces interaction of APPL1 with AdipoR1 or AdipoR2 leading to the downstream activation of multiple signaling via AMPK, PPARα, and p38MAPK [140], Ca^{2+}, and SIRT1 [44]. Fig. 4. Adiponectin binding to AdipoR1 and AdipoR2 also modulates ceramidase activity Activation of AMPK

suppresses lipogenesis and inflammation and promotes autophagy, and fatty acid oxidation. Adiponectin-stimulated PPARα signaling inhibits endoplasmic reticulum stress and increases fatty acid oxidation. In addition to AMPK and PPARα, adiponectin signaling involves other downstream effectors Ca^{2+}, and SIRT1 [44]. The multiple adiponectin signaling via AMPK, PPARα, and p38MAPK mediates its antidiabetic, anti-inflammatory, and antiatherogenic functions.

In addition to the canonical adiponectin receptors, AdipoR1 and AdipoR2, adiponectin binds to T-cadherin, a cell surface-anchored glycoprotein. T-cadherin is highly expressed in skeletal muscle, smooth muscle, and endothelial cells. T-cadherin lacks both cytoplasmic and transmembrane domains required for intracellular adiponectin signaling, provides a docking site for the binding of HMW adiponectin, and may serve as a regulator of adiponectin bioavailability [24, 40].

Metabolic Effects of Adiponectin

Adiponectin deficiency has been linked to obesity, insulin resistance, and metabolic syndrome

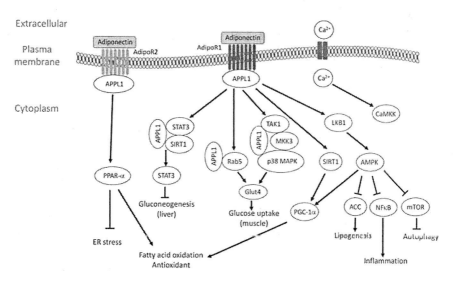

Fig. 4 Adiponectin signaling pathways. Adiponectin binds to AdipoR1 and AdipoR2 leading to interaction with APPL1 and downstream signaling via AMPK, PPARα, and p38MAPK and other molecules.

Adiponectin-induced signaling enhances glucose homeostasis, fatty acid oxidation, and autophagy, inhibits endoplasmic reticulum stress, and exerts potent antioxidant, antiatherogenic, and anti-inflammatory effects

[124, 146]. AdipoR1 and AdipoR2 levels are reduced in livers of obese mice, and this has been related to attenuation of AMPK activity and insulin resistance [144]. Adenovirus-mediated expression of AdipoR1 and AdipoR2 reverses these defects. AdipoR1 and AdipoR2 may have different roles since ablation of AdipoR1 in the liver prevents the ability of adiponectin to activate AMPK while ablation of AdipoR2 decreases PPARα signaling [144]. Deficiency of both AdipoR1 and AdipoR2 prevents adiponectin binding and induces steatosis, inflammation, oxidative stress, and insulin resistance. AdipoR1 deficiency decreases energy expenditure, increases body fat, and induces insulin resistance, while AdipoR2 deficiency increases energy expenditure, decreases body weight and fat, and improves glucose metabolism.

AdipoR1 and AdipoR2 are widely distributed in the brain, and some studies indicate that adiponectin affects energy and glucose metabolism by targeting the brain [96]. Trimeric and LMW forms of adiponectin are present in cerebrospinal fluid [26, 51, 53], and the concentration of adiponectin in cerebrospinal fluid increases after intravenous injection, consistent with blood-to-brain transport [51, 96]. Intracerebroventricular administration of adiponectin increases energy expenditure and fatty acid oxidation, and these effects may be mediated through Corticotropin Releasing Hormone and melanocortin signaling [96]. Other studies suggest an opposite effect of adiponectin on energy balance. Overexpression of adiponectin in wild-type and $Lep^{ob/ob}$ mice resulted in obesity; however, insulin resistance and inflammation were reduced in these obese mice. Systemic administration of adiponectin increased AMPK activity in the arcuate nucleus through AdipoR1 signaling, resulting in hyperphagia and weight gain [51]. In contrast, adiponectin-deficient mice displayed reduced AMPK activation in the hypothalamus, associated with reduced food intake, increased energy expenditure, and resistance to obesity. Adiponectin levels in cerebrospinal fluid are increased in response to fasting and decreased after refeeding, suggesting that adiponectin may act as a starvation signal [51].

AdipoR1 and AdipoR2 are expressed in pancreatic β-cells, and adiponectin enhances glucose-stimulated insulin secretion and prevents apoptosis of β-cells. PPARγ, MEK–ERK, and PI3K–Akt signaling mediate the effects of adiponectin on insulin secretion, while activation of ERK and Akt mediates the antiapoptotic effects of adiponectin. Adiponectin decreases blood glucose by inhibiting hepatic glucose production [11, 18]. Studies have shown that adiponectin inhibits hepatic lipogenesis in mice [142] by suppressing the expression of SREBP1c via AdipoR1–LKB1–AMPK signaling. Adiponectin may also modulate hepatic insulin signaling via IRS2–IL6–STAT3 signaling.

Adiponectin stimulates differentiation, glucose uptake, and triglyceride accumulation in 3T3-L1 adipocytes. Leptin-deficient ob/ob mice overexpressing adiponectin developed excessive fat storage in subcutaneous depots, but they were protected from visceral adiposity, steatosis, and inflammation, indicative of metabolically healthy phenotype. High plasma adiponectin levels are also associated with metabolically healthy obesity in humans, a condition characterized by increased subcutaneous fat, preservation of insulin sensitivity, reduced oxidative stress and inflammation, and lower cardiovascular risk.

Earlier studies demonstrated potent effects of the globular (head) form of adiponectin on fatty acid oxidation in skeletal muscle (Fig. 3). Adiponectin stimulates AMPK phosphorylation and activity, inhibits acetyl-CoA carboxylase [131, 143], increases expression of acetyl-CoA oxidase, Uncoupling Protein-2, and Uncoupling Protein-3, and activates p38 MAPK and PPARα [145]. Adiponectin also signals through calcium-mediated pathway via AMPK to affect mitochondrial function in myocytes [44]. Adiponectin acting through AdipoR1 in skeletal muscle triggers extracellular Ca^{2+} influx, leading to activation of Ca^{2+}/calmodulin-dependent protein kinase kinase β (CaMKKβ), AMPK, SIRT1, and PGC-1α, which enhances mitochondrial function and fatty acid oxidation [44].

Effects of Adiponectin on Inflammation and Cardiovascular Risk

Adiponectin exerts major cardioprotective effects by modulating LDL, HDL, and total cholesterol and glucose levels and inflammation [84, 94, 106, 113, 146]. Adiponectin knockout mice are more vulnerable to vascular and myocardial injury, while adenovirus overexpression of adiponectin protects adiponectin knockout and wild-type mice from myocardial ischemia [116]. These effects may be mediated through AdipoR1 and AdipoR2 acting via ceramidase activity [38]. T-cadherin binds adiponectin in cardiomyocytes and may be involved in cardioprotection, as evident by the increased susceptibility of T-cadherin knockout mice to myocardial injury [24].

Adiponectin reduces oxidative stress and improves endothelial function through activation of AMPK–eNOS and PKA signaling [139]. Calreticulin/CD91-PI3K-Akt-COX2 signaling also serves as a downstream mediator of adiponectin in blood vessels (Ohashi et al. 2009). Population studies have demonstrated associations of adiponectin and proteinuria in patients with chronic kidney disease. In mice, adiponectin decreases oxidative injury and albumin permeability in podocytes and ameliorates renal interstitial fibrosis. Adiponectin has direct anti-inflammatory effects on macrophages in adipose tissue, promoting a switch from pro-inflammatory M1 to anti-inflammatory M2 macrophages. Adiponectin stimulates transcription of IL-6, and this has been linked to elevated plasma IL-6 levels and IRS-2 expression and hepatic insulin signaling.

Role of Adiponectin in Cancer

Epidemiological studies have established a strong association of adiponectin and cancer [20], particularly endometrium [91, 123], breast [12, 60], colon [137], and kidney [120]. Adiponectin levels are also associated with leukemia [92], lymphoma [93], myeloma (Dalamaga et al. 2009), and chronic lymphocytic leukemia. The underlying mechanisms are unclear and may involve effects of adiponectin on other tumorigenic factors or direct AdipoR-mediated cellular signaling regulating insulin sensitivity, tumor growth, and angiogenesis. Some in vitro studies have shown potent proangiogenic and tumorigenic effects of adiponectin mediated partly by local changes in sphingosine levels and ceramidase activity.

Resistin

Resistin is a cysteine-rich protein that was discovered during a search for genes downregulated by thiazolidinedione drugs [121]. Murine resistin is mainly expressed in mature white adipocytes, suppressed by thiazolidinediones and insulin treatment and upregulated by glucose [98]. Resistin expression in mouse adipocytes is also inhibited by inflammatory cytokines, e.g., TNF-α. Resistin is decreased in the adipose tissue during fasting and increased in response to refeeding in mice [98, 100, 121]. Obese mice have high plasma resistin levels; however, resistin mRNA expression is suppressed in adipose tissue in these mice [100]. Unlike murine resistin, human resistin is expressed in monocytes and macrophages and is induced by TNF-α. The lack of resistin expression in human adipocytes may be due to loss of a genomic binding site for PPARγ which controls resistin gene (retn) expression in mouse adipocytes [130].

Murine resistin circulates mainly as a disulfide-linked hexamer, but a smaller trimeric protein is also detected. The trimeric form of resistin is more potent in decreasing hepatic insulin sensitivity in mice. However, oligomerization is necessary for the inhibitory action of resistin on glucose uptake in cardiomyocytes. Human resistin also circulates as trimeric and oligomeric forms, and the latter is thought to be more potent in stimulating the production of inflammatory cytokines [6, 31, 32].

Resistin Signaling

The resistin receptor has not yet been clarified; however, studies indicate that decorin and tyrosine kinase-like orphan receptor 1 resistin receptors may mediate effects of resistin on WAT expansion or modulate glucose homeostasis [107]. Murine resistin decreases the phosphorylation of AMPK in the liver, skeletal muscle, and WAT [10]. Resistin inhibits the phosphorylation of insulin receptor substrates and activation of phosphatidylinositol-3-kinase (PI3K) and protein kinase B/Akt in the liver, muscle, and WAT [122]. Resistin induces SOCS3, a known inhibitor of insulin signaling, in the liver, muscle, and WAT [54, 75, 122].

Adenylyl cyclase-associated protein 1 (CAP1) has been identified as a functional resistin receptor. Human resistin binds directly to CAP1 in monocytes and increases cAMP, PKA activity, and NF-κB-mediated transcription of inflammatory cytokines. CAP1 overexpression in monocytes enhances the effects of resistin treatment. In contrast, a reduction of CAP1 expression reduced the effects of resistin on inflammatory activity in monocytes as well as in transgenic mice expressing human resistin.

Metabolic Effects of Resistin in Rodents

Earlier studies demonstrated potent effects of resistin on glucose homeostasis in mice. Neutralization of resistin with antiresistin antibody enhanced insulin sensitivity in obese mice [121]. CNS or systemic resistin treatment or transgenic overexpression of resistin induced hepatic insulin resistance in mice [99, 121]. In contrast, the deletion or knockdown of resistin increased hepatic insulin sensitivity in obese mice [10]. Resistin knockout mice developed hypoglycemia during fasting, associated with suppression of gluconeogenic enzymes in the liver [10]. Resistin treatment of 3 T3-L1 adipocytes, murine cardiomyocytes, and skeletal muscle cells decreased insulin-stimulated glucose uptake [121], indicating that resistin plays an important role in glucose homeostasis in rodents. Resistin also promotes fatty liver in mouse models [119].

Biological Effects of Human Resistin

The expression of human resistin is increased in peripheral mononuclear cells as they differentiate into macrophages [108, 128]. Thiazolidinedione drugs suppress the expression of human resistin in macrophages. Resistin is also detectable in the stromal vascular fraction in the WAT, cirrhotic liver, and atherosclerotic lesions, consistent with the view that macrophages are the main source of human resistin [47, 108]. Given the potent metabolic effects of murine resistin, there are questions concerning the biological actions of human resistin.

Epidemiological studies have revealed conflicting associations of resistin and obesity in humans (Azuma et al. 2003; [45, 63, 72, 102]). However, some studies have suggested positive associations of resistin and inflammation, insulin resistance, and cardiovascular diseases. Several single-nucleotide polymorphisms (SNPs) are associated with resistin levels [65]. The $-638\ \mathrm{G} > \mathrm{A}$, $-420\ \mathrm{C} > \mathrm{G}$, and $-358\ \mathrm{G} > \mathrm{A}$ polymorphisms in the promoter region of human resistin gene (*RETN*) were associated with resistin levels in Japanese obese individuals [8]. The G/G genotype at SNP -420 in *RETN* was associated with susceptibility to type 2 diabetes and also was correlated with monocyte resistin expression and plasma resistin levels [82]. A cross-sectional study in Japanese subjects showed that plasma resistin was associated with SNP -420 and also correlated with insulin resistance [83]. The $-420\mathrm{G}$ and $-537\mathrm{A}$ alleles were associated with increased resistin levels but not with T2DM in a Korean cohort. Among Chinese, both $-420\mathrm{G}$ and $+62\mathrm{A}$ alleles were strongly predictive of glucose levels [141]. A study in Italy showed that the presence of -420 C/G SNP in *RETN* was associated with obesity and metabolic syndrome [80]. In the Framingham Offspring Study, SNPs in the 3$'$ region of *RETN* were associated with resistin levels [37]. El-Shal et al. [27] found that both $-420\ \mathrm{C} > \mathrm{G}$ and $+299\ \mathrm{G} > \mathrm{A}$ SNP were significantly associated with resistin, obesity, and insulin resistance in obese people in Egypt.

Tang et al. [127] have reported that −420 C/G SNP in *RETN* is associated with coronary artery disease, but studies of the −420 variant in Europeans and Caucasians found no correlation with atherosclerosis [80]. How may resistin affect the development of atherosclerosis? Human resistin increases the proliferation and migration of human endothelial and vascular smooth muscle cells, mediated through PI3K or p38 mitogen-activated protein kinase signaling pathways. Resistin attenuates insulin signaling, inhibits endothelial nitric oxide synthase, and increases oxidative stress in endothelial cells. In addition, resistin increases intercellular adhesion molecule-1, vascular cell adhesion molecule-1, P-selectin, fractalkine, Monocyte Chemoattractant Protein-1, PAI-1, endothelin-1, matrix metalloproteinases, and vascular endothelial growth factor receptors, which increase monocyte adhesion in vascular endothelial cells [47, 134]. Resistin promotes foam cell transformation [47] and induces thrombosis via tissue factor expression in human coronary artery endothelial cells [46].

Plasma resistin levels correlate with inflammatory and fibrinolytic markers such as C-reactive protein (CRP), TNF-α, IL-6, or plasminogen activator inhibitor (PAI)-1 in type 2 diabetes, coronary artery disease, chronic kidney disease, and sepsis [63, 102, 115, 125] as well as the general population ([28, 52, 83, 97, 102]; Konrad et al. 2007). Hyper-resistinemia has been observed in patients with rheumatoid arthritis and inflammatory bowel disease and tracks well with disease activity [31]. Elevated resistin levels are related to disease severity of sepsis and acute pancreatitis and predictive of mortality in critically ill patients [125].

To understand the molecular pathways mediating the biology of human resistin, Qatanani et al. [95] produced a transgenic mouse expressing human resistin via a macrophage promoter and bred them with resistin knockout mice. The "humanized" resistin mice developed inflammation and insulin resistance consistent with epidemiological studies [17, 114]. To further elucidate the biology of human resistin, Park et al. [89] generated mice lacking murine resistin but transgenic for a bacterial artificial chromosome containing human resistin (BAC-Retn).

Lipopolysaccharide treatment increased resistin levels in this model and resulted in mild hypoglycemia. The BAC-Retn mice developed hepatic insulin resistance under chronic endotoxemia, accompanied by inflammation in the liver and skeletal muscle [89]. These results are in agreement with a study showing that resistin competes with lipopolysaccharide (LPS) for binding to Toll-like receptor 4 (TLR4) to mediate the pro-inflammatory action of resistin [129].

Batokines

Brown adipose tissue (BAT) is abundant in neonatal humans, regresses in adults, and is restricted to the cervical, paravertebral, and perirenal regions. Beige or brite adipose tissue is composed of adipocytes with BAT characteristics interspersed within white adipose tissue (WAT). In addition to its thermogenic function, emerging research shows that BAT secretes molecular mediators known as "batokines" [4, 110, 135, 136] (Table 2).

FGF21 is produced and secreted by the liver and mediates several functions. In rodents, Fgf21 is produced and secreted from BAT in response to thermogenic stimulation. Human brown adipocytes express minimal FGF21 mRNA and protein levels; however, FGF21 enhances thermogenesis in human brown adipocytes. FGF21-mediated browning of WAT is associated with weight loss in mice. Further studies are needed to delineate the specific functions of liver-derived versus BAT-derived FGF21.

Interleukin (IL)-6 is a cytokine with multiple functions including acute inflammatory response, and as a myokine promoting muscle growth and glucose uptake. IL-6 has also been shown to promote exercise-induced browning of WAT. Interleukin-6 (IL6) is synthesized and secreted by BAT in response β-adrenergic stimuli. Acute release of IL-6 from BAT enhances hepatic gluconeogenesis, suggesting a BAT-liver crosstalk in glucose metabolism.

Myocytes and brown adipocytes are derived from mesenchymal stem cells and share similarities in precursor transcriptome profile. In mice, BAT is the main thermogenic organ, while in humans skeletal muscle is the major site of thermogenesis after infancy. Myostatin expressed in skeletal muscle in mice and humans acts via autocrine mechanism to inhibit muscle growth. Myostatin is expressed in mouse BAT, and upregulation of BAT myostatin modulates muscle function and insulin sensitivity. These findings suggest crosstalk between BAT and skeletal muscle, and possibly other organs.

BAT has resident immune cells which regulate BAT thermogenic activity and exert systemic effects. CXCL14 is synthesized in BAT in response to thermogenic activation, recruits alternatively activated macrophages into BAT, and promotes adaptive thermogenesis and M2-mediated browning of inguinal WAT in mice.

Conclusion

This review highlights the roles of adipose tissue in energy homeostasis and the biology of adipokines and other secreted proteins that mediate a variety of local and systemic functions. A better understanding of the production and signaling pathways of adipokines will benefit the diagnosis and treatment of diabetes, lipid disorders, cardiovascular diseases, cancer, and other diseases associated with obesity. Future research requires systematic approaches in human and animal models to elucidate how adipokines specifically affect energy homeostasis and other physiological processes via hormonal, paracrine, or autocrine mechanisms and how these affect the pathogenesis of various diseases.

Cross-References

▷ Adipose Structure (White, Brown, Beige)
▷ Brain Regulation of Feeding and Energy Homeostasis
▷ Insulin Resistance in Obesity
▷ Linking Inflammation, Obesity, and Diabetes
▷ Overview of Metabolic Syndrome

Acknowledgments This chapter was supported by grants R01DK135751 and RF1 AG059621 from the US National Institutes of Health, American Heart Association Obesity Research Network, and Cardiometabolic Health and Type 2 Diabetes Research Network.

References

1. Ahima RS, Osei SY. Leptin signaling. Physiol Behav. 2004;81(2):223–41. https://doi.org/10.1016/j.physbeh.2004.02.014.
2. Ahima RS, Prabakaran D, Mantzoros C, et al. Role of leptin in the neuroendocrine response to fasting. Nature. 1996;382(6588):250–2. https://doi.org/10.1038/382250a0.
3. Ahima RS, Kelly J, Elmquist JK, et al. Distinct physiologic and neuronal responses to decreased leptin and mild hyperleptinemia. Endocrinology. 1999;140(11):4923–31. https://doi.org/10.1210/endo.140.11.7105.
4. Ahmad B, Vohra MS, Saleemi MA, Serpell CJ, Fong IL, Wong EH. Brown/beige adipose tissues and the emerging role of their secretory factors in improving metabolic health: the batokines. Biochimie. 2021;184:26–39. https://doi.org/10.1016/j.biochi.2021.01.015. Epub 2021 Feb 4. PMID: 33548390
5. Arita Y, Kihara S, Ouchi N, et al. Paradoxical decrease of an adipose-specific protein, adiponectin, in obesity. Biochem Biophys Res Commun. 1999;257(1):79–83.
6. Aruna B, Islam A, Ghosh S, et al. Biophysical analyses of human resistin: oligomer formation suggests novel biological function. Biochemistry. 2008;47(47):12457–66. https://doi.org/10.1021/bi801266k.
7. Asilmaz E, Cohen P, Miyazaki M, et al. Site and mechanism of leptin action in a rodent form of congenital lipodystrophy. J Clin Invest. 2004;113(3):414–24. https://doi.org/10.1172/JCI19511.
8. Azuma K, Oguchi S, Matsubara Y, et al. Novel resistin promoter polymorphisms: association with serum resistin level in Japanese obese individuals. Horm Metab Res. 2004;36(8):564–70. https://doi.org/10.1055/s-2004-825762.
9. Balland E, Dam J, Langlet F, et al. Hypothalamic tanycytes are an ERK-gated conduit for leptin into the brain. Cell Metab. 2014;19(2):293–301. https://doi.org/10.1016/j.cmet.2013.12.015.
10. Banerjee RR, Rangwala SM, Shapiro JS, et al. Regulation of fasted blood glucose by resistin. Science. 2004;303(5661):1195–8. https://doi.org/10.1126/science.1092341.
11. Berg AH, Combs TP, Du X, et al. The adipocyte-secreted protein Acrp30 enhances hepatic insulin action. Nat Med. 2001;7(8):947–53. https://doi.org/10.1038/90992.
12. Brown JC, Ligibel JA, Crane TE, Kontos D, Yang S, Conant EF, Mack JA, Ahima RS, Schmitz KH. Obesity and metabolic dysfunction correlate with background parenchymal enhancement in

premenopausal women. Obesity (Silver Spring). 2023;31(2):479–86. https://doi.org/10.1002/oby. 23649. Epub 2023 Jan 11. PMID: 36628617

13. Carbone F, La Rocca C, Matarese G. Immunological functions of leptin and adiponectin. Biochimie. 2012;94(10):2082–8. https://doi.org/10.1016/j. biochi.2012.05.018.

14. Chan JL, Mantzoros CS. Role of leptin in energy-deprivation states: normal human physiology and clinical implications for hypothalamic amenorrhoea and anorexia nervosa. Lancet. 2005;366(9479):74–85. https://doi.org/10.1016/S0140-6736(05)66830-4.

15. Chan JL, Heist K, DePaoli AM, et al. The role of falling leptin levels in the neuroendocrine and metabolic adaptation to short-term starvation in healthy men. J Clin Invest. 2003;111(9):1409–21. https://doi.org/10.1172/JCI17490.

16. Chan JL, Lutz K, Cochran E, et al. Clinical effects of long-term metreleptin treatment in patients with lipodystrophy. Endocr Pract Off J Am Coll Endocrinol Am Assoc Clin Endocrinol. 2011;17(6):922–32. https://doi.org/10.4158/EP11229.OR.

17. Chen BH, Song Y, Ding EL, et al. Circulating levels of resistin and risk of type 2 diabetes in men and women: results from two prospective cohorts. Diabetes Care. 2009;32(2):329–34. https://doi.org/10.2337/dc08-1625.

18. Combs TP, Berg AH, Obici S, et al. Endogenous glucose production is inhibited by the adipose-derived protein Acrp30. J Clin Invest. 2001;108(12):1875–81. https://doi.org/10.1172/JCI14120.

19. Considine RV, Sinha MK, Heiman ML, et al. Serum immunoreactive-leptin concentrations in normal-weight and obese humans. N Engl J Med. 1996;334(5):292–5. https://doi.org/10.1056/NEJM199602013340503.

20. Dalamaga M, Diakopoulos KN, Mantzoros CS. The role of adiponectin in cancer: a review of current evidence. Endocr Rev. 2012;33(4):547–94. https://doi.org/10.1210/er.2011-1015.

21. Dalamaga M, Chou SH, Shields K, et al. Leptin at the intersection of neuroendocrinology and metabolism: current evidence and therapeutic perspectives. Cell Metab. 2013;18(1):29–42. https://doi.org/10.1016/j. cmet.2013.05.010.

22. Davis C, Mudd J, Hawkins M. Neuroprotective effects of leptin in the context of obesity and metabolic disorders. Neurobiol Dis. 2014; https://doi.org/10.1016/j.nbd.2014.04.012.

23. Depaoli A, Long A, Fine GM, Stewart M, Rahilly S. Efficacy of metreleptin for weight loss in overweight and obese adults with low leptin levels. Diabetes. 2018;67:296–LB. https://doi.org/10.2337/db18-296-LB.

24. Denzel MS, Scimia MC, Zumstein PM, et al. T-cadherin is critical for adiponectin-mediated cardioprotection in mice. J Clin Invest. 2010;120(12):4342–52. https://doi.org/10.1172/JCI43464.

25. Doherty G, Holiday A, Malekizadeh Y, Manolescu C, Duncan S, Flewitt I, Hamilton K, MacLeod B, Ainge JA, Harvey J. Leptin-based hexamers facilitate memory and prevent amyloid-driven AMPA receptor internalization and neuronal degeneration. J Neurochem. 2023;165(6):809–26. https://doi.org/10.1111/jnc. 15733. Epub 2022 Dec 14. PMID: 36444683

26. Ebinuma H, Miida T, Yamauchi T, et al. Improved ELISA for selective measurement of adiponectin multimers and identification of adiponectin in human cerebrospinal fluid. Clin Chem. 2007;53(8):1541–4. https://doi.org/10.1373/clinchem.2007. 085654.

27. El-Shal AS, Pasha HF, Rashad NM. Association of resistin gene polymorphisms with insulin resistance in Egyptian obese patients. Gene. 2013;515(1):233–8. https://doi.org/10.1016/j.gene.2012.09.136.

28. Fargnoli JL, Sun Q, Olenczuk D, et al. Resistin is associated with biomarkers of inflammation while total and high-molecular weight adiponectin are associated with biomarkers of inflammation, insulin resistance, and endothelial function. Eur J Endocrinol/Eur Fed Endocr Soc. 2010;162(2):281–8. https://doi.org/10.1530/EJE-09-0555.

29. Farooqi IS, Jebb SA, Langmack G, et al. Effects of recombinant leptin therapy in a child with congenital leptin deficiency. N Engl J Med. 1999;341(12):879–84. https://doi.org/10.1056/NEJM199909163411204.

30. Farooqi IS, Matarese G, Lord GM, et al. Beneficial effects of leptin on obesity, T cell hyporesponsiveness, and neuroendocrine/metabolic dysfunction of human congenital leptin deficiency. J Clin Invest. 2002;110(8):1093–103. https://doi.org/10.1172/JCI15693.

31. Filkova M, Haluzik M, Gay S, et al. The role of resistin as a regulator of inflammation: implications for various human pathologies. Clin Immunol. 2009;133(2):157–70. https://doi.org/10.1016/j.clim. 2009.07.013.

32. Gerber M, Boettner A, Seidel B, et al. Serum resistin levels of obese and lean children and adolescents: biochemical analysis and clinical relevance. J Clin Endocrinol Metab. 2005;90(8):4503–9. https://doi. org/10.1210/jc.2005-0437.

33. Hamilton MP, Gore MO, Ayers CR, et al. Adiponectin and cardiovascular risk profile in patients with type 2 diabetes mellitus: parameters associated with adiponectin complex distribution. Diab Vasc Dis Res. 2011;8(3):190–4. https://doi.org/10.1177/1479164111407784.

34. Hamilton K, Harvey J. Leptin regulation of hippocampal synaptic function in health and disease. Vitam Horm. 2021;115:105–27. https://doi.org/10.1016/bs. vh.2020.12.006. Epub 2021 Jan 30. PMID: 33706945

35. Hausman GJ, Barb CR, Lents CA. Leptin and reproductive function. Biochimie. 2012;94(10):2075–81. https://doi.org/10.1016/j.biochi.2012.02.022.

36. Heymsfield SB, Greenberg AS, Fujioka K, Dixon RM, Kushner R, Hunt T, et al. Recombinant leptin

for weight loss in obese and lean adults: a randomized, controlled, dose-escalation trial. JAMA. 1999;282:1568–75. https://doi.org/10.1001/jama.282.16.1568.

37. Hivert MF, Manning AK, McAteer JB, et al. Association of variants in RETN with plasma resistin levels and diabetes-related traits in the Framingham Offspring Study. Diabetes. 2009;58(3):750–6. https://doi.org/10.2337/db08-1339.

38. Holland WL, Miller RA, Wang ZV, et al. Receptor-mediated activation of ceramidase activity initiates the pleiotropic actions of adiponectin. Nat Med. 2011;17(1):55–63. https://doi.org/10.1038/nm.2277.

39. Hu E, Liang P, Spiegelman BM. AdipoQ is a novel adipose-specific gene dysregulated in obesity. J Biol Chem. 1996;271:10697–703. [PubMed] [Google Scholar]

40. Hug C, Wang J, Ahmad NS, et al. T-cadherin is a receptor for hexameric and high-molecular-weight forms of Acrp30/adiponectin. Proc Natl Acad Sci U S A. 2004;101(28):10308–13. https://doi.org/10.1073/pnas.0403382101.

41. Hukshorn CJ, van Dielen FM, Buurman WA, et al. The effect of pegylated recombinant human leptin (PEG-OB) on weight loss and inflammatory status in obese subjects. Int J Obes Relat Metab Disord J Int Assoc Study Obes. 2002;26(4):504–9.

42. Hukshorn CJ, Saris WH, Westerterp-Plantenga MS, Farid AR, Smith FJ, Campfield LA. Weekly subcutaneous pegylated recombinant native human leptin (PEG-OB) administration in obese men. J Clin Endocrinol Metab. 2000;85:4003–9. https://doi.org/10.1210/jcem.85.11.6955.

43. Hukshorn CJ, Westerterp-Plantenga MS, Saris WH. Pegylated human recombinant leptin (PEG-OB) causes additional weight loss in severely energy-restricted, overweight men. Am J Clin Nutr. 2003;77:771–6. https://doi.org/10.1093/ajcn/77.4.771.

44. Iwabu M, Yamauchi T, Okada-Iwabu M, et al. Adiponectin and AdipoR1 regulate PGC-1alpha and mitochondria by Ca(2+) and AMPK/SIRT1. Nature. 2010;464(7293):1313–9. https://doi.org/10.1038/nature08991.

45. Jain SH, Massaro JM, Hoffmann U, et al. Cross-sectional associations between abdominal and thoracic adipose tissue compartments and adiponectin and resistin in the Framingham Heart Study. Diabetes Care. 2009;32(5):903–8. https://doi.org/10.2337/dc08-1733.

46. Jamaluddin MS, Weakley SM, Yao Q, et al. Resistin: functional roles and therapeutic considerations for cardiovascular disease. Br J Pharmacol. 2012;165(3):622–32. https://doi.org/10.1111/j.1476-5381.2011.01369.x.

47. Jung HS, Park KH, Cho YM, et al. Resistin is secreted from macrophages in atheromas and promotes atherosclerosis. Cardiovasc Res. 2006;69(1):76–85. https://doi.org/10.1016/j.cardiores.2005.09.015.

48. Kim YW, Kim JY, Park YH, et al. Metformin restores leptin sensitivity in high-fat-fed obese rats with leptin resistance. Diabetes. 2006;55(3):716–24.

49. Kissileff HR, Thornton JC, Torres MI, et al. Leptin reverses declines in satiation in weight-reduced obese humans. Am J Clin Nutr. 2012;95(2):309–17. https://doi.org/10.3945/ajcn.111.012385.

50. Korner J, Conroy R, Febres G, McMahon DJ, Conwell I, Karmally W, et al. Randomized double-blind placebo-controlled study of leptin administration after gastric bypass. Obes (Silver Spring). 2013;21:951–6. https://doi.org/10.1002/oby.20433.

51. Kubota N, Yano W, Kubota T, et al. Adiponectin stimulates AMP-activated protein kinase in the hypothalamus and increases food intake. Cell Metab. 2007;6(1):55–68. https://doi.org/10.1016/j.cmet.2007.06.003.

52. Kunnari A, Ukkola O, Paivansalo M, et al. High plasma resistin level is associated with enhanced highly sensitive C-reactive protein and leukocytes. J Clin Endocrinol Metab. 2006;91(7):2755–60. https://doi.org/10.1210/jc.2005-2115.

53. Kusminski CM, McTernan PG, Schraw T, et al. Adiponectin complexes in human cerebrospinal fluid: distinct complex distribution from serum. Diabetologia. 2007;50(3):634–42. https://doi.org/10.1007/s00125-006-0577-9.

54. Lazar MA. Resistin- and obesity-associated metabolic diseases. Horm Metab Res. 2007;39(10):710–6. https://doi.org/10.1055/s-2007-985897.

55. Lee JH, Chan JL, Sourlas E, et al. Recombinant methionyl human leptin therapy in replacement doses improves insulin resistance and metabolic profile in patients with lipoatrophy and metabolic syndrome induced by the highly active antiretroviral therapy. J Clin Endocrinol Metab. 2006;91(7):2605–11. https://doi.org/10.1210/jc.2005-1545.

56. Licinio J, Mantzoros C, Negrao AB, et al. Human leptin levels are pulsatile and inversely related to pituitary-adrenal function. Nat Med. 1997;3(5):575–9.

57. Lieb W, Beiser AS, Vasan RS, et al. Association of plasma leptin levels with incident Alzheimer disease and MRI measures of brain aging. JAMA. 2009;302(23):2565–72. https://doi.org/10.1001/jama.2009.1836.

58. Lord GM, Matarese G, Howard JK, et al. Leptin modulates the T-cell immune response and reverses starvation-induced immunosuppression. Nature. 1998;394(6696):897–901. https://doi.org/10.1038/29795.

59. Maeda K, et al. cDNA cloning and expression of a novel adipose specific collagen-like factor, apM1 (AdiPose Most abundant Gene transcript 1). Biochem Biophys Res Commun. 1996;221:286–9. [PubMed] [Google Scholar].

60. Mantzoros C, Petridou E, Dessypris N, et al. Adiponectin and breast cancer risk. J Clin Endocrinol

Metab. 2004;89(3):1102–7. https://doi.org/10.1210/jc.2003-031804.

61. Matarese G, La Rocca C, Moon HS, et al. Selective capacity of metreleptin administration to reconstitute CD4+ T-cell number in females with acquired hypoleptinemia. Proc Natl Acad Sci U S A. 2013;110(9): E818–27. https://doi.org/10.1073/pnas.1214554110.

62. Matochik JA, London ED, Yildiz BO, et al. Effect of leptin replacement on brain structure in genetically leptin-deficient adults. J Clin Endocrinol Metab. 2005;90(5):2851–4. https://doi.org/10.1210/jc.2004-1979.

63. McTernan PG, Fisher FM, Valsamakis G, et al. Resistin and type 2 diabetes: regulation of resistin expression by insulin and rosiglitazone and the effects of recombinant resistin on lipid and glucose metabolism in human differentiated adipocytes. J Clin Endocrinol Metab. 2003;88(12):6098–106. https://doi.org/10.1210/jc.2003-030898.

64. Mejido DCP, Peny JA, Vieira MNN, Ferreira ST, De Felice FG. Insulin and leptin as potential cognitive enhancers in metabolic disorders and Alzheimer' disease. Neuropharmacology. 2020;171:108115. https://doi.org/10.1016/j.neuropharm.2020.108115. Epub 2020 Apr 25. PMID: 32344008

65. Menzaghi C, Coco A, Salvemini L, et al. Heritability of serum resistin and its genetic correlation with insulin resistance-related features in nondiabetic Caucasians. J Clin Endocrinol Metab. 2006;91(7):2792–5. https://doi.org/10.1210/jc.2005-2715.

66. Miller KK, Parulekar MS, Schoenfeld E, et al. Decreased leptin levels in normal weight women with hypothalamic amenorrhea: the effects of body composition and nutritional intake. J Clin Endocrinol Metab. 1998;83(7):2309–12. https://doi.org/10.1210/jcem.83.7.4975.

67. Mittendorfer B, Horowitz JF, DePaoli AM, et al. Recombinant human leptin treatment does not improve insulin action in obese subjects with type 2 diabetes. Diabetes. 2011;60(5):1474–7. https://doi.org/10.2337/db10-1302.

68. Montague CT, Prins JB, Sanders L, et al. Depot- and sex-specific differences in human leptin mRNA expression: implications for the control of regional fat distribution. Diabetes. 1997;46(3):342–7.

69. Moon HS, Chamberland JP, Diakopoulos KN, et al. Leptin and amylin act in an additive manner to activate overlapping signaling pathways in peripheral tissues: in vitro and ex vivo studies in humans. Diabetes Care. 2011a;34(1):132–8. https://doi.org/10.2337/dc10-0518.

70. Moon HS, Matarese G, Brennan AM, et al. Efficacy of metreleptin in obese patients with type 2 diabetes: cellular and molecular pathways underlying leptin tolerance. Diabetes. 2011b;60(6):1647–56. https://doi.org/10.2337/db10-1791.

71. Moon HS, Dalamaga M, Kim SY, et al. Leptin's role in lipodystrophic and nonlipodystrophic insulin-resistant and diabetic individuals. Endocr Rev. 2013;34(3):377–412. https://doi.org/10.1210/er.2012-1053.

72. Moschen AR, Molnar C, Wolf AM, et al. Effects of weight loss induced by bariatric surgery on hepatic adipocytokine expression. J Hepatol. 2009;51(4):765–77. https://doi.org/10.1016/j.jhep.2009.06.016.

73. Muller TD, Sullivan LM, Habegger K, et al. Restoration of leptin responsiveness in diet-induced obese mice using an optimized leptin analog in combination with exendin-4 or FGF21. J Pept Sci Off Publ Eur Pept Soc. 2012;18(6):383–93. https://doi.org/10.1002/psc.2408.

74. Mulligan K, Khatami H, Schwarz JM, et al. The effects of recombinant human leptin on visceral fat, dyslipidemia, and insulin resistance in patients with human immunodeficiency virus-associated lipoatrophy and hypoleptinemia. J Clin Endocrinol Metab. 2009;94(4):1137–44. https://doi.org/10.1210/jc.2008-1588.

75. Muse ED, Lam TK, Scherer PE, et al. Hypothalamic resistin induces hepatic insulin resistance. J Clin Invest. 2007;117(6):1670–8. https://doi.org/10.1172/JCI30440.

76. Musso C, Cochran E, Javor E, et al. The long-term effect of recombinant methionyl human leptin therapy on hyperandrogenism and menstrual function in female and pituitary function in male and female hypoleptinemic lipodystrophic patients. Metab Clin Exp. 2005;54(2):255–63. https://doi.org/10.1016/j.metabol.2004.08.021.

77. Myers MG Jr, Heymsfield SB, Haft C, et al. Challenges and opportunities of defining clinical leptin resistance. Cell Metab. 2012;15(2):150–6. https://doi.org/10.1016/j.cmet.2012.01.002.

78. Nakano Y, Tobe T, Choi-Miura NH, Mazda T, Tomita M. Isolation and characterization of GBP28, a novel gelatin-binding protein purified from human plasma. J Biochem (Tokyo). 1996;120:803–12. [PubMed] [Google Scholar]

79. Nawrocki AR, Rajala MW, Tomas E, et al. Mice lacking adiponectin show decreased hepatic insulin sensitivity and reduced responsiveness to peroxisome proliferator-activated receptor gamma agonists. J Biol Chem. 2006;281(5):2654–60. https://doi.org/10.1074/jbc.M505311200.

80. Norata GD, Ongari M, Garlaschelli K, et al. Effect of the -420C/G variant of the resistin gene promoter on metabolic syndrome, obesity, myocardial infarction and kidney dysfunction. J Intern Med. 2007;262(1):104–12. https://doi.org/10.1111/j.1365-2796.2007.01787.x.

81. Oral EA, Simha V, Ruiz E, et al. Leptin-replacement therapy for lipodystrophy. N Engl J Med. 2002;346 (8):570–8. https://doi.org/10.1056/NEJMoa012437.

82. Osawa H, Yamada K, Onuma H, et al. The G/G genotype of a resistin single-nucleotide polymorphism at −420 increases type 2 diabetes mellitus susceptibility by inducing promoter activity through

specific binding of Sp1/3. Am J Hum Genet. 2004;75 (4):678–86. https://doi.org/10.1086/424761.

83. Osawa H, Tabara Y, Kawamoto R, et al. Plasma resistin, associated with single nucleotide polymorphism −420, is correlated with insulin resistance, lower HDL cholesterol, and high-sensitivity C-reactive protein in the Japanese general population. Diabetes Care. 2007;30(6):1501–6. https://doi.org/10.2337/dc06-1936.

84. Otsuka F, Sugiyama S, Kojima S, et al. Plasma adiponectin levels are associated with coronary lesion complexity in men with coronary artery disease. J Am Coll Cardiol. 2006;48(6):1155–62. https://doi.org/10.1016/j.jacc.2006.05.054.

85. Pajvani UB, Du X, Combs TP, et al. Structure-function studies of the adipocyte-secreted hormone Acrp30/adiponectin. Implications for metabolic regulation and bioactivity. J Biol Chem. 2003;278(11): 9073–85. https://doi.org/10.1074/jbc.M207198200.

86. Pajvani UB, Hawkins M, Combs TP, et al. Complex distribution, not absolute amount of adiponectin, correlates with thiazolidinedione-mediated improvement in insulin sensitivity. J Biol Chem. 2004;279(13): 12152–62. https://doi.org/10.1074/jbc.M311113200.

87. Park HK, Ahima RS. Leptin signaling. F1000Prime Rep. 2014;6:73. https://doi.org/10.12703/P6-73. eCollection 2014

88. Park HK, Ahima RS. Physiology of leptin: energy homeostasis, neuroendocrine function and metabolism. Metabolism. 2015;64(1):24–34. https://doi.org/10.1016/j.metabol.2014.08.004. Epub 2014 Aug 15

89. Park HK, Qatanani M, Briggs ER, et al. Inflammatory induction of human resistin causes insulin resistance in endotoxemic mice. Diabetes. 2011;60(3):775–83. https://doi.org/10.2337/db10-1416.

90. Peake PW, Kriketos AD, Campbell LV, et al. The metabolism of isoforms of human adiponectin: studies in human subjects and in experimental animals. Eur J Endocrinol/Eur Fed Endocr Soc. 2005;153(3): 409–17. https://doi.org/10.1530/eje.1.01978.

91. Petridou E, Mantzoros C, Dessypris N, et al. Plasma adiponectin concentrations in relation to endometrial cancer: a case–control study in Greece. J Clin Endocrinol Metab. 2003;88(3):993–7. https://doi.org/10.1210/jc.2002-021209.

92. Petridou E, Mantzoros CS, Dessypris N, et al. Adiponectin in relation to childhood myeloblastic leukaemia. Br J Cancer. 2006;94(1):156–60. https://doi.org/10.1038/sj.bjc.6602896.

93. Petridou ET, Sergentanis TN, Dessypris N, et al. Serum adiponectin as a predictor of childhood non-Hodgkin's lymphoma: a nationwide case–control study. J Clin Oncol Off J Am Soc Clin Oncol. 2009;27(30):5049–55. https://doi.org/10.1200/JCO.2008.19.7525.

94. Pischon T, Girman CJ, Hotamisligil GS, et al. Plasma adiponectin levels and risk of myocardial infarction in men. JAMA. 2004;291(14):1730–7. https://doi.org/10.1001/jama.291.14.1730.

95. Qatanani M, Szwergold NR, Greaves DR, et al. Macrophage-derived human resistin exacerbates adipose tissue inflammation and insulin resistance in mice. J Clin Invest. 2009;119(3):531–9. https://doi.org/10.1172/JCI37273.

96. Qi Y, Takahashi N, Hileman SM, et al. Adiponectin acts in the brain to decrease body weight. Nat Med. 2004;10(5):524–9. https://doi.org/10.1038/nm1029.

97. Qi Q, Wang J, Li H, et al. Associations of resistin with inflammatory and fibrinolytic markers, insulin resistance, and metabolic syndrome in middle-aged and older Chinese. Eur J Endocrinol/Eur Fed Endocr Soc. 2008;159(5):585–93. https://doi.org/10.1530/EJE-08-0427.

98. Rajala MW, Lin Y, Ranalletta M, et al. Cell type-specific expression and coregulation of murine resistin and resistin-like molecule-alpha in adipose tissue. Mol Endocrinol. 2002;16(8):1920–30. https://doi.org/10.1210/me.2002-0048.

99. Rajala MW, Obici S, Scherer PE, et al. Adipose-derived resistin and gut-derived resistin-like molecule-beta selectively impair insulin action on glucose production. J Clin Invest. 2003;111(2):225–30. https://doi.org/10.1172/JCI16521.

100. Rajala MW, Qi Y, Patel HR, et al. Regulation of resistin expression and circulating levels in obesity, diabetes, and fasting. Diabetes. 2004;53(7):1671–9.

101. Ravussin E, Smith SR, Mitchell JA, et al. Enhanced weight loss with pramlintide/metreleptin: an integrated neurohormonal approach to obesity pharmacotherapy. Obesity. 2009;17(9):1736–43. https://doi.org/10.1038/oby.2009.184.

102. Reilly MP, Lehrke M, Wolfe ML, et al. Resistin is an inflammatory marker of atherosclerosis in humans. Circulation. 2005;111(7):932–9. https://doi.org/10.1161/01.CIR.0000155620.10387.43.

103. Rosenbaum M, Goldsmith R, Bloomfield D, et al. Low-dose leptin reverses skeletal muscle, autonomic, and neuroendocrine adaptations to maintenance of reduced weight. J Clin Invest. 2005;115(12):3579–86. https://doi.org/10.1172/JCI25977.

104. Rosenbaum M, Sy M, Pavlovich K, et al. Leptin reverses weight loss-induced changes in regional neural activity responses to visual food stimuli. J Clin Invest. 2008;118(7):2583–91. https://doi.org/10.1172/JCI35055.

105. Roth JD, Roland BL, Cole RL, et al. Leptin responsiveness restored by amylin agonism in diet-induced obesity: evidence from nonclinical and clinical studies. Proc Natl Acad Sci U S A. 2008;105(20):7257–62. https://doi.org/10.1073/pnas.0706473105.

106. Rothenbacher D, Brenner H, Marz W, et al. Adiponectin, risk of coronary heart disease and correlations with cardiovascular risk markers. Eur Heart J. 2005;26(16):1640–6. https://doi.org/10.1093/eurheartj/ehi340.

107. Sanchez-Solana B, Laborda J, Baladron V. Mouse resistin modulates adipogenesis and glucose uptake in 3T3-L1 preadipocytes through the ROR1 receptor.

Mol Endocrinol. 2012;26(1):110–27. https://doi.org/10.1210/me.2011-1027.

108. Savage DB, Sewter CP, Klenk ES, et al. Resistin/Fizz3 expression in relation to obesity and peroxisome proliferator-activated receptor-gamma action in humans. Diabetes. 2001;50(10):2199–202.

109. Scarpace PJ, Matheny M, Pollock BH, et al. Leptin increases uncoupling protein expression and energy expenditure. Am J Phys. 1997;273(1 Pt 1):E226–30.

110. Scheele C, Wolfrum C. Brown adipose crosstalk in tissue plasticity and human metabolism. Endocr Rev. 2020;41(1):53–65. https://doi.org/10.1210/endrev/bnz007. PMID: 31638161

111. Scherer PE, Williams S, Fogliano M, Baldini G, Lodish HF. A novel serum protein similar to C1q, produced exclusively in adipocytes. J Biol Chem. 1995;270:26746–9. [PubMed] [Google Scholar]

112. Schraw T, Wang ZV, Halberg N, et al. Plasma adiponectin complexes have distinct biochemical characteristics. Endocrinology. 2008;149(5):2270–82. https://doi.org/10.1210/en.2007-1561.

113. Schulze MB, Shai I, Rimm EB, et al. Adiponectin and future coronary heart disease events among men with type 2 diabetes. Diabetes. 2005;54(2):534–9.

114. Schwartz DR, Lazar MA. Human resistin: found in translation from mouse to man. Trends Endocrinol Metab TEM. 2011;22(7):259–65. https://doi.org/10.1016/j.tem.2011.03.005.

115. Shetty GK, Economides PA, Horton ES, et al. Circulating adiponectin and resistin levels in relation to metabolic factors, inflammatory markers, and vascular reactivity in diabetic patients and subjects at risk for diabetes. Diabetes Care. 2004;27(10):2450–7.

116. Shibata R, Sato K, Pimentel DR, et al. Adiponectin protects against myocardial ischemia-reperfusion injury through AMPK- and COX-2-dependent mechanisms. Nat Med. 2005;11(10):1096–103. https://doi.org/10.1038/nm1295.

117. Shimomura I, Hammer RE, Ikemoto S, et al. Leptin reverses insulin resistance and diabetes mellitus in mice with congenital lipodystrophy. Nature. 1999;401(6748):73–6. https://doi.org/10.1038/43448.

118. Sienkiewicz E, Magkos F, Aronis KN, et al. Long-term metreleptin treatment increases bone mineral density and content at the lumbar spine of lean hypoleptinemic women. Metab Clin Exp. 2011;60(9):1211–21. https://doi.org/10.1016/j.metabol.2011.05.016.

119. Singhal NS, Patel RT, Qi Y, et al. Loss of resistin ameliorates hyperlipidemia and hepatic steatosis in leptin-deficient mice. Am J Physiol Endocrinol Metab. 2008;295(2):E331–8. https://doi.org/10.1152/ajpendo.00577.2007.

120. Spyridopoulos TN, Petridou ET, Skalkidou A, et al. Low adiponectin levels are associated with renal cell carcinoma: a case–control study. Int J Cancer. 2007;120(7):1573–8. https://doi.org/10.1002/ijc.22526.

121. Steppan CM, Bailey ST, Bhat S, et al. The hormone resistin links obesity to diabetes. Nature. 2001;409(6818):307–12. https://doi.org/10.1038/35053000.

122. Steppan CM, Wang J, Whiteman EL, et al. Activation of SOCS-3 by resistin. Mol Cell Biol. 2005;25(4):1569–75. https://doi.org/10.1128/MCB.25.4.1569-1575.2005.

123. Stępień S, Olczyk P, Gola J, Komosińska-Vassev K, Mielczarek-Palacz A. The role of selected adipocytokines in ovarian cancer and endometrial cancer. Cells. 2023;12(8):1118. https://doi.org/10.3390/cells12081118. PMID: 37190027

124. Straub LG, Scherer PE. Metabolic messengers: adiponectin. Nat Metab. 2019;1(3):334–9. https://doi.org/10.1038/s42255-019-0041-z. Epub 2019 Mar 14. PMID: 32661510

125. Sunden-Cullberg J, Nystrom T, Lee ML, et al. Pronounced elevation of resistin correlates with severity of disease in severe sepsis and septic shock. Crit Care Med. 2007;35(6):1536–42. https://doi.org/10.1097/01.CCM.0000266536.14736.03.

126. Takeda S, Karsenty G. Molecular bases of the sympathetic regulation of bone mass. Bone. 2008;42(5):837–40. https://doi.org/10.1016/j.bone.2008.01.005.

127. Tang NP, Wang LS, Yang L, et al. A polymorphism in the resistin gene promoter and the risk of coronary artery disease in a Chinese population. Clin Endocrinol. 2008;68(1):82–7. https://doi.org/10.1111/j.1365-2265.2007.03003.x.

128. Taouis M, Benomar Y. Is resistin the master link between inflammation and inflammation-related chronic diseases? Mol Cell Endocrinol. 2021;533:111341. https://doi.org/10.1016/j.mce.2021.111341. Epub 2021 May 31. PMID: 34082045

129. Tarkowski A, Bjersing J, Shestakov A, et al. Resistin competes with lipopolysaccharide for binding to toll-like receptor 4. J Cell Mol Med. 2010;14(6B):1419–31. https://doi.org/10.1111/j.1582-4934.2009.00899.x.

130. Tomaru T, Steger DJ, Lefterova MI, et al. Adipocyte-specific expression of murine resistin is mediated by synergism between peroxisome proliferator-activated receptor gamma and CCAAT/enhancer-binding proteins. J Biol Chem. 2009;284(10):6116–25. https://doi.org/10.1074/jbc.M808407200.

131. Tomas E, Tsao TS, Saha AK, et al. Enhanced muscle fat oxidation and glucose transport by ACRP30 globular domain: acetyl-CoA carboxylase inhibition and AMP-activated protein kinase activation. Proc Natl Acad Sci U S A. 2002;99(25):16309–13. https://doi.org/10.1073/pnas.222657499.

132. Trevaskis JL, Coffey T, Cole R, et al. Amylin-mediated restoration of leptin responsiveness in diet-induced obesity: magnitude and mechanisms. Endocrinology. 2008;149(11):5679–87. https://doi.org/10.1210/en.2008-0770.

133. Vatier C, Gautier JF, Vigouroux C. Therapeutic use of recombinant methionyl human leptin. Biochimie. 2012;94(10):2116–25. https://doi.org/10.1016/j.biochi.2012.03.013.

134. Verma S, Li SH, Wang CH, et al. Resistin promotes endothelial cell activation: further evidence of adipokine-endothelial interaction. Circulation. 2003;108(6):736–40. https://doi.org/10.1161/01. CIR.0000084503.91330.49.

135. Villarroya F, Cereijo R, Villarroya J, Giralt M. Brown adipose tissue as a secretory organ. Nat Rev Endocrinol. 2017;13(1):26–35. https://doi.org/10.1038/ nrendo.2016.136. Epub 2016 Sep 12. PMID: 27616452

136. Villarroya J, Cereijo R, Gavaldà-Navarro A, Peyrou M, Giralt M, Villarroya F. New insights into the secretory functions of brown adipose tissue. J Endocrinol. 2019;243(2):R19–27. https://doi.org/10. 1530/JOE-19-0295. PMID: 31419785

137. Wei EK, Giovannucci E, Fuchs CS, et al. Low plasma adiponectin levels and risk of colorectal cancer in men: a prospective study. J Natl Cancer Inst. 2005;97(22):1688–94. https://doi.org/10.1093/jnci/ dji376.

138. Welt CK, Chan JL, Bullen J, et al. Recombinant human leptin in women with hypothalamic amenorrhea. N Engl J Med. 2004;351(10):987–97. https:// doi.org/10.1056/NEJMoa040388.

139. Wong WT, Tian XY, Xu A, et al. Adiponectin is required for PPARgamma-mediated improvement of endothelial function in diabetic mice. Cell Metab. 2011;14(1):104–15. https://doi.org/10.1016/j.cmet. 2011.05.009.

140. Xin X, Zhou L, Reyes CM, et al. APPL1 mediates adiponectin-stimulated p38 MAPK activation by scaffolding the TAK1-MKK3-p38 MAPK pathway. Am J Physiol Endocrinol Metab. 2011;300(1):

E103–10. https://doi.org/10.1152/ajpendo.00427. 2010.

141. Xu JY, Sham PC, Xu A, et al. Resistin gene polymorphisms and progression of glycaemia in southern Chinese: a 5-year prospective study. Clin Endocrinol. 2007;66(2):211–7. https://doi.org/10.1111/j. 1365-2265.2006.02710.x.

142. Yamauchi T, Kamon J, Waki H, et al. The fat-derived hormone adiponectin reverses insulin resistance associated with both lipoatrophy and obesity. Nat Med. 2001;7(8):941–6. https://doi.org/10.1038/90984.

143. Yamauchi T, Kamon J, Minokoshi Y, et al. Adiponectin stimulates glucose utilization and fatty-acid oxidation by activating AMP-activated protein kinase. Nat Med. 2002;8(11):1288–95. https://doi. org/10.1038/nm788.

144. Yamauchi T, Nio Y, Maki T, et al. Targeted disruption of AdipoR1 and AdipoR2 causes abrogation of adiponectin binding and metabolic actions. Nat Med. 2007;13(3):332–9. https://doi.org/10.1038/ nm1557.

145. Yoon MJ, Lee GY, Chung JJ, et al. Adiponectin increases fatty acid oxidation in skeletal muscle cells by sequential activation of AMP-activated protein kinase, p38 mitogen-activated protein kinase, and peroxisome proliferator-activated receptor alpha. Diabetes. 2006;55(9):2562–70. https://doi.org/10.2337/ db05-1322.

146. Zhao S, Kusminski CM, Scherer PE. Adiponectin, leptin and cardiovascular disorders. Circ Res. 2021;128(1):136–49. https://doi.org/10.1161/ CIRCRESAHA.120.314458. Epub 2021 Jan 7. PMID: 33411633

Gut Hormones and Metabolic Syndrome

19

Salman Zahoor Bhat, Hyeong-Kyu Park, and Rexford S. Ahima

Contents

S. Z. Bhat · R. S. Ahima (✉)
Department of Medicine, Division of Endocrinology, Diabetes and Metabolism, Johns Hopkins University School of Medicine, Baltimore, MD, USA
e-mail: sbhat13@jhmi.edu; ahima@jhmi.edu

H.-K. Park
Department of Internal Medicine, Soonchunhyang University College of Medicine, Seoul, South Korea
e-mail: hkpark@schmc.ac.kr

Abstract

The gastrointestinal tract has a critical role in energy homeostasis as the site of food ingestion, digestion, and absorption of nutrients. Neural and humoral signals from the gastrointestinal tract control food ingestion, digestion and transit of food, satiety, nutrient partitioning, and energy homeostasis. Enteroendocrine cells distributed throughout the gastrointestinal tract sense nutrients and

© Springer Nature Switzerland AG 2023
R. S. Ahima (ed.), *Metabolic Syndrome*,
https://doi.org/10.1007/978-3-031-40116-9_25

synthesize and secrete peptides that act via autocrine, paracrine, and endocrine mechanisms to regulate nutrient processing and metabolism. Ghrelin is produced by the stomach and acts as a meal initiator. Cholecystokinin, Peptide YY, pancreatic polypeptide, and glucagon-like peptide 1 are satiety signals. This chapter reviews the biological actions of gut hormones with an emphasis on mechanisms of action, roles in the pathophysiology of diabetes and obesity, and gut hormone-based therapies.

Keywords

Obesity · Diabetes · Gastrointestinal tract · Enteroendocrine · Hormone · Incretin

Introduction

Energy homeostasis is mediated via communication between the gut, nervous system, and neuroendocrine system. Long-term signals of energy balance, such as leptin and insulin, communicate the status of energy stores in adipose tissue to the brain through neuronal and endocrine pathways to regulate feeding, energy expenditure, and various systems. The gastrointestinal tract plays a crucial role in energy homeostasis as the site of food ingestion, digestion and absorption, and partitioning of nutrients. Gut hormones are produced by enteroendocrine cells widely dispersed throughout the gastrointestinal epithelium. Enteroendocrine cells form the largest endocrine system and have receptors on their apical pole that sense nutrients in the gut lumen and secrete regulatory peptides at the basolateral pole into the blood.

Gut hormones regulate various aspects of *feeding behavior* by influencing meal intake, the interval between meals, and the frequency of meals. The initiation of a meal is triggered by *hunger signals* related to energy deficit as well as external factors such as social setting, memory, and cognitive and sensory cues. When food is ingested through the mouth, information about the taste, temperature, and texture of the food is conveyed from the oropharynx by the facial, glossopharyngeal, and vagal nerves to the brainstem where palatability of food is perceived. After the food transits to the stomach, the mechanical distension is relayed to the nucleus tractus solitarius (NTS) in the brainstem by the vagus nerve, eliciting inhibitory signals to control the rate of meal ingestion from the oral cavity and the transit of digested food in the intestine. Nutrients and various chemical signals in the gut lumen stimulate the secretion of neurotransmitters and peptides from the pancreas and enteroendocrine cells that inform the brain about the status of the meal. Ghrelin is secreted by the stomach and stimulates feeding, i.e., *orexigenic*. In contrast, most gut-derived hormones are *anorexigenic*. They inhibit *appetite* and/or elicit *satiation*, i.e., within-meal inhibition of food intake. The net effect of satiation signals results in meal termination, i.e., *satiety*, which persists from the end of one meal to the next meal.

In the next sections, we discuss gut hormones, their physiological actions, changes in obesity and diabetes, therapeutic uses in diabetes and obesity, and potential for future treatment of metabolic disorders (Table 1).

Ghrelin

Ghrelin is produced primarily in the P/D1 cells of the stomach and exists as des-acyl ghrelin and acylated forms [1]. Acylation of ghrelin is regulated by the enzyme ghrelin *O*-acyltransferase (GOAT) [2]. Plasma acyl-ghrelin concentration is lower than des-acyl ghrelin [1, 3]. The orexigenic action of ghrelin is mostly mediated via the acylated hormone [4]. Ghrelin levels are increased during fasting [5], plasma ghrelin peaks at the onset of feeding [6], and ghrelin levels decline after meals. The postprandial reduction in ghrelin is more pronounced following ingestion of high dietary carbohydrates than fats or proteins [7, 8]. Ghrelin secretion is stimulated by low blood glucose levels [9].

Ghrelin binds and activates the growth hormone secretagogue receptor (GHS-R1a) [10], a G protein-coupled receptor, predominantly to the

Table 1 Sources and actions of gut hormones

Gut hormone	Source and regulation	Targets	Physiology	Obesity
Amylin	Pancreatic ß cell. Amylin is cosecreted with insulin in response to nutrients and incretin hormones	Amylin receptors in the nucleus accumbens, dorsal raphe, and area postrema	Inhibits postprandial glucagon secretion, feeding, and gastric emptying	Increased in obesity. Amylin receptor agonist, Pramlintide, is FDA-approved for diabetes and also reduces body weight
Ghrelin	P/D1-type cell in gastric antrum and fundus, and duodenum	GHSR1a on vagus nerve and in arcuate hypothalamus and other brain areas. Acyl-ghrelin is the active hormone	Stimulates feeding, gastric emptying, gastric acid production, and reduces insulin secretion	Increased in Prader-Willi Syndrome, and in the preprandial state, and following weight loss. Decreased in the postprandial state. Diet-induced obesity in rodents is associated with ghrelin resistance
Gastrin	Enteroendocrine G cells. Stimulated by low acid, suppressed by high acid and somatostatin	CCK2R in the stomach and intestine	Gastric acid secretion	Incretin-like effect
Cholecystokinin (CCK)	Enteroendocrine I cell. Stimulated by nutrient intake, especially dietary lipids and protein	CCK1R receptors in the gut, and CCK2R receptors in the brain	Inhibits feeding via CCK1R on vagal afferents. Inhibits gastric secretion, and increases insulin secretion	Satiety effect of CCK is attenuated in obesity
Glucose-dependent insulinotropic polypeptide (GIP)	Enteroendocrine K cell. Stimulated by dietary lipids	GIP receptor in pancreatic islet cells, hypothalamus, and adipose tissue	Stimulates insulin secretion, has antiapoptotic function in pancreatic ß cell, and reduces energy intake	Plasma levels may be higher in obesity. GIP increases secretion of insulin, glucagon, and somatostatin. GIP has antidiabetic and antiobesity effects when combined with GLP-1R agonist
Peptide YY	Enteroendocrine L cell, pancreas, and brainstem	PYY exerts its anorexigenic action through Y2R in the arcuate nucleus of hypothalamus	Reduces appetite and energy intake, delays gastric emptying, promotes insulin secretion, and stimulates vagus nerve	Individuals with obesity have attenuated nutrient-stimulated PYY levels compared to normal weight individuals
Neurotensin (NT)	Enteroendocrine L cell and CNS. Released in response to nutrient intake, in particular dietary lipids	NT receptors: NTR1, NTR2, and NTR3 widely distributed in the brain and peripheral organs	Reduces gut motility and gastric secretion and stimulates pancreatic and biliary secretion	People with severe obesity have lower plasma concentration of NT than normal weight individuals
Uroguanylin	Intestinal epithelial cell. Released in response to nutrient ingestion. Secreted as prouroguanylin and	Activates guanylyl cyclase 2C (GUCY2C) receptors on intestinal epithelial	Promotes satiety and reduces food intake	Plasma levels are reduced in obesity

(continued)

Table 1 (continued)

Gut hormone	Source and regulation	Targets	Physiology	Obesity
	undergoes enzymatic conversion to uroguanylin	cells and the hypothalamus		
Glucagon-like-peptide 1 (GLP-1)	Enteroendocrine L cell and brainstem neurons. Gut-derived GLP-1 is secreted in response to nutrients and bile acids	GLP-1 receptors (GLP-1R) are distributed in the brain, gut, liver, and pancreatic islets	Reduces appetite and food intake, delays gastric emptying, promotes insulin secretion, enhances pancreatic islet β cell proliferation, and suppresses glucagon secretion	Nutrient-stimulated GLP-1 is attenuated in obesity and type 2 diabetes. DDP4 inhibitors protect native GLP-1 from degradation, increase insulin stimulation, and reduce blood glucose. GLP-1R agonists enhance insulin secretion, reduce glucagon and blood glucose, and are potent antidiabetic and antiobesity drugs
Oxyntomodulin (OXM)	Enteroendocrine L cell; cosecreted with GLP-1	GLP-1R, and glucagon receptors in brain and gut	Decreases food intake, delays gastric emptying, and causes glucose-dependent insulin secretion	Exogenous administration of OXM reduces food intake

G_q pathway [11, 12]. The GHSR1a is widely distributed in the brain and peripheral tissues [13, 14]. Ghrelin crosses the blood-brain barrier [15], and the hyperphagic effect of ghrelin is mediated via GHSR1a expressed on neuropeptide Y (NPY)/agouti-related peptide (AgRP) neurons in the arcuate nucleus of the hypothalamus [16]. In addition to directly stimulating food intake via NPY/AgRP neurons, ghrelin acting on NPY/AgRP neurons stimulates the release of GABA on proopiomelanocortin (POMC) neurons within the arcuate nucleus [17], resulting in inhibition of the anorectic action of these neurons. Thus, ghrelin boosts food intake directly via NPY/AgRP and indirectly via POMC.

Ghrelin targets other CNS sites, including the dorsal vagal complex [18], paraventricular nucleus of the hypothalamus [19, 20], lateral hypothalamic area [21], hippocampus [22], and amygdala [23]. Ghrelin regulates the mesolimbic dopamine pathway, including the ventral tegmental area [24–26], providing a link to food reward and hedonic (pleasurable) eating [27]. Ghrelin also decreases energy expenditure [28], increases glucose oxidation, and promotes fat storage [29, 30].

Acyl-ghrelin is also produced in ε cell in the pancreatic islets. Blocking the GHSR enhances insulin secretion during a glucose tolerance test. Genetic deletion of GHSR results in severe hypoglycemia [31]. Moreover, exogenous ghrelin administration increases blood glucose and reduces insulin in rodents, and ghrelin directly inhibits insulin secretion in vitro [32]. These data suggest a role for ghrelin in the control of pancreatic ß-cell function and glucose homeostasis.

While acyl-ghrelin administration increases food intake and body weight in rodents, deletion of ghrelin or ghrelin receptors (GHSR) does not reduce body weight or adiposity, raising the possibility of a complex regulation involving multiple organs. Ghrelin resistance has been demonstrated in obesity. A study showed that liver-enriched antimicrobial peptide-2 (LEAP2) is an endogenous GHSR antagonist that attenuates ghrelin action in the postprandial and obese states [33]. Plasma LEAP2 levels are elevated in obesity and in response to acute hyperglycemia, and

LEAP2 is decreased with fasting, weight loss from bariatric surgery, or in response to hypoglycemia [33]. LEAP2 prevents acyl-ghrelin from activating NPY/AgRP neurons in the arcuate nucleus of the hypothalamus. The interaction of LEAP2 and acyl-ghrelin is likely to play an important role in modulating acyl-ghrelin activity in obesity and related disorders [34].

People with obesity have a blunted suppression of postprandial ghrelin levels compared to lean individuals [5, 35, 36]. Weight loss results in an increase in ghrelin levels [6, 37]. Presumably, the rise in plasma ghrelin during weight loss stimulates hunger and weight gain following calorically restricted weight loss. Blockade of plasma ghrelin with antighrelin immunoglobulins reduces feeding and body weight in rodent models [38, 39]. Inhibition of GOAT, the enzyme that generates acyl-ghrelin, reduces food intake and body weight in rodents [40]. Moreover, treatment with a desacylated ghrelin analogue decreased hunger and body fat in patients with Prader-Willi syndrome, a condition characterized by hyperphagia, morbid obesity, and elevated plasma ghrelin levels [41]. These data suggest that ghrelin is a potential therapeutic target for obesity and eating disorders.

Motilin

Motilin shares 36% sequence homology with ghrelin, and it is produced by M cells located mostly in the proximal duodenum [42]. Motilin secretion is stimulated by gastric acid, bile salts, and dietary fat, while somatostatin, pancreatic polypeptide, and secretin inhibit motilin release. Motilin regulates a characteristic gastrointestinal contraction pattern known as *migrating motor complex* which occurs in the fasting state [43]. A plasma motilin peak initiates contraction of the gastric antrum which then migrates caudally throughout the small intestine [43].

Motilin controls the lower esophageal sphincter (LES), a high-pressure zone located between the esophagus and stomach. The LES pressure increases when the stomach is most acidic and decreases when the stomach is less acidic [43]. Administration of motilin or motilin receptor agonist increases the LES pressure, thus preventing reflux of gastric content into the esophagus. Motilin also affects the gastric capacity. After meal intake, the gastric fundus relaxes to increase the gastric volume and accommodate the food. Administration of motilin or a motilin receptor agonist, erythromycin A, increases the proximal gastric tone and reduces the gastric accommodation. Motilin increases gastric emptying and stimulates gall bladder contraction and bile secretion. Exogenous administration of motilin increases insulin levels via vagal-mediated pathway but does not affect blood glucose.

Low-dose erythromycin A acts as a motilin receptor agonist, but due to concerns about the emergence of antimicrobial resistance strains, there are efforts to develop erythromycin derivatives lacking antibacterial activity but possessing enhanced motilin receptor agonist activity [42]. Mitemcinal (erythromycin derivative) and camicinal (small molecule motilin receptor agonist) are under investigation for gastroparesis treatment [42]. There is also interest in clinical applications of motilin for obesity therapy based on its ability to regulate appetite, gastric emptying, and satiety. Noncaloric foods and bitter substances reduce motilin levels and suppress appetite. Modulation of gastric acid, bile, and dietary macronutrients has varying effects on motilin levels and may provide novel therapeutic targets.

Cholecystokinin (CCK)

CCK is synthesized and secreted by enteroendocrine I cells in response to ingestion of nutrients [44]. CCK controls gallbladder contraction and pancreatic and gastric acid secretion and was the first gut hormone shown to potently reduce meal size [45]. CCK acts via CCK1 receptors (CCK1R) localized on afferent terminals of the vagus nerve and in various regions of the CNS. Endogenous CCK or systemic administration of CCK acts via the vagal afferents [46]. Blockade of CCK1R with selective antagonists increases food intake [47]. Genetic deletion of CCK1R results in hyperphagia and obesity [48]. Gastric distension enhances the ability of CCK to suppress food intake [49]. CCK1R activation also reduces gastric emptying and increases gastric distension during feeding [50, 51]. CCK interacts with other signals, e.g., leptin potentiates the anorectic effects of CCK via vagal afferents, NTS, parabrachial nucleus, and hypothalamic nuclei [52–54].

Despite the convincing evidence of the role of CCK in the control of feeding, the pharmaceutical development of CCK has been unsuccessful due to diminished CCK sensitivity in obesity and tachyphylaxis that develops in response to repeated CCK administration [55, 56]. Furthermore, there is concern that CCK1R agonists may result in pancreatitis [57, 58]. A CCK agonist, GI181771X (GlaxoSmithKline), had no adverse effects on the pancreas in overweight or obese subjects, but it did not reduce food intake and body weight [59].

CCK affects glucose homeostasis by signaling through CCK2R. CCK stimulates glucagon and insulin release, and infusion of a CCK fragment containing 8 amino acids (CCK-8) increases insulin and decreases glucose in subjects with or without type 2 diabetes following a meal ingestion [60]. CCK-8 promotes regeneration of pancreatic islet β cells in type 1 diabetes rodent models, and genetic disruption of CCK exacerbates hyperglycemia in *ob/ob* mice [61].

Gastrin

Gastrin was discovered in 1905, based on its function to stimulate meal-related gastric secretion [62]. Gastrin is produced mostly in G cells of the gastric antrum, and smaller amounts are produced in the rest of the stomach, duodenum, jejunum, ileum, and pancreas. The precursor preprogastrin is processed into progastrin and gastrin peptide fragments by sequential enzymatic cleavage. Secretion of bioactive gastrin peptides, mainly G-34 and G-17, is affected by gastric pH. An increase in gastric acid inhibits gastrin release, whereas a reduction in gastric acid or high pH stimulates gastric secretion. Mild gastric

distention inhibits gastrin secretion, and greater gastric distension increases gastrin. These changes in gastrin levels are related to somatostatin secretion. Gastrin secretion is stimulated by dietary amino acids and a neurotransmitter, gastrin-releasing peptide (GRP), and inhibited by somatostatin via a paracrine mechanism. In humans, the plasma gastrin in the fasted state consists mainly of G-34, and the rise in plasma gastrin after a mixed meal consists mainly of G-17 [62].

Gastrin and CCK both signal though the CCK/gastrin receptor family [62, 63]. Gastrin binds to CCK2R, which is abundant in the stomach, brain, and pancreatic islets. The major function of gastrin is to stimulate gastric acid secretion via CNS and enteric nervous systems mediated via GRP and acetylcholine. As expected, CCK2R knockout mice have reduced gastric acid secretion. Gastrin regulates pepsinogen secretion from chief cells for protein digestion. Gastrin also enhances the ability of GLP-1 to increase insulin secretion and reduce glucose levels in rodent models, suggesting an incretin-like function.

The role of gastrin in obesity and diabetes is unknown, and there are few clinical uses of gastrin-based therapies. A gastrin analog, pentagastrin, is used clinically to stimulate histamine and gastric acid secretion when evaluating gastric acid secretory capacity. Pentagastrin is also used as a diagnostic tool to stimulate 5-hydroxytryptamine release in the carcinoid syndrome under careful medical monitoring. Gastrin receptor antagonists may have a role in treatment of CCK2R-expressing gastrointestinal cancer, gastric carcinoids, and Barrett esophagus.

Peptide YY (PYY)

PYY is a member of a peptide family that includes NPY and pancreatic polypeptide (PP), named for the presence of two tyrosine residues (YY) flanking the peptide sequence [64]. PYY is coreleased with GLP-1 from the enteroendocrine L cells in response to nutrient stimulation. PYY is secreted as a longer inactive peptide, PYY_{1-36}, and rapidly cleaved by the enzyme dipeptidyl peptidase 4 (DPP4) into PYY_{3-36}. The two circulating isoforms, PYY_{1-36} and PYY_{3-36}, bind to Y1, Y2, and Y5 receptors with different affinities. The bioactive form, PYY_{3-36}, has highest affinity for the Y2 receptor.

Peripheral administration of PYY_{3-36} reduces food intake and body weight in mice and humans [65, 66]. PYY_{3-36} crosses the blood-brain barrier [67] and acts via Y2R expressed on NPY/AgRP neurons in the arcuate nucleus of the hypothalamus [68]. Pharmacological blockade of Y2R prevents the ability of peripherally administered PYY_{3-36} to inhibit feeding [68]. However, PYY_{3-36} acts on other CNS neurons to increase food intake [69–71].

Plasma levels of PYY_{1-36} and PYY_{3-36} are low during fasting and increase rapidly after meals. PYY acts as a satiety signal together with GLP-1 resulting in meal termination [72]. PYY_{3-36} also reduces gastric emptying and increases vagal-induced satiation [73, 74]. The development of diet-induced obesity in mice is associated with reduction in PYY_{3-36} levels, and obese subjects display reduced fasting PYY_{3-36} levels and attenuation of postprandial PYY_{3-36} release following a meal [66, 75]. While the reduction in PYY_{3-36} levels in obesity has led to efforts to develop PYY replacement or agonist therapies, the development of $PYY_{(3-36)}$ as an antiobesity pharmacotherapy has been limited by poor efficacy and side effects [76, 77].

Amylin (Islet Amyloid Polypeptide)

Amylin is produced in pancreatic islet β cells and cosecreted with insulin in response to a meal. Amylin is a satiation signal, delays gastric emptying, inhibits glucagon release, and lowers blood glucose [78]. Amylin receptors are composed of calcitonin receptor (CTa/CTb; a G protein-coupled receptor) that heterodimerizes with receptor activity modifying proteins RAMP 1, RAMP2, or RAMP3, and widely distributed in the brain and peripheral tissues. The anorectic action of amylin is mediated via the area postrema of the hindbrain [79]. Amylin exerts a potent effect in the ventral tegmental area to suppress meal palatability [80] and also interacts with leptin in the hypothalamus to inhibit feeding [81].

Chronic amylin administration reduces body weight in rodent models by inhibiting food intake and increasing energy expenditure [78]. An amylin agonist, pramlintide, is approved by the US FDA for the treatment of diabetes. Pramlintide treatment reduces appetite and body weight in patients with obesity and diabetes [82–84]. There is interest in combining amylin-based pharmaceuticals with leptin to overcome leptin resistance in obesity [83].

Incretin Hormones

Incretin hormones secreted in response to nutrients in the lumen of the gastrointestinal tract stimulate insulin secretion to reduce blood glucose levels. Glucose-dependent insulinotropic polypeptide (GIP) and glucagon-like peptide-1 (GLP-1) are responsible for the *incretin effect*, i.e., producing a two- to threefold higher insulin-secretory response to oral glucose administration compared to intravenous glucose administration. In people with type 2 diabetes, the incretin effect is diminished or absent.

Glucose-Dependent Insulinotropic Polypeptide (GIP)

GIP was originally discovered as a 42–amino acid peptide that inhibited gastric motility, and it was later shown to enhance glucose-stimulated insulin secretion [85, 86]. GIP is expressed in the stomach and proximal small intestinal K cells. GIP acts via GIP receptor (GIPR) that is widely expressed in the brain, pancreas, stomach, small intestine, and other tissues [86, 87]. GIP secretion is stimulated by dietary carbohydrates in rodents and by dietary fat in humans. The main action of GIP is the stimulation of glucose-dependent insulin secretion. Blockage of endogenous GIP leads to defective insulin secretion after oral glucose ingestion [88–90]. Mice lacking GIPR have reduced adiposity [89, 90]. The effects of GIP on adiposity are likely to be mediated directly via GIPR expressed in adipose tissue.

Proglucagon-Derived Peptides

Proglucagon-derived peptides are derived from the posttranslational processing of the precursor proglucagon in the pancreatic islets, intestine, and brain [91]. Glucagon is produced in α cells of the islets, and glucagon-like peptide-1 (GLP1), glucagon-like peptide-2 (GLP2), glicentin, and oxyntomodulin are produced from proglucagon in enteroendocrine L cells.

GLP1 has two forms in the plasma, GLP_{17-37} and GLP_{17-36} amide, mostly GLP_{17-36} amide in humans. GLP1 is stimulated by meal intake, and this response is blunted in people with obesity or type 2 diabetes. GLP1 acts via GLP1R distributed in the brain and pancreatic islets. GLP1 stimulates insulin secretion in a glucose-dependent manner [92, 93] and also increases insulin synthesis in rodent models. The function of endogenous GLP1 has been demonstrated using *Glp1r* knockout mice and pharmacological agents [89]. Treatment with GLP1R antagonist, $exendin_{9-39}$, a truncated form of GLP1-related peptide, exendin-4, isolated from Gila monster, resulted in a reduction in glucose-stimulated insulin secretion and impaired glucose tolerance in rodents and humans [89, 94–96]. Similarly, *Glp1r* knockout mice display glucose-stimulated insulin secretion and hyperglycemia [97]. In rodents, GLP1 reduces pancreatic islet β cell proliferation and neogenesis, and inhibits apoptosis, while the lack of GLP1R reduces β cell mass and blunts the islet-regenerative response to partial pancreatectomy [98–102].

GLP2 is cosecreted with GLP1 from enteroendocrine L cells in a nutrient-dependent manner. GLP2 stimulates expansion of the small intestinal mucosal epithelium in rodents with intestinal injury and in patients with short bowel syndrome [103–106]. Acute GLP2 administration increases the postprandial levels of glucagon, triglycerides, and fatty acids, but there is no evidence that GLP2 affects insulin secretion or blood glucose levels [106]. Glicentin is cosecreted with GLP1 and GLP2 from enteroendocrine L cells, but it has not been shown to regulate glucose homeostasis. Oxyntomodulin inhibits food intake, meal-induced gastric acid secretion, and gastric emptying and stimulates glucose absorption in the small intestine and insulin secretion in rodents [107, 108]. Oxyntomodulin suppresses appetite, induces satiety, and increases energy expenditure in humans [109, 110]. Oxyntomodulin binds to GLP1R, and the anorectic action of oxyntomodulin is blocked by $exendin_{9-39}$ and is absent in *Glp1r* knockout mice [111, 112].

GLP1 Therapy for Diabetes and Obesity

Endogenous GLP1 is rapidly cleaved and inactivated by the enzyme DPP4, which is widely expressed and catalyzes the cleavage and inactivation of GIP as well as GLP1. DPP4-deficient rodents exhibit elevated levels of GLP1 and GIP and enhanced insulin secretion and glucose tolerance [113, 114], consistent with a physiologic role of these incretins in glucose homeostasis. Similarly, DPP4 inhibitors improved glycemia in patients with type 2 diabetes [115]. The development of DPP4 inhibitors was a major milestone in harnessing the clinical utility of endogenous GLP1 for the treatment of type 2 diabetes. DPP4 inhibitors, known as gliptins, are oral medications approved for treatment of type 2 diabetes. These drugs can be used as monotherapy or combined with other diabetes medications, e.g., metformin, sulfonylureas, thiazolidinediones, or insulin [116–120].

Potent GLP1 agonists have been developed based on structural modifications of GLP1 to improve its stability and efficacy. The discovery of exendin-4, a GLP1 agonist in Gila monster, led to the development of exenatide, which was approved for treatment of type 2 diabetes in 2005 [121]. Other GLP1 analogues have been developed [122]. Liraglutide was the first GLP1 analogue approved for type 2 diabetes, and later at a higher dose for obesity treatment [123]. The Satiety and Clinical Adiposity – Liraglutide Evidence (SCALE) trial assessed the efficacy of 3 mg liraglutide injected once daily in people with BMI >27 and one comorbid condition or in people with obesity (BMI >30). The mean weight loss in the liraglutide group was 8.4 kg after 56 weeks, and discontinuation from the study due to adverse events (nausea, vomiting, and diarrhea) was 9.9% for liraglutide and 3.8% for placebo, respectively. Liraglutide improved blood glucose, blood pressure, and inflammatory markers [123]. In the SCALE maintenance study, people who achieved >5% weight loss from liraglutide therapy over 52 weeks were followed on a low-calorie diet for 12 weeks, and then randomized to either diet alone or liraglutide therapy. Liraglutide treatment resulted in 6.2% greater loss of body weight compared to low-calorie diet alone [124]. The SCALE diabetes trial studied people with obesity and type 2 diabetes. Liraglutide (3 mg daily) treatment reduced body weight by 6% over 52 weeks [125]. The SCALE sleep apnea trial assessed the effectiveness of liraglutide versus placebo, in addition to diet and lifestyle intervention, in people with sleep apnea [126]. A mean weight loss of 5.7% and a significant reduction in the apnea-hypoapneic index (AHI) were observed in subjects treated with liraglutide.

Semaglutide, an acylated long-acting GLP1R agonist, was approved by the US FDA for treatment of type 2 diabetes in doses of 0.5, 1 and 2 mg, to be administered subcutaneously once weekly. Semaglutide is also available in 7 or 14 mg doses administered once daily in a tablet. The Semaglutide Treatment Effect in People with Obesity (STEP) study compared the effects of 2.4 mg semaglutide once weekly versus placebo in subjects with BMI >27 and at least one obesity-related comorbid condition [127]. Semaglutide was started at the dose of 0.25 mg, and escalated weekly to a final dose of 2.4 mg over 16 weeks. The trial duration was 68 weeks. The mean weight loss in semaglutide-treated group was 16.9% and 2.4% in the placebo group [127]. Semaglutide improved the blood glucose, blood pressure, lipids, and inflammatory markers. Similar to liraglutide, the side effects of semaglutide were nausea, vomiting, diarrhea, and gallbladder-related events.

In the STEP 3 trial, semaglutide was administered to subjects on an initial low-calorie diet for 8 weeks and intensive behavioral therapy and physical activity over 68 weeks [128]. The mean weight loss in semaglutide group was 17.6% versus 5% in the placebo group [128]. Semaglutide treatment improved the blood glucose, blood pressure, and lipids [128]. The STEP 4 trial compared the effects of an initial 20 weeks of injection of semaglutide 2.4 mg once weekly followed by continuation of semaglutide versus placebo. The participants were maintained on a low-calorie diet, increased physical activity, and intensive behavioral therapy for the 68 weeks duration of the study [129]. The subjects maintained on semaglutide treatment had an additional 7.9% weight loss compared to 6.9% weight gain in the placebo group. A continuation of semaglutide treatment improved blood glucose, blood pressure, lipids, and physical activity [129].

Because people with type 2 diabetes have a higher risk for the development of cardiovascular diseases, the effects of GLP1R agonists have been studied [130, 131]. The results show significant benefits of long-acting GLP1R agonist therapy on cardiovascular events in people with overweight or obesity and type 2 diabetes. Liraglutide (1.8 mg) reduced the rates of major adverse cardiovascular events (MACE) in people with type 2 diabetes. Other GLP1R agonists, e.g., albiglutide and efpeglenatide, reduce MACE in people with type 2 diabetes despite modest weight loss [132, 133]. Once weekly semaglutide injection has also been associated with a reduction in rates of MACE in people with type 2 diabetes [134].

Combining Gut Hormones for Diabetes and Obesity Treatment

In addition to its classical action in regulating blood glucose, glucagon has potent anorexigenic, lipolytic, and thermogenic effects [135]. Thus, there is growing interest to combine glucagon, GLP1, GIP, and gut hormones to achieve better efficacy for the treatment of diabetes and obesity [136, 137]. A glucagon receptor/GLP1R dual agonist was first developed in 2009 [138]. A phase II trial of a glucagon receptor/GLP1R dual agonist, cotadutide, resulted in slight weight loss [139].

GIPR/GLP1R coagonists were developed and shown to be highly efficacious and safe in humans

[140]. Tirzepatide, a novel GIP/GLP1R coagonist, was the first to be approved for treatment of type 2 diabetes, and recently for weight loss in people with obesity [141]. In the SUR-MOUNT-1 study, subjects with obesity (BMI >30) or BMI >27 and at least one weight-related condition, excluding diabetes, were randomized to receive once-weekly subcutaneous tirzepatide (5 mg, 10 mg, or 15 mg) or placebo for 72 weeks. The mean percentage weight loss was 15.0% with 5 mg tirzepatide, 19.5% with 10 mg tirzepatide, and 20.9% with 15 mg tirzepatide, compared with placebo. Tirzepatide is more potent than either GIPR agonist or GLP1R agonist alone (Fig. 1).

Amylin analogs, e.g., pramlintide, were originally developed for treatment of diabetes, found to produce significant weight loss. A combination of pramlintide and metreleptin produced substantial weight loss [83]. The efficacy and safety of the cagrilintide (an acylated long-acting nonselective human amylin receptor agonist) and semaglutide

is under investigation in clinical trials for obesity [142, 143]. Other gut hormone combinations are in the drug development pipeline for obesity, type 2 diabetes, NAFLD, and other diseases [137].

Conclusion

The gastrointestinal tract is the most abundant source of peptides that control gut functions, as well as diverse hormones, appetite regulation, and energy homeostasis. We are increasing our understanding of the complexities of gut hormones and their actions in normal physiology and disease pathogenesis. Until recently, the pharmacotherapy for obesity had limited efficacy and side effects that constrained wider use. However, the development of novel GLP1R agonists, e.g., liraglutide and semaglutide, and GIP/GLP1R coagonists, e.g., tirzepatide, has opened a new era. The challenge is to turn the knowledge into effective

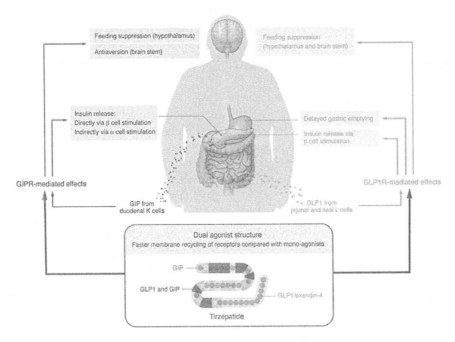

Fig. 1 Putative mechanisms underlying the antidiabetic and antiobesity effects of GIP/GLP1R coagonism. Two hypotheses have been proposed to explain the synergy of GIP and GLP1R coagonism: (i) Tirzepatide induces faster recycling of the internalized GLP1R compared to GLP1R alone, hence increasing signaling; (ii) GIPR enhances GLP1R signaling while minimizing gastrointestinal side effects that limit the tolerability of GLP1R agonist treatment. (The figure is reproduced from Ref. [137]: Bass J, Tschöp MH, Beutler LR. J Clin Invest 2023;133. The JCI is a Gold Open Access journal. Users can use the content without asking prior permission from the publisher or the author)

strategies for prevention, diagnosis, and therapies to better manage the epidemics of obesity, diabetes, and related diseases.

Cross-References

▷ Adipose Structure (White, Brown, Beige)
▷ Brain Regulation of Feeding and Energy Homeostasis
▷ Overview of Metabolic Syndrome
▷ Pharmacotherapy of Obesity and Metabolic Syndrome

Acknowledgments This chapter was supported by grants R01DK135751 and RF1 AG059621 from the US National Institutes of Health, American Heart Association Obesity Research Network, and Cardiometabolic Health and Type 2 Diabetes Research Network.

References

1. Hosoda H, Kojima M, Matsuo H, Kangawa K. Ghrelin and des-acyl ghrelin: two major forms of rat ghrelin peptide in gastrointestinal tissue. Biochem Biophys Res Commun. 2000;279:909–13.
2. Yang J, Brown MS, Liang G, Grishin NV, Goldstein JL. Identification of the acyltransferase that octanoylates ghrelin, an appetite-stimulating peptide hormone. Cell. 2008;132:387–96.
3. Murakami N, Hayashida T, Kuroiwa T, Nakahara K, Ida T, Mondal MS, et al. Role for central ghrelin in food intake and secretion of stomach ghrelin in rats. J Endocrinol. 2002;174:283–8.
4. Asakawa A, Inui A, Fujimiya M, Sakamaki R, Shinfuku N, Ueta Y, et al. Stomach regulates energy balance via acylated ghrelin and desacyl ghrelin. Gut. 2005;54:18–24.
5. Tschöp M, Wawarta R, Riepl RL, Friedrich S, Bidlingmaier M, Landgraf R, et al. Post-prandial decrease of circulating human ghrelin levels. J Endocrinol Investig. 2001;24:Rc19–21.
6. Cummings DE, Weigle DS, Frayo RS, Breen PA, Ma MK, Dellinger EP, et al. Plasma ghrelin levels after diet-induced weight loss or gastric bypass surgery. N Engl J Med. 2002;346:1623–30.
7. Overduin J, Frayo RS, Grill HJ, Kaplan JM, Cummings DE. Role of the duodenum and macronutrient type in ghrelin regulation. Endocrinology. 2005;146:845–50.
8. Erdmann J, Töpsch R, Lippl F, Gussmann P, Schusdziarra V. Postprandial response of plasma ghrelin levels to various test meals in relation to

food intake, plasma insulin, and glucose. J Clin Endocrinol Metab. 2004;89:3048–54.
9. Lauritzen ES, Voss T, Kampmann U, Mengel A, Vendelbo MH, Jørgensen JO, et al. Circulating acylghrelin levels are suppressed by insulin and increase in response to hypoglycemia in healthy adult volunteers. Eur J Endocrinol. 2015;172:357–62.
10. Shuto Y, Shibasaki T, Otagiri A, Kuriyama H, Ohata H, Tamura H, et al. Hypothalamic growth hormone secretagogue receptor regulates growth hormone secretion, feeding, and adiposity. J Clin Invest. 2002;109:1429–36.
11. Falls HD, Dayton BD, Fry DG, Ogiela CA, Schaefer VG, Brodjian S, et al. Characterization of ghrelin receptor activity in a rat pituitary cell line RC-4B/C. J Mol Endocrinol. 2006;37:51–62.
12. Cuellar JN, Isokawa M. Ghrelin-induced activation of cAMP signal transduction and its negative regulation by endocannabinoids in the hippocampus. Neuropharmacology. 2011;60:842–51.
13. Dass NB, Munonyara M, Bassil AK, Hervieu GJ, Osbourne S, Corcoran S, et al. Growth hormone secretagogue receptors in rat and human gastrointestinal tract and the effects of ghrelin. Neuroscience. 2003;120:443–53.
14. Gnanapavan S, Kola B, Bustin SA, Morris DG, McGee P, Fairclough P, et al. The tissue distribution of the mRNA of ghrelin and subtypes of its receptor, GHS-R, in humans. J Clin Endocrinol Metab. 2002;87:2988.
15. Banks WA, Tschöp M, Robinson SM, Heiman ML. Extent and direction of ghrelin transport across the blood-brain barrier is determined by its unique primary structure. J Pharmacol Exp Ther. 2002;302:822–7.
16. Shintani M, Ogawa Y, Ebihara K, Aizawa-Abe M, Miyanaga F, Takaya K, et al. Ghrelin, an endogenous growth hormone secretagogue, is a novel orexigenic peptide that antagonizes leptin action through the activation of hypothalamic neuropeptide Y/Y1 receptor pathway. Diabetes. 2001;50:227–32.
17. Cowley MA, Smith RG, Diano S, Tschöp M, Pronchuk N, Grove KL, et al. The distribution and mechanism of action of ghrelin in the CNS demonstrates a novel hypothalamic circuit regulating energy homeostasis. Neuron. 2003;37:649–61.
18. Faulconbridge LF, Cummings DE, Kaplan JM, Grill HJ. Hyperphagic effects of brainstem ghrelin administration. Diabetes. 2003;52:2260–5.
19. Currie PJ, Mirza A, Fuld R, Park D, Vasselli JR. Ghrelin is an orexigenic and metabolic signaling peptide in the arcuate and paraventricular nuclei. Am J Physiol Regul Integr Comp Physiol. 2005;289:R353–8.
20. Olszewski PK, Grace MK, Billington CJ, Levine AS. Hypothalamic paraventricular injections of ghrelin: effect on feeding and c-Fos immunoreactivity. Peptides. 2003;24:919–23.
21. Olszewski PK, Li D, Grace MK, Billington CJ, Kotz CM, Levine AS. Neural basis of orexigenic effects of

ghrelin acting within lateral hypothalamus. Peptides. 2003;24:597–602.

22. Kanoski SE, Fortin SM, Ricks KM, Grill HJ. Ghrelin signaling in the ventral hippocampus stimulates learned and motivational aspects of feeding via PI3K-Akt signaling. Biol Psychiatry. 2013;73:915–23.

23. Alvarez-Crespo M, Skibicka KP, Farkas I, Molnár CS, Egecioglu E, Hrabovszky E, et al. The amygdala as a neurobiological target for ghrelin in rats: neuroanatomical, electrophysiological and behavioral evidence. PLoS One. 2012;7:e46321.

24. Skibicka KP, Hansson C, Alvarez-Crespo M, Friberg PA, Dickson SL. Ghrelin directly targets the ventral tegmental area to increase food motivation. Neuroscience. 2011;180:129–37.

25. King SJ, Isaacs AM, O'Farrell E, Abizaid A. Motivation to obtain preferred foods is enhanced by ghrelin in the ventral tegmental area. Horm Behav. 2011;60:572–80.

26. Cone JJ, McCutcheon JE, Roitman MF. Ghrelin acts as an interface between physiological state and phasic dopamine signaling. J Neurosci. 2014;34:4905–13.

27. Narayanan NS, Guarnieri DJ, DiLeone RJ. Metabolic hormones, dopamine circuits, and feeding. Front Neuroendocrinol. 2010;31:104–12.

28. Yasuda T, Masaki T, Kakuma T, Yoshimatsu H. Centrally administered ghrelin suppresses sympathetic nerve activity in brown adipose tissue of rats. Neurosci Lett. 2003;349:75–8.

29. Tschöp M, Smiley DL, Heiman ML. Ghrelin induces adiposity in rodents. Nature. 2000;407:908–13.

30. Wren AM, Small CJ, Abbott CR, Dhillo WS, Seal LJ, Cohen MA, et al. Ghrelin causes hyperphagia and obesity in rats. Diabetes. 2001;50:2540–7.

31. Gray SM, Page LC, Tong J. Ghrelin regulation of glucose metabolism. J Neuroendocrinol. 2019;31:e12705.

32. Dezaki K, Hosoda H, Kakei M, Hashiguchi S, Watanabe M, Kangawa K, et al. Endogenous ghrelin in pancreatic islets restricts insulin release by attenuating Ca^{2+} signaling in beta-cells: implication in the glycemic control in rodents. Diabetes. 2004;53:3142–51.

33. Shankar K, Takemi S, Gupta D, Varshney S, Mani BK, Osborne-Lawrence S, et al. Ghrelin cell-expressed insulin receptors mediate meal- and obesity-induced declines in plasma ghrelin. JCI Insight. 2021;6:e146983.

34. Gupta D, Ogden SB, Shankar K, Varshney S, Zigman JM. A LEAP 2 conclusions? Targeting the ghrelin system to treat obesity and diabetes. Mol Metab. 2021;46:101128.

35. English PJ, Ghatei MA, Malik IA, Bloom SR, Wilding JP. Food fails to suppress ghrelin levels in obese humans. J Clin Endocrinol Metab. 2002;87:2984.

36. Tschöp M, Weyer C, Tataranni PA, Devanarayan V, Ravussin E, Heiman ML. Circulating ghrelin levels are decreased in human obesity. Diabetes. 2001;50:707–9.

37. Hansen TK, Dall R, Hosoda H, Kojima M, Kangawa K, Christiansen JS, et al. Weight loss increases circulating levels of ghrelin in human obesity. Clin Endocrinol. 2002;56:203–6.

38. Takagi K, Legrand R, Asakawa A, Amitani H, François M, Tennoune N, et al. Anti-ghrelin immunoglobulins modulate ghrelin stability and its orexigenic effect in obese mice and humans. Nat Commun. 2013;4:2685.

39. Shearman LP, Wang SP, Helmling S, Stribling DS, Mazur P, Ge L, et al. Ghrelin neutralization by a ribonucleic acid-SPM ameliorates obesity in diet-induced obese mice. Endocrinology. 2006;147:1517–26.

40. Abizaid A, Hougland JL. Ghrelin signaling: GOAT and GHS-R1a take a LEAP in complexity. Trends Endocrinol Metab. 2020;31:107–17.

41. Cardona Cano S, Merkestein M, Skibicka KP, Dickson SL, Adan RA. Role of ghrelin in the pathophysiology of eating disorders: implications for pharmacotherapy. CNS Drugs. 2012;26:281–96.

42. Mori H, Verbeure W, Tanemoto R, Sosoranga ER, Jan T. Physiological functions and potential clinical applications of motilin. Peptides. 2023;160:170905.

43. Deloose E, Tack J. Redefining the functional roles of the gastrointestinal migrating motor complex and motilin in small bacterial overgrowth and hunger signaling. Am J Physiol Gastrointest Liver Physiol. 2016;310:G228–33.

44. Moran TH. Gut peptide signaling in the controls of food intake. Obesity (Silver Spring). 2006;14(Suppl 5):250s–3s.

45. Gibbs J, Young RC, Smith GP. Cholecystokinin decreases food intake in rats. J Comp Physiol Psychol. 1973;84:488–95.

46. Smith GP, Jerome C, Norgren R. Afferent axons in abdominal vagus mediate satiety effect of cholecystokinin in rats. Am J Phys. 1985;249:R638–41.

47. Moran TH, Ameglio PJ, Schwartz GJ, McHugh PR. Blockade of type A, not type B, CCK receptors attenuates satiety actions of exogenous and endogenous CCK. Am J Phys. 1992;262:R46–50.

48. Moran TH, Katz LF, Plata-Salaman CR, Schwartz GJ. Disordered food intake and obesity in rats lacking cholecystokinin A receptors. Am J Phys. 1998;274:R618–25.

49. Schwartz GJ, McHugh PR, Moran TH. Gastric loads and cholecystokinin synergistically stimulate rat gastric vagal afferents. Am J Phys. 1993;265:R872–6.

50. Moran TH, McHugh PR. Cholecystokinin suppresses food intake by inhibiting gastric emptying. Am J Phys. 1982;242:R491–7.

51. Schwartz GJ, Netterville LA, McHugh PR, Moran TH. Gastric loads potentiate inhibition of food intake produced by a cholecystokinin analogue. Am J Phys. 1991;261:R1141–6.

52. Peters JH, Ritter RC, Simasko SM. Leptin and CCK selectively activate vagal afferent neurons innervating the stomach and duodenum. Am J Physiol Regul Integr Comp Physiol. 2006;290:R1544–9.

53. Emond M, Schwartz GJ, Ladenheim EE, Moran TH. Central leptin modulates behavioral and neural responsivity to CCK. Am J Phys. 1999;276:R1545–9.

54. Flak JN, Patterson CM, Garfield AS, D'Agostino G, Goforth PB, Sutton AK, et al. Leptin-inhibited PBN neurons enhance responses to hypoglycemia in negative energy balance. Nat Neurosci. 2014;17:1744–50.

55. Duca FA, Zhong L, Covasa M. Reduced CCK signaling in obese-prone rats fed a high fat diet. Horm Behav. 2013;64:812–7.

56. Crawley JN, Beinfeld MC. Rapid development of tolerance to the behavioural actions of cholecystokinin. Nature. 1983;302:703–6.

57. Lampel M, Kern HF. Acute interstitial pancreatitis in the rat induced by excessive doses of a pancreatic secretagogue. Virchows Arch A Pathol Anat Histol. 1977;373:97–117.

58. Makovec F, Bani M, Cereda R, Chistè R, Revel L, Rovati LC, et al. Protective effect of CR 1409 (cholecystokinin antagonist) on experimental pancreatitis in rats and mice. Peptides. 1986;7:1159–64.

59. Jordan J, Greenway FL, Leiter LA, Li Z, Jacobson P, Murphy K, et al. Stimulation of cholecystokinin-A receptors with GI181771X does not cause weight loss in overweight or obese patients. Clin Pharmacol Ther. 2008;83:281–7.

60. Ahrén B, Holst JJ, Efendic S. Antidiabetogenic action of cholecystokinin-8 in type 2 diabetes. J Clin Endocrinol Metab. 2000;85:1043–8.

61. Boushey RP, Abadir A, Flamez D, Baggio LL, Li Y, Berger V, et al. Hypoglycemia, defective islet glucagon secretion, but normal islet mass in mice with a disruption of the gastrin gene. Gastroenterology. 2003;125:1164–74.

62. Chen D, Hagen SJ, Boyce M, Zhao CM. Neuroendocrine mechanism of gastric acid secretion: Historical perspectives and recent developments in physiology and pharmacology. J Neuroendocrinol. 2023;18: e13305. https://doi.org/10.1111/jne.13305. Epub ahead of print. PMID: 37317882.

63. Bugge A, Jansen PG, Maria L, Sanni SJ, Clausen TR. Cloning and characterization of the porcine gastrin/cholecystokinin type 2 receptor. Eur J Pharmacol. 2018;833:357–63.

64. Manning S, Batterham RL. The role of gut hormone peptide YY in energy and glucose homeostasis: twelve years on. Annu Rev Physiol. 2014;76:585–608.

65. Batterham RL, Cowley MA, Small CJ, Herzog H, Cohen MA, Dakin CL, et al. Gut hormone PYY (3-36) physiologically inhibits food intake. Nature. 2002;418:650–4.

66. Batterham RL, Cohen MA, Ellis SM, Le Roux CW, Withers DJ, Frost GS, et al. Inhibition of food intake in obese subjects by peptide YY3-36. N Engl J Med. 2003;349:941–8.

67. Nonaka N, Shioda S, Niehoff ML, Banks WA. Characterization of blood-brain barrier permeability to PYY3-36 in the mouse. J Pharmacol Exp Ther. 2003;306:948–53.

68. Abbott CR, Small CJ, Kennedy AR, Neary NM, Sajedi A, Ghatei MA, et al. Blockade of the neuropeptide Y Y2 receptor with the specific antagonist BIIE0246 attenuates the effect of endogenous and exogenous peptide YY(3-36) on food intake. Brain Res. 2005;1043:139–44.

69. Morley JE, Levine AS, Grace M, Kneip J. Peptide YY (PYY), a potent orexigenic agent. Brain Res. 1985;341:200–3.

70. Corp ES, Melville LD, Greenberg D, Gibbs J, Smith GP. Effect of fourth ventricular neuropeptide Y and peptide YY on ingestive and other behaviors. Am J Phys. 1990;259:R317–23.

71. Raposinho PD, Pierroz DD, Broqua P, White RB, Pedrazzini T, Aubert ML. Chronic administration of neuropeptide Y into the lateral ventricle of C57BL/6J male mice produces an obesity syndrome including hyperphagia, hyperleptinemia, insulin resistance, and hypogonadism. Mol Cell Endocrinol. 2001;185:195–204.

72. Stadlbauer U, Arnold M, Weber E, Langhans W. Possible mechanisms of circulating PYY-induced satiation in male rats. Endocrinology. 2013;154:193–204.

73. Allen JM, Fitzpatrick ML, Yeats JC, Darcy K, Adrian TE, Bloom SR. Effects of peptide YY and neuropeptide Y on gastric emptying in man. Digestion. 1984;30:255–62.

74. Chen CH, Rogers RC, Stephens RL Jr. Intracisternal injection of peptide YY inhibits gastric emptying in rats. Regul Pept. 1996;61:95–8.

75. Meyer-Gerspach AC, Wölnerhanssen B, Beglinger B, Nessenius F, Napitupulu M, Schulte FH, et al. Gastric and intestinal satiation in obese and normal weight healthy people. Physiol Behav. 2014;129:265–71. https://doi.org/10.1016/j.physbeh.2014.02.043. Epub 2014 Feb 28. PMID: 24582673.

76. Gantz I, Erondu N, Mallick M, Musser B, Krishna R, Tanaka WK, et al. Efficacy and safety of intranasal peptide YY3-36 for weight reduction in obese adults. J Clin Endocrinol Metab. 2007;92:1754–7.

77. Troke RC, Tan TM, Bloom SR. The future role of gut hormones in the treatment of obesity. Ther Adv Chronic Dis. 2014;5:4–14.

78. Lutz TA. Creating the amylin story. Appetite. 2022,172.105965.

79. Lutz TA. The role of amylin in the control of energy homeostasis. Am J Physiol Regul Integr Comp Physiol. 2010;298:R1475–84.

80. Mietlicki-Baase EG, Hayes MR. Amylin activates distributed CNS nuclei to control energy balance. Physiol Behav. 2014;136:39–46.

81. Turek VF, Trevaskis JL, Levin BE, Dunn-Meynell AA, Irani B, Gu G, et al. Mechanisms of amylin/leptin synergy in rodent models. Endocrinology. 2010;151: 143–52.

82. Chapman I, Parker B, Doran S, Feinle-Bisset C, Wishart J, Strobel S, et al. Effect of pramlintide on satiety and food intake in obese subjects and subjects with type 2 diabetes. Diabetologia. 2005;48:838–48.

83. Ravussin E, Smith SR, Mitchell JA, Shringarpure R, Shan K, Maier H, et al. Enhanced weight loss with pramlintide/metreleptin: an integrated neurohormonal approach to obesity pharmacotherapy. Obesity (Silver Spring). 2009;17:1736–43.

84. Smith SR, Blundell JE, Burns C, Ellero C, Schroeder BE, Kesty NC, et al. Pramlintide treatment reduces 24-h caloric intake and meal sizes and improves control of eating in obese subjects: a 6-wk translational research study. Am J Physiol Endocrinol Metab. 2007;293:E620–7.

85. Dupre J, Ross SA, Watson D, Brown JC. Stimulation of insulin secretion by gastric inhibitory polypeptide in man. J Clin Endocrinol Metab. 1973;37:826–8.

86. Pederson RA, Schubert HE, Brown JC. Gastric inhibitory polypeptide. Its physiologic release and insulinotropic action in the dog. Diabetes. 1975;24: 1050–6.

87. Yip RG, Boylan MO, Kieffer TJ, Wolfe MM. Functional GIP receptors are present on adipocytes. Endocrinology. 1998;139:4004–7.

88. Tseng CC, Kieffer TJ, Jarboe LA, Usdin TB, Wolfe MM. Postprandial stimulation of insulin release by glucose-dependent insulinotropic polypeptide (GIP). Effect of a specific glucose-dependent insulinotropic polypeptide receptor antagonist in the rat. J Clin Invest. 1996;98:2440–5.

89. Baggio L, Kieffer TJ, Drucker DJ. Glucagon-like peptide-1, but not glucose-dependent insulinotropic peptide, regulates fasting glycemia and nonenteral glucose clearance in mice. Endocrinology. 2000;141:3703–9.

90. Miyawaki K, Yamada Y, Yano H, Niwa H, Ban N, Ihara Y, et al. Glucose intolerance caused by a defect in the entero-insular axis: a study in gastric inhibitory polypeptide receptor knockout mice. Proc Natl Acad Sci U S A. 1999;96:14843–7.

91. Drucker DJ. GLP-1 physiology informs the pharmacotherapy of obesity. Mol Metab. 2022;57:101351.

92. Kreymann B, Williams G, Ghatei MA, Bloom SR. Glucagon-like peptide-1 7-36: a physiological incretin in man. Lancet. 1987;2:1300–4.

93. Mojsov S, Weir GC, Habener JF. Insulinotropin: glucagon-like peptide I (7-37) co-encoded in the glucagon gene is a potent stimulator of insulin release in the perfused rat pancreas. J Clin Invest. 1987;79:616–9.

94. D'Alessio DA, Vogel R, Prigeon R, Laschansky E, Koerker D, Eng J, et al. Elimination of the action of glucagon-like peptide 1 causes an impairment of glucose tolerance after nutrient ingestion by healthy baboons. J Clin Invest. 1996;97:133–8.

95. Edwards CM, Todd JF, Mahmoudi M, Wang Z, Wang RM, Ghatei MA, et al. Glucagon-like peptide 1 has a physiological role in the control of postprandial glucose in humans: studies with the antagonist exendin 9-39. Diabetes. 1999;48:86–93.

96. Wang Z, Wang RM, Owji AA, Smith DM, Ghatei MA, Bloom SR. Glucagon-like peptide-1 is a physiological incretin in rat. J Clin Invest. 1995;95:417–21.

97. Scrocchi LA, Brown TJ, MaClusky N, Brubaker PL, Auerbach AB, Joyner AL, et al. Glucose intolerance but normal satiety in mice with a null mutation in the glucagon-like peptide 1 receptor gene. Nat Med. 1996;2:1254–8.

98. Xu G, Stoffers DA, Habener JF, Bonner-Weir S. Exendin-4 stimulates both beta-cell replication and neogenesis, resulting in increased beta-cell mass and improved glucose tolerance in diabetic rats. Diabetes. 1999;48:2270–6.

99. Stoffers DA, Kieffer TJ, Hussain MA, Drucker DJ, Bonner-Weir S, Habener JF, et al. Insulinotropic glucagon-like peptide 1 agonists stimulate expression of homeodomain protein IDX-1 and increase islet size in mouse pancreas. Diabetes. 2000;49:741–8.

100. Perfetti R, Zhou J, Doyle ME, Egan JM. Glucagon-like peptide-1 induces cell proliferation and pancreatic-duodenum homeobox-1 expression and increases endocrine cell mass in the pancreas of old, glucose-intolerant rats. Endocrinology. 2000;141: 4600–5.

101. Ling Z, Wu D, Zambre Y, Flamez D, Drucker DJ, Pipeleers DG, et al. Glucagon-like peptide 1 receptor signaling influences topography of islet cells in mice. Virchows Arch. 2001;438:382–7.

102. De León DD, Deng S, Madani R, Ahima RS, Drucker DJ, Stoffers DA. Role of endogenous glucagon-like peptide-1 in islet regeneration after partial pancreatectomy. Diabetes. 2003;52:365–71.

103. Boushey RP, Yusta B, Drucker DJ. Glucagon-like peptide 2 decreases mortality and reduces the severity of indomethacin-induced murine enteritis. Am J Phys. 1999;277:E937–47.

104. Boushey RP, Yusta B, Drucker DJ. Glucagon-like peptide (GLP)-2 reduces chemotherapy-associated mortality and enhances cell survival in cells expressing a transfected GLP-2 receptor. Cancer Res. 2001;61:687–93.

105. Jeppesen PB, Hartmann B, Thulesen J, Graff J, Lohmann J, Hansen BS, et al. Glucagon-like peptide 2 improves nutrient absorption and nutritional status in short-bowel patients with no colon. Gastroenterology. 2001;120:806–15.

106. Jeppesen PB. Clinical significance of GLP-2 in short-bowel syndrome. J Nutr. 2003;133:3721–4.

107. Collie NL, Zhu Z, Jordan S, Reeve JR Jr. Oxyntomodulin stimulates intestinal glucose uptake in rats. Gastroenterology. 1997;112:1961–70.

108. Jarrousse C, Bataille D, Jeanrenaud B. A pure enteroglucagon, oxyntomodulin (glucagon 37), stimulates insulin release in perfused rat pancreas. Endocrinology. 1984;115:102–5.

109. Wynne K, Park AJ, Small CJ, Meeran K, Ghatei MA, Frost GS, et al. Oxyntomodulin increases energy expenditure in addition to decreasing energy intake in overweight and obese humans: a randomised controlled trial. Int J Obes. 2006;30:1729–36.

110. Wynne K, Park AJ, Small CJ, Patterson M, Ellis SM, Murphy KG, et al. Subcutaneous oxyntomodulin reduces body weight in overweight and obese subjects: a double-blind, randomized, controlled trial. Diabetes. 2005;54:2390–5.

111. Dakin CL, Gunn I, Small CJ, Edwards CM, Hay DL, Smith DM, et al. Oxyntomodulin inhibits food intake in the rat. Endocrinology. 2001;142:4244–50.

112. Baggio LL, Huang Q, Brown TJ, Drucker DJ. Oxyntomodulin and glucagon-like peptide-1 differentially regulate murine food intake and energy expenditure. Gastroenterology. 2004;127:546–58.

113. Mitani H, Takimoto M, Hughes TE, Kimura M. Dipeptidyl peptidase IV inhibition improves impaired glucose tolerance in high-fat diet-fed rats: study using a Fischer 344 rat substrain deficient in its enzyme activity. Jpn J Pharmacol. 2002;88:442–50.

114. Ahrén B, Holst JJ, Mårtensson H, Balkan B. Improved glucose tolerance and insulin secretion by inhibition of dipeptidyl peptidase IV in mice. Eur J Pharmacol. 2000;404:239–45. https://doi.org/10.1016/s0014-2999(00)00600-2. PMID: 10980284.

115. Ahrén B, Simonsson E, Larsson H, Landin-Olsson M, Torgeirsson H, Jansson PA, et al. Inhibition of dipeptidyl peptidase IV improves metabolic control over a 4-week study period in type 2 diabetes. Diabetes Care. 2002;25:869–75. https://doi.org/10.2337/diacare.25.5.869. PMID: 11978683.

116. Bosi E, Camisasca RP, Collober C, Rochotte E, Garber AJ. Effects of vildagliptin on glucose control over 24 weeks in patients with type 2 diabetes inadequately controlled with metformin. Diabetes Care. 2007;30:890–5.

117. DeFronzo RA, Hissa MN, Garber AJ, Luiz Gross J, Yuyan Duan R, Ravichandran S, et al. The efficacy and safety of saxagliptin when added to metformin therapy in patients with inadequately controlled type 2 diabetes with metformin alone. Diabetes Care. 2009;32:1649–55.

118. Hermansen K, Kipnes M, Luo E, Fanurik D, Khatami H, Stein P. Efficacy and safety of the dipeptidyl peptidase-4 inhibitor, sitagliptin, in patients with type 2 diabetes mellitus inadequately controlled on glimepiride alone or on glimepiride and metformin. Diabetes Obes Metab. 2007;9:733–45.

119. Rosenstock J, Brazg R, Andryuk PJ, Lu K, Stein P. Efficacy and safety of the dipeptidyl peptidase-4 inhibitor sitagliptin added to ongoing pioglitazone therapy in patients with type 2 diabetes: a 24-week, multicenter, randomized, double-blind, placebo-controlled, parallel-group study. Clin Ther. 2006;28:1556–68.

120. Fonseca V, Schweizer A, Albrecht D, Baron MA, Chang I, Dejager S. Addition of vildagliptin to insulin improves glycaemic control in type 2 diabetes. Diabetologia. 2007;50:1148–55.

121. Göke R, Fehmann HC, Linn T, Schmidt H, Krause M, Eng J, et al. Exendin-4 is a high potency agonist and truncated exendin-(9-39)-amide an antagonist at the glucagon-like peptide 1-(7-36)-amide receptor of insulin-secreting beta-cells. J Biol Chem. 1993;268:19650–5.

122. Knudsen LB, Lau J. The discovery and development of liraglutide and semaglutide. Front Endocrinol (Lausanne). 2019;10:155.

123. Pi-Sunyer X, Astrup A, Fujioka K, Greenway F, Halpern A, Krempf M, et al. A randomized, controlled trial of 3.0 mg of liraglutide in weight management. N Engl J Med. 2015;373:11–22.

124. Wadden TA, Hollander P, Klein S, Niswender K, Woo V, Hale PM, et al. Weight maintenance and additional weight loss with liraglutide after low-calorie-diet-induced weight loss: the SCALE Maintenance randomized study. Int J Obes. 2013;37:1443–51.

125. Davies MJ, Bergenstal R, Bode B, Kushner RF, Lewin A, Skjøth TV, et al. Efficacy of liraglutide for weight loss among patients with type 2 diabetes: the SCALE diabetes randomized clinical trial. JAMA. 2015;314:687–99.

126. Blackman A, Foster GD, Zammit G, Rosenberg R, Aronne L, Wadden T, et al. Effect of liraglutide 3.0 mg in individuals with obesity and moderate or severe obstructive sleep apnea: the SCALE Sleep Apnea randomized clinical trial. Int J Obes. 2016;40:1310–9.

127. Wilding JPH, Batterham RL, Calanna S, Davies M, Van Gaal LF, Lingvay I, et al. Once-weekly semaglutide in adults with overweight or obesity. N Engl J Med. 2021;384:989–1002.

128. Wadden TA, Bailey TS, Billings LK, Davies M, Frias JP, Koroleva A, et al. Effect of subcutaneous semaglutide vs placebo as an adjunct to intensive behavioral therapy on body weight in adults with overweight or obesity: the STEP 3 randomized clinical trial. JAMA. 2021;325:1403–13.

129. Rubino D, Abrahamsson N, Davies M, Hesse D, Greenway FL, Jensen C, et al. Effect of continued weekly subcutaneous semaglutide vs placebo on weight loss maintenance in adults with overweight or obesity: the STEP 4 randomized clinical trial. JAMA. 2021;325:1414–25.

130. Kristensen SL, Rørth R, Jhund PS, Docherty KF, Sattar N, Preiss D, et al. Cardiovascular, mortality, and kidney outcomes with GLP-1 receptor agonists in patients with type 2 diabetes: a systematic review and meta-analysis of cardiovascular outcome trials. Lancet Diabetes Endocrinol. 2019;7:776–85.

131. Sattar N, Lee MMY, Kristensen SL, Branch KRH, Del Prato S, Khurmi NS, et al. Cardiovascular, mortality, and kidney outcomes with GLP-1 receptor agonists in patients with type 2 diabetes: a systematic review and meta-analysis of randomised trials. Lancet Diabetes Endocrinol. 2021;9:653–62.

132. Hernandez AF, Green JB, Janmohamed S, D'Agostino RB Sr, Granger CB, Jones NP, et al. Albiglutide and cardiovascular outcomes in patients with type 2 diabetes and cardiovascular disease (Harmony Outcomes): a double-blind, randomised placebo-controlled trial. Lancet. 2018;392:1519–29.

133. Gerstein HC, Sattar N, Rosenstock J, Ramasundarahettige C, Pratley R, Lopes RD, et al. Cardiovascular and renal outcomes with efpeglenatide in type 2 diabetes. N Engl J Med. 2021;385:896–907.

134. Marso SP, Bain SC, Consoli A, Eliaschewitz FG, Jódar E, Leiter LA, et al. Semaglutide and cardiovascular outcomes in patients with type 2 diabetes. N Engl J Med. 2016;375:1834–44.

135. Müller TD, Finan B, Clemmensen C, DiMarchi RD, Tschöp MH. The new biology and pharmacology of glucagon. Physiol Rev. 2017;97:721–66.

136. Müller TD, Blüher M, Tschöp MH, DiMarchi RD. Anti-obesity drug discovery: advances and challenges. Nat Rev Drug Discov. 2022;21:201–23.

137. Bass J, Tschöp MH, Beutler LR. Dual gut hormone receptor agonists for diabetes and obesity. J Clin Invest. 2023;133:e167952.

138. Day JW, Ottaway N, Patterson JT, Gelfanov V, Smiley D, Gidda J, et al. A new glucagon and GLP-1 co-agonist eliminates obesity in rodents. Nat Chem Biol. 2009;5:749–57.

139. Nahra R, Wang T, Gadde KM, Oscarsson J, Stumvoll M, Jermutus L, et al. Effects of cotadutide on metabolic and hepatic parameters in adults with overweight or obesity and type 2 diabetes: a 54-week randomized phase 2b study. Diabetes Care. 2021;44: 1433–42.

140. Frias JP, Bastyr EJ 3rd, Vignati L, Tschöp MH, Schmitt C, Owen K, et al. The sustained effects of a dual GIP/GLP-1 receptor agonist, NNC0090-2746, in patients with type 2 diabetes. Cell Metab. 2017;26: 343–52.e2.

141. Jastreboff AM, Aronne LJ, Ahmad NN, Wharton S, Connery L, Alves B, et al. Tirzepatide once weekly for the treatment of obesity. N Engl J Med. 2022;387: 205–16.

142. Kruse T, Hansen JL, Dahl K, Schäffer L, Sensfuss U, Poulsen C, et al. Development of cagrilintide, a long-acting amylin analogue. J Med Chem. 2021;64: 11183–94.

143. Enebo LB, Berthelsen KK, Kankam M, Lund MT, Rubino DM, Satylganova A, et al. Safety, tolerability, pharmacokinetics, and pharmacodynamics of concomitant administration of multiple doses of cagrilintide with semaglutide 2·4 mg for weight management: a randomised, controlled, phase 1b trial. Lancet. 2021;397:1736–48.

Gut Microbiome, Obesity, and Metabolic Syndrome

20

Herbert Tilg and Alexander R. Moschen

Contents

H. Tilg (✉)
Department of Internal Medicine I, Gastroenterology, Endocrinology & Metabolism, Medical University Innsbruck, Innsbruck, Austria
e-mail: herbert.tilg@i-med.ac.at

A. R. Moschen
Department of Internal Medicine 2 and Christian Doppler Laboratory for Mucosal Immunology, Faculty of Medicine, Johannes Kepler University, Linz, Austria
e-mail: alexander.moschen@jku.at

Abstract

Obesity, metabolic syndrome, and type 2 diabetes (T2D) reflect a major disease burden throughout the world. In all these disorders, low-grade chronic inflammation is commonly observed. The origin of this type of inflammation is currently unknown. Recent studies, however, suggest that the gastrointestinal tract with its enormous microbial world, i.e., the intestinal microbiota, not only could play a role in these disorders but also contribute to low-grade chronic inflammation. The gut microbiota affects many biological functions throughout the body including many immune and metabolic features. Data from animal models and humans support that obesity and associated disorders are characterized by a so-called dysbiosis. Human metagenome-wide association studies mainly in obesity and T2D have demonstrated that there exists a "gut microbiotal signature" in these diseases.

© Springer Nature Switzerland AG 2023
R. S. Ahima (ed.), *Metabolic Syndrome*,
https://doi.org/10.1007/978-3-031-40116-9_26

Further evidence for a major role of the gut microbiome has been derived from studies in pregnancy and after Cesarean section. Antibiotic use in early-life also affects the microbiota in a profound manner and might contribute to the development of childhood obesity, T2D, and immune-mediated disorders in later life. Therefore, as a "gut" signature became evident in the last years in these diseases, a better understanding of these aspects is mandatory to gain further insights and define a basis for new therapeutic approaches.

Keywords

Adipokines · Inflammation · Innate immunity · Metagenomics · Microbiota

Abbreviations

AMPK	AMP-activated protein kinase
FFAR	free fatty acid receptor
FIAF	fasting-induced adipose factor
FXR	farnesoid X receptor
GLP-1	glucagon-like peptide 1
GPCR	G-protein coupled receptor
HFD	high-fat diet
HGC	high gene count
ILC	innate lymphoid cells
LGC	low gene count
LPL	lipoprotein lipase
MLG	metagenomic linkage group
mTORC1	mechanistic target of rapamycin complex 1
SCFA	short-chain fatty acid
T2D	type 2 diabetes
TLR5	toll-like receptor 5

Introduction

The human intestinal tract harbors an immense number of **microorganisms**, i.e., the intestinal microbiota consisting of at least 10^{14} bacteria, archaea, and viruses. These microorganisms generate a biomass of up to 1,0 kg, and their genomes (i.e., microbiome) exceed the human genome more than 100-fold [1, 2]. Initial studies suggested that these genes encode mainly functions directing immune pathways and such ones needed for digestion of complex carbohydrates. Recent investigations, however, convincingly demonstrated that the microbiota may have key functions in regulating **metabolic pathways** in health and disease [2–5]. High-throughput sequencing technologies have allowed in the past years to increase the understanding of the complexity and diversity of the microbiota [6]. Importantly, many of the more than 5000 assumed bacterial species cannot be cultured currently [7, 8].

An altered intestinal microbiota in metabolic diseases might play a role in initiating inflammatory processes throughout the organism. Such an altered microbiota might not only act "locally" but via an impaired **mucosal barrier** also systemically. This is in accordance with the recently proposed concept of "**metabolic infection,**" where parts of the intestinal microbiota might act systemically and affect systemic including adipose tissue **inflammation** [9]. In many disorders such as inflammatory bowel disease, obesity, or type 2 diabetes (T2D), a "microbiotal signature" has been identified [10, 11]. In this chapter, we will discuss the current evidence for a role of the intestinal microbiota in obesity and T2D and thereby could contribute to the phenotype of these disorders.

Role of the Intestinal Microbiota in Obesity

Many studies from the last years, particularly using animal models, have shown that the microbiota might reflect one major player in the development of obesity [12–15]. A landmark study by Turnbaugh and colleagues in 2006 observed that colonizing **germ-free mice** with the intestinal microbiota from *ob/ob* mice, genetically obese mice, caused a higher fat mass compared with gut microbes from lean mice independent from consumption of food [14]. Ridaura and colleagues also showed that the microbiota derived from discordant obese twins affects metabolism in mice [16]. These investigators transferred the microbiota collected from human female twin pairs discordant for obesity into germ-free mice showing that obesity can again be transferred to rodents. Importantly, co-housing of mice containing cultured bacteria from an obese twin with mice containing bacteria from a lean twin prohibited development of the obese phenotype. Diet appeared as a critical co-founder in these experiments highlighting the dominant role of diet on the microbial community. When mice were treated with a low-fat, high-fiber diet even when harboring the obese microbiota and were co-housed with mice containing the lean microbiota, the lean microbiota dominated in the obese mice preventing adiposity.

The gene count of the intestinal microbiota might be important in human obesity [17]. Le Chatalier and colleagues observed that in case of low **bacterial richness** (low gene count, LGC), obesity and related disorders such as insulin resistance, fatty liver, and **low-grade inflammation** were more common compared to subjects characterized by high gene count (HGC). Individuals with this LGC in their microbiota gained more weight and had a higher rate of systemic inflammation as demonstrated by higher levels of high-sensitive **C-reactive protein**, a higher rate of insulin resistance, and dyslipidemia. Whereas *Bacteroides* and some *Ruminococcus* species were more dominant in LGC, ***Faecalibacterium prausnitzii***, *Bifidobacterium*, *Lactobacillus*, *Alistipes*, ***Akkermansia***, and others were significantly associated with HGC. At phylum levels, *Bacteroidetes* and Proteobacteria were more commonly observed in LGC, whereas *Verrucomicrobia* (e.g., *Akkermansia muciniphila*) and *Actinobacter* were more dominant in HGC. Findings of this study overall support a concept that in case of obesity potential pro-inflammatory bacteria may dominate. e.g., *Ruminococcus gnavus* or *Bacteroides* and anti-inflammatory such as *F. prausnitzii* are less prevalent. Further studies from this cohort of patients showed that LGC subjects contained a more pro-inflammatory microbiotal profile accompanied by an increase in oxidative stress. Dietary interventions by using an energy-restricted diet improved this microbial richness and clinical phenotype in LGC subjects, although subjects with an already high microbial richness responded less well to dietary treatment [18]. These studies support the current belief that microbial composition and potentially the richness of these bacterial genes in our gut might be able to define obese people with metabolic and inflammatory complications.

It has been less well studied until recently how the gut microbiota changes in obese subjects after weight loss. Remely and colleagues investigated obese people receiving a **dietary intervention** proposed by the German, Austrian, and Swiss Society of Nutrition over 3 months [19]. Here, fecal microbiota and bioelectrical impedance analysis were performed before, during, and after the dietary intervention. After weight loss, the ratio of *Firmicutes/Bacteroidetes* significantly decreased, whereas *Lactobacilli*, *Clostridium cluster IV*, *F. prausnitzii*, and *Akkermansia muciniphila* increased significantly. Increase in these bacteria is of relevance, as these strains have been demonstrated to exert beneficial and anti-inflammatory properties [20, 21]. The use of **pre-** and **probiotics** besides weight loss reflect another important treatment approach as they might be able to cause beneficial shifts in the intestinal microbiota. Dewulf and colleagues recently demonstrated that the administration of certain prebiotics (i.e., inulin-type fructans) changed the gut microbiota composition in obese women with an increase in *Lactobacilli*, *Bifidobacteria*, and *Clostridium* cluster IV resulting in modest changes in **host metabolism** [22]. Many preclinical studies have also focused on the use of certain probiotics to affect an obese phenotype. *Lactobacillus casei*, *Lactobacillus rhamnosus*, and *Bifidobacterium animalis subsp. lactis* are able to shift the microbiotal structure in mice after receiving a high-fat diet (HFD) toward a lean phenotype [23]. Whereas ***Lactobacillus casei*** and *Lactobacillus rhamnosus* in this study mainly increased the concentration of the short-chain fatty acid acetate, *Bifidobacterium animalis subsp. lactis* failed such an effect but still was able to decrease adipose tissue inflammation.

Overall, all many studies have gathered convincing evidence that the gut microbiota plays a role in human obesity and intervention via **weight-loss** strategies and/or pre-/probiotics might not only affect phenotype but also composition of this microbiota. Despite these insights, it remains unclear until today what is the clinical relevance of dysbiosis in humans. Various metabolic pathways might be affected by manifest dysbiosis in human obesity. Many gut microbiota driven metabolites might be either detrimental such as endotoxin or beneficial in protecting the host from obesity-related inflammation such as short-chain fatty acids (SCFAs), indoles, bile acids, or various amino acids, and a dysbalance in these metabolites might contribute to the obesity phenotype. It has to be stated though that some reports in the past years have shown different findings by suggesting that *Bacteroides* are more abundant in obese subjects compared to lean counterparts [24, 25]. Several of described discrepant findings so far are based on the fact that many analyses were phyla-oriented which are overall too simplistic and superficial [26]. Within the phylum Bacteroidetes, for example, the Prevotella to *Bacteroides* ratio seems important as *Bacteroides* dominance is associated with a dominantly Western diet. The Prevotella enterotype is linked with lower BMI values, and a *Bacteroides* 2-enterotype is more prevalent among obese subjects and positively correlated with BMI. Many relevant changes might take place at the level of species. *Christenellaceae* is again positively associated with increased α-diversity and lower BMI values [27, 28]. *Dysosmobacter welbionis* is another recently identified human commensal bacterium having the capacity to prevent diet-induced obesity and to prevent metabolic diseases in mice [29]. To summarize, there are many preclinical findings and clinical studies supporting an important role for the gut microbiome in obesity. To figure out and to identify key players remain a challenge and especially to translate these findings toward clinical improvements and benefits for our obese patients.

Gut Microbiota and Diabetes

As most of **T2D** patients are obese, it has been expected that also in this condition a "microbiotal signature" might exist. The first study using high-throughput sequencing was performed by analyzing stool samples from Chinese T2D patients, and metagenomic analysis was combined with clinical data [30]. T2D patients showed a modest **intestinal dysbiosis** characterized by a decrease in butyrate-producing *Roseburia intestinalis* and *F. prausnitzii*. In this study, the concept of metagenomic linkage group (MLG) analysis has been applied, and thereby, they observed that in the healthy control samples especially various butyrate-producing bacteria were enriched (e.g., *Clostridiales* sp. SS3/4, *Eubacterium rectale*, *F. prausnitzii*, *Roseburia intestinalis*), whereas in T2D most MLGs belonged to more opportunistic pathogens such as *Bacteroides caccae*, various *Clostridiales, and Escherichia coli*. When assessing potential associated functions of this gut dysbiosis in T2D, T2D microbiota showed enrichment in membrane transport of sugars, branched-chain amino acid transport and sulfate reduction and decreased **butyrate biosynthesis** but even more importantly also an increase in oxidative stress response. This could become of special relevance as one could speculate that the gastrointestinal tract with its microbiota could reflect a starting point for the observed low-grade inflammation in T2D. Overall more than 3% of the gut microbial genes differed between T2D patients and healthy subjects. Another important study came from Sweden [11]. Here, the authors applied shotgun sequencing studying only postmenopausal female T2D patients. T2D patients showed increases in the abundance of four *Lactobacillus* species including *L. gasseri*, *Streptococcus mutans,* and certain *Clostridiales* such as *Clostridium clostridioforme* and again decreases in at least five other *Clostridium* species. **Roseburia intestinalis** and *F. prausnitzii*, both prototypic butyrate producers, were highly discriminant for T2D. It has to be stated that the number of analyzed T2D patients in the Scandinavian study was rather low and study design was not able to detect whether a diabetes-specific drug might have influenced microbiota composition. These two studies reflect an important initiative in this field and support the notion that not only a "gut signature" might exist, but more importantly functional analysis also revealed that a **pro-inflammatory** tone might be initiated in the intestine which could reflect the starting point of low-grade systemic inflammation as commonly observed in T2D and related disorders such as nonalcoholic fatty liver disease (Fig. 1). Importantly, Wu and colleagues observed that drugs might contribute to observed gut microbiota alterations in T2D demonstrating that metformin indeed had a substantial impact on the gut microbiome in a double-blind study in humans [31]. In this study, the investigators even found that the altered gut microbiota mediated some of proposed metformin's effects as an anti-diabetic drug. Wu and colleagues furthermore showed in large populations of treatment naïve T2D patients that indeed an altered gut micro-biome exists in T2D [32]. In a further elegant study from Fredrik Bäckhed's group, it could be demonstrated that the microbiota-derived metab-olite imidazole propionate is able to affect insulin signaling through activation of mechanistic target of rapamycin complex 1 (mTORC1) [33]. In sum-mary, the results from the here presented studies clearly suggest that T2D patients show evidence of a gut dysbiosis independent of confounding drugs. More mechanistic studies are needed to understand potential pathways contributing to this phenotype.

Involved Immunometabolic Pathways and Role of Certain Bacteria

Short-Chain Fatty Acids

One important activity of the gut's microbiota is to digest dietary fibers [34]. The main end products of this digestion by enzymes derived from the gut microbiota reflect **short-chain fatty acids** (SCFAs) such as **acetate**, butyrate, and **propio-nate**. SCFA constitute 5–10% of energy source in healthy people. There is certain evidence that lean subjects exhibit higher stool levels of SCFA com-pared to obese people. Interestingly, fiber-enriched diets are also able to improve insulin sensitivity in lean and obese diabetic subjects [35]. Furthermore, dietary fibers have been shown to alleviate T2D in a randomized clinical trial observing that fiber-driven bacteria-producing SCFAs were present in greater diversity and these patients had better improvements in hemoglobin A1c levels [36]. SCFAs diffuse passively are recovered via mono-carboxylic acid transporters or act as signaling molecules by binding to **G-protein-coupled receptors (GPCRs)** such as Gpr41 (free fatty acid receptor 3, FFAR3) and Gpr43 (FFAR2) [37]. These GPCRs are expressed by many cell

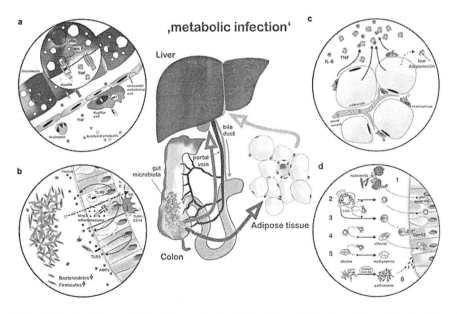

Fig. 1 Gut-derived factors drive metabolic inflammation in the liver (**a**), gut (**b**), adipose tissue (**c**) and besides microbes certain nutrients are able to act pro-inflammatory

types including gut epithelial cells, adipocytes, and immune cells. Gpr43-deficient mice are obese even when consuming a normal diet, whereas mice over-expressing this receptor specifically in the adipose tissue remain lean independent of calorie consumption [38]. In this study, when mice were raised germ-free or were treated with certain antibiotics both types of mice exhibited a normal phenotype. Gpr43 activation also enhances insulin sensitivity by promoting **GLP-1 secretion** in the gut [39]. Gpr43 is neither expressed in liver nor in muscle, and therefore, it seems that adipose tissue-derived Gpr43 is able to modulate all the metabolic effects after engagement with microbiota-derived products such as SCFAs. Therefore, SCFAs are not only an important energy source for the host, but also act as signaling molecules especially in the adipose tissue thereby maintaining energy balance. Data also suggest that the microbiota is the major source for **Gpr43 agonists** and biological functions of Gpr43 are completely dependent on the gut's microbiota.

Therefore, SCFAs could reflect a missing link between the microbiota and systemic inflammatory diseases as they (especially butyrate) regulate the development of extrathymic anti-inflammatory regulatory T cells [40]. SCFAs also control the generation of colonic **regulatory T cells** and protect against colitis in a Gpr43-dependent manner [41]. Trompette and colleagues have demonstrated that mice fed a high-fiber diet, have an altered microbiota, and are protected from allergic airway inflammation [42]. These data are supportive for the current notion that microbiota-derived products are important players in the generation of local and systemic immunity/inflammation. As studies in T2D revealed that production of SCFAs, especially butyrate, is impaired, it sounds reasonable to assume that such mechanisms might contribute to low-grade inflammation observed in those disorders.

Several other mechanisms may allow the microbiota to interact with the host. The gut microbiota affects the composition and abundance of certain bile acid species through a variety of mechanisms resulting commonly in low levels of various **bile acids** in case of obesity [43]. Obese mice demonstrate increased expression of **farnesoid X receptor** (FXR) and fibroblast growth factor 15, which expression is regulated by bile acids, and directly regulate various metabolic effects. Conventionally raised mice contain much more total body fat compared to those raised under germ-free conditions [12]. Conventionalization of mice suppresses intestinal expression of **fasting-induced adipose factor** (FIAF) specifically in differentiated villous epithelial cells in the ileum. FIAF acts as a circulating lipoprotein lipase (LPL) inhibitor [44]. Another metabolic pathway apart from FIAF involves **AMP-activated protein kinase (AMPK)** [45]. Germ-free mice remain lean despite high-calorie intake, and this state is accompanied by increased activity of phosphorylated AMPK levels both in liver and skeletal muscle and enhanced insulin sensitivity, in the liver [45]. In summary, several pathomechanisms have been identified in the past years which could help to explain how the microbiota directs metabolic processes in health and disease (Fig. 1).

Innate Immunity

Metabolic syndrome might develop through the interaction of various genetic and environmental factors and includes a complex and yet poorly understood interaction between the intestinal microbiota and the **innate immune system** [46]. **Toll-like receptors** might play an important role in the development of a metabolic syndrome as demonstrated for the pattern recognition receptor **TLR5** [47]. TLR5$^{-/-}$ mice exhibit hyperphagia, developed hyperlipidemia, hypertension, insulin resistance and obesity, and an altered microbiota. Transfer of intestinal microbiota of TLR5$^{-/-}$ mice into germ-free mice led to metabolic syndrome. These data suggest that innate immune signaling is critical in the development of the metabolic syndrome and alterations in the intestinal microbiota are able to induce the metabolic syndrome. Inflammasomes consist of an upstream sensor NLR protein, the adaptor protein Asc, and the effector protein caspase-1. Various groups have recently shown that the inflammasome may play an important role in metabolic inflammation and some inflammasomes might affect the intestinal microbiota, metabolic syndrome, and fatty liver disease [48]. Whether similar phenomena are also relevant in human disease is currently unclear (Fig. 1).

"Metabolic Cytokines": A Role for Interleukin-22

It has long been assumed that certain cytokines might be crucially involved in the crosstalk between metabolic processes and inflammation. Interleukin-22 (IL-22) is an IL-10 family cytokine and mainly expressed by certain lymphoid cells (innate lymphoid cells, ILCs) and specialized T helper (Th) cells such as Th17 or Th22 [49]. IL-10 family cytokines exert mainly anti-inflammatory actions, and the biological functions of IL-22 are focused on control of innate immune defense, tissue protection and regenerative functions. Furthermore, IL-22 maintains epithelial integrity and homeostasis of commensals [50], as mice deficient in IL-22 show evidence of systemic dissemination of bacteria and chronic inflammation [51, 52]. Importantly, conditions of obesity are associated with a "**leaky gut**" and an impaired epithelial integrity suggesting that certain mediators might be involved in this process [53]. A recent elegant study investigated the role of IL-22 in metabolic disorders and **mucosal immunity** [54]. Here, the authors observed that IL-22 production in ILCs and CD4$^+$ T cells is impaired in obese mice and after challenge with a HFD. Interestingly, infection with *Citrobacter rodentium* resulted in a dramatic reduction of peak IL-22 synthesis in the colon of *ob/ob* mice or in animals after HFD feeding. IL-22 is dispensable for a successful mucosal defense of *C. rodentium* [51], and administration of exogenous IL-22-Tc reduced mortality, restored epithelial damage and inflammation, and inhibited dissemination of *C. rodentium* in leptin receptor-deficient (*db/db*) mice. Surprisingly, exogenous IL-22-Fc treatment of obese mice reduced body weight and epididymal fat mass, decreased blood glucose levels, and improved insulin resistance under both fed and fasting conditions clearly proving that IL-22 is a metabolically beneficial cytokine. In addition, IL-22-Fc therapy improved metabolic functions in *db/db* mice with hyperglycemia. As IL-22 reflects a prototypic barrier cytokine, the authors investigated in their models effects of IL-22-Fc administration on the intestinal microbiota and could indeed observe that this therapy increased the *Firmicutes/Bacteroidetes* ratio although beneficial effects of this treatment could not be transferred to control mice via **fecal transplant**. Furthermore, IL-22-Fc also regulates lipid metabolism in liver [55] and adipose tissue. These studies clearly highlight that certain cytokines such as IL-22, which are mainly active at barriers such as in the gut, link various aspects observed in obesity, and related disorders such as impaired epithelial integrity, mucosal inflammation, systemic inflammation, and metabolic dysfunction.

Role of Certain Commensals: *Akkermansia muciniphila*

Akkermansia muciniphila has been recently characterized as a mucin-degrading bacterium residing in the mucus layer [56]. *A. muciniphila*, a Gram-negative bacterium, is highly prevalent and constitutes 3–5% of the gut's microbiota, and its concentrations are inversely correlated with the presence of overweight and diabetes in murine and human studies [57]. Dietary supplementation with **fibers**, i.e., oligofructose to genetically obese mice dramatically increases abundance of *A. muciniphila* [57]. Several studies have shown that *A. muciniphila* might play a key role in the integrity of the mucous layer and has the potential to reduce inflammation and offer protection against the development of obesity and T2D. The most convincing report suggesting such a function for *Akkermansia* was recently presented by Everard et al. [21]. The authors demonstrated that both in genetic and dietary models of murine obesity concentrations of *A. muciniphila* were highly decreased. A prebiotic therapy with **oligofructose** restored levels of *A. muciniphila* and improved metabolic functions including metabolic endotoxemia. Endotoxemia has been demonstrated to be of importance in metabolic dysfunction [58], and recent studies have corroborated this as increased levels of **lipopolysaccharide** binding protein, an indirect surrogate of increased endotoxin activity, correlated with later development of metabolic syndrome in middle-aged and older Chinese individuals [59]. Metformin, an antidiabetic drug results in an increase in *Akkermansia* concentrations and also in this study administration of *A. muciniphila* resulted in an improvement of various metabolic functions including glucose tolerance and adipose tissue inflammation [60]. NOD mice treated with vancomycin exhibit an increase in the abundance of *Akkermansia* accompanied by improved metabolic parameters further supporting a protective function for this bacterium [61]. Several studies have now demonstrated that *A. muciniphila* is of major importance in metabolic health and fecal concentrations were correlated with better clinical outcomes after calorie restriction and weight loss [62]. Even early human studies administering *A. muciniphila* in subjects with overweight and obesity showed improvement in several metabolic parameters proposing that this bacterium could reflect an attractive "metabolic probiotic" in such diseases [63]. Again dietary components might be highly relevant as, e.g., consumption of polyphenols enriched in grapes promotes substantially growth of this bacterium in rodents [64]. *A. muciniphila* might exert anti-inflammatory functions also in other disease models as it has been shown that administration of this bacterium improves DSS-induced colitis [65], this bacterium is massively depleted by excessive alcohol consumption, and the use of it in an experimental model of alcoholic liver injury was highly beneficial [66].

Early-Life Manipulation of the Microbiota: Role of Antibiotics

As stated, obese and lean humans differ in their microbiota, and disease phenotypes can be transferred to germ-free mice [16]. A seminal study from 1963 by Dubos and colleagues described that antibiotic therapy might affect body weight of mice [67]. This was paralleled by the observation and practice of farmers to expose livestocks to low doses of antibiotics to promote growth of respective animals [68]. All these facts have been rather ignored by medicine namely that these effects can be pronounced and especially are dependent on the time of use, e.g., in early life as interventions might have a profound impact in later life. Antibiotic therapy causes dramatic shifts in the microbiota with certain long-term effects [69]. Especially, exposure in early life might have a major impact [70]. Several large prospective clinical studies have now also shown that "disturbance" of the intestinal microbiota by either mode of delivery or **antibiotic usage** might lead to childhood obesity [71]. Elegant experimental studies have demonstrated that early-life subtherapeutic antibiotic therapy not only affected the intestinal microbiome but also resulted in obesity [72]. In this study, this intervention also resulted in a significant increase of SCFA, important energy substrates for the organism. A study by Martin Balser's group has brought further insight into this topic. Low-dose penicillin (LDP) therapy initiated at birth induced major metabolic alterations in the host accompanied by changes in the expression of ileal innate immunity genes finally resulting in a substantially perturbed microbiota [73]. Early penicillin exposure especially already to adult mice before birth resulted in enhanced metabolic phenotypes including total abdominal, visceral, and liver adiposity. LDP treatment had a major impact on the intestinal microbiota, and it suppressed multiple taxa that typically peak early in life. Furthermore, LDP and a **HFD** had independent selective effects, with LDP consistently affecting specific microbial strains. This important study overall clearly shows that at least in mice early life is the critical window with respect to host–microbe metabolic interactions and even exposure limited to infancy resulted in adiposity later in early to mid-adulthood. Importantly, they also observed that the altered microbiota alone, not continued LDP exposure showed causality. Interestingly, this fits with this study, germ-free chickens do not demonstrate weight gain when treated with low-dose penicillin [74], and animals were especially responsive to a HFD, and importantly, this "disease" phenotype was transferrable via antibiotic-selected microbiota to a healthy host. All these studies clearly suggest that interference with the microbiota in early life especially antibiotic therapy may have a profound effect finally resulting in an increased risk for obesity and metabolic dysfunction in later life. Further studies are needed to define key members of the early-life microbiota and also to prove whether similar mechanisms take place in humans.

Gut Microbiome and Pregnancy

Pregnancy is accompanied by massive hormonal, immunological, and metabolic changes. Metabolic alterations during pregnancy are substantial and approximately 20% of patients develop prediabetes or manifest T2D. Earlier studies have revealed that the composition of the gut microbiota is changing over the course of gestation [75]. A major study providing robust insights into the relationship between microbiotal evolution and pregnancy and associated metabolic consequences has been recently reported [76]. During pregnancy, many metabolic parameters changed significantly with an increase in serum leptin levels, cholesterol, insulin, and HbA1c levels. From the first trimester (T1) to the third trimester (T3), the relative abundance from *Proteobacteria* and *Actinobacteria* increased in approximately 2/3 of women. Levels of *Bacteroidetes* and *Firmicutes* were not significantly different between trimesters. T1 was characterized by a high rate of the *Clostridiales* order of the *Firmicutes* (e.g., butyrate producers *F. prausnitzii* and *Eubacterium*), whereas T3 was characterized by members of the *Enterobacteriaceae* and *Streptococcus* genus. *Proteobacteria*, enriched in T3 stools, have been shown to exert pro-inflammatory effects [77]. The authors transferred T1/3 microbiota to germ-free wild-type mice, and only after 2 weeks of inoculation, inflammatory mediators in the stool and cecal samples including lipocalin were significantly higher in the T3 versus T1 recipients. This was paralleled by more adiposity and an **impaired glucose tolerance**. Overall, this fascinating translational work clearly suggests that pregnancy is associated with major shifts in the gut's microbiota characterized by a switch toward a pro-inflammatory tonus.

Mode of delivery might be crucial as a vaginal birth has been demonstrated to have a major impact on the establishment and development of the intestinal flora [78]. In contrast, **Caesarian section** results in a markedly altered child microbiota, and this may have consequences with respect to disease patterns [79]. Indeed, studies suggest an increased risk of childhood obesity after Cesarean section [80]. Investigators have tried to compensate for this "altered microbiota" by exposing infants delivered by Cesarean section to maternal vaginal fluids at birth [81]. Indeed, the gut, oral, and skin bacterial microflora of these infants during the first month of life were enriched in vaginal bacteria. However, a much larger study published recently could not prove a beneficial effect of vaginal seeding as authors did not observe an impact on gut microbiota, growth, or allergy risks during the first 2 years of life [82]. The key effect of Cesarean section on the gut microbiome has been questioned by a large study [83]. An exciting topic remains when and how is the gut colonized by bacteria in early life. One report recently proposed that viable bacteria are highly limited in the fetal intestine at mid-gestation with *Micrococcaceae* and *Lactobacillus* being the most abundant [84]. In summary, pregnancy might indeed be associated with a disturbed microbiota, thereby affecting metabolic pathways including insulin resistance although mechanisms remain unclear and probably also involving various gestational hormones. Furthermore, although initially "hyped," the effects of Cesarean section on development of gut microbiota might be only moderate as suggested by more recent studies.

Conclusions

Host phenotypes are dependent on interactions between diet, intestinal microbiota, and immunity. Until recently, it appeared that the direct interaction between food and immunity drives health and disease and only recently evidence accumulated that "the big elefant" in us; i.e., the intestinal microbiota has been ignored and has now been recognized as crucial player at this interphase. Over the past years, the intestinal microbiota has been defined as a fascinating "new organ" which affects many biological systems throughout the body including the immune system, metabolic functions, and development and programming of the nervous system. Fascinating recent data have now demonstrated an important role for this microbiota in metabolic diseases such as obesity and T2D. A "microbiotal gut signature" is present not only in human obesity but also in T2D, and it will become fascinating to define bacterial species in the near future which are metabolically beneficial or detrimental. Several interesting candidates have already been defined and *A. muciniphila* reflects such a promising candidate. Mechanistically SCFAs, especially butyrate and propionate, have evolved as attractive pathways shaping immunological and metabolic functions. An exciting new area has been started in medicine bringing metabolic inflammation, food, and microbiota research to the forefront of biomedical research.

References

1. Lozupone CA, Stombaugh JI, Gordon JI, Jansson JK, Knight R. Diversity, stability and resilience of the human gut microbiota. Nature. 2012;489(7415):220–30.
2. Tremaroli V, Backhed F. Functional interactions between the gut microbiota and host metabolism. Nature. 2012;489(7415):242–9.
3. Eckburg PB, Bik EM, Bernstein CN, et al. Diversity of the human intestinal microbial flora. Science. 2005;308(5728):1635–8.
4. Costello EK, Lauber CL, Hamady M, Fierer N, Gordon JI, Knight R. Bacterial community variation in human body habitats across space and time. Science. 2009;326(5960):1694–7.
5. Human Microbiome Project C. Structure, function and diversity of the healthy human microbiome. Nature. 2012;486(7402):207–14.
6. Qin J, Li R, Raes J, et al. A human gut microbial gene catalogue established by metagenomic sequencing. Nature. 2010;464(7285):59–65.
7. Pasolli E, Asnicar F, Manara S, et al. Extensive unexplored human microbiome diversity revealed by over 150,000 genomes from metagenomes spanning age, geography, and lifestyle. Cell. 2019;176(3):649–62. e620

8. Valles-Colomer M, Menni C, Berry SE, Valdes AM, Spector TD, Segata N. Cardiometabolic health, diet and the gut microbiome: a meta-omics perspective. Nat Med. 2023;29(3):551–61.
9. Amar J, Chabo C, Waget A, et al. Intestinal mucosal adherence and translocation of commensal bacteria at the early onset of type 2 diabetes: molecular mechanisms and probiotic treatment. EMBO Mol Med. 2011;3(9):559–72.
10. Breen DM, Rasmussen BA, Cote CD, Jackson VM, Lam TK. Nutrient-sensing mechanisms in the gut as therapeutic targets for diabetes. Diabetes. 2013;62(9):3005–13.
11. Karlsson FH, Tremaroli V, Nookaew I, et al. Gut metagenome in European women with normal, impaired and diabetic glucose control. Nature. 2013;498(7452):99–103.
12. Backhed F, Ding H, Wang T, et al. The gut microbiota as an environmental factor that regulates fat storage. Proc Natl Acad Sci U S A. 2004;101(44):15718–23.
13. Ley RE, Turnbaugh PJ, Klein S, Gordon JI. Microbial ecology: human gut microbes associated with obesity. Nature. 2006;444(7122):1022–3.
14. Turnbaugh PJ, Ley RE, Mahowald MA, Magrini V, Mardis ER, Gordon JI. An obesity-associated gut microbiome with increased capacity for energy harvest. Nature. 2006;444(7122):1027–31.
15. Turnbaugh PJ, Hamady M, Yatsunenko T, et al. A core gut microbiome in obese and lean twins. Nature. 2009;457(7228):480–4.
16. Ridaura VK, Faith JJ, Rey FE, et al. Gut microbiota from twins discordant for obesity modulate metabolism in mice. Science. 2013;341(6150):1241214.
17. Le Chatelier E, Nielsen T, Qin J, et al. Richness of human gut microbiome correlates with metabolic markers. Nature. 2013;500(7464):541–6.
18. Cotillard A, Kennedy SP, Kong LC, et al. Dietary intervention impact on gut microbial gene richness. Nature. 2013;500(7464):585–8.
19. Remely M, Tesar I, Hippe B, Gnauer S, Rust P, Haslberger AG. Gut microbiota composition correlates with changes in body fat content due to weight loss. Benefic Microbes. 2015;6:431–9.
20. Sokol H, Pigneur B, Watterlot L, et al. *Faecalibacterium prausnitzii* is an anti-inflammatory commensal bacterium identified by gut microbiota analysis of Crohn disease patients. Proc Natl Acad Sci U S A. 2008;105(43):16731–6.
21. Everard A, Belzer C, Geurts L, et al. Cross-talk between *Akkermansia muciniphila* and intestinal epithelium controls diet-induced obesity. Proc Natl Acad Sci U S A. 2013;110(22):9066–71.
22. Dewulf EM, Cani PD, Claus SP, et al. Insight into the prebiotic concept: lessons from an exploratory, double blind intervention study with inulin-type fructans in obese women. Gut. 2013;62(8):1112–21.
23. Wang J, Tang H, Zhang C, et al. Modulation of gut microbiota during probiotic-mediated attenuation of

metabolic syndrome in high fat diet-fed mice. ISME J. 2015;9(1):1–15.

24. Wu GD, Chen J, Hoffmann C, et al. Linking long-term dietary patterns with gut microbial enterotypes. Science. 2011;334(6052):105–8.

25. De Filippo C, Cavalieri D, Di Paola M, et al. Impact of diet in shaping gut microbiota revealed by a comparative study in children from Europe and rural Africa. Proc Natl Acad Sci U S A. 2010;107(33):14691–6.

26. Sankararaman S, Noriega K, Velayuthan S, Sferra T, Martindale R. Gut microbiome and its impact on obesity and obesity-related disorders. Curr Gastroenterol Rep. 2023;25(2):31–44.

27. Goodrich JK, Waters JL, Poole AC, et al. Human genetics shape the gut microbiome. Cell. 2014;159(4):789–99.

28. Peters BA, Shapiro JA, Church TR, et al. A taxonomic signature of obesity in a large study of American adults. Sci Rep. 2018;8(1):9749.

29. Le Roy T, Moens de Hase E, Van Hul M, et al. *Dysosmobacter welbionis* is a newly isolated human commensal bacterium preventing diet-induced obesity and metabolic disorders in mice. Gut. 2022;71(3): 534–43.

30. Qin J, Li Y, Cai Z, et al. A metagenome-wide association study of gut microbiota in type 2 diabetes. Nature. 2012;490(7418):55–60.

31. Wu H, Esteve E, Tremaroli V, et al. Metformin alters the gut microbiome of individuals with treatment-naive type 2 diabetes, contributing to the therapeutic effects of the drug. Nat Med. 2017;23(7):850–8.

32. Wu H, Tremaroli V, Schmidt C, et al. The gut microbiota in prediabetes and diabetes: a population-based cross-sectional study. Cell Metab. 2020;32(3): 379–90. e373

33. Koh A, Molinaro A, Stahlman M, et al. Microbially produced imidazole propionate impairs insulin signaling through mTORC1. Cell. 2018;175(4): 947–61. e917

34. Flint HJ, Bayer EA, Rincon MT, Lamed R, White BA. Polysaccharide utilization by gut bacteria: potential for new insights from genomic analysis. Nat Rev Microbiol. 2008;6(2):121–31.

35. Robertson MD, Bickerton AS, Dennis AL, Vidal H, Frayn KN. Insulin-sensitizing effects of dietary resistant starch and effects on skeletal muscle and adipose tissue metabolism. Am J Clin Nutr. 2005;82(3): 559–67.

36. Zhao L, Zhang F, Ding X, et al. Gut bacteria selectively promoted by dietary fibers alleviate type 2 diabetes. Science. 2018;359(6380):1151–6.

37. Brown AJ, Goldsworthy SM, Barnes AA, et al. The orphan G protein-coupled receptors GPR41 and GPR43 are activated by propionate and other short chain carboxylic acids. J Biol Chem. 2003;278(13): 11312–9.

38. Kimura I, Ozawa K, Inoue D, et al. The gut microbiota suppresses insulin-mediated fat accumulation via the short-chain fatty acid receptor GPR43. Nat Commun. 2013;4:1829.

39. Tolhurst G, Heffron H, Lam YS, et al. Short-chain fatty acids stimulate glucagon-like peptide-1 secretion via the G-protein-coupled receptor FFAR2. Diabetes. 2012;61(2):364–71.

40. Arpaia N, Campbell C, Fan X, et al. Metabolites produced by commensal bacteria promote peripheral regulatory T-cell generation. Nature. 2013;504(7480): 451–5.

41. Smith PM, Howitt MR, Panikov N, et al. The microbial metabolites, short-chain fatty acids, regulate colonic Treg cell homeostasis. Science. 2013;341(6145): 569–73.

42. Trompette A, Gollwitzer ES, Yadava K, et al. Gut microbiota metabolism of dietary fiber influences allergic airway disease and hematopoiesis. Nat Med. 2014;20(2):159–66.

43. Swann JR, Want EJ, Geier FM, et al. Systemic gut microbial modulation of bile acid metabolism in host tissue compartments. Proc Natl Acad Sci U S A. 2011;108(Suppl 1):4523–30.

44. Yoon JC, Chickering TW, Rosen ED, et al. Peroxisome proliferator-activated receptor gamma target gene encoding a novel angiopoietin-related protein associated with adipose differentiation. Mol Cell Biol. 2000;20(14):5343–9.

45. Backhed F, Manchester JK, Semenkovich CF, Gordon JI. Mechanisms underlying the resistance to diet-induced obesity in germ-free mice. Proc Natl Acad Sci U S A. 2007;104(3):979–84.

46. Tilg H, Kaser A. Gut microbiome, obesity, and metabolic dysfunction. J Clin Invest. 2011;121(6):2126–32.

47. Vijay-Kumar M, Aitken JD, Carvalho FA, et al. Metabolic syndrome and altered gut microbiota in mice lacking toll-like receptor 5. Science. 2010;328(5975): 228–31.

48. Stienstra R, Joosten LA, Koenen T, et al. The inflammasome-mediated caspase-1 activation controls adipocyte differentiation and insulin sensitivity. Cell Metab. 2010;12(6):593–605.

49. Colonna M. Interleukin-22-producing natural killer cells and lymphoid tissue inducer-like cells in mucosal immunity. Immunity. 2009;31(1):15–23.

50. Tilg H. Diet and intestinal immunity. N Engl J Med. 2012;366(2):181–3.

51. Zheng Y, Valdez PA, Danilenko DM, et al. Interleukin-22 mediates early host defense against attaching and effacing bacterial pathogens. Nat Med. 2008;14(3): 282–9.

52. Sugimoto K, Ogawa A, Mizoguchi E, et al. IL-22 ameliorates intestinal inflammation in a mouse model of ulcerative colitis. J Clin Invest. 2008;118(2): 534–44.

53. Bischoff SC, Barbara G, Buurman W, et al. Intestinal permeability–a new target for disease prevention and therapy. BMC Gastroenterol. 2014;14:189.

54. Wang X, Ota N, Manzanillo P, et al. Interleukin-22 alleviates metabolic disorders and restores mucosal

immunity in diabetes. Nature. 2014;514(7521): 237–41.

55. Yang L, Zhang Y, Wang L, et al. Amelioration of high fat diet induced liver lipogenesis and hepatic steatosis by interleukin-22. J Hepatol. 2010;53(2):339–47.

56. Derrien M, Vaughan EE, Plugge CM, de Vos WM. *Akkermansia muciniphila* gen. nov., sp. nov., a human intestinal mucin-degrading bacterium. Int J Syst Evol Microbiol. 2004;54(Pt 5):1469–76.

57. Everard A, Lazarevic V, Derrien M, et al. Responses of gut microbiota and glucose and lipid metabolism to prebiotics in genetic obese and diet-induced leptin-resistant mice. Diabetes. 2011;60(11):2775–86.

58. Cani PD, Amar J, Iglesias MA, et al. Metabolic endotoxemia initiates obesity and insulin resistance. Diabetes. 2007;56(7):1761–72.

59. Liu X, Lu L, Yao P, et al. Lipopolysaccharide binding protein, obesity status and incidence of metabolic syndrome: a prospective study among middle-aged and older Chinese. Diabetologia. 2014;57(9):1834–41.

60. Shin NR, Lee JC, Lee HY, et al. An increase in the Akkermansia spp. population induced by metformin treatment improves glucose homeostasis in diet-induced obese mice. Gut. 2014;63(5):727–35.

61. Hansen CH, Krych L, Nielsen DS, et al. Early life treatment with vancomycin propagates *Akkermansia muciniphila* and reduces diabetes incidence in the NOD mouse. Diabetologia. 2012;55(8):2285–94.

62. Dao MC, Everard A, Aron-Wisnewsky J, et al. *Akkermansia muciniphila* and improved metabolic health during a dietary intervention in obesity: relationship with gut microbiome richness and ecology. Gut. 2016;65(3):426–36.

63. Depommier C, Everard A, Druart C, et al. Supplementation with *Akkermansia muciniphila* in overweight and obese human volunteers: a proof-of-concept exploratory study. Nat Med. 2019;25(7):1096–103.

64. Roopchand DE, Carmody RN, Kuhn P, et al. Dietary polyphenols promote growth of the gut bacterium *Akkermansia muciniphila* and attenuate high-fat diet-induced metabolic syndrome. Diabetes. 2015;64(8): 2847–58.

65. Kang CS, Ban M, Choi EJ, et al. Extracellular vesicles derived from gut microbiota, especially *Akkermansia muciniphila*, protect the progression of dextran sulfate sodium-induced colitis. PLoS One. 2013;8(10): e76520.

66. Grander C, Adolph TE, Wieser V, et al. Recovery of ethanol-induced *Akkermansia muciniphila* depletion ameliorates alcoholic liver disease. Gut. 2018;67(5): 891–901.

67. Dubos R, Schaedler RW, Costello RL. The effect of antibacterial drugs on the weight of mice. J Exp Med. 1963;117(2):245–57.

68. Cromwell GL. Why and how antibiotics are used in swine production. Anim Biotechnol. 2002;13(1):7–27.

69. Morgun A, Dzutsev A, Dong X, et al. Uncovering effects of antibiotics on the host and microbiota using transkingdom gene networks. Gut. 2015;64:1732–43.

70. Greenwood MR, Hirsch J. Postnatal development of adipocyte cellularity in the normal rat. J Lipid Res. 1974;15(5):474–83.

71. Trasande L, Blustein J, Liu M, Corwin E, Cox LM, Blaser MJ. Infant antibiotic exposures and early-life body mass. Int J Obes. 2013;37(1):16–23.

72. Cho I, Yamanishi S, Cox L, et al. Antibiotics in early life alter the murine colonic microbiome and adiposity. Nature. 2012;488(7413):621–6.

73. Cox LM, Yamanishi S, Sohn J, et al. Altering the intestinal microbiota during a critical developmental window has lasting metabolic consequences. Cell. 2014;158(4):705–21.

74. Coates ME, Fuller R, Harrison GF, Lev M, Suffolk SF. A comparison of the growth of chicks in the Gustafsson germ-free apparatus and in a conventional environment, with and without dietary supplements of penicillin. Br J Nutr. 1963;17:141–50.

75. Collado MC, Isolauri E, Laitinen K, Salminen S. Distinct composition of gut microbiota during pregnancy in overweight and normal-weight women. Am J Clin Nutr. 2008;88(4):894–9.

76. Koren O, Goodrich JK, Cullender TC, et al. Host remodeling of the gut microbiome and metabolic changes during pregnancy. Cell. 2012;150(3):470–80.

77. Mukhopadhya I, Hansen R, El-Omar EM, Hold GL. IBD-what role do Proteobacteria play? Nat Rev Gastroenterol Hepatol. 2012;9(4):219–30.

78. Dominguez-Bello MG, Costello EK, Contreras M, et al. Delivery mode shapes the acquisition and structure of the initial microbiota across multiple body habitats in newborns. Proc Natl Acad Sci U S A. 2010;107(26):11971–5.

79. Pandey PK, Verma P, Kumar H, Bavdekar A, Patole MS, Shouche YS. Comparative analysis of fecal microflora of healthy full-term Indian infants born with different methods of delivery (vaginal vs cesarean): Acinetobacter sp. prevalence in vaginally born infants. J Biosci. 2012;37(6):989–98.

80. Blustein J, Attina T, Liu M, et al. Association of caesarean delivery with child adiposity from age 6 weeks to 15 years. Int J Obes. 2013;37(7):900–6.

81. Dominguez-Bello MG, De Jesus-Laboy KM, Shen N, et al. Partial restoration of the microbiota of cesarean-born infants via vaginal microbial transfer. Nat Med. 2016;22(3):250–3.

82. Liu Y, Li HT, Zhou SJ, et al. Effects of vaginal seeding on gut microbiota, body mass index, and allergy risks in infants born through cesarean delivery: a randomized clinical trial. Am J Obstet Gynecol MFM. 2023;5(1):100793.

83. Chu DM, Ma J, Prince AL, Antony KM, Seferovic MD, Aagaard KM. Maturation of the infant microbiome community structure and function across multiple body sites and in relation to mode of delivery. Nat Med. 2017;23(3):314–26.

84. Rackaityte E, Halkias J, Fukui EM, et al. Viable bacterial colonization is highly limited in the human intestine in utero. Nat Med. 2020;26(4):599–607.

Pancreatic Islet Adaptation and Failure in Obesity

21

Yumi Imai, Dalal El Ladiki, and Spencer J. Peachee

Contents

Y. Imai (✉)
Division of Endocrinology and Metabolism, Department
of Internal Medicine, University of Iowa, Iowa City, IA,
USA

Fraternal Order of Eagles Diabetes Research Center,
University of Iowa, Iowa City, IA, USA

Iowa City Veterans Affairs Medical Center, Iowa City, IA,
USA
e-mail: yumi-imai@uiowa.edu

D. El Ladiki · S. J. Peachee
Division of Endocrinology and Metabolism, Department
of Internal Medicine, University of Iowa, Iowa City, IA,
USA

Fraternal Order of Eagles Diabetes Research Center,
University of Iowa, Iowa City, IA, USA

© Springer Nature Switzerland AG 2023
R. S. Ahima (ed.), *Metabolic Syndrome*,
https://doi.org/10.1007/978-3-031-40116-9_27

Abstract

Type 2 diabetes is the major comorbidity associated with metabolic syndrome and compromises health and quality of life for those incurred the disease. Metabolic syndrome is considered to increase the risk of type 2 diabetes by causing insulin resistance and increasing the influx of nutrition to pancreatic islets. This chapter summarizes evidence indicating that the adaptability of pancreatic islets to insulin resistance is critical to prevent the development of type 2 diabetes and describes how pancreatic islets transition from adaptive to maladaptive status during the development of type 2 diabetes. In brief, pancreatic islets increase the efficiency of insulin secretion and beta cell mass to meet increased demand from insulin resistance. Functional adaptation occurs early and is robust compared with a mild increase in beta cell mass. However, functional adaptation to increase insulin output itself contributes to beta cell dysfunction if prolonged. In addition, nutritional load (gluco-, glucolipotoxicity) and signals from other tissues affected by metabolic syndrome activate stress responses in pancreatic islets. Evidence indicates the presence of multiple stress and maladaptive responses in human islets affected by type 2 diabetes (e.g., ER stress, mitochondrial dysfunction, oxidative stress, inflammation, amyloid deposition, and autophagy dysfunction). Expansion of beta cell mass compensates for beta cell dysfunction, but beta cell mass declines when stress continues leading to overt hyperglycemia and type 2 diabetes. Glucagon secretion is also dysregulated in metabolic syndrome and type 2 diabetes. However, it is currently unclear how the alteration in glucagon modifies pathogenesis of type 2 diabetes.

Keywords

Type 2 diabetes · Insulin resistance · Insulin secretion · Beta cell mass

Introduction

The incidence of type 2 diabetes (T2D) has been increasing steadily for the last 50 years eliciting significant burden to those affected. Metabolic syndrome increases the risk of T2D due to insulin resistance, nutritional overload, and derangement in lipid metabolism. However, not all subjects with metabolic syndrome develop T2D. Thus, there is a coping mechanism to prevent the development of hyperglycemia, which eventually fails in the subgroup of the population who develops T2D. This chapter addresses the importance of pancreatic islets for the maintenance of glucose homeostasis in metabolic syndrome. Then, we will discuss how maladaptation of pancreatic islets occurs and leads to the development of T2D in metabolic syndrome. The emphasis is on data whose validity in humans is supported or tested considering a number of differences in pancreatic islets between human and rodents [1]. Due to the space limitation, review articles are primarily cited, and original studies is cited for those with high significance or published recently.

Adaptation of Pancreatic Islets to Metabolic Syndrome

Adaptation of Pancreatic Islets to Insulin Resistance Is Critical for Normoglycemia

Pancreatic Islets Play a Central Role in Glucose Homeostasis

Pancreatic islets contain a cluster of endocrine cells (beta, alpha, delta, pancreatic polypeptide (PP), and epsilon cells) and play a key role in glucose and energy homeostasis. Intricately regulated hormone secretion from pancreatic islets maintains blood glucose levels tightly between 60 and 100 mg/dl in humans [2]. The beta cells secrete insulin which is, the sole hormone in the body with a glucose-lowering action. Insulin is an anabolic hormone to retain nutrients such as glycogen, lipids, and proteins in insulin target tissues (i.e., the liver, muscle, and adipose tissues). On the other end, hypoglycemia under nutritional deprivation is prevented by suppressing insulin secretion and promoting glucagon secretion. Species' specific blood glucose set point is determined by paracrine communication between alpha cells and beta cells within islets [2].

Insulin Output Needs to be Increased to Adapt to Insulin Resistance

Excessive nutritional load increases adiposity and causes insulin resistance, the condition that raises insulin requirement. Human studies indicate that the lowering of insulin sensitivity drives insulin secretion and that the ability to increase insulin secretion is needed to maintain normoglycemia [3, 4]. When assessed in non-diabetic humans, insulin secretion and insulin sensitivity show hyperbolic relations indicating that pancreatic islets adjust insulin secretion to match insulin sensitivity (Fig. 1a) [3]. Reduced ability to enhance insulin secretion to the level appropriate for insulin sensitivity appears to confer the risk for developing

diabetes, further supporting the notion that an adaptive increase in insulin secretion prevents diabetes development. Insulin secretion for given insulin sensitivity falls in a low percentile in relatives of T2D, women with polycystic ovary syndrome (PCO), subjects with impaired glucose tolerance (IGT), subjects with a history of gestational diabetes (GDM), and the elderly population (Fig. 1a) [3]. Longitudinal study of Pima Indians who are insulin-resistant and have a high propensity to develop T2D also indicates that the ability of pancreatic islets to increase insulin secretion is the primary determinant for the prevention of T2D [4]. This observational study tested insulin sensitivity and insulin secretion at the beginning and after ~5 years in non-diabetic, IGT, and diabetic subjects. While insulin sensitivity progressively dropped in all groups, those who were non-diabetic at the end of the 5 years increased insulin secretion, while those who failed to increase insulin secretion became diabetic (Fig. 1b) [4]. In genome-wide association studies (GWAS), T2D risk loci are enriched in beta cell-specific genes and open chromatin regions specific for beta cells, further highlighting islet failure as the key determinant of T2D development [5].

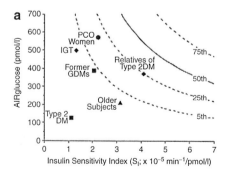

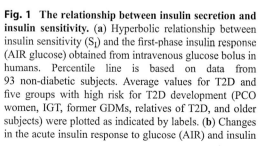

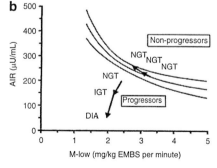

Fig. 1 **The relationship between insulin secretion and insulin sensitivity.** (**a**) Hyperbolic relationship between insulin sensitivity (S_I) and the first-phase insulin response (AIR glucose) obtained from intravenous glucose bolus in humans. Percentile line is based on data from 93 non-diabetic subjects. Average values for T2D and five groups with high risk for T2D development (PCO women, IGT, former GDMs, relatives of T2D, and older subjects) were plotted as indicated by labels. (**b**) Changes in the acute insulin response to glucose (AIR) and insulin

sensitivity measured by the clamp technique at a low insulin concentration (M-low) during ~5 years of observation are shown in arrows for 11 Pima Indians who progressed from normal glucose tolerance (NGT) to IGT and diabetes and 23 subjects who maintained NGT. The lines represent predicted average and the 95% confidence intervals of the regression between AIR and M-low determined from 277 Pima Indians with NGT. (Both panels are reprinted from Ref. [3] with permission of Springer Nature)

Hypersecretion of Insulin May Contribute to the Development of Obesity and Insulin Resistance

While upregulation of insulin secretion is an important adaptive response to insulin resistance, the relationship between the two may not be uni-directional. Some propose that hypersecretion of insulin drives obesity and insulin resistance. While a hyperbolic relationship exists between insulin secretion and insulin sensitivity in non-diabetic subjects, there is a range of variation in insulin secretion for the given level of insulin resistance, indicating that some show highly efficient upregulation of insulin secretion than others [3], due to genetics or environmental factors such as food additive and the gut microbiome [6]. There is evidence that augmented secretion of insulin may increase adiposity and insulin resistance. In mice that have two insulin genes (*Ins1* and *Ins2*), the knockdown of three out of 4 insulin gene loci reduces circulating insulin levels and adiposity [7]. However, there are still mixed opinions regarding the extent by which hypersecretion of insulin contributes to obesity [6, 8]. A reduction in insulin genes in *ob/ob* mice reduced adipose mass but caused overt hyperglycemia. Thus, to consider therapeutic implication, it will be important to determine whether there is a level of insulin secretion that prevents obesity without causing hyperglycemia in humans [6, 8]. Also, it is of note that insulin clearance affects blood insulin levels and tissue insulin availability besides the rate of insulin secretion [9].

Functional Adaptation of Pancreatic Islets in Metabolic Syndrome

Pancreatic Islets Adapt to Insulin Resistance by Increasing Insulin Secretion and Beta Cell Mass

To meet increased demand for insulin due to insulin resistance, pancreatic islets upregulate the efficiency of insulin secretion (functional adaptation) and beta cell mass (morphological adaptation). In humans, functional adaptation likely plays a more significant role in beta cell adaptation to insulin resistance, considering that a several fold increase in insulin secretion is often seen in obesity while the increase in beta cell mass reported is only 30~50% [10]. Longitudinal study in mice also showed a dominant contribution of functional adaptation that occurred quickly upon an increase in insulin demand [11]. In a study by Chen et al, C57Bl/6J mouse islets genetically expressing green fluorescent protein (GFP) and GCaMP in beta cells were transplanted into an anterior chamber of an eye to monitor beta cell mass (GFP) and calcium signaling (GCaMP) in a live mouse fed 60% kcal high fat diet (HFD) [11]. The increase in beta cell mass was slow, showing statistical significance after 4 weeks, reaching a modest 1.88-fold by 16 weeks. In contrast, plasma insulin level upon glucose load was significantly elevated by 1 week on HFD. There are at least two components in the functional adaption of beta cells: the increase in insulin granules available for exocytosis and the effectiveness of nutrient sensing for insulin secretion (Fig. 2). In a human islet study comparing non-obese to mildly obese donors (body mass index (BMI) 18.8 to 33), both insulin contents and glucose-, tolbutamide-, and forskolin-stimulated insulin secretion corrected for insulin contents correlated positively with BMI [12].

Physiological Regulation of Insulin Production and Secretion

Pancreatic beta cells are highly specialized in the production and secretion of insulin. By dedicating ~30% of protein synthesis for insulin, a single beta cell maintains ~20 pg of insulin packed into 10,000 granules [13, 14]. Insulin granule formation and secretion can be briefly summarized as follows. Proinsulin peptide undergoes three disulfide bonding (folding) in the endoplasmic reticulum (ER), then transported through the Golgi apparatus to pack into a dense core secretory granule that contains 200,000 molecules of insulin crystalized with Zn^{2+}. Glucose metabolism in beta cells is programmed to sense glucose effectively to secrete insulin in proportion to blood glucose level [15]. After entering beta cells via glucose transporter (Glut) 1 (human beta cells) and 2 (human and mouse beta cells), glucose is

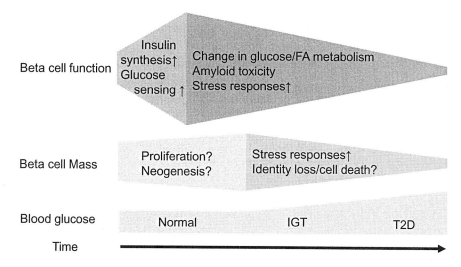

Fig. 2 **Compensation and decompensation of pancreatic islets during the development of type 2 diabetes in metabolic syndrome.** Insulin resistance associated with metabolic syndrome increases demand for insulin. Functional adaptation increases insulin output early and robustly. Beta cell mass may increase up to ~50% in humans. Beta cell proliferation is increased in rodent models but not decisively shown to be increased in obese humans. Neogenesis is reported to be increased in pancreas of obese humans. Demand for insulin secretion combined with nutritional stress starts to compromise beta cell function even before development of hyperglycemia. During this period, normoglycemia is likely maintained by sustaining beta cell mass. However, stress responses eventually reduce beta cell mass causing the elevation of glucose

phosphorylated to glucose-6-phosphate (G6P) by glucokinase, that is the rate-limiting enzyme for glycolysis. Beta cell glucokinase allows glucose metabolism in proportion to glucose availability above ~4 mM [16]. Glucokinase has Km of 8 mM and the inflection point at ~4 mM for glucose. Unlike other hexokinases, glucokinase lacks feedback inhibition by its product, G6P, and thus can continue to produce G6P with the increase in glucose availability. In addition, the activity of lactate dehydrogenase is low in beta cells. As lactate dehydrogenase disperses glycolytic product as lactate and regenerates NAD^+ for GAPDH, low lactate dehydrogenase activity connects glycolysis to the tricarboxylic (TCA) cycle tightly for ATP production [17]. Glycolysis eventually triggers $[Ca^{2+}]$ influx which is the major signal for exocytosis of insulin granules [15]. It has long been believed that ATP produced in mitochondria through the TCA cycle is responsible for the closure of membrane K_{ATP} channel to initiate depolarization and $[Ca^{2+}]$ influx through voltage-gated calcium channel. Recently, the initial closure of K_{ATP} channel is shown to be mediated by ATP

produced by pyruvate kinase locally at the plasma membrane adjacent to K_{ATP} channel (Mitosynth). Initially, ATP production by pyruvate kinase suppresses oxidative phosphorylation in mitochondria (Mitoox) [18]. Once the workload associated with exocytosis consumes ATP and generates ADP, ATP production in mitochondria becomes active, driven by ADP availability. The model proposes that cycling between Mitosynth and Mitoox creates an oscillation in insulin secretion [18]. In addition to glycolysis leading to K_{ATP} channel closure, termed "triggering pathway," glucose metabolism increases insulin secretion independent from K_{ATP} channel closure termed "amplification pathway" [15]. The amplification pathway may account for 50% of glucose-stimulated insulin secretion (GSIS) [19]. In addition to glucose, amino acids (AA) such as arginine, glutamine, and leucine stimulate insulin secretion on their own (secretagogues). Fatty acids (FA) augment GSIS but do not trigger insulin secretion at glucose below threshold level (~4 mM). As FAs serve as primary fuels and are elevated in circulation during fasting, the inability of FA to trigger insulin secretion below the threshold glucose level avoids hypoglycemia.

Increase in the Production of Insulin Granules

Insulin production is reported to be upregulated in islets of obese/insulin-resistant rodents [20]. The increase depended on nutritional stimulus as promoting exocytosis by glibenclamide was insufficient to promote proinsulin synthesis in rat islets [20, 21]. Nutritional load can increase insulin production within hours. The acute (<4 h) increase in proinsulin production occurs by activating insulin mRNA translation. Prolonged glucose stimulation (>12 h) enhances the transcription of insulin and other proteins required for mature insulin granule formation [22]. It is important to note that insulin granules in beta cells are heterogenous for affinity to calcium, association with exocytosis machinery, and protein/lipid compositions [23]. Beta cells preferentially secrete newly synthesized insulin granules over old granule. Thus, despite the large reserve of insulin granules in the face value (usually less than 5% of insulin granules are secreted in a single day), proinsulin translation and insulin granule formation are critical to support insulin secretion from beta cells [22].

Left Shift of Glucose Responsiveness of Insulin Secretion

Raising the sensitivity of insulin secretion to glucose is another early adaptive response to meet the increased demand for insulin. The left shift of GSIS elevates insulin secretion at the given concentration of glucose and reduces the threshold glucose level for insulin secretion [24]. This left shift of GSIS is seen in human and rodent islets cultured under high glucose and FA as well. Higher sensitivity to glucose is demonstrated not only at the level of insulin secretion but also for other glucose-responsive parameters, including NAD(P)H production and $[Ca^{2+}]_i$ oscillation [25, 26]. Several mechanisms are proposed to mediate changes in glucose responsiveness. Glucose metabolism is reported to be accelerated at glycolysis and TCA cycle [27, 28]. The reduction

in K_{ATP} channel at the plasma membrane is also reported [26]. Activation of transcription factors (e.g., PPARγ, HIF1α) [29] and epigenetic modifications start to contribute when nutritional load is prolonged. An increase in glucose responsiveness occurs both at the levels of an individual beta cell and a cluster of cells. In C57/BL6J female mice on HFD, glucose sensitivity of an individual beta cell and the proportion of glucose-responsive beta cells within an islet are increased [30].

Increasing Beta Cells Mass as an Adaptation to Metabolic Syndrome

Factors that Determine Beta Cell Mass

Pancreatic islets undergo rapid expansion and turnover in early life, but islets have relatively low proliferation and cell death at the rate of <1% in adults in adult humans [31]. The change in beta cell mass defined by insulin positivity could occur when the number or size of beta cells is altered. The increase in beta cell number could occur by beta cell proliferation, transformation of non-beta endocrine cells to beta cell (transdifferentiation), or emergence of beta cells from non-endocrine cells such as acinar and ductal cells in pancreas (neogenesis). The loss of beta cell could occur either by cell death (necrosis, apoptosis, ferroptosis), changing to non-beta endocrine cells (transdifferentiation), or losing hormone production (dedifferentiation).

Increase in Beta Cell Mass Under Insulin Resistance in Rodent Models

It is well established that systemic insulin resistance causes a marked increase in beta cell mass in rodents, that is generally associated with the increased in beta cell proliferation, especially in young rodents [31]. Lineage tracing study [32] and labeling of previously proliferated beta cells [33] indicated that beta cell number increases primarily by replicating of existing beta cells in rodents. However, hypertrophy of beta cells and enhanced beta cell survival may also contribute to increase beta cell mass in rodents.

Does Metabolic Syndrome Increase Beta Cell Mass in Humans?

As there is no reliable method to determine beta cell mass in vivo, it is challenging to monitor beta cell mass longitudinally in humans. Thus, the impact of metabolic syndrome on beta cell mass in humans is primarily assessed using histological analysis of pancreatectomy or autopsy specimens. The extent of beta cell mass expansion is subtle in humans compared with rodents. Human studies summarized in recent reviews report a 30~50% increase in beta cell mass in obese humans, although the increase is less clear in Asians [31, 34]. Both increases in the size and number of beta cells are reported [31, 34]. However, it has been difficult to identify proliferating beta cells in human islets to establish beta cell proliferation in obese humans [31]. Proliferation using Ki67 as a cell proliferation marker may have underestimated beta cell proliferation in published studies as immunoreactivity of Ki67 is not preserved well unless fresh samples are used [13]. Some report the increase in neogenesis but not proliferation in obese, insulin-resistant humans [35].

Mechanisms Responsible for the Increase in Beta Cell Mass in Metabolic Syndrome

Nutritional load and insulin resistance in metabolic syndrome could increase beta cell proliferation directly or indirectly through humoral or neuronal cues from tissues that are altered in metabolic syndrome. Most of the information we have on this subject is based on rodent studies. In mice, acute and chronic systemic insulin resistance increases beta cell mass dramatically in the absence of nutritional load. Acute systemic insulin resistance provoked by an insulin receptor (IR) antagonist (S961) [36] or an IGF-1 receptor/IR inhibitor (OSI-906) [37] increased beta cell mass and proliferation in mice. Normalization of glucose by co-treatment with a SGLT2 inhibitor did not prevent beta cell proliferation, excluding the possibility that hyperglycemia is driving beta cell proliferation in this model [37]. Beta cell proliferation induced by S961 or OSI-906 depends on circulatory mitogens for beta cells. Serum from S961 or OSI-906 treated mice is sufficient to stimulate beta cell proliferation in culture [36, 37]. The identity of circulatory factors that stimulate beta cell proliferation in acute insulin-resistant status has not been elucidated, but adipocytes are a possible source of mitogens [36]. In the case of chronic hepatic insulin resistance in liver-specific IR knockout, beta cell proliferation depends on SerpinB1 secreted by the liver [38].

Among nutrients, glucose is a well-established beta cell mitogen in rodents [37, 39]. Elevated influx of glucose without hyperglycemia is proposed to be sufficient to increase glucose metabolism within beta cells and stimulate beta cell proliferation in rodents [40] and possibly in humans. In humans, gain-of-function mutation of glucokinase (V91L) causes hypoglycemia due to inappropriate insulin secretion at low glucose level. Pancreatectomy performed for therapeutic purpose showed hypertrophic islets and beta cell replication (and apoptosis) when control subjects did not show any beta cell replication [41]. Glucose metabolism is proposed to promote beta cell proliferation by number of downstream effectors, including insulin receptor substrate 2 (IRS2)/mammalian target of rapamycin (mTOR) signaling, calcineurin, and transcription factors such as carbohydrate-responsive element-binding protein β (ChREBPβ) [42, 43]. Lipids are commonly increased in metabolic syndrome, but it is unclear whether lipids promote beta cell proliferation. Positive, neutral, and negative effects of lipids on beta cell mass and proliferation are reported indicating that the effect of FA on beta cell proliferation differs depending on settings [44]. It is important to recognize that raising FA levels in circulation increases insulin resistance and makes it hard to separate an indirect effect of insulin resistance from the direct effect of lipids on beta cell proliferation in vivo [45]. AA, especially branch chain AA, increase in circulation under overnutrition and are known to activate mTOR, a well-known stimulator of beta cell proliferation. However, it has not been shown whether AA contributes to beta cell proliferation in the setting of metabolic syndrome. Epigenetic modification due to changes in carbohydrates, FA, and AA is an additional pathway that could promote beta cell proliferation in response to nutritional load [42].

Except for a case study of glucokinase mentioned above, it is unclear whether any of the pathways activated in rodents regulate beta cell mass in humans with metabolic syndrome. Considering the significant difference in the ability to expand beta cell mass between rodents and humans [1], further studies using human models are required to determine a mechanism responsible for beta cell mass expansion in humans with metabolic syndrome.

Inputs from Other Organs Contribute to Adaptation and Decompensation of Pancreatic Islets in Metabolic Syndrome

Multiple organs, including the liver, adipose tissue, skeletal muscle, and immune system, show lipid accumulation, insulin resistance, and other abnormalities in metabolic syndrome. The changes in these organs affect beta cell function and health through many factors (e.g., peptides, FA, mi-RNA, neurotransmitters, and exosome vesicles (EV)) during the process of islet adaptation and eventual decompensation [46, 47]. Incretins such as glucagon-like peptide-1 (GLP-1) and gastric inhibitory polypeptide (GIP) are prime examples of gut-secreted factors that augment insulin secretion upon nutritional intake. Experimental models of insulin resistance in mice (S961, OSI-906, and liver IR knockout, discussed above) revealed the presence of beta cell mitogens secreted from insulin-resistant adipose tissue and the liver [36, 37, 38]. In recent years, the list of factors mediating positive and negative crosstalk with pancreatic islets is growing (Table 1). For example, adipsin/complement factor D is an adipokine that augments insulin secretion and preserves beta cell mass by blocking beta cell dedifferentiation and death in *db/db* mice. A higher level of adipsin is reported to decrease the risk of T2D development in humans, indicating that adipsin may promote beta cell adaptation to nutritional stress [48]. Adipose tissue macrophage from obese mice secretes EV that reduces insulin secretion but increases beta cell proliferation by delivering miR-155 to beta cells [49]. Short-chain FA produced by the gut

Table 1 Factors that mediate inter-organ crosstalk with pancreatic islets

Organs	Factors
Brain	VIP, GRP, Ach, PACAP
Adipose tissue	Adiponectin, Adipsin, Asprosin, Leptin, FA
Liver	Kisspeptin, SerpinB1, IGFBP1, FGF21, Selenoprotein p, miR-375, Follistatin, HGF, miR7218-5p
Skeletal muscle	IL-6, OPG, Follistatin
Gastrointestinal system/microbiota	GLP-1, GIP, short-chain FA, bile acids, Ghrelin, Galanin, NMU
Immune system	IL-1β, MCP-1, SDF1, TNFα
Bone	Osteocalcin

VIP, *vasoactive intestinal polypeptide*; GRP, gastrin-releasing *peptide*; Ach, acetylcholine; PACAP, pituitary adenylate-cyclase-activating *polypeptide;* IGFBP1, insulin-like growth factor binding protein 1; FGF21, fibroblast growth factor 21; HGF, hepatocyte growth factor; OPG, osteoprotegerin; NMU, Neuromedin U; SDF1, stromal cell-derived factor 1; TNFα, tumor necrosis factor α

microbiota affect beta cell function through G protein-coupled receptor (GPR) 41/43 and epigenetic modification of histones [50].

Failure of Islet Adaptation and the Development of T2D in Metabolic Syndrome

Functional Defect of Pancreatic Islets Occurs Early During the Development of T2D

Both functional and morphological defects ensue during the transition from beta cell compensation to decompensation (Fig. 2). The loss of first-phase insulin secretion is the most prominent early sign of human beta cell dysfunction [13, 24]. First-phase insulin secretion is the rapid rise of insulin secretion lasting a few minutes in response to intravenous glucose loading in vivo. Human islets ex vivo also show first-phase insulin secretion indicating the islet intrinsic nature of the response (Fig. 3) [51]. In the study of partial pancreatectomy (~50%) that reduced beta cell mass acutely, low preoperative first-phase insulin secretion predicted postoperative conversion from normoglycemia to

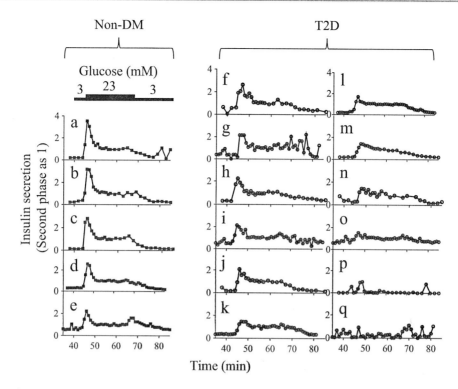

Fig. 3 First-phase insulin secretion is blunted in human islets from T2D donors. Insulin secretion in response to the indicated concentration of glucose was measured in human islets from non-diabetic (non-DM, a-e) and type 2 diabetic (T2D, f-q) organ donors by perfusion. (Reprinted from Ref. [51] with the permission of Springer Nature)

IGT or diabetes [52]. The finding agrees with cross-sectional studies that detected the low first-phase insulin secretion in subjects at risk of developing T2D (Fig. 1a) [3, 53]. In a study of pancreas slices that allowed the simultaneous assessment of beta cell function and beta cell mass, first-phase insulin secretion was reduced in IGT subjects compared with non-diabetic subjects. T2D subjects showed advanced functional defect with the loss of the first and second phases of GSIS. In contrast, beta cell mass was not different between non-diabetic, IGT, and T2D subjects [54]. The longitudinal rodent studies also noted functional defects in beta cells from an early stage when beta cell mass is still expanding [10, 11]. Collectively, beta cell dysfunction ensues well before the manifestation of T2D and is compensated by beta cell mass during the prediabetic stage (Fig. 2). Indeed, cross-sectional studies of the human pancreas report roughly 50% reduction in beta cell mass in T2D subjects [13]. With heterogeneity in

the pathogenesis of T2D, there likely is not a universal tipping point of beta cell mass for the development of T2D. However, low beta cell mass due to genetic factors or nutritional deprivation during early life (in utero and early childhood) may increase the risk for T2D in later life due to a low reserve of beta cell mass [31, 34].

Changes Reported in Pancreatic Islets in T2D

Histological Characteristics of Pancreatic Islets in T2D

In T2D, the reduction of beta cell mass appears to be progressive and is estimated to occur at 1.6%/ year [34]. As adult beta cell proliferation is low, especially in humans, accelerated death of beta cells is often suspected, but has not been demonstrated decisively. One mechanism for beta cell loss without beta cell death is the loss of beta cell identity (dedifferentiation). First demonstrated by lineage tracing in mice [55], beta cells under stress may lose expression of differentiated beta cell markers, including insulin, and gain expression of progenitor markers, including neurogenin 3 (NEUROG3). Although lineage tracing is challenging in humans, hormone-negative (insulin, glucagon, somatostatin, or PP) and chromogranin A positive endocrine cells are increased in human T2D islets and speculated to be dedifferentiated beta cells [56]. Increase in glucagon-positive cells is reported in several studies (3–4% in T2D versus 0.5–3% in non-diabetic islets), which may reflect the transdifferentiation of beta cells to alpha cells [57]. Some report the increase in polyhormonal endocrine cells such as insulin and glucagon double-positive cells in T2D islets [56, 58]. Although it still is speculative, the emergence of dedifferentiated or transdifferentiated cells may be an adaptive response to allow cell survival under stress and preserve a pool of cells with the ability to differentiate back to beta cells [59]. The loss of mature beta cell phenotype may reduce ER stress by decreasing insulin secretion (see ER stress below) [59]. It was also shown that insulin and glucagon double-positive cells were less prone to apoptosis induced by interleukin 1β (IL-1β) and interferon γ (INFγ) in cultured human islets [60].

Signs of inflammation, represented by increase in islet macrophages, has been reported in rodent model of diabetes and human T2D [61, 62]. Recently, multi-spectral image mass cytometry allowed detailed characterization of immune cells and revealed that HLA-DR$^+$ macrophages and CD8 T cells are increased in human T2D islets. Type 1 collagen was also increased in T2D islets in this study [61]. Other morphological changes associated with human T2D islets include amyloid deposition that is formed by aggregates of islet amyloid polypeptide (IAPP), a protein co-secreted with insulin [58]. Due to sequence differences, human IAPP but not mouse IAPP is amyloidogenic, which may be one factor that increases the vulnerability of human beta cells to nutritional stress compared with mouse beta cells [63].

The Insight Gained from Transcriptome and Proteome Analyses of Human Islets

The application of omics to islet biology has yielded a large volume of information in recent years. Wiggler et al. performed transcriptome and proteome analysis of islets from partial pancreatectomy samples of living humans. Donors were well characterized for metabolic parameters and included non-diabetic, IGT, and T2D [64]. Differential expression of islet genes was already seen at the stage of IGT. Some gene sets (i.e., immune response, cell-extracellular matrix response, RNA processing, protein translation, and oxidative phosphorylation) are dysregulated in T2D islets as well, implicating that these may be responsible for the progression to T2D. However, this analysis did not see cell type drifting indicative of the change in beta cell identity. While the proteome of non-diabetic donors showed similar profiles across donors, the proteome of T2D islets was highly heterogenous indicating that complex pathology of beta cell failure in T2D. They did not see reduction in PDX1, MAFA, NKX6.1, or UNC3 in beta cells. They concluded that human T2D beta cells do not have a clear linear trajectory toward precursor cells or transdifferentiation. The major reduction in proteins related to ER and mitochondria indicated significant alterations in these organelles. ALDOB, an enzyme in the pathway of glycolysis, was increased in both transcriptome and proteome data [64].

A recent review summarizes the status quo of single-cell RNA sequences (sc seq) of human islet cells and cites seven studies comparing T2D and non-diabetic islets [65]. One key finding is heterogeneity and plasticity in gene expression, even in non-diabetic beta cells. The major challenge in deducing the pathogenesis of T2D from sc seq data is that very few beta cell genes are differentially expressed reproducibly in T2D across multiple sc seq analyses. FXYD2 (a regulating subunit of Na$^+$-K$^+$-ATPase 2) is differentially expressed most persistently in four out of five studies. Ghrelin cells are underrepresented in T2D islets in the majority of studies [65]. Further technical refinement will likely yield information with higher clarity in the future, but it is unsettled whether there are specific gene sets in beta cells affected by T2D at this point. Below, we highlight studies relevant to beta cell adaptation and failure in T2D.

Avrahami et al. first performed a sc seq of human islet cells from youth to elderly (18 days to 65 years old). They found that beta cells show maturity in gene expression over several years by increasing expression of beta cell-specific genes [66]. Interestingly, the gene expression profile of T2D beta cells showed the similarity to juvenile beta cells, including re-expression of genes characteristically seen in juvenile but not in adult beta cells such as G6PC2, PCK1, and FABP5. However, typical progenitor markers (NEUROG3, POU5F1, NANOG) were not reactivated in T2D beta cells. Also, inflammatory genes and stress genes were increased [66]. Combined with the study by Wiggler et al., "immaturity" in T2D beta cells may represent juvenile status but not progenitor status. However, sc seq may not detect hormone-negative cells efficiently and underscore the presence of progenitor-like cells.

The study by Fang et al. [67] obtained 39,905 sc seq from 9 human islets, including 3 obese and 3 T2D donors. They developed RePact, an algorithm to determine disease-related genes from a relatively limited number of donors, and defined gene signatures associated with obesity and T2D. They found several genes with known roles in metabolism are downregulated in both obesity and T2D (GAPDH for glycolysis, IAPP, and CPE for insulin processing). In gene set enrichment analysis (GSEA), upregulation of hypoxia, glycolysis, and HIF1A target genes and downregulation of aerobic respiration pathways were seen in both obesity and T2D. However, more gene sets were unique or showed the opposite direction of changes between obesity and T2D. INS was upregulated in obesity and reduced in T2D, while two ferritin genes (FTL and FTH1) were increased in obesity and reduced in T2D. The proteosome pathway was upregulated in T2D and downregulated in obesity.

The study by Son et al. [68] applied reverse engineering to obtain the activity of gene expression regulatory proteins from sc seq data of non-diabetic and T2D human islets. Based on

characteristics of regulatory proteins, non-diabetic islets were enriched with metabolically flexible, high insulin-expressing beta cells (MI^{-1}) and metabolically inflexible, weak glucagon expressing alpha cells (MI^{+5}). In comparison, T2D islets were dominated by metabolically inflexible beta cells (MI^{+2}) that also showed high activity of stress response regulatory proteins. For alpha cells, T2D islets were enriched with metabolically flexible cells that showed progenitor/stem-cell-like features (MI^{-5}), a cluster that may reflect beta to alpha cell transition. Furthermore, BACH2 emerged as a potential transcription factor that drives the activation of T2D-associated regulatory proteins in human islets.

Although each study reports a unique set of T2D-associated genes, it is of note that stress responses and glycolysis-related genes are often implicated in T2D islets in above studies.

Are Pathways Involved in Islet Compensation Also Responsible for Islet Decompensation in Metabolic Syndrome?

Unfortunately, some pathways activated to increase insulin output may be detrimental to beta cells if activated chronically or excessively. Upregulation of insulin production inevitably leads to ER stress (discussed below). Accelerating glucose metabolism can cause glucotoxicity and oxidative stress. There also is evidence that the overactivation of the insulin secretion may paradoxically reduce insulin secretion. Although the closure of K_{ATP} channel is a crucial step of GSIS, lowering K_{ATP} channel activity does not progressively increase insulin secretion. K_{ATP} activity below 30% paradoxically impairs insulin secretion (termed crossover) [69]. Hyperglycemia and insulin resistance have been shown to reduce K_{ATP} channel density, which may augment insulin secretion at the beginning but may impair insulin secretion if the reduction passes the point of crossover. Sulphonyl urea (SU) augments insulin secretion by closing K_{ATP} channel independent from glucose metabolism and is widely used to treat T2D. However, the use of SU is associated with accelerated loss of beta cell function and secondary medication failure in humans with T2D. In contrast, a K_{ATP} channel opener diazoxide was shown to improve islet function, possibly by increasing K_{ATP} activity above the threshold of crossover or by "resting" beta cells from the excessive workload of insulin secretion [69]. Similar transition from hypersecretion to impaired secretion of insulin is seen when a glucokinase activator is used to increase glucose metabolism.

Transcription factor ChREBPβ is another example that aids beta cell adaptation acutely but could accelerate beta cell demise after chronic activation [43]. ChREBPβ is activated in beta cells in response to prolonged hyperglycemia and is necessary for glucose-responsive expansion of beta cell mass. However, chronic overexpression of ChREBPβ leads to the loss of beta cell identity, apoptosis, and hyperglycemia in mice.

Mechanisms Proposed for Beta Cell Demise in T2D

Glucotoxicity

While glucose promotes beta cell compensation by increasing beta cell mass and insulin secretion, exposure to excess glucose for a prolonged time is considered detrimental for beta cells and contributes to beta cell demise during the development of T2D [13]. Clinically, overt hyperglycemia impairs beta cell function, and the correction of hyperglycemia improves insulin secretion in uncontrolled diabetic subjects [70]. To clarify the impact of subtle hyperglycemia in humans in vivo, 72-h glucose infusion was performed to raise fasting glucose mildly (~50 mg/dl) in non-diabetic subjects. In the study, the absolute value of plasma insulin level was elevated, but insulin sensitivity and clearance were reduced. The study concluded that beta cell function corrected for insulin resistance was reduced [70]. Overall, it still is unsettled whether mild hyperglycemia or increased glucose utilization by beta cells at normoglycemia is sufficient to trigger beta cell failure in humans.

In vitro, high glucose (above ~8 mM) reduces insulin contents, blunts GSIS, and impairs mitochondrial function in human islets [17]. The alteration in glycolysis was recently highlighted as one culprit for glucose-induced beta cell dysfunction. GAPDH activity was markedly reduced in beta cell models exposed to chronic hyperglycemia. This led to hyperactivate of mechanistic target of rapamycin complex 1 (mTORC1) by glycolytic metabolites upstream of GAPDH. mTORC1 reduces the entrance of pyruvate into the TCA cycle by suppressing pyruvate dehydrogenase, thus impairing mitochondrial function and decreasing insulin secretion. The contribution of mTORC1 hyperactivation to beta cell dysfunction in T2D is supported by another study that showed hyperactivation of mTORC1 in non-diabetic islets exposed to high glucose and T2D islets [71]. The inhibition of mTORC1-S6K1 improved GSIS from human T2D islets further implicating that mTORC1 hyperactivation plays a role in beta cell dysfunction in T2D.

The expression of the thioredoxin-interacting protein (TXNIP) is markedly induced in human islets cultured at high glucose [72]. TXNIP expression is elevated in diabetic islets, although glucose may not be the sole driver considering ER stress also increases TXNIP. TXNIP is proposed to impair beta cell function and survival through several pathways: it alters redox status through binding to thioredoxin in the cytosol, activates caspase 3 by promoting phosphorylation of ASK1 in mitochondria, modulates gene expression in nuclei, and activates inflammasome. Verapamil reduces TXNIP expression by decreasing intracellular calcium and may improve beta cell survival and function in T2D [72]. ALDOB is a glycolytic enzyme whose expression is upregulated by glucose and reported to correlate with beta cell dysfunction in human T2D [73]. As discussed, chronic overexpression of ChREBPβ by glucose is another potential pathway by which glucose impairs beta cell survival and function [43].

(Gluco)Lipotoxicity

Organ dysfunction in metabolic syndrome is often attributed to lipid overload in adipose tissue, the liver, skeletal muscle, the heart, and others. In vitro, culturing human islets with FA, especially saturated FA, impairs GSIS and cell viability [44]. As the detrimental effect of FA on human islets usually requires an elevated level of glucose, the term glucolipotoxicity is often preferred. The increase in cytotoxic metabolites (e.g., ceramides, superoxide, acylcarnitine) and the activation of multiple stress pathways (e.g., ER stress, mitochondrial dysfunction, and inflammation) are reported in beta cells and islets exposed to FA in culture [44]. However, there is unresolved debate on whether culture models provide sufficient evidence that lipid overload contributes to beta cell demise in human T2D [74, 75]. While palmitic acid (C16:0) is often used in culture models, toxic effects demonstrated by saturated FA may not translate into a condition in vivo where islets are exposed to a mixture of FA including unsaturated FA that reduces toxic effect of saturated FA [44]. At the same time, volume of evidence points to the contribution of lipid overload to beta cell failure in T2D. In addition to lipids from the blood supply, adipose tissue locally infiltrating the pancreas can increase the exposure of pancreatic islets to lipids. Pancreatic fat contents measured by magnetic resonance imaging, computer tomography, and ultrasound are increased in human T2D and negatively correlate with parameters of beta cell function [44]. When obese T2D subjects were placed on a very low calory diet, the improvement in insulin secretion was associated with the reduction in pancreatic fats [76]. When human and mouse islets were transplanted into an immune-deficient mouse, HFD caused beta cell dysfunction and lipid droplet accumulation in human but not mouse beta cells [63]. Although the transplant study did not directly test an isolated effect of lipids, it supports that nutritional overload increases lipid accumulation in human beta cells in vivo and causes beta cell dysfunction. It is important to recognize species-specific differences in lipid handling between human and mouse beta cells as the contribution of lipid overload to beta cell failure might be underestimated in mouse studies [44, 75]. Notably, the increase in lipid deposition in human T2D islets is recently reported, indicating that the influx of lipids is increased and/or clearance of lipids is impaired in human beta cells affected by T2D [77].

ER Stress

When demand for protein synthesis exceeds its capacity, ER activates a stress response (unfolded protein response, UPR) to mitigate pressure from protein synthesis by lowering protein translation, increasing ER chaperon production, and degrading misfolded proteins (ER-associated protein degradation (ERAD)) [57]. If the stress is prolonged or overwhelming, the activation of ER stress pathway leads to inflammation, oxidative stress response, and apoptosis [57]. Importance of ER homeostasis for insulin secretion in humans is inferred from monogenic diabetes that occurs with mutations in insulin synthesis (e.g., proinsulin, translation factor Ssr1, tRNA methylthio-transferase Cdkal1), PERK-eIF2a branch of ER stress signaling, and ER membrane protein WFS1 [19, 57]. Multiple signs of ER stress are reported in human islets affected by T2D. ER stress genes are upregulated in human T2D islets [57]. The ER is swollen in both alpha and beta cells of human T2D islets [57]. Proinsulin/insulin is increased in T2D, indicating reduced efficiency of proinsulin processing [78].

Increased demand for insulin production is one likely trigger of ER stress in T2D islets [19, 57]. In a study of human islets isolated from partial pancreatectomy, the expression of ER stress markers (GRP78, XBP-1, PDIAI) in islets negatively correlated with insulin sensitivity of donors that ranged from non-diabetic, and IGT to T2D [78]. FA are well-known inducers of ER stress in many types of cells in culture and provide another potential link between nutritional load and ER stress in islets [57]. FA deplete ER calcium that is maintained at ~200–500 µM, a concentration much higher than that of cytosolic calcium at 100 nM [19].

Interestingly, there is a strong correlation between the activation of ER stress and change in the differentiated status of beta cells. When ER stress is provoked acutely and reversibly by depleting ER calcium using a sarcoendoplasmic reticulum calcium transport ATPase (SERCA) inhibitor, beta cells reduce expression of mature beta cell markers (e.g., insulin, MafA, Glut2) transiently. However, repetitive ER stress resulted in chronic loss of beta cell maturity and function [59]. Beta cells may reduce beta cell markers and mature function, including insulin secretion, to create a window to recover from ER stress [79].

Oxidative Stress

Although low levels of reactive oxygen species (ROS) are important signaling molecules for insulin secretion [62], oxidative stress occurs when the accumulation of ROS exceeds the antioxidant capacity of the cells. Beta cells are susceptible to oxidative stress due to low levels of anti-oxidative enzymes [62]. In beta cells, mitochondrial metabolism of glucose/FA and peroxisome activity can produce ROS. Activation of NADPH oxidase (NOX), which cytokines could trigger, is another source of ROS that is proposed to play a role in beta cell failure [80]. Peroxidation of lipids, proteins, and nucleic acids by ROS will disrupt their function and have detrimental effects on cells [80]. Evidence of oxidative stress is reported in human T2D islets [62, 80]. NRF2 is a transcription factor activated by oxidative stress to aid the resolution of the stress and its activation was shown to improve beta cell function in *db/db* mice and INS1 cells treated by H_2O_2 [81].

Mitochondrial Dysfunction

Mitochondria participate in glucose sensing in beta cells by coupling glucose metabolism with the TCA cycle. Also, mitochondria support energetic needs for insulin production and secretion. Not surprisingly, mitochondrial mutations (such as tRNA (Leu)) are known causes of a genetic form of diabetes [82]. In beta cells affected by T2D, mitochondria are functionally impaired [17] and morphologically swollen and fragmented [83, 84]. Detrimental effects of FA and glucose on beta cells are at least partially mediated through mitochondrial dysfunction. FA and glucose exposure increases ROS production and fragments mitochondria in beta cells in culture. As discussed above [17], glucose overload impairs mitochondrial function through glycolysis-mTORC1 pathway. Incomplete oxidation of FA at the mitochondria produces acylcarnitine that negatively affects insulin synthesis and secretion

[85]. In-site metabolome of islets in prediabetic and diabetic TallyHo and *db/db* mice showed that the accumulation of acylcarnitine is one of the early changes in islets during the development of diabetes [85]. Acylcarnitines (stearoyl, palmitoyl, and acetyl) were also increased in human T2D islets compared with non-diabetic controls [85].

Inflammation

As in adipose tissue in metabolic syndrome, chronic inflammation occurs in human T2D islets. Infiltration of leukocytes, including macrophages, increase in inflammatory mediators (e.g., IL-1β, monocyte chemoattractant protein-1 (MCP1)), and activation of nuclear factor kappa B (NF-κB) are reported in human T2D islets [62]. During the development of beta cell demise in T2D, inflammatory pathways can be activated by nutritional stress and other stress associated with T2D, such as ER stress, oxidative stress, amyloid, and mitochondrial dysfunction [62]. Among proposed mediators of inflammation, anti-IL-1β agents and salsalate (NF-κB inhibitor) targeted therapies have been tested in T2D humans and both showed small but significant reduction in hemoglobin A1C (HbA1C) [86, 87]. However, it is not clear whether they reduced HbA1C by improving beta cell function [86, 87]. Targeting a single molecule may not be sufficient to resolve beta cell inflammation and stress response in beta cells in T2D subjects.

Other Pathways Implicated

Numerous other pathways and targets are proposed to play a role in beta cell demise in T2D. Amyloidogenic IAPP seen in T2D islets is known to be cytotoxic [88]. Autophagy–lysosome system, important for the clearance of damaged cell components under stress, is reportedly dysfunctional in beta cell models of T2D [89]. In support, polymorphisms/mutations of autophagy-related proteins increase the risk for diabetes [90]. Senescent beta cells are increased in human T2D islets and islets of insulin-resistant and HFD-fed mice [91]. The removal of senescent cells (senolysis) improves secretory function and expression of cell-specific markers in beta cells [91].

Interaction between Stress Pathways

It is very common to see that one stress pathway activates additional stress pathways to amplify the stress response [62]. The interaction between stress pathways occurs in multiple layers. Homeostasis of one organelle depends on the health of other organelles. For example, the disulfide bond formation of insulin depends on the oxidizing environment of ER that is supported by mitochondria. The mitochondrial TCA cycle regulates the redox cycling of glutathione and thioredoxin which is important for the replenishment of reducing equivalents to keep redox homeostasis of ER [22]. Molecules implicated in beta cell stress often participate in multiple stress pathways. In addition to reducing reduce TCA cycle activity in mitochondria [17], hyperactivation of mTORC1 could impair autophagy considering that mTORC1 is a negative regulator of autophagy [89].

It also occurs that the activation of a stress pathway is counteracted by a response to mitigate the stress. Mice expressing amyloidogenic human IAPP activates the HIF1α/PFKFB3 stress/repair signaling pathway that is also increased in beta cells of human T2D islets. This protects beta cells against the detrimental increase in $[Ca^{2+}]$ at the expense of mitochondrial fragmentation and reduction of oxidative phosphorylation [92]. Thus, at any given moment, beta cells show heterogeneous pathology from combination of compensatory and maladaptive responses based on the duration of stress, type of stressor, environmental input, and genetic background.

A Role of Alpha Cells in the Development of T2D

Physiology of Alpha Cells

Comprising 30–60% of endocrine cells in human islets, alpha cells are distributed throughout human islets and make frequent contact with beta cells. Mouse alpha cells occupy 10–15% of endocrine cells at the periphery of islets [93]. Alpha cells predominantly produce glucagon from the pre-pro-glucagon gene through the action of proprotein convertase 2 (PCSK2), but also produce GLP-1 via PCSK1/3 under stress conditions [94]. It is well recognized that hypoglycemia increases glucagon secretion, a process initiated by opening of K_{ATP} channel that ultimately opens P/Q Ca^{2+} channel [94]. However, it is important to note that AA, especially gluconeogenic AA (alanine, glutamine, and glycine), are strong stimulus for glucagon secretion. GIP is known to synergize with AA to increase glucagon secretion. In addition to cell autonomous regulation by glucose and AA, glucagon secretion is controlled by juxtracrine (cell-cell interaction) and neural input. Insulin, GABA, serotonin, and zinc from beta cells and somatostatin from delta cells reduce glucagon secretion in a paracrine manner. Beta cells communicate with alpha cells by presenting ephrin ligand to ephrin receptor on alpha cells [94]. Thus, glucagon secretion is not solely determined by glucose and induced postprandially when AA levels are increased. Although glucagon has been classically viewed as a hormone to elevate glucose level, a wider action of glucagon is now recognized that may seem the opposite of historically known action [93]. Under hypoglycemia, glucagon acts on the liver to increase gluconeogenesis and glycogenolysis and thus prevents dangerous hypoglycemia. However, in postprandial status, glucagon mitigates hyperglycemia by increasing GSIS primarily through GLP-1 receptor (GLP-1R) and to a lesser extent by activating glucagon receptor (GcgR). As an augmentation of GSIS by GLP-1R does not occur below the permissive level of glucose, glucagon positively affects insulin secretion only when glucose is above the threshold level. Antagonism of GLP-1R/GcgR reduces GSIS by ~80% in mouse and human islets supporting the significant contribution of glucagon in the augmentation of GSIS [93]. Interestingly, incretin action of GIP requires alpha cell GIP receptor indicating upregulation of glucagon secretion is a key pathway by which GIP augments GSIS [93].

Does Hyperglucagonemia Contribute to Hyperglycemia in T2D?

Elevation of glucagon at fasting and impaired suppression of glucagon upon glucose loading are reported in obesity, insulin-resistant status, and T2D in humans [35, 93]. An absolute or relative (to beta cell mass) increase in alpha cell mass is reported for both obese and T2D human islets [35]. Thus, there are functional and morphological changes in alpha cells associated with T2D. Historically, the elevation in glucagon in diabetes (both T1D and T2D) has been proposed to worsen hyperglycemia. However, with recent findings of the insulinotropic action of glucagon, the origin and consequence of hyperglucagonemia in T2D require reassessment as reviewed recently [93]. Capozzi et al propose that hyperglucagonemia in obesity and diabetes is driven by the increase in the circulatory AA, due to altered AA metabolism in the liver and muscle, and an appropriate compensatory response [93]. It is of note that hyperglucagonemia is seen in T2D with NAFLD but not in those without NAFLD supporting that the liver-alpha cell axis may drive hyperglucagonemia.

At intracellular level, there is number of changes in alpha cells from T2D humans that implicate alpha cell intrinsic damages that dysregulate glucagon secretion in response to glucose [93, 94]. One potential mechanism is the reduced expression of somatostatin 2 receptor that weakens paracrine suppression by somatostatin [95]. Also, transcriptome analysis of human islets indicated that alpha cells affected by T2D show immaturity [66]. By combining patch clamp and single-cell sequencing, Dai et al reported that Ca^{2+} channel activity in response to glucose is impaired in a subset of diabetic alpha cells and this impairment correlates with transcriptome changes in mitochondrial respiratory chain complex, cell surface receptor, and maturity [96].

Collectively, alpha cells likely play an important role in pathogenesis of T2D. However, we still do not know whether hyperglucagonemia serves as an adaptive response or accelerates hyperglycemia in obesity and T2D. Further complicating the picture, glucagon improves energy homeostasis by reducing food intake, increasing energy expenditure, increasing lipid oxidation, and slowing gastric emptying [93]. The complexity of glucagon action is reflected by the fact that both glucagon antagonists and agonists are showing promising results in clinical trials for the treatment of diabetes [93].

Conclusion

To meet increased demand from insulin resistance, pancreatic islets increase insulin secretion by upregulating insulin production, raising efficiency of metabolism secretion coupling, and expanding beta cell mass (Fig. 2). Functional adaptation appears to play an important role in sustaining insulin secretion due to limited ability of beta cells to proliferate in adults. However, an effort to increase insulin production and secretion can become a stressor to beta cells if prolonged. The increased workload and nutritional overload start to impair beta cell function well before the development of hyperglycemia, which is likely prevented by increasing beta cell mass at the beginning. However, with the activation of multiple stress pathways, both the mass and function of beta cells decline during the development of T2D. Multiple stress pathways interact with each other and amplify stress response. Thus, islet failure in T2D is generally progressive and makes T2D subjects insulin dependent. However, recent studies indicate that remission of T2D could occur with bariatric surgery or calory restriction, especially for those with less advanced islet failure [97]. Clearly, resolving insulin resistance and nutritional load are the key to prevent the development and progression of islet failure in T2D. Among multiple stress pathways and targeted implicated, it is important to identify a target that effectively blocks the amplification of stress response to prevent progressive decline in islet mass and function.

References

1. Hart NJ, Powers AC. Use of human islets to understand islet biology and diabetes: progress, challenges and suggestions. Diabetologia. 2019;62(2):212–22.
2. Rodriguez-Diaz R, Molano RD, Weitz JR, Abdulreda MH, Berman DM, Leibiger B, et al. Paracrine interactions within the pancreatic islet determine the glycemic set point. Cell Metab. 2018;27(3):549–58. e4
3. Kahn SE. The relative contributions of insulin resistance and beta-cell dysfunction to the pathophysiology of type 2 diabetes. Diabetologia. 2003;46(1):3–19.
4. Weyer C, Bogardus C, Mott DM, Pratley RE. The natural history of insulin secretory dysfunction and insulin resistance in the pathogenesis of type 2 diabetes mellitus. J Clin Invest. 1999;104(6):787–94.
5. Rai V, Quang DX, Erdos MR, Cusanovich DA, Daza RM, Narisu N, et al. Single-cell ATAC-Seq in human pancreatic islets and deep learning upscaling of rare cells reveals cell-specific type 2 diabetes regulatory signatures. Mol Metab. 2020;32:109–21.
6. Johnson JD. On the causal relationships between hyperinsulinaemia, insulin resistance, obesity and dysglycaemia in type 2 diabetes. Diabetologia. 2021;64(10):2138–46.
7. Page MM, Johnson JD. Mild suppression of hyperinsulinemia to treat obesity and insulin resistance. Trends Endocrinol Metab. 2018;29(6):389–99.
8. Esser N, Utzschneider KM, Kahn SE. Early beta cell dysfunction vs insulin hypersecretion as the primary event in the pathogenesis of dysglycaemia. Diabetologia. 2020;63(10):2007–21.
9. Koh HE, Cao C, Mittendorfer B. Insulin clearance in obesity and type 2 diabetes. Int J Mol Sci. 2022;23(2):596.
10. Chen C, Cohrs CM, Stertmann J, Bozsak R, Speier S. Human beta cell mass and function in diabetes: recent advances in knowledge and technologies to understand disease pathogenesis. Mol Metab. 2017;6(9):943–57.
11. Chen C, Chmelova H, Cohrs CM, Chouinard JA, Jahn SR, Stertmann J, et al. Alterations in beta-cell calcium dynamics and efficacy outweigh islet mass adaptation in compensation of insulin resistance and prediabetes onset. Diabetes. 2016;65(9):2676–85.
12. Henquin JC. Influence of organ donor attributes and preparation characteristics on the dynamics of insulin secretion in isolated human islets. Physiol Rep. 2018;6(5):e13646.
13. Weir GC, Butler PC, Bonner-Weir S. The beta-cell glucose toxicity hypothesis: attractive but difficult to prove. Metabolism. 2021;124:154870.
14. Holman RR, Clark A, Rorsman P. beta-cell secretory dysfunction: a key cause of type 2 diabetes. Lancet Diabetes Endocrinol. 2020;8(5):370.
15. Prentki M, Matschinsky FM, Madiraju SR. Metabolic signaling in fuel-induced insulin secretion. Cell Metab. 2013;18(2):162–85.
16. Matschinsky FM. Regulation of pancreatic beta-cell glucokinase: from basics to therapeutics. Diabetes. 2002;51(Suppl 3):S394–404.
17. Haythorne E, Lloyd M, Walsby-Tickle J, Tarasov AI, Sandbrink J, Portillo I, et al. Altered glycolysis triggers impaired mitochondrial metabolism and mTORC1 activation in diabetic beta-cells. Nat Commun. 2022;13(1):6754.
18. Merrins MJ, Corkey BE, Kibbey RG, Prentki M. Metabolic cycles and signals for insulin secretion. Cell Metab. 2022;34(7):947–68.
19. Kalwat MA, Scheuner D, Rodrigues-Dos-Santos K, Eizirik DL, Cobb MH. The pancreatic ss-cell response to secretory demands and adaption to stress. Endocrinology. 2021;162(11):bqab173.
20. Boland BB, Rhodes CJ, Grimsby JS. The dynamic plasticity of insulin production in beta-cells. Mol Metab. 2017;6(9):958–73.
21. Alarcon C, Wicksteed B, Rhodes CJ. Exendin 4 controls insulin production in rat islet beta cells predominantly by potentiation of glucose-stimulated proinsulin biosynthesis at the translational level. Diabetologia. 2006;49(12):2920–9.
22. Rohli KE, Boyer CK, Blom SE, Stephens SB. Nutrient regulation of pancreatic islet beta-cell secretory capacity and insulin production. Biomol Ther. 2022;12(2):335.
23. Kreutzberger AJB, Kiessling V, Doyle CA, Schenk N, Upchurch CM, Elmer-Dixon M, et al. Distinct insulin granule subpopulations implicated in the secretory pathology of diabetes types 1 and 2. elife. 2020;9:e62506.
24. Weir GC, Laybutt DR, Kaneto H, Bonner-Weir S, Sharma A. Beta-cell adaptation and decompensation during the progression of diabetes. Diabetes. 2001;50(Suppl 1):S154–9.
25. Irles E, Neco P, Lluesma M, Villar-Pazos S, Santos-Silva JC, Vettorazzi JF, et al. Enhanced glucose-induced intracellular signaling promotes insulin hypersecretion: pancreatic beta-cell functional adaptations in a model of genetic obesity and prediabetes. Mol Cell Endocrinol. 2015;404:46–55.
26. Glynn E, Thompson B, Vadrevu S, Lu S, Kennedy RT, Ha J, et al. Chronic glucose exposure systematically shifts the oscillatory threshold of mouse islets: experimental evidence for an early intrinsic mechanism of compensation for hyperglycemia. Endocrinology. 2016;157(2):611–23.
27. Liu YQ, Jetton TL, Leahy JL. beta-Cell adaptation to insulin resistance. Increased pyruvate carboxylase and malate-pyruvate shuttle activity in islets of nondiabetic Zucker fatty rats. J Biol Chem. 2002;277(42):39163–8.
28. Liu YQ, Tornheim K, Leahy JL. Fatty acid-induced beta cell hypersensitivity to glucose. Increased phosphofructokinase activity and lowered glucose-6-phosphate content. J Clin Invest. 1998;101(9):1870–5.
29. Gupta D, Jetton TL, LaRock K, Monga N, Satish B, Lausier J, et al. Temporal characterization of beta cell-adaptive and -maladaptive mechanisms during chronic

high-fat feeding in C57BL/6NTac mice. J Biol Chem. 2017;292(30):12449–59.

30. Gonzalez A, Merino B, Marroqui L, Neco P, Alonso-Magdalena P, Caballero-Garrido E, et al. Insulin hypersecretion in islets from diet-induced hyperinsulinemic obese female mice is associated with several functional adaptations in individual beta-cells. Endocrinology. 2013;154(10):3515–24.

31. Alejandro EU, Gregg B, Blandino-Rosano M, Cras-Meneur C, Bernal-Mizrachi E. Natural history of beta-cell adaptation and failure in type 2 diabetes. Mol Asp Med. 2015;42:19–41.

32. Dor Y, Brown J, Martinez OI, Melton DA. Adult pancreatic beta-cells are formed by self-duplication rather than stem-cell differentiation. Nature. 2004;429(6987): 41–6.

33. Teta M, Rankin MM, Long SY, Stein GM, Kushner JA. Growth and regeneration of adult beta cells does not involve specialized progenitors. Dev Cell. 2007;12 (5):817–26.

34. Sasaki H, Saisho Y, Inaishi J, Itoh H. Revisiting regulators of human beta-cell mass to achieve beta-cell-centric approach toward type 2 diabetes. J Endocr Soc. 2021;5(10):bvab128.

35. Mezza T, Muscogiuri G, Sorice GP, Clemente G, Hu J, Pontecorvi A, et al. Insulin resistance alters islet morphology in nondiabetic humans. Diabetes. 2014;63(3): 994–1007.

36. Shirakawa J, Togashi Y, Basile G, Okuyama T, Inoue R, Fernandez M, et al. E2F1 transcription factor mediates a link between fat and islets to promote beta cell proliferation in response to acute insulin resistance. Cell Rep. 2022;41(1):111436.

37. Shirakawa J, Tajima K, Okuyama T, Kyohara M, Togashi Y, De Jesus DF, et al. Luseogliflozin increases beta cell proliferation through humoral factors that activate an insulin receptor- and IGF-1 receptor-independent pathway. Diabetologia. 2020;63(3):577–87.

38. El Ouaamari A, Dirice E, Gedeon N, Hu J, Zhou JY, Shirakawa J, et al. SerpinB1 promotes pancreatic beta cell proliferation. Cell Metab. 2016;23(1):194–205.

39. Bonner-Weir S, Deery D, Leahy JL, Weir GC. Compensatory growth of pancreatic beta-cells in adult rats after short-term glucose infusion. Diabetes. 1989;38(1):49–53.

40. Porat S, Weinberg-Corem N, Tornovsky-Babaey S, Schyr-Ben-Haroush R, Hija A, Stolovich-Rain M, et al. Control of pancreatic beta cell regeneration by glucose metabolism. Cell Metab. 2011;13(4):440–9.

41. Kassem S, Bhandari S, Rodriguez-Bada P, Motaghedi R, Heyman M, Garcia-Gimeno MA, et al. Large islets, beta-cell proliferation, and a glucokinase mutation. N Engl J Med. 2010;362(14):1348–50.

42. Moulle VS, Ghislain J, Poitout V. Nutrient regulation of pancreatic beta-cell proliferation. Biochimie. 2017;143:10–7.

43. Katz LS, Brill G, Zhang P, Kumar A, Baumel-Alterzon S, Honig LB, et al. Maladaptive positive feedback production of ChREBPbeta underlies

glucotoxic beta-cell failure. Nat Commun. 2022;13 (1):4423.

44. Imai Y, Cousins RS, Liu S, Phelps BM, Promes JA. Connecting pancreatic islet lipid metabolism with insulin secretion and the development of type 2 diabetes. Ann N Y Acad Sci. 2020;1461(1):53–72.

45. Moulle VS, Vivot K, Tremblay C, Zarrouki B, Ghislain J, Poitout V. Glucose and fatty acids synergistically and reversibly promote beta cell proliferation in rats. Diabetologia. 2017;60(5):879–88.

46. Langlois A, Dumond A, Vion J, Pinget M, Bouzakri K. Crosstalk communications between islets cells and insulin target tissue: the hidden face of iceberg. Front Endocrinol (Lausanne). 2022;13:836344.

47. Evans RM, Wei Z. Interorgan crosstalk in pancreatic islet function and pathology. FEBS Lett. 2022;596(5): 607–19.

48. Gomez-Banoy N, Guseh JS, Li G, Rubio-Navarro A, Chen T, Poirier B, et al. Adipsin preserves beta cells in diabetic mice and associates with protection from type 2 diabetes in humans. Nat Med. 2019;25(11):1739–47.

49. Gao H, Luo Z, Jin Z, Ji Y, Ying W. Adipose tissue macrophages modulate obesity-associated beta cell adaptations through secreted miRNA-containing extracellular vesicles. Cell. 2021;10(9):2451.

50. Fernandez-Millan E, Guillen C. Multi-organ crosstalk with endocrine pancreas: a focus on how gut microbiota shapes pancreatic beta-cells. Biomol Ther. 2022;12(1):104.

51. Butcher MJ, Hallinger D, Garcia E, Machida Y, Chakrabarti S, Nadler J, et al. Association of pro-inflammatory cytokines and islet resident leucocytes with islet dysfunction in type 2 diabetes. Diabetologia. 2014;57(3):491–501.

52. Mezza T, Ferraro PM, Di Giuseppe G, Moffa S, Cefalo CM, Cinti F, et al. Pancreaticoduodenectomy model demonstrates a fundamental role of dysfunctional beta cells in predicting diabetes. J Clin Invest. 2021;131 (12):e146788.

53. Ferrannini E, Gastaldelli A, Miyazaki Y, Matsuda M, Pettiti M, Natali A, et al. Predominant role of reduced beta-cell sensitivity to glucose over insulin resistance in impaired glucose tolerance. Diabetologia. 2003;46 (9):1211–9.

54. Cohrs CM, Panzer JK, Drotar DM, Enos SJ, Kipke N, Chen C, et al. Dysfunction of persisting beta cells is a key feature of early type 2 diabetes pathogenesis. Cell Rep. 2020;31(1):107469.

55. Talchai C, Xuan S, Lin HV, Sussel L, Accili D. Pancreatic beta cell dedifferentiation as a mechanism of diabetic beta cell failure. Cell. 2012;150(6): 1223–34.

56. Amo-Shiinoki K, Tanabe K, Hoshii Y, Matsui H, Harano R, Fukuda T, et al. Islet cell dedifferentiation is a pathologic mechanism of long-standing progression of type 2 diabetes. JCI Insight. 2021;6(1): e143791.

57. Eizirik DL, Pasquali L, Cnop M. Pancreatic beta-cells in type 1 and type 2 diabetes mellitus: different

pathways to failure. Nat Rev Endocrinol. 2020;16(7): 349–62.

58. Spijker HS, Song H, Ellenbroek JH, Roefs MM, Engelse MA, Bos E, et al. Loss of beta-cell identity occurs in type 2 diabetes and is associated with islet amyloid deposits. Diabetes. 2015;64(8):2928–38.

59. Chen CW, Guan BJ, Alzahrani MR, Gao Z, Gao L, Bracey S, et al. Adaptation to chronic ER stress enforces pancreatic beta-cell plasticity. Nat Commun. 2022;13(1):4621.

60. Tesi M, Bugliani M, Ferri G, Suleiman M, De Luca C, Bosi E, et al. Pro-inflammatory cytokines induce insulin and glucagon double positive human islet cells that are resistant to apoptosis. Biomol Ther. 2021;11(2): 320.

61. Wu M, Lee MYY, Bahl V, Traum D, Schug J, Kusmartseva I, et al. Single-cell analysis of the human pancreas in type 2 diabetes using multi-spectral imaging mass cytometry. Cell Rep. 2021;37(5): 109919.

62. Imai Y, Dobrian AD, Morris MA, Nadler JL. Islet inflammation: a unifying target for diabetes treatment? Trends Endocrinol Metab. 2013;24(7):351–60.

63. Dai C, Kayton NS, Shostak A, Poffenberger G, Cyphert HA, Aramandla R, et al. Stress-impaired transcription factor expression and insulin secretion in transplanted human islets. J Clin Invest. 2016;126(5): 1857–70.

64. Wigger L, Barovic M, Brunner AD, Marzetta F, Schoniger E, Mehl F, et al. Multi-omics profiling of living human pancreatic islet donors reveals heterogeneous beta cell trajectories towards type 2 diabetes. Nat Metab. 2021;3(7):1017–31.

65. Ngara M, Wierup N. Lessons from single-cell RNA sequencing of human islets. Diabetologia. 2022;65(8): 1241–50.

66. Avrahami D, Wang YJ, Schug J, Feleke E, Gao L, Liu C, et al. Single-cell transcriptomics of human islet ontogeny defines the molecular basis of beta-cell dedifferentiation in T2D. Mol Metab. 2020;42:101057.

67. Fang Z, Weng C, Li H, Tao R, Mai W, Liu X, et al. Single-cell heterogeneity analysis and CRISPR screen identify key beta-cell-specific disease genes. Cell Rep. 2019;26(11):3132–44. e7

68. Son J, Ding HX, Farb TB, Efanov AM, Sun JJ, Core JL, et al. BACH2 inhibition reverses beta cell failure in type 2 diabetes models. J Clin Investig. 2021;131(24): e153876.

69. Nichols CG, York NW, Remedi MS. ATP-sensitive potassium channels in hyperinsulinism and type 2 diabetes: inconvenient paradox or new paradigm? Diabetes. 2022;71(3):367–75.

70. Merovci A, Tripathy D, Chen X, Valdez I, Abdul-Ghani M, Solis-Herrera C, et al. Effect of mild physiologic hyperglycemia on insulin secretion, insulin clearance, and insulin sensitivity in healthy glucose-tolerant subjects. Diabetes. 2021;70(1):204–13.

71. Yuan T, Rafizadeh S, Gorrepati KD, Lupse B, Oberholzer J, Maedler K, et al. Reciprocal regulation

of mTOR complexes in pancreatic islets from humans with type 2 diabetes. Diabetologia. 2017;60(4):668–78.

72. Shalev A. Minireview: thioredoxin-interacting protein: regulation and function in the pancreatic beta-cell. Mol Endocrinol. 2014;28(8):1211–20.

73. Gerst F, Jaghutriz BA, Staiger H, Schulte AM, Lorza-Gil E, Kaiser G, et al. The expression of aldolase B in islets is negatively associated with insulin secretion in humans. J Clin Endocrinol Metab. 2018;103(12): 4373–83.

74. Prentki M, Peyot ML, Masiello P, Madiraju SRM. Nutrient-induced metabolic stress, adaptation, detoxification, and toxicity in the pancreatic beta-cell. Diabetes. 2020;69(3):279–90.

75. Weir GC. Glucolipotoxicity, beta-cells, and diabetes: the emperor has no clothes. Diabetes. 2020;69(3):273–8.

76. Al-Mrabeh A, Zhyzhneuskaya SV, Peters C, Barnes AC, Melhem S, Jesuthasan A, et al. Hepatic lipoprotein export and remission of human type 2 diabetes after weight loss. Cell Metab. 2020;31(2):233–49. e4

77. Horii T, Kozawa J, Fujita Y, Kawata S, Ozawa H, Ishibashi C, et al. Lipid droplet accumulation in beta cells in patients with type 2 diabetes is associated with insulin resistance, hyperglycemia and beta cell dysfunction involving decreased insulin granules. Front Endocrinol (Lausanne). 2022;13:996716.

78. Brusco N, Sebastiani G, Di Giuseppe G, Licata G, Grieco GE, Fignani D, et al. Intra-islet insulin synthesis defects are associated with endoplasmic reticulum stress and loss of beta cell identity in human diabetes. Diabetologia. 2023;66(2):354–66.

79. Xin Y, Dominguez Gutierrez G, Okamoto H, Kim J, Lee AH, Adler C, et al. Pseudotime ordering of single human beta-cells reveals states of insulin production and unfolded protein response. Diabetes. 2018;67(9): 1783–94.

80. Kulkarni A, Muralidharan C, May SC, Tersey SA, Mirmira RG. Inside the beta cell: molecular stress response pathways in diabetes pathogenesis. Endocrinology. 2022;164(1):bqac184.

81. Dodson M, Shakya A, Anandhan A, Chen J, Garcia JGN, Zhang DD. NRF2 and diabetes: the good, the bad, and the complex. Diabetes. 2022;71(12):2463–76.

82. Las G, Oliveira MF, Shirihai OS. Emerging roles of beta-cell mitochondria in type-2-diabetes. Mol Asp Med. 2020;71:100843.

83. Stiles L, Shirihai OS. Mitochondrial dynamics and morphology in beta-cells. Best Pract Res Clin Endocrinol Metab. 2012;26(6):725–38.

84. Anello M, Lupi R, Spampinato D, Piro S, Masini M, Boggi U, et al. Functional and morphological alterations of mitochondria in pancreatic beta cells from type 2 diabetic patients. Diabetologia. 2005;48(2): 282–9.

85. Aichler M, Borgmann D, Krumsiek J, Buck A, MacDonald PE, Fox JEM, et al. N-acyl taurines and acylcarnitines cause an imbalance in insulin synthesis

and secretion provoking beta cell dysfunction in type 2 diabetes. Cell Metab. 2017;25(6):1334–47 e4.

86. Goldfine AB, Fonseca V, Jablonski KA, Chen YD, Tipton L, Staten MA, et al. Salicylate (salsalate) in patients with type 2 diabetes: a randomized trial. Ann Intern Med. 2013;159(1):1–12.

87. Kataria Y, Ellervik C, Mandrup-Poulsen T. Treatment of type 2 diabetes by targeting interleukin-1: a meta-analysis of 2921 patients. Semin Immunopathol. 2019;41(4):413–25.

88. Gupta D, Leahy JL. Islet amyloid and type 2 diabetes: overproduction or inadequate clearance and detoxification? J Clin Invest. 2014;124(8):3292–4.

89. Lee YH, Kim J, Park K, Lee MS. Beta-cell autophagy: mechanism and role in beta-cell dysfunction. Mol Metab. 2019;27S:S92–S103.

90. Pearson GL, Gingerich MA, Walker EM, Biden TJ, Soleimanpour SA. A selective look at autophagy in pancreatic beta-cells. Diabetes. 2021;70(6):1229–41.

91. Aguayo-Mazzucato C, Andle J, Lee TB Jr, Midha A, Talemal L, Chipashvili V, et al. Acceleration of beta cell aging determines diabetes and senolysis improves disease outcomes. Cell Metab. 2019;30(1):129–42. e4

92. Montemurro C, Nomoto H, Pei L, Parekh VS, Vongbunyong KE, Vadrevu S, et al. IAPP toxicity activates HIF1alpha/PFKFB3 signaling delaying beta-cell loss at the expense of beta-cell function. Nat Commun. 2019;10(1):2679.

93. Capozzi ME, D'Alessio DA, Campbell JE. The past, present, and future physiology and pharmacology of glucagon. Cell Metab. 2022;34(11):1654–74.

94. Martinez MS, Manzano A, Olivar LC, Nava M, Salazar J, D'Marco L, et al. The role of the alpha cell in the pathogenesis of diabetes: a world beyond the mirror. Int J Mol Sci. 2021;22(17):9504.

95. Omar-Hmeadi M, Lund PE, Gandasi NR, Tengholm A, Barg S. Paracrine control of alpha-cell glucagon exocytosis is compromised in human type-2 diabetes. Nat Commun. 2020;11(1):1896.

96. Dai XQ, Camunas-Soler J, Briant LJB, Dos Santos T, Spigelman AF, Walker EM, et al. Heterogenous impairment of alpha cell function in type 2 diabetes is linked to cell maturation state. Cell Metab. 2022;34(2):256–68 e5.

97. Suleiman M, Marselli L, Cnop M, Eizirik DL, De Luca C, Femia FR, et al. The role of beta cell recovery in type 2 diabetes remission. Int J Mol Sci. 2022;23(13):7435.

Insulin Resistance in Obesity

22

Wanbao Yang, Jeffrey Guo, and Shaodong Guo

Contents

W. Yang · J. Guo · S. Guo (✉)
Department of Nutrition, College of Agriculture and Life Sciences, Texas A&M University, College Station, TX, USA
e-mail: wanbao.yang@ag.tamu.edu;
shaodong.guo@ag.tamu.edu

Abstract

Insulin resistance is a hallmark of obesity and a forerunner of type 2 diabetes mellitus (T2DM). Obesity-induced lipotoxicity and inflammation

© Springer Nature Switzerland AG 2023
R. S. Ahima (ed.), *Metabolic Syndrome*,
https://doi.org/10.1007/978-3-031-40116-9_28

impair insulin sensitivity through activation of intracellular protein kinases. Sexual dimorphism in insulin resistance has been observed in young women versus men. Premenopausal women with a normal menstrual cycle show higher insulin sensitivity than age-matched men. Estrogen plays a key role in regulating the sexual dimorphism in insulin resistance. Estrogen binds to estrogen receptor (ER) α to control glucose and energy homeostasis in brain, liver, adipose tissue, skeletal muscle, pancreas, and immune system. Estrogen action on insulin sensitivity is mainly mediated by its non-genomic mechanism. Estrogen stimulates interaction of ERα with key components of insulin signaling, such as phosphatidylinositol 3-kinase (PI3K), thereby enhancing insulin sensitivity. This chapter discusses the contribution of the sex hormone estrogen to sexual dimorphism in insulin resistance and focuses on the molecular mechanism by which estrogen improves insulin resistance via the forkhead/winged helix transcription factor FoxO1, with emphasis on the genomic versus non-genomic actions as well as the role of ERα and β in estrogen action.

Keywords

Insulin resistance · Diabetes mellitus · Sexual dimorphism · Estrogen · Estrogen receptor · The forkhead/winged helix transcription factor FoxO1

Introduction

Type 2 diabetes mellitus (T2DM) is an increasing global health issue, which is highly associated with the epidemic of obesity. T2DM is caused by systemic insulin resistance and impaired insulin secretion, leading to dysregulation of carbohydrate, lipid, and protein metabolism. Insulin resistance is a hallmark of obesity and a forerunner of T2DM. Insulin resistance refers to a decrease in the target tissues' glucose-lowering response to insulin. Increased insulin secretion compensates for insulin resistance. Thus, fasting plasma insulin increases, and hyperinsulinemia progressively develops. Insulin resistance and

hyperinsulinemia are linked and culminate in β-cell failure, leading to hyperglycemia.

At the cellular level, insulin receptor (IR), a protein tyrosine kinase, is activated to recruit downstream substrates, such as insulin receptor substrate (IRS), upon insulin binding, thereby initiating proximal insulin signaling cascade. Phosphorylated IRS activates phosphoinositide 3-kinase (PI3K)→protein kinase B (AKT) signaling cascade and regulates the activity of the distal downstream targets, including forkhead box protein O1 (FoxO1), mammalian target of rapamycin complex 1 (mTORC1), and glucose transporter type 4 (GLUT4), thereby controlling energy homeostasis. Insulin resistance develops at multiple levels in cells, including desensitizing insulin receptor at cellular surface, inhibiting IRS function through degradation, suppressing PI3K activity, failing to restrain FoxO1-induced transcriptional profile, and reduction of insulin clearance from blood circulation. Overnutrition is associated with insulin resistance through multiple mechanisms. During overnutrition, accumulated toxic metabolites, such as nonesterified fatty acid (NEFA), diacylglycerol (DAG), and ceramides, stimulate protein kinase C (PKC) and regulate Ser/Thr phosphorylation of IRS1 and IR to inhibit proximal insulin signaling cascade. Nutrient excess increases the branched-chain amino acid levels in circulation, leading to activation of mTORC1 that inhibits IRS function. Increased proinflammatory cytokines during overnutrition stimulate IRS protein phosphorylation at Ser/Thr and inhibit insulin receptor signaling through activation of JNK1 and IKKβ. Hyperinsulinemia developing during obesity enhances insulin resistance through inhibition of IRS activity.

Sexual dimorphism in insulin resistance and T2DM has been well-documented. Premenopausal women with a normal menstrual history show better insulin sensitivity compared to age-matched men, which potentially contributes to the lower incidence of T2DM in premenopausal women. Estrogen replacement therapy protects against insulin resistance in humans and rodents induced by high-fat diet or fatty acids. Therefore, estrogen plays a key role in sexual dimorphism in insulin resistance. Understanding estrogen action on insulin resistance and its underlying molecular mechanisms would provide new therapeutic strategies to treat insulin resistance and T2DM. In this chapter, we will focus on how estrogen action improves insulin sensitivity and protects against T2DM.

Insulin Action, Insulin Resistance, and the Forkhead Transcription Factor FoxO1

Insulin is a peptide hormone secreted by the pancreatic β-cells and orchestrates the anabolic response to nutrient intake. The discovery of insulin more than a century ago, the studies of insulin signal transduction, and its application to the treatment of diabetic patients have led to breakthroughs in the history of medicine (Fig. 1). Insulin action is mediated by the insulin receptor (IR) and its intrinsic tyrosine kinase activity. Insulin-induced conformational changes and autophosphorylation of IR stimulate the recruitment and phosphorylation of insulin receptor substrates, including IRS and SH3-containing protein (Shc). IRS proteins activate PI3K→AKT pathway to regulate the metabolic actions of insulin, whereas Shc activates Ras→MAPK pathway to mediate the cellular and organismal growth and differentiation. In addition to the canonical insulin signaling pathways, IR also regulates cell cycle, senescence, and apoptosis in a ligand and tyrosine kinase-independent manner [50].

The molecular basis of insulin resistance has been well reviewed [31, 57, 80]. In obesity, lipotoxicity, chronic inflammation, hyperglycemia, hyperinsulinemia, mitochondrial dysfunction, and ER stress activate Ser/Thr kinases and inhibit the activity of IR, IRS proteins, and AKT through Ser/Thr phosphorylation, leading to insulin resistance. Insulin resistance is an important underlying mechanism that causes metabolic diseases. Studies from our lab and others show that FoxO1 promotes hepatic glucose production (HGP) through upregulation of the gene expression of gluconeogenic enzymes, such *as glucose-6-phosphatase (G6pase)* and *phosphoenolpyruvate carboxykinase 1 (Pck1)* [34, 91]. Insulin

suppresses FoxO1 activity through the activated AKT-mediated phosphorylation of FoxO1 at T24, S253, and S316, thereby inhibiting HGP [32, 64]. Hepatic IRS1 and 2 deletion induces insulin resistance in mice, which leads to diabetic phenotypes, including hyperglycemia and hyperinsulinemia; these diabetic phenotypes are normalized by hepatic FoxO1 deficiency [17]. We found that glucagon stimulates FoxO1 phosphorylation at S273 through cAMP→PKA signaling pathway, enhancing FoxO1 protein stability, promoting its nuclear distribution, and increasing its transcriptional activity. The phosphorylation of FoxO1 at S273 attenuates insulin-induced FoxO1 degradation in cells and leads to glucose intolerance in mice [82, 89]. These results indicate that FoxO1 is a key mediator that connects insulin and glucagon signaling in control of glucose homeostasis. FoxO1 activation impairs mitochondrial function through regulating heme homeostasis, thereby mediating insulin resistance-induced mitochondrial dysfunction [8, 88]. Activation of heme oxygenase-1 (HO-1), a target of FoxO1, in the liver induces inflammation through the generation of ferrous iron [42], suggesting that FoxO1→HO-1 signaling pathway potentially mediates insulin resistance-induced ferrous iron overload and metabolic inflammation. Cardiac IRS1 and IRS2 deletion-induced insulin resistance leads to heart failure and death in male mice. Cardiac FoxO1 ablation rescues the cardiac insulin resistance-induced heart failure [60, 62]. FoxO1 regulates hepatic angiotensinogen gene expression and controls serum angiotensinogen and angiotensin II levels, thereby modulating blood pressure in mice [61]. In addition, FoxO1 is a major target of estrogen in the regulation of glucose homeostasis and insulin resistance-induced heart failure [86, 87], which contributes to the sexual dimorphism in diabetes and cardiovascular diseases. Taken together, these studies suggest that FoxO1 is a key player in insulin resistance-induced hyperglycemia, metabolic inflammation, mitochondrial dysfunction, heart failure, and hypertension. Therefore, FoxO1 is a potential therapeutic target for the treatment of insulin resistance-induced metabolic and chronic diseases. Indeed,

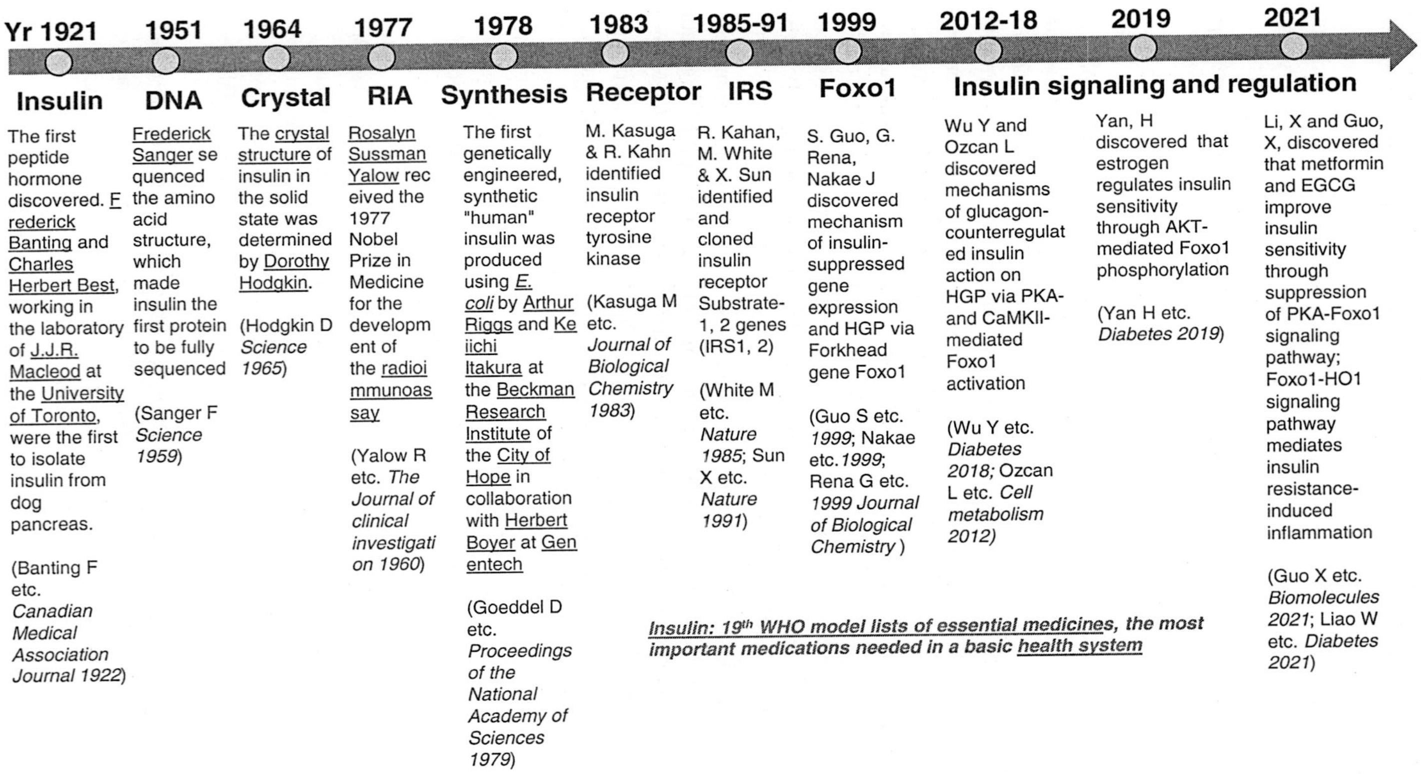

Yr 1921	1951	1964	1977	1978	1983	1985-91	1999	2012-18	2019	2021
Insulin	**DNA**	**Crystal**	**RIA**	**Synthesis**	**Receptor**	**IRS**	**Foxo1**	**Insulin signaling and regulation**		
The first peptide hormone discovered. Frederick Banting and Charles Herbert Best, working in the laboratory of J.J.R. Macleod at the University of Toronto, were the first to isolate insulin from dog pancreas. (Banting F etc. *Canadian Medical Association Journal 1922*)	Frederick Sanger sequenced the amino acid structure, which made insulin the first protein to be fully sequenced (Sanger F *Science 1959*)	The crystal structure of insulin in the solid state was determined by Dorothy Hodgkin. (Hodgkin D *Science 1965*)	Rosalyn Sussman Yalow received the 1977 Nobel Prize in Medicine for the development of the radioimmunoassay (Yalow R etc. *The Journal of clinical investigation 1960*)	The first genetically engineered, synthetic "human" insulin was produced using *E. coli* by Arthur Riggs and Keiichi Itakura at the Beckman Research Institute of the City of Hope in collaboration with Herbert Boyer at Genentech (Goeddel D etc. *Proceedings of the National Academy of Sciences 1979*)	M. Kasuga & R. Kahn identified insulin receptor tyrosine kinase (Kasuga M etc. *Journal of Biological Chemistry 1983*)	R. Kahan, M. White & X. Sun identified and cloned insulin receptor Substrate-1, 2 genes (IRS1, 2) (White M etc. *Nature 1985*; Sun X etc. *Nature 1991*)	S. Guo, G. Rena, Nakae J discovered mechanism of insulin-suppressed gene expression and HGP via Forkhead gene Foxo1 (Guo S etc. *Nature 1999*; Nakae J etc. *1999*; Rena G etc. *1999 Journal of Biological Chemistry*)	Wu Y and Ozcan L discovered mechanisms of glucagon-counterregulated insulin action on HGP via PKA- and CaMKII-mediated Foxo1 activation (Wu Y etc. *Diabetes 2018*; Ozcan L etc. *Cell metabolism 2012*)	Yan, H discovered that estrogen regulates insulin sensitivity through AKT-mediated Foxo1 phosphorylation (Yan H etc. *Diabetes 2019*)	Li, X and Guo, X, discovered that metformin and EGCG improve insulin sensitivity through suppression of PKA-Foxo1 signaling pathway; Foxo1-HO1 signaling pathway mediates insulin resistance-induced inflammation (Guo X etc. *Biomolecules 2021*; Liao W etc. *Diabetes 2021*)

Insulin: 19th WHO model lists of essential medicines, the most important medications needed in a basic health system

Fig. 1 **Milestones of insulin discovery and insulin signaling studies.** The discovery of insulin and its application to the treatment of diabetes have resulted in a breakthrough in the history of medicine. The insulin signal transduction studies have provided several potential therapeutic strategies for the treatment of diabetes. *RIA* radioimmunoassay, *HGP* hepatic glucose production, *FoxO1* forkhead/winged helix transcription factor O-class member 1, *PKA* protein kinase A, *AKT* protein kinase B, *HO-1* heme oxygenase 1, *EGCG* epigallocatechin-3-gallate, *CaMKII* Ca^{2+}/calmodulin-dependent protein kinase II

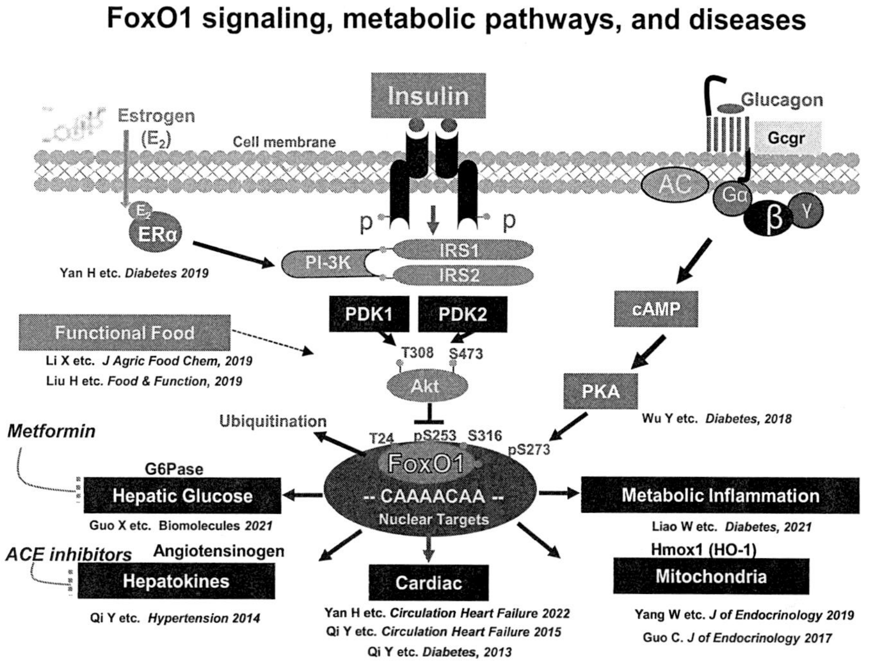

FoxO1 signaling, metabolic pathways, and diseases

Fig. 2 **FoxO1 acts as a key metabolic regulator in hormonal signaling, metformin, and bioactive functional food in physiology and disease.** Insulin and estrogen inhibit FoxO1 activity through PI3K→AKT signaling pathway-stimulated FoxO1 phosphorylation at T24, S253, and S316, whereas glucagon increases FoxO1 activity through cAMP→PKA signaling pathway-stimulated FoxO1 phosphorylation at S273, thereby controlling glucose homeostasis, metabolic inflammation, mitochondrial function, cardiac function, and hypertension. Abbreviations: *IRS* insulin receptor substrate, *PI3K* phosphatidylinositol 3-kinase, *PDK* phosphoinositide-dependent protein kinase, *AKT* protein kinase B, *FoxO1* forkhead/winged helix transcription factor O-class member 1, *Gcgr* glucagon receptor, *AC* adenylyl cyclase, *cAMP* cyclic adenosine monophosphate, *PKA* protein kinase A, *HO-1* heme oxygenase 1, *G6Pase* glucose-6-phosphatase, *Pck1* phosphoenolpyruvate carboxykinase 1, *ER* estrogen receptor

metformin, a first-line drug for the treatment of T2DM, and epigallocatechin gallate (EGCG), a polyphenol from green tea, both suppress FoxO1 activity through inhibition of cAMP/PKA-stimulated FoxO1 phosphorylation at S273, contributing to the improvement of hyperglycemia [33, 41] (Fig. 2).

Contribution of Sex Hormones to Insulin Resistance

Sex Difference in Insulin Resistance and Diabetes Mellitus

Diabetes mellitus is an expanding global health problem, with around 415 million people having diabetes and an estimated 193 million people with undiagnosed diabetes worldwide. T2DM that is characterized by relative insulin deficiency and insulin resistance in metabolic organs accounts for more than 90% of diabetic patients [15]. Sex has an important effect on the pathogenesis of T2DM. It has been shown that diabetes is more prevalent in young men than in young women. The analysis of data from 751 population-based studies shows that from 1980 to 2014, age-standardized adult diabetes prevalence increased in men (from 4.3% to 9.0%) compared to that in women (5.0–7.9%) [92]. Consistently, the data from the National Health and Nutrition Examination Survey (NHANES) show that the prevalence of diabetes mellitus is lower in women as compared to men, from 2013 to 2016 (11% vs. 13%) [56]. International Diabetes Federation (IDF) reports that the worldwide prevalence of diabetes is lower in women (8.4%, 18–99 years) than that in men (8.9%) in 2017. It is estimated that around 12.3 million more men (231.7 million) than women (219.3 million) live with diabetes. It is noteworthy that there is a delay in peak of the diabetes prevalence in women (men: peak at 65–69-year-old versus women: peak at 70–79-year-old) [9]. In studies of systemic screening procedures for diabetes, men have a higher diabetes prevalence when the diagnosis is based on fasting plasma glucose (FPG) and hemoglobin A1c (HbA1c) parameters. However, when diagnosis of diabetes is based on 2 h plasma glucose after an OGTT (2 h PG-OGTT), male predominance in diabetes is not observed. Studies from 9 European countries with 7680 men and 9251 women (30–89 years old) show that the prevalence of undiagnosed diabetes and impaired fasting glycemia is higher in men than that in women based on isolated fasting hyperglycemia, whereas the prevalence of impaired glucose tolerance is higher in women [30]. In the Inter99 study with 13,016 inhabitants living in Copenhagen County, the proportion of men diabetic individuals aged 60 years is higher than that in women (63% vs. 52%). The prevalence of IFG in men is higher than that in women. However, impaired glucose tolerance is more frequent in young women than that in young men [26]. The differences in 2 h PG after an OGTT may be due to challenging both men and women with similar amount of glucose, without considering the sex differences in body size, muscle mass, and physical fitness. Instead, sex differences in FPG and HbA1c may reflect the physiology.

Estrogen Regulates Blood Glucose and Sexual Dimorphism in Insulin Resistance

Sex differences are attributed to the role of sex chromosomes, the organizational role of testosterone in the perinatal period, and the activation role of sex hormones at puberty. The main contributors of sexual dimorphisms in diabetes and insulin resistance are sex hormone-mediated stimulatory effect, including androgens and estrogens. In this chapter, we will focus on the effect of estrogen on sexual dimorphism in insulin resistance and its associated diseases.

In healthy premenopausal women, there are three endogenous estrogens, including estrone (E1), 17β-estradiol (E2), and estriol (E3). In the circulation, 17β-estradiol (E2) is the predominant estrogen; in ovaries, it is converted from E1 that is aromatized from androstenedione. During normal menstrual cycles, E2 acts as an endocrine hormone to regulate distant target organs. However, E2 does not function as an endocrine hormone in postmenopausal women and men; instead, the major source of E2 originates from several extragonadal sites, including brain, breast, muscle, bone, and adipose tissue, where E2 functions as a paracrine or intracrine factor. Therefore, circulating E2 is not the main determinant for estrogen signaling in postmenopausal women and men; in contrast, E2 biosynthesized in the extragonadal tissues is the major driver for estrogen function. In the extragonadal tissues, aromatase catalyzes the estrogen biosynthesis from androgens (it catalyzes androstenedione to estrone and testosterone to estradiol). Estrogen sulfotransferase (EST) conjugates a sulfonate group to estrogens, preventing its binding to estrogen receptors and enhancing urinary excretion. Therefore, cellular action of estrogens is regulated by: (i) estrogen receptor signaling and sensitivity; (ii) activity of aromatase or other key enzymes involved in biosynthesis of estrogen from androgenic precursors; and (iii) activity of estrogen sulfotransferases that inhibits estrogenic action through sulfonate group conjugation.

Although sex differences in diabetes are observed in young women, the prevalence of diabetes becomes comparable in men and women during postmenopause when circulated estrogen level declines. Hormone replacement therapy (HRT) provides evidence that estrogen is important in the low risk of diabetes incidence in young women. Clinical studies conducted in postmenopausal women show that postmenopausal estrogen replacement therapy significantly improves insulin resistance and glucose tolerance. Meta-analysis of 107 clinical trials about HRT in postmenopausal women shows that HRT reduces homeostatic model assessment for insulin resistance (HOMA-IR) by 12.9% and abdominal fat by 6.8% in women without diabetes; HRT reduces fasting glucose by 11.5% and HOMA-IR by

35.8% in women with diabetes [70]. Further evidence in human shows that mutations in aromatase genes dramatically decrease estrogen release as well as result in physiological dysregulation and insulin resistance indicated by hyperinsulinemia in both sexes [12, 49]. Consistently, in mouse models, the females show better insulin sensitivity and glucose tolerance than that in the males under both regular and high-fat diet feeding. The protective effect in females on diet-induced obesity and insulin resistance is diminished by bilateral ovariectomy and restored by estrogen supplementation [65, 75]. Global knockout of aromatase or ERα in female mice triggers obesity, insulin resistance, and glucose intolerance [36, 38]. Thus, sex hormone estrogen plays an important role in the regulation of insulin sensitivity in both humans and mice.

Molecular Mechanisms of Estrogen-Estrogen Receptor (ER) Signaling

More than 60 years ago, it was concluded that the biological effects of estrogen were mediated by receptor proteins based on its binding specificity in the uterus. During the past several decades, genetically engineered mouse models for estrogen receptors (ERs) have provided solid evidence that ERs mediate the effect of estrogen on metabolic diseases. There are two main forms of ERs, ERα and ERβ. ERα was cloned by both Pierre Chambon and John Shine groups in 1986 [28, 29]. After 10 years, ERβ was cloned from the rat prostate and ovary by Gustafsson group [39]. ERα and ERβ, as the nuclear receptors of steroid/thyroid hormone superfamily, consist of NH_2-terminal domain (NTD or A/B), DNA-binding domain (DBD or C), and ligand-binding domain (LBD or E).

The NTD of ERs encompasses a ligand-independent activation function 1 (AF1) domain that mediates protein-protein interactions and transcription activation of the downstream target genes. The AF1 in ERα shows high activity in stimulating transcriptional activation of the reporter gene from the estrogen response element

(ERE) reporter plasmid. However, the activity of AF1 in ERβ is negligible. There is only 16% similarity in AF1 domain between ERα and ERβ, which may explain the significant differences in AF1-mediated transcriptional activity. The DBDs in ERα and ERβ are highly conserved, with 97% amino acid identity. There is a two-zinc finger structure in DBD, which has an effect on receptor dimerization and binding to specific DNA elements. Therefore, ERα and ERβ are expected to show similar specificity and affinity to bind to different EREs. The "D" domain nearby DBD is known as a hinge region that acts as a flexible region to connect DBD and LBD; it includes a nuclear localization signal that is unmasked when ligand binds to receptors. The COOH-terminal domain that contains LBD is responsible for ligand binding, receptor dimerization, and transactivation of the target genes. The LBD contains an activation function 2 (AF2) domain whose function is regulated by the ligand binding. The LBDs in ERα and ERβ show a high homology in both their primary amino acids and tertiary architecture, which may also explain that ERα and ERβ have similar ERE-mediated transcriptional activation potencies. The "F" domain that follows LBD contains 42 amino acids; this domain is involved in modulating transactivation, protein-protein interaction, and receptor dimerization.

Estrogen, as a steroid hormone, enters the cell membrane and regulates biological process through binding to ERα and ERβ. There are two molecular mechanisms of E2-ERs signaling cascades: genomic action and non-genomic action. In genomic action, estrogen or other related ligand binding induces a conformational change of ERs and then dissociation from their chaperones heat-shock proteins. As a result, the ERs complexes translocate into the cell nucleus and bind either directly to an ERE in the promoter regions of target genes or indirectly to specificity protein 1 (SP-1), activator protein 1 (AP-1), or activating transcription factor 2 (ATF-2) response elements through protein tethering to DNA, thereby regulating target gene expression. The classical genomic action of E2-ERs mainly mediates the reproductive function and normally occurs within hours, resulting in activation or repression of target genes. In non-genomic action, estrogen triggers rapid signaling within seconds or minutes through cytosolic and membrane-associated ERs. The extranuclear and membrane-associated ERs congregate with other signaling molecules, thereby initiating rapid intracellular signaling transduction and regulating gene expression. Upon estrogen binding, ERs interact or crosstalk with G protein coupled receptors (GPCRs), cellular membrane ion channels, and protein kinase signaling pathways (such as MPAKs, tyrosine kinases, and PI3K) to mediate the non-genomic action. In addition to traditional estrogen receptors, ERα and ERβ, abundant evidence shows that G protein-coupled estrogen receptor (GPER) is involved in metabolic regulation, immune responses, nervous system, cardiovascular physiology, and reproduction. GPER responds to E2 in a non-genomic manner through activating multiple downstream signaling pathways, including MAPK, PI3K, PKC, calcium mobilization, and adenylyl cyclase. However, the function of GPER on energy metabolism is controversial. Therefore, we mainly discuss the roles of ERα and ERβ in the regulation of insulin resistance and glucose homeostasis.

Crosstalk Between Insulin and E2-ER Signaling

Both ERα and ERβ play an important role in the regulation of cancer development and reproduction. The evidence from transgenic mice shows that ERα, but not ERβ, mediates the effect of estrogen on glucose homeostasis and insulin sensitivity. In diet-induced obesity mouse model, global ERα deficiency leads to significant increases in body weight, insulin resistance, and glucose intolerance [36]. Although global ERβ deletion mice have a significant increase in body weight under high-fat diet feeding, global ERβ deletion improves insulin sensitivity and glucose tolerance in diet-induced obesity mouse model [20]. Therefore, ERα is the major estrogen receptor that mediates the beneficial effect of estrogen

on insulin sensitivity and glucose homeostasis. The Levine lab showed that genetic rescue of non-genomic ERα signaling normalizes ERα deficiency-induced insulin resistance, glucose intolerance, and obesity [54], suggesting that the non-genomic action of E2-ERα signaling predominantly mediates the beneficial effects of estrogen on energy metabolism and glucose homeostasis. Mauvais-Jarvis' lab reported that nuclear ERα, but not membrane ERα, predominantly controls insulin sensitivity and glucose homeostasis in female mice [1]. Taken together, nuclear ERα-mediated non-genomic action of estrogen potentially plays a key role in the regulation of energy metabolism and insulin sensitivity.

In type 2 diabetes, insulin fails to suppress glucose production but reserves the ability to regulate lipid metabolism in peripheral tissues, which is called "selective insulin resistance." Insulin-regulated glucose homeostasis is mainly mediated by Insulin receptor (IR)→Insulin receptor substrate 1/2 (IRS1/2) → Phosphoinositide 3-kinase (PI3K) →Protein kinase B (AKT) →FoxO1 signaling pathway [31]. The non-genomic mechanism of E2-ERα signaling is mediated through the interaction of ERα with associated kinases and receptors. Therefore, the interaction of ERα with molecules in insulin signaling likely contributes to positive effect of E2-ERα signaling on insulin sensitivity. In COS7 and L6 cells, E2 stimulates the binding of ERα to insulin-like-growth factor 1 receptor (IGF-1R) to activate IGF-1R signaling cascade. It is also reported that ERs interact with IGF-1R to regulate neuronal survival and neuroprotection in brain [6]. IGF-1R, as a class II receptor tyrosine kinase, belongs to the insulin receptor family, exerting an important role in cell growth and differentiation. IGF-1R and IR are closely associated with a high structure identity. Although there is no direct evidence that ERα interacts with IR, it is plausible that E2 induces the interaction between ERα and IR systems, thereby involving insulin signaling activity. Future studies are needed to determine whether E2-ERα signaling affects the tyrosine kinase activity of IR. In breast cancer cells, ERα interacts with IRS1/2 and increases their protein abundance through inhibiting ubiquitination independent of E2 [48]. Therefore, IRS proteins may be one of the key nodes that connect ERα and insulin signaling. However, E2 improves hyperglycemia and suppresses gluconeogenesis in the liver IRS1 and IRS2 double gene knockout mice [86], which indicates that E2-ERα signaling can control the insulin action partially in an IRS1/2-independent manner. E2 promotes the binding of ERα to p85α and stimulates PI3K activity, thereby increasing downstream AKT activity [73]. ERα also interacts with FoxO1 through the forkhead domain and carboxyl terminus of FoxO1 in a ligand-dependent manner, thereby attenuating FoxO1 transactivation ability [72] (Fig. 3). The direct interaction of ERα with PI3K and FoxO1 may contribute to the fact that E2-ERα signaling bypasses IRS1 and 2 to enhance insulin action. ERα tightly interacts with insulin signaling molecules such as IR, IRS, PI3K, and FoxO1, forming an ERα-insulin signaling complex system and

mediating signal transduction in control of glucose homeostasis and beyond. In addition, ER-α-insulin signaling complex system may intervene the spatial distances among proteins and then increase kinase-substrate availability, contributing to insulin sensitivity.

Nuclear ERα overexpression rescues ERα deletion-induced insulin resistance in female mice [1], suggesting that ERα-regulated nuclear insulin signaling contributes to the improvement of insulin sensitivity. Insulin-mediated AKT activation stimulates FoxO1 phosphorylation at T24, S253, and S316, thereby promoting FoxO1 nuclear exclusion and inhibiting its transcriptional activity. Therefore, nuclear insulin signaling plays an important role in the regulation of glucose homeostasis through control of nuclear FoxO1 distribution. Moreover, IR can internalize and translocate to the nucleus, interacting with DNA through co-regulator host cell factor-1 (HCF-1) and associated transcription factors [35]. IRS1

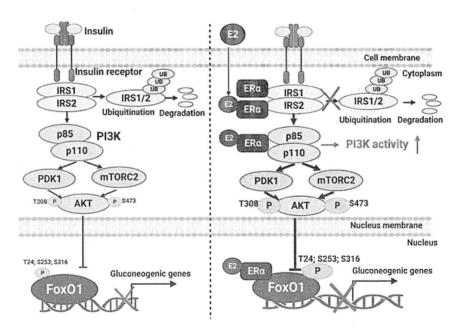

Fig. 3 Crosstalk between estrogen and insulin signaling. Activated estrogen receptor α (ERα) by 17β-estradiol (E2) or unoccupied ER interacts with insulin receptor substrate (IRS) 1 and 2, increasing IRS1 and IRS2 protein abundance through inhibition of their ubiquitination. E2 stimulates the binding of ERα to p85, increasing the activity of phosphatidylinositol 3-kinase (PI3K). The increased IRS proteins levels and PI3K activity enhance activation of

protein kinase B (AKT), thereby stimulating FoxO1 phosphorylation (T24, S253, and S316) and inhibiting its activity. E2 also stimulates the interaction between ERα and FoxO1, attenuating its transactivation ability. Abbreviation: *PDK1* 3-phosphoinositide-dependent kinase 1, *mTORC2* mammalian target of rapamycin complex-2, *UB* ubiquitination, *P* phosphorylation. This diagram is created using BioRender

shows nuclear distribution and activates the promoters of cell cycle genes through binding to their DNA regions in cancer cell lines. The p110β catalytic isoform of PI3K has been found in the nucleus and it may control cell cycle S-phase progression. AKT also shows nuclear distribution, which may be due to native localization or translocation from cytosol. Thus, nuclear IR and IRS1 regulate cell cycle-related genes expression by directly binding to the corresponding promoter regions. We expect that nuclear insulin signaling machinery, including IR, IRS, PI3K, and AKT, controls glucose homeostasis through regulating the activity of nuclear FoxO1. In our unpublished data (W Yang and S Guo), ERα deletion attenuates nuclear insulin sensitivity, suggesting that nuclear ERα increases insulin sensitivity potentially through interaction with nuclear insulin signaling components. However, it is unknown whether ERα is capable of acting as a chaperon protein to interact with insulin signaling molecules and mediate their nuclear translocation.

E2-ERs Signaling in Control of Insulin Resistance and Energy Expenditure

The pathophysiological development of T2DM is characterized by insulin resistance and β-cell dysfunction which progressively impairs glucose homeostasis. T2DM is a multifactorial disease caused by both genetic and environmental factors. Insulin resistance and hyperglycemia during T2DM involve dysfunction of multiple organs, including brain, adipose tissue, liver, skeletal muscle, pancreas, and immune system. The activation of E2-ERs signaling in these organs or systems contributes to the improvement of insulin resistance and uncontrolled glycemia.

E2-ERs Signaling Controls Energy Homeostasis in the Brain

The natural menopause accompanied by a decline in circulating estrogens in women is associated with increased abdominal fat accumulation, reduced energy expenditure, and decreased physical activity. In animal models, ovariectomy increases body weight and food intake, promotes abdominal fat accumulation, and decreases energy expenditure, which is rescued by E2 administration. ERα deficiency leads to increases in body weight and adiposity and decreases in energy expenditure [37]; these data suggest that ERα plays a key role in mediating the effect of estrogen on energy metabolism. The hypothalamus is an important area in the central nervous system (CNS) that regulates the homeostasis of food intake, energy expenditure, and body weight. It is composed of different hypothalamic nuclei, including the arcuate nucleus (ARC), the paraventricular nucleus (PVN), the lateral hypothalamic area (LHA), the dorsomedial nucleus (DMN), and the ventromedial nucleus (VMN). Lesion of specific hypothalamic nuclei induces dramatic dysregulation of energy homeostasis. In rodent brain, ERα is dominantly expressed in the ventrolateral region of VMN, ARC, the medial preoptic area, and PVN. Although ERβ shows a similar expression pattern to ERα in rodent brain, its expression level is significantly lower than ERα. Therefore, ERα is the major isoform of estrogen receptor to mediate the effect of E2 on energy homeostasis.

Loss of ERα in CNS results in increases in body weight, adiposity, as well as decreases in energy expenditure and physical activity in both male and female mice [84]. POMC neurons in ARC modulate food intake, energy expenditure, and reproduction. E2 administration robustly increases the number of excitatory inputs into POMC neurons [24]. ERα deficiency in POMC neurons in females significantly increases food intake but has no direct effect on energy expenditure and fat distribution [84]. The ERα→PI3K signaling cascade in POMC neurons mediates the action of estrogen on suppression of food intake and improvement of insulin sensitivity. The hypothalamic VMN plays an important role in the regulation of energy expenditure and glucose homeostasis. Lesions of the VMN increase food intake and decrease energy expenditure, which contributes to obesity. Steroidogenic factor 1 (SF1) deletion-induced VMN dysfunction induces obesity in mice. Estrogen can directly regulate the electrophysiological properties of VMN neurons, suggesting VMN is one of the targets by estrogen in control of energy homeostasis. ERα deficiency in VMN SF1 neurons increases body weight and adiposity, decreases energy expenditure, and attenuates brown adipose tissue (BAT) thermogenesis in female mice, without affecting food intake. 5-hydroxytryptamine expressed in dorsal raphe nucleus (DRN) neurons mediates the stimulatory action of ERα in VMN ventrolateral subdivision on energy expenditure. ERα expressing neurons in the ventrolateral subdivision of VMH also sense glucose fluctuations and maintain euglycemia in female mice. Activation of E2-ERα signaling in the nucleus of solitary tract (NTS) of brainstem, preoptic anterior hypothalamus (POAH), or serotonin neurons in DRN decreases food intake in female rodents. ERα is highly expressed in the medial amygdala (MeA). E2-ERα signaling activates MeA neurons to stimulate physical activity and prevent body weight gain. Therefore, brain E2-ERα signaling plays an important role in regulation of glucose and energy homeostasis.

E2-ERs Signaling Improves Insulin Sensitivity in the Liver

The liver is an important metabolic organ and controls body energy metabolism. Hepatic insulin resistance induced by loss of hepatic IR or IRS1/2 genes in mice results in systemic insulin resistance. Therefore, hepatic insulin signaling plays a dominant role in the pathogenesis of systemic insulin resistance and hyperglycemia. E2 replacement suppresses endogenous glucose production (EGP) in both male and ovariectomized female mice, and E2 treatment stimulates insulin signaling in primary hepatocytes [86]. These data suggest that estrogen can directly target the liver to suppress gluconeogenesis and increase hepatic insulin sensitivity. ERα, but not ERβ, is the predominant estrogen receptor expressed in the liver. The euglycemic-hyperinsulinemic clamp in global ERα but not ERβ knockout mice showed that the insulin-induced suppression of EGP is significantly attenuated [5], indicating that global

ERα deletion mediates hepatic insulin resistance. ERα agonist PPT dramatically increases insulin sensitivity and suppresses glucose production in primary hepatocytes. ERα gain-of-function in liver cancer cell line enhances insulin sensitivity [86]. Thus, liver E2-ERα signaling activation enhances hepatic insulin sensitivity to suppress hepatic glucose production. It has been reported that hepatic ERα deletion increases hepatic gluconeogenic activity in mice. ERα-mediated transcription of gluconeogenic genes by directly binding to their promoter regions may contribute to the effect of ERα on hepatic gluconeogenesis [63]. However, it is reported that non-genomic action of E2-ERα signaling plays a key role in the regulation of glucose homeostasis and insulin resistance [54]. These data suggest that ERα regulates hepatic gluconeogenic activity mainly through enhancing insulin sensitivity. Previous studies provided evidence that ERα interacts with key components of the insulin signaling pathway, thereby potentially enhancing hepatic insulin sensitivity [48]. ERα action can be stimulated in the absence of estrogen or other ERα agonists. ERα prevents IRS1/2 from ubiquitin-mediated degradation through direct binding independent of E2 [48], suggesting that IRS1/2 protein abundance is regulated by ERα in a ligand-independent manner. E2 or ERα agonist PPT activates insulin signaling in primary mouse hepatocytes, which is potentially independent of IRS1 and 2 [86]. E2 treatment increases ERα-associated PI3K activity, subsequently stimulating downstream AKT activation [73]. These results indicate that ERα also enhances insulin signaling through direct activation of PI3K in a ligand-dependent manner. Thus, we propose two potential mechanisms by which ERα regulates hepatic insulin sensitivity: (i) ligand-independent effect: ERα-increased IRS1 and 2 protein abundance and (ii) ligand-dependent effect: ERα-associated PI3K activation.

In addition to enhancing hepatic insulin sensitivity directly, hepatic ERα improves liver lipid homeostasis, thereby contributing to insulin sensitivity indirectly. Ablation of ERα increases hepatic triglyceride accumulation and ERα gain-of-function ameliorates hepatosteatosis in diet-induced obesity female mice [78]. Liver ERα controls hepatic cholesterol balance through regulation of expression of genes responsible for cholesterol transport, lipoprotein remodeling, and cholesterol uptake in female mice [16, 93]. Taken together, these data suggest that liver ERα activation prevents ectopic liver lipid accumulation, thereby protecting against hepatic insulin resistance. It seems that the effect of E2-ERα signaling on hepatic lipid is mediated by both genomic and non-genomic action. Genome-wide identification of ERα binding elements in the mouse liver reveals that ERα binding sites are mainly clustered into the promoter regions of genes responsible for lipid metabolism [23]; this result indicates that genomic action of E2-ERα signaling plays a key role in regulating hepatic lipid metabolism. Indeed, activation of E2-ERα signaling increases *small heterodimer partner* (*SHP*) gene expression through directly binding to its promoter region, thereby suppressing SREBP-1c activity and decreasing liver triglyceride [78]. However, it also has been reported that ERα interacts with liver X receptor α (LXRα) to regulate hepatic lipid metabolism [16]. Therefore, it is possible that E2-ERα signaling controls hepatic lipid metabolism through both genomic and non-genomic action. Future studies are warranted to distinguish which mechanism plays a dominant role in regulation of hepatic lipid metabolism.

E2-ERs Signaling in Adipose Tissue

Adipose tissue controls whole-body energy and glucose homeostasis through energy storage and endocrine function. Excessive accumulation of visceral fat is highly associated with incidence of metabolic diseases, such as T2DM, hyperlipidemia, and hypertension. Subcutaneous adipose tissue shows enhanced ability to expand and store excessive caloric intake. It has been believed that visceral fat is more deleterious, whereas subcutaneous adipose tissue is protective from development of obesity and T2DM. In support of this, transplantation of subcutaneous fat to visceral cavity but not visceral fat to subcutaneous

compartment reduces adiposity and improves glucose homeostasis [21, 77]. Therefore, the fat distribution plays an important role in the development of metabolic syndromes, such as hyperglycemia and insulin resistance.

It is well known that there is a sexual dimorphism of body fat. Compared to men, young women tend to have more subcutaneous fat and less visceral fat. However, postmenopausal women have a significant increase in visceral fat, shifting to a phenotype of fat distribution similar to that in men, which is prevented by estrogen replacement therapy. In rodents, ovariectomy increases body weight, promotes visceral fat accumulation, and results in insulin resistance, which is normalized by E2 replacement. These results suggest that estrogen signaling plays a key role in regulating fat distribution. Adipose tissue expresses both ERα and ERβ. Global ERα deletion leads to insulin resistance and increases adiposity in both male and female mice, with a significant accumulation of visceral fat [37]. Clinical evidence showed that a man with disruptive mutation in ERα has obesity, glucose intolerance, and hyperinsulinemia. The adipose tissue-specific ERα knockout mice provide direct evidence of the effect of ERα on adipose tissue function. Adipose tissue ERα deletion results in enlarged adipocytes as well as increased adipose tissue inflammation and fibrosis in both males and females. Glucose tolerance and insulin sensitivity are largely impaired in the adipose tissue ERα knockout male mice. Body weight gain is largely increased in the adipose tissue ERα knockout female mice [13]. These results suggest that E2-ERα plays an important role in the regulation of adipose tissue function and fat distribution. In contrast to ERα, ERβ deletion has no significant effect on visceral fat deposition in male mice under regular diet [53]. In diet-induced obesity mouse model, ERβ deletion decreases liver triglyceride level, improves insulin resistance, and increases adiposity; this result suggests that ERβ exerts a pro-diabetic function. However, selective ERβ agonist reduces adiposity and improves glucose tolerance [90]. Although these results suggest that ERβ activation improves fat accumulation, more direct evidence of the effect of ERβ on adipose tissue function from adipose tissue-specific ERβ knockout mouse model should be warranted.

Estrogen decreases lipogenesis in adipose tissue through downregulation of lipogenic gene expression in mice, which partially contributes to reduced adiposity by estrogen treatment [76]. In postmenopausal women, estrogen replacement also significantly decreases lipogenic gene expression in abdominal adipose tissue [47]. It has been shown that ERα mediates the suppressive effect of estrogen on lipogenic gene expression through direct binding to the promoter regions of lipogenic genes, such as *fatty acid synthase* (*Fasn*) and *acetyl-CoA carboxylase 1* (*ACC1*) [63]. On the other hand, E2-ERα signaling regulates mRNA expression of lipogenic genes through controlling the activity of transcriptional factor SREBP1-c [78]. In addition, ERβ selective agonist significantly decreases expression of lipogenic genes in the adipose tissue of ovariectomized female rats [79]. These results demonstrate that both ERα and ERβ mediate the anti-lipogenic effect of estrogen in adipose tissue. Estrogen has disparate effects on lipolysis in adipose tissue. A previous study showed that E2-ERα signaling attenuates lipolysis through upregulating anti-lipolytic α2A-adrenergic receptor expression in subcutaneous fat but not in visceral fat tissues [55]. Greenberg's lab reported that estrogen decreases lipolysis at basal level and enhances lipolysis upon epinephrine stimulation in visceral fat tissue-derived adipocytes [76]. It has been convincingly shown that estrogen suppresses the activity of lipoprotein lipase (LPL) in both human and mouse adipose tissues. Therefore, estrogen may regulate lipid homeostasis by maintaining the equilibrium between lipogenesis and lipolysis in adipose tissue. Adipocyte-specific knockout of ERα leads to increases in inflammation and fibrosis in the adipose tissue [13]. Although the molecular mechanism remains unknown, these results suggest that E2-ERα signaling may control secretum of adipocytes, such as adipokines, thereby regulating inflammation status of immune cells in adipose tissue. Adipocyte ERα deficiency-induced inflammation potentially impairs adipocyte insulin sensitivity, which decreases glucose uptake and induces lipid metabolism dysregulation in adipose tissue. Taken together, E2-ERα signaling plays an important role in regulation of healthy adipogenesis.

E2-ERs Signaling Regulates Insulin-Induced Glucose Uptake in the Skeletal Muscle

Skeletal muscle accounts for 75% of glucose uptake in response to insulin. In skeletal muscle, glucose transporter 1 (GLUT1) is responsible for basal glucose transport and GLUT4 mediates insulin-induced glucose uptake. Activation of insulin signaling stimulates translocation of GLUT4 from cytosol to the cellular membrane, facilitating the transportation of glucose into the cell. In type 2 diabetic patients, insulin-stimulated glucose transport in skeletal muscle is severely impaired.

E2 action modulates insulin sensitivity in skeletal muscle. In rat soleus, E2 stimulates phosphorylation of AKT, AMP-activated protein kinase (AMPK), and TBC1 domain family member 1 (TBC1D1). In diet-induced obesity mice, E2 administration significantly increases IRS1 protein level as well as insulin-induced AKT and AMPKα phosphorylation in skeletal muscle. During aging, chronic E2 treatment increases plasma membrane GLUT4 localization in the skeletal muscle from OVX female rats. These results suggest that E2, to some extent, increases insulin sensitivity and promotes glucose uptake through mobilizing GLUT4 membrane translocation in skeletal muscle. Both ERα and ERβ show expression in skeletal muscle. Global ERα knockout mice show hyperglycemia, insulin resistance, and decreased GLUT4 expression in skeletal muscle [4]. ERα deficiency induces significant skeletal muscle insulin resistance and attenuates insulin-mediated glucose uptake in skeletal muscle [5, 67]. The studies with the selective estrogen receptor modulators show that ERα selective agonist increases membrane GLUT4 localization and silencing of ERα decreases membrane GLUT4 abundance in L6 myoblast [22]. In OVX rats, administration of ERα selective agonist increases insulin-stimulated glucose uptake and GLUT4 expression level in skeletal muscle [27]. In muscle-specific ERα knockout mice, insulin-stimulated glucose disposal is significantly reduced but GLUT4 expression level is not changed in skeletal muscle [66]. ERα-increased glucose uptake in skeletal muscle is mainly mediated through promoting insulin-induced GLUT4 membrane localization. Global ERβ knockout has no significant effect on insulin sensitivity but increases skeletal muscle GLUT4 level [4]. Administration of ERβ selective agonist in OVX rats has no significant effect on insulin-induced glucose uptake in skeletal muscle. These results indicate that ERα plays a dominant role in regulation of insulin sensitivity and glucose disposal in skeletal muscle.

Healthy young women are protected against acute lipid-induced insulin resistance as compared to men, which might be explained by the fact that women rely more on fatty acid oxidation as a fuel source. E2 supplementation enhances lipid oxidation in men in vivo and stimulates palmitate oxidation in myotubes ex vivo. These results indicate that E2 plays a role in controlling lipid oxidation in skeletal muscle. In human skeletal muscle, E2 treatment significantly increases expression of lipid oxidation-related genes, including *peroxisome proliferator-activated receptors α/γ (PPAR α/γ)*, *carnitine palmitoyltransferase 1 (CPT 1)*, and *fatty acid-binding protein c (FABPc)*, which contributes to E2-induced lipid oxidation. In global ERα knockout mice, skeletal muscle shows accumulation of lipid intermediates and inflammation, which is accompanied by a decreased *PPARα* expression. AMPK regulates cellular energy homeostasis through activation of glucose and fatty acid uptake and oxidation. It has been shown that E2 activates AMPK in both skeletal muscle tissue and C2C12 myotubes. Impaired AMPK activation is also observed in skeletal muscle from global ERα knockout mice. Further evidence showed that E2-induced AMPK activation is mediated through direct interaction between AMPK βγ-binding domain and ERα but not ERβ [44]. In muscle-specific ERα knockout mice, lipid oxidation in skeletal muscle is significantly impaired; however, AMPK activity and *PPARα* expression level are not affected

[66]. The impaired mitochondrial function in skeletal muscle may be attributed to the diminished lipid oxidation in muscle-specific ERα knockout mice. ERα knockdown reduces oxygen consumption rate in C2C12 myotube. The activity of respiratory complex 1 in skeletal muscle is significantly decreased in muscle-specific ERα knockout mice. Taken together, E2-ERα signaling stimulates lipid oxidation and improves lipid accumulation in skeletal muscle, thereby increasing muscle insulin sensitivity. Of note is that the cardiac muscle deficient for IRS1/2 gene results in myocardial mitochondrial dysfunction and death of mice in males rather than females, underscoring that estrogen or the female-derived hormone plays critical roles in cardiac protection from dilated diabetic cardiomyopathy or loss of insulin sensitivity in the heart of mice [60, 87].

E2-ERs Signaling Preserves β-Cell Function in the Pancreas

It is well-documented that E2 promotes insulin release in pancreas. Glucose-stimulated insulin release is significantly reduced in the islets isolated from OVX mice, which is normalized in the OVX mice treated with E2. E2 regulates both insulin biosynthesis and insulin secretion, thereby stimulating glucose-induced insulin release. ERα selective agonist increases insulin content in β-cells of islets, whereas ERβ selective agonist has no significant effect on insulin content [2]. Pancreas-specific ERα knockout abolishes E2-induced insulin synthesis, which is mediated by the non-genomic action of E2-ERα signaling. ERα interacts with tyrosine kinase Src, activates extracellular signal-regulated kinase$_{1/2}$ (ERK), and increases NeuroD1 nuclear localization, thereby promoting NeuroD1 binding to the insulin promoter region and increasing insulin transcription [81]. E2 controls insulin secretion through regulating ATP-sensitive potassium (K_{ATP}) channels in β-cells. Closure of K_{ATP} channels depolarizes β-cell membrane and induces insulin release. The acute inhibitory effect of E2 on K_{ATP} channels is reduced in β-cells from global ERβ but not ERα knockout mice. Activation of ERβ by its selective agonist enhances glucose-induced Ca^{2+} signaling and insulin release [74]. Global ERβ knockout leads to a delayed first-phase insulin release upon glucose stimulation in pancreas [4], suggesting ERβ deletion impairs insulin release. The suppressive effect of ERβ on K_{ATP} channels is mediated by atrial natriuretic peptide receptor in β-cells [74]. Thus, ERα is responsible for the action of E2 on insulin biosynthesis and E2-mediated insulin secretion depends on ERβ in β-cells; these effects of E2 are mainly mediated by its non-genomic action.

Pancreatic β-cells are protected by E2 against oxidative stress, lipotoxicity, and apoptosis. E2 suppresses fatty acid and glycerolipid synthesis in pancreatic islets and protects against β-cell failure in type 2 diabetic mouse models. This anti-lipogenic effect of E2 is recapitulated by pharmacological activation of either ERα or ERβ in β-cells. E2-ERs signaling-mediated anti-lipogenic effect in pancreas majorly depends on the non-genomic action. It has been reported that chronic activation of LXR leads to lipotoxicity-induced β-cell failure [10]. E2-ERs signaling activates phosphorylation of signal transducer and activator of transcription 3 (STAT3) through SRC, which downregulates expression of *LXRβ*, a key regulator of lipogenesis, and expression of its downstream targets, such as *SREBP1c* and *carbohydrate response element-binding protein (ChREBP)*. E2-ERs signaling-mediated suppression of LXR expression in pancreas may contribute to the prevention of islet lipotoxicity and β-cell failure. Activation of E2-ERs signaling stimulates AMPK activity, thereby suppressing S*REBP1c* expression. Therefore, E2-ERs signaling inhibits the activity of SREBP1c and ChREBP through AMPK and STAT3-mediated non-genomic action, thereby reducing fatty acid synthesis and lipid accumulation in pancreatic islets. Pancreatic β-cell failure is a key feature in both type 1 and 2 diabetes mellitus. E2 protects β-cells against apoptosis in diabetic condition and promotes β-cell survival. In E2-deficient mouse model (global aromatase knockout), the β-cell is vulnerable to develop apoptosis when exposed to streptozotocin, which is rescued by E2 supplementation. ERα deficiency diminishes the

protective effect of E2 against apoptosis in the pancreatic islets [40]. By knocking in a mutated ERα, it was discovered that E2-ERα signaling protects against apoptosis in islets through a non-genomic action. ERβ deletion mildly predisposes islets to apoptosis upon streptozotocin treatment [46]. Thus, ERα mediates the beneficial effect of E2 on prevention of β-cell apoptosis in islets, preserving β-cell function and protecting against diabetes.

E2-ERs Signaling Regulates Metabolic Inflammation

Metabolic inflammation is a low-grade inflammatory state induced by metabolic surplus and a feature of obesity-related metabolic diseases, which is highly associated with insulin resistance and T2DM. Metabolic inflammation can be initiated by several events, such as increased free fatty acids (FFA) released from adipose tissue and elevated lipopolysaccharides (LPS) from gut microbiome. E2 regulates immune responses and inflammatory processes during metabolic stress. Postmenopausal women show increasing trend of proinflammatory cytokines in circulation, such as IL-6, IL-1, and TNFα. In OVX female mice, expression of proinflammatory markers is significantly increased in the adipose tissue; this result suggests that immune cell infiltration and initiation of inflammation in the adipose tissue are enhanced by ovary removal [69]. The previous in vitro studies in the immune cells show that E2 can directly target immune cells to regulate inflammatory processes. In human peripheral blood mononuclear cells (PBMCs), E2 inhibits LPS-induced TNF secretion in both male and female subjects. In human promonocytic and monocytic cells, E2 attenuates LPS-stimulated TNF, IL-1β, and IL-6 secretion, which is potentially mediated through regulation of CD16 cross-linking. In mouse splenic or bone marrow-derived macrophages, E2 pretreatment inhibits LPS-induced TNF release through modulating NF-κB binding activity. E2 also decreases TNF, IFNγ, and IL-12 production in mature dendritic cells. It is noteworthy that the effect of E2 on

LPS-induced proinflammatory cytokines secretion depends on the concentration of E2. High level of E2 at pregnancy level tends to exert a suppressive role in LPS stimulation, whereas relatively low concentration of E2 enhances LPS stimulation. In the brain of chronic inflammatory experimental autoimmune encephalomyelitis (EAE) mouse model, E2 administration markedly decreases the recruitment of total inflammatory cells as well as TNFα$^+$ macrophage and T cells into the central nervous system. This protective effect of E2 on EAE was abolished in ERα knockout but not ERβ knockout mice [45, 58]. In hepatic fibrosis rodent models, E2 treatment significantly improves liver fibrosis and inflammation [83]. In the ovariectomized mouse liver, proinflammatory cytokine IL-1β treatment induces around 75 genes expression. Ethinyl estradiol pretreatment reduces expression of one third of genes induced by cytokine IL-1β, which is dependent of ERα but not ERβ [18].

Macrophages are critical in both innate and adaptive immunity. Adipose tissue from obese subjects shows a significant increase in macrophage population. Macrophages are major sources of inflammatory mediators that are associated with insulin resistance during obesity development. Mature immune cells in murine lymphoid organs show ERα expression but limited ERβ expression. Murine lymphocytes, including B-cells, T-cells, and natural killer (NK) cells express ERα. ERβ is reported to be expressed in B-cells and NK-cells. Bone marrow-derived and peritoneal macrophages show expression of ERα but not ERβ. Therefore, ERα predominantly mediates the effect of E2 on immune responses in macrophage. The significance of macrophage ERα in metabolic disorders is revealed in hematopoietic or myeloid-specific ERα knockout mice from Hevener group [68]. Hematopoietic or myeloid-specific ERα deletion decreases plasma adipokines, increases plasma cytokine levels, impairs glucose tolerance, induces insulin resistance, and increases adipose tissue mass in female mice. In isolated macrophages, ERα is required by repression of inflammation, maintenance of oxidative metabolism, IL-4-induced alternative activation, and LPS-mediated phagocytic capacity. Coculture of ERα-deficient macrophage with

C2C12 myotubes or 3T3L1 adipocytes shows that insulin sensitivity is impaired in both myotubes and adipocytes. These results indicate that ERα may regulate secretum of macrophages, thereby controlling insulin sensitivity in metabolic tissues. However, the underlying mechanisms by which E2-ERα signaling regulates macrophage features need to be further investigated in the future.

Estrogen Therapy for Insulin Resistance and Diabetes

Estrogen Replacement Therapy

During estrogen replacement therapy, the type of estrogen and route of administration affect clinical outcomes. There are two steroidal formulations: natural and synthetic. The naturally occurring estrogens are several different forms of steroidal components that are recovered from animal sources, such as conjugated equine estrogens (CEE). All natural estrogen products are composed of several chemically different estrogens. The synthetic steroidal estrogens show similar structure with the natural estrogens. Synthetic estrogens can be either a single entity estrogen, such as estrace, or a combination of chemically different estrogens, such as cenestin. They have a high binding affinity to estrogen receptor and stimulate estrogenic action. The combination of either naturally derived estrogens or synthetic derivatives is used in hormone replacement therapy (HRT). There are two major delivery methods of estrogen, oral and transdermal delivery. Compared to oral administration, transdermal delivery avoids first entry to liver metabolism, which maintains serum estrogen at a stable level without supraphysiological estrogen exposure to liver. A meta-analysis study compared the effects of oral delivery-based and transdermal delivery-based hormone replacement therapies on metabolic syndrome in postmenopausal women [70]. They found that in postmenopausal women without diabetes, both oral and transdermal estrogens improve insulin resistance, reduce abdominal fat, and decrease new-onset diabetes. In postmenopausal women with diabetes, both oral and transdermal estrogens reduce fasting glucose, improve insulin resistance, decrease low-density/high-density lipoprotein ratio, and decrease blood pressure. Although oral delivery shows larger beneficial effects than transdermal delivery, oral delivery leads to a significant increase in C-reactive protein level and decrease in protein S [70]. A previous short-term study shows that oral estrogen may worsen insulin resistance and adipocytokine parameters, increasing cardiovascular risk. However, transdermal estrogen has minimal effects on insulin resistance and increases adiponectin level [11]. The better effect of oral estrogen HRT on insulin resistance and lipid profile may be due to better bioavailability of estrogen to liver. Oral estrogen HRT potentially induces inflammation and decreases coagulation inhibitor protein S [70], which could increase cardiovascular risk. These results suggest that transdermal estrogen delivery could be a preferable strategy for HRT.

Selective Estrogen Receptor Modulators (SERMs)

SERMs are nonsteroidal drugs that act as ERs agonist or antagonist in a tissue-dependent manner. There are several SERMs in clinical practice, including tamoxifen, raloxifene, toremifene, bazedoxifene, lasofoxifene, ospemifene, and fulvestrant. Tamoxifen acts as an ERα antagonist in breast but acts as an ERα agonist in bone. Therefore, tamoxifen is used to treat breast cancer and prevents osteoporosis. However, tamoxifen treatment increases the risk of fatty liver incidence. The exact mechanism by which tamoxifen leads to fatty liver is not clear. Raloxifene acts as ER agonist in bone and is approved by FDA to treat postmenopausal osteoporosis. Raloxifene reversed OVX-induced increases in food intake, body weight, and fat mass content; this result suggests that raloxifene potentially targets hypothalamus and adipose tissue to control metabolic homeostasis. In insulin-secreting INS-1 cells, raloxifene acts as an ER agonist to suppress triglyceride accumulation. In osteoporotic postmenopausal women, 3-year raloxifene treatment significantly decreases total cholesterol, low-density lipoprotein cholesterol, and

fibrinogen, without affecting glycemic control [3]. These data suggest that raloxifene mainly regulates lipid homeostasis potentially through targeting hypothalamus and adipose tissue. Bazedoxifene is a third-generation SERM for the treatment of postmenopausal osteoporosis. Although bazedoxifene has no significant effect on glucose metabolism in Japanese postmenopausal women with type 2 diabetes, bazedoxifene reduces the incidence and severity of streptozotocin-induced type 1 diabetes. It is also reported that bazedoxifene protects from diet-induced obesity and type 2 diabetes in OVX mice. However, further studies are warranted to confirm the effect of bazedoxifene on metabolic syndrome.

Phytoestrogens and Dietary Interventions

Phytoestrogens are botanical products with natural sterols that bind to estrogen receptors. Their binding affinity to estrogen receptors is lower than E2. However, emerging evidence from preclinical models suggests that phytoestrogens have antidiabetic function through both estrogen-dependent and estrogen-independent pathways. There are three groups of phytoestrogens: (1) isoflavones (soy, lentils, and other legumes); (2) ligans (flaxseed and other seed oils); and (3) coumestans (red clover, sunflower seeds, and bean sprouts). A previous study shows that dietary soy supplement prevents obesity and increases insulin sensitivity partially through activation of AMPK in the adipose tissue from mice [7]. Considering traditional HRT increases risk of breast cancer, diet-derived phytoestrogens would be a promising strategy to treat metabolic diseases.

Other Considerations

Insulin Clearance and Insulin Resistance

In addition to insulin secretion from pancreatic β-cells, insulin clearance plays an important role in regulating the homeostatic level of insulin that initiates normal insulin signaling pathway. Liver is the major site where endogenously released insulin is removed. Hepatic insulin clearance is triggered by the activation of IR upon insulin exposure. Carcinoembryonic antigen-related cell adhesion molecule 1 (CEACAM1) is a key player in the regulation of receptor-mediated insulin endocytosis and degradation in the liver [14, 25, 59]. Insulin-induced activation of tyrosine kinase of IR stimulates its autophosphorylation at tyrosine 1316 (Y1316), resulting in the phosphorylation of CEACAM1 at Y488. Phosphorylated CEACAM1 (Y488) interacts with Shc that binds to IR. Thus, Shc mediates the formation of a complex between IR and CEACAM1, thereby CEACAM1 promotes IR-mediated insulin endocytosis and degradation processes [51]. Both global and liver-specific Ceacam1 knockout mice display chronic hyperinsulinemia and hepatic insulin resistance [14, 25]. These results indicate that impaired insulin clearance causes progressive insulin resistance potentially through development of chronic hyperinsulinemia. The data from clinical studies show that reduced hepatic insulin clearance is associated with increased incidence of T2DM. The down-regulation of hepatic CEACAM1 potentially contributes to the impaired hepatic insulin clearance in obese humans. It has been shown that women display higher insulin clearance than that in men. Estrogen replacement significantly increases insulin clearance in postmenopausal women. These results suggest that E2-ERs signaling may regulate insulin clearance, thereby controlling insulin sensitivity. However, the underlying mechanism needs to be further investigated.

Androgen and Insulin Resistance

Androgens, the male sex hormones, also play a pivotal role in regulating insulin resistance and energy homeostasis. In males, low testosterone is associated with insulin resistance. On one hand, aromatization of testosterone into estrogen mediates the beneficial effect of androgens on insulin sensitivity. On the other hand, androgen receptor (AR) mediates the antidiabetic properties of testosterone. AR deletion in male mice leads to late-onset obesity, hepatic steatosis, and decrease in insulin secretion in β-cells, which contributes to insulin resistance [19, 43, 52, 85]. In females, hyperandrogenism predisposes to T2DM, whereas AR deficiency has no significant effect on energy metabolism [71]. Polycystic ovary syndrome (PCOS), a common endocrine disorder in women, is characterized by hyperandrogenism. Women with PCOS are at high risk of developing insulin resistance. Hyperandrogenism leads to skeletal muscle insulin resistance, visceral adiposity, and β-cell dysfunction in females. However, whether AR mediates the detrimental effects of hyperandrogenism on insulin sensitivity in females need to be further determined. Therefore, androgen deficiency in males and androgen excess in females lead to insulin resistance.

Conclusions

Estrogen improves insulin sensitivity and protects against development of T2DM, which contributes to sexual dimorphism in insulin resistance. Estrogen targets both CNS and peripheral tissues to regulate energy homeostasis. The estrogenic action in insulin sensitivity and energy metabolism is mainly mediated through ERα. Activation of E2-ERα signaling in hypothalamus decreases body weight and adiposity through suppression of food intake and induction of energy expenditure, thereby contributing to insulin sensitivity indirectly. In metabolic tissues, such as liver, skeletal muscle, and adipose tissue, activation of E2-ERα signaling increases local insulin sensitivity directly, contributing to the improvement of systemic insulin resistance. Macrophage E2-ERα signaling activation induces anti-inflammatory function, thereby attenuating chronic inflammation in obesity and improving insulin resistance. In the pancreas, E2-ERα signaling protects against β-cell failure through inhibition of lipotoxicity and apoptosis (Fig. 4). The protective role of E2-ERα signaling in insulin sensitivity is mediated mainly through non-genomic action. ERα interacts with IRS proteins and increases IRS protein abundance in a ligand-independent manner. ERα also stimulates PI3K activity in a

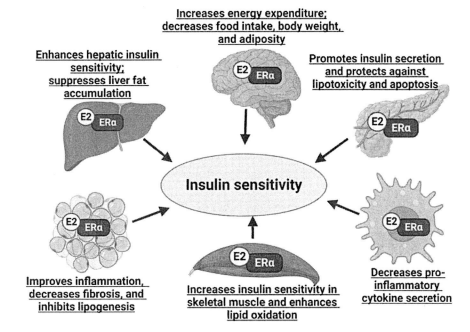

Fig. 4 **Activation of E2-estrogen receptor α (ERα) signaling in brain, liver, adipose tissue, skeletal muscle, pancreas, and macrophage regulates insulin sensitivity.** Hypothalamic E2-ERα signaling activation increases energy expenditure and decreases adiposity, contributing to insulin sensitivity. Activation of E2-ERα signaling in metabolic tissues including liver, skeletal muscle, and adipose tissue enhances local insulin sensitivity and improves lipid metabolism. Pancreatic E2-ERα signaling activation promotes insulin secretion and attenuates lipotoxicity as well as apoptosis in β-cells, maintaining the homeostatic level of insulin and regulating insulin sensitivity. In macrophage, E2-ERα signaling activation decreases its pro-inflammatory features, thereby improving insulin sensitivity. This diagram is created using BioRender

ligand-dependent manner, thereby triggering downstream AKT→FoxO1 signaling cascades. Targeting E2-ERα signaling could be a therapeutic strategy for the treatment of insulin resistance and T2DM.

References

1. Allard C, Morford JJ, Xu B, Salwen B, Xu W, Desmoulins L, Zsombok A, Kim JK, Levin ER, Mauvais-Jarvis F. Loss of nuclear and membrane estrogen receptor-α differentially impairs insulin secretion and action in male and female mice. Diabetes. 2019;68: 490–501.
2. Alonso-Magdalena P, Ropero AB, Carrera MP, Cederroth CR, Baquie M, Gauthier BR, Nef S, Stefani E, Nadal A. Pancreatic insulin content regulation by the estrogen receptor ERα. PloS One. 2008;3: e2069.
3. Barrett-Connor E, Ensrud KE, Harper K, Mason TM, Sashegyi A, Krueger KA, Anderson PW. Post hoc analysis of data from the Multiple Outcomes of Raloxifene Evaluation (MORE) trial on the effects of three years of raloxifene treatment on glycemic control and cardiovascular disease risk factors in women with and without type 2 diabetes. Clin Ther. 2003;25:919–30.
4. Barros RP, Gabbi C, Morani A, Warner M, Gustafsson J-A. Participation of ERα and ERβ in glucose homeostasis in skeletal muscle and white adipose tissue. Am J Physiol Endocrinol Metab. 2009;297:E124–33.
5. Bryzgalova G, Gao H, Ahrén B, Zierath J, Galuska D, Steiler T, Dahlman-Wright K, Nilsson S, Gustafsson J-Å, Efendic S. Evidence that oestrogen receptor-α plays an important role in the regulation of glucose homeostasis in mice: insulin sensitivity in the liver. Diabetologia. 2006;49:588–97.
6. Cardona-Gómez GP, Mendez P, Doncarlos LL, Azcoitia I, Garcia-Segura LM. Interactions of estrogens and insulin-like growth factor-I in the brain: implications for neuroprotection. Brain Res Rev. 2001;37:320–34.
7. Cederroth CR, Vinciguerra M, Gjinovci A, Kuhne F, Klein M, Cederroth M, Caille D, Suter M, Neumann D, James RW. Dietary phytoestrogens activate AMP-activated protein kinase with improvement in lipid and glucose metabolism. Diabetes. 2008;57: 1176–85.
8. Cheng Z, Guo S, Copps K, Dong X, Kollipara R, Rodgers JT, Depinho RA, Puigserver P, White

MF. Foxo1 integrates insulin signaling with mitochondrial function in the liver. Nat Med. 2009;15:1307–11.

9. Cho NH, Shaw J, Karuranga S, Huang Y, Da Rocha Fernandes J, Ohlrogge A, Malanda B. IDF Diabetes Atlas: Global estimates of diabetes prevalence for 2017 and projections for 2045. Diabetes Res Clin Pract. 2018;138:271–81.

10. Choe SS, Choi AH, Lee J-W, Kim KH, Chung J-J, Park J, Lee K-M, Park K-G, Lee I-K, Kim JB. Chronic activation of liver X receptor induces β-cell apoptosis through hyperactivation of lipogenesis: liver X receptor–mediated lipotoxicity in pancreatic β-cells. Diabetes. 2007;56:1534–43.

11. Chu MC, Cosper P, Nakhuda GS, Lobo RA. A comparison of oral and transdermal short-term estrogen therapy in postmenopausal women with metabolic syndrome. Fertil Steril. 2006;86:1669–75.

12. Conte FA, Grumbach MM, Ito Y, Fisher CR, Simpson ER. A syndrome of female pseudohermaphrodism, hypergonadotropic hypogonadism, and multicystic ovaries associated with missense mutations in the gene encoding aromatase (P450arom). J Clin Endocrinol Metab. 1994;78:1287–92.

13. Davis KE, Neinast MD, Sun K, Skiles WM, Bills JD, Zehr JA, Zeve D, Hahner LD, Cox DW, Gent LM. The sexually dimorphic role of adipose and adipocyte estrogen receptors in modulating adipose tissue expansion, inflammation, and fibrosis. Mol Metab. 2013;2:227–42.

14. Deangelis AM, Heinrich G, Dai T, Bowman TA, Patel PR, Lee SJ, Hong E-G, Jung DY, Assmann A, Kulkarni RN. Carcinoembryonic antigen-related cell adhesion molecule 1: a link between insulin and lipid metabolism. Diabetes. 2008;57:2296–303.

15. Defronzo RA, Ferrannini E, Groop L, Henry RR, Herman WH, Holst JJ, Hu FB, Kahn CR, Raz I, Shulman GI. Type 2 diabetes mellitus. Nat Rev Dis Primers. 2015;1:1–22.

16. Della Torre S, Mitro N, Fontana R, Gomaraschi M, Favari E, Recordati C, Lolli F, Quagliarini F, Meda C, Ohlsson C. An essential role for liver ERα in coupling hepatic metabolism to the reproductive cycle. Cell Rep. 2016;15:360–71.

17. Dong XC, Copps KD, Guo S, Li Y, Kollipara R, Depinho RA, White MF. Inactivation of hepatic Foxo1 by insulin signaling is required for adaptive nutrient homeostasis and endocrine growth regulation. Cell Metab. 2008;8:65–76.

18. Evans MJ, Lai K, Shaw LJ, Harnish DC, Chadwick CC. Estrogen receptor α inhibits IL-1β induction of gene expression in the mouse liver. Endocrinology. 2002;143:2559–70.

19. Fan W, Yanase T, Nomura M, Okabe T, Goto K, Sato T, Kawano H, Kato S, Nawata H. Androgen receptor null male mice develop late-onset obesity caused by decreased energy expenditure and lipolytic activity but show normal insulin sensitivity with high adiponectin secretion. Diabetes. 2005;54:1000–8.

20. Foryst-Ludwig A, Clemenz M, Hohmann S, Hartge M, Sprang C, Frost N, Krikov M, Bhanot S, Barros R, Morani A. Metabolic actions of estrogen receptor beta (ERβ) are mediated by a negative cross-talk with PPARγ. PLoS Genet. 2008;4:e1000108.

21. Foster MT, Softic S, Caldwell J, Kohli R, Dekloet AD, Seeley RJ. Subcutaneous adipose tissue transplantation in diet-induced obese mice attenuates metabolic dysregulation while removal exacerbates it. Phys Rep. 2013;1:e00015.

22. Galluzzo P, Rastelli C, Bulzomi P, Acconcia F, Pallottini V, Marino M. 17β-Estradiol regulates the first steps of skeletal muscle cell differentiation via ER-α-mediated signals. Am J Phys Cell Phys. 2009;297:C1249–62.

23. Gao H, Fält S, Sandelin A, Gustafsson J-A, Dahlman-Wright K. Genome-wide identification of estrogen receptor α-binding sites in mouse liver. Mol Endocrinol. 2008;22:10–22.

24. Gao Q, Mezei G, Nie Y, Rao Y, Choi CS, Bechmann I, Leranth C, Toran-Allerand D, Priest CA, Roberts JL. Anorectic estrogen mimics leptin's effect on the rewiring of melanocortin cells and Stat3 signaling in obese animals. Nat Med. 2007;13:89–94.

25. Ghadieh HE, Russo L, Muturi HT, Ghanem SS, Manaserh IH, Noh HL, Suk S, Kim JK, Hill JW, Najjar SM. Hyperinsulinemia drives hepatic insulin resistance in male mice with liver-specific Ceacam1 deletion independently of lipolysis. Metabolism. 2019;93:33–43.

26. Glumer C, Jørgensen T, Borch-Johnsen K. Prevalences of diabetes and impaired glucose regulation in a Danish population: the Inter99 study. Diabetes Care. 2003;26:2335–40.

27. Gorres BK, Bomhoff GL, Morris JK, Geiger PC. In vivo stimulation of oestrogen receptor α increases insulin-stimulated skeletal muscle glucose uptake. J Physiol. 2011;589:2041–54.

28. Green S, Walter P, Kumar V, Krust A, Bornert J-M, Argos P, Chambon P. Human oestrogen receptor cDNA: sequence, expression and homology to v-erb-A. Nature. 1986;320:134–9.

29. Greene GL, Gilna P, Waterfield M, Baker A, Hort Y, Shine J. Sequence and expression of human estrogen receptor complementary DNA. Science. 1986;231:1150–4.

30. Group DS. Age-and sex-specific prevalences of diabetes and impaired glucose regulation in 13 European cohorts. Diabetes Care. 2003;26:61–9.

31. Guo S. Insulin signaling, resistance, and the metabolic syndrome: insights from mouse models to disease mechanisms. J Endocrinol. 2014;220:T1.

32. Guo S, Rena G, Cichy S, He X, Cohen P, Unterman T. Phosphorylation of serine 256 by protein kinase B disrupts transactivation by FKHR and mediates effects of insulin on insulin-like growth factor-binding protein-1 promoter activity through a conserved insulin response sequence. J Biol Chem. 1999;274:17184–92.

33. Guo X, Li X, Yang W, Liao W, Shen JZ, Ai W, Pan Q, Sun Y, Zhang K, Zhang R. Metformin targets foxo1 to control glucose homeostasis. Biomolecules. 2021;11: 873.

34. Haeusler RA, Kaestner KH, Accili D. FoxOs function synergistically to promote glucose production. J Biol Chem. 2010;285:35245–8.

35. Hancock ML, Meyer RC, Mistry M, Khetani RS, Wagschal A, Shin T, Sui SJH, Näär AM, Flanagan JG. Insulin receptor associates with promoters genome-wide and regulates gene expression. Cell. 2019;177(722-736):e22.

36. Handgraaf S, Riant E, FaBRE A, Waget A, Burcelin R, Lière P, Krust A, Chambon P, Arnal J-F, Gourdy P. Prevention of obesity and insulin resistance by estrogens requires ERα activation function-2 (ERαAF-2), whereas ERαAF-1 is dispensable. Diabetes. 2013;62: 4098–108.

37. Heine P, Taylor J, Iwamoto G, Lubahn D, Cooke P. Increased adipose tissue in male and female estrogen receptor-α knockout mice. Proc Natl Acad Sci. 2000;97:12729–34.

38. Jones ME, Thorburn AW, Britt KL, Hewitt KN, Wreford NG, Proietto J, Oz OK, Leury BJ, Robertson KM, Yao S. Aromatase-deficient (ArKO) mice have a phenotype of increased adiposity. Proc Natl Acad Sci. 2000;97:12735–40.

39. Kuiper G, Enmark E, Pelto-Huikko M, Nilsson S, Gustafsson J. Cloning of a novel receptor expressed in rat prostate and ovary. Proc Natl Acad Sci. 1996;93: 5925–30.

40. Le May C, Chu K, Hu M, Ortega CS, Simpson ER, Korach KS, Tsai M-J, Mauvais-Jarvis F. Estrogens protect pancreatic β-cells from apoptosis and prevent insulin-deficient diabetes mellitus in mice. Proc Natl Acad Sci. 2006;103:9232–7.

41. Li X, Chen Y, Shen JZ, Pan Q, Yang W, Yan H, Liu H, Ai W, Liao W, Guo S. Epigallocatechin gallate inhibits hepatic glucose production in primary hepatocytes via downregulating PKA signaling pathways and transcriptional factor FoxO1. J Agric Food Chem. 2019;67:3651–61.

42. Liao W, Yang W, Shen Z, Ai W, Pan Q, Sun Y, Guo S. Heme oxygenase-1 regulates ferrous iron and foxo1 in control of hepatic gluconeogenesis. Diabetes. 2021;70:696–709.

43. Lin HY, Yu IC, Wang RS, Chen YT, Liu NC, Altuwaijri S, Hsu CL, Ma WL, Jokinen J, Sparks JD. Increased hepatic steatosis and insulin resistance in mice lacking hepatic androgen receptor. Hepatology. 2008;47:1924–35.

44. Lipovka Y, Chen H, Vagner J, Price TJ, Tsao T-S, Konhilas JP. Oestrogen receptors interact with the α-catalytic subunit of AMP-activated protein kinase. Biosci Rep. 2015;35:e00264.

45. Liu H-B, Loo KK, Palaszynski K, Ashouri J, Lubahn DB, Voskuhl RR. Estrogen receptor α mediates estrogen's immune protection in autoimmune disease. J Immunol. 2003;171:6936–40.

46. Liu S, Le May C, Wong WP, Ward RD, Clegg DJ, Marcelli M, Korach KS, Mauvais-Jarvis F. Importance of extranuclear estrogen receptor-α and membrane G protein–coupled estrogen receptor in pancreatic islet survival. Diabetes. 2009;58:2292–302.

47. Lundholm L, Zang H, Hirschberg AL, Gustafsson J-Å, Arner P, Dahlman-Wright K. Key lipogenic gene expression can be decreased by estrogen in human adipose tissue. Fertil Steril. 2008;90:44–8.

48. Morelli C, Garofalo C, Bartucci M, Surmacz E. Estrogen receptor-α regulates the degradation of insulin receptor substrates 1 and 2 in breast cancer cells. Oncogene. 2003;22:4007–16.

49. Morishima A, Grumbach MM, Simpson ER, Fisher C, Qin K. Aromatase deficiency in male and female siblings caused by a novel mutation and the physiological role of estrogens. J Clin Endocrinol Metab. 1995;80: 3689–98.

50. Nagao H, Jayavelu AK, Cai W, Pan H, Dreyfuss JM, Batista TM, Brandão BB, Mann M, Kahn CR. Unique ligand and kinase-independent roles of the insulin receptor in regulation of cell cycle, senescence and apoptosis. Nat Commun. 2023;14:57.

51. Najjar SM, Perdomo G. Hepatic insulin clearance: mechanism and physiology. Physiology. 2019;34: 198–215.

52. Navarro G, Allard C, Xu W, Mauvais-Jarvis F. The role of androgens in metabolism, obesity, and diabetes in males and females. Obesity. 2015;23:713–9.

53. Ohlsson C, Hellberg N, Parini P, Vidal O, Bohlooly M, Rudling M, Lindberg MK, Warner M, Angelin B, Gustafsson J-Å. Obesity and disturbed lipoprotein profile in estrogen receptor-α-deficient male mice. Biochem Biophys Res Commun. 2000;278:640–5.

54. Park CJ, Zhao Z, Glidewell-Kenney C, Lazic M, Chambon P, Krust A, Weiss J, Clegg DJ, Dunaif A, Jameson JL. Genetic rescue of nonclassical ERα signaling normalizes energy balance in obese Erα-null mutant mice. J Clin Invest. 2011;121:604–12.

55. Pedersen SB, Kristensen K, Hermann PA, Katzenellenbogen JA, Richelsen B. Estrogen controls lipolysis by up-regulating α2A-adrenergic receptors directly in human adipose tissue through the estrogen receptor α. Implications for the female fat distribution. J Clin Endocrinol Metab. 2004;89:1869–78.

56. Peters SA, Muntner P, Woodward M. Sex differences in the prevalence of, and trends in, cardiovascular risk factors, treatment, and control in the United States, 2001 to 2016. Circulation. 2019;139:1025–35.

57. Petersen MC, Shulman GI. Mechanisms of insulin action and insulin resistance. Physiol Rev. 2018;98: 2133–223.

58. Polanczyk M, Zamora A, Subramanian S, Matejuk A, Hess DL, Blankenhorn EP, Teuscher C, Vandenbark AA, Offner H. The protective effect of 17β-estradiol on experimental autoimmune encephalomyelitis is mediated through estrogen receptor-α. Am J Pathol. 2003;163:1599–605.

59. Poy MN, Yang Y, Rezaei K, Fernström MA, Lee AD, Kido Y, Erickson SK, Najjar SM. CEACAM1 regulates insulin clearance in liver. Nat Genet. 2002;30: 270–6.

60. Qi Y, Xu Z, Zhu Q, Thomas C, Kumar R, Feng H, Dostal DE, White MF, Baker KM, Guo S. Myocardial loss of IRS1 and IRS2 causes heart failure and is controlled by p38α MAPK during insulin resistance. Diabetes. 2013;62:3887–900.

61. Qi Y, Zhang K, Wu Y, Xu Z, Yong QC, Kumar R, Baker KM, Zhu Q, Chen S, Guo S. Novel mechanism of blood pressure regulation by Forkhead box class O1–Mediated transcriptional control of hepatic angiotensinogen. Hypertension. 2014;64:1131–40.

62. Qi Y, Zhu Q, Zhang K, Thomas C, Wu Y, Kumar R, Baker KM, Xu Z, Chen S, Guo S. Activation of Foxo1 by insulin resistance promotes cardiac dysfunction and β–myosin heavy chain gene expression. Circ Heart Fail. 2015;8:198–208.

63. Qiu S, Vazquez JT, Boulger E, Liu H, Xue P, Hussain MA, Wolfe A. Hepatic estrogen receptor α is critical for regulation of gluconeogenesis and lipid metabolism in males. Sci Rep. 2017;7:1–12.

64. Rena G, Guo S, Cichy SC, Unterman TG, Cohen P. Phosphorylation of the transcription factor forkhead family member FKHR by protein kinase B. J Biol Chem. 1999;274:17179–83.

65. Riant E, Waget A, Cogo H, Arnal J-F, Burcelin R, Gourdy P. Estrogens protect against high-fat diet-induced insulin resistance and glucose intolerance in mice. Endocrinology. 2009;150:2109–17.

66. Ribas V, Drew B, Soleymani T, Daraei P, Hevener A. Skeletal Muscle Specific ERα Deletion Is Causal for the Metabolic Syndrome. Endocr Rev. 2010a;31: S5.

67. Ribas V, Nguyen MA, Henstridge DC, Nguyen A-K, Beaven SW, Watt MJ, Hevener AL. Impaired oxidative metabolism and inflammation are associated with insulin resistance in ERα-deficient mice. Am J Physiol Endocrinol Metab. 2010b;298:E304–19.

68. Ribas V, Drew BG, Le JA, Soleymani T, Daraei P, Sitz D, Mohammad L, Henstridge DC, Febbraio MA, Hewitt SC. Myeloid-specific estrogen receptor α deficiency impairs metabolic homeostasis and accelerates atherosclerotic lesion development. Proc Natl Acad Sci. 2011;108:16457–62.

69. Rogers NH, Perfield JW, Strissel KJ, Obin MS, Greenberg AS. Reduced energy expenditure and increased inflammation are early events in the development of ovariectomy-induced obesity. Endocrinology. 2009;150:2161–8.

70. Salpeter S, Walsh J, Ormiston T, Greyber E, Buckley N, Salpeter E. Meta-analysis: effect of hormone-replacement therapy on components of the metabolic syndrome in postmenopausal women. Diabetes Obes Metab. 2006;8:538–54.

71. Sato T, Matsumoto T, Yamada T, Watanabe T, Kawano H, Kato S. Late onset of obesity in male

72. Schuur ER, Loktev AV, Sharma M, Sun Z, Roth RA, Weigel RJ. Ligand-dependent interaction of estrogen receptor-α with members of the forkhead transcription factor family. J Biol Chem. 2001;276:33554–60.

73. Simoncini T, Hafezi-Moghadam A, Brazil DP, Ley K, Chin WW, Liao JK. Interaction of oestrogen receptor with the regulatory subunit of phosphatidylinositol-3-OH kinase. Nature. 2000;407:538–41.

74. Soriano S, Ropero AB, Alonso-Magdalena P, Ripoll C, Quesada I, Gassner B, Kuhn M, Gustafsson J-A, Nadal A. Rapid regulation of KATP channel activity by 17-β-estradiol in pancreatic β-cells involves the estrogen receptor β and the atrial natriuretic peptide receptor. Mol Endocrinol. 2009;23:1973–82.

75. Stubbins RE, Holcomb VB, Hong J, Núñez NP. Estrogen modulates abdominal adiposity and protects female mice from obesity and impaired glucose tolerance. Eur J Nutr. 2012;51:861–70.

76. Tara M, Souza SC, Aronovitz M, Obin MS, Fried SK, Greenberg AS. Estrogen regulation of adiposity and fuel partitioning: evidence of genomic and non-genomic regulation of lipogenic and oxidative pathways. J Biol Chem. 2005;280:35983–91.

77. Tran TT, Yamamoto Y, Gesta S, Kahn CR. Beneficial effects of subcutaneous fat transplantation on metabolism. Cell Metab. 2008;7:410–20.

78. Wang X, Lu Y, Wang E, Zhang Z, Xiong X, Zhang H, Lu J, Zheng S, Yang J, Xia X. Hepatic estrogen receptor α improves hepatosteatosis through upregulation of small heterodimer partner. J Hepatol. 2015;63:183–90.

79. Weigt C, Hertrampf T, Kluxen FM, Flenker U, Hülsemann F, Fritzemeier KH, Diel P. Molecular effects of ER alpha-and beta-selective agonists on regulation of energy homeostasis in obese female Wistar rats. Mol Cell Endocrinol. 2013;377:147–58.

80. White MF, Kahn CR. Insulin action at a molecular level–100 years of progress. Mol Metab. 2021;52: 101304.

81. Wong WP, Tiano JP, Liu S, Hewitt SC, Le May C, Dalle S, Katzenellenbogen JA, Katzenellenbogen BS, Korach KS, Mauvais-Jarvis F. Extranuclear estrogen receptor-α stimulates NeuroD1 binding to the insulin promoter and favors insulin synthesis. Proc Natl Acad Sci. 2010;107:13057–62.

82. Wu Y, Pan Q, Yan H, Zhang K, Guo X, Xu Z, Yang W, Qi Y, Guo CA, Hornsby C. Novel mechanism of Foxo1 phosphorylation in glucagon signaling in control of glucose homeostasis. Diabetes. 2018;67:2167–82.

83. Xu J-W, Gong J, Chang X-M, Luo J-Y, Dong L, Hao Z-M, Jia A, Xu G-P. Estrogen reduces CCL4-induced liver fibrosis in rats. World J Gastroenterol. 2002;8: 883.

84. Xu Y, Nedungadi TP, Zhu L, Sobhani N, Irani BG, Davis KE, Zhang X, Zou F, Gent LM, Hahner LD. Distinct hypothalamic neurons mediate estrogenic effects on energy homeostasis and reproduction. Cell Metab. 2011;14:453–65.

androgen receptor-deficient (AR KO) mice. Biochem Biophys Res Commun. 2003;300:167–71.

85. Xu W, Niu T, Xu B, Navarro G, Schipma MJ, Mauvais-Jarvis F. Androgen receptor-deficient islet β-cells exhibit alteration in genetic markers of insulin secretion and inflammation. A transcriptome analysis in the male mouse. J Diabetes Complicat. 2017;31:787–95.

86. Yan H, Yang W, Zhou F, Li X, Pan Q, Shen Z, Han G, Newell-Fugate A, Tian Y, Majeti R. Estrogen improves insulin sensitivity and suppresses gluconeogenesis via the transcription factor Foxo1. Diabetes. 2019;68:291–304.

87. Yan H, Yang W, Zhou F, Pan Q, Allred K, Allred C, Sun Y, Threadgill D, Dostal D, Tong C. Estrogen protects cardiac function and energy metabolism in dilated cardiomyopathy induced by loss of cardiac IRS1 and IRS2. Circ Heart Fail. 2022;15:e008758.

88. Yang W, Yan H, Pan Q, Shen JZ, Zhou F, Wu C, Sun Y, Guo S. Glucagon regulates hepatic mitochondrial function and biogenesis through FOXO1. J Endocrinol. 2019;241:265–78.

89. Yang W, Liao W, Li X, Ai W, Pan Q, Shen Z, Jiang W, Guo S. Hepatic p38α MAPK controls gluconeogenesis

90. Yepuru M, Eswaraka J, Kearbey JD, Barrett CM, Raghow S, Veverka KA, Miller DD, Dalton JT, Narayanan R. Estrogen receptor-β-selective ligands alleviate high-fat diet-and ovariectomy-induced obesity in mice. J Biol Chem. 2010;285:31292–303.

91. Zhang K, Li L, Qi Y, Zhu X, Gan B, Depinho RA, Averitt T, Guo S. Hepatic suppression of Foxo1 and Foxo3 causes hypoglycemia and hyperlipidemia in mice. Endocrinology. 2012;153:631–46.

92. Zhou B, Lu Y, Hajifathalian K, Bentham J, Di Cesare M, Danaei G, Bixby H, Cowan MJ, Ali MK, Taddei C. Worldwide trends in diabetes since 1980: a pooled analysis of 751 population-based studies with 4· 4 million participants. Lancet. 2016;387:1513–30.

93. Zhu L, Shi J, Luu TN, Neuman JC, Trefts E, Yu S, Palmisano BT, Wasserman DH, Linton MF, Stafford JM. Hepatocyte estrogen receptor alpha mediates estrogen action to promote reverse cholesterol transport during Western-type diet feeding. Mol Metab. 2018;8:106–16.

via FOXO1 phosphorylation at S273 during glucagon signalling in mice. Diabetologia. 2023;66:1–18.

Linking Inflammation, Obesity, and Diabetes

23

Maeve A. McArdle, Elaine B. Kennedy, and Helen M. Roche

Contents

M. A. McArdle (✉) · E. B. Kennedy · H. M. Roche
University College Dublin, Dublin, Ireland
e-mail: maeve.mc-ardle@ucdconnect.ie;
elaine.kennedy.1@ucdconnect.ie; helen.roche@ucd.ie

Abstract

Overnutrition disrupts normal adipose tissue function. Dysfunctional lipid metabolism leads to an increase in circulating free fatty acids, initiating inflammatory signaling cascades and increased immune cell activity in metabolic tissue. A feedback loop of pro-inflammatory cytokines exacerbates this

© Springer Nature Switzerland AG 2023
R. S. Ahima (ed.), *Metabolic Syndrome*,
https://doi.org/10.1007/978-3-031-40116-9_29

chronic inflammatory state, driving further immune cell infiltration, cytokine secretion, and activation of inflammasome complexes. This disrupts the insulin signaling cascade and is causative of defects in hepatic and skeletal muscle glucose homeostasis, resulting in systemic insulin resistance and ultimately the development of type 2 diabetes. This chapter will focus on the initiation of the inflammatory response in obesity and describe the impact of this on metabolic tissue, with a particular emphasis on the development of insulin resistance and type 2 diabetes. We will also review current and prospective treatment and intervention strategies and the biological mechanisms through which these function.

Keywords

Inflammation · Insulin resistance · Adipose tissue · Macrophage · Inflammasome

Abbreviations

ADP	Adenosine diphosphate
AMP	Adenosine monophosphate
AMPK	AMP-activated protein kinase
ASC	Apoptosis-associated speck-like protein containing a CARD
ATM	Adipose tissue macrophages
ATP	Adenosine triphosphate
BAT	Brown adipose tissue
BMI	Body mass index
BMM	Bone marrow macrophages
CCR	C–C chemokine receptor
CLS	Crown-like structures
DAG	Diacylglycerols
DAMPs	Danger-associated molecular patterns
DC	Dendritic cell
DGAT	Diacylglycerol acyltransferase
DHA	Docosahexaenoic acid
DIO	Diet-induced obesity
ECM	Extracellular matrix
EPA	Eicosapentaenoic acid
FA	Fatty acids
FFA	Free fatty acids
Fiaf	Fasting-induced adipocyte factor
GLUT	Glucose transporter type

GPR	G protein-coupled receptor
HFD	High-fat diet
ICAM	Intercellular adhesion molecule
IKK	IκB kinase
IL	Interleukin
IR	Insulin resistance
IRS	Insulin receptor substrate
IS	Insulin sensitivity
IκB	Inhibitor of κB
JNK	c-Jun N-terminal kinase
LPS	Lipopolysaccharide
MAPK	Mitogen-activated protein kinase
MCP	Monocyte chemoattractant protein
MetS	Metabolic syndrome
MHC	Major histocompatibility complex
MUFA	Monounsaturated fatty acids
NF-κB	Nuclear factor kappa B
NLR	NOD-like receptor
PI3K	Phosphatidylinositol 3-kinase
PKB	Protein kinase B
PKC	Protein kinase C
PPAR	Peroxisome proliferator-activated receptor
PUFA	Polyunsaturated fatty acids
R	Receptor
RA	Receptor antagonist
SCFA	Short-chain fatty acid
SFA	Saturated fatty acids
SOCS	Suppressor of cytokine signaling
SVF	Stromal vascular fraction
T2D	Type 2 diabetes
TAG	Triacylglycerol
T_H	T helper
TLR	Toll-like receptor
TNF	Tumor necrosis factor
TNFR	Tumor necrosis factor receptor
Treg	Regulatory T cell
TZDs	Thiazolidinediones
UCP-1	Uncoupling protein 1
WAT	White adipose tissue

Introduction

Metabolic syndrome (MetS) is a health condition that encompasses a number of factors including obesity and high blood glucose concentrations, which both are risk factors for the development of type 2 diabetes (T2D). It is projected that >420 million people will have prediabetes worldwide by 2030 [146], with 5–10% of prediabetic individuals progressing to develop T2D annually [129]. As prevalence figures continue on this upward trajectory, examination of the pathophysiological determinants underlying this condition is required.

The obese state is linked to the development of insulin resistance (IR), through the induction of an inflammatory response in insulin-sensing organs. Obesity-associated inflammation is described as being chronic, in that it fails to be resolved. A number of events can initiate this state of chronic inflammation, and these act synergistically to maintain an inflammatory environment. Such an inflammatory response can result from increased cell exposure to free fatty acids (FFA) which initiate inflammatory signaling, a shift in the cell population types present in metabolic tissues and changes in the gut microbiome (Fig. 1).

The immune system is necessary in promoting and resolving inflammation. This paradigm is also true for obesity-associated inflammation. Immune cells, including macrophages and T cells, infiltrate metabolic tissue during the development of obesity. These immune cells secrete chemokines and cytokines. Chemokines function to attract additional immune cells into metabolic tissues. With obesity, there is increased production of the pro-inflammatory cytokines, tumor necrosis factor (TNF)-α (alpha), interleukin (IL)-6 and IL-1β (beta). These cytokines induce inflammatory signaling pathways in neighboring inflammatory and metabolic cells and impede insulin signaling. Insulin is a critical hormone that regulates glucose, lipid, and energy metabolism, in the liver, adipose tissue, and skeletal muscle. With IR, glucose is not taken up by metabolic tissues, circulating glucose levels increase, and this is an early indicator of T2D.

This chapter will focus on the link between obesity and inflammation. We will explore early

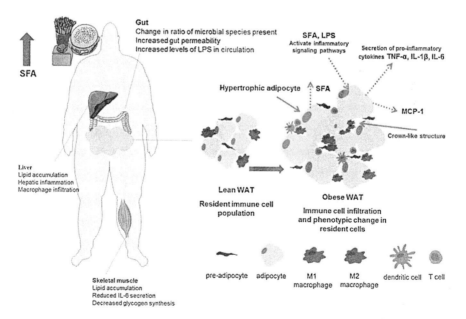

Fig. 1 Obesity – the impact on metabolic tissues and the gut. Excessive caloric intake has a negative impact on metabolic tissue. Increased exposure of metabolic cell types to circulating fatty acids results in lipid accumulation, the influx of immune cells, and a phenotypic switch in resident immune cell populations (M2 to M1 macrophages). Saturated fatty acids and LPS derived from the gut activate inflammatory pathways in metabolic tissue.

This results in the production of pro-inflammatory cytokines (TNF-α (alpha), IL-1β (beta), IL-6); these signal within the tissue to sustain an inflammatory environment and promote the infiltration of immune cells. The release of FFA from adipocytes that have reached their expansion capacity further stimulates inflammatory signaling and thus chronic inflammation propagates

events that initiate this process, from expanding adipocytes and increased levels of FFA to the deleterious impact of an altered gut microbiome. We examine how these factors alter metabolic tissue composition, cytokine secretion, insulin signaling, and glucose uptake. Finally, this chapter will highlight both nutritional and pharmacological strategies to counteract obesity-induced inflammation, IR, and T2D.

Metabolic Tissues

Multiple pathogenic factors have been implicated in the development of "metaflammation," a term coined to describe the synergy between metabolic and inflammatory pathways [49]. These pathways interact within the context of obesity, IR, and T2D, resulting in the deleterious effect of obesity at a systemic level [86].

Adipose Tissue

There are different subtypes of adipose tissue: white adipose tissue (WAT), brown adipose tissue (BAT), and the recently identified beige adipose tissue. White adipose tissue is responsible for the storage of excess energy as triacylglycerol (TAG). These fatty acids (FA) can be oxidized by BAT and released as heat; however, the decreased BAT levels associated with obesity cause dysregulation in this response [117]. Overproduction of WAT-derived TNF-α (alpha) has become a hallmark of obesity-induced IR and is associated with impaired insulin signaling [62]. Chronic low-grade inflammation in WAT is characterized by increased inflammatory macrophage and T cell number [130]. Conversely, lower levels of WAT-derived adiponectin are associated with IR [150] and are inversely related to ectopic lipid accumulation [119]. Interestingly, despite WAT inflammation having unfavorable effects on IR, Asterholm et al. demonstrate that pro-inflammatory signaling is necessary for WAT functionality [145]. If

adipocytes fail to expand, then excess FA may end up being deposited in other cell types. Inflammation is also important for proper extracellular matrix (ECM) remodeling which facilitates adipogenesis [32]. Both processes are likely mechanisms through which inflammation promotes WAT functionality [145].

Brown adipose tissue represents a small fat depot located in the neck and upper chest of adults [132], and it has been associated with a protective effect against metabolic diseases such as T2D [27]. The protective effect of BAT has been attributed to the presence of uncoupling protein 1 (UPC-1) which is involved in the conversion of energy from food into heat [19]. Beige adipocytes express a distinct gene expression profile that distinguishes them from WAT and BAT. In the basal state, beige cells resemble WAT, demonstrating low levels of UCP-1; however, upon stimulation with cyclic adenosine monophosphate (AMP), UCP-1 levels increase, and these adipocytes demonstrate a BAT-like phenotype [148]. It is suggested that BAT depots in adults may be composed of beige adipocytes. Beige and brown adipocytes exert a similar beneficial effect in terms of metabolic regulation [57], and manipulation of these may open new opportunities for promoting metabolic health.

Liver

Hepatic steatosis refers to the accumulation of lipid in the liver; it is associated with obesity-induced inflammation and is a hallmark of nonalcoholic fatty liver disease [5]. Accumulation of FA metabolites such as diacylglycerols (DAG), FFA, ceramides, and acylcarnitines, within insulin-sensitive tissues is one mechanism through which obesity causes IR [119]. Hepatic FA accumulation activates protein kinase C (PKC)-δ (delta); this interferes with insulin signaling by blocking insulin receptor substrate (IRS)-associated phosphatidylinositol (PI) 3-kinase activity [76]. Similar to WAT, hepatic macrophage number increases with obesity [101]. Excess lipid derivatives in the liver induce endoplasmic reticulum stress and hepatic inflammation, evident by increased secretion of pro-inflammatory cytokines, acute-phase reactants, and activation of nuclear factor kappa B (NF-κ (kappa) B) and c-Jun N-terminal kinase (JNK)-mediated pathways [15, 134]. Specific deletion of *Ikbkb* from hepatocytes, the gene that encodes IKKβ (beta), showed an important role for this gene in the development of HFD-induced IR. Obese HFD-fed hepatic *Ikbkb$^{-/-}$* mice maintained hepatic insulin sensitivity (IS) but developed IR in muscle and WAT, with no overall improvement peripheral IS [6]. In contrast, myeloid-specific deletion of *Ikbkb* improved systemic IS.

Skeletal Muscle

Skeletal muscle is the main site for glucose uptake in the body, and muscle IR represents a core defect in T2D [34]. Numerous defective mechanisms contribute to IR in skeletal muscle. These include impaired glycogen synthesis [124] and glucose transport [2], elevated IL-6 [126] and FFA levels [115], with reduced AMP-activated protein kinase (AMPK) activity [150]. Skeletal muscle dysregulation plays a critical role in the development of IR, and glycogen synthesis is reduced by up to 50% in T2D [124]. Defects in glucose transport are also critical in the development of skeletal muscle IR [116]. Lower glucose-6-phosphate levels in diabetic individuals link defective glucose transport and decreased glycogen synthesis in skeletal muscle [116].

Lipotoxicity with obesity is associated with the development of skeletal muscle IR. Myocyte lipid accumulation as FFA, fatty acyl-coenzyme A (CoA), DAG, and ceramides is a mechanism which potentiates skeletal muscle IR [1]. The pleiotropic cytokine IL-6 is considered a myokine; levels of IL-6 secretion from skeletal muscle increase following exercise, which promotes IS [109]. However, increased IL-6 expression is unfavorable in WAT and liver, and elevated plasma levels of IL-6 are predictive of T2D [112, 126].

Instigators of Inflammation

Traditionally, inflammation is considered to stem from infection and tissue injury. More recently, the impact of metabolic stress is considered to promote inflammation also. Weight gain places additional metabolic stress on the body initiating an inflammatory response. While the metabolic stressors are only beginning to be identified and understood, saturated fatty acids (SFA), lipotoxicity, and the altered gut microbiome are implicated in obesity-induced inflammation.

Lipotoxicity and Adipose Health

With increasing weight gain, adipocytes are faced with two fates, hypertrophy or hyperplasia, an increase in cell size or cell number, respectively. Hypertrophy naturally occurs prior to hyperplasia, in response to increasing adiposity [64]. When excessive dietary intake persists over time, the expansion capacity of adipocytes is exceeded, and FFA are released [122].

Circulating SFA can induce an inflammatory response similar to infectious agents. Both SFA and microbial lipopolysaccharide (LPS) signal via toll-like receptor (TLR) 4 and TLR2 present on the surface of adipocytes and immune cells [52, 78, 123]. Circulating FFA increase with obesity and promote IR through induction of inflammatory signaling pathways and downstream serine/threonine kinase phosphorylation of IRS-1 [124]. The profound effect of SFA on IS has been confirmed through studies that induce transient IR within hours of TAG emulsions plus heparin infusion which elicits FFA release [14, 52].

Intracellular accumulation of TAG and other FA metabolites such as fatty acyl-Co-A, DAG, and ceramides interferes with insulin signaling and leads to IR [124]. Intracellular accumulation of DAG activates PKC and initiates serine/threonine phosphorylation of IRS [119]. With obesity, inflammatory signaling induces the expression of genes involved in lipid metabolism, including enzymes that synthesize ceramide [59, 88]. Ceramide is a sphingolipid that has been shown to accumulate in response to HFD or infusion of SFA. Ceramides suppress insulin action by inhibiting phosphorylated protein kinase B (PKB) [24]. Pharmacological inhibition of ceramide by myriocin improves glucose tolerance [88]. Data from studies investigating lipodystrophy in human and mouse models show that ectopic lipid accumulation may be a factor which potentiates IR, irrespective of peripheral and visceral adiposity [119]. This places intracellular lipid accumulation as an early instigator of chronic low-grade inflammation and IR.

Altered Gut Microbiome

The gut microbiome can modulate immune responses and therefore impact an inflammatory response [70]. The gut flora of obese individuals differs markedly from their lean counterparts, with circulating levels of LPS being significantly higher in the obese state [9]. In murine and human studies, a change in the ratio of bacteroidetes/firmicutes has been shown with weight gain, and this may impact the levels of microbiome-derived LPS [45, 56, 92]. Transport of LPS from the gut lumen to circulation is upregulated in response to HFD feeding [44]. High-fat diet feeding also increases gut permeability and reduces tight-junction integrity allowing for movement of LPS across the gut epithelium [18]. The composition of the gut microbiome has been directly linked to the development of metabolic disorders associated with obesity [9, 33, 70]. It has been established that the NLRP3 and NLRP6 inflammasomes and caspase-1 play a role in regulating gut microbiota. Deficiencies in these inflammasome components lead to gut microbiota dysregulation [58]. This interaction also provides a mechanism through which changes in gut microbiota exert a regulatory effect on obesity-associated inflammation [33].

Gut microbiota also affects energy absorption via short-chain fatty acid (SCFA) metabolism and storage by inhibition of fasting-induced adipocyte factor (Fiaf) [8]. Elevated levels of the lipoprotein lipase inhibitor Fiaf is one mechanism responsible for the resistance to diet-induced obesity (DIO) in germ-free mice. The obese microbiome has increased energy absorption potential [135], and the suppression of Fiaf plays a critical role in this [33]. Additionally, suppression of Fiaf is vital for gut microbiota-associated deposition of TAG in adipocytes [7].

The influence of TLRs on the gut microbiota also represents another important factor linking inflammation and obesity. Ablation of TLR5 alters gut microbiota and leads to metabolic complications such as IR [140]. Whereas the absence of TLR4 exerts positive effects on metabolic health, reducing inflammatory signaling required for the development of obesity-associated IR [9]. The influential function of the gut microbiota makes it an interesting target for future therapies aimed at reducing the inflammation associated with obesity.

"Metaflammation": Cells and Signaling

With obesity, the changes evident at a metabolic tissue level result from alterations in tissue composition and secretory profile. Increased circulating concentrations of TNF-α (alpha), IL-1β (beta), and monocyte chemoattractant protein-1 (MCP-1/CCL2) have been observed in T2D and are indicative of future disease risk [88].

Adipocytes and the Stromal Vascular Fraction

Adipose tissue is composed of adipocytes and a stromal vascular fraction (SVF). At a fundamental level, adipocytes function in the uptake and release of FA; however, they are more complex than simply lipid storage cells. They secrete proteins and hormones which influence satiety and immune cell infiltration. Proteins secreted from adipocytes are often referred to as adipokines and include MCP-1 and IL-6 in addition to the hormones leptin and adiponectin. Additionally, adipocytes are involved in insulin signaling and glycemic control.

The SVF in turn is composed of adipose-derived stem cells, precursor preadipocytes, and immune cells that are crucial for normal tissue function. With obesity, the secretory profile of these cell types is altered toward an inflammatory response. The presence of inflammatory cytokines TNF-α (alpha), IL-1β (beta), and IL-6 halts the maturation of preadipocytes in vitro, characterized by reduced lipid accumulation [55]. Additionally, TNF-α (alpha) treatment of preadipocytes results in increased secretion of IL-6 and MCP-1 [28]. Collagenase digestion of WAT separates the floating adipocyte layer from a SVF pellet. Analysis of the adipocyte layer from obese mice has shown that lipid-laden macrophages closely surround adipocytes [40].

Adipogenesis is the process through which precursor preadipocyte cells become adipocytes, and it is crucial for the expansion of WAT. Once committed to differentiation, preadipocytes undergo growth arrest, and there is a concurrent increase in the expression of mature adipocyte genes such as fatty acid-binding protein and lipid-metabolizing enzymes [53]. The transcription factor peroxisome proliferator-activated receptor (PPAR)-γ (gamma) is an important driver of this process, and for this reason (PPAR)-γ (gamma) is the target of the thiazolidinediones (TZDs) family of medication, used in the treatment of T2D.

Crucial to WAT function, adipocytes undergo hypertrophy and hyperplasia, which together contribute to an overall increase in WAT mass. When adipocytes become dysfunctional, cell death follows. The occurrence of adipocyte death is correlated with cell size, and adipocyte death is a pathologic marker of obesity [29]. These dying cells leak FFA, which are taken up by local adipose tissue macrophages (ATM) [29]. It has been demonstrated that lipolysis, the hydrolysis of TAG, acts in the recruitment of macrophages into obese WAT [73].

Macrophages

It has been estimated that up to 50% of obese WAT is comprised of macrophages, a fivefold increase from the lean state [75, 142]. Three research papers are crucial to our current understanding of the role of macrophages in metaflammation. First, in 1993, Hotamisgil et al. published research that showcased the role of WAT-derived TNF-α (alpha) in obesity [61]. A decade later, two research papers published in the Journal of Clinical Investigation highlighted that macrophages were crucial to obesity-associated inflammation and identified these cells as the main source of TNF-α (alpha) in obese WAT [142, 149]. Xu et al. demonstrate that inflammatory and macrophage-specific genes including *MCP-1* and macrophage markers F4/80 and CD11b were significantly upregulated in *ob/ob*, *db/db*, and high-fat diet (HFD)-fed murine SVF [149].

Additionally, TNF-α (alpha) acts to stimulate adipocyte lipolysis, thus contributing to elevated FFA concentrations in the serum [22]. In vitro treatment of 3T3-L1 adipocyte cells with TNF-α (alpha) leads to reduced expression of *Pparg* gene [153]. Circulating levels of TNF-α (alpha) have been shown to be increased in obese and T2D subjects, and expression is also increased in WAT and skeletal muscle [62, 71, 155].

Lumeng et al. investigated the inflammatory profile of ATM from lean and obese mice [83]. This research demonstrated a distinct difference in cell surface marker expression. Macrophages from obese mice have significantly increased expression of the cell surface marker CD11c. This CD11c population has greater *Il6* and *Nos2* gene expression than lean ATM, and these genes are associated with inflammation. In contrast, CD11c negative cell populations were shown to express anti-inflammatory genes such as *Il10*.

The chemokine MCP-1 is a key instigator of macrophage recruitment. In murine models of obesity, WAT and BAT *MCP-1* expression is increased [69], and this is coincident with IR, macrophage infiltration of WAT and hepatic TAG accumulation [67, 69]. Such features are absent in HFD-fed $MCP-1^{-/-}$ mice. Overexpression of *MCP-1* increases WAT and plasma, TNF-α (alpha), and IL-6 levels, concomitant with reduced hepatic and skeletal muscle pPKB, suggesting a role for circulating MCP-1 in systemic IR [67]. Recently it has been demonstrated that TNF-α (alpha) treatment increased *MCP-1* expression in 3T3-L1 preadipocytes [66], but this induction did not occur when mature 3T3-L1 cells were treated with TNF-α (alpha). Thus in experimental models, TNF-α (alpha) can halt pre-adipocyte maturation while increasing pre-adipocytes MCP-1 production. Genetic manipulation of the MCP-1 receptor has a positive impact on IS. MCP-1 signals via the C–C chemokine receptor (CCR)2 receptor and *Ccr2* expression are increased in HFD-fed WAT [143]. High levels of CCR2 have been shown in macrophages that are located in regions of WAT where there are crown-like structures (CLS), a description given to a group of macrophages that surround dying adipocytes [84]. The presence of CLS in WAT is associated with obesity.

The origin of ATM however is not certain. There is evidence to suggest that the obese environment draws monocytes from the circulation into WAT. The monocytes then differentiate into macrophages which express distinct cell surface markers, behavior, and secretory patterns from the resident ATM population [84]. Lumeng et al. labeled ATM from lean and HFD-fed mice in order to determine if there were distinct localization patterns in the obese environment [84]. This research showed that in obese WAT, ATM with pro-inflammatory characteristics preferentially localized in CLS clusters. This study also highlighted that resident ATM localization occurs independently of MCP-1 signaling. Importantly, despite the presence of these CLS, resident ATM populations remain in interstitial spaces between adipocytes, as is the case in lean WAT. Approximately 90% of ATM in both obese mice and humans are localized to CLS [29]. The role of hematopoietic IL-1R has also been demonstrated to be involved in monocytosis. Nagareddy et al. performed bone marrow transplants and fat pad transplants on *ob/ob* and HFD-fed murine models to highlight a positive feedback loop between ATM and bone marrow myeloid progenitor cells in obesity [97]. The results of this study show that in inflamed WAT, an increase in inflammatory mediators is accompanied by increased cross talk with hematopoietic progenitor cells. The IL-1R plays an important role in this signaling which the researchers suggest, ultimately leads to an increase in circulating monocytes and increased WAT infiltration.

Alternatively, the obese environment may initiate a phenotypic change in resident ATM causing these cells to act in a pro-inflammatory manner. New research demonstrated that tissue resident macrophages originate during embryonic development rather than from infiltration of circulating monocytes [43]. Fate-mapping techniques track embryonic macrophage populations into adulthood and allow comparative functional relationships of resident macrophages and circulating monocytes [43]. Further, a separate study demonstrated that macrophage populations' resident in the WAT undergo local cell differentiation in response to MCP-1 treatment ex vivo, independently of monocyte recruitment [4]. It is likely that a combination of events takes place in the obese environment, including the recruitment of monocytes into the WAT and a shift in the phenotype of the resident ATM when weight gain promotes aberrant cytokine and chemokine secretion in WAT.

Recently there have been discussions around the naming conventions of macrophages in obesity-induced inflammation [96]. At present, the inflammatory macrophages that increase with obesity are considered M1 or classically activated ATM, while resident macrophages, with a regulatory or anti-inflammatory phenotype, are classified as M2 or alternatively activated macrophages. This M1–M2 split has since been further subdivided as research demonstrates subpopulations of M1 and M2 cells, with unique characteristics. It is likely that in obese WAT, ATM phenotypes lie along a spectrum ranging from M1–M2 [95].

Resident macrophages from different organs have been shown to be as distinct from each other as they are from circulating macrophages [51]. This suggests that tissue-specific factors drive macrophage differentiation. In the liver, resident macrophages called Kupffer cells play a role in tissue homeostasis. However with obesity, additional macrophages are present within the liver, recruited by MCP-1 signaling. Depletion of all macrophages from the liver is protective against HFD-induced IR. Recently, hepatic macrophage content was shown to decrease by 80% when $Ccr2^{-/-}$ monocytes were injected into obese WT mice [103]. Kupffer cells mediate the recruitment of hepatic macrophages in obesity [93]. These recruited macrophages are six times more prevalent in obese vs. lean mice and demonstrate greater *Il6*, *Tnfa*, and *MCP-1* expression [93]. The presence of hepatic macrophages impacts on hepatic IS rather than systemic IS [15].

Further Inflammatory Cells Types

Other immune cell types are also drawn into the chronic inflammatory tissue environment. These include cells of the innate and adaptive immune response. Dendritic cells (DC) are hematopoietic-derived cells, and function in antigen-presenting, an important process in initiating a T cell response [118]. Murine models of DIO have demonstrated an increase in DC number in bone marrow, WAT, and liver [25, 113, 127]. A comparison of DC isolated from the SVF of lean and obese mice demonstrated a difference in population subsets [13]. Dendritic cells derived from obese SVF have a greater propensity to drive the differentiation of a T-helper (T_H)17 cell population, which in turn produce high levels of pro-inflammatory IL-17 [13, 25]. The DC-derived pro-inflammatory cytokine IL-12 has been shown to be increased with obesity, and elevated serum levels of IL-12 have been noted in human T2D studies [90, 98, 141]. This cytokine can drive T cells to differentiate to pro-inflammatory T_H1 cells.

T cells make up approximately 30% of the SVF in HFD-fed mice [88]. T cell infiltration of WAT occurs before ATM expansion [100, 147]. In addition to increased numbers of T_H17 cells, obesity results in a change in other T cell populations such as a reduction in regulatory T cell (T_{reg}) number [47, 147]. These T cells promote alternative activated macrophage responses to inflammation [105], and when depleted, there is reduced tyrosine phosphorylation of IRS-1 [47]. With HFD feeding, there is an increase in WAT T_H1 cell number [147], and these cells activate pro-inflammatory macrophages and increase

IL-1β (beta), IL-6, and TNF-α (alpha) secretion. Thus the secretory profile of T cell populations becomes skewed with obesity, further promoting the inflammatory environment. T cells are traditionally thought to be activated by antigen-presenting cells such as DC, via interaction with the major histocompatibility complex (MHC). Recent research suggests a new role for the MHC II in obesity. Deng et al. demonstrated that within 2 weeks of HFD feeding, murine subcutaneous and visceral adipocytes upregulate genes involved in MHC II presentation and processing [35]. A similar set of genes was also upregulated in a cohort of obese female subjects [35]. In HFD-fed MHC II$^{-/-}$ mice, there was reduced T_H cell number, reduced expression of *Nlrp3* and *Tnf*, and improved IS. However, Morris et al. and follow-up research by Cho et al. describe the ATM MHC II–T cell interactions as an important driver of WAT inflammation, through T cell proliferation and WAT inflammation [26, 94] but did not support the finding of MHC II protein expression in WAT [26]. This research revealed that macrophage cell-specific deletion of *MHC II* improved IS in HFD-fed mice.

The NLRP3 Inflammasome

The pro-inflammatory cytokine IL-1β (beta) is secreted by macrophages [83], as immature pro--IL1β (beta). It is processed to an active mature state via an inflammasome complex. Inflammasomes are multicomponent structures that assemble in response to danger-associated molecular patterns (DAMPs) and pathogen-associated molecular patterns, in order to activate an immune response [128]. Such DAMPs include obesity-related metabolic stressors (monosodium urate, FA, ceramides, cholesterol crystals). There has been a particular focus on the NLRP3 inflammasome in relation to IL-1β (beta) processing [89]. This inflammasome is comprised of an NLRP3 NOD-like receptor (NLR), an apoptosis-associated speck-like protein, containing a CARD (ASC) adaptor protein and caspase-1. The complex functions to activate caspase-1, which in turn cleaves immature pro-IL-1 family members to their active form [3, 36]. Activation of the NLRP3 inflammasome itself is required for cytokine processing to proceed; in vitro, this can be achieved through a two-step process of priming followed by activation. Firstly, TLR4 is activated by a ligand such as LPS or SFA, and this initiates pro-IL-1β (beta) production [113, 144] and is considered a first "hit." A second activation signal results in the assembly of the inflammasome complex. Exogenous adenosine triphosphate (ATP) may be used as a second activation stimulus in experimental models.

NLRP3 activation by FA is variable upon FA saturation [49]. Whereas SFA prime the NLRP3 inflammasome, monounsaturated fatty acids (MUFA) have a reduced ability to prime the complex. Consequently, in MUFA-HFD-fed mice, there is reduced WAT *Nlrp3, caspase-1*, and *Il1β* (beta) expression ex vivo relative to SFA-HFD. Research has shown a role for the metabolic sensor AMPK in NLRP3 activation [86]. This complex is involved in energy balance and FA metabolism, and it is activated by threonine phosphorylation [86, 156]. Treatment with the SFA, palmitate, reduces AMPK activation in bone marrow macrophages (BMM) and is coincident with increased IL-1β (beta) secretion [144]. Finucane et al. demonstrated a significant reduction in SFA-HFD-fed WAT pAMPK levels relative to a chow and MUFA-HFD group. Oleic acid, a MUFA, induces BMM AMPK activity in vitro which in turn reduces the IL-1β (beta) response to ATP stimulation [49]. Ex vivo analysis of LPS-treated monocyte-derived macrophages (MDM) from T2D patients demonstrates increased expression in *Nlrp3* and *Asc* [79] and following stimulation with DAMPs increased IL-1β (beta) secretion. Metformin treatment of T2D patients prevented maturation of MDM-derived IL-1β (beta), through enhanced AMPK phosphorylation. Together these studies highlight a link between AMPK and NLRP3 inflammasome activity (Fig. 2) and point to AMPK activation as an attractive target to attenuate "metaflammation."

Linking Inflammatory and Insulin Signaling Pathways

Toll-like receptor-4 has a central role in inflammatory signaling in the context of obesity. This receptor is present on the cell surface of adipocytes and macrophages and can induce inflammation in response to diverse stimuli including LPS and SFA. Hematopoietic cell depletion of TLR4 protects mice from diet-induced IR and results in a reduction in *Tnfa* and *Il6* expression in WAT and liver [104]. Signaling via the TLR4 receptor can activate either the MyD88-dependent pathway or the TRIF-dependent pathway, and these pathways converge at the protein kinase TAK-1. Activation of TAK-1 results in downstream activation of the NF-κ (kappa) B and mitogen-activated protein kinase (MAPK)signaling pathways [72].

The NF-κ (kappa) B pathway is downstream of receptors TLR4, TNFR, and IL1R. This pathway has a major role in a number of inflammatory conditions [11, 12]. Activation of NF-κ (kappa) B signaling drives secretion of TNF-α (alpha), IL-1β (beta), and IL-6, thus propagating the inflammatory environment [38]. Upon receptor engagement, a signaling cascade is initiated, resulting in the phosphorylation and thus activation of the Iκ (kappa) B kinase (IKK) complex and subsequently phosphorylation of inhibitor of κ (kappa) B (Iκ (kappa) B), marking this molecule for degradation and releasing the NF-κ (kappa) B transcription factor. Once released, NF-κ (kappa) B translocates to the nucleus and initiates expression of cytokines.

With obesity, there is increased expression of suppressor of cytokine signaling (SOCS) proteins, and members of this family act to inhibit insulin signaling [41, 42, 137]. The SOCS-1 and SOCS-3 proteins function to control cytokine action through feedback loops. These proteins also partially block tyrosine phosphorylation of the insulin receptor, and downstream from this, phosphorylation of IRS-1 and IRS-2 is almost entirely inhibited [137]. Preferential phosphorylation of serine/threonine residues on IRS-1 over tyrosine residues results in abrogation of the insulin receptor signaling cascade [54, 108]. Factors that promote

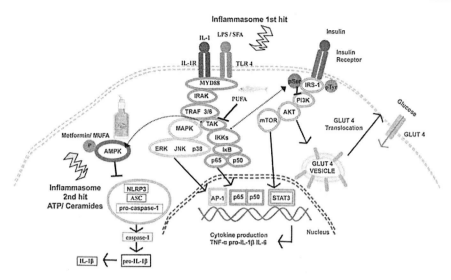

Fig. 2 Metaflammation – interaction between inflammatory and insulin signaling pathways. With obesity, the interaction between inflammatory signaling pathways and the insulin signaling pathway results in diminished insulin signaling and, if the inflammatory state persists, insulin resistance and reduced insulin-stimulated glucose uptake. Inflammatory signaling results in preferential serine/threonine phosphorylation of IRS-1, and this halts the signaling cascade and prevents GLUT4 trafficking to the cell surface. Research into the role of the NLRP3 inflammasome in pro-inflammatory IL-1β (beta) processing has emphasized the cross talk between inflammatory signaling and insulin resistance and highlighted this inflammasome complex as a therapeutic target. Metformin and oleic acid, a monounsaturated fatty acid, reduce NLRP3 inflammasome activity via activation of the metabolic sensor AMPK. Blocking of NF-κ (kappa) B signaling by the dietary fatty acids EPA and DHA has shown antiinflammatory potential in vitro models, but data on this effect is contentious in human studies

aberrant serine/threonine IRS-1 phosphorylation include SOCS-3 but also FFA and inflammatory mediators such as TNF-α (alpha), via NF-κ (kappa) B, JNK, and MAPK pathways [54, 131]. Tyrosine phosphorylation of IRS-1 allows for continuation of insulin signaling. Downstream of IRS-1 lie the molecules phosphoinositide-3-kinase (PI3K) and AKT, and these function in glucose uptake into the WAT, liver, and muscle. In normal physiological conditions, insulin-dependent signaling results in AKT-stimulating glucose transporter type (GLUT) 4 translocation to the cell surface via PKC phosphorylation of AS160 [63, 99]; GLUT4 functions in the transport of glucose into the cell.

Therapeutic Approaches

There is sound evidence showing that an obesity-induced inflammatory state promotes the progression of IR. Therefore, therapeutic approaches which attenuate this state and/or promote the resolution of inflammation may impact favorably upon obesity-induced IR. Several pharmacological agents and lifestyle interventions have an impact on both metabolism and inflammation. In reviewing the concept of resolution of metabolic inflammation, it is clear that exact processes involved are not completely understood. Thus more research is required to identify and assess effective anti-inflammatory treatment strategies.

Drug Therapies

As IR can precede the development of T2D by decades, therapies that target inflammation associated with IR are central to halting the progression toward overt T2D. If IR progresses to T2D, there are a variety of treatments available. Some pharmacological approaches which show potential include metformin, TZDs, and anakinra. While these therapies have potential in terms of clinical efficacy, they are limited by their side effects. Anti-inflammatory therapies also have potential adverse effects, linked to long-term usage and immune suppression.

At present, guidelines recommend metformin as a first-line treatment for T2D [23]. The biomarker HbA1c gives a measure of average plasma glucose concentrations over the previous weeks and therefore indicates loss of glycemic control associated with T2D. Metformin leads to an initial drop in HbA1C, after which patients exhibit a loss of glycemic control and HbA1C levels increase [136]. Metformin regulates lipid and glucose metabolism through increased phosphorylation and activation of AMPK [157]. This antidiabetic drug inhibits mitochondrial function, leading to elevated AMP and ADP levels, thus stimulating AMPK activation [86]. Given the role of metabolic stress on IL-1 β (beta) activation and IR, this has important implications with respect to attenuating the inflammatory response associated with obesity and T2D. Therapies which inhibit pro-inflammatory responses offer an opportunity to correct the metabolic consequences of obesity.

The insulin-sensitizing class of drugs, TZDs, are selective ligands of PPAR-γ (gamma) and target IR [154]. These PPAR-γ (gamma) ligands function by increasing both peripheral glucose disposal and adiponectin levels while also decreasing FFA and pro-inflammatory cytokine levels [60]. Insulin signaling is enhanced through increased IRS-1 expression and inhibition of the MAPK pathway [91]. Therapies that regulate PPAR-γ (gamma) activity by targeting posttranslational modifications of its receptor have the potential to preserve the treatment effect of TZDs while minimizing the side effects associated with their use [80]. Nevertheless the cross talk between PPARγ activation and inflammation requires further investigation.

In obese WAT, macrophage number correlates with the extent of tissue IR. Therefore, therapies which target macrophage accumulation are of particular interest. With obesity, pro-inflammatory macrophages are characterized by the expression of CD11c. Depletion of CD11c macrophages results in reduced WAT inflammation and improved IS in obese mice [107].

Clodronate liposomes that ablate macrophages in a tissue-specific manner offer another potential approach [46]. In a murine model, macrophage ablation specific to WAT improved glucose homeostasis, increased adiponectin levels, reduced TAG levels, and significantly altered cytokine expression levels [46]. While this type of therapy is not yet suitable for clinical use, it presents an interesting proof of concept.

Increased TNF-α (alpha) levels are well documented in obesity; however, inhibition of TNF-α (alpha) provided limited success in humans with T2D [33]. Certain TNF-α (alpha) inhibitors such as etanercept that have beneficial effects in other inflammatory conditions such as rheumatoid arthritis and psoriasis, are associated with a decreased risk of developing T2D but are not currently used in the treatment of T2D [88]. Targeting another pro-inflammatory cytokine, IL-1β (beta) has shown some positive results. Anakinra is an IL-1 receptor antagonist (RA) that improves glycemic control, preserves β (beta)-cell function, and reduces markers of inflammation [77]. Use of the monoclonal antibody XOMA 052 also targets IL-1β (beta), resulting in improved glycemic management and β (beta)-cell function in a murine model of DIO [106]. As the IL-1 family is key to the inflammatory response in metabolic dysregulation, IL-1 antagonism has therapeutic potential [38]. However, global anti-inflammatory therapies such as TNF-α (alpha), IL-1 RA, and MAPK inhibitors are not without side effects [68]. The chronic nature of obesity-associated inflammation requires long-term treatment which raises concern for potential interference with inflammatory-mediated immune responses and key cellular processes [37].

Co-stimulatory interactions have been implicated in obesity-associated inflammation. One such pair is the co-stimulatory protein CD40 and its ligand CD40L, members of the tumor necrosis factor receptor (TNFR) family. The positive correlations between increased body mass index (BMI) and CD40 and the implication of CD40 ligation in activation of pro-inflammatory pathways such as JNK, MAPK, and NF-κ (kappa) B make it an interesting therapeutic target [121]. In HFD-fed mice, small molecule-mediated inhibition of the CD40-TRAF6 interaction improved glucose tolerance [138]. However, immunosuppressive side effects prevent long-term use of antibody treatment against co-stimulatory molecules and cytokine inhibition. Therapies which inhibit the NLRP3 inflammasome offer a more targeted approach rather than global immunosuppressive agents. Recently, the small molecule inhibitor MCC950 was shown to inhibit the NLRP3 inflammasome activation and reduce serum IL-1β (beta) levels in a murine model of inflammatory disease [30]. Existing therapies that decrease NLRP3 activation have shown clinical efficacy. The success of metformin [79], anakinra [77], and the sulfonylurea glyburide [85] highlights the potential for NLRP3 inhibitors as targets for the treatment of metabolic disorders [86].

Lifestyle Interventions

From the lifestyle perspective, weight loss is one strategy that reduces inflammation and halts the development of IR. Dietary and lifestyle modifications that attain significant weight loss attenuate inflammation and improve IS by lowering metabolic stress and reducing ATM number [74]. However, achieving and maintaining weight loss is challenging [49, 50]. Exercise improves insulin IS, and it increases IL-6 and diacylglycerol acyltransferase (DGAT) 1 expression in skeletal muscle [120]. Skeletal muscle-derived-IL-6 induces the production of IL-1 RA and IL-10, inhibits TNF-α (alpha) secretion, and functions to promote glucose uptake [110]. DGAT induces TAG formation from DAG, thereby reducing DAG concentrations, which otherwise impede insulin signaling [31]. Even a single bout of exercise can reduce the lipotoxic and potentially pro-inflammatory effect of elevated DAG levels to improve IS. Presently, there is lack of firm evidence as to whether anti-inflammatory strategies are the most efficacious therapy within the context of obesity. Further work is needed in this area to understand fully their mechanism of action.

Nutrient-Based Approaches: Reducing Inflammation

Inflammatory signaling through several kinases, namely, MAPK, PKC, and NF-κ (kappa) B, drives obesity-induced inflammation [60]. Therapies which target NF-κ (kappa) B, TLR4, and PPAR-γ (gamma) are of clinical importance.

Long-chain n-3 polyunsaturated fatty acids (LC n-3 PUFA), particularly eicosapentaenoic acid (EPA) and docosahexaenoic acid (DHA), exert anti-inflammatory effects [16]. Animal studies provide convincing mechanistic evidence that LC n-3 PUFA stimulate G protein-coupled receptor 120 (GPR120) [102, 151], resulting in inhibition of TAK phosphorylation, and this halts further signaling [102]. Additionally, a role for EPA and DHA has been proposed in ameliorating the pro-inflammatory effects of SFA which activate TLR4 and increase NF-κ (kappa) B transcriptional activity [113]. LC n-3 PUFA also inhibit the production of pro-inflammatory eicosanoids [16], due to a combination of reduced arachidonic acid, the precursor of pro-inflammatory eicosanoids [21], and enhanced DHA-derived resolvin and protectin synthesis [16].

Despite consistent in vitro data demonstrating the benefits of LC n-3 PUFA on metabolic health, these effects have translated to only a modest effect in vivo [65, 133]. Long-term LC n-3 supplementation did not show the positive effects on IS observed in short-term high-dose studies or in in vitro models [133]. Some cross-sectional and epidemiological data suggests that high LC n-3 PUFA status is associated with a reduced risk of obesity-associated inflammation and IR [82]. Human LC n-3 PUFA interventions provide conflicting evidence on the efficacy of n-3 PUFA supplementation, and these show little or no effect on inflammatory markers or IR [87] and only modestly alter lipoprotein risk factor profile; TAG levels are significantly altered, while there was no significant impact on LDL or HDL levels [39, 48]. It is possible that LC n-3 PUFA may be ineffective when the metabolic stress associated with obesity goes beyond a certain level, after which the potential efficacy-associated LC n-3 PUFA are negated by the adverse metabolic phenotype. Alternatively, an individual's responsiveness to LC n-3 PUFA interventions may be due to age, gender, genetic variability, variations in treatment duration, dose, or the populations studied [17]. For example, in the case of gender-specific effects, LIPGENE demonstrated that LC n-3 PUFA were only effective in men but not in women with MetS [133]. A similar gender effect was also observed in the FINGEN study [20].

A number of additional nutrients impact on the NF-κ (kappa) B pathway, including the polyphenols epigallocatechin gallate, found in green tea, which also suppresses ERK phosphorylation, and resveratrol present in red wine [10, 81, 152]. Curcumin is a known anti-inflammatory and anti-carcinogenic agent that has also been shown to inhibit NF-κ (kappa) B activation [125].

Combinations of anti-inflammatory nutritional therapies may offer a more robust effect, capable of targeting multiple inflammatory signaling pathways. A dietary intervention which included resveratrol, lycopene, epigallocatechin gallate, α (alpha)-tocopherol, vitamin C, EPA, and DHA given over 5 weeks elicited anti-inflammatory effects on healthy overweight subjects [10]. This anti-inflammatory dietary mix increased adiponectin levels; however, C-reactive protein and pro-inflammatory cytokines remained largely unchanged [10]. A similar anti-inflammatory dietary mix in mice reduced plasma cholesterol, TAG, and serum amyloid A and improved inflammatory risk factors of cardiovascular disease such as intercellular adhesion molecule-1 (ICAM-1) and E-selectin [139]. Despite the potential of an anti-inflammatory dietary mix for disease prevention, their impact to date has resulted in only subtle improvements in inflammatory biomarkers, and future work in this area is required to maximize this potential.

Pharmacological therapies such as co-stimulatory molecule and cytokine inhibitors, clodronate liposomes, PPAR-γ (gamma) ligands, and therapies which stimulate AMPK activation have been shown to effectively reduce obesity-associated inflammation thus providing treatment opportunities for conditions such as IR and T2D. However, from a nutritional perspective, although some prospective and cross-sectional data is potentially promising, results from interventions are mixed. Perhaps nutritional status can prevent development but not treat inflammation or IR once established. Certain individuals may respond more favorably to interventions based on age, gender, and genetics.

Conclusion

The past two decades have seen a drastic increase in obesity levels; however, our understanding of the underlying mechanism of action has also greatly increased. Greater knowledge of the underlying pathology of obesity-induced inflammation and IR may reveal new treatment options. A good lifestyle and metabolic phenotype can attenuate the risk of developing IR [111, 114]. Nevertheless, there is lack of clarity in relation to dietary/lifestyle/pharmaceutical intervention strategy efficacy. Therefore, greater knowledge in relation to potential therapies which target the chronic low-grade inflammation associated with obesity and metabolic disorders such as IR and T2D is vitally important.

Cross-References

References

1. Abdul-Ghani MA, Defronzo RA. Pathogenesis of insulin resistance in skeletal muscle. J Biomed Biotechnol. 2010;2010:1.

2. Abel ED, Peroni O, Kim JK, et al. Adipose-selective targeting of the GLUT4 gene impairs insulin action in muscle and liver. Nature. 2001;409(6821):729–33.

3. Agostini L, Martinon F, Burns K, et al. NALP3 forms an IL-1B -processing inflammasome with increased activity in Muckle-Wells autoinflammatory disorder. Immunity. 2004;20:319–25.

4. Amano SU, Cohen JL, Vangala P, et al. Local proliferation of macrophages contributes to obesity-associated adipose tissue inflammation. Cell Metab. 2014;19(1):162–71. Elsevier Inc.

5. Angulo P. Nonalcoholic fatty liver disease. N Engl J Med. 2002;15(16):7–10. Mass Medical Soc.

6. Arkan MC, Hevener AL, Greten FR, et al. IKK-beta links inflammation to obesity-induced insulin resistance. Nat Med. 2005;11(2):191–8.

7. Backhed F, Ding H, Wang T, et al. The gut microbiota as an environmental factor that regulates fat storage. Proc Natl Acad Sci U S A. 2004;101(44):15718–23.

8. Backhed F, Manchester JK, Semenkovich CF, et al. Mechanisms underlying the resistance to diet-induced obesity in germ-free mice. Proc Natl Acad Sci U S A. 2007;104(3):979–84.

9. Baker RG, Hayden MS, Ghosh S. NF-kB, inflammation, and metabolic disease. Cell Metab. 2011;13(1):11–22.

10. Bakker GCM, Van Erk MJ, Pellis L, et al. An anti-inflammatory dietary mix modulates inflammation and oxidative and metabolic stress in overweight men: a nutrigenomics approach. Am J Clin Nutr. 2010;91(4):1044–59.

11. Baltimore D. NF-kB is 25. Nat Immunol. 2011;12(8):683–5.

12. Ben-Neriah Y, Karin M. Inflammation meets cancer, with NF-kB as the matchmaker. Nat Immunol. 2011;12(8):715–23.

13. Bertola A, Ciucci T, Rousseau D, et al. Identification of adipose tissue dendritic cells correlated with obesity-associated insulin-resistance and inducing Th17 responses in mice and patients. Diabetes. 2012;61(9):2238–47.

14. Boden G, Jadali F, White J, et al. Effects of fat on insulin-stimulated carbohydrate metabolism in normal men indirect calorimetry respiratory gas exchange. J Clin Investig. 1991;88(September):960–6.

15. Cai D, Yuan M, Frantz DF, et al. Local and systemic insulin resistance resulting from hepatic activation of IKK-beta and NF-kappaB. Nat Immunol. 2005;11(2):183–90.

16. Calder PC. n-3 polyunsaturated fatty acids, inflammation, and inflammatory diseases. Am J Clin Nutr. 2006;83(6 Suppl):1505S–19S.

17. Calder PC, Ahluwalia N, Brouns F, et al. Dietary factors and low-grade inflammation in relation to overweight and obesity. Br J Nutr. 2011;106(Suppl):S5–S78.

18. Cani PD, Bibiloni R, Knauf C, et al. Changes in gut microbiota control metabolic endotoxemia-induced inflammation in high-fat diet-induced obesity and diabetes in mice. Diabetes. 2008;57(6):1470–81.

19. Cannon B, Nedergaard J. Brown adipose tissue: function and physiological significance. Physiol Rev. 2004;84(1):277–359.

20. Caslake MJ, Miles EA, Kofler BM, et al. Effect of sex and genotype on cardiovascular biomarker response to fish oils: the FINGEN Study. Am J Clin Nutr. 2008;88(3):618–29.

21. Caughey GE, Mantzioris E, Gibson RA, et al. The effect on human tumor necrosis factor alpha and interleukin 1 beta production of diets enriched in n-3 fatty acids from vegetable oil or fish oil. Am J Clin Nutr. 1996;63:116–22.

22. Cawthorn WP, Sethi JK. TNF-alpha and adipocyte biology. FEBS Lett. 2008;582(1):117–31.

23. Centre for Clinical Practice at NICE. Type 2 diabetes: newer agents for blood glucose control in type 2 diabetes. London: National Institute for Health and Clinical Excellence; 2009.

24. Chavez JA, Summers SA. A ceramide-centric view of insulin resistance. Cell Metab. 2012;15(5):585–94.

25. Chen Y, Tian J, Tian X, et al. Adipose tissue dendritic cells enhances inflammation by prompting the generation of Th17 cells. PLoS One. 2014;9(3):e92450.

26. Cho KW, Morris DL, DelProposto JL, et al. An MHC class II dependent activation loop between adipose tissue macrophages and CD4+ Tcells controls obesity- induced inflammation. Cell Rep. 2014;9(2):605–17.

27. Chondronikola M, Volpi E, Børsheim E, et al. Brown adipose tissue improves whole body glucose homeostasis and insulin sensitivity in humans. Diabetes. 2014;63:4089–99.

28. Chung S, Lapoint K, Martinez K, et al. Preadipocytes mediate lipopolysaccharide-induced inflammation and insulin resistance in primary cultures of newly differentiated human adipocytes. Endocrinology. 2006;147(11):5340–51.

29. Cinti S, Mitchell G, Barbatelli G, et al. Adipocyte death defines macrophage localization and function in adipose tissue of obese mice and humans. J Lipid Res. 2005;46(11):2347–55.

30. Coll RC, Robertson AAB, Chae JJ, et al. A small-molecule inhibitor of the NLRP3 inflammasome for the treatment of inflammatory diseases. Nat Med. 2015;21:248–55.

31. Corcoran MP, Lamon-Fava S, Fielding RA. Skeletal muscle lipid deposition and insulin resistance: effect of dietary fatty acids and exercise. Am J Clin Nutr. 2007;85:662–77.

32. Cristancho AG, Lazar MA. Forming functional fat: a growing understanding of adipocyte differentiation. Nat Rev Mol Cell Biol. 2011;12(11):722–34.

33. Dali-Youcef N, Mecili M, Ricci R, et al. Metabolic inflammation: connecting obesity and insulin resistance. Ann Med Engl. 2013;45(3):242–53.

34. DeFronzo RA, Tripathy D. Skeletal muscle insulin resistance is the primary defect in type 2 diabetes. Diabetes Care. 2009;32(Suppl 2):S157–63.

35. Deng T, Lyon CJ, Minze LJ, et al. Class II major histocompatibility complex plays an essential role in obesity-induced adipose inflammation. Cell Metab. 2013;17(3):411–22.

36. Dinarello CA. Immunological and inflammatory functions of the interleukin-1 family. Annu Rev Immunol. 2009;27:519–50.

37. Dinarello CA. Anti-inflammatory agents: present and future. Cell. 2010;140(6):935–50.

38. Donath MY, Shoelson SE. Type 2 diabetes as an inflammatory disease. Nat Rev Immunol. 2011;11(2):98–107. Nature Publishing Group.

39. Dyerberg J, Eskesen DC, Andersen PW, et al. Effects of trans- and n-3 unsaturated fatty acids on cardiovascular risk markers in healthy males. An 8 weeks dietary intervention study. Eur J Clin Nutr. 2004;58(7):1062–70.

40. Ebke LA, Nestor-Kalinoski AL, Slotterbeck BD, et al. Tight association between macrophages and adipocytes in obesity: implications for adipocyte preparation. Obesity (Silver Spring). 2014;22(5):1246–55.

41. Emanuelli B. SOCS-3 is an insulin-induced negative regulator of insulin signaling. J Biol Chem. 2000;275(21):15985–91.

42. Emanuelli B, Macotela Y, Boucher J, et al. SCOS-1 deficiency does not prevent diet-induced insulin resistance. Biochem Biophys Res Commun. 2008;377(2):447–52.

43. Epelman S, Lavine KJ, Randolph GJ. Origin and functions of tissue macrophages. Immunity. 2014;41(1):21–35. Elsevier Inc.

44. Erridge C, Attina T, Spickett CM, et al. A high-fat meal induces low-grade endotoxemia: evidence of a novel mechanism of postprandial inflammation. Am J Clin Nutr. 2007;86(5):1286–92.

45. Everard A, Lazarevic V, Gaïa N, et al. Microbiome of prebiotic-treated mice reveals novel targets involved in host response during obesity. ISME J. 2014;8:2116–30.

46. Feng B, Jiao P, Nie Y, et al. Clodronate liposomes improve metabolic profile and reduce visceral adipose macrophage content in diet-induced obese mice. PLoS One. 2011;6(9):e24358.

47. Feuerer M, Herrero L, Cipolletta D, et al. Lean, but not obese, fat is enriched for a unique population of regulatory T cells that affect metabolic parameters. Nat Med. 2009;15(8):930–9. Nature Publishing Group.

48. Finnegan YE, Minihane AM, Leigh-Firbank EC, et al. Plant- and marine-derived n-3 polyunsaturated fatty acids have differential effects on fasting and postprandial blood lipid concentrations and on the susceptibility of LDL to oxidative modification in moderately hyperlipidemic subjects. Am J Clin Nutr. 2003;77(4):783–95.

49. Finucane OM, Lyons CL, Murphy AM, et al. Monounsaturated fatty acid enriched high fat-diets impede adipose NLRP3 inflammasome mediated IL-1beta secretion and insulin resistance despite obesity. Diabetes. 2015;64:2116.

50. Gage D. Weight loss/maintenance as an effective tool for controlling type 2 diabetes: novel methodology to sustain weight reduction. Diabetes Metab Res Rev. 2012;28(3):214–8.

51. Gautier EL, Shay T, Miller J, et al. Gene-expression profiles and transcriptional regulatory pathways that underlie the identity and diversity of mouse tissue macro-phages. Nat Immunol. 2012;13(11):1118–28.

52. Glass CK, Olefsky JM. Inflammation and lipid signaling in the etiology of insulin resistance. Cell Metab. 2012;15(5):635–45.

53. Gregoire FM, Smas CM, Sul HS. Understanding adipocyte differentiation. Physiol Rev. 1998;78(3):783–809.

54. Gual P, Le Marchand-Brustel Y, Tanti J-FF. Positive and negative regulation of insulin signaling through IRS-1 phosphorylation. Biochimie. 2005;87(1):99–109.

55. Gustafson B, Smith U. Cytokines promote Wnt signaling and inflammation and impair the normal differentiation and lipid accumulation in 3T3-L1 preadipocytes. J Biol Chem. 2006;281(14):9507–16.

56. Harley ITW, Karp CL. Obesity and the gut microbiome: striving for causality. Mol Metab. 2012;1(1–2):21–31.

57. Harms M, Seale P. Brown and beige fat: development, function and therapeutic potential. Nat Med. 2013;19(10):1252–63.

58. Henao-Mejia J, Elinav E, Jin C, et al. Inflammasome-mediated dysbiosis regulates progression of NAFLD and obesity. Nature. 2012;482(7384):179–85. Nature Publishing Group.

59. Holland WL, Bikman BT, Wang LP, et al. Lipid-induced insulin resistance mediated by the pro-inflammatory receptor TLR4 requires saturated fatty acid-induced ceramide biosynthesis in mice. J Clin Invest. 2011;121(5):1858–70.

60. Hotamisligil GS. Role of endoplasmic reticulum stress and c-Jun NH2-terminal kinase pathways in inflammation and origin of obesity and diabetes. Diabetes. 2005;54(Suppl 2):S73–8.

61. Hotamisligil GS, Shargill NS, Spiegelman BM, et al. Adipose expression of tumor necrosis factor-alpha: direct role in obesity-linked insulin resistance. Science. 1993;259(5091):87–91.

62. Hotamisligil GS, Arner P, Caro JF, et al. Increased adipose tissue expression of tumor necrosis factor-alpha in human obesity and insulin resistance. J Clin Invest. 1995;95(5):2409–15.

63. Imamura T, Huang J, Usui I, et al. Insulin-induced GLUT4 translocation involves protein kinase C-λ-mediated functional coupling between Rab4 and the motor protein kinesin. Mol Cell Biol. 2003;23(14):4892–900.

64. Jo J, Gavrilova O, Pack S, et al. Hypertrophy and/or hyperplasia: dynamics of adipose tissue growth. PLoS Comput Biol. 2009;5(3):e1000324.

65. Kabir M, Skurnik G, Naour N, et al. Treatment for 2 mo with n 3 polyunsaturated fatty acids reduces adiposity and some atherogenic factors but does not improve insulin sensitivity in women with type 2 diabetes: a randomized controlled study. Am J Clin Nutr. 2007;86(6):1670–9.

66. Kabir SM, Lee E-S, Son D-S. Chemokine network during adipogenesis in 3T3-L1 cells: differential response between growth and proinflammatory factor in preadipocytes vs. adipocytes. Adipocytes. 2014;3(2):97–106.

67. Kamei N, Tobe K, Suzuki R, et al. Overexpression of monocyte chemoattractant protein-1 in adipose tissues causes macrophage recruitment and insulin resistance. J Biol Chem. 2006;281(36):26602–14.

68. Kaminska B. MAPK signalling pathways as molecular targets for anti-inflammatory therapy – from molecular mechanisms to therapeutic benefits. Biochim Biophys Acta. 2005;1754(1–2):253–62.

69. Kanda H, Tateya S, Tamori Y, et al. MCP-1 contributes to macrophage infiltration into adipose tissue, insulin resistance, and hepatic steatosis in obesity. J Clin Invest. 2006;116(6):1494.

70. Kanneganti T-D, Dixit VD. Immunological complications of obesity. Nat Immunol. 2012;13(8):707–12. Nature Publishing Group.

71. Kern PA, Saghizadeh M, Ong JM, et al. The expression of tumor necrosis factor in human adipose tissue. Regulation by obesity, weight loss, and relationship to lipoprotein lipase. J Clin Invest. 1995;95(5):2111–9.

72. Könner AC, Brüning JC. Toll-like receptors: linking inflammation to metabolism. Trends Endocrinol Metab. 2011;22(1):16–23.

73. Kosteli A, Sugaru E, Haemmerle G, et al. Weight loss and lipolysis promote a dynamic immune response in murine adipose tissue. J Clin Invest. 2010;120(10):3466–79.

74. Kovacikova M, Sengenes C, Kovacova Z, et al. Dietary intervention-induced weight loss decreases macrophage content in adipose tissue of obese women. Int J Obes. 2011;35(1):91–8.

75. Kraakman MJ, Murphy AJ, Jandeleit-Dahm K, et al. Macrophage polarization in obesity and type 2 diabetes: weighing down our understanding of macrophage function? Front Immunol. 2014;5(September):470.

76. Lam TK, Yoshii H, Haber CA, et al. Free fatty acid-induced hepatic insulin resistance: a potential role for protein kinase C-delta. Am J Physiol Endocrinol Metab. 2002;283(4):E682–91.

77. Larsen CM, Faulenbach M, Vaag A, et al. Interleukin-1-receptor antagonist in type 2 diabetes mellitus. N Engl J Med. 2007;357(3):302–3.

78. Lee JY, Sohn KH, Rhee SH, et al. Saturated fatty acids, but not unsaturated fatty acids, induce the expression of cyclooxygenase-2 mediated through Toll-like receptor 4. J Biol Chem. 2001;276(20):16683–9.

79. Lee H-M, Kim J-J, Kim HJ, et al. Upregulated NLRP3 inflammasome activation in patients with type 2 diabetes. Diabetes. 2013;62:1–11.

80. Lefterova MI, Haakonsson AK, Lazar MA, et al. PPARg and the global map of adipogenesis and beyond. Trends Endocrinol Metab. 2014;25(6):293–302.

81. Liu H-S, Chen Y-H, Hung P-F, et al. Inhibitory effect of green tea(−)-epigallocatechin gallate on resistin gene expression in 3T3-L1 adipocytes depends on the ERK pathway. Am J Physiol Endocrinol Metab. 2006;290(2):E273–81.

82. Lopez-Garcia E, Schulze MB, Manson JE, et al. Consumption of (n-3) fatty acids is related to plasma biomarkers of inflammation and endothelial activation in women. J Nutr. 2004;134(7):1806–11.

83. Lumeng CN, Bodzin JL, Saltiel AR. Obesity induces a phenotypic switch in adipose tissue macrophage polarization. J Clin Invest. 2007;117(1):175–84.

84. Lumeng CN, DelProposto JB, Westcott DJ, et al. Phenotypic switching of adipose tissue macro-phages with obesity is generated by spatiotemporal differences in macrophage subtypes. Diabetes. 2008;57(12):3239–46.

85. Masters SL, Dunne A, Subramanian SL, et al. Activation of the NLRP3 inflammasome by islet amyloid polypeptide provides a mechanism for enhanced IL-1b in type 2 diabetes. Nat Immunol. 2010;11(10):8–11.

86. McGettrick AF, O'Neill LAJ. NLRP3 and IL-1beta in macrophages as critical regulators of metabolic diseases. Diabetes Obes Metab. 2013;15(Suppl 3):19–25.

87. McMorrow AM, Connaughton RM, Lithander FE, et al. Adipose tissue dysregulation and metabolic consequences in childhood and adolescent obesity: potential impact of dietary fat quality. Proc Nutr Soc. 2015;74(1):67–82.

88. McNelis JC, Olefsky JM. Macrophages, immunity, and metabolic disease. Immunity. 2014;41(1):36–48.

89. Mills KH, Dunne A. Immune modulation: IL-1, master mediator or initiator of inflammation. Nat Med. 2009;15(12):1363–4.

90. Mishra M, Kumar H, Bajpai S, et al. Level of serum IL-12 and its correlation with endothelial dysfunction, insulin resistance, proinflammatory cytokines and lipid profile in newly diagnosed type 2 diabetes. Diabetes Res Clin Pract. 2011;94(2):255–61.

91. Miyazaki Y, He H, Mandarino LJ, et al. Rosiglitazone improves downstream insulin receptor signaling in

type 2 diabetic patients. Diabetes. 2003;52(8): 1943–50.

92. Moreno-Indias I, Cardona F, Tinahones FJ, et al. Impact of the gut microbiota on the development of obesity and type 2 diabetes mellitus. Front Microbiol. 2014;5(April):1–10.

93. Morinaga H, Mayoral R, Heinrichsdorff J, et al. Characterization of distinct subpopulations of hepatic macrophages in HFD/obese mice. Diabetes. 2014;64(4): 1120. epub ahead.

94. Morris DL, Cho KW, Delproposto JL, et al. Adipose tissue macrophages function as antigen-presenting cells and regulate adipose tissue CD4+ T cells in mice. Diabetes. 2013;62(8):2762–72.

95. Mosser DM, Edwards JP. Exploring the full spectrum of macrophage activation. Nat Rev Immunol. 2008;8(12):958–69. Nature Publishing Group.

96. Murray PJ, Allen JE, Biswas SK, et al. Macrophage activation and polarization: nomenclature and experimental guidelines. Immunity. 2014;41(1):14–20. Elsevier.

97. Nagareddy PR, Kraakman M, Masters SL, et al. Adipose tissue macrophages promote myelopoiesis and monocytosis in obesity. Cell Metab. 2014;19(5): 821–35. Cell Press.

98. Nam H, Ferguson BS, Stephens JM, Morrison RF. Impact of obesity on IL-12 family gene expression in insulin responsive tissues. Biochim Biophys Acta. 2013;1832(1):11. ePub.

99. Ng Y, Ramm G, Burchfield JG, et al. Cluster analysis of insulin action in adipocytes reveals a key role for Akt at the plasma membrane. J Biol Chem. 2010;285(4):2245–57.

100. Nishimura S, Manabe I, Nagasaki M, et al. CD8+ effector T cells contribute to macrophage recruitment and adipose tissue inflammation in obesity. Nat Med. 2009;15(8):914–20.

101. Obstfeld AE, Sugaru E, Thearle M, et al. Recruitment of myeloid cells that promote obesity-induced hepatic steatosis. Diabetes. 2010;59:916.

102. Oh DY, Talukdar S, Bae EJ, et al. GPR120 is an omega-3 fatty acid receptor mediating potent anti-inflammatory and insulin-sensitizing effects. Cell. 2010;142(5):687–98. Elsevier Ltd.

103. Oh DY, Morinaga H, Talukdar S, et al. Increased macrophage migration into adipose tissue in obese mice. Diabetes. 2012;61(2):346–54.

104. Orr JS, Puglisi MJ, Ellacott KLJ, et al. Toll-like receptor 4 deficiency promotes the alternative activation of adipose tissue macrophages. Diabetes. 2012;61(11):2718–27.

105. Osborn O, Olefsky JM. The cellular and signaling networks linking the immune system and metabolism in disease. Nat Med. 2012;18(3):363–74. Nature Publishing Group.

106. Owyang AM, Maedler K, Gross L, et al. XOMA 052, an anti-IL-1{beta} monoclonal antibody, improves glucose control and {beta}-cell function in the diet-induced obesity mouse model. Endocrinology. 2010;151(6):2515–27.

107. Patsouris D, Li PP, Thapar D, et al. Ablation of CD11c-positive cells normalizes insulin sensitivity in obese insulin resistant animals. Cell Metab. 2008;8(4):301–9.

108. Paz K, Hemi R, LeRoith D, et al. A molecular basis for insulin resistance: elevated serine/threonine phosphorylation of IRS-1 and IRS-2 inhibits their binding to the juxtamembrane region of the insulin receptor and impairs their ability to undergo insulin-induced tyrosine phosphorylation. J Biol Chem. 1997;272(47):29911–8.

109. Pedersen BK, Febbraio MA. Muscle as an endocrine organ: focus on muscle-derived interleukin-6. Physiol Rev. 2008;88(4):1379–406.

110. Petersen AMW, Pedersen BK. The anti-inflammatory effect of exercise. J Appl Physiol. 2005;98(4): 1154–62.

111. Phillips CM, Dillon C, Harrington JM, et al. Defining metabolically healthy obesity: role of dietary and lifestyle factors. PLoS One. 2013;8(10):e76188.

112. Pradhan AD, Manson JE, Buring JE, et al. C-reactive protein, interleukin 6, and risk of developing type 2 diabetes mellitus. JAMA. 2001;286(3):327–34.

113. Reynolds CM, McGillicuddy FC, Harford KA, et al. Dietary saturated fatty acids prime the NLRP3 inflammasome via TLR4 in dendritic cells-implications for diet-induced insulin resistance. Mol Nutr Food Res. 2012;56(8):1212–22.

114. Rhee EJ, Lee MK, Kim JD, et al. Metabolic health is a more important determinant for diabetes development than simple obesity: a 4-year retrospective longitudinal study. PLoS One. 2014;9(5):1–8.

115. Roden M, Price TB, Perseghin G, et al. Mechanism of free fatty acid-induced insulin resistance in humans. J Clin Invest. 1996;97(12):2859–65.

116. Rothman DL, Shulman RG, Shulman GI. 31P nuclear magnetic resonance measurements of muscle glucose-6-phosphate: evidence for reduced insulin-dependent muscle glucose transport or phosphorylation activity in non-insulin-dependent diabetes mellitus. J Clin Invest. 1992;89(4):1069–75.

117. Saito M, Okamatsu-ogura Y, Matsushita M, et al. High incidence of metabolically active brown adipose effects of cold exposure and adiposity. Diabetes. 2009;58(July):1526–31.

118. Sallusto F, Lanzavecchia A. Efficient presentation of soluble antigen by cultured human dendritic cells is maintained by granulocyte/macrophage colony-stimulating factor plus interleukin 4 and down-regulated by tumor necrosis factor A. J Exp Med. 1994;179(4):1109–18.

119. Samuel VT, Petersen KF, Shulman GI. Lipid-induced insulin resistance: unravelling the mechanism. Lancet. 2010;375:2267–77.

120. Schenk S, Horowitz JF. Acute exercise increases triglyceride synthesis in skeletal muscle and prevents

fatty acid-induced insulin resistance. J Clin Invest. 2007;117(6):1690–8.

121. Seijkens T, Kusters P, Chatzigeorgiou A, et al. Immune cell crosstalk in obesity: a key role for costimulation? Diabetes. 2014;63(12):3982–91.

122. Sethi JK, Vidal-Puig AJ. Thematic review series: adipocyte biology. Adipose tissue function and plasticity orchestrate nutritional adaptation. J Lipid Res. 2007;48(6):1253–62.

123. Shi H, Kokoeva MV, Inouye K, et al. TLR4 links innate immunity and fatty acid-induced insulin resistance. J Clin Invest. 2006;116(11):3015–25.

124. Shulman GI. On diabetes: insulin resistance cellular mechanisms of insulin resistance. J Clin Invest. 2000;106(2):171–6.

125. Singh S, Aggarwal BB. Activation of transcription factor NF-kappa B is suppressed by curcumin (diferuloylmethane) [corrected]. J Biol Chem. 1995;270(42):24995–5000.

126. Spranger J, Kroke A, Mohlig M, et al. Inflammatory cytokines and the risk to develop type 2 diabetes: results of the prospective population-based European Prospective Investigation into Cancer and Nutrition (EPIC)-Potsdam Study. Diabetes. 2003;52(3):812–7.

127. Stefanovic-Racic M, Yang X, Turner MS, et al. Dendritic cells promote macrophage infiltration and comprise a substantial proportion of obesity-associated increases in CD11c+ cells in adipose tissue and liver. Diabetes. 2012;61(9):2330–9.

128. Strowig T, Henao-Mejia J, Elinav E, et al. Inflammasomes in health and disease. Nature. 2012;481(7381):278–86.

129. Tabak AG, Herder C, Rathmann W, Brunner EJ, Kivimaki M. Prediabetes: a high-risk state for diabetes development. Lancet. 2012;379(9833):2279–90. England.

130. Talukdar S, Oh DY, Bandyopadhyay G, et al. Neutrophils mediate insulin resistance in mice fed a high-fat diet through secreted elastase. Nat Med. 2012;18(9): 1407–12. Nature Publishing Group.

131. Tanti J-F, Jager J. Cellular mechanisms of insulin resistance: role of stress-regulated serine kinases and insulin receptor substrates (IRS) serine phosphorylation. Curr Opin Pharmacol. 2009;9(6):753–62.

132. Tchkonia T, Tchoukalova YD, Giorgadze N, et al. Abundance of two human preadipocyte subtypes with distinct capacities for replication, adipogenesis, and apoptosis varies among fat depots. Am J Physiol Endocrinol Metab. 2005;288(1):E267–77.

133. Tierney AC, McMonagle J, Shaw DI, et al. Effects of dietary fat modification on insulin sensitivity and on other risk factors of the metabolic syndrome – LIPGENE: a European randomized dietary intervention study. Int J Obes (Lond). 2011;35(6):800–9. England.

134. Tuncman G, Hirosumi J, Solinas G, et al. Functional in vivo interactions between JNK1 and JNK2

isoforms in obesity and insulin resistance. Proc Natl Acad Sci U S A. 2006;103(28):10741–6.

135. Turnbaugh PJ, Ley RE, Mahowald MA, et al. An obesity-associated gut microbiome with increased capacity for energy harvest. Nature. 2006;444(7122):1027–31. England.

136. Turner RC, Cull CA, Frighi V, et al. Glycemic control with diet, sulfonylurea, metformin, or insulin in patients with type 2 diabetes mellitus: progressive requirement for multiple therapies (UKPDS 49). UK Prospective Diabetes Study (UKPDS) Group. JAMA. 1999;281:2005–12.

137. Ueki K, Kondo T, Kahn CR. Suppressor of cytokine signaling 1 (SOCS-1) and SOCS-3 cause insulin resistance through inhibition of tyrosine phosphorylation of insulin receptor substrate proteins by discrete mechanisms. Mol Cell Biol. 2004;24(12):5434–46.

138. Van den Berg SM, Seijkens TTP, Kusters PJH, et al. Blocking CD40-TRAF6 interactions by small-molecule inhibitor 6860766 ameliorates the complications of diet-induced obesity in mice. Int J Obes. 2014;39(5):782.

139. Verschuren L, Wielinga PY, van Duyvenvoorde W, et al. A dietary mixture containing fish oil, resveratrol, lycopene, catechins, and vitamins E and C reduces atherosclerosis in transgenic mice. J Nutr. 2011;141(5):863–9. United States.

140. Vijay-Kumar M, Aitken JD, Carvalho FA, et al. Metabolic syndrome and altered gut microbiota in mice lacking Toll-like receptor 5. Science. 2010;328(5975):228–31.

141. Wegner M, Winiarska H, Bobkiewicz-Kozłowska T, et al. IL-12 serum levels in patients with type 2 diabetes treated with sulphonylureas. Cytokine. 2008;42(3):312–6.

142. Weisberg SP, McCann D, Desai M, et al. Obesity is associated with macrophage accumulation. J Clin Invest. 2003;112(12):1796–808.

143. Weisberg SP, Hunter D, Huber R, et al. CCR2 modulates inflammatory and metabolic effects of high-fat feeding. J Clin Invest. 2006;116(1):115–24.

144. Wen H, Gris D, Lei Y, et al. Fatty acid-induced NLRP3-ASC inflammasome activation interferes with insulin signaling. Nat Immunol. 2011;12(5): 408–15.

145. Wernstedt Asterholm I, Tao C, Morley TS, et al. Adipocyte inflammation is essential for healthy adipose tissue expansion and remodeling. Cell Metab. 2014;20(1):103–18.

146. WHO/IDF. Definition and diagnosis of diabetes mellitus and intermediate hyperglycaemia: report of a WHO/IDF consultation. Geneva: World Health Organization; 2006.

147. Winer S, Chan Y, Paltser G, et al. Normalization of obesity-associated insulin resistance through immunotherapy. Nat Med. 2009;15(8):921–9.

148. Wu J, Boström P, Sparks LM, et al. Beige adipocytes are a distinct type of thermogenic fat cell in mouse and human. Cell. 2012;150(2):366–76.

149. Xu H, Barnes GT, Yang Q, et al. Chronic inflammation in fat plays a crucial role in the development of obesity-related insulin resistance. J Clin Invest. 2003;112(12):1821–30.

150. Yamauchi T, Kamon J, Waki H, et al. The fat-derived hormone adiponectin reverses insulin resistance associated with both lipoatrophy and obesity. Nat Med. 2001;7(8):941–6.

151. Yan Y, Jiang W, Spinetti T, et al. Omega-3 fatty acids prevent inflammation and metabolic disorder through inhibition of NLRP3 inflammasome activation. Immunity. 2013;38(6):1154–63.

152. Yang F, Oz HS, Barve S, et al. The green tea polyphenol(−)-epigallocatechin-3-gallate blocks nuclear factor-kappa B activation by inhibiting I kappa B kinase activity in the intestinal epithelial cell line IEC-6. Mol Pharmacol. 2001;60(3):528–33.

153. Ye J. Regulation of PPARy function by TNF-alpha. Biochem Biophys Res Commun. 2009;374(3):405–8.

154. Yki-Järvinen H. Thiazolidinediones. N Engl J Med. 2004;351:1106–18.

155. Zahorska-Markiewicz B, Janowska J, Olszanecka-Glinianowicz M, et al. Serum concentrations of TNF- a and soluble TNF- a receptors in obesity. Int J Obes. 2000;24:1392–5.

156. Zeng L, Tang WJ, Yin JJ, et al. Signal transductions and nonalcoholic fatty liver: a mini-review. Int J Clin Exp Med. 2014;7(7):1624–31.

157. Zhou G, Myers R, Li Y, et al. Role of AMP-activated protein kinase in mechanism of metformin action. J Clin Invest. 2001;108(8):1167–74.

Circadian Rhythms and Metabolism

24

Edith Grosbellet and Etienne Challet

Contents

Abstract

The circadian system relies on a master clock in the suprachiasmatic nucleus (SCN) of the hypothalamus, synchronizing a multitude of brain and peripheral oscillators that set physiological and metabolic functions in phase with the light-dark cycle. The SCN functions as a relay integrating environmental signals before sending appropriate neuronal and hormonal signals to the brain and peripheral tissues to control, among others, sleep/wake and feeding/fasting cycles. Studies show that the circadian system and metabolism are tightly

E. Grosbellet · E. Challet (✉)
Institute of Cellular and Integrative Neurosciences,
UPR3212, CNRS, University of Strasbourg, Strasbourg,
France
e-mail: challet@inci-cnrs.unistra.fr

© Springer Nature Switzerland AG 2023
R. S. Ahima (ed.), *Metabolic Syndrome*,
https://doi.org/10.1007/978-3-031-40116-9_32

interconnected. Peripheral oscillators in the liver and adipose tissue can be shifted by meal timing. In contrast, feeding signals do not affect the master clock under light-dark conditions, although nutritional cues affect its functioning under metabolic challenges, such as calorie restriction and high-fat diet. Circadian desynchronization, such as shift-work and chronic jet-lag, is now recognized as a determinant of metabolic disturbances. Therefore, chronotherapeutic approaches of daily dieting to avoid circadian misalignment are important for the management of obesity and type 2 diabetes.

Keywords

Circadian rhythm · Clock gene · Feeding time · Desynchronization · Metabolic disturbances · Obesity · Diabetes

Introduction

Every day we experience rhythms of our physiological functions and behaviors, which follow the 24-h light-dark cycle due to the rotation of Earth around its axis. For instance, we are awake and eat during daytime, while we sleep during the night. Our body temperature drops every night and most of our hormones are secreted at particular times of day, e.g., melatonin released from the pineal gland during the night, and peak cortisol levels in the morning. As detailed in this chapter, daily rhythms are not passive responses to the changing outside world, but are controlled by a network of endogenous circadian clocks and oscillators. Here, we will focus on the relationships between circadian system and metabolism. After presenting the organization of the circadian system and its involvement in metabolism, we will describe the nature of signals synchronizing peripheral oscillators, thus ensuring the circadian control of metabolism. The last section presents pathological situations in which circadian disruption lead to metabolic dysfunction, and vice versa.

A Network of Clocks and Oscillators Ensuring the Circadian Control of Metabolism

The Master Clock in the Suprachiasmatic Nucleus

In mammals, the daily variations of physiological functions and behaviors are controlled by a multi-oscillatory network that generates internal daily oscillations and adjusts their timing to external temporal cues, such as the 24-h variations in ambient light. At the top of this circadian network, a master clock, located in the suprachiasmatic nucleus of the hypothalamus (SCN), adjusts the timing of secondary clocks and oscillators in other brain regions and peripheral tissues, via neural and hormonal signals [1].

The clock mechanism in the SCN involves 24-h oscillations of core clock components, called clock genes and defined as genes whose protein products are necessary for the generation and regulation of circadian rhythms within individual cells [2]. The heterodimer CLOCK/BMAL1 stimulates expression of essential clock components PERs and CRYs which, after a delay, repress the transcriptional activity of the CLOCK/BMAL1 heterodimer by inhibiting its binding to their own promoters. This main loop is responsible for oscillations of PER and CRY proteins. CLOCK/BMAL1 also stimulates expression of other clock-related proteins, such as REV-ERBα and RORα, which create auxiliary loops that help stabilizing the main loop (Fig. 1). The circadian transcription factors control the temporal transcription of numerous downstream, clock-controlled genes, which constitute outputs of the molecular clock and are involved in a large variety of biological processes. Many levels of regulation are important for the proper functioning of the circadian clock, including epigenetic, transcriptional, post-transcriptional and post-translational mechanisms. Together, these regulatory mechanisms provide robust oscillations, resilient to large fluctuations in temperature (the so-called temperature compensation) and overall transcriptions rates [1].

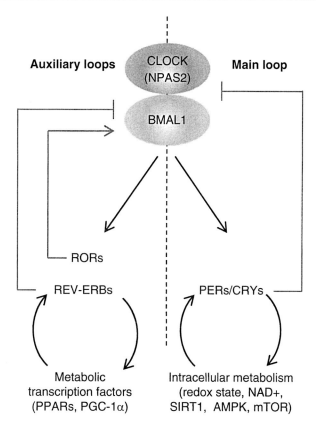

Fig. 1 Molecular clockwork and its interactions with cellular metabolism

The mammalian molecular clockwork consists of a set of clock genes and their protein products that generate 24-h feedback loops of transcription and translation. Main loop: The heterodimer CLOCK/BMAL1 stimulates the expression of core clock components *Pers* and *Crys*, which in turn repress the transcriptional activity of the CLOCK/BMAL1 heterodimer by inhibiting its binding to the E-box response elements located in their own promoters, through formation of a complex with the casein kinase 1ε and δ. Auxiliary loop: CLOCK/BMAL1 also stimulates expression of other clock-related proteins, such as REV–ERBs and RORs, which create an auxiliary loop that helps stabilize the main regulatory loop. Ouputs of the clock: These circadian transcription factors control numerous clock-controlled genes to influence a variety of biological activities. The molecular clockwork interacts with intracellular metabolism via redox changes, PPARs, SIRT1, AMPK, and mTOR. AMPK: 5′ adenosine monophosphate-activated protein kinase; BMAL1: brain-muscle-arnt-like protein 1; CLOCK circadian locomotor output cycle kaput, CRY cryptochrome, mTOR mammalian/mechanistic target of rapamycin, NAD+ nicotinamide adenine dinucleotide, NPAS2 neuronal PAS domain protein 2, PER period, PGC-1α (alpha) PPARγ (gamma) coactivator-1α (alpha), PPAR peroxisome proliferator-activated receptor, ROR retinoic acid receptor-related orphan nuclear receptor REV–ERB reverse viral erythroblastis oncogene product, SIRT1 sirtuin 1. (Data from [2, 45, 94, 96, 97, 101])

In the absence of environmental inputs, the master clock "free-runs" with a period close to, but not exactly, 24 h. Therefore, biological rhythms need to be synchronized to the day-night cycle, which represents the most important environmental cue for the majority of living organisms. The resetting effects of light on circadian rhythms depend on the time of light exposure. For a nocturnal rodent, light in early and late night produces phase delays and advances, respectively, while light during most of day has no effect on the phase of the SCN clock.

Light is perceived in the retina by classical photoreceptors and a subset of ganglion cells that are photosensitive because they express a photopigment called the melanopsin, highly responsive to blue light stimulation [3]. These ganglion cells project via the retino-hypothalamic tract to the ventral SCN, where they release mainly glutamate and the neuropeptide pituitary adenylate cyclase-activating protein (PACAP) [4]. The downstream signaling pathway in ventral SCN cells induces acute expression of clock genes *Per1* and *Per2*, together with several immediate early genes such as *c-fos* [4].

The retino-hypothalamic tract also projects to the thalamic intergeniculate leaflets (IGL). From the IGL, the geniculohypothalamic tract projects to the SCN and can thus indirectly convey light information by releasing neuropeptide Y (NPY), γ-aminobutyric acid (GABA), and enkephalin [5]. Other structures can also convey indirect light information to the SCN. Arousal-promoting orexigenic neurons of the lateral hypothalamic area (LH), for instance, are a target of retinal projections [3] and project in turn to the immediate vicinity of the SCN [6].

Even if the light is the most important time-giver (also called *Zeitgeber* in chronobiology), other temporal cycling cues called "non-photic," such as food availability, temperature, or stimulated locomotor activity, are putative synchronizers. Two major input pathways convey non-photic messages to the SCN: the NPY-ergic

projection from the IGL, also transmitting photic information, and the serotonergic input from the midbrain raphe nuclei [5, 7]. Beside a possible direct action of metabolic cues on SCN cells, the pathways conveying feeding and metabolic cues to the SCN may involve nuclei of the mediobasal hypothalamus, such as arcuate nucleus (ARC) and ventromedial hypothalamic nucleus (VMH), which could integrate metabolic information and energy status before projecting to the SCN [8] (Fig. 2).

In summary, the SCN is a robust clock, whose self-sustained rhythmicity, relying on molecular transcriptional-translational feedback loops, is synchronized by photic and non-photic synchronizers and distributed to the whole organism.

Central Clocks and Oscillators

SCN and Extra-SCN Oscillators

Many brain areas exhibit daily oscillations of clock genes [1, 9]. Retina and olfactory bulb are extra-SCN oscillators fulfilling all the criteria to be considered as circadian clocks [10], i.e., self-sustained oscillations compensated for

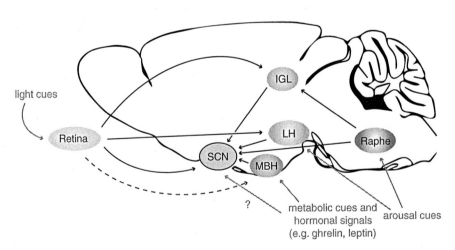

Fig. 2 Main afferent pathways to the master clock in rodents

Structures conveying directly or indirectly light information to the SCN are in yellow (retina) and orange (IGL and LH). The raphe nuclei (red) convey non-photic information to the master clock, while the IGL receives both photic and non-photic cues. The MBH (green) integrates metabolic signals and possibly photic cues. IGL intergeniculatse leaflet of the thalamus, LH lateral hypothalamic area, SCN suprachiasmatic nucleus, MBH mediobasal hypothalamus (i.e., arcuate and ventromedial hypothalamic nuclei). (Data from [3, 7, 8, 115])

temperature and reset by environmental inputs, and outputs distributed out of the structure. Some other brain areas have been classified as semiautonomous, such as ARC and dorsomedial hypothalamic nucleus (DMH), both structures of the medial hypothalamus involved in feeding and energy metabolism [10]. Cells of these oscillators exhibit independent circadian rhythms but appear less coupled in vitro than SCN cells. Moreover, their timing of clock gene oscillations differ from SCN. For example, in rat, the peak of *Per1* mRNA in ARC occurs at dusk, i.e., 6 h later than in SCN, while *Per2* mRNA is delayed by 4 h [11]. The slave oscillators are independently arrhythmic but can provide a circadian output totally dependent on inputs from clocks or semiautonomous oscillators [10]. For example, the LH and hypothalamic paraventricular nucleus (PVN) display a rapid dampening of rhythmicity of *Per1-luc* expression in vitro [12]. Of note, the core clock mechanism in brain oscillators is similar to the SCN. However, NPAS2, a paralog of CLOCK that dimerizes with BMAL1, may replace CLOCK in the mammalian forebrain [13].

Entrainment of Brain Oscillators by Inputs from SCN

The SCN efferents terminate in few brain sites, mainly limited to hypothalamus and thalamus. Within the hypothalamus, the SCN projects most densely to the subparaventricular zone (sPVZ). Of interest for the present topic are the projections of the SCN on hypothalamic nuclei involved in energy balance, referred as "metabolic hypothalamus," receiving SCN input directly or via polysynaptic relays (principally via the sPVZ). Pre-autonomic neurons in PVN and arousal-promoting orexin neurons in the LH are controlled by a daily balance between glutamatergic and GABAergic inputs from the SCN [14]. Neurosecretory corticotrophin-releasing factor neurons in PVN, involved in hypothalamic-pituitary-adrenal regulation, are inhibited by vasopressinergic SCN inputs in nocturnal rodents. GABAergic and vasopressinergic SCN neurons project also on DMH, a key site for integration of circadian timing into numerous physiological processes [14] (Fig. 3). Moreover, dopaminergic neurons of the semiautonomous oscillator ARC, which

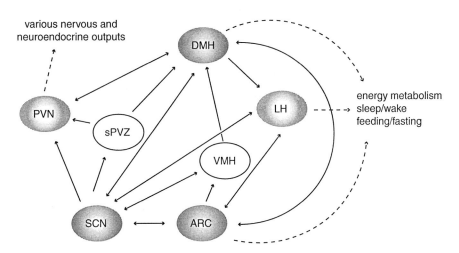

Fig. 3 Intra-hypothalamic network connecting the master clock and nuclei involved in the regulation of energy metabolism and feeding rhythm
Nuclei of metabolic hypothalamus are interconnected and share reciprocal connections with the SCN. This network of hypothalamic oscillators is supposed to be involved in circadian control of feeding and energy metabolism. The SCN clock is in red, semiautonomous oscillators are in blue and slave oscillators in green. Solid arrows represent direct neuronal connections, while dashed arrows represent indirect outputs. SCN suprachiasmatic nucleus, ARC arcuate nucleus, VMH ventromedial hypothalamic nucleus, DMH dorsomedial hypothalamic nucleus, sPVZ subparaventricular zone, PVN paraventricular hypothalamic nucleus, LH lateral hypothalamic area. (Data from [8, 27, 115, 151])

express rhythmic clock genes, are directly regulated by SCN neurons containing vasoactive intestinal peptide [15, 16]. Finally, it is also noteworthy that nervous outputs from the SCN are not required for the establishment of locomotor activity rhythms [17], suggesting the presence of paracrine factors diffusing from SCN cells and controlling rhythmic activity. At least three diffusible circadian factors have been identified, i.e., transforming growth factor-α, prokineticin 2, and cardiotropin-like cytokine [18].

Outputs of Brain Oscillators for the Feeding/Fasting Cycle

Circadian oscillations in the hypothalamus influence many physiological processes and behaviors such as reproductive cycle, thermoregulation, sexual and maternal behavior, stress-related responses, and food intake. Circadian oscillations in hypothalamic nuclei may ensure the expression of appropriate behaviors at appropriate times of the day, thus avoiding the disadvantageous expression of multiple and incompatible behaviors at the same time, like sleep and food intake [10].

Lesions in the SCN abolish rhythmic behaviors, including the feeding rhythm [19]. However, the feeding/fasting cycle is not a passive consequence of the sleep/wake cycle and likely involves the circadian timing of nuclei in the metabolic hypothalamus. The direct projections from SCN to these nuclei may provide a first gating of feeding responses. We will further focus on the ARC and DMH, key structures for regulation of energy balance and food intake [20]. The ARC contains neurons sensitive to circulating nutrients (e.g., glucose-sensing neurons)[21] and to feeding-related hormones, e.g., leptin, secreted from adipose tissue [22]. This integration of peripheral energetic information constitutes a homeostatic feedback loop (Fig. 3). Moreover, the ARC oscillator is involved in the daily variations in hunger feeling and the integration of leptinergic signals [23].

Two populations of ARC neurons express neuropeptides oppositely involved in regulation of feeding. Neuropeptide Y (NPY) and agouti-related peptide (AgRP) are orexigenic, while pro-opiomelanocortin (POMC) and cocaine and amphetamine regulated transcript (CART) are anorexigenic. These neuropeptides are rhythmically synthesized in the ARC [24–26]. The DMH is important for the integration of circadian rhythms into various physiological functions and behaviors, due to its wide afferent and efferent connections to hypothalamic (e.g., PVN, ARC, and LH) and extra-hypothalamic sites [27]. By its circadian oscillations, sensitivity to feeding-related cues and involvement in homeostatic regulation of food intake, the DMH could thus be a key structure in the hypothalamic network controlling rhythms in feeding behavior (Fig. 3). In addition, the PVN oscillator participates in the daily rhythmicity of energy metabolism [28].

Because peripheral tissues involved in metabolism harbor circadian oscillators, it is essential for the circadian regulation of energy balance to consider their oscillatory characteristics and their crosstalk with the CNS circuits.

Peripheral Oscillators

The vast majority of cells in peripheral tissues contain the molecular clock machinery [29, 30]. Bioluminescent constructs allowed the real-time visualization of clock genes oscillations, both in vitro [31] and in vivo [32]. Some peripheral tissues can exhibit self-sustained oscillations for several days, but the coupling is weaker than in the SCN clock. Moreover, as in the SCN clock, the period of peripheral oscillators is resilient to large fluctuations in temperature and overall transcription rates, as shown in cultured fibroblasts [33]. They also exhibit circadian outputs, as exemplified below. Circadian transcriptome profiling studies reveal that around 10% of a tissue's transcriptome has a circadian pattern of expression [34]. Moreover, the peripheral oscillators are entrained by neuronal and endocrine signals emanating from the SCN, or indirectly by SCN-controlled behavioral rhythms, e.g., feeding/fasting and sleep/wake cycles.

Outputs of Peripheral Oscillators

Rhythmically expressed genes control a multitude of physiological functions. For example, they encode key enzymes involved in hepatic metabolism of fatty acids, cholesterol, bile acids, amino acids and xenobiotics [35], and control adipogenesis and lipid metabolism in adipose tissue [36]. The rhythmic physiological outputs of peripheral tissues result from signals emanating from the SCN and/or from local peripheral oscillators. Specific inactivation of the clock gene *Bmal1* in the liver of mice (L-*Bmal1*$^{-/-}$) disrupts rhythmic expression of genes involved in glucose metabolism, as well as rhythmic circulating glucose levels. During their resting phase, L-*Bmal1*$^{-/-}$ mice display mild hypoglycemia, suggesting that the daily rhythm of hepatic glucose export driven by the liver clock counterbalances the brain-driven fasting–feeding cycle [37].

Adipose tissue also exhibits robust oscillations of core clock components, controlling the circadian expression of many transcription factors [38, 39]. Moreover, adipose tissue secretes several hormones termed adipokines, including leptin and adiponectin, involved in the regulation of energy balance [22]. Ando et al. [39] showed a rhythmic expression of several adipokine genes. Circulating levels of leptin display clear diurnal variations in both rodents and humans [40–42]. Moreover, leptin secretion is rhythmic in cultured adipocytes [43]. These results strongly suggest that rhythmic expression of adipokines is under control of the adipose clock, although the underlying mechanisms are still unclear.

Another example is the pancreas in which specific inactivation of the clock gene *Bmal1* leads to glucose intolerance and hyposecretion of insulin, highlighting the importance of the pancreatic clock in glucose homeostasis [44].

Circadian Control of Metabolism at Molecular Level

The link between molecular clock and metabolism may be provided either by metabolic functions of clock genes (i.e., pleiotropy of clock genes) or by the involvement of clock-controlled genes. Both mechanisms seem to exist, involving many nuclear receptors, such as REV-ERBs and RORs (components of the molecular clockwork) and peroxisome proliferator-activated receptors (PPARs, clock-controlled proteins)[45]. RORα (alpha) directly regulates genes involved in the fatty acid metabolism of skeletal muscles [46]. Moreover, REV-ERBα (alpha) is important for the daily variations of fuel utilization [47] and plays a pivotal role in the interface between liver clock and lipid metabolism. PPARs are members of the steroid/nuclear receptor superfamily, acting as ligand-activated transcription factors. *Ppara* (alpha), a clock-controlled gene whose activation requires CLOCK, is rhythmically expressed in tissues with a high rate of fatty acid catabolism (e.g., muscles, heart or liver), and is involved in lipoprotein and lipid metabolism [48, 49]. *Ppara* is therefore recognized as a strong link between circadian clocks and lipid metabolism in peripheral tissues [45]. Furthermore, as demonstrated by lipidomic profiling in adipose tissue, PER2 is important for normal lipid metabolism. This effect is mediated by PPARγ (gamma), a master regulator of adipogenesis and lipid metabolism in adipose tissue, whose transcriptional activity is directly inhibited by PER2 [50] (Fig. 1). To ensure a proper control of circadian metabolism, central and peripheral clocks need to be phase-adjusted. The next section describes the nature of signals synchronizing peripheral oscillators. First, we consider neural and hormonal signals emanating from the SCN, acting as a relay between environmental synchronizers and peripheral tissues. Then, we present the resetting effects of nutritional cues.

Nature of Signals Synchronizing Peripheral Oscillators

Entrainment by Nervous Outputs from the SCN

SCN Controls Glucose Metabolism

The daily rhythmicity of plasma glucose, peaking before the onset of activity in rats, is not a passive response to the feeding/fasting cycle [51]. The liver plays a pivotal role in glycemic regulation, as a site of glucose uptake and a major source of glucose production [52]. Glucose homeostasis requires both functional hepatic and SCN clocks [37, 51]. Besides SCN lesion, glucose rhythm can also be disturbed by inactivation of either sympathetic or parasympathetic inputs [53], underlying the importance of balanced inputs from the SCN via the autonomous nervous system (ANS). The actual model is that rhythmic GABAergic input from the SCN inhibits the sympathetic and parasympathetic pre-autonomic neurons of the PVN, predominantly during the day. In contrast, glutamatergic projections from the SCN stimulate sympathetic pre-autonomic neurons of the PVN [52]. Thus, the entrainment of circadian glucose rhythm is controlled by the SCN, fine-tuning the balance between both branches of the ANS innervating the liver clock (Fig. 4). Moreover, hypothalamic orexin is a key regulator of plasma glucose, being particularly the main effector of the peak occurring before the activity phase. Sympathetic denervation of the liver prevented the stimulatory effect of orexin on glucose levels,

suggesting that orexin translates SCN-derived GABAergic rhythms into glucose rhythm via the sympathetic nervous system [54].

SCN and the Adipose Tissue

Adipose tissue is densely innervated by sympathetic fibers whose activation stimulates lipolysis. Parasympathetic innervation of adipose tissue has been shown more recently [55]. As for the liver, the SCN controls both branches of ANS innervating adipose tissues, modulating the rhythmic outputs of the adipose clock. For example, the activity of hormone-sensitive lipase, exhibiting a daily rhythmicity, is increased by 50% in adipose tissue selectively denervated for the parasympathetic input [55]. Moreover, leptin rhythm is under the control of both local adipose clock [43] and the master SCN clock since SCN lesions suppress the daily rhythm of plasma leptin in rats [41].

By modulating the autonomous innervation of liver and adipose clocks, the SCN controls the circadian rhythmicity of metabolites (carbohydrates

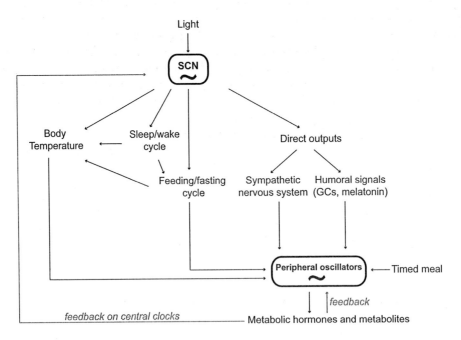

Fig. 4 Functional organization of the circadian timing system

The master clock in the SCN is mostly reset by ambient light. Extra-SCN oscillators in the brain (not shown) and in peripheral tissues are phase-controlled by cues from the SCN and by timed feeding. The SCN clock transmits temporal cues to peripheral oscillators via "direct" outputs

using nervous and hormonal pathways, and indirectly via behavioral (i.e., feeding/fasting and sleep/wake cycles) and physiological (i.e., body temperature cycle) rhythmic signals. In turn, peripheral oscillators release rhythmically metabolic hormones and metabolites that feedback to central and peripheral oscillatory structures. SCN suprachiasmatic nucleus, GCs glucocorticoids. (Based on [1, 8])

and lipids) and metabolic hormones (e.g., leptin). However, some peripheral clocks do not respond directly or only to nervous cues. Glucocorticoids (GC) and melatonin, whose rhythmic release is driven by the SCN via nervous pathways, can in turn entrain many peripheral oscillators.

Entrainment by Hormonal Outputs: Glucocorticoids and Melatonin

Glucocorticoids (GCs) show a strong circadian rhythm, their secretion from the adrenal glands peaking around wake-up time (morning in humans and evening in nocturnal rodents). Different actors are involved in the circadian rhythmicity of GCs secretion. The SCN drives GCs rhythm via the hypothalamo-pituitary-adrenal axis and modulates the daily sensitivity of adrenal gland to ACTH via splanchnic fibers [56]. Furthermore, the local adrenal clock gates the sensitivity of the adrenal gland to ACTH, therefore modulating the secretion of GCs throughout the day [57]. The GC nuclear receptor is expressed in virtually all cell types in periphery and the brain, except in adult SCN cells [58]. Activated GC receptors act as transcription factors, via direct activation or repression of various target genes [59]. Around 60% of rhythmic transcriptome in mouse liver, mostly genes involved in metabolism, lose their rhythmicity after adrenalectomy, while expression of clock genes is hardly affected [60]. Dexamethasone, a glucocorticoid receptor agonist, activates *Per1* expression and synchronizes rat fibroblasts in vitro [61]. In the same study, dexamethasone was shown to phase-shift peripheral clocks (liver, kidney, and heart), but not SCN clock, in vivo. Thus, glucocorticoids possess clock-resetting properties and represent a robust phase-entrainment signal from the SCN (Fig. 4).

Melatonin is derived from the amino acid tryptophan and secreted from the pineal gland always during the dark phase, either in nocturnal or diurnal mammals. The rhythmic release of melatonin is driven by SCN clock and acts an internal daily time-giver [62] (Fig. 4). Of interest for the circadian control of metabolism, MT1 and MT2 melatonin receptors are present in pancreatic islets [63].

Simple and double knock-out mice for MT1 and MT1/MT2 exhibit an upregulation of insulin secretion, highlighting a negative action of melatonin signaling on insulin secretion [64]. Moreover, melatonin applied on isolated islets, for 2 h at the maximum of the circadian insulin rhythm, induces a 9-h phase-advance of the insulin rhythm [65]. Genetic studies in humans have correlated the presence of an allele variant of the melatonin receptor in the pancreatic islets, hyperglycemia, and impaired early-phase insulin secretion [66]. Thus, the homeostatic and circadian effects of melatonin on insulin secretion provide a framework for further investigations into type 2 diabetes.

Coupling the SCN to Peripheral Oscillators in Diurnal and Nocturnal Species

At the cellular level in peripheral clocks involved in metabolism, anticipation of metabolic pathways optimizes food processing. Peripheral clocks also sequester chemically incompatible reactions (e.g., gluconeogenesis and glycolysis in liver) to different time windows and limit metabolic processes with adverse side effects to times when they are needed. At physiological level, the subtle differences in how peripheral clocks are phased by the master clock allow different organs to synchronize their functions. At behavioral level, circadian rhythms allow organisms to anticipate and thus adapt to daily environmental variations. Of interest, phases of clock genes oscillations and their photic entrainment in the SCN are similar between nocturnal and diurnal species [67, 68], while their respective phase of circadian gene expression in peripheral tissues is opposite, for example, in the liver [69]. Therefore, the signals emanating from the SCN are differentially interpreted at downstream targets. One possible mechanism would be differences in polysynaptic relays conveying SCN outputs to peripheral targets. The SCN releases vasopressin on inter-neurons of PVN during daytime. The targeted interneurons are excitatory in nocturnal rodents, while inhibitory in diurnal rodents (such as Sudanian grass rat, *Arvicanthis ansorgei*), leading to an opposite phased release of GCs between nocturnal and diurnal species [70]. Furthermore, several species can even switch between nocturnal and diurnal patterns of behaviors. These switches may rely on modifications of polysynaptic relays from SCN to periphery, highlighting the adaptive value of the multistage organization of circadian timing.

Adjusting Clocks with Metabolism

Extra-SCN Clocks Are Entrained by Feeding Time

Among the different ways used by the SCN to synchronize peripheral clocks, the daily rhythm in spontaneous food intake is a strong *Zeitgeber* for many tissues. In normal conditions, food ingestion is in phase with activity period. Daytime restricted feeding in nocturnal rodents (i.e., when food is available few hours during the day, corresponding to the usual resting period) inverts the phase of gene expression in peripheral organs within about a week, thereby uncoupling peripheral clocks from the SCN [71, 72] (Fig. 4).

In the brain, food restriction entrains the activity of numerous oscillating structures. For example, the multineuronal activity in LH and VMH of rats under restricted feeding shows a peak entrained to the time of feeding [73]. Moreover, daily oscillations of clock genes and proteins in various brain areas, such as the cerebral cortex or the striatum, from mice entrained to daytime restricted feeding also show phase-shifts with peaks around mealtime, different from the nocturnal peaks of expression in animals fed *ad libitum* [9, 74]. These data suggest that clocks within and outside of the brain are affected by restricted feeding schedules.

The effects of food on the circadian system involve a specific clock mechanism, the food-entrainable oscillator (FEO). Under restricted feeding, several components of physiological and metabolic functions become entrained to the availability of food (e.g., anticipatory bouts of locomotor activity, and rises in body temperature and GC release), and some of them, such as the food-anticipatory activity, are still evident in SCN-lesioned animals. This implies the existence of the FEO, located outside of the SCN. The location and mechanisms of the FEO have been the subject of much controversy. Most evidence supports the fact that FEO is a network of neural sites in the hypothalamus and brainstem, which interact to provide timing and behavioral entrainment of feeding [75].

Mechanisms of Entrainment of Extra-SCN Clocks by Food

The nature of signals that arise from feeding and entrain peripheral clocks has been an area of intense research. It is now established that feeding cues include food itself, the increase of postprandial temperature, food-derived metabolites, metabolic hormones, and energetic status of cells.

Temperature Fluctuations

Variations in ambient temperature can entrain behavioral rhythms in ectothermic organisms such as flies, and temperature fluctuations mimicking body temperature rhythms sustain previously induced oscillations in cultured rat fibroblasts. In vivo, inverted environmental temperature cycles reverse circadian rhythms of clock genes (*Per2* and *Cry1*) in the liver without affecting the SCN in most mammals [76]. Thus, postprandial temperature elevation could be an entrainment pathway from feeding/fasting cycle in homeothermic organisms. Hepatic heat-shock factor 1 (HSF1), which exhibits a highly rhythmic activity that drives the expression of heat-shock proteins in liver, could be a key component linking temperature fluctuations to the phase of molecular clocks [77, 78] (Fig. 4).

Food-Related Hormones

Anorexigenic hormones (e.g., insulin, leptin) and orexigenic hormones (e.g., ghrelin) may participate in the entrainment of peripheral clocks by food intake. For example, insulin and insulin-like growth factor 1 (IGF1) cause an acute induction of *Per* mRNA and protein levels and phase-shift peripheral oscillators [79–82]. *Ob/ob* mice, genetically obese mice lacking functional leptin, display alterations in clock gene oscillations of peripheral clocks but not in SCN. Of interest, impairments of peripheral clocks appear in young 3-wk-old *ob/ob* mice, before appearance of metabolic disorders, and are partially improved by leptin treatment [83]. The mechanisms by which leptin would modulate peripheral clocks need further investigations. It may involve a direct action of leptin on peripheral oscillators, or a central action of leptin affecting peripheral tissues. For example, leptin is known to modulate various physiological processes in peripheral tissues via activation of sympathetic innervations [84, 85].

Other hormones that could participate in feeding entrainment in rodents are GCs. Restricted feeding in rats triggers an anticipatory rise of corticosterone in addition to the nocturnal rise controlled by the SCN [86], and corticosterone is known to entrain peripheral clocks. However, corticosterone injection failed to mimic the phase-shifting effects of feeding in rats [71]. Gene expression rhythm in the liver of adrenalectomized or GC receptor deficient mice is still entrained under food restriction, the phase-shifts being even faster in the absence of GCs [87]. Hence, the specific role of GCs in feeding entrainment is still unclear.

Metabolites (Lipids and Glucose)

In addition to their role in metabolism, nuclear receptors can regulate clock components, therefore participating in the pathway by which food intake entrains peripheral oscillators. The transcription factor PPARα is essential for lipid metabolism. After activation by fatty acids, PPARα directly binds to a response element in *Bmal1* promoter [88]. PPARα can also directly activate *Rev-erbα* expression, and PER2 is able to recruit PPARα and REV-ERBα to modulate *Bmal1* expression, highlighting the intimate reciprocal interactions between clock components and metabolism [89, 90]. Additionally, a coactivator of PPAR (PPARγ (gamma) coactivator-1α, stimulates *Bmal1* expression through coactivation of ROR proteins. Since PGC-1α (alpha) is sensitive to various signals including nutritional status, activity and temperature, and regulates energy metabolism in peripheral tissues, it could be a key component in the coupling of metabolism and clocks [91] (Fig. 1).

Per1 and *Per2* mRNA levels are downregulated after the addition of glucose in the culture medium of rat fibroblasts, while the expression of many other genes, including transcription factors, is upregulated. The glucose-induced decrease of *Per* mRNA levels seems to be mediated via glucose metabolism (involving transcriptional regulators) rather than glucose itself [92]. Thus, lipids and glucose can reset peripheral clocks and provide a mechanism for entrainment of peripheral clocks by feeding time.

Intracellular Redox State

CLOCK (or its paralog NPAS2), BMAL1, and/or PERs may directly sense energy-related signals through their PAS domain, by detecting the reduced or oxidized environment within the cell. Redox signals, closely tied to the energy status, are transduced by PAS domains, which modulate the functional state of the protein [93]. In vitro, the DNA-binding activity of the dimers CLOCK-BMAL1 and NPAS2-BMAL1 is altered by cellular redox status [94]. The reduced forms of the nicotinamide adenine dinucleotide, NADH and NADPH, activate DNA-binding of CLOCK (or NPAS2)-BMAL1, whereas their oxidized forms inhibit it. NAD(P)H/NAD(P)$^+$ ratio reflects mitochondrial activity and the switch between activation and inhibition of DNA-binding is very sensitive, providing a rapid mechanism, which could convey changes in feeding to the cellular clocks [94]. Sirtuin 1 (SIRT1), another energy sensor, links metabolism to circadian physiology. SIRT1 catalyzes the deacetylation of various substrates in NAD$^+$-dependent manner. By deacetylating histones, SIRT1 participates to epigenetic silencing by chromatin condensation. By deacetylating metabolic enzymes and transcription factors, SIRT1 contributes to multiple metabolic pathways, including gluconeogenesis, lipid metabolism, insulin secretion, and thermogenesis. Besides being a critical component of the longevity response to calorie restriction [95], SIRT1 is circadianly regulated. A specific deletion of SIRT1 in liver of mice shows its participation to circadian control in vivo [96]. SIRT1 influences the transcription of a number of clock genes and promotes deacetylation of PER2, thus modulating the phase of the clockwork [97]. In addition, 5′ adenosine monophosphate-activated protein kinase (AMPK) is another important metabolic fuel gauge, sensing changes in the AMP/ATP ratio. AMPK detects nutritional and hormonal signals in peripheral tissues and the hypothalamus [98]. As SIRT1, AMPK can directly impact the clockwork by phase-shifting peripheral oscillators [99, 100]. Furthermore, another essential intracellular factor, namely, mammalian/mechanistic target of rapamycin (mTOR), also regulates the period of the circadian clocks in the SCN and peripheral organs [101] (Fig. 1).

Coupling of cellular metabolism to the molecular clockwork in peripheral tissues has been intensely investigated, while less is known in central extra-SCN oscillators. Many mechanisms could be similar, including aforementioned sensors of energy and redox states. In particular, AMPK is a potent regulator of energy balance within the hypothalamus. For example, leptin inhibits specifically AMPK in ARC and PVN, and this inhibition is required to mediate anorexigenic and weight loss effects of leptin [98]. AMPK signaling is thus a likely route through which circadian and feeding signals are integrated in the hypothalamus [27].

Nutritional Cues and the Master Clock

Effects of Metabolic Signals on the Master Clock

While peripheral clocks are entrained by feeding time with great efficiency, the SCN clock seems impervious to the synchronizing effects of mealtime, provided that animals are exposed to a light-dark cycle and ingest enough daily energy [71, 72]. However, SCN can respond to feeding cues under specific calorie conditions. In particular, rats exposed to a light-dark cycle and entrained to restricted feeding coupled with a hypocaloric diet display phase advances for circadian rhythms of locomotor activity, body temperature, and melatonin in comparison to ad libitum

fed animals [102]. Entrainment to light-dark cycle is also altered in mice submitted to a timed hypocaloric feeding and their SCN clockwork is phase-advanced [103]. Conditions of low glucose availability can alter the circadian responses to light [104]. In the absence of photic cues (i.e., constant darkness), the mouse SCN can also entrain to regular scheduled feeding [105]. Under constant light conditions, leading to behavioral arrhythmicity in albino rats, scheduled feeding rescues both locomotor activity rhythm and clock gene oscillation in the SCN [106]. Free access to high fat also impacts on the master clock, as evidenced by lengthened free-running period in mice housed under constant darkness [107, 108]. In mice with free access to chow diet, a palatable food (chocolate) given every day at the same time entrains the SCN clock in constant darkness and reduces its circadian responses to light [109]. Together, these results highlight that the SCN function can be changed by various nutritional cues.

The pathways conveying metabolic signals to the SCN are not well identified. It is possible that timed calorie changes the redox status of SCN cells. Of note, redox signals in SCN exhibit circadian rhythm, which modulates the excitability of SCN neurons [110]. This result demonstrates the close connection between cellular metabolism and dynamic regulation of SCN functioning. Another possibility would involve relays from brain structures sensitive to nutrients. Lesion experiments suggest an involvement of IGL in the transmission of metabolic information to the SCN [111, 112]. Moreover, orexigenic and anorexigenic neurons in the hypothalamus controlling feeding behavior respond to fluctuations in circulating nutrients (e.g., glucose, fatty acids, amino-acids) levels that reflect nutritional status [20]. Since SCN receives numerous projections from hypothalamic nuclei, the metabolic hypothalamus could integrate and transmit information from circulating nutrients to the SCN.

Feedback of Metabolic Hormones

Since receptors of leptin and ghrelin are present on SCN cells, these hormones are plausible candidates to provide metabolic information to the SCN [113, 114]. Leptin and ghrelin receptors are also present on several hypothalamic structures that project on the SCN, such as ARC [115], raising the possibility of either a direct or indirect effect on the master clock. Ghrelin is predominantly synthesized by the stomach. Ghrelin receptors are present in hypothalamus, including SCN and mediobasal hypothalamic nuclei involved in food intake [114]. Ghrelin levels exhibit a circadian rhythm and closely follow feeding schedules, making this peptide a putative candidate for food-related entraining signals. In vitro, ghrelin phase-advanced the electrical rhythm of SCN slices and the *PER2: LUC* expression in cultured SCN explants [116], suggesting a direct action of ghrelin on the SCN. In vivo experiment shows that besides increasing food intake, ghrelin treatment only causes phase-shifts in fasted mice, but not in *ad libitum* fed mice [116]. The shifting effects of ghrelin on the SCN and its reducing effects of photic responses in the SCN could be mediated by the ARC [115, 117].

Leptin is produced and secreted by the white adipose tissue, and consequently, its circulating levels are closely related to body fat mass. Among all its targets, leptin signals to hypothalamus, where it promotes satiety and stimulates energy expenditure [22]. The mediobasal hypothalamus lies within close proximity to the median eminence, a circumventricular structure containing specialized hypothalamic glial cells called tanycytes. It has recently been shown that circulating leptin enters the brain via the median eminence, through internalization by tanycytes, which release leptin in the mediobasal hypothalamus [118]. In addition to its effects on energy balance, leptin can affect the circadian system. Indeed, expression of leptin receptors has been detected in the SCN [113]. Leptin in vitro can phase-advance the SCN oscillations [119] and modulate firing rates of SCN neurons [120]. In vivo injections of leptin modulate the photic synchronization of the master clock in micez, this effect being likely mediated by the mediobasal hypothalamus [121].

Feedback of Other Hormones: Glucocorticoids and Melatonin

While the GC agonist dexamethasone can phase-shift circadian gene expression in peripheral clocks, it does not affect clock gene expression in the SCN [61]. However, mice with genetic ablation of adrenal clock, as well as adrenalectomized rats re-entrain faster to a new light-dark cycle than control animals, suggesting that the adrenal clock feeds back to the SCN, probably via indirect effect of GCs [122, 123]. At least midbrain raphe nuclei are identified relays mediating feedback effects of GCs on the SCN via the serotonergic system. Indeed, daily variations of circulating GCs trigger the daily rhythm of tryptophan hydroxylase mRNA, a limiting enzyme for serotonin synthesis [124].

Melatonin is known for its sedative (i.e., sleep-promoting) effect in humans [125]. Beyond its effect on sleep, melatonin has been shown to directly influence the SCN, where melatonin receptors MT1 and MT2 are present. Daily perfusions of supraphysiological doses of melatonin can entrain the free-running activity of rats. Melatonin also accelerates the re-entrainment of circadian rhythms after a shift in the light-dark cycle [62]. Together, melatonin and glucocorticoid rhythms appear to stabilize the functioning of the circadian system.

The above sections showed the crosstalk between circadian system and metabolism, leading to a finely tuned regulation of circadian and energy physiology. Disruption in the circadian system results in metabolism dysfunction, and vice versa.

Circadian Disruption and Metabolic Disturbances

Circadian Disruption Affects Metabolism

Since clock genes and clock-controlled genes determine the circadian organization of metabolism, genetic clock disruptions affect metabolism in rodents. For example, *Bmal1* deletion in mice impairs glucose metabolism and triglycerides rhythms in addition to increased body fat [37]. Moreover, *Clock* mutant mice are hyperphagic, with increased food intake during the resting period and decreased energy expenditure at night, leading to fat excess. *Clock* mutant mice show severe metabolic alterations, including disruptions in lipid (e.g., hypercholesterolemia and hypertriglyceridemia) and glucose (hyperglycemia) homeostasis [126].

The circadian rhythmicity can also be altered by environmental factors, such as chronic changes in timing of light-dark cycles (chronic jetlag) or work occurring during the usual resting period (shift-work). Numerous epidemiological studies in different countries link the circadian desynchronization induced by shift-work with increased risks for the metabolic syndrome. These observations lead to the concept of "chronobesity," defined as obesity induced or aggravated by circadian desynchronization. The metabolic disturbances resulting from shift-work include impairments in lipid and glucose metabolism and hypertension [127, 128]. Moreover, recurrent sleep debt is also a risk factor for obesity and diabetes [129], indicating that it is likely an aggravating factor for metabolic disturbances in shift workers.

In nocturnal rats, repeated weekly light-dark shifts increase food intake and reduce activity, resulting in weight gain [130] or impaired insulin regulation [131]. Moreover, nocturnal rats forced to work during daytime show no alteration in clock protein oscillations in the SCN, which remain in phase with the light-dark cycle, while temporal patterns of activity and food intake are altered together with a loss of glucose rhythmicity and a reversed rhythm of triglycerides. These results reveal an internal desynchronization, in which activity combined with feeding uncouples metabolic functions from the master clock [132]. Furthermore, diurnal Sudanian grass rats challenged with weekly light-dark shifts display impaired glucose tolerance and accelerated cellular aging [133].

Metabolic Disruptions Induce Circadian Disturbances

Diet-Induced Obesity

Obesity in rodents can be induced by a high-fat diet. In nocturnal mice, high-fat diet attenuates the daily pattern of locomotor activity, concomitantly with a hypoactivity, due to a reduction of activity during the dark phase. The daily pattern of food intake is also dampened, with increased feeding during the resting phase and a relative decrease during the active phase at night [107]. A high-fat diet lengthens the free-running period of mice under dark conditions [107], slows the resynchronization after shifts of the light-dark cycle, and decreases light-induced phase-shifts [108]. Moreover, high-fat feeding is accompanied by changes in neuropeptide expression in the mediobasal hypothalamus, despite no major modification in clock gene oscillations in that region [107]. In the brainstem, more precisely in the nucleus of the solitary tract, a high-fat diet alters the daily patterns of clock gene expression, including downregulated *Rev-erbα*, and upregulated *Bmal1* and *Clock* mRNA levels [134]. These results suggest that CNS dysfunction of circadian system contributes to the development of diet-induced obesity.

Short-term high-fat feeding reduces circadian variations of leptin levels in rats [135]. High-fat feeding also alters the daily variation in glucose tolerance and insulin sensitivity in mice [47]. Since metabolites, food-related hormones, and feeding rhythms are potent synchronizers for peripheral clocks, it would not be surprising that peripheral clocks are altered in high-fat-fed mice. High-fat feeding can attenuate the amplitude of clock gene expression and alters the rhythmic patterns of nuclear receptors, such as PPARγ (gamma) and RORα (alpha), in adipose tissue and liver of mice [107], while other studies found that high-fat diet fails to markedly alter peripheral clock gene oscillations [47, 136, 137]. Several hepatic transcripts were shown to gain rhythmicity in mice fed a high-fat diet [137]. In humans, oscillations of clock genes in adipose tissue do not differ between lean, obese, and diabetic patients [138], suggesting that excess adiposity does not impact peripheral clocks.

Genetic Obesity

Genetic obesity and diabetes in rodents provides experimental models for studying the connection between the circadian system and metabolism. Obese Zucker rats (*fa/fa* rats) that carry a mutation in the leptin receptor gene display phase-advance in feeding [139] and locomotor activity rhythms [140]. The amplitude of the activity-rest cycle is dampened in genetically obese rats and mice, due to increased activity during the resting light phase and decreased activity during night-time [140–142]. Both *ob/ob* and *db/db* mice show altered photic resetting of the master clock [142–144], albeit neither *ob/ob* nor *db/db* mice exhibit major alterations of molecular clockwork in the SCN [83, 141, 144].

In contrast, the daily variations of clock gene expression are clearly reduced in liver and adipose tissue of obese *ob/ob* mice and in liver of *db/db* mice [83, 141]. Of interest, impairments of peripheral clocks in *ob/ob* mice precede the appearance of metabolic disorders, suggesting that the circadian disturbances are due to the lack of leptin and not to obesity. Accordingly, leptin injection partially restores clock gene oscillations in peripheral clocks [83]. The relationship between obesity and circadian disturbances appears often to be a chicken-and-egg problem, since in most cases, it is difficult to determine which problem appears first and disturbs the other system. Notwithstanding, circadian desynchrony could be an aggravating factor for the development of obesity and/or diabetes and as such, deserves careful examination.

Preventive Therapies for Internal Desynchronization and Its Metabolic Consequences

One possibility to improve circadian alignment in individuals exposed to shift-work or jetlag is timed exposure to light, since light is able to reset circadian rhythms and also directly improves alertness in humans [145]. Because feeding time is a potent synchronizer of peripheral oscillators, it is a possible resynchronizer in case of altered circadian rhythmicity. Obese Zucker rats (*fa/fa*) ingest a larger proportion of food during the light phase (i.e., the resting phase) than wild-type rats [140]. In this study, *ad libitum*-fed Zucker rats gained 23% more weight than animals with access to food limited to nighttime (i.e., the normal period of feeding in nocturnal rats), despite similar amounts of daily food intake. This suggests that excessive diurnal feeding may contribute to body weight gain. Moreover, the negative effects of unbalanced high-fat diet are limited if high-fat feeding is restricted to the dark phase in mice [146].

In humans, eating during late evening is associated with higher daily energy intake, a major risk factor for weight gain [147]. Furthermore, nocturnal feeding is correlated with an increased risk of overweight in some, but not all, epidemiological studies [148, 149]. Although shift-workers often report normal total energy intake, there is commonly an altered temporal distribution of feeding characterized by more irregular eating times, more snacking, and fewer substantial meals [150]. These results show that studies on obesity should not focus exclusively on food intake and energy expenditure. The timing of food intake itself plays a significant role in weight gain. Feeding at the right time might attenuate weight gain by normalizing the phase relation between circadian rhythms of food intake and metabolic processes involved in utilization and storage of ingested fuels.

Conclusion

In conclusion, this chapter shows that energy metabolism and circadian rhythmicity interact at multiple (i.e., molecular, cellular and systemic) levels. The daily temporal regulation of energy metabolism is controlled by a multi-oscillatory network comprising a master clock in the SCN and numerous secondary clocks and oscillators in the brain and peripheral tissues. Furthermore, core clock components interact closely with molecular regulators of intracellular metabolism. While the ambient light detected by the retina is the most powerful synchronizer of the master clock, the SCN is also sensitive to metabolic signals associated with metabolic challenges. Meal timing can adjust the phase of many brain and peripheral oscillators outside the SCN. From a pathophysiological point of view, metabolic diseases are associated with circadian alterations. Conversely, induction of circadian disturbances by genetic alterations in the clock or by desynchronizing conditions (e.g., shift work, chronic jet-lag) affects metabolism. Because altered circadian rhythm is recognized as a determinant of metabolic dysfunction, chronotherapeutic approaches of daily dieting should be taken into consideration for the management of metabolic health.

Cross-References

▶ Adipokines and Metabolism
▶ Brain Regulation of Feeding and Energy Homeostasis
▶ Diet, Exercise, and Behavior Therapy
▶ Overview of Metabolic Syndrome

References

1. Dibner C, Schibler U, Albrecht U. The mammalian circadian timing system: organization and coordination of central and peripheral clocks. Annu Rev Physiol. 2010;72:517–49. https://doi.org/10.1146/annurev-physiol-021909-135821.
2. Ko CH, Takahashi JS. Molecular components of the mammalian circadian clock. Hum Mol Genet. 2006;15(Spec 2):R271–7. https://doi.org/10.1093/hmg/ddl207. 15/suppl_2/R271 [pii]
3. Hattar S, Kumar M, Park A, Tong P, Tung J, Yau KW, Berson DM. Central projections of melanopsin-expressing retinal ganglion cells in the mouse. J Comp Neurol. 2006;497(3):326–49. https://doi.org/10.1002/cne.20970.
4. Golombek DA, Rosenstein RE. Physiology of circadian entrainment. Physiol Rev. 2010;90(3):1063–102. https://doi.org/10.1152/physrev.00009.2009. 90/3/1063 [pii]
5. Harrington ME. The ventral lateral geniculate nucleus and the intergeniculate leaflet: interrelated structures in the visual and circadian systems. Neurosci Biobehav Rev. 1997;21(5):705–27. S0149-7634(96)00019-X [pii]
6. Brown TM, Coogan AN, Cutler DJ, Hughes AT, Piggins HD. Electrophysiological actions of orexins on rat suprachiasmatic neurons in vitro. Neurosci Lett. 2008;448(3):273–8. https://doi.org/10.1016/j.neulet.2008.10.058. S0304-3940(08)01459-6 [pii]
7. Morin LP. Serotonin and the regulation of mammalian circadian rhythmicity. Ann Med. 1999;31(1):12–33.
8. Challet E. Interactions between light, mealtime and calorie restriction to control daily timing in mammals. J Comp Physiol B. 2010;180(5):631–44. https://doi.org/10.1007/s00360-010-0451-4.
9. Feillet CA, Mendoza J, Albrecht U, Pevet P, Challet E. Forebrain oscillators ticking with different clock hands. Mol Cell Neurosci. 2008;37(2):209–21. https://doi.org/10.1016/j.mcn.2007.09.010. S1044-7431(07)00221-7 [pii]
10. Guilding C, Piggins HD. Challenging the omnipotence of the suprachiasmatic timekeeper: are circadian oscillators present throughout the mammalian brain? Eur J Neurosci. 2007;25(11):3195–216. https://doi.org/10.1111/j.1460-9568.2007.05581.x. EJN5581 [pii]
11. Shieh KR, Yang SC, Lu XY, Akil H, Watson SJ. Diurnal rhythmic expression of the rhythm-related genes, rPeriod1, rPeriod2, and rClock, in the rat brain. J Biomed Sci. 2005;12(1):209–17. https://doi.org/10.1007/s11373-004-8176-6.
12. Abe M, Herzog ED, Yamazaki S, Straume M, Tei H, Sakaki Y, Menaker M, Block GD. Circadian rhythms in isolated brain regions. J Neurosci. 2002;22(1):350–6. 22/1/350 [pii]
13. Reick M, Garcia JA, Dudley C, McKnight SL. NPAS2: an analog of clock operative in the mammalian forebrain. Science. 2001;293(5529):506–9. https://doi.org/10.1126/science.1060699.
14. Kalsbeek A, Palm IF, La Fleur SE, Scheer FA, Perreau-Lenz S, Ruiter M, Kreier F, Cailotto C, Buijs RM. SCN outputs and the hypothalamic balance of life. J Biol Rhythms. 2006;21(6):458–69. https://doi.org/10.1177/0748730406293854. 21/6/458 [pii]
15. Sellix MT, Egli M, Poletini MO, McKee DT, Bosworth MD, Fitch CA, Freeman ME. Anatomical and functional characterization of clock gene expression in neuroendocrine dopaminergic neurons. Am J Physiol Regul Integr Comp Physiol. 2006;290(5):R1309–23. https://doi.org/10.1152/ajpregu.00555.2005. 00555.2005 [pii]
16. Gerhold LM, Horvath TL, Freeman ME. Vasoactive intestinal peptide fibers innervate neuroendocrine dopaminergic neurons. Brain Res. 2001;919(1):48–56. S0006-8993(01)02993-6 [pii]
17. Silver R, LeSauter J, Tresco PA, Lehman MN. A diffusible coupling signal from the transplanted suprachiasmatic nucleus controlling circadian locomotor rhythms. Nature. 1996;382(6594):810–3. https://doi.org/10.1038/382810a0.

18. Li JD, Hu WP, Zhou QY. The circadian output signals from the suprachiasmatic nuclei. Prog Brain Res. 2012;199:119–27. https://doi.org/10.1016/B978-0-444-59427-3.00028-9. B978-0-444-59427-3.00028-9 [pii]

19. Nagai K, Nishio T, Nakagawa H, Nakamura S, Fukuda Y. Effect of bilateral lesions of the suprachiasmatic nuclei on the circadian rhythm of food-intake. Brain Res. 1978;142(2):384–9. 0006-8993(78)90648-0 [pii]

20. Williams KW, Elmquist JK. From neuroanatomy to behavior: central integration of peripheral signals regulating feeding behavior. Nat Neurosci. 2012;15(10):1350–5. https://doi.org/10.1038/nn.3217.

21. Burdakov D, Luckman SM, Verkhratsky A. Glucose-sensing neurons of the hypothalamus. Philos Trans R Soc Lond B Biol Sci. 2005;360(1464):2227–35. https://doi.org/10.1098/rstb.2005.1763. L238W86787251W54 [pii]

22. Ahima RS, Lazar MA. Adipokines and the peripheral and neural control of energy balance. Mol Endocrinol. 2008;22(5):1023–31. https://doi.org/10.1210/me.2007-0529.

23. Cedernaes J, Huang W, Ramsey KM, Waldeck N, Cheng L, Marcheva B, Omura C, Kobayashi Y, Peek CB, Levine DC, Dhir R, Awatramani R, Bradfield CA, Wang XA, Takahashi JS, Mokadem M, Ahima RS, Bass J. Transcriptional basis for rhythmic control of hunger and metabolism within the AgRP neuron. Cell Metab. 2019;29(5):1078–91. e1075. https://doi.org/10.1016/j.cmet.2019.01.023.

24. Xu B, Kalra PS, Farmerie WG, Kalra SP. Daily changes in hypothalamic gene expression of neuropeptide Y, galanin, proopiomelanocortin, and adipocyte leptin gene expression and secretion: effects of food restriction. Endocrinology. 1999;140(6):2868–75. https://doi.org/10.1210/endo.140.6.6789.

25. Steiner RA, Kabigting E, Lent K, Clifton DK. Diurnal rhythm in proopiomelanocortin mRNA in the arcuate nucleus of the male rat. J Neuroendocrinol. 1994;6(6):603–8.

26. Akabayashi A, Levin N, Paez X, Alexander JT, Leibowitz SF. Hypothalamic neuropeptide Y and its gene expression: relation to light/dark cycle and circulating corticosterone. Mol Cell Neurosci. 1994;5(3):210–8. https://doi.org/10.1006/mcne.1994.1025. S1044-7431(84)71025-6 [pii]

27. Bechtold DA, Loudon AS. Hypothalamic clocks and rhythms in feeding behaviour. Trends Neurosci. 2013;36(2):74–82. https://doi.org/10.1016/j.tins.2012.12.007. S0166-2236(12)00222-6 [pii]

28. Kim ER, Xu Y, Cassidy RM, Lu Y, Yang Y, Tian J, Li DP, Van Drunen R, Ribas-Latre A, Cai ZL, Xue M, Arenkiel BR, Eckel-Mahan K, Xu Y, Tong Q. Paraventricular hypothalamus mediates diurnal rhythm of metabolism. Nat Commun. 2020;11(1):3794. https://doi.org/10.1038/s41467-020-17578-7.

29. Balsalobre A, Damiola F, Schibler U. A serum shock induces circadian gene expression in mammalian tissue culture cells. Cell. 1998;93(6):929–37. S0092-8674(00)81199-X [pii]

30. Yagita K, Tamanini F, van Der Horst GT, Okamura H. Molecular mechanisms of the biological clock in cultured fibroblasts. Science. 2001;292(5515):278–81. https://doi.org/10.1126/science.1059542. 292/5515/278

31. Yoo SH, Yamazaki S, Lowrey PL, Shimomura K, Ko CH, Buhr ED, Siepka SM, Hong HK, Oh WJ, Yoo OJ, Menaker M, Takahashi JS. PERIOD2::LUCIFER-ASE real-time reporting of circadian dynamics reveals persistent circadian oscillations in mouse peripheral tissues. Proc Natl Acad Sci U S A. 2004;101(15):5339–46. https://doi.org/10.1073/pnas.0308709101.

32. Tahara Y, Kuroda H, Saito K, Nakajima Y, Kubo Y, Ohnishi N, Seo Y, Otsuka M, Fuse Y, Ohura Y, Komatsu T, Moriya Y, Okada S, Furutani N, Hirao A, Horikawa K, Kudo T, Shibata S. In vivo monitoring of peripheral circadian clocks in the mouse. Curr Biol. 2012;22(11):1029–34. https://doi.org/10.1016/j.cub.2012.04.009. S0960-9822(12)00396-X [pii]

33. Dibner C, Sage D, Unser M, Bauer C, d'Eysmond T, Naef F, Schibler U. Circadian gene expression is resilient to large fluctuations in overall transcription rates. EMBO J. 2009;28(2):123–34. https://doi.org/10.1038/emboj.2008.262.

34. Panda S, Antoch MP, Miller BH, Su AI, Schook AB, Straume M, Schultz PG, Kay SA, Takahashi JS, Hogenesch JB. Coordinated transcription of key pathways in the mouse by the circadian clock. Cell. 2002;109(3):307–20. S0092867402007225 [pii]

35. Gachon F, Olela FF, Schaad O, Descombes P, Schibler U. The circadian PAR-domain basic leucine zipper transcription factors DBP, TEF, and HLF modulate basal and inducible xenobiotic detoxification. Cell Metab. 2006;4(1):25–36. https://doi.org/10.1016/j.cmet.2006.04.015. S1550-4131(06)00155-0 [pii]

36. Gimble JM, Sutton GM, Ptitsyn AA, Floyd ZE, Bunnell BA. Circadian rhythms in adipose tissue: an update. Curr Opin Clin Nutr Metab Care. 2011;14(6):554–61. https://doi.org/10.1097/MCO.0b013e32834ad94b.

37. Lamia KA, Storch KF, Weitz CJ. Physiological significance of a peripheral tissue circadian clock. Proc Natl Acad Sci U S A. 2008;105(39):15172–7. https://doi.org/10.1073/pnas.0806717105.

38. Zvonic S, Ptitsyn AA, Conrad SA, Scott LK, Floyd ZE, Kilroy G, Wu X, Goh BC, Mynatt RL, Gimble JM. Characterization of peripheral circadian clocks in adipose tissues. Diabetes. 2006;55(4):962–70. 55/4/962 [pii]

39. Ando H, Yanagihara H, Hayashi Y, Obi Y, Tsuruoka S, Takamura T, Kaneko S, Fujimura A. Rhythmic messenger ribonucleic acid expression of clock genes and adipocytokines in mouse visceral

adipose tissue. Endocrinology. 2005;146(12): 5631–6. https://doi.org/10.1210/en.2005-0771.

40. Sinha MK, Ohannesian JP, Heiman ML, Kriauciunas A, Stephens TW, Magosin S, Marco C, Caro JF. Nocturnal rise of leptin in lean, obese, and non-insulin-dependent diabetes mellitus subjects. J Clin Invest. 1996;97(5):1344–7. https://doi.org/10.1172/JCI118551.

41. Kalsbeek A, Fliers E, Romijn JA, La Fleur SE, Wortel J, Bakker O, Endert E, Buijs RM. The suprachiasmatic nucleus generates the diurnal changes in plasma leptin levels. Endocrinology. 2001;142(6): 2677–85. https://doi.org/10.1210/endo.142.6.8197.

42. Cuesta M, Clesse D, Pevet P, Challet E. From daily behavior to hormonal and neurotransmitters rhythms: comparison between diurnal and nocturnal rat species. Horm Behav. 2009;55(2):338–47. https://doi.org/10.1016/j.yhbeh.2008.10.015. S0018-506X(08)00306-1 [pii]

43. Otway DT, Frost G, Johnston JD. Circadian rhythmicity in murine pre-adipocyte and adipocyte cells. Chronobiol Int. 2009;26(7):1340–54. https://doi.org/10.3109/07420520903412368.

44. Marcheva B, Ramsey KM, Buhr ED, Kobayashi Y, Su H, Ko CH, Ivanova G, Omura C, Mo S, Vitaterna MH, Lopez JP, Philipson LH, Bradfield CA, Crosby SD, JeBailey L, Wang X, Takahashi JS, Bass J. Disruption of the clock components CLOCK and BMAL1 leads to hypoinsulinaemia and diabetes. Nature. 2010;466(7306):627–31. https://doi.org/10.1038/nature09253.

45. Teboul M, Guillaumond F, Grechez-Cassiau A, Delaunay F. The nuclear hormone receptor family round the clock. Mol Endocrinol. 2008;22(12): 2573–82. https://doi.org/10.1210/me.2007-0521.

46. Lau P, Nixon SJ, Parton RG, Muscat GE. RORalpha regulates the expression of genes involved in lipid homeostasis in skeletal muscle cells: caveolin-3 and CPT-1 are direct targets of ROR. J Biol Chem. 2004;279(35):36828–40. https://doi.org/10.1074/jbc.M404927200.

47. Delezie J, Dumont S, Dardente H, Oudart H, Grechez-Cassiau A, Klosen P, Teboul M, Delaunay F, Pevet P, Challet E. The nuclear receptor REV-ERBalpha is required for the daily balance of carbohydrate and lipid metabolism. FASEB J. 2012;26(8):3321–35. https://doi.org/10.1096/fj.12-208751.

48. Yoon M. The role of PPARalpha in lipid metabolism and obesity: focusing on the effects of estrogen on PPARalpha actions. Pharmacol Res. 2009;60(3): 151–9. https://doi.org/10.1016/j.phrs.2009.02.004. S1043-6618(09)00057-7 [pii]

49. Oishi K, Shirai H, Ishida N. CLOCK is involved in the circadian transactivation of peroxisome-proliferator-activated receptor alpha (PPARalpha) in mice. Biochem J. 2005;386(Pt 3):575–81. https://doi.org/10.1042/BJ20041150.

50. Grimaldi B, Bellet MM, Katada S, Astarita G, Hirayama J, Amin RH, Granneman JG, Piomelli D, Leff T, Sassone-Corsi P. PER2 controls lipid metabolism by direct regulation of PPARgamma. Cell Metab. 2010;12(5):509–20. https://doi.org/10.1016/j.cmet.2010.10.005. S1550-4131(10)00357-8 [pii]

51. La Fleur SE, Kalsbeek A, Wortel J, Buijs RM. A suprachiasmatic nucleus generated rhythm in basal glucose concentrations. J Neuroendocrinol. 1999;11(8):643–52. jne373 [pii]

52. Kalsbeek A, Yi CX, La Fleur SE, Fliers E. The hypothalamic clock and its control of glucose homeostasis. Trends Endocrinol Metab. 2010;21(7):402–10. https://doi.org/10.1016/j.tem.2010.02.005. S1043-2760(10)00040-8 [pii]

53. Cailotto C, van Heijningen C, van der Vliet J, van der Plasse G, Habold C, Kalsbeek A, Pevet P, Buijs RM. Daily rhythms in metabolic liver enzymes and plasma glucose require a balance in the autonomic output to the liver. Endocrinology. 2008;149(4): 1914–25. https://doi.org/10.1210/en.2007 0816.

54. Yi CX, Serlie MJ, Ackermans MT, Foppen E, Buijs RM, Sauerwein HP, Fliers E, Kalsbeek A. A major role for perifornical orexin neurons in the control of glucose metabolism in rats. Diabetes. 2009;58(9): 1998–2005. https://doi.org/10.2337/db09-0385.

55. Kreier F, Fliers E, Voshol PJ, Van Eden CG, Havekes LM, Kalsbeek A, Van Heijningen CL, Sluiter AA, Mettenleiter TC, Romijn JA, Sauerwein HP, Buijs RM. Selective parasympathetic innervation of subcutaneous and intra-abdominal fat – functional implications. The Journal of clinical investigation. 2002;110(9):1243–50. https://doi.org/10.1172/JCI15736.

56. Ulrich-Lai YM, Arnhold MM, Engeland WC. Adrenal splanchnic innervation contributes to the diurnal rhythm of plasma corticosterone in rats by modulating adrenal sensitivity to ACTH. Am J Physiol Regul Integr Comp Physiol. 2006;290(4):R1128–35. https://doi.org/10.1152/ajpregu.00042.2003.

57. Oster H, Damerow S, Kiessling S, Jakubcakova V, Abraham D, Tian J, Hoffmann MW, Eichele G. The circadian rhythm of glucocorticoids is regulated by a gating mechanism residing in the adrenal cortical clock. Cell Metab. 2006;4(2):163–73.

58. Rosenfeld P, Van Eekelen JA, Levine S, De Kloet ER. Ontogeny of the type 2 glucocorticoid receptor in discrete rat brain regions: an immunocytochemical study. Brain Res. 1988;470(1):119–27.

59. Surjit M, Ganti KP, Mukherji A, Ye T, Hua G, Metzger D, Li M, Chambon P. Widespread negative response elements mediate direct repression by agonist-liganded glucocorticoid receptor. Cell. 2011;145(2):224–41. https://doi.org/10.1016/j.cell.2011.03.027. S0092-8674(11)00304-7 [pii]

60. Oishi K, Amagai N, Shirai H, Kadota K, Ohkura N, Ishida N. Genome-wide expression analysis reveals 100 adrenal gland-dependent circadian genes in the mouse liver. DNA Res. 2005;12(3):191–202. https://doi.org/10.1093/dnares/dsi003. 12/3/191 [pii]

61. Balsalobre A, Brown SA, Marcacci L, Tronche F, Kellendonk C, Reichardt HM, Schutz G, Schibler U. Resetting of circadian time in peripheral tissues by glucocorticoid signaling. Science. 2000;289(5488):2344–7. 8856 [pii]

62. Pevet P, Challet E. Melatonin: both master clock output and internal time-giver in the circadian clocks network. J Physiol Paris. 2011;105(4-6):170–82. https://doi.org/10.1016/j.jphysparis.2011.07.001. S0928-4257(11)00004-0 [pii]

63. Mulder H, Nagorny CL, Lyssenko V, Groop L. Melatonin receptors in pancreatic islets: good morning to a novel type 2 diabetes gene. Diabetologia. 2009;52(7):1240–9. https://doi.org/10.1007/s00125-009-1359-y.

64. Mühlbauer E, Gross E, Labucay K, Wolgast S, Peschke E. Loss of melatonin signalling and its impact on circadian rhythms in mouse organs regulating blood glucose. Eur J Pharmacol. 2009;606(1-3):61–71. https://doi.org/10.1016/j.ejphar.2009.01.029. S0014-2999(09)00098-3 [pii]

65. Peschke E, Peschke D. Evidence for a circadian rhythm of insulin release from perifused rat pancreatic islets. Diabetologia. 1998;41(9):1085–92. https://doi.org/10.1007/s001250051034.

66. Bouatia-Naji N, Bonnefond A, Cavalcanti-Proenca C, Sparso T, Holmkvist J, Marchand M, Delplanque J, Lobbens S, Rocheleau G, Durand E, De Graeve F, Chevre JC, Borch-Johnsen K, Hartikainen AL, Ruokonen A, Tichet J, Marre M, Weill J, Heude B, Tauber M, Lemaire K, Schuit F, Elliott P, Jorgensen T, Charpentier G, Hadjadj S, Cauchi S, Vaxillaire M, Sladek R, Visvikis-Siest S, Balkau B, Levy-Marchal-C, Pattou F, Meyre D, Blakemore AI, Jarvelin MR, Walley AJ, Hansen T, Dina C, Pedersen O, Froguel P. A variant near MTNR1B is associated with increased fasting plasma glucose levels and type 2 diabetes risk. Nat Genet. 2009;41(1):89–94. https://doi.org/10.1038/ng.277.

67. Caldelas I, Poirel VJ, Sicard B, Pevet P, Challet E. Circadian profile and photic regulation of clock genes in the suprachiasmatic nucleus of a diurnal mammal Arvicanthis ansorgei. Neuroscience. 2003;116(2):583–91. S0306452202006541 [pii]

68. Mrosovsky N, Edelstein K, Hastings MH, Maywood ES. Cycle of period gene expression in a diurnal mammal (Spermophilus tridecemlineatus): implications for nonphotic phase shifting. J Biol Rhythms. 2001;16(5):471–8.

69. Lambert CM, Weaver DR. Peripheral gene expression rhythms in a diurnal rodent. J Biol Rhythms. 2006;21(1):77–9. https://doi.org/10.1177/0748730405281843. 21/1/77 [pii]

70. Kalsbeek A, Verhagen LA, Schalij I, Foppen E, Saboureau M, Bothorel B, Buijs RM, Pevet P. Opposite actions of hypothalamic vasopressin on circadian corticosterone rhythm in nocturnal versus diurnal species. Eur J Neurosci. 2008;27(4):818–27.

71. https://doi.org/10.1111/j.1460-9568.2008.06057.x. EJN6057 [pii]

72. Stokkan KA, Yamazaki S, Tei H, Sakaki Y, Menaker M. Entrainment of the circadian clock in the liver by feeding. Science. 2001;291(5503):490–3. https://doi.org/10.1126/science.291.5503.490.

73. Damiola F, Le Minh N, Preitner N, Kornmann B, Fleury-Olela F, Schibler U. Restricted feeding uncouples circadian oscillators in peripheral tissues from the central pacemaker in the suprachiasmatic nucleus. Genes Dev. 2000;14(23):2950–61.

74. Kurumiya S, Kawamura H. Damped oscillation of the lateral hypothalamic multineuronal activity synchronized to daily feeding schedules in rats with suprachiasmatic nucleus lesions. J Biol Rhythms. 1991;6(2):115–27.

75. Wakamatsu H, Yoshinobu Y, Aida R, Moriya T, Akiyama M, Shibata S. Restricted-feeding-induced anticipatory activity rhythm is associated with a phase-shift of the expression of mPer1 and mPer2 mRNA in the cerebral cortex and hippocampus but not in the suprachiasmatic nucleus of mice. Eur J Neurosci. 2001;13(6):1190–6. ejn1483 [pii]

76. Mistlberger RE. Neurobiology of food anticipatory circadian rhythms. Physiol Behav. 2011;104(4):535–45. https://doi.org/10.1016/j.physbeh.2011.04.015. S0031-9384(11)00174-0 [pii]

77. Brown SA, Zumbrunn G, Fleury-Olela F, Preitner N, Schibler U. Rhythms of mammalian body temperature can sustain peripheral circadian clocks. Curr Biol. 2002;12(18):1574–83. S0960982202011454 [pii]

78. Buhr ED, Yoo SH, Takahashi JS. Temperature as a universal resetting cue for mammalian circadian oscillators. Science. 2010;330(6002):379–85. https://doi.org/10.1126/science.1195262. 330/6002/379 [pii]

79. Saini C, Morf J, Stratmann M, Gos P, Schibler U. Simulated body temperature rhythms reveal the phase-shifting behavior and plasticity of mammalian circadian oscillators. Genes Dev. 2012;26(6):567–80. https://doi.org/10.1101/gad.183251.111. gad.183251.111 [pii]

79. Tahara Y, Otsuka M, Fuse Y, Hirao A, Shibata S. Refeeding after fasting elicits insulin-dependent regulation of Per2 and Rev-erbalpha with shifts in the liver clock. J Biol Rhythms. 2011;26(3):230–40. https://doi.org/10.1177/0748730411405958. 26/3/230 [pii]

80. Sato M, Murakami M, Node K, Matsumura R, Akashi M. The role of the endocrine system in feeding-induced tissue-specific circadian entrainment. Cell Rep. 2014;8(2):393–401. https://doi.org/10.1016/j.celrep.2014.06.015. S2211-1247(14)00483-5 [pii]

81. Balsalobre A, Marcacci L, Schibler U. Multiple signaling pathways elicit circadian gene expression in cultured Rat-1 fibroblasts. Curr Biol. 2000;10(20):1291–4. S0960-9822(00)00758-2 [pii]

82. Crosby P, Hamnett R, Putker M, Hoyle NP, Reed M, Karam CJ, Maywood ES, Stangherlin A, Chesham JE, Hayter EA, Rosenbrier-Ribeiro L, Newham P,

Clevers H, Bechtold DA, O'Neill JS. Insulin/IGF-1 drives PERIOD synthesis to entrain circadian rhythms with feeding time. Cell. 2019;177(4): 896–909. e820. https://doi.org/10.1016/j.cell.2019. 02.017.

83. Ando H, Kumazaki M, Motosugi Y, Ushijima K, Maekawa T, Ishikawa E, Fujimura A. Impairment of peripheral circadian clocks precedes metabolic abnormalities in ob/ob mice. Endocrinology. 2011;152(4): 1347–54. https://doi.org/10.1210/en.2010-1068.

84. Haynes WG, Morgan DA, Walsh SA, Mark AL, Sivitz WI. Receptor-mediated regional sympathetic nerve activation by leptin. J Clin Invest. 1997;100(2): 270–8. https://doi.org/10.1172/JCI119532.

85. Takeda S, Elefteriou F, Levasseur R, Liu X, Zhao L, Parker KL, Armstrong D, Ducy P, Karsenty G. Leptin regulates bone formation via the sympathetic nervous system. Cell. 2002;111(3):305–17. S00928674020-10498 [pii]

86. Honma KI, Honma S, Hiroshige T. Feeding-associated corticosterone peak in rats under various feeding cycles. Am J Physiol. 1984;246(5 Pt 2): R721–6.

87. Le Minh N, Damiola F, Tronche F, Schutz G, Schibler U. Glucocorticoid hormones inhibit food-induced phase-shifting of peripheral circadian oscillators. EMBO J. 2001;20(24):7128–36. https://doi.org/10. 1093/emboj/20.24.7128.

88. Canaple L, Rambaud J, Dkhissi-Benyahya O, Rayet B, Tan NS, Michalik L, Delaunay F, Wahli W, Laudet V. Reciprocal regulation of brain and muscle Arnt-like protein 1 and peroxisome proliferator-activated receptor alpha defines a novel positive feedback loop in the rodent liver circadian clock. Mol Endocrinol. 2006;20(8):1715–27. https://doi.org/10. 1210/me.2006-0052.

89. Gervois P, Chopin-Delannoy S, Fadel A, Dubois G, Kosykh V, Fruchart JC, Najib J, Laudet V, Staels B. Fibrates increase human REV-ERBalpha expression in liver via a novel peroxisome proliferator-activated receptor response element. Mol Endocrinol. 1999;13(3):400–9. https://doi.org/10.1210/mend.13. 3.0248.

90. Schmutz I, Ripperger JA, Baeriswyl-Aebischer S, Albrecht U. The mammalian clock component PERIOD2 coordinates circadian output by interaction with nuclear receptors. Genes Dev. 2010;24(4): 345–57. https://doi.org/10.1101/gad.564110. 24/4/ 345 [pii]

91. Liu C, Li S, Liu T, Borjigin J, Lin JD. Transcriptional coactivator PGC-1alpha integrates the mammalian clock and energy metabolism. Nature. 2007;447(7143): 477–81. https://doi.org/10.1038/nature05767.

92. Hirota T, Okano T, Kokame K, Shirotani-Ikejima H, Miyata T, Fukada Y. Glucose down-regulates Per1 and Per2 mRNA levels and induces circadian gene expression in cultured Rat-1 fibroblasts. J Biol Chem. 2002;277(46):44244–51. https://doi.org/10.1074/jbc. M206233200.

93. Gu YZ, Hogenesch JB, Bradfield CA. The PAS super-family: sensors of environmental and developmental signals. Annu Rev Pharmacol Toxicol. 2000;40: 519–61. https://doi.org/10.1146/annurev.pharmtox. 40.1.519.

94. Rutter J, Reick M, Wu LC, McKnight SL. Regulation of clock and NPAS2 DNA binding by the redox state of NAD cofactors. Science. 2001;293(5529):510–4. https://doi.org/10.1126/science.1060698.

95. Yu J, Auwerx J. The role of sirtuins in the control of metabolic homeostasis. Ann N Y Acad Sci. 2009;1173(Suppl 1):E10–9. https://doi.org/10.1111/ j.1749-6632.2009.04952.x. NYAS4952 [pii]

96. Nakahata Y, Kaluzova M, Grimaldi B, Sahar S, Hirayama J, Chen D, Guarente LP, Sassone-Corsi P. The NAD+-dependent deacetylase SIRT1 modulates CLOCK-mediated chromatin remodeling and circadian control. Cell. 2008;134(2):329–40. https:// doi.org/10.1016/j.cell.2008.07.002. S0092 8674(08) 00879-9 [pii]

97. Asher G, Gatfield D, Stratmann M, Reinke H, Dibner C, Kreppel F, Mostoslavsky R, Alt FW, Schibler U. SIRT1 regulates circadian clock gene expression through PER2 deacetylation. Cell. 2008;134(2):317–28. https://doi.org/10.1016/j.cell. 2008.06.050. S0092-8674(08)00837-4 [pii]

98. Kahn BB, Alquier T, Carling D, Hardie DG. AMP-activated protein kinase: ancient energy gauge provides clues to modern understanding of metabolism. Cell Metab. 2005;1(1):15–25. https:// doi.org/10.1016/j.cmet.2004.12.003. S1550-4131(04)00009-9 [pii]

99. Um JH, Yang S, Yamazaki S, Kang H, Viollet B, Foretz M, Chung JH. Activation of 5′-AMP-activated kinase with diabetes drug metformin induces casein kinase Iepsilon (CKIepsilon)-dependent degradation of clock protein mPer2. J Biol Chem. 2007;282(29):20794–8. https://doi.org/ 10.1074/jbc.C700070200.

100. Lamia KA, Sachdeva UM, DiTacchio L, Williams EC, Alvarez JG, Egan DF, Vasquez DS, Juguilon H, Panda S, Shaw RJ, Thompson CB, Evans RM. AMPK regulates the circadian clock by cryptochrome phosphorylation and degradation. Science. 2009;326(5951):437–40. https://doi.org/10. 1126/science.1172156. 326/5951/437 [pii]

101. Ramanathan C, Kathale ND, Liu D, Lee C, Freeman DA, Hogenesch JB, Cao R, Liu AC. mTOR signaling regulates central and peripheral circadian clock function. PLoS Genet. 2018;14(5):e1007369. https://doi. org/10.1371/journal.pgen.1007369.

102. Challet E, Pevet P, Vivien-Roels B, Malan A. Phase-advanced daily rhythms of melatonin, body temperature, and locomotor activity in food-restricted rats fed during daytime. J Biol Rhythms. 1997;12(1):65–79.

103. Mendoza J, Graff C, Dardente H, Pevet P, Challet E. Feeding cues alter clock gene oscillations and photic responses in the suprachiasmatic nuclei of mice exposed to a light/dark cycle. J Neurosci.

2005;25(6):1514–22. https://doi.org/10.1523/JNEUROSCI.4397-04.2005. 25/6/1514 [pii]

104. Challet E, Losee-Olson S, Turek FW. Reduced glucose availability attenuates circadian responses to light in mice. Am J Physiol. 1999;276(4 Pt 2):R1063–70.

105. Castillo MR, Hochstetler KJ, Tavernier RJ Jr, Greene DM, Bult-Ito A. Entrainment of the master circadian clock by scheduled feeding. Am J Physiol Regul Integr Comp Physiol. 2004;287(3):R551–5. https://doi.org/10.1152/ajpregu.00247.2004.

106. Lamont EW, Diaz LR, Barry-Shaw J, Stewart J, Amir S. Daily restricted feeding rescues a rhythm of period2 expression in the arrhythmic suprachiasmatic nucleus. Neuroscience. 2005;132(2):245–8. https://doi.org/10.1016/j.neuroscience.2005.01.029. S0306-4522(05)00133-8 [pii]

107. Kohsaka A, Laposky AD, Ramsey KM, Estrada C, Joshu C, Kobayashi Y, Turek FW, Bass J. High-fat diet disrupts behavioral and molecular circadian rhythms in mice. Cell Metab. 2007;6(5):414–21. https://doi.org/10.1016/j.cmet.2007.09.006. S1550-4131(07)00266-5 [pii]

108. Mendoza J, Pevet P, Challet E. High-fat feeding alters the clock synchronization to light. J Physiol. 2008;586(Pt 24):5901–10. https://doi.org/10.1113/jphysiol.2008.159566.

109. Mendoza J, Clesse D, Pevet P, Challet E. Food-reward signalling in the suprachiasmatic clock. J Neurochem. 2010;112(6):1489–99. https://doi.org/10.1111/j.1471-4159.2010.06570.x. JNC6570 [pii]

110. Wang TA, Yu YV, Govindaiah G, Ye X, Artinian L, Coleman TP, Sweedler JV, Cox CL, Gillette MU. Circadian rhythm of redox state regulates excitability in suprachiasmatic nucleus neurons. Science. 2012;337(6096):839–42. https://doi.org/10.1126/science.1222826.

111. Challet E, Pevet P, Malan A. Intergeniculate leaflet lesion and daily rhythms in food-restricted rats fed during daytime. Neurosci Lett. 1996;216(3):214–8. S0304394096130123 [pii]

112. Saderi N, Cazarez-Marquez F, Buijs FN, Salgado-Delgado RC, Guzman-Ruiz MA, del Carmen BM, Escobar C, Buijs RM. The NPY intergeniculate leaflet projections to the suprachiasmatic nucleus transmit metabolic conditions. Neuroscience. 2013;246:291–300. https://doi.org/10.1016/j.neuroscience.2013.05.004. S0306-4522(13)00415-6 [pii]

113. Guan XM, Hess JF, Yu H, Hey PJ, van der Ploeg LH. Differential expression of mRNA for leptin receptor isoforms in the rat brain. Mol Cell Endocrinol. 1997;133(1):1–7. S0303-7207(97)00138-X [pii]

114. Zigman JM, Jones JE, Lee CE, Saper CB, Elmquist JK. Expression of ghrelin receptor mRNA in the rat and the mouse brain. J Comp Neurol. 2006;494(3):528–48. https://doi.org/10.1002/cne.20823.

115. Yi CX, van der Vliet J, Dai J, Yin G, Ru L, Buijs RM. Ventromedial arcuate nucleus communicates peripheral metabolic information to the suprachiasmatic nucleus. Endocrinology. 2006;147(1):283–94. https://doi.org/10.1210/en.2005-1051.

116. Yannielli PC, Molyneux PC, Harrington ME, Golombek DA. Ghrelin effects on the circadian system of mice. J Neurosci. 2007;27(11):2890–5. https://doi.org/10.1523/JNEUROSCI.3913-06.2007. 27/11/2890 [pii]

117. Yi CX, Challet E, Pevet P, Kalsbeek A, Escobar C, Buijs RM. A circulating ghrelin mimetic attenuates light-induced phase delay of mice and light-induced Fos expression in the suprachiasmatic nucleus of rats. Eur J Neurosci. 2008;27(8):1965–72. https://doi.org/10.1111/j.1460-9568.2008.06181.x. EJN6181 [pii]

118. Balland E, Dam J, Langlet F, Caron E, Steculorum S, Messina A, Rasika S, Falluel-Morel A, Anouar Y, Dehouck B, Trinquet E, Jockers R, Bouret SG, Prevot V. Hypothalamic tanycytes are an ERK-gated conduit for leptin into the brain. Cell Metab. 2014;19(2):293–301. https://doi.org/10.1016/j.cmet.2013.12.015. S1550-4131(14)00004-7 [pii]

119. Prosser RA, Bergeron HE. Leptin phase-advances the rat suprachiasmatic circadian clock in vitro. Neurosci Lett. 2003;336(3):139–42. S030439400201234X [pii]

120. Inyushkin AN, Bhumbra GS, Dyball RE. Leptin modulates spike coding in the rat suprachiasmatic nucleus. J Neuroendocrinol. 2009;21(8):705–14. https://doi.org/10.1111/j.1365-2826.2009.01889.x. JNE1889 [pii]

121. Grosbellet E, Gourmelen S, Pevet P, Criscuolo F, Challet E. Leptin normalizes photic synchronization in male ob/ob mice, via indirect effects on the suprachiasmatic nucleus. Endocrinology. 2015;156(3):1080–90. https://doi.org/10.1210/en.2014-1570.

122. Sage D, Ganem J, Guillaumond F, Laforge-Anglade-G, Francois-Bellan AM, Bosler O, Becquet D. Influence of the corticosterone rhythm on photic entrainment of locomotor activity in rats. J Biol Rhythms. 2004;19(2):144–56.

123. Kiessling S, Eichele G, Oster H. Adrenal glucocorticoids have a key role in circadian resynchronization in a mouse model of jet lag. J Clin Invest. 2010;120(7):2600–9. https://doi.org/10.1172/JCI41192.

124. Malek ZS, Sage D, Pevet P, Raison S. Daily rhythm of tryptophan hydroxylase-2 messenger ribonucleic acid within raphe neurons is induced by corticoid daily surge and modulated by enhanced locomotor activity. Endocrinology. 2007;148(11):5165–72. https://doi.org/10.1210/en.2007-0526.

125. Sack RL, Hughes RJ, Edgar DM, Lewy AJ. Sleep-promoting effects of melatonin: at what dose, in whom, under what conditions, and by what mechanisms? Sleep. 1997;20(10):908–15.

126. Turek FW, Joshu C, Kohsaka A, Lin E, Ivanova G, McDearmon E, Laposky A, Losee-Olson S, Easton A, Jensen DR, Eckel RH, Takahashi JS, Bass J. Obesity and metabolic syndrome in circadian Clock mutant mice. Science. 2005;308(5724):1043–5. https://doi.org/10.1126/science.1108750.

127. Karlsson BH, Knutsson AK, Lindahl BO, Alfredsson LS. Metabolic disturbances in male workers with rotating three-shift work. Results of the WOLF study. Int Arch Occup Environ Health. 2003;76(6): 424–30. https://doi.org/10.1007/s00420-003-0440-y.

128. Dochi M, Suwazono Y, Sakata K, Okubo Y, Oishi M, Tanaka K, Kobayashi E, Nogawa K. Shift work is a risk factor for increased total cholesterol level: a 14-year prospective cohort study in 6886 male workers. Occup Environ Med. 2009;66(9):592–7. https://doi.org/10.1136/oem.2008.042176. 66/9/592 [pii]

129. Spiegel K, Tasali E, Leproult R, Van Cauter E. Effects of poor and short sleep on glucose metabolism and obesity risk. Nat Rev Endocrinol. 2009;5(5):253–61. https://doi.org/10.1038/nrendo.2009.23.

130. Tsai LL, Tsai YC, Hwang K, Huang YW, Tzeng JE. Repeated light-dark shifts speed up body weight gain in male F344 rats. Am J Physiol Endocrinol Metab. 2005;289(2):E212–7. https://doi.org/10.1152/ajpendo.00603.2004.

131. Bartol-Munier I, Gourmelen S, Pevet P, Challet E. Combined effects of high-fat feeding and circadian desynchronization. Int J Obes (Lond). 2006;30(1): 60–7. https://doi.org/10.1038/sj.ijo.0803048.

132. Salgado-Delgado R, Angeles-Castellanos M, Buijs MR, Escobar C. Internal desynchronization in a model of night-work by forced activity in rats. Neuroscience. 2008;154(3):922–31. https://doi.org/10.1016/j.neuroscience.2008.03.066.

133. Grosbellet E, Zahn S, Arrive M, Dumont S, Gourmelen S, Pevet P, Challet E, Criscuolo F. Circadian desynchronization triggers premature cellular aging in a diurnal rodent. FASEB J. 2015;29(12):4794–803. https://doi.org/10.1096/fj.14-266817.

134. Kaneko K, Yamada T, Tsukita S, Takahashi K, Ishigaki Y, Oka Y, Katagiri H. Obesity alters circadian expressions of molecular clock genes in the brainstem. Brain Res. 2009;1263:58–68. https://doi.org/10.1016/j.brainres.2008.12.071. S0006-8993(09)00003-1 [pii]

135. Cha MC, Chou CJ, Boozer CN. High-fat diet feeding reduces the diurnal variation of plasma leptin concentration in rats. Metabolism. 2000;49(4):503–7. S0026-0495(00)80016-5 [pii]

136. Yanagihara H, Ando H, Hayashi Y, Obi Y, Fujimura A. High-fat feeding exerts minimal effects on rhythmic mRNA expression of clock genes in mouse peripheral tissues. Chronobiol Int. 2006;23(5):905–14. https://doi.org/10.1080/07420520600827103. M6X0146501105014 [pii]

137. Eckel-Mahan KL, Patel VR, de Mateo S, Orozco-Solis R, Ceglia NJ, Sahar S, Dilag-Penilla SA, Dyar KA, Baldi P, Sassone-Corsi P. Reprogramming of the circadian clock by nutritional challenge. Cell. 2013;155(7):1464–78. https://doi.org/10.1016/j.cell.2013.11.034.

138. Otway DT, Mantele S, Bretschneider S, Wright J, Trayhurn P, Skene DJ, Robertson MD, Johnston JD. Rhythmic diurnal gene expression in human adipose tissue from individuals who are lean, overweight, and type 2 diabetic. Diabetes. 2011;60(5): 1577–81. https://doi.org/10.2337/db10-1098.

139. Fukagawa K, Sakata T, Yoshimatsu H, Fujimoto K, Uchimura K, Asano C. Advance shift of feeding circadian rhythm induced by obesity progression in Zucker rats. Am J Physiol. 1992;263(6 Pt 2): R1169–75.

140. Mistlberger RE, Lukman H, Nadeau BG. Circadian rhythms in the Zucker obese rat: assessment and intervention. Appetite. 1998;30(3):255–67. S0195-6663(97)90134-3 [pii]. https://doi.org/10.1006/appe.1997.0134.

141. Kudo T, Akiyama M, Kuriyama K, Sudo M, Moriya T, Shibata S. Night-time restricted feeding normalises clock genes and Pai-1 gene expression in the db/db mouse liver. Diabetologia. 2004;47(8): 1425–36. https://doi.org/10.1007/s00125-004-1461-0.

142. Sans-Fuentes MA, Diez-Noguera A, Cambras T. Light responses of the circadian system in leptin deficient mice. Physiol Behav. 2010;99(4):487–94. https://doi.org/10.1016/j.physbeh.2009.12.023. S0031-9384(09)00410-7 [pii]

143. Grosbellet E, Gourmelen S, Pevet P, Criscuolo F, Challet E. Leptin normalizes photic synchronization in male ob/ob mice, via indirect effects on the suprachiasmatic nucleus. Endocrinology. 2015: en20141570. https://doi.org/10.1210/en.2014-1570.

144. Grosbellet E, Dumont S, Schuster-Klein C, Guardiola-Lemaitre B, Pevet P, Criscuolo F, Challet E. Circadian phenotyping of obese and diabetic db/db mice. Biochimie. 2016;124:198–206. https://doi.org/10.1016/j.biochi.2015.06.029. S0300-9084(15)00208-4 [pii]

145. Chellappa SL, Gordijn MC, Cajochen C. Can light make us bright? Effects of light on cognition and sleep. Prog Brain Res. 2011;190:119–33. https://doi.org/10.1016/B978-0-444-53817-8.00007-4. B978-0-444-53817-8.00007-4 [pii]

146. Hatori M, Vollmers C, Zarrinpar A, DiTacchio L, Bushong EA, Gill S, Leblanc M, Chaix A, Joens M, Fitzpatrick JA, Ellisman MH, Panda S. Time-restricted feeding without reducing caloric intake prevents metabolic diseases in mice fed a high-fat diet. Cell Metab. 2012;15(6):848–60. https://doi.org/10.1016/j.cmet.2012.04.019. S1550-4131(12)00189-1 [pii]

147. Reid KJ, Baron KG, Zee PC. Meal timing influences daily caloric intake in healthy adults. Nutr Res. 2014;34(11):930–5. https://doi.org/10.1016/j.nutres.2014.09.010. S0271-5317(14)00195-X [pii]

148. Colles SL, Dixon JB, O'Brien PE. Night eating syndrome and nocturnal snacking: association with obesity, binge eating and psychological distress. Int J Obes (Lond). 2007;31(11):1722–30. https://doi.org/10.1038/sj.ijo.0803664.

149. Striegel-Moore RH, Rosselli F, Wilson GT, Perrin N, Harvey K, DeBar L. Nocturnal eating: association with binge eating, obesity, and psychological distress. Int J Eat Disord. 2010;43(6):520–6. https://doi.org/10.1002/eat.20735.

150. Lowden A, Moreno C, Holmback U, Lennernas M, Tucker P. Eating and shift work – effects on habits, metabolism and performance. Scand J Work Environ Health. 2010;36(2):150–62. 2898 [pii]

151. Chou TC, Scammell TE, Gooley JJ, Gaus SE, Saper CB, Lu J. Critical role of dorsomedial hypothalamic nucleus in a wide range of behavioral circadian rhythms. J Neurosci. 2003;23(33):10691–702. 23/33/10691 [pii]

Obesity, Myokines, and Metabolic Health

25

Noemi Malandrino and Rexford S. Ahima

Contents

Abstract

Skeletal muscle is a major determinant of energy expenditure and glucose disposal. Muscle fibers express and secrete several peptides, defined as myokines, which act through autocrine, paracrine or endocrine mechanisms to regulate skeletal muscle growth and regeneration, energy homeostasis, and glucose and lipid metabolism. Obesity and aging are associated with dysregulated myokine secretion and signaling, which may contribute to skeletal muscle loss and development of metabolic disease. Studies investigating the effects of myokines may help identify potential targets for the

N. Malandrino · R. S. Ahima (✉)
Department of Medicine, Division of Endocrinology,
Diabetes and Metabolism, Johns Hopkins University
School of Medicine, Baltimore, MD, USA
e-mail: nmaland2@jh.edu; ahima@jhmi.edu

© Springer Nature Switzerland AG 2023
R. S. Ahima (ed.), *Metabolic Syndrome*,
https://doi.org/10.1007/978-3-031-40116-9_56

prevention and treatment of obesity, diabetes, and aging-related metabolic diseases.

Keywords

Myokines · Exercise · Obesity · Aging · Myostatin · Interleukin-6 · Irisin · Interleukin-15

Introduction

The prevalence of obesity among adults in the United States increased from 30.5% in 1999–2000 to 41.9% in 2017–2020 [1]. Even more concerning is the increase in prevalence of severe obesity (defined as a body mass index [BMI] $\geq$ 40 kg/m^2) from 4.7% to 9.2% during the same period [1]. The rapidly increasing prevalence of obesity poses significant public health concerns. Obesity is an established risk factor for chronic diseases, disability, and premature death. The Global Burden of Diseases, Injuries and Risk Factors Study, which systematically collects mortality data worldwide, has shown that, among the spectrum of metabolic diseases (i.e., obesity, type 2 diabetes, hypertension, hyperlipidemia, non-alcoholic fatty liver disease), obesity is associated with the largest proportion of metabolic-related mortality and disability-adjusted life years [2]. Furthermore, sarcopenic obesity, primarily affecting older adults and characterized by the coexistence of increased adiposity and sarcopenia (age-related decrease in muscle mass and function), is associated with a higher degree of cardiovascular risk factors and an increased mortality risk compared to not having sarcopenia or obesity, or either obesity or sarcopenia alone [3].

Lifestyle interventions, including healthy diet, exercise, and behavioral modification, are recommended as the first step in the management of obesity and metabolic disease [4, 5]. Several studies have shown the beneficial effects of regular physical activity and exercise on the prevention and treatment of obesity, sarcopenic obesity, and the related complications, including type 2 diabetes, cardiovascular disease, cognitive decline and cancer, as well as on the promotion of health span and longevity [6–8]. Skeletal muscle accounts for up to 40% of the total body weight in nonobese adults and is a major determinant of energy expenditure and glucose disposal, playing a critical role in the maintenance of metabolic health [9, 10]. The well-established benefits of exercise are partly attributed to the expression and secretion of muscle-derived peptides known as myokines (reviewed in [11]). These peptides are released from muscle cells during proliferation and differentiation or in response to muscle contraction [11]. Myokines can exert their effects through autocrine or paracrine mechanisms in skeletal muscle, or endocrine mechanisms mediating crosstalk between skeletal muscle and other organs, including adipose tissue, liver, brain, and pancreas, thus mediating some of the effects of exercise on these organs (reviewed in [7, 11]) (Fig. 1).

Dysregulated secretion and signaling of several myokines have been described both in the presence of obesity and aging, which may be related to the decline in physical activity and skeletal muscle mass associated with these conditions, contributing to the development of related metabolic dysregulation [12, 13]. A deeper understanding of the actions of myokines may help identify potential pharmacological targets for the treatment of obesity, diabetes, and aging-related diseases. This chapter reviews the current knowledge on the biology of some of the myokines involved in metabolism.

Myostatin

Myostatin, also known as growth differentiation factor 8 (GDF-8), is a member of the transforming growth factor β superfamily and the first identified muscle-derived peptide to fulfill the criteria of "myokine" [14]. Myostatin is expressed and secreted predominantly by skeletal muscle, and functions as a negative regulator of skeletal muscle growth in an autocrine manner [14]. Myostatin function is strongly conserved in many species, as shown by the development of muscle cell

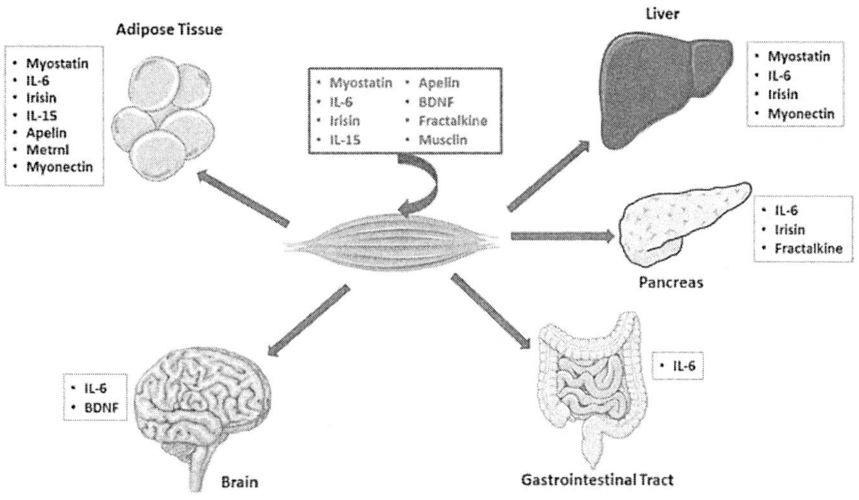

Fig. 1 Myokines act via autocrine, paracrine (red color), or endocrine pathways (black color) to regulate skeletal muscle mass, energy metabolism, glucose homeostasis, and other functions. IL-6: interleukin-6; IL-15: interleukin-15; BDNF: brain-derived neurotrophic factor; Metrnl: meteorin-like. The figure was partly generated using Servier Medical Art, provided by Servier, licensed under a Creative Commons Attribution 3.0 unported license

hyperplasia and hypertrophy with targeted or naturally occurring mutations affecting myostatin gene activation in mice, sheep, cattle, dog, rabbit, rat, goat, and humans (reviewed in [15]).

During early postnatal development, myostatin inhibits the hyperplastic growth of myoblasts by inducing cell cycle arrest via upregulation of p21, a cyclin-dependent kinase (Cdk) inhibitor, resulting in reduction of Cdk 2 and Cdk 4 levels [16]. By preventing myoblast proliferation, myostatin signaling also leads to a reduction in the number of cells differentiating into mature myofibers [16]. Studies in mammals suggest that myostatin delays the differentiation of myoblasts by inducing cellular quiescence via reduced expression of myogenic regulatory factors, such as Pax3, MyoD, Myf5 [16]. Furthermore, in postnatal mature muscle fibers, myostatin reduces myofiber protein synthesis and myosatellite cell activation and renewal, inhibiting the hypertrophic growth of mature muscle [16]. Human obesity and sarcopenia are associated with increased expression of myostatin at the level of muscle tissue [17, 18]. Conversely, endurance exercise training decreases myostatin expression [19].

Myostatin Signaling

Myostatin is synthesized as a precursor protein, subsequently cleaved by furin proteases into an N-terminal propeptide and a C-terminal disulfide-linked dimer, which is the biologically active signaling molecule. After proteolytic processing, the N-terminal propeptide and C-terminal dimer remain noncovalently bound, maintaining myostatin in an inactive latent state [15]. Activation of latent myostatin occurs via proteolytic cleavage of the propeptide, immediately N-terminal to aspartate 76, by four members of the bone morphogenetic protein (BMP)-1/tolloid (TLD) family of metalloproteases (BMP-1, TLD, TLL-1, TLL-2). This major mechanism of myostatin activation in vivo has been supported by studies in mice carrying mutations consisting of either substitution of aspartate with alanine in position 76 of the propeptide or loss-of-function in TLL2, both resulting in a phenotype characterized by increased muscle mass [15].

In addition to the N-terminal propeptide, other proteins are involved in the regulation of myostatin action at the extracellular level. Among these proteins, follistatin, follistatin like-3 (FSTL3), and growth and differentiation factor-associated serum protein-1 and 2 (GASP-1, GASP-2) are capable of inhibiting myostatin action by preventing the binding to its receptor [15]. The role of these proteins in myostatin inhibition is supported by studies in mice carrying deletions at the genes encoding for follistatin, GASP-1 and GASP-2, characterized by decreased muscle mass and regeneration ability. Similarly, overexpression of follistatin, FSTL-3, and GASP-1 results in muscle mass growth [15]. Interestingly, transgenic overexpression of follistatin in myostatin knockout mice is still associated with a dramatic increase in muscle mass. This observation has suggested the existence of at least one additional TGF-β family member with partially redundant function, later identified as activin A, which cooperates with myostatin in inhibiting muscle growth [15].

Within the skeletal muscle fibers, when not bound to inhibitory proteins, myostatin signals through the binding of the C-terminal dimer to the activin type 2 receptors ActRIIA and ActRIIB (also called ACVR2 and ACVR2B). While myostatin binds to ActRIIB with higher affinity than ActRIIA, an increase in muscle growth is observed in mice carrying deletion mutations in either receptor, indicating that both activin type 2 receptors are involved in myostatin's ability to regulate muscle mass. ActRIIA and ActRIIB are partially functionally redundant with each other, as shown by a more significant increase in muscle mass when targeting the two receptors simultaneously rather than targeting either alone [15]. Binding of myostatin to ActRIIA and ActRIIB results into the recruitment, phosphorylation, and activation of the type 1 receptors activin receptor-like kinase (ALK) 4 and ALK5, then leading to phosphorylation and activation of Smad2 and Smad3. Genetic studies have shown that ALK4 and ALK5 are partially functionally redundant with each other, as targeting these receptors simultaneously in myofibers leads to a more dramatic muscle growth compared to targeting either receptor alone. Once phosphorylated, Smad2 and Smad3 form a heterodimeric complex with Smad4, which in turn functions as a transcription factor regulating gene expression

and resulting in inhibition of muscle growth [15] (Fig. 2).

Metabolic Effects of Myostatin Inhibition

Studies in animals have shown that the anabolic effects on muscle mass secondary to the blockade of myostatin signaling are associated with beneficial effects on adipose tissue and glucose and lipid metabolism. Indeed, in addition to increased skeletal muscle mass, myostatin knockout mice have reduced white adipose tissue (WAT), which becomes more prominent with increasing age and appears to be related to decreased adipogenesis, rather than decreased fat deposition in mature adipocytes [20, 21]. In agouti lethal yellow and leptin-deficient mice, two mouse models of obesity and diabetes, loss of myostatin results in decreased WAT content [20]. Myostatin signaling is also involved in the regulation of glucose metabolism, as shown by improved glucose utilization and insulin sensitivity in myostatin knockout mice, as well as improved hyperglycemia in myostatin-null agouti lethal yellow and leptin deficient mice [20, 22]. Similarly, in mice fed chow or high-fat diets, pharmacological inhibition of myostatin signaling induced by treatment with a soluble activin receptor type IIB (ActRIIB-Fc) results in increased muscle mass and functional parameters (grip strength and contractile force), decreased WAT, and improved glucose and lipid metabolism, including enhanced hepatic and peripheral insulin sensitivity [23]. It has been suggested that the changes in WAT and glucose homeostasis secondary to myostatin blockade are indirectly driven by the anabolic effects on skeletal muscle, rather than a direct effect on adipose tissue. This is supported by findings in mice carrying a dominant negative ActRIIB receptor expressed in either skeletal muscle or WAT, where the absence of myostatin signaling in skeletal muscle, but not in adipocytes, results in a metabolic phenotype similar to the one observed in myostatin knockout mice, characterized by hypermuscularity, reduced body fat, and increased insulin sensitivity [22].

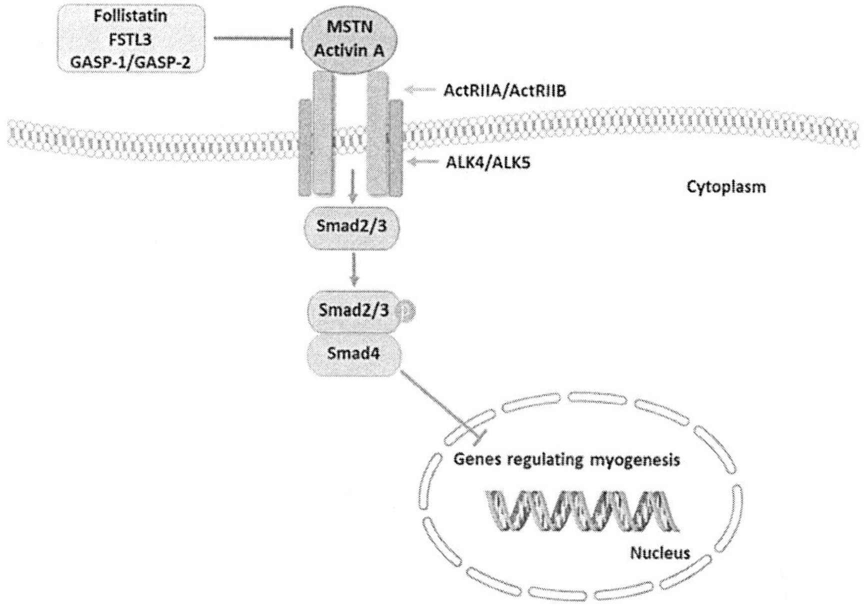

Fig. 2 Myostatin signaling pathway in skeletal muscle. Myostatin and activin A signal via the activin receptors II (ActRIIA, ActRIIB) and the activin receptor-like kinases (ALK4, ALK5), leading to phosphorylation and activation of Smad2 and Smad3. Smad2 and Smad3 bind to Smad4 to inhibit muscle growth. Follistatin, follistatin like-3 (FSTL3) and growth and differentiation factor-associated serum protein-1 and 2 (GASP-1, GASP-2) inhibit myostatin action. The figure was partly generated using Servier Medical Art, provided by Servier, licensed under a Creative Commons Attribution 3.0 unported license

Myostatin signaling appears to be involved also in WAT browning and regulation of brown adipose tissue (BAT). Myostatin knockout mice show features of WAT browning, such as increased expression of thermogenic genes, i.e., uncoupling protein 1 (UCP1) and peroxisomal proliferator-activated receptor-γ coactivator 1α (PGC1α), as well as beige adipocyte markers, Tmem26 and CD137 [24]. Likewise, studies in rodents treated with ActRIIB-Fc have shown not only increased skeletal muscle mass, but also induction of WAT browning and thermogenesis, in addition to enhancement of BAT differentiation, growth, and activation [25, 26]. The mechanisms linking myostatin blockade to the observed changes in WAT and BAT are unclear. Another myokine, irisin, has been suggested to contribute to the browning of WAT in myostatin knockout mice, where inhibition of myostatin signaling results in increased expression and phosphorylation of AMPK, which in turn activates PGC1α and irisin [24]. However, irisin does not appear to play a role in the enhancement of BAT resulting from ActRIIB-Fc treatment [26].

Clinical Applications of Myostatin Inhibition

The identification of key mechanisms regulating myostatin signaling and the related changes in body composition and metabolism in mice, in addition to the findings of increased myostatin levels in plasma and muscle tissue of women with obesity compared to those with normal weight, as well as reduced myostatin levels following exercise, have laid the foundation for clinical trials testing the blockade of myostatin as a possible treatment for a wide range of diseases, including obesity, metabolic disorders, and sarcopenia [15, 17, 19, 22–27].

Two classes of biologics have been tested as myostatin inhibitors in clinical trials. One class of these biologics specifically targets myostatin, with some cross-reactivity to the myostatin-related protein GDF-11. The second class, which includes the myostatin inhibitors bimagrumab, ACE-031, and ACE-083, is able to block activin A in addition to myostatin and GDF-11 [15]. The average increase in muscle mass observed in humans after treatment with myostatin inhibitors ranges between 3% and 9% in trials for different clinical indications, with larger increases seen with drugs targeting both myostatin and activin A (5–9%), compared to those targeting only myostatin (3–5%) [28–30]. This increase in muscle mass, though significant, is lower than the changes observed in mice, where compounds targeting myostatin alone resulted in 10–30% muscle mass increase, while those targeting both myostatin and activin A resulted in 25–50% muscle mass increase [15]. In humans, a larger contribution of activin A to muscle mass regulation, compared to myostatin, may partly explain the lower response to myostatin inhibitors observed in clinical studies. This hypothesis is supported by differences in circulating levels of myostatin and activin A in humans, which are seven- to eightfold lower and three- to fourfold higher, respectively, compared with mice [31].

Similar to studies in mice, clinical studies in individuals with either obesity or sarcopenia have confirmed additional beneficial effects of myostatin inhibitors on adipose tissue and glucose metabolism. In a double-blind, placebo-controlled study, after 10 weeks of a single intravenous dose of bimagrumab, a monoclonal antibody binding to the ActRII receptor, healthy individuals with insulin resistance showed not only increased muscle mass, but significantly decreased total adipose tissue (by 7.9%) and improved insulin sensitivity (by 20–40%) [32]. Furthermore, in healthy postmenopausal women, a single subcutaneous dose of ACE-031, a decoy ActRIIB receptor, did not affect the adipose tissue amount, but resulted in significant changes in adipose tissue biomarkers, i.e., 51.3% increase in adiponectin and 27.7% decrease in leptin, consistent with a favorable metabolic profile [29]. The strongest effects of myostatin blockade on adipose tissue have been shown in a double-blind placebo-controlled randomized study in overweight and obese adults

with type 2 diabetes receiving bimagrumab or placebo for 48 weeks. Treatment with bimagrumab compared to placebo resulted in a reduction in total fat mass by 20%, an increase in lean mass by 4.4%, a reduction in waist circumference by 9.5 cm, and a reduction in hemoglobin A1c by 0.72 percentage points [33]. Likewise, an increase in muscle mass and function is associated with favorable adipose tissue changes in clinical trials of older individuals affected by sarcopenia [28, 30, 34]. For example, a randomized, double-blind, placebo-controlled, proof-of-concept study showed a significant reduction in total fat mass, intermuscular thigh adipose tissue, and subcutaneous thigh fat in community-dwelling adults with sarcopenia aged 65 and older, after 24 weeks of treatment with bimagrumab compared to placebo [30]. Whether the changes in body composition observed with myostatin inhibitors significantly affect the development and progression of metabolic disease in individuals with obesity or sarcopenic obesity needs further investigation.

Interleukin-6

Interleukin-6 (IL-6) is a member of the granulocyte colony-stimulating factor-like protein family of cytokines, which includes many cytokines sharing the membrane glycoprotein gp130 as signal transducing receptor. Conventionally defined as a pro-inflammatory cytokine, IL-6 plays a main role in the regulation of the immune system at sites of inflammation, favoring the transition from innate to acquired immunity, the recruitment and differentiation of immune cells, and the promotion of antibody production from B-cells (reviewed in [35]). Increased plasma levels of IL-6 have been implicated in the development of insulin resistance in individuals with obesity and type 2 diabetes, conditions known to be associated with chronic low-grade inflammation [11]. Similarly, older age and sarcopenia are associated with higher plasma levels of IL-6, which is positively correlated with a higher risk for muscle strength loss (reviewed in [36]). However, studies in models of exercise and skeletal muscle contraction identify an additional opposite role of IL-6 as a myokine with anti-inflammatory and insulin-sensitizing properties [11]. The notion of skeletal muscle being the source of production of IL-6 in response to exercise has been supported by transcriptional analysis of IL-6 mRNA levels during exercise, in situ hybridization and immunohistochemistry of IL-6, microdialysis of contracting skeletal muscle, and measurement of arteriovenous IL-6 concentrations and blood flow across an exercising leg [11]. During acute exercise, the increased secretion of IL-6 from muscle cells is associated with an exponential increase of its plasma levels, in proportion to the muscle mass involved in the exercise and the duration of exercise [11]. On the other hand, epidemiological studies have shown that basal plasma IL-6 levels are negatively associated with the amount of physical activity, and positively associated with physical inactivity, obesity, and metabolic syndrome [37–39]. Indeed, chronic exercise results in a reduction of basal IL-6 levels, in addition to a blunted increase in IL-6 plasma and muscle tissue levels during exercise. Conversely, the basal IL-6 receptor α (IL-6Rα) mRNA content increases, possibly to counteract the reduction in IL-6 [11].

IL-6 Signaling

The dual roles of IL-6 in inflammation and metabolism seem to be related to its complex signaling mechanisms [35]. IL-6 can exert its function via classical signaling or a trans-signaling pathways. The classical pathway is initiated by IL-6 binding to the membrane-bound form of the IL-6Rα, which triggers its association with the signal transducing gp130 receptor. This pathway occurs in few cell types that express the IL-6Rα on their cell surface, e.g., macrophages, neutrophils, hepatocytes, and myocytes [35]. The trans-signaling pathway is initiated by IL-6 binding to a soluble form of IL-6Rα (sIL-6Rα), allowing for IL-6 to exert its effects on cells expressing gp130, but not IL-6Rα. The sIL-6Rα is predominantly made by proteolytic cleavage of the membrane-bound IL-6Rα, and, to a lesser extent, by alternative splicing of the IL-6Rα gene. As gp130 is ubiquitously expressed, the IL6 trans-signaling pathway may occur in a wider range of cells [35].

Binding of IL-6 to its specific α-receptor results into the recruitment of two gp130 molecules to form a hexameric complex. This complex transmits the IL-6 signal into the cells via the recruitment and activation of multiple intracellular signaling pathways, including the Jak-STAT pathway, the Ras-MAPK pathway, the p38 and JNK MAPK pathways, the PI 3-K-Akt pathway, and the MEK-ERK5 pathway [35, 40]. Although both the classic and trans-signaling pathways activate similar intracellular signals, studies have suggested that the proinflammatory effects of IL-6 are mediated by the trans-signaling pathway in inflammatory cells via the sIL-6Rα. Conversely, the anti-inflammatory effects of IL-6 are mediated by the classical pathway via the IL-6Rα constitutively expressed on the cell surface [35].

Metabolic Effects of IL-6

Mouse models have shown the role of IL-6 as an anabolic factor promoting myogenesis and hypertrophic muscle growth via autocrine and paracrine mechanisms. Indeed, IL-6 appears to be a major regulator of satellite cell proliferation-mediated muscle growth via the STAT3 pathway [41]. However, the main effects of IL-6 as a myokine are related to regulation of glucose and lipid metabolism in muscle and adipose tissue. Through a mechanism at least partially mediated by AMP-activated protein kinase (AMPK), treatment of rat L6 myotubes with IL-6 results in increased basal glucose uptake via glucose transporter 4 translocation, as well as increased insulin-stimulated glucose uptake [42]. In healthy resting humans, the acute administration of recombinant human IL-6 (rhIL-6) to achieve physiological plasma IL-6 concentrations did not affect whole-body glucose disposal, muscle glucose uptake, or endogenous glucose production [43]. In contrast, infusion of rhIL-6 into healthy volunteers during low-intensity exercise resulted in increased endogenous glucose production, suggesting an IL-6-mediated muscle-liver crosstalk for the regulation of plasma glucose levels during exercise

[42]. Furthermore, the infusion of rhIL-6 to achieve plasma IL-6 concentrations similar to those of high-intensity exercise resulted in enhanced whole-body glucose disposal during a hyperinsulinemic-euglycemic clamp. These findings may provide a mechanism explaining the increased insulin action observed after a single exercise bout [42].

The role of IL-6 as a regulator of lipid metabolism through stimulation of intra-myocellular and whole-body fatty acid oxidation as well as lipolysis, has been described in vitro, in rodents, and human studies [42, 44–46]. In healthy young and older men, enhanced fat oxidation and lipolysis were observed after infusion of rhIL-6 [45, 46]. Conversely, blockade of IL-6 signaling may increase fat accumulation in adipose tissue due to impaired lipolysis. This notion is supported by a randomized placebo-controlled trial in adults with central obesity receiving either tocilizumab (IL-6 receptor antibody) or placebo, during a 12-week intervention with either bicycle exercise or no exercise. In this study, aerobic exercise reduced visceral adipose tissue, and this effect was abolished by IL-6 receptor blockade [47]. Studies have shown an association between physical inactivity and increased visceral adipose tissue, as well as exercise training and decreased visceral adipose tissue [7].

IL-6 is also involved in browning of WAT. In mice receiving daily intraperitoneal injections of IL-6 for 1 week, an increase in UCP-1 mRNA in the inguinal WAT was observed [36]. Exercise training increased UCP1 mRNA in the inguinal WAT of wild-type mice, but not in IL-6 knockout mice [36]. Experiments have also shown lower mitochondrial density, thermogenic gene expression, and phosphorylation of STAT3 in white adipocytes derived from IL-6 knockout mice compared to wild-type mice. The subsequent treatment of IL-6 knockout white adipocytes with exogenous IL-6 results in increased transcription of peroxisome proliferator-activated receptor gamma (PPARγ), PGC1α, and UCP-1 via induction of STAT3 phosphorylation, in turn leading to enhanced browning of white adipocytes [36]. Additional in vivo experiments from the same study have confirmed the findings of

decreased browning of white adipocytes and STAT3 phosphorylation in IL-6 knockout mice that are further characterized by deranged glucose metabolism and accelerated hepatic steatosis [36]. Moreover, during differentiation of human beige adipocytes, the blockade of IL-6 receptor by a specific antibody results in downregulation of brown marker genes and an increase in morphological changes characteristic of white adipocytes, suggesting that beige adipocytes regulate IL-6 production to enhance browning in an autocrine manner [36]. Whether exercise-induced browning of white adipose tissue is caused by IL-6 requires further investigation.

Additional proposed effects of the myokine IL-6 on the regulation of appetite and pancreatic α- and β-cell function, as well as its anti-inflammatory properties, may play a role in promoting metabolic health. Administration of the same dose of IL-6 centrally, but not intraperitoneally, results in improved glucose tolerance and suppressed feeding in mice. On the other hand, a fourfold higher dose of IL-6 injected peripherally results in significantly decreased food intake. These findings suggest that the increased plasma IL-6 concentration observed during exercise may regulate appetite centrally, by crossing the blood–brain barrier [7]. In humans, an acute increase in IL-6 plasma concentrations, via infusion of rhIL-6, leads to delayed gastric emptying and reduction in postprandial glucose levels [7]. However, these findings are not replicated in physically inactive individuals with obesity after 12 weeks of exercise training [48]. In vitro studies have shown that IL-6 released by skeletal muscle during exercise stimulates the secretion of glucagon-like peptide-1 (GLP-1) from pancreatic α-cells and intestinal L-cells. The release of GLP-1 leads to increased insulin secretion and improved glucose homeostasis. These findings were not replicated in GLP-1 receptor knockout mice, despite increased IL-6 levels, suggesting that GLP-1 is an essential mediator of IL-6 actions on β-cell function and glucose homeostasis [7]. In mouse islet cells, IL-6 also stimulates α- and β-cell proliferation, while exerting distinct effects on α- and β-cell apoptosis, i.e., inhibition of α-cell apoptosis and enhancement of β-cell apoptosis in the presence of elevated glucose and palmitate [7]. Exercise-induced release of IL-6 inhibits monocyte production of tumor necrosis factor-α (TNF- α) and IL-1β, while increasing the expression of anti-inflammatory cytokines IL-10, IL-1 receptor antagonist and soluble TNF receptor [7].

Irisin

Irisin is a 112 amino acid peptide, highly homologous between mouse and humans. Irisin is secreted from the skeletal muscle as the extracellular N-terminal portion of the transmembrane protein fibronectin type III domain-containing protein 5 (FNDC5) [49]. FNDC5 is a gene target of PGC1α, which is a transcriptional co-activator induced by exercise in the skeletal muscle and regulating several beneficial effects of exercise, including mitochondrial biogenesis, angiogenesis, and fiber-type switching. Boström et al. have shown that, under the regulation of PGC1α, muscle FNDC5 expression and plasma irisin levels are increased in mice and humans after short-term exercise [49]. Also, this study identified the role of irisin as a myokine promoting thermogenic gene expression and browning of the subcutaneous WAT, as well as increasing energy expenditure and improving glucose tolerance in mice fed a high fat diet. The metabolic effects mediated by muscle-derived irisin result in protection against obesity and insulin resistance, suggesting that irisin may drive at least some of the beneficial effects of exercise [49]. In vitro studies with 3T3-L1 preadipocytes and subcutaneous human adipocytes have further demonstrated the capacity of irisin to stimulate lipolysis and inhibit lipogenesis and fat storage, via the regulation of adipose triglyceride lipase and hormone-sensitive lipase, and fatty acid-binding protein 4 and the Wnt signaling [36]. Similar findings of enhanced lipolysis are observed in obese mice overexpressing FNDC5 or receiving persistent subcutaneous infusion of irisin, resulting in increased hormone-sensitive lipase expression and phosphorylation and reduced perilipin levels, and leading to improved metabolic derangements [36]. In diabetic mice fed a high fat diet, treatment with irisin also increases skeletal muscle fatty acid oxidation and glucose uptake and decreases liver gluconeogenesis [36]. A study with mouse islets has shown the protective effects of irisin under glucolipotoxic conditions, including suppression of lipogenesis, improvement of insulin secretion, inhibition of apoptosis, and restoration of β-cell function-related gene expression [50].

While in vitro and rodent studies are supportive of a protective role of muscle-derived irisin against metabolic disease, the biological role of irisin is controversial in humans. First, it is unclear whether irisin is truly a myokine since human WAT also expresses FNDC5 and secretes irisin [51]. Second, although plasma irisin levels generally increase with acute exercise in humans, the changes in irisin following chronic aerobic or resistance exercise are highly variable in individuals of different age and level of obesity [52–56]. Even decreased circulating irisin concentrations have been described after chronic exercise training [57]. Third, the current literature describes contradictory results regarding measured irisin levels in individuals with low-grade inflammatory metabolic states, such as obesity and type 2 diabetes, in older individuals and in those with or without sarcopenia. Several studies have shown that individuals with obesity or type 2 diabetes have decreased baseline plasma irisin levels compared to controls [58, 59]. On the other hand, some studies have suggested an upregulation of circulating irisin in individuals who are overweight or obese, with a positive correlation between irisin levels and the BMI [60]. A decline in irisin concentrations has been reported both in older and sarcopenic individuals, suggesting that the decline of irisin with age may contribute to the aging-associated metabolic disease [54, 61–63]. However, there have also been clinical studies showing no significant difference in circulating irisin levels in older adults with and without sarcopenia, with a lack of association between irisin levels and sarcopenia-related parameters, such as skeletal muscle index, grip strength, gait speed [64].

The reasons for these conflicting results in humans are unclear. In individuals with obesity, it has been suggested that the elevation of irisin levels may be a compensatory response to the metabolic derangements and insulin resistance observed in this population or may be related to the development of irisin resistance [60]. Differences in study populations and sample size, level of exercise training, or assays used to measure irisin, as well as suboptimal storage of tissue samples and differences in the function of irisin in rodents versus humans can further contribute to the divergent results observed in human studies.

Interleukin-15

Interleukin-15 (IL-15) is a 14-kDa protein belonging to the IL-2 superfamily. While IL-15 is expressed in several tissues, a particularly high expression has been observed in skeletal muscle (reviewed in [65]). An in vitro model supports the notion that secretion of IL-15 from the skeletal muscle occurs in response to contraction [66]. In individuals at rest, IL-15 levels in skeletal muscle interstitium are ten times higher than plasma IL-15 levels, suggesting that muscle-derived IL-15 can exert its effects locally in an autocrine or paracrine fashion [67].

Data on plasma IL-15 levels after exercise are mixed. Acute and chronic aerobic and resistance exercise have been associated with an increase in circulating IL-15 levels in studies enrolling different populations, including untrained and trained young and old individuals and individuals with normal weight and obesity [65]. Other studies have shown no changes in IL-15 after either resistance or aerobic exercise. These discrepancies could be related to the timing of blood sampling, since in the latter studies IL-15 was collected immediately after or more than 1 h after the end of exercise. Since the half-life of free IL-15 is estimated to be 30–60 min, it has been suggested that collecting IL-15 more than 1 h after exercise may result in missing the acute increase in IL-15 [65].

The role of IL-15 as an anabolic factor for the skeletal muscle is controversial [12], though several animal studies support a role of IL-15 in the regulation of glucose and lipid metabolism. Studies in rats treated with supraphysiological doses of IL-15 or in mice overexpressing IL-15 show enhanced whole body insulin sensitivity and decreased adiposity, likely mediated by an increased skeletal muscle glucose uptake, increased adipose tissue lipolysis, decreased lipogenesis and glucose incorporation into fat, and upregulation of calcineurin leading to inhibition of adipocyte differentiation [65].

The associations of IL-15 with insulin resistance, glucose metabolism, and adiposity are less clear in human studies. While single-nucleotide polymorphisms (SNPs) of the IL-15 gene have been associated with measures of insulin resistance and fasting blood glucose, other studies have shown no relationship between plasma IL-15 levels and insulin resistance [68, 69]. Moreover, both increased and decreased circulating IL-15 levels have been observed in individuals with type 2 diabetes compared to controls [70, 71]. Similarly, SNPs in human IL-15 and IL-15Rα genes have been associated with markers of adiposity, while conflicting results on the association between obesity and levels of plasma IL-15 and skeletal muscle IL-15 mRNA have been described [67–70]. Specifically, increased, decreased, or similar plasma IL-15 and skeletal muscle IL-15 mRNA levels have been described in individuals with obesity compared to lean controls [67, 69, 70]. The reasons for these discrepant results in humans are unknown. Differences in age and physical activity level have been suggested as possible contributors to the variable findings observed in prior studies [65].

In rodents treated with IL-15 or overexpressing IL-15, a shift toward a more oxidative skeletal muscle phenotype is observed [72, 73]. This shift results in increased endurance capacity and decreased adiposity and appears to be secondary to the activation of PPARδ by IL-15 [72, 73]. PPARδ is a nuclear hormone receptor highly expressed in the skeletal muscle and induced by exercise. Of note, the overexpression or activation of PPARδ results in an oxidative skeletal muscle phenotype similar to that observed with IL-15 overexpression [74].

IL-15 exerts its effects by binding to a plasma membrane receptor composed of three subunits: an IL-15 receptor α (IL-15Rα) chain, which specifically binds IL-15; a β subunit, which is common with the IL-2 receptor; and a gamma chain (γc), which is common to the receptors for other cytokines [12]. Animal studies have suggested a role of IL-15Rα in determining the muscle phenotype in mice. In the IL-15Rα knockout mouse, loss of IL-15Rα leads to remodeling of skeletal muscle toward a more oxidative phenotype associated with increased spontaneous locomotor activity and exercise capacity, fatigue resistance, and a substantial increase in mitochondrial density [75, 76]. IL-15Rα knockout mice are also characterized by elevated IL-15 expression in the skeletal muscle, as well as increased levels of circulating IL-15 [76, 77]. These findings led to the hypothesis that loss of IL-15Rα in the skeletal muscle of IL-15Rα knockout mice stimulates an increase in muscle IL-15 secretion, which in turn leads to a pro-oxidative remodeling of muscle tissue in an autocrine manner, independently of IL-15Rα. However, this hypothesis is not supported by a subsequent in vitro study showing that, in myotubes lacking IL-15Rα, acute treatment with IL-15 does not induce the expected increase in markers of oxidative metabolism, including PPARδ and PGC1α mRNA levels [78]. Further studies are needed to better understand the role of IL-15 as a regulator of adiposity and metabolism in humans and to evaluate whether IL-15Rα can be targeted specifically for obesity treatment by increasing energy expenditure and fatty acid oxidation.

Other Myokines

Apelin

Until recently, apelin was described as an adipokine whose circulating levels are elevated in obesity [79]. However, further evidence supports an additional role of apelin as a myokine released during muscle contraction and affecting muscle function and glucose and lipid metabolism [80–84]. Animal and human models have shown that exercise increases mRNA levels of apelin in the muscle and possibly plasma apelin levels [80, 85]. Both muscle and plasma apelin levels

decline with aging [85]. Studies in old mice treated with daily injections of apelin or overexpressing apelin at the level of the skeletal muscle have shown that, through the activation of AMPK signaling, apelin promotes mitochondrial biogenesis, muscle protein synthesis, and muscle regeneration via enhancement of muscle stem cells [85]. In addition, apelin treatment in insulin resistant mice fed a high fat diet resulted in decreased fat mass, improved insulin sensitivity and increased lipid utilization secondary to increased fatty acid oxidation, mitochondrial biogenesis, and oxidative capacity at the level of the skeletal muscle [84]. Based on the evidence from these studies, apelin has recently been proposed as a pharmacological target for improvement of age-associated muscle weakness and for the treatment of metabolic disease associated with obesity and sarcopenic obesity (reviewed in [86]). Phase I trials have assessed the safety, tolerability, pharmacokinetics, and pharmacodynamics of a novel apelin receptor agonist, AMG 986, in healthy individuals and patients with heart failure [87]. Human studies targeting the apelin pathway are needed to assess the potential beneficial effects of this myokine on metabolic health.

Brain-Derived Neurotrophic Factor

Brain-derived neurotrophic factor (BDNF) is a growth factor belonging to the neurotrophin family and mostly expressed in the brain. Chronic exercise increases BDNF in the hippocampus, where it plays a major role in adult neurogenesis and neural plasticity [88]. Several studies have shown that *BDNF* is also expressed in skeletal muscle. Rodent and human studies have described an induction of *BDNF* expression in the muscle tissue with both exercise and electrical stimulation of skeletal muscle [89, 90]. In humans, acute exercise increases plasma levels of BDNF, whereas an increase, decrease, or no change in plasma BDNF have been reported with chronic exercise (reviewed in [91]). BDNF levels are decreased in patients with obesity and type 2 diabetes and related to multiple metabolic parameters [86]. Muscle-derived BDNF is not released into the circulation, but instead exerts its effects in an autocrine or paracrine manner, enhancing AMPK activation and in turn fat oxidation within the skeletal muscle [90]. Moreover, BDNF released from the skeletal muscle is involved in muscle repair, regeneration, and differentiation [86].

Fractalkine

Fractalkine, also known as CX3CL1, is a chemokine which signals via the G protein-coupled receptor CX3CR1. Both plasma and muscle levels of fractalkine are increased in humans after an acute exercise bout, but unchanged after chronic exercise [91]. By attracting macrophages and other immune cells, fractalkine may play a role in promoting skeletal muscle regeneration physiologically occurring after acute exercise. Infiltration of macrophages is believed to be crucial for exercise-induced hypertrophy [92].

Fractalkine has been shown to positively regulate both glucose-stimulated and GLP-1-stimulated insulin secretion by enhancing β-cell function [93]. A significant defect in insulin secretion is observed in fractalkine knockout mice compared to wild-type mice, which may be related to the reduced expression of genes necessary for maintaining an appropriate β-cell differentiated state. In vivo treatment with fractalkine increased insulin secretion and improved glucose tolerance in wild type but not in knockout mice. Consistent with these findings, in vitro treatment of pancreatic islets with fractalkine is associated with increased intracellular calcium, in turn leading to enhanced insulin secretion in both mouse and human islets [93]. Lee et al. further showed that aging and obesity are associated with decreased fractalkine in pancreatic islets, and that disruption of the fractalkine signaling may play a role in inducing β-cell dysfunction in type 2 diabetes [93]. These findings are in contrast with human studies showing increased circulating fractalkine in individuals with type 2 diabetes [94]. Proposed explanations for these opposite findings include impairment in the CX3CR1 signaling or decreased CX3CR1 expression in diabetic β-cells, leading to fractalkine resistance [93]. Future studies will be necessary to explore whether the beneficial effects of fractalkine on β-cell function are related to its role as a myokine, and whether fractalkine may play a role as a treatment target for type 2 diabetes.

Meteorin-Like

Meteorin-like (Metrnl) was first identified by the Spiegelman lab in 2014 [95]. Expression of Metrnl is induced in the skeletal muscle after both acute and chronic exercise [91]. Animal and human models support a role of Metrnl in beige fat thermogenesis, stimulation of energy expenditure, and improvement of glucose tolerance [95]. However, similar to other myokines, results on Metrnl are mixed in humans, where clinical studies have reported increased, decreased, or unchanged plasma Metrnl levels in individuals with obesity [96]. Therefore, the role of Metrnl as a biomarker or therapeutic agent for metabolic disease in humans remains to be proven.

Musclin

Musclin is expressed in skeletal muscle, bone, and brain. Acute exercise induces an increase in musclin levels, whereas chronic exercise decreases musclin levels [91]. Animal studies have shown that musclin enhances skeletal muscle oxidative capacity and physical endurance via the promotion of mitochondrial biogenesis [86]. On the other hand, musclin mRNA expression is increased in the skeletal muscle of obese insulin-resistant mice, and treatment with recombinant musclin inhibits insulin-stimulated glucose uptake and glycogen synthesis in myocytes via inhibition of GLUT-4 expression [86]. Plasma musclin levels are increased in obesity and type 2 diabetes, and positively associated with obesity-related insulin resistance [86]. These data suggest that musclin may be involved in the development of obesity-related insulin resistance. However, additional research is required to investigate the specific metabolic role of musclin in humans.

Myonectin

Myonectin is expressed mainly in skeletal muscle and stimulated by exercise and intake of nutrients [86]. Current studies support a role of myonectin in the regulation of lipid metabolism via a crosstalk between skeletal muscle, liver, and adipose tissue. In animal studies, treatment with recombinant myonectin decreases circulating free fatty acids and increases fatty acid uptake in cultured adipocytes and hepatocytes, partially due to increased expression of genes involved in lipid uptake (CD36, FATP1, Fabp1, and Fabp4). On the other hand, genetic deletion of myonectin in mice fed a high fat diet leads to impaired handling of acute oral lipid loading, resulting in hyperlipidemia, hepatic steatosis, and significantly increased adiposity secondary to larger lipid storage in hypertrophic adipocytes [86]. In humans, plasma myonectin is positively associated with insulin resistance, impaired glucose tolerance, and type 2 diabetes, maybe as a compensatory mechanism against insulin resistance [86]. Whether myonectin is a specific biomarker or therapeutic target for metabolic disease requires further investigation.

Conclusions

Since the discovery of skeletal muscle as an endocrine organ that secretes peptides during proliferation and differentiation or in response to muscle contraction, the number of putative myokines keeps increasing. Specific biological functions have been described for very few myokines. The identification and characterization of myokines may provide information on how the skeletal muscle exerts exercise-induced effects through autocrine, paracrine, or endocrine mechanisms. Some limitations that need to be taken into account when investigating myokines include: (i) specific expression and secretion from skeletal muscle; (ii) lack of consistency in the response to acute and chronic exercise; (iii) divergent results between animals and humans; (iv) variability of assays in tissues and plasma; (v) specific signaling

pathways mediating biological actions [91]. Despite these limitations, studying the role of myokines as mediators of muscle growth and exercise-induced effects on glucose and lipid metabolism can provide information on the physiology of exercise and pathophysiology and treatment of sarcopenia, obesity, diabetes, and other metabolic diseases.

References

1. Stierman BAJ, Carroll MD, Chen T, Davy O, Fink S, Fryar CD, Gu Q, Hales CM, Hughes JP, Ostchega Y, Storandt RJ, Akinbami LJ, National Center for Health Statistics (U.S.). National Health and Nutrition Examination Survey 2017–March 2020 prepandemic data files – development of files and prevalence estimates for selected health outcomes. Series: NHSR No. 158. Source: National Health Statistics Reports. Published 14 June 2021. https://stacks.cdc.gov/view/cdc/106273.
2. Chew NWS, Ng CH, Tan DJH, Kong G, Lin C, Chin YH, et al. The global burden of metabolic disease: data from 2000 to 2019. Cell Metab. 2023;35(3):414–28 e3.
3. Atkins JL, Wannamathee SG. Sarcopenic obesity in ageing: cardiovascular outcomes and mortality. Br J Nutr. 2020;124(10):1102–13.
4. ElSayed NA, Aleppo G, Aroda VR, Bannuru RR, Brown FM, Bruemmer D, et al. 8. Obesity and weight management for the prevention and treatment of type 2 diabetes: standards of care in diabetes-2023. Diabetes Care. 2023;46(Suppl 1):S128–S39.
5. Garvey WT, Mechanick JI, Brett EM, Garber AJ, Hurley DL, Jastreboff AM, et al. American Association of Clinical Endocrinologists and American College of endocrinology comprehensive clinical practice guidelines for medical care of patients with obesity. Endocr Pract. 2016;22(Suppl 3):1–203.
6. Piercy KL, Troiano RP, Ballard RM, Carlson SA, Fulton JE, Galuska DA, et al. The physical activity guidelines for Americans. JAMA. 2018;320(19):2020–8.
7. Severinsen MCK, Pedersen BK. Muscle-organ crosstalk: the emerging roles of myokines. Endocr Rev. 2020;41(4):594–609.
8. Williams MA, Haskell WL, Ades PA, Amsterdam EA, Bittner V, Franklin BA, et al. Resistance exercise in individuals with and without cardiovascular disease: 2007 update: a scientific statement from the American Heart Association Council on Clinical Cardiology and Council on Nutrition, Physical Activity, and Metabolism. Circulation. 2007;116(5):572–84.
9. Janssen I, Heymsfield SB, Wang ZM, Ross R. Skeletal muscle mass and distribution in 468 men and women aged 18–88 yr. J Appl Physiol (1985). 2000;89(1):81–8.
10. Friedrichsen M, Mortensen B, Pehmoller C, Birk JB, Wojtaszewski JF. Exercise-induced AMPK activity in

skeletal muscle: role in glucose uptake and insulin sensitivity. Mol Cell Endocrinol. 2013;366(2):204–14.

11. Pedersen BK, Febbraio MA. Muscles, exercise and obesity: skeletal muscle as a secretory organ. Nat Rev Endocrinol. 2012;8(8):457–65.

12. Ahima RS, Park HK. Connecting myokines and metabolism. Endocrinol Metab (Seoul). 2015;30(3):235–45.

13. Zamboni M, Mazzali G, Brunelli A, Saatchi T, Urbani S, Giani A, et al. The role of crosstalk between adipose cells and myocytes in the pathogenesis of sarcopenic obesity in the elderly. Cell. 2022;11(21):3361.

14. McPherron AC, Lawler AM, Lee SJ. Regulation of skeletal muscle mass in mice by a new TGF-beta superfamily member. Nature. 1997;387(6628):83–90.

15. Lee SJ. Targeting the myostatin signaling pathway to treat muscle loss and metabolic dysfunction. J Clin Invest. 2021;131(9):e148372.

16. Rodgers BD, Garikipati DK. Clinical, agricultural, and evolutionary biology of myostatin: a comparative review. Endocr Rev. 2008;29(5):513–34.

17. Hittel DS, Berggren JR, Shearer J, Boyle K, Houmard JA. Increased secretion and expression of myostatin in skeletal muscle from extremely obese women. Diabetes. 2009;58(1):30–8.

18. Ryan AS, Li G. Skeletal muscle myostatin gene expression and sarcopenia in overweight and obese middle-aged and older adults. JCSM Clin Rep. 2021;6(4):137–42.

19. Hittel DS, Axelson M, Sarna N, Shearer J, Huffman KM, Kraus WE. Myostatin decreases with aerobic exercise and associates with insulin resistance. Med Sci Sports Exerc. 2010;42(11):2023–9.

20. McPherron AC, Lee SJ. Suppression of body fat accumulation in myostatin-deficient mice. J Clin Invest. 2002;109(5):595–601.

21. Lin J, Arnold HB, Della-Fera MA, Azain MJ, Hartzell DL, Baile CA. Myostatin knockout in mice increases myogenesis and decreases adipogenesis. Biochem Biophys Res Commun. 2002;291(3):701–6.

22. Guo T, Jou W, Chanturiya T, Portas J, Gavrilova O, McPherron AC. Myostatin inhibition in muscle, but not adipose tissue, decreases fat mass and improves insulin sensitivity. PLoS One. 2009;4(3):e4937.

23. Akpan I, Goncalves MD, Dhir R, Yin X, Pistilli EE, Bogdanovich S, et al. The effects of a soluble activin type IIB receptor on obesity and insulin sensitivity. Int J Obes. 2009;33(11):1265–73.

24. Shan T, Liang X, Bi P, Kuang S. Myostatin knockout drives browning of white adipose tissue through activating the AMPK-PGC1alpha-Fndc5 pathway in muscle. FASEB J. 2013;27(5):1981–9.

25. Koncarevic A, Kajimura S, Cornwall-Brady M, Andreucci A, Pullen A, Sako D, et al. A novel therapeutic approach to treating obesity through modulation of TGFbeta signaling. Endocrinology. 2012;153(7):3133–46.

26. Fournier B, Murray B, Gutzwiller S, Marcaletti S, Marcellin D, Bergling S, et al. Blockade of the activin

receptor IIb activates functional brown adipogenesis and thermogenesis by inducing mitochondrial oxidative metabolism. Mol Cell Biol. 2012;32(14):2871–9.

27. Allen DL, Hittel DS, McPherron AC. Expression and function of myostatin in obesity, diabetes, and exercise adaptation. Med Sci Sports Exerc. 2011;43(10):1828–35.

28. Rooks D, Petricoul O, Praestgaard J, Bartlett M, Laurent D, Roubenoff R. Safety and pharmacokinetics of bimagrumab in healthy older and obese adults with body composition changes in the older cohort. J Cachexia Sarcopenia Muscle. 2020;11(6):1525–34.

29. Attie KM, Borgstein NG, Yang Y, Condon CH, Wilson DM, Pearsall AE, et al. A single ascending-dose study of muscle regulator ACE-031 in healthy volunteers. Muscle Nerve. 2013;47(3):416–23.

30. Rooks D, Praestgaard J, Hariry S, Laurent D, Petricoul O, Perry RG, et al. Treatment of sarcopenia with bimagrumab: results from a phase II, randomized, controlled. Proof-of-Concept Study J Am Geriatr Soc. 2017;65(9):1988–95.

31. Latres E, Mastaitis J, Fury W, Miloscio L, Trejos J, Pangilinan J, et al. Activin a more prominently regulates muscle mass in primates than does GDF8. Nat Commun. 2017;8:15153.

32. Garito T, Roubenoff R, Hompesch M, Morrow L, Gomez K, Rooks D, et al. Bimagrumab improves body composition and insulin sensitivity in insulin-resistant individuals. Diabetes Obes Metab. 2018;20(1):94–102.

33. Heymsfield SB, Coleman LA, Miller R, Rooks DS, Laurent D, Petricoul O, et al. Effect of bimagrumab vs placebo on body fat mass among adults with type 2 diabetes and obesity: a phase 2 randomized clinical trial. JAMA Netw Open. 2021;4(1):e2033457.

34. Rooks D, Swan T, Goswami B, Filosa LA, Bunte O, Panchaud N, et al. Bimagrumab vs optimized standard of care for treatment of sarcopenia in community-dwelling older adults: a randomized clinical trial. JAMA Netw Open. 2020;3(10):e2020836.

35. Pal M, Febbraio MA, Whitham M. From cytokine to myokine: the emerging role of interleukin-6 in metabolic regulation. Immunol Cell Biol. 2014;92(4):331–9.

36. Fang P, She Y, Yu M, Min W, Shang W, Zhang Z. Adipose-muscle crosstalk in age-related metabolic disorders: the emerging roles of adipo-myokines. Ageing Res Rev. 2023;84:101829.

37. Colbert LH, Visser M, Simonsick EM, Tracy RP, Newman AB, Kritchevsky SB, et al. Physical activity, exercise, and inflammatory markers in older adults: findings from the Health, Aging and Body Composition Study. J Am Geriatr Soc. 2004;52(7):1098–104.

38. Platat C, Wagner A, Klumpp T, Schweitzer B, Simon C. Relationships of physical activity with metabolic syndrome features and low-grade inflammation in adolescents. Diabetologia. 2006;49(9):2078–85.

39. Hamer M, Sabia S, Batty GD, Shipley MJ, Tabak AG, Singh-Manoux A, et al. Physical activity and

inflammatory markers over 10 years: follow-up in men and women from the Whitehall II cohort study. Circulation. 2012;126(8):928–33.

40. Wunderlich CM, Hovelmeyer N, Wunderlich FT. Mechanisms of chronic JAK-STAT3-SOCS3 signaling in obesity. JAKSTAT. 2013;2(2):e23878.

41. Serrano AL, Baeza-Raja B, Perdiguero E, Jardi M, Munoz-Canoves P. Interleukin-6 is an essential regulator of satellite cell-mediated skeletal muscle hypertrophy. Cell Metab. 2008;7(1):33–44.

42. Carey AL, Steinberg GR, Macaulay SL, Thomas WG, Holmes AG, Ramm G, et al. Interleukin-6 increases insulin-stimulated glucose disposal in humans and glucose uptake and fatty acid oxidation in vitro via AMP-activated protein kinase. Diabetes. 2006;55(10):2688–97.

43. Steensberg A, Fischer CP, Sacchetti M, Keller C, Osada T, Schjerling P, et al. Acute interleukin-6 administration does not impair muscle glucose uptake or whole-body glucose disposal in healthy humans. J Physiol. 2003;548(Pt 2):631–8.

44. Pedersen BK, Febbraio MA. Muscle as an endocrine organ: focus on muscle-derived interleukin-6. Physiol Rev. 2008;88(4):1379–406.

45. van Hall G, Steensberg A, Sacchetti M, Fischer C, Keller C, Schjerling P, et al. Interleukin-6 stimulates lipolysis and fat oxidation in humans. J Clin Endocrinol Metab. 2003;88(7):3005–10.

46. Petersen EW, Carey AL, Sacchetti M, Steinberg GR, Macaulay SL, Febbraio MA, et al. Acute IL-6 treatment increases fatty acid turnover in elderly humans in vivo and in tissue culture in vitro. Am J Physiol Endocrinol Metab. 2005;288(1):E155–62.

47. Wedell-Neergaard AS, Lang Lehrskov L, Christensen RH, Legaard GE, Dorph E, Larsen MK, et al. Exercise-induced changes in visceral adipose tissue mass are regulated by IL-6 signaling: a randomized controlled trial. Cell Metab. 2019;29(4):844–55 e3.

48. Lehrskov LL, Christensen RH, Wedell-Neergaard AS, Legaard GE, Dorph E, Larsen MK, et al. Effects of exercise training and IL-6 receptor blockade on gastric emptying and GLP-1 secretion in obese humans: secondary analyses from a double blind randomized clinical trial. Front Physiol. 2019;10:1249.

49. Bostrom P, Wu J, Jedrychowski MP, Korde A, Ye L, Lo JC, et al. A PGC1-alpha-dependent myokine that drives brown-fat-like development of white fat and thermogenesis. Nature. 2012;481(7382):463–8.

50. Zhang D, Xie T, Leung PS. Irisin ameliorates glucolipotoxicity-associated beta-cell dysfunction and apoptosis via AMPK signaling and anti-inflammatory actions. Cell Physiol Biochem. 2018;51(2):924–37.

51. Moreno-Navarrete JM, Ortega F, Serrano M, Guerra E, Pardo G, Tinahones F, et al. Irisin is expressed and produced by human muscle and adipose tissue in association with obesity and insulin resistance. J Clin Endocrinol Metab. 2013;98(4):E769–78.

52. Fox J, Rioux BV, Goulet EDB, Johanssen NM, Swift DL, Bouchard DR, et al. Effect of an acute exercise

bout on immediate post-exercise irisin concentration in adults: a meta-analysis. Scand J Med Sci Sports. 2018;28(1):16–28.

53. Colpitts BH, Rioux BV, Eadie AL, Brunt KR, Senechal M. Irisin response to acute moderate intensity exercise and high intensity interval training in youth of different obesity statuses: a randomized crossover trial. Physiol Rep. 2022;10(4):e15198.

54. Miyamoto-Mikami E, Sato K, Kurihara T, Hasegawa N, Fujie S, Fujita S, et al. Endurance training-induced increase in circulating irisin levels is associated with reduction of abdominal visceral fat in middle-aged and older adults. PLoS One. 2015;10(3):e0120354.

55. Cosio PL, Crespo-Posadas M, Velarde-Sotres A, Pelaez M. Effect of chronic resistance training on circulating irisin: systematic review and meta-analysis of randomized controlled trials. Int J Environ Res Public Health. 2021;18(5):2476.

56. Tsai CL, Pan CY, Tseng YT, Chen FC, Chang YC, Wang TC. Acute effects of high-intensity interval training and moderate-intensity continuous exercise on BDNF and irisin levels and neurocognitive performance in late middle-aged and older adults. Behav Brain Res. 2021;413:113472.

57. Qiu S, Cai X, Sun Z, Schumann U, Zugel M, Steinacker JM. Chronic exercise training and circulating irisin in adults: a meta-analysis. Sports Med. 2015;45(11):1577–88.

58. Jedrychowski MP, Wrann CD, Paulo JA, Gerber KK, Szpyt J, Robinson MM, et al. Detection and quantitation of circulating human irisin by tandem mass spectrometry. Cell Metab. 2015;22(4):734–40.

59. Song R, Zhao X, Zhang DQ, Wang R, Feng Y. Lower levels of irisin in patients with type 2 diabetes mellitus: a meta-analysis. Diabetes Res Clin Pract. 2021;175:108788.

60. Park KH, Zaichenko L, Brinkoetter M, Thakkar B, Sahin-Efe A, Joung KE, et al. Circulating irisin in relation to insulin resistance and the metabolic syndrome. J Clin Endocrinol Metab. 2013;98(12):4899–907.

61. McCormick JJ, King KE, Notley SR, Fujii N, Boulay P, Sigal RJ, et al. Exercise in the heat induces similar elevations in serum irisin in young and older men despite lower resting irisin concentrations in older adults. J Therm Biol. 2022;104:103189.

62. Chang JS, Kim TH, Nguyen TT, Park KS, Kim N, Kong ID. Circulating irisin levels as a predictive biomarker for sarcopenia: a cross-sectional community-based study. Geriatr Gerontol Int. 2017;17(11):2266–73.

63. Oguz A, Sahin M, Tuzun D, Kurutas EB, Ulgen C, Bozkus O, et al. Irisin is a predictor of sarcopenic obesity in type 2 diabetes mellitus: a cross-sectional study. Medicine (Baltimore). 2021;100(26):e26529.

64. Baek JY, Jang IY, Jung HW, Park SJ, Lee JY, Choi E, et al. Serum irisin level is independent of sarcopenia

and related muscle parameters in older adults. Exp Gerontol. 2022;162:111744.

65. Nadeau L, Aguer C. Interleukin-15 as a myokine: mechanistic insight into its effect on skeletal muscle metabolism. Appl Physiol Nutr Metab. 2019;44(3): 229–38.

66. Raschke S, Eckardt K, Bjorklund Holven K, Jensen J, Eckel J. Identification and validation of novel contraction-regulated myokines released from primary human skeletal muscle cells. PLoS One. 2013;8(4): e62008.

67. Pierce JR, Maples JM, Hickner RC. IL-15 concentrations in skeletal muscle and subcutaneous adipose tissue in lean and obese humans: local effects of IL-15 on adipose tissue lipolysis. Am J Physiol Endocrinol Metab. 2015;308(12):E1131–9.

68. Pistilli EE, Devaney JM, Gordish-Dressman H, Bradbury MK, Seip RL, Thompson PD, et al. Interleukin-15 and interleukin-15R alpha SNPs and associations with muscle, bone, and predictors of the metabolic syndrome. Cytokine. 2008;43(1):45–53.

69. Nielsen AR, Hojman P, Erikstrup C, Fischer CP, Plomgaard P, Mounier R, et al. Association between interleukin-15 and obesity: interleukin-15 as a potential regulator of fat mass. J Clin Endocrinol Metab. 2008;93(11):4486–93.

70. Perez-Lopez A, Valades D, Vazquez Martinez C, de Cos Blanco AI, Bujan J, Garcia-Honduvilla N. Serum IL-15 and IL-15Ralpha levels are decreased in lean and obese physically active humans. Scand J Med Sci Sports. 2018;28(3):1113–20.

71. Al-Shukaili A, Al-Ghafri S, Al-Marhoobi S, Al-Abri S, Al-Lawati J, Al-Maskari M. Analysis of inflammatory mediators in type 2 diabetes patients. Int J Endocrinol. 2013;2013:976810.

72. Almendro V, Busquets S, Ametller E, Carbo N, Figueras M, Fuster G, et al. Effects of interleukin-15 on lipid oxidation: disposal of an oral [(14)C]-triolein load. Biochim Biophys Acta. 2006;1761(1):37–42.

73. Quinn LS, Anderson BG, Conner JD, Wolden-Hanson T. IL-15 overexpression promotes endurance, oxidative energy metabolism, and muscle PPARdelta, SIRT1, PGC-1alpha, and PGC-1beta expression in male mice. Endocrinology. 2013;154(1):232–45.

74. Luquet S, Lopez-Soriano J, Holst D, Fredenrich A, Melki J, Rassoulzadegan M, et al. Peroxisome proliferator-activated receptor delta controls muscle development and oxidative capability. FASEB J. 2003;17(15):2299–301.

75. Pistilli EE, Bogdanovich S, Garton F, Yang N, Gulbin JP, Conner JD, et al. Loss of IL-15 receptor alpha alters the endurance, fatigability, and metabolic characteristics of mouse fast skeletal muscles. J Clin Invest. 2011;121(8):3120–32.

76. Pistilli EE, Guo G, Stauber WT. IL-15Ralpha deficiency leads to mitochondrial and myofiber differences in fast mouse muscles. Cytokine. 2013;61(1):41–5.

77. Quinn LS, Anderson BG, Conner JD, Wolden-Hanson T, Marcell TJ. IL-15 is required for postexercise

78. induction of the pro-oxidative mediators PPARdelta and SIRT1 in male mice. Endocrinology. 2014;155 (1):143–55.

78. O'Connell GC, Pistilli EE. Interleukin-15 directly stimulates pro-oxidative gene expression in skeletal muscle in-vitro via a mechanism that requires interleukin-15 receptor alpha. Biochem Biophys Res Commun. 2015;458(3):614–9.

79. Boucher J, Masri B, Daviaud D, Gesta S, Guigne C, Mazzucotelli A, et al. Apelin, a newly identified adipokine up-regulated by insulin and obesity. Endocrinology. 2005;146(4):1764–71.

80. Besse-Patin A, Montastier E, Vinel C, Castan-Laurell I, Louche K, Dray C, et al. Effect of endurance training on skeletal muscle myokine expression in obese men: identification of apelin as a novel myokine. Int J Obes. 2014;38(5):707–13.

81. Higuchi K, Masaki T, Gotoh K, Chiba S, Katsuragi I, Tanaka K, et al. Apelin, an APJ receptor ligand, regulates body adiposity and favors the messenger ribonucleic acid expression of uncoupling proteins in mice. Endocrinology. 2007;148(6):2690–7.

82. Son JS, Kim HJ, Son Y, Lee H, Chae SA, Seong JK, et al. Effects of exercise-induced apelin levels on skeletal muscle and their capillarization in type 2 diabetic rats. Muscle Nerve. 2017;56(6):1155–63.

83. Yue P, Jin H, Aillaud M, Deng AC, Azuma J, Asagami T, et al. Apelin is necessary for the maintenance of insulin sensitivity. Am J Physiol Endocrinol Metab. 2010;298(1):E59–67.

84. Attane C, Foussal C, Le Gonidec S, Benani A, Daviaud D, Wanecq E, et al. Apelin treatment increases complete fatty acid oxidation, mitochondrial oxidative capacity, and biogenesis in muscle of insulin-resistant mice. Diabetes. 2012;61(2):310–20.

85. Vinel C, Lukjanenko L, Batut A, Deleruyelle S, Pradere JP, Le Gonidec S, et al. The exerkine apelin reverses age-associated sarcopenia. Nat Med. 2018;24 (9):1360–71.

86. Guo A, Li K, Xiao Q. Sarcopenic obesity: myokines as potential diagnostic biomarkers and therapeutic targets? Exp Gerontol. 2020;139:111022.

87. Winkle P, Goldsmith S, Koren MJ, Lepage S, Hellawell J, Trivedi A, et al. A first-in-human study of AMG 986, a novel apelin receptor agonist, in healthy subjects and heart failure patients. Cardiovasc Drugs Ther. 2023;37(4):743–755.

88. Liu PZ, Nusslock R. Exercise-mediated neurogenesis in the hippocampus via BDNF. Front Neurosci. 2018;12:52.

89. Copray S, Liem R, Brouwer N, Greenhaff P, Habens F, Fernyhough P. Contraction-induced muscle fiber damage is increased in soleus muscle of streptozotocin-diabetic rats and is associated with elevated expression of brain-derived neurotrophic factor mRNA in muscle fibers and activated satellite cells. Exp Neurol. 2000;161(2):597–608.

90. Matthews VB, Astrom MB, Chan MH, Bruce CR, Krabbe KS, Prelovsek O, et al. Brain-derived

neurotrophic factor is produced by skeletal muscle cells in response to contraction and enhances fat oxidation via activation of AMP-activated protein kinase. Diabetologia. 2009;52(7):1409–18.

91. Chow LS, Gerszten RE, Taylor JM, Pedersen BK, van Praag H, Trappe S, et al. Exerkines in health, resilience and disease. Nat Rev Endocrinol. 2022;18(5):273–89.

92. Catoire M, Mensink M, Kalkhoven E, Schrauwen P, Kersten S. Identification of human exercise-induced myokines using secretome analysis. Physiol Genomics. 2014;46(7):256–67.

93. Lee YS, Morinaga H, Kim JJ, Lagakos W, Taylor S, Keshwani M, et al. The fractalkine/CX3CR1 system regulates beta cell function and insulin secretion. Cell. 2013;153(2):413–25.

94. Shah R, Hinkle CC, Ferguson JF, Mehta NN, Li M, Qu L, et al. Fractalkine is a novel human adipochemokine associated with type 2 diabetes. Diabetes. 2011;60(5):1512–8.

95. Rao RR, Long JZ, White JP, Svensson KJ, Lou J, Lokurkar I, et al. Meteorin-like is a hormone that regulates immune-adipose interactions to increase beige fat thermogenesis. Cell. 2014;157(6):1279–91.

96. Alizadeh H. Meteorin-like protein (Metrnl): a metabolic syndrome biomarker and an exercise mediator. Cytokine. 2022;157:155952.

Body Composition Assessment

26

Roshan Dinparastisaleh, Sara Atiq Khan, and
Prasanna Santhanam

Contents

R. Dinparastisaleh
College of Medicine, Division of Pulmonary and Critical
Care, University of Florida, Jacksonville, FL, USA

S. A. Khan
Division of Endocrinology, Diabetes, & Metabolism,
Department of Medicine, University of Maryland School
of Medicine, Baltimore, MD, USA

P. Santhanam (✉)
Division of Endocrinology, Diabetes, & Metabolism,
Department of Medicine, Johns Hopkins University
School of Medicine, Baltimore, MD, USA
e-mail: psantha1@jhmi.edu

© Springer Nature Switzerland AG 2023
R. S. Ahima (ed.), *Metabolic Syndrome*,
https://doi.org/10.1007/978-3-031-40116-9_33

Abstract

Obesity is characterized by excess fat accumulation in adipose tissues and ectopically in liver, muscle, and other organs. However, the measurement techniques for the fat have widely varied with poor standardization and generalization. As a result, many techniques have been developed to assess the actual mass of adipose tissue in proportion to muscle, bone, water, and the rest of the human tissue. In this chapter, we discuss the different techniques to measure body composition and relevance to metabolic health and discuss the accuracy and cost-effectiveness of the methods.

Keywords

Body fat · Lean mass · Fat-free mass · Obesity · Diabetes · Cardiovascular

Introduction

The Need to Measure the Composition of the Human Body

Obesity imposes enormous metabolic disease burden on the global population and is associated with chronic diseases – diabetes, cardiovascular disease, and cancer. Body composition measurement began in human fetuses and expanded to involve the cadavers of adults [1–3]. Over the years, measures of the shape and size of the human body evolved into the standardization of the body mass index (body mass index (BMI), calculated as weight $(kg)/height(m)^2$) as the most popular measure of body fat [4, 5]. A high BMI is associated with diabetes and cardiometabolic risk; however, the health outcomes differ between subtypes of people with obesity. Healthy persons may have a high BMI characterized by higher muscle mass, higher fat in the appendages and lower visceral fat, and less likelihood of fatty liver disease. These individuals have less insulin resistance and a lower risk for poor cardiovascular outcomes. On the other hand, high amounts of visceral adipose tissue (characterized by increased waist circumference and increased amount of hepatic fat) are associated with insulin resistance, type 2 diabetes mellitus, and cardiovascular disease. Subsequently, other measures like waist circumference (in cm, an estimation of abdominal obesity) and skin fold thickness (obtained by anthropometry that measures body fat percentage) have been used as practical, cost-effective, and reasonably accurate methods for body composition. However, there was a need for more precise methods.

The Compartment Model for Body Composition Analysis

Body composition measurement can be visualized as the estimation of individual compartments, the body's total weight being the sum total of the individual compartments. The fundamental premise of these measurements pertains to the differing densities of fat, water, bone and other tissues, and the determination of these densities.

The Multiple-Compartment (Two, Three, and Four) Approaches to Body Composition

Two-Compartment Model

The body compartment is broken down into fat mass (FM) and fat-free mass (FFM). In 1987,

Forbes showed a nonlinear relationship between FFM and FM data and postulated that changes in body composition moved along a functional curve and derived a mathematical equation for the FFM proportion of body weight (BW) as a dependent of FM [6, 7].

Three-Compartment Model

The three-compartment body composition model partitions the FFM into lean body mass (LBM) and bone mineral content (BMC). This helps in the direct measurement of the BMC, thereby aiding in the diagnosis of osteopenia [8]. Direct measurement of LBM helps diagnose sarcopenia, which is widely considered an independent risk factor for mortality and morbidity [9]. Dual-energy X-ray absorptiometry (DXA) is the technique most used for LBM and BMC estimation. DXA can be used effectively to diagnose sarcopenia [10, 11].

Four-Compartment Model

The four-compartment body composition model further partitions the LBM into water (TBW), protein, and BMC. TBW, protein (non-aqueous material), mineral content, and fat mass form the four components of the human body. The TBW is estimated using isotope dilution (total body density is estimated using underwater weighing), and then, the four components are derived using complex mathematical calculations [12, 13]. The four-component model was derived from accounting for the differences in hydration levels of different tissues across individuals and climate/weather while calculating the LBM [14, 15].In the future, these techniques might help improve and standardize human hydration levels.

The Clinical Implications of Measurement of Body Composition

Studies have evaluated the relative benefits of different body composition measurement techniques for cardiovascular outcomes. The components measured in each of the techniques are shown in Table 1 (adapted from Weber et al.) [16]. Table 2 shows the advantages and

Table 1 Body composition components measured using different techniques

Method	Measured metric
Anthropometry	
Weight	Weight
BMI	BMI
Waist circumference Skinfold thickness	Visceral fat estimation Body fat estimation
Bioelectric impedance	Fat-free mass, TBW
Isotope dilution for body water	Fat mass and TBW
Anatomical imaging	
DXA	Fat mass, lean body mass, bone mineral content
CT	Fat mass, lean body mass, visceral adiposity, muscle mass, hepatic fat, and bone mineral content
MRI	Fat mass, lean body mass, visceral adiposity, muscle mass, hepatic fat, and bone mineral content
Molecular imaging	
PET	Fat mass, lean body mass, visceral adiposity, muscle mass, hepatic fat, bone mineral content, and brown adipose tissue

disadvantages of the conventional methods and associated evidence in relation to cardiovascular disease [17–22]. Finally, some of the more intensive and expensive techniques (risks and benefits) are shown in Table 3 [23–27].

Body Composition Analysis Methods for Clinical Assessment

Anthropometry

The components of anthropometry are height, weight, head circumference, body mass index (BMI), body circumferences (waist, hip, and limbs), and skinfold thickness to assess adiposity. Anthropometric methods are safe, cost-effective, and more feasible for providers and are implemented in research and clinical guidelines to assess cardiometabolic risk factors.

Table 2 The relatively easy-to-measure metrics of body composition and research evidence

Technique	Advantages	Disadvantages	Research Studies
Body height (in cm)	Simplest method	Overestimation in shorter individuals and underestimation in taller individuals	Genetically determined shorter height is associated with an increased risk of CVD (Nelson et al.)
Weight (kg)	Performed routinely during clinical care	There are substantial racial and ethnic variations	Longitudinal studies like the Framingham Heart Study have shown that an increase in weight is associated with higher cardiovascular disease risk (Kennel et al.)
BMI (kg/m^2)	Computed as an index using height and weight. A simple derivation of two techniques	BMI cannot capture all three components (LBM, FM, BMC), although it does correlate with fat mass. There is substantial variation in its predictive ability across race and ethnicity (especially in persons with higher muscle mass)	Body mass index has a U/J-shaped relationship to cardiovascular disease (Ortega et al.; Bastian et al.)
Skin fold thickness	Easy to measure	Not standardized across the different body sites	Skinfold thicknesses taken at various sites correlates with total body fat and percentage body fat (Roche et al.)
Waist circumference	Relatively easy	There might be interoperator and intraoperator variability	Waist circumference is an independent predictor of cardiovascular mortality (Posterino et al.)

However, anthropometric measures have significant interoperator variability that can potentially lead to the misclassification of the patients [28]. Therefore, quality control checks and standardized protocols are essential in the training of the operators.

Body Mass Index (BMI)

The BMI calculated as body weight (kg)/[height (meters)]^2 was introduced in the early nineteenth century by a Belgian statistician, Lambert Adolphe Jacques Quetelet [29]. Since then, the BMI has been the most used measure in identifying obesity. Table 4 shows the United States Centers for Disease Control and Prevention's (CDC) definitions of nutritional status based on the BMI in adult (above 20 years old) and pediatric (under 20 years old) populations [30].

The diagnosis of obesity in children is defined by comparing the measurements with a reference population due to BMI's variability with age. Table 5 demonstrates different definitions of obesity in children [31–34].

Although BMI is considered the best available index of obesity in the pediatric population, it does have limitations, including its nonlinear relationship with adiposity [35]. Nevertheless, BMI is still the standard diagnostic tool to assess nutritional status in the child and adolescents.

Waist Circumference (WC)

A strong link exists between obesity and visceral fat (fat deposition near abdominal tissue). Visceral fat (measured usually by WC) is as an independent cardiovascular risk factor [21]. Cardiometabolic disease in those with "normal-BMI obesity" leads to misclassification and underdiagnosis of metabolic risk in clinical practice [36]. Higher WC in individuals with regular weight/BMI implies higher cardiometabolic risk [37]. Therefore, WC as a measure of abdominal obesity adds critical information along with BMI, as per expert opinion [38, 39]. To measure WC (National Heart, Lung, and Blood Institute (NHLBI) and CDC recommendations), localize the top of the right iliac crest. Place a measuring

Table 3 Newer body composition techniques: visceral adipose tissue (VAT)

Newer techniques	Advantages	Disadvantages	Research studies
Bioimpedance assay	Inexpensive and no- radiation	Measurement conditions have not been standardized across different settings.	Body fat % (measured by bioimpedance) cutoffs for CVD risk factors correctly risk stratified 3.43% more subjects compared to BMI in a cohort of over 10,000 middle-aged Japanese men (Yamashita et al.)
DXA (dual-energy X-ray absorptiometry)	All three compartments (BMC, LBM, and FM) can be assessed with a high degree of accuracy. It involves very minimal radiation exposure	Technicians need training; the software is expensive and varies across the machines, and substantial inter and intraoperator variability.	Sarcopenic obesity has been shown to be associated with incident CVD in studies involving DXA-measured muscle mass (Fukuda et al.)
CT scan	Improves upon DXA by obtaining a three-dimensional, accurate estimation of different tissue components	More expensive than DXA and involves a higher amount of radiation	VAT obtained from automated measurements of abdominal CTs predicted MI or stroke independent of other usual obesity metrics like weight and BMI (Magudia et al.)
MRI/MRS (magnetic resonance spectroscopy)	Highly precise quantification of abdominal fat including hepatic fat possible	Very expensive	Studies have shown associations between MRI-quantified VAT volume and MRI-quantified brain white matter lesional volume in patients with ischemic stroke (Seabolt et al.; Karcher et al.)

Table 4 CDC definitions of various weight categories in adults and children

BMI (kg/m^2)	Category
Adult population	
<18.5	Underweight
18.5–24.99	Normal weight
25–29.99	Overweight
≥30	Obese
30–34.9	Class I obesity
35–39.9	Class II obesity
≥40	Class III obesity
Pediatric population	
[a] Based-on comparison to CDC reference curves	
<5th percentile	Underweight
5th–84th percentile	Normal weight
85th–94th percentile	Overweight
≥95th percentile	Obese

tape in a horizontal plane around the abdomen at the level of the superior edge of the iliac crest. Before reading the tape measure, ensure that the tape is snug but does not compress the skin and is parallel to the floor. The measurement is made at the end of a normal expiration [40]. WHO has a slightly different measurement approach (midpoint between the lower margin of the last palpable rib and the top of the iliac crest); however, there is no evidence to suggest the use of one technique over the other as long as there is unanimity and standardization in multiple measurements [41].

The NIH was the first to use the cutoff values for WC [≥88 cm (35 in.) in women and ≥102 cm (40 in.) in men] [42]. The WHO and International Diabetes Federation (IDF) recommend the use of racial/ethnic-specific thresholds, which vary in males from ≥85 cm in Asian populations to ≥94 cm in Europeans and ≥80 cm in females [43]. The WC can be further adjusted for height and hip circumference (waist-to-height ratio, waist divided by height$^{0.5}$, waist-hip ratio).

Table 5 Commonly used definitions of children (under 20 years of age) according to BMI and percentile

Definitions of childhood obesity	CDC	WHO	IOTF
Overweight	85th–95th	85th–97th	91st
Obesity	>95th	>97th	99th

CDC Center for Disease Control and Prevention, *WHO* World Health Organization, *IOTF* International Obesity Task Force

Skinfold Thickness

Skinfold thickness is one of the anthropometric measures used to predict body fat percentage. The body density is first calculated in adults using the Jackson & Pollock equations [44, 45]. Subsequently, the level of percent body fat can be determined using the Siri equation [46].

Radiology-Based Techniques

Dual-Energy X-Ray Absorptiometry (DXA)

DXA is a spectral imaging modality that requires special beam filtering and spatial registration of the two attenuations [47]. It provides whole-body and regional estimates of the three major body compartments: fat, lean body mass (LBM), and bone mineral content [48]. DXA exposes the patient and operator to minimal ionizing radiation. The effective radiation dose from a single whole-body DXA is almost equivalent to the average background radiation received over one day at sea level (< 10 micro Sieverts) [47]. Large body size has historically limited the use of DXA scans, but new technologies have made it easier to integrate partial measurements [49]. An example of a DXA body composition report is shown in Fig. 1.

Individuals with metal surgical implants or those who cannot lay flat due to muscle contractures are not ideal candidates for DXA scanning. Furthermore, the measurement of LBM is affected by volume status, which may be an important limiting factor when evaluating patients/participants with chronic disease. Hydration changes may affect the attenuation of LBM. There are substantial variations in body composition measurements comparing DXA scanners from different manufacturers, different models of the same manufacturer, or even the same model.

Imaging: CT, MRI, Ultrasound, and PET

Imaging modalities, such as computed tomography (CT) and magnetic resonance imaging (MRI), are the most accurate in vivo body composition measurement methods. After segmentation into different compartments, these modalities can measure total adipose tissue, subcutaneous adipose tissue (SAT), visceral adipose tissue (VAT), skeletal muscle, and bone mineral content [50].

CT imaging involves an X-ray beam attenuated as it passes through the tissues, and the slides are reconstructed mathematically through iteration. The measurement of attenuation is the Hounsfield unit (HU), a surrogate for tissue density. The HU number is a measure of the attenuation relative to water (HU water = 0, HU air $\approx$ −1000). The HU value for body fat and skeletal muscle is between −190 and −30 and 30–100 HU, respectively. To calculate the surface area (cm^2) for various tissues, segmentation techniques (either automatic or manual) discriminated by HU values can be applied [51].

Consequently, the calculation of organ volumes is based on the sum of cross-sectional areas multiplied by slice thickness and the distance between slices [52]. Various studies have shown the accuracy, validity, and interobserver correlation of body composition analysis from CT compared with the direct morphometric method in human cadavers for measuring visceral and subcutaneous adipose tissue [53]. This is also true for muscle mass [54]. The reproducibility of volume assessments compared with masses determined from postmortem cadaver morphometric analyses was within the range of ±5% [55]. Exposure to ionizing radiation is the primary concern while using CT for whole-body composition.

MRI signal is derived from the hydrogen molecules as they move back into alignment with the external magnetic field and fall out of phase with each other. Tissue segmentation is performed either manually or automatically based on signal

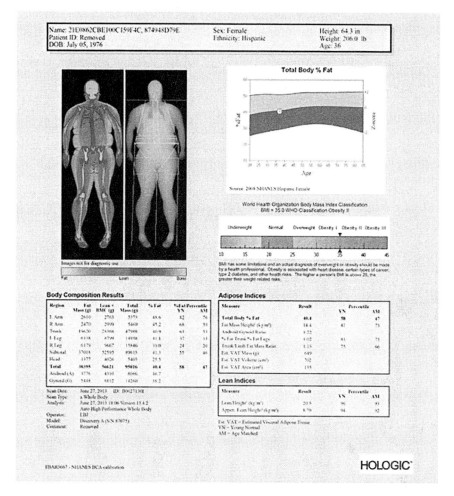

Fig. 1 DXA body composition report. Integrated software allows for calculating measures such as percentage body fat and for the individual's data to be converted into a standard deviation score and compared to a reference population, as shown above. The scan was obtained on a Hologic Horizon scanner (Hologic, Inc., Bedford MA). (https://www.hologic.com/hologic-products/body-composition/horizon-dxa-system)

intensity, semi-automated tagging, or morphology [56–58]. A semi-automatic approach is often preferred since it is time-saving and precise but allows manual correction to enhance accuracy [57]. Similar to CT scans, MRI has shown an acceptable correlation with values produced by cadaver dissection and chemical analysis [59, 60]. The reproducibility of MRI-based body composition analysis is dependent on the technique used for segmentation, but the CV% varies from 0.3% to 1.7% in measurements of subcutaneous adipose tissue and 3.5–9.4% in visceral adipose tissue [61, 62]. However, the cost and long scan times prohibit the widespread applicability of MRI.

Ultrasound is a modality complementary to anthropometric methods. It helps measure the thickness of subcutaneous adipose tissue, skeletal muscle, and intra-abdominal depth – ultrasound benefits obese subjects at anatomical sites where caliper use is not feasible [63]. However, the accuracy and reproducibility of the B-mode (a two-dimensional image of the tissue displaying tissue discontinuity) depend on the appropriate selection of the anatomical area for measurement and the correct placement of the probe [63].

PET (positron emission tomography) is a type of nuclear medicine procedure that measures the metabolic activity of the cells of body tissues. A common practice is to attach a positron-emitting tracer to ^{18}F-fluorodeoxyglucose, the concentration of measured tracer activity reflects glucose uptake, and therefore metabolic activity of the cells [64]. PET is especially beneficial for the quantification and localization of brown adipose tissue. PET is commonly combined with MRI or CT to incorporate metabolic and anatomic information.

Other Techniques

Bioimpedance Analysis

Bioelectrical impedance analysis (BIA) is a method for the assessment of body composition, especially body fat and muscle mass, in which an electrical current passes through a compartment of interest, and the voltage is measured to calculate the impedance (resistance) of the tissue [65]. However, body composition measurement by BIA is prone to errors in relation to previous physical activity, body position, skin temperature, and dietary and fluid intake [66, 67]. Therefore, it is critical to follow the recommendations regarding standardized measurement conditions, subject preparation, and the compared reference population.

Densitometry (Hydrostatic Weighing and Air Displacement Plethysmography)

Measurement of body density is part of body composition analysis. Hydrostatic weighing is considered the gold standard for body volume measurement. The body density is calculated from the measured body volume and weight and can be used to estimate body fat percentage from Siri and Brozek equations [68, 69]. However, hydrostatic weighing is expensive and requires ample space, and the method could be more subject-friendly. Therefore, air displacement plethysmography (ADP) emerged as an alternative to hydrostatic weighing for body density analysis for a broader range of participants, including infants, elderly, and debilitated patients [69].

Isotope Dilution

Another unique method of estimating the total body water (TBW) and fat-free mass (FFM) is the isotope dilution technique in which stable isotopes such as deuterium oxide (^2H_2O) are administered, and the concentration of administered isotope is measured after an equilibration phase [70]. This modality is low risk but not popular due to its high cost and a detailed protocol.

Whole-Body Counting and Neutron Activation

Whole-body counting (e.g., of potassium) and neutron activation are methods used to assess body composition at the molecular and atomic levels [71, 72]. However, their application in cardiometabolic risk assessment is limited.

Correlation Between the Methods

All methods of body composition assessments rely on certain assumptions that vary with subject characteristics – age, gender, nutrition, volume status, etc. These assumptions are important to consider, as violations may cause imprecise results.

Compared to a standard four-compartment model, body composition assessment by DXA has a good correlation between the two approaches with a reported bias in the determination of percentage body fat ranging from 2% to 4%. In general, there has been a tendency for DXA to underestimate fat mass in lean individuals [73]. The precision of DXA measurement expressed as a coefficient of variation (CV%) ranges from 0.8% to 2.7% (SEM 0.39–0.5 kg) for whole body fat mass and 0.4–1.3% (SEM 0.35–0.54 kg) for lean tissue in sequential measurements [74, 75]. Reproducibility of CT-based sequential measurements of visceral adipose tissue reported as CV% fluctuates between 0.6% and 12.3% [76, 77]. The reproducibility of MRI-based measurements varies between 0.3% and 1.7% for the quantification of subcutaneous adipose tissue and 3.5–9.4% for visceral adipose tissue [61, 62].

Body Composition and Cardiometabolic Disease

Cardiovascular Disease

Obesity is a risk factor for cardiovascular diseases, promoting atherosclerosis is associated pathology. As discussed before, although obesity definition is often based on the BMI, a growing body of evidence shows that other indices of regional adiposity, such as waist circumference and waist-hip ratio, are better predictors of cardiovascular disease (CVD) [78, 79]. Within the same BMI range, Asian populations have total body fat and more abdominal fat. In contrast, African Americans tend to have higher fat-free mass and lower body fat than European Americans [80]. A higher fat-free mass reflects more muscle mass and has been linked to a reduced risk of CVD.

In comparison, sarcopenic obesity (lower fat-free mass together with a high-fat mass) is hypothesized to be a more sensitive predictor of CVD risk, carrying the cumulative risk derived from each of the two individual body composition phenotypes [80]. When compared to visceral adipocytes, subcutaneous fat tissue has low catecholamine-stimulated lipolysis rates and is more sensitive to insulin [81–83]. It has been proposed that subcutaneous adipose tissue may act as a metabolic sink, metabolizing and storing excess free fatty acids in fasting and postprandial states.

Diabetes Mellitus

Park et al. studied a cohort of 2600 patients followed for 6 years and showed that appendicular lean mass (skeletal muscle mass) declined in older adults with type 2 diabetes and was independent of weight changes over time [84]. There is also an independent negative relationship between hyperglycemia and lean body mass in older persons, even without diabetes [85]. Research has shown that aerobic exercise is associated with losing fat and lean mass in diabetic adults; however, adding resistance training might preserve and increase lean mass [86]. Bariatric procedures have been shown to have significant improvements in diabetes control. The estimation of body composition shows a concomitant detrimental loss of muscle mass after bariatric procedures, and nutritional interventions are needed to address this issue.

Hypertension

Studies have shown that higher BMI and waist circumference are related to elevated blood pressure (BP) [87]. There appears to be a positive association between lean body mass and elevated BP and hypertension in young adults or postmenopausal women [88–90]. Adolescents with primary hypertension have increased fat mass and an imbalanced relationship between body weight, fat mass, and lean body mass [91].

Metabolic Syndrome

The metabolic syndrome includes metrics for central obesity, type 2 diabetes mellitus or glucose intolerance, elevated blood pressure, and dyslipidemia. It is well-known that a higher fat mass and visceral fat accumulation significantly increase the risk of metabolic syndrome, type 2 diabetes, and cardiovascular disease. Sarcopenia, a state of age-related reduced fat-free mass (FFM), is associated with adverse metabolic health, insulin resistance, type 2 diabetes, and cardiovascular diseases. A higher baseline FFM, relative to total body weight, was linked to more favorable metabolic health after a 4-year follow-up [92]. A higher FFM percentage (FFM/total body weight $\times$ 100) is shown to be a protective factor against metabolic syndrome [93].

There are two reasons why higher FFM implies a better cardiometabolic profile. First, FFM is involved in insulin-stimulated glucose uptake, leading to better glucose homeostasis. Second, a better FFM may protect individuals from accumulating fat through elevation of the resting energy expenditure.

Therefore, one can safely conclude that body composition assessments offer greater potential to predict the metabolic health of subtypes of people with obesity and offer appropriate risk treatment.

Use of Artificial Intelligence for Assessment of Body Composition

Accurate body composition assessment is a time-consuming process that can be significantly enhanced using automation and artificial intelligence (AI). This application is rapidly expanding in medical imaging and diagnostic radiology. Deep learning methods like neural networks can help determine metabolic changes related to obesity and resting energy expenditure and predict body fat percentage changes.

AI Methods for Cardiometabolic Health

Automatic segmentation of body composition has been performed to quantify subcutaneous, visceral adipose tissue, bone, and muscle mass from low-dose CT scans. MRI studies involving whole-body adipose tissue segmentation from proton density fat fraction MRI images have used automation algorithms [94]. Automatic adipose tissue segmentation has also been performed in children with nonalcoholic fatty liver disease employing MRI images and neural networks [95].

AI Methods for Muscle and Bone Health

Deep learning algorithms can enhance fracture risk prediction from traditional risk factors and measured bone density. Sarcopenia may be assessed from CT scans using neural network algorithms [96, 97]. Automated lean body imaging metrics from CT scans accurately predict osteoporotic fractures [98].

Potential Applications of Body Composition Assessment by Clinicians

Cardiovascular Risk Stratification

Studies have shown that the BMI, waist circumference, waist-to-hip ratio, and adiposity index can augment and enhance the predictive capabilities of different scoring systems for cardiovascular risk stratification. Body composition analysis better identifies the metabolically healthy phenotype in persons with high BMI. It may help the clinician to apply individualized therapeutic interventions.

Pharmacotherapy Dosing

Obesity imposes significant challenges on dosing of different pharmacological agents, including antibiotics, hormones, and cancer chemotherapy. Different formulas and equations to calculate the lean body weight from total body weight and BMI have been proposed for drug dosing [99]. Chemotherapy toxicity in cancer therapy is strongly linked to sarcopenia, while low muscle mass changes are associated with varied insulin sensitivity. In the future, body composition measurements are likely to be critical if not indispensable, for drug dosing that maximizes therapeutic effects and minimizes adverse reactions.

Identification of Sarcopenic Obesity

In the elderly population, the identification of sarcopenic obesity is being increasingly recognized as an essential factor contributing to drug toxicity, mental health and cognition issues, and overall poor outcomes. Geriatricians are likely to have numerous applications of body composition assessments.

Sports/Athletic Performance

Sports performance and training are strongly influenced by body composition, especially strength and weight class sports. Highly precise and affordable methods would enhance selection and performance assessments.

Summary

As we are facing a global health crisis in the form of increasing rates of obesity and related diseases, it is essential to have reliable and standardized means of measuring body composition, particularly as it relates to health outcomes such as diabetes and cardiovascular risk. Having a comprehensive understanding of available tools used to measure body composition will assist clinicians in assessing disease risk and treatment.

Although the BMI is widely used to assess adiposity and is used for the definition of normal weight, overweight, and obesity, it has some limitations, including its generalizability across different ages, races, and sex. Other anthropometric tools to assess body fat, e.g., waist circumference, are also limited in accuracy, though they are cost-effective and readily available for most providers. Imaging tools like DXA, CT, and MRI using a compartmental model of body composition help define the fat mass of an individual concerning the total body water (TBW), protein, and mineral content. However, the widespread use of these methods is limited by their practicability and cost. Other methods have limitations; e.g., bioimpedance analysis is subject to errors based on fluid intake and physical activity, and densitometry requires expensive equipment and is impractical.

Moreover, it has become apparent that it is not only the absolute amount of body fat that is important in determining cardiometabolic risk, but, more importantly, fat distribution (visceral vs. subcutaneous) and fat proportion in relation to muscle mass (FM vs. FFM) are more accurate predictors of cardiometabolic health. With expanding interest in the application of artificial intelligence in the health sector, deep learning methods may serve a distinctive role in predicting cardiometabolic health when paired with the expanding utilization of various imaging modalities like CT and MRI in the future. This could help streamline the process to allow physicians to make more efficient body composition assessments and more accurate risk assessments. The ultimate goal is to allow for easier clinical decision-making based on practical and affordable measures of body composition.

References

1. Ellis KJ. Human body composition: in vivo methods. Physiol Rev. 2000;80(2):649–80.
2. Fee B, Weil W Jr. Body composition of infants of diabetic mothers by direct analysis. Ann N Y Acad Sci. 1963;110(2):869–97.
3. Givens MH, Macy IG. The chemical composition of the human fetus. J Biol Chem. 1933;102:7–17.
4. Adab P, Pallan M, Whincup PH. Is BMI the best measure of obesity? BMJ. 2018;360:k1274.
5. Aune D, Sen A, Prasad M, Norat T, Janszky I, Tonstad S, et al. BMI and all cause mortality: systematic review and non-linear dose-response meta-analysis of 230 cohort studies with 3.74 million deaths among 30.3 million participants. BMJ (Clin Res Ed). 2016;353:i2156.
6. Forbes GB. Lean body mass-body fat interrelationships in humans. Nutr Rev (USA). 1987;45:225–31.
7. Hall KD. Body fat and fat-free mass inter-relationships: Forbes's theory revisited. Br J Nutr. 2007;97(6):1059–63.
8. Finkelstein JS, Cleary RL, Butler JP, Antonelli R, Mitlak BH, Deraska DJ, et al. A comparison of lateral versus anterior-posterior spine dual energy x-ray absorptiometry for the diagnosis of osteopenia. J Clin Endocrinol Metabol. 1994;78(3):724–30.
9. Xu J, Wan CS, Ktoris K, Reijnierse EM, Maier AB. Sarcopenia is associated with mortality in adults: a systematic review and meta-analysis. Gerontology. 2022;68(4):361–76.
10. Guglielmi G, Ponti F, Agostini M, Amadori M, Battista G, Bazzocchi A. The role of DXA in sarcopenia. Aging Clin Exp Res. 2016;28(6):1047–60.
11. Sinclair M, Hoermann R, Peterson A, Testro A, Angus PW, Hey P, et al. Use of dual X-ray absorptiometry in men with advanced cirrhosis to predict sarcopenia-associated mortality risk. Liver Int. 2019;39(6):1089–97.
12. Heymsfield SB, Lichtman S, Baumgartner RN, Wang J, Kamen Y, Aliprantis A, et al. Body composition of humans: comparison of two improved four-compartment models that differ in expense, technical complexity, and radiation exposure. Am J Clin Nutr. 1990;52(1):52–8.
13. Withers RT, LaForgia J, Pillans R, Shipp N, Chatterton B, Schultz C, et al. Comparisons of two-, three-, and four-compartment models of body composition analysis in men and women. J Appl Physiol. 1998;85(1):238–45.
14. Wells JC, Williams JE, Chomtho S, Darch T, Grijalva-Eternod C, Kennedy K, et al. Pediatric reference data for lean tissue properties: density and hydration from age 5 to 20 y. Am J Clin Nutr. 2010;91(3):610–8.
15. Wells JC, Williams JE, Chomtho S, Darch T, Grijalva-Eternod C, Kennedy K, et al. Body-composition reference data for simple and reference techniques and a

4-component model: a new UK reference child. Am J Clin Nutr. 2012;96(6):1316–26.

16. Weber DR, Leonard MB, Zemel BS. Body composition analysis in the pediatric population. Pediatr Endocrinol Rev PER. 2012;10(1):130.

17. Bastien M, Poirier P, Lemieux I, Després J-P. Overview of epidemiology and contribution of obesity to cardiovascular disease. Prog Cardiovasc Dis. 2014;56(4): 369–81.

18. Kannel WB, d'Agostino R, Cobb JL. Effect of weight on cardiovascular disease. Am J Clin Nutr. 1996;63(3): 419S–22S.

19. Nelson CP, Hamby SE, Saleheen D, Hopewell JC, Zeng L, Assimes TL, et al. Genetically determined height and coronary artery disease. N Engl J Med. 2015;372(17):1608–18.

20. Ortega FB, Lavie CJ, Blair SN. Obesity and cardiovascular disease. Circ Res. 2016;118(11):1752–70.

21. Postorino M, Marino C, Tripepi G, Zoccali C, Group CW. Abdominal obesity and all-cause and cardiovascular mortality in end-stage renal disease. J Am Coll Cardiol. 2009;53(15):1265–72.

22. Roche AF, Sievogel R, Chumlea WC, Webb P. Grading body fatness from limited anthropometric data. Am J Clin Nutr. 1981;34(12):2831–8.

23. Fukuda T, Bouchi R, Takeuchi T, Tsujimoto K, Minami I, Yoshimoto T, et al. Sarcopenic obesity assessed using dual energy X-ray absorptiometry (DXA) can predict cardiovascular disease in patients with type 2 diabetes: a retrospective observational study. Cardiovasc Diabetol. 2018;17(1):1–12.

24. Karcher HS, Holzwarth R, Mueller HP, Ludolph AC, Huber R, Kassubek J, et al. Body fat distribution as a risk factor for cerebrovascular disease: an MRI-based body fat quantification study. Cerebrovasc Dis (Basel, Switzerland). 2013;35(4):341–8.

25. Magudia K, Bridge CP, Bay CP, Farah S, Babic A, Fintelmann FJ, et al. Utility of normalized body composition areas, derived from outpatient abdominal CT using a fully automated deep learning method, for predicting subsequent cardiovascular events. Am J Roentgenol. 2023;220(2):236–244.

26. Seabolt LA, Welch EB, Silver HJ. Imaging methods for analyzing body composition in human obesity and cardiometabolic disease. Ann N Y Acad Sci. 2015;1353:41–59.

27. Yamashita K, Kondo T, Osugi S, Shimokata K, Maeda K, Okumura N, et al. The significance of measuring body fat percentage determined by bioelectrical impedance analysis for detecting subjects with cardiovascular disease risk factors. Circ J. 2012;76(10):2435–42.

28. Panoulas VF, Ahmad N, Fazal AA, Kassamali RH, Nightingale P, Kitas GD, et al. The inter-operator variability in measuring waist circumference and its potential impact on the diagnosis of the metabolic syndrome. Postgrad Med J. 2008;84(993):344–7.

29. Eknoyan G. Adolphe Quetelet (1796–1874) – the average man and indices of obesity. Nephrol Dial Transplant. 2008;23(1):47–51.

30. WHO. Obesity: preventing and managing the global epidemic. Report of a WHO consultation. Geneva: World Health Organization; 2000. p. 1–253.

31. Tyson N, Frank M. Childhood and adolescent obesity definitions as related to BMI, evaluation and management options. Best Pract Res Clin Obstet Gynaecol. 2018;48:158–64.

32. Shields M, Tremblay MS. Canadian childhood obesity estimates based on WHO, IOTF and CDC cut-points. Int J Pediatr Obes IJPO. 2010;5(3):265–73.

33. Secker D. Promoting optimal monitoring of child growth in Canada: using the new WHO growth charts. Can J Diet Pract Res. 2010;71(1):e1–3.

34. Cole TJ, Bellizzi MC, Flegal KM, Dietz WH. Establishing a standard definition for child overweight and obesity worldwide: international survey. BMJ (Clin Res Ed). 2000;320(7244):1240–3.

35. Centre for Public Health Excellence at N, National Collaborating Centre for Primary C. National Institute for health and clinical excellence: guidance. Obesity: the prevention, identification, assessment and Management of Overweight and Obesity in adults and children. London: National Institute for Health and Clinical Excellence (UK); 2006. Copyright © 2006, National Institute for Health and Clinical Excellence.

36. Gómez-Ambrosi J, Silva C, Galofré JC, Escalada J, Santos S, Millán D, et al. Body mass index classification misses subjects with increased cardiometabolic risk factors related to elevated adiposity. Int J Obes (2005). 2012;36(2):286–94.

37. Sahakyan KR, Somers VK, Rodriguez-Escudero JP, Hodge DO, Carter RE, Sochor O, et al. Normal-weight central obesity: implications for total and cardiovascular mortality. Ann Intern Med. 2015;163(11):827–35.

38. Bray GA, Heisel WE, Afshin A, Jensen MD, Dietz WH, Long M, et al. The science of obesity management: an endocrine society scientific statement. Endocr Rev. 2018;39(2):79–132.

39. Jensen MD, Ryan DH, Apovian CM, Ard JD, Comuzzie AG, Donato KA, et al. 2013 AHA/ACC/TOS guideline for the management of overweight and obesity in adults: a report of the American College of Cardiology/American Heart Association Task Force on Practice Guidelines and The Obesity Society. Circulation. 2014;129(25 Suppl 2):S102–38.

40. NHLBI Obesity Education Initiative Expert Panel on the Identification, Evaluation, and Treatment of Obesity in Adults (US) Clinical guidelines on the identification, evaluation, and treatment of overweight and obesity in adults – the evidence report. National Institutes of Health. Obes Res. 1998;6(Suppl 2):51s–209s.

41. Ross R, Berentzen T, Bradshaw AJ, Janssen I, Kahn HS, Katzmarzyk PT, et al. Does the relationship between waist circumference, morbidity and mortality depend on measurement protocol for waist circumference? Obes Rev. 2008;9(4):312–25.

42. Lean ME, Han TS, Morrison CE. Waist circumference as a measure for indicating need for weight management. BMJ (Clin Res Ed). 1995;311(6998):158–61.

43. Alberti KG, Eckel RH, Grundy SM, Zimmet PZ, Cleeman JI, Donato KA, et al. Harmonizing the metabolic syndrome: a joint interim statement of the International Diabetes Federation Task Force on Epidemiology and Prevention; National Heart, Lung, and Blood Institute; American Heart Association; World Heart Federation; International Atherosclerosis Society; and International Association for the Study of Obesity. Circulation. 2009;120(16):1640–5.

44. Jackson AS, Pollock ML. Generalized equations for predicting body density of men. Br J Nutr. 1978;40(3): 497–504.

45. Jackson AS, Pollock ML, Ward A. Generalized equations for predicting body density of women. Med Sci Sports Exerc. 1980;12(3):175–81.

46. Siri WE. Body composition from fluid spaces and density: analysis of methods. In: Techniques for measuring body composition. Washington, DC: National Academy of Science, National Research Council; 1961.

47. Shepherd JA, Ng BK, Sommer MJ, Heymsfield SB. Body composition by DXA. Bone. 2017;104:101–5.

48. Laskey MA. Dual-energy X-ray absorptiometry and body composition. Nutrition (Burbank, Los Angeles County, Calif). 1996;12(1):45–51.

49. Rothney MP, Brychta RJ, Schaefer EV, Chen KY, Skarulis MC. Body composition measured by dual-energy X-ray absorptiometry half-body scans in obese adults. Obesity (Silver Spring, Md). 2009;17(6):1281–6.

50. Ross R, Janssen I. Computed tomography and magnetic resonance imaging. Human Body Composition. In: Heymsfield SB, Lohman TG, Wang Z, Going SB (eds) (pp.89–108). Human Kinetics. 2005. https://doi.org/10.5040/9781492596950.ch-007

51. Chowdhury B, Sjöström L, Alpsten M, Kostanty J, Kvist H, Löfgren R. A multicompartment body composition technique based on computerized tomography. Int J Obes Relat Metab Disord. 1994;18(4):219–34.

52. Shen W, Wang Z, Tang H, Heshka S, Punyanitya M, Zhu S, et al. Volume estimates by imaging methods: model comparisons with visible woman as the reference. Obes Res. 2003;11(2):217–25.

53. Rössner S, Bo WJ, Hiltbrandt E, Hinson W, Karstaedt N, Santago P, et al. Adipose tissue determinations in cadavers – a comparison between cross-sectional planimetry and computed tomography. Int J Obes. 1990;14(10):893–902.

54. Engstrom CM, Loeb GE, Reid JG, Forrest WJ, Avruch L. Morphometry of the human thigh muscles. A comparison between anatomical sections and computer tomographic and magnetic resonance images. J Anat. 1991;176:139–56.

55. Muller MJ, Braun W, Pourhassan M, Geisler C, Bosy-Westphal A. Application of standards and models in body composition analysis. Proc Nutr Soc. 2016;75(2): 181–7.

56. Arif H, Racette SB, Villareal DT, Holloszy JO, Weiss EP. Comparison of methods for assessing abdominal adipose tissue from magnetic resonance images. Obesity (Silver Spring, Md). 2007;15(9):2240–4.

57. Shen W, Chen J. Application of imaging and other noninvasive techniques in determining adipose tissue mass. Methods Mol Biol (Clifton, NJ). 2008;456:39–54.

58. Gray C, MacGillivray TJ, Eeley C, Stephens NA, Beggs I, Fearon KC, et al. Magnetic resonance imaging with k-means clustering objectively measures whole muscle volume compartments in sarcopenia/cancer cachexia. Clin Nutr (Edinburgh, Scotland). 2011;30 (1):106–11.

59. Fowler PA, Fuller MF, Glasbey CA, Foster MA, Cameron GG, McNeill G, et al. Total and subcutaneous adipose tissue in women: the measurement of distribution and accurate prediction of quantity by using magnetic resonance imaging. Am J Clin Nutr. 1991;54(1): 18–25.

60. Ross R, Léger L, Guardo R, De Guise J, Pike BG. Adipose tissue volume measured by magnetic resonance imaging and computerized tomography in rats. J Appl Physiol (1985). 1991;70(5):2164–72.

61. Kullberg J, Ahlström H, Johansson L, Frimmel H. Automated and reproducible segmentation of visceral and subcutaneous adipose tissue from abdominal MRI. Int J Obes (2005). 2007;31(12):1806–17.

62. Wald D, Teucher B, Dinkel J, Kaaks R, Delorme S, Boeing H, et al. Automatic quantification of subcutaneous and visceral adipose tissue from whole-body magnetic resonance images suitable for large cohort studies. J Magn Reson Imaging JMRI. 2012;36(6): 1421–34.

63. Müller W, Horn M, Fürhapter-Rieger A, Kainz P, Kröpfl JM, Ackland TR, et al. Body composition in sport: interobserver reliability of a novel ultrasound measure of subcutaneous fat tissue. Br J Sports Med. 2013;47(16):1036–43.

64. Wang H, Chen YE, Eitzman DT. Imaging body fat: techniques and cardiometabolic implications. Arterioscler Thromb Vasc Biol. 2014;34(10):2217–23.

65. Kyle UG, Bosaeus I, De Lorenzo AD, Deurenberg P, Elia M, Gómez JM, et al. Bioelectrical impedance analysis--part I: review of principles and methods. Clin Nutr (Edinburgh, Scotland) 2004;23(5):1226–1243.

66. Gudivaka R, Schoeller D, Kushner RF. Effect of skin temperature on multifrequency bioelectrical impedance analysis. J Appl Physiol (1985). 1996;81(2): 838–45.

67. Kushner RF, Gudivaka R, Schoeller DA. Clinical characteristics influencing bioelectrical impedance analysis measurements. Am J Clin Nutr. 1996;64 (3 Suppl):423s–7s.

68. Siri WE. The gross composition of the body. Adv Biol Med Phys. 1956;4:239–80.

69. Brozek J, Grande F, Anderson JT, Keys A. Densitometric analysis of body composition:

revision of some quantitative assumptions. Ann N Y Acad Sci. 1963;110:113–40.

70. Wells JC, Davies PS, Fewtrell MS, Cole TJ. Body composition reference charts for UK infants and children aged 6 weeks to 5 years based on measurement of total body water by isotope dilution. Eur J Clin Nutr. 2020;74(1):141–8.

71. Harvey T, Dykes P, Chen N, Ettinger K, Jain S, James H, et al. Measurement of whole-body nitrogen by neutron-activation analysis. Lancet. 1973;302 (7826):395–9.

72. Kotler DP, Rosenbaum K, Allison DB, Wang J, Pierson RN Jr. Validation of bioimpedance analysis as a measure of change in body cell mass as estimated by whole-body counting of potassium in adults. J Parenter Enter Nutr. 1999;23(6):345–9.

73. Fosbøl M, Zerahn B. Contemporary methods of body composition measurement. Clin Physiol Funct Imaging. 2015;35(2):81–97.

74. Fosbøl M, Dupont A, Alslev L, Zerahn B. The effect of 99mTc on dual-energy X-ray absorptiometry measurement of body composition and bone mineral density. J Clin Densitom. 2013;16(3):297–301.

75. Hind K, Oldroyd B, Truscott JG. In vivo precision of the GE Lunar iDXA densitometer for the measurement of total body composition and fat distribution in adults. Eur J Clin Nutr. 2011;65(1):140–2.

76. Yoon DY, Moon JH, Kim HK, Choi CS, Chang SK, Yun EJ, et al. Comparison of low-dose CT and MR for measurement of intra-abdominal adipose tissue: a phantom and human study. Acad Radiol. 2008;15(1): 62–70.

77. Maurovich-Horvat P, Massaro J, Fox CS, Moselewski F, O'Donnell CJ, Hoffmann U. Comparison of anthropometric, area- and volume-based assessment of abdominal subcutaneous and visceral adipose tissue volumes using multi-detector computed tomography. Int J Obes (2005). 2007;31(3):500–6.

78. Srikanthan P, Seeman TE, Karlamangla AS. Waist-hip-ratio as a predictor of all-cause mortality in high-functioning older adults. Ann Epidemiol. 2009;19 (10):724–31.

79. Staiano AE, Reeder BA, Elliott S, Joffres MR, Pahwa P, Kirkland SA, et al. Body mass index versus waist circumference as predictors of mortality in Canadian adults. Int J Obes (2005). 2012;36(11):1450–4.

80. Rao G, Powell-Wiley TM, Ancheta I, Hairston K, Kirley K, Lear SA, et al. Identification of obesity and cardiovascular risk in ethnically and racially diverse populations: a scientific statement from the American Heart Association. Circulation. 2015;132(5):457–72.

81. Busetto L, Digito M, Dalla Montá P, Carraro R, Enzi G. Omental and epigastric adipose tissue lipolytic activity in human obesity. Effect of abdominal fat distribution and relationship with hyperinsulinemia. Horm Metab Res. 1993;25(7):365–71.

82. Edens NK, Fried SK, Kral JG, Hirsch J, Leibel RL. In vitro lipid synthesis in human adipose tissue from three abdominal sites. Am J Phys. 1993;265(3 Pt 1):E374–9.

83. Mauriège P, Prud'homme D, Lemieux S, Tremblay A, Després JP. Regional differences in adipose tissue lipolysis from lean and obese women: existence of postreceptor alterations. Am J Phys. 1995;269(2 Pt 1):E341–50.

84. Park SW, Goodpaster BH, Lee JS, Kuller LH, Boudreau R, de Rekeneire N, et al. Excessive loss of skeletal muscle mass in older adults with type 2 diabetes. Diabetes Care. 2009;32(11):1993–7.

85. Kalyani RR, Tra Y, Egan JM, Ferrucci L, Brancati F. Hyperglycemia is associated with relatively lower lean body mass in older adults. J Nutr Health Aging. 2014;18(8):737–43.

86. Al-Sofiani ME, Ganji SS, Kalyani RR. Body composition changes in diabetes and aging. J Diabetes Complicat. 2019;33(6):451–9.

87. Deng WW, Wang J, Liu MM, Wang D, Zhao Y, Liu YQ, et al. Body mass index compared with abdominal obesity indicators in relation to prehypertension and hypertension in adults: the CHPSNE study. Am J Hypertens. 2013;26(1):58–67.

88. Sidoti A, Nigrelli S, Rosati A, Bigazzi R, Caprioli R, Fanelli R, et al. Body mass index, fat free mass, uric acid, and renal function as blood pressure levels determinants in young adults. Nephrology (Carlton). 2017;22(4):279–85.

89. Peppa M, Koliaki C, Boutati E, Garoflos E, Papaefstathiou A, Siafakas N, et al. Association of lean body mass with cardiometabolic risk factors in healthy postmenopausal women. Obesity (Silver Spring, Md). 2014;22(3):828–35.

90. Ye S, Zhu C, Wei C, Yang M, Zheng W, Gan D, et al. Associations of body composition with blood pressure and hypertension. Obesity (Silver Spring, Md). 2018;26(10):1644–50.

91. Pludowski P, Litwin M, Sladowska J, Antoniewicz J, Niemirska A, Wierzbicka A, et al. Bone mass and body composition in children and adolescents with primary hypertension: preliminary data. Hypertension (Dallas, Tex: 1979). 2008;51(1):77–83.

92. Lee MJ, Kim EH, Bae SJ, Choe J, Jung CH, Lee WJ, et al. Protective role of skeletal muscle mass against progression from metabolically healthy to unhealthy phenotype. Clin Endocrinol. 2019;90(1):102–13.

93. Atlantis E, Martin SA, Haren MT, Taylor AW, Wittert GA. Inverse associations between muscle mass, strength, and the metabolic syndrome. Metab Clin Exp. 2009;58(7):1013–22.

94. Wang Z, Cheng C, Peng H, Qi Y, Wan Q, Zhou H, et al. Automatic segmentation of whole-body adipose tissue from magnetic resonance fat fraction images based on machine learning. Magma (New York, NY). 2021. https://doi.org/10.2214/AJR.22.27977. Epub 2022 Aug 31.

95. Delgado T, Wang K, Wolfson T, Mamidipalli A, Schwimmer JB, Hsiao AM, et al. Automated quantification in children of visceral and subcutaneous adipose tissue from routine MRI using a convolutional neural network. Hepatology. 2018;68:612A.

96. Belharbi S, Chatelain C, Hérault R, Adam S, Thureau S, Chastan M, et al. Spotting L3 slice in CT scans using deep convolutional network and transfer learning. Comput Biol Med. 2017;87:95–103.

97. Nerot A, Betry C, Fontaine E, Moreau-gaudry A, Bricault I. Automated measurement of cross-sectional muscle area for diagnosis of sarcopenia in any tomodensitometry. Clin Nutr ESPEN. 2020;40:489.

98. Pickhardt PJ, Graffy PM, Zea R, Lee SJ, Liu J, Sandfort V, et al. Automated abdominal CT imaging biomarkers for opportunistic prediction of future major osteoporotic fractures in asymptomatic adults. Radiology. 2020;297(1):64–72.

99. Han P, Duffull S, Kirkpatrick C, Green B. Dosing in obesity: a simple solution to a big problem. Clin Pharmacol Ther. 2007;82(5):505–8.

Type 2 Diabetes: Etiology, Epidemiology, Pathogenesis, and Treatment

27

Carrie Burns and Nnenia Francis

Contents

Abstract

Diabetes is one of the largest health problems facing the world today. It is estimated that by the year 2030 over 7% of the world's adult population will have diabetes. Several risk factors play into an individual's risk of developing diabetes. Some are modifiable such as obesity, diet, and exercise. Other risk factors including genetic and environmental factors are topics of ongoing research. The physiology of diabetes is a complex interplay between pancreatic beta-cell function and insulin resistance. Other hormones such as GLP-1 and leptin also play a role. The classic presentation of type 2 diabetes is polyuria, polydipsia, and unintentional weight loss. However, many people with diabetes are asymptomatic and diagnosed with routine screening either with a hemoglobin A1c test or an oral glucose tolerance test. The treatment of type 2 diabetes is multifaceted. Patient education regarding diet and exercise and adjustment of modifiable risk factors remain the cornerstone of treatment. Patients should be screened for microvascular and macrovascular complications. While studies have shown a benefit of intensive glycemic control for type 2 diabetes in reducing

C. Burns (✉)
Division of Endocrinology, Diabetes, and Metabolism, Perelman School of Medicine, Department of Medicine, University of Pennsylvania, Philadelphia, PA, USA
e-mail: Carrie.Burns@uphs.upenn.edu

N. Francis
Division of Endocrinology, Diabetes and Metabolism, Department of Medicine, University of Kentucky, Lexington, KY, USA
e-mail: Nnenia.Francis@uky.edu

© Springer Nature Switzerland AG 2023
R. S. Ahima (ed.), *Metabolic Syndrome*,
https://doi.org/10.1007/978-3-031-40116-9_34

microvascular complications, the effect on macrovascular complications has been less clear. Long-term studies suggest that optimal glycemic control at the onset of diabetes can have beneficial impact decades later.

Keywords

Obesity · Beta-cell dysfunction · Insulin · Insulin resistance · Incretin · Adipocytokines · Hemoglobin A1c · Oral glucose tolerance test · Diabetes complications

Etiology

The etiology of type 2 diabetes is multifactorial and spans a wide range of factors from genetic to lifestyle to environmental (see Box 1). There is clearly an association between obesity and type 2 diabetes. Analysis of large observational cohorts of men in the Health Professionals' Study and women in the Nurses' Health Study demonstrated that increased body mass index (BMI) is associated with an increased risk of developing diabetes [17, 43]. Population data in the United States showed that the lifetime risk of diabetes for men beginning at 18 years of age increased from 7.6% for a BMI of <18.5 to 70.3% for a BMI of 35 or higher. For women, the increase was similar, 12.2% versus 74.4% between lowest and highest BMI, respectively [70].

Box 1 Risk Factors for Type 2 Diabetes
Modifiable
- Obesity
- Diet
- Physical inactivity
- Smoking
- Environmental

Non-modifiable
- Age
- Ethnicity
- Family history
- Gestational diabetes
- Intrauterine environment/birth weight

There are several lifestyle factors that, when modified, can lower the risk of type 2 diabetes. This includes a diet high in fiber and polyunsaturated fats and low in trans-fat. Maintaining regular exercise and abstaining from smoking and consuming alcohol moderately also lower risk the risk of diabetes. Men who followed a healthy diet (characterized by higher consumption of vegetables, fruit, fish, poultry, and whole grains) had a modestly decreased risk of developing diabetes. Conversely, men who followed a "western" diet (characterized by higher consumption of red meat, processed meat, French fries, high-fat dairy products, refined grains, and sweets and desserts) had a significantly increased risk of diabetes (RR 1.6, 95% CI 1.3–1.9) [92]. This risk was independent of body mass index (BMI), physical activity, or family history. Similar results were found in women [36].

Sugar-sweetened beverages (SSB) have been studied as an independent risk factor for diabetes. Women who consumed one or more sugar-sweetened soft drinks per day had almost twice the risk of developing diabetes compared to those who consumed less than one of these beverages a month (RR 1.8, 95% CI 1.42–2.36). The risk remained significant even after adjustment for changes in BMI and caloric intake, suggesting that sweetened beverages may increase the risk of diabetes due to rapid absorption rate of carbohydrates [85]. Individuals who drink 1–2 servings/day of SSB had a 26% (RR 1.26, 95% CI 1.12–1.41) greater risk of developing type 2 diabetes compared to those who drink none or < 1 per month [61]. Replacing one daily serving of SSB with water, coffee, or tea was associated with a 2–10% lower diabetes risk [27].

Meat consumption appears to be related to the incidence of type 2 diabetes. Individuals that reported an increase in red meat consumption over 4 years had a higher subsequent risk of developing diabetes, though this association was partly mediated by body weight [74]. However, in a meta-analysis of meat consumption, consumption of processed meat was associated with a statistically significant increase in the risk of diabetes, whereas unprocessed red meat consumption showed a nonsignificant trend toward increased risk [67].

Physical activity significantly impacts type 2 diabetes and cardiovascular outcomes. Moderate-intensity exercise is associated with a lower risk of developing type 2 diabetes. The association persists even after adjustment for BMI, suggesting that exercise can reduce the risk of developing diabetes independent of weight loss [46]. Additional studies have examined associations between the development of diabetes and sedentary behavior. A meta-analysis analyzed television viewing as a risk factor for development of diabetes and found that the viewing duration was associated with a higher risk of type 2 diabetes (pooled RR, 1.20 95% CI 1.14–1.27) [38]. Retrospective analysis of prediabetic patients showed a 3.4% increased risk of diabetes for every hour spent watching television ($p < 0.01$) [78].

Smoking is postulated to be a risk factor for type 2 diabetes. In a meta-analysis of 25 prospective cohort studies, active smoking was associated with an increased risk for type 2 diabetes, although only a few of the studies adjusted for other unhealthy behaviors were associated with smoking, such as poor diet and lack of physical activity [96]. There is some evidence that smoking acutely affects glucose metabolism. Subjects who smoked prior to an oral glucose tolerance test showed a significant increase in plasma glucose levels compared with those who did not smoke [35].

Sleep patterns are associated with an increased risk of diabetes. A large meta-analysis of sleep and incidence of type 2 diabetes showed an increased risk for diabetes in both people who had a short duration of sleep (≤5–6 h a night) and a long duration of sleep (>8–9 h a night) [14]. By extending the sleep duration of short sleepers, it is possible to improve insulin sensitivity and reduce energy intake [23]. However, it is difficult to determine if sleep duration is causal or indirectly associated with obesity and comorbidities such as obstructive sleep apnea. Melatonin has been postulated to affect a person's risk of developing diabetes. Melatonin is regulated by light exposure, and its secretion peaks 3–5 h after sleep onset in darkness, with almost no production during the daytime hours. A study that measured urinary excretion of melatonin metabolites showed that lower melatonin secretion was independently associated with a higher risk of developing type 2 diabetes [64].

Building on observational studies of obesity and lifestyle as a risk factor for diabetes, large prevention trials have investigated lifestyle interventions to reduce the risk of developing diabetes. The Finnish Diabetes Prevention Study included a population of 522 middle-aged overweight subjects with impaired glucose tolerance and randomized them to an intervention group or control. The intervention group received intensive individualized counseling aimed at reducing weight and total intake of fat and increasing fiber and physical activity. The mean weight lost at 2 years was 3.5 ± 5.5 kg in the intervention group and 0.8 ± 4.4 kg in the control group. The cumulative incidence of diabetes after 4 years was 11% in the intervention group compared with 23% in the control group, which translated to a 58% reduction in the incidence of diabetes between the two groups [89].

The Diabetes Prevention Program (DPP) trial was a multicenter trial in the United States that addressed prevention of diabetes in a high-risk and ethnically diverse population. The DPP was a comparative effectiveness trial that recruited 3224 participants with prediabetes and assigned them to one of three interventions: intensive lifestyle intervention, metformin, and a control group, which received standard lifestyle recommendations and placebo. The intensive lifestyle intervention included an individualized curriculum covering diet, exercise, and behavior modification intended to achieve a 7% weight loss through a healthy low-calorie, low-fat diet, and 150 min of exercise a week. Over 2 years, those assigned to the lifestyle intervention had greater weight loss and a greater increase in physical activity than participants in the other groups (weight loss of 0.1, 2.1, and 5.6 kg in the placebo, metformin, and lifestyle intervention groups, respectively). The lifestyle intervention also decreased the incidence of diabetes by 58%, compared to metformin treatment (31%) or placebo. Subgroup analyses showed that lifestyle intervention was effective regardless of gender, ethnicity, or genetic predisposition to diabetes [56].

Subsequently participants in the DPP were unmasked to their group and placebo was stopped. All participants were then offered a group-administered version of the curriculum. The Diabetes Prevention Program Outcomes Study (DPPOS) followed participants for 10 years and showed that the cumulative incidence of diabetes remained lowest in the lifestyle group with a reduction in diabetes incidence of 34% (95% CI 24–42) versus 18% (7–28) in the metformin group compared with placebo [26].

Although previous guidelines focused on a *low-fat diet*, this has not been shown to reduce the risk of diabetes [88], and subsequent studies suggest the type of dietary fat may be more important than the amount of fat per se. Salmerón et al. reported that an increase in the intake of total fat and saturated fat was not associated with an increased risk of type 2 diabetes. However, increased trans-fats were associated with increased risk of diabetes while polyunsaturated fatty acids were associated with reduced risk of diabetes [82].

Mediterranean diet is characterized by high consumption of vegetables and legumes with moderate consumption of fish and wine and low consumption of red and processed meat. The Mediterranean diet contains high levels of mono-unsaturated and polyunsaturated fatty acids from sources like virgin olive oil and nuts. Adherence to a Mediterranean diet among nondiabetic subjects with at least one cardiovascular risk factor was associated with >50% lower incidence of diabetes when compared with a low-fat diet [81]. A meta-analysis comparing nine dietary approaches (low-fat, vegetarian, Mediterranean, high-protein, moderate-carbohydrate, low-carbohydrate, control, low GI/GL, Paleolithic) showed that the Mediterranean diet is the most effective dietary approach to improve glycemic control in patients with type 2 diabetes [101]. In a study in persons with high cardiovascular risk, the incidence of major cardiovascular events was lower among those assigned to a Mediterranean diet supplemented with extra-virgin olive oil or nuts compared to those assigned to a reduced-fat diet [30].

Nut consumption is inversely associated with risk of type 2 diabetes. Women eating five or more ounce servings of nuts per week had a lower incidence of diabetes compared with women who did not consume any nuts [47]. High *coffee consumption* has been associated with a decreased risk of diabetes. A recent 2018 systematic review and meta-analysis identified an inverse association of coffee consumption with the risk of type 2 diabetes and suggested that both caffeinated and decaffeinated coffee have favorable metabolic effects [15]. However, there is currently not enough evidence to recommend increased coffee intake as a prevention strategy for diabetes [91].

Certain medical conditions are associated with an increased risk of type 2 diabetes. *Gestational diabetes* is associated with a subsequent increased risk of developing type 2 diabetes. Studies of a large population-based cohort showed that 9 years after gestational diabetes, 19% of women had developed type 2 diabetes compared with only 2% in women who did not have gestational diabetes [32]. *Polycystic ovarian syndrome* (PCOS) [59], metabolic syndrome [34], and cardiovascular disease [69] have also been associated with increased risk of diabetes.

While obesity, lifestyle choices, and medical history are clearly strong risk factors for the development of diabetes, a person's risk of developing diabetes is affected by factors starting before conception.

Family history is clearly a risk factor of diabetes. Identical twins have a high concordance rate of type 2 diabetes [12]. Individuals with one parent with type 2 diabetes are two to three times more likely to have type 2 diabetes themselves. Individuals with both parents with diabetes have five times the risk of developing diabetes [65]. Even when controlling for potential confounding factors such as body weight, diet, education, and genetic risk, the family history remained a significant risk factor for developing diabetes [45]. Ethnicity is also a risk factor for diabetes as evidenced by the substantially higher rates of diabetes in certain ethnic groups, such as African Americans, Hispanic and native populations in North America.

Genetic factors contribute to an individual's risk of developing diabetes. *Monogenic diabetes* is a result of a genetic defect that leads to diabetes. The defect has a high penetrance, which leads to inherited diabetes in a classical Mendelian fashion (e.g., dominant or recessive). However, monogenic diabetes accounts for approximately 1–5% of diabetes. Genome-wide association studies (GWAS) look for associations between specific genetic variations (most commonly, single-nucleotide polymorphisms) and a particular disease. While some genetic variants have been identified that are associated with an increased risk of type 2 diabetes, such as TCF7L2 in Europeans and KCNQ1 in Asians, genetic screening is not commonly used except for cases where monogenic diabetes is suspected [63]. Current research is ongoing on how best to integrate genetic and clinical risk factors to precisely predict a person's risk for developing type 2 diabetes.

Intrauterine factors affect an individual's risk of diabetes. Poor fetal nutrition has been associated with greater susceptibility to obesity and diabetes later in life. This was demonstrated through studies of the Dutch Hunger Famine birth cohort, which showed that adults who had been exposed to famine during fetal life had more glucose intolerance than unexposed people [77]. This finding led to the *thrifty genotype* hypothesis that insulin resistance develops as a protective mechanism in response to intrauterine growth restriction, and rapid weight gain in adulthood when exposed to caloric excess, thereby increasing the risk of developing type 2 diabetes.

Low birth weight has been associated with increased risk of developing type 2 diabetes later in life. A large meta-analysis showed that in most populations a 1 kg increase in birth weight corresponds to a 20% reduction in type 2 diabetes risk [95]. It is unclear whether the relevant causal exposure is body weight itself or metabolic alterations linked to fetal health and nutrition. Native North American populations, e.g., Pima Indians, showed opposite results – higher birth weight was associated with a greater risk of type 2 diabetes. These groups have very high prevalence of type 2 diabetes and gestational diabetes, which may explain the increased incidence of diabetes in their offspring. It is possible that as the rates of diabetes in other ethnic groups continue to increase, the relationship between birth weight and diabetes risk may start to mimic that seen in native North American populations [95].

There is growing evidence that environmental factors also affect an individual's risk of developing diabetes. The Endocrine Society defines an *endocrine disruptor* as an exogenous chemical, or mixture of chemicals, that interferes with aspects of hormone action [100]. Exposure to endocrine disruptors has been associated with an increased risk of metabolic disorders. One of the most studied endocrine disruptors is *bisphenol A (BPA)*, a chemical used extensively in the lining of food and beverage containers, BPA is detectable in urine of 90% of the US population. Research into endocrine disruptors has mostly revolved around rodent studies and epidemiological studies. In a study by Alonso-Magdalena et al., when mice were exposed to BPA injections of 10 µg/kg per day during early pregnancy, at 6 months of age, males prenatally exposed to BPA developed glucose intolerance, insulin resistance, hyperinsulinemia, and altered insulin release from pancreatic β-cells as compared with control mice. Exposure of pregnant mice to a higher dose of BPA (100 µg/kg per day) during the same period showed male offspring with glucose intolerance but normal insulin sensitivity and only a mild alteration in β-cell function. Moreover, the pregnant mice that were exposed to BPA developed glucose intolerance and obesity [5]. In 2008 the US National Health and Nutrition Examination Survey (NHANES) 2003–2004 released the first large-scale data on BPA, and in a study by Lang et al. higher BPA urine concentrations were associated with a diagnosis of diabetes and cardiovascular disease [57]. When the subsequent NHANES data from 2005 to 2006 was evaluated, higher BPA concentrations were not associated with a diagnosis of diabetes. However, when the data from 2003–2004 to 2005–2006 were pooled, there was a statistically significant association between BPA and diabetes [66].

Epidemiology

The prevalence of diabetes is rapidly increasing in both the United States and throughout the world. This increase comes at a great cost to not only the individual but also the community and the health system. The estimated cost in the United States of diabetes in 2012 was $245 billion, of which $176 billion (72%) represented direct health expenditures attributed to diabetes and $69 billion (28%) represented lost productivity from absence in the workplace and premature mortality [6]. It is estimated that in 2012, 29.1 million people or 9.3% of the US population had diabetes and over 27% of this group was undiagnosed, proving that type 2 diabetes is a public health crisis. Certain ethnic groups have a higher incidence of diabetes. In the United States, the highest incidence rate is in American Indians/Alaska natives (15.9% 2010–2012). Non-Hispanic blacks, Hispanics, and Asian Americans also have a higher incidence rate than non-Hispanic whites [16]. Worldwide, the number of people with diabetes has doubled over the past three decades increasing from an estimated 153 million in 1980 to 347 million in 2008 [22]. The number of people worldwide with diabetes is projected to increase even further to an estimated 439 million people by 2030, which represents 7.7% of the world population aged 20–79 [87].

The increase in diabetes largely parallels the increased rates of obesity seen in the United States and throughout the world (Fig. 1). The concomitant rise in diabetes and obesity worldwide is a result of a complex interplay between genetic, environmental, and behavioral factors that have led to more sedentary behavior and an excess of calorie-rich food [99]. While there is clearly an association between obesity and diabetes, there are individuals who are normal weight but have metabolic characteristics similar to obese people, such as hyperinsulinemia, insulin resistance, predisposition to type 2 diabetes, and high triglycerides [80]. This *metabolically unhealthy normal weight* phenotype may explain why Asians tend to develop type 2 diabetes at lower BMI than people of European origin [98].

While diabetes was once rare in developing countries, it is now growing rapidly, and Asia has emerged as the diabetes epicenter of the world [18]. India and China have the largest number of patients with diabetes, and this is expected to continue to increase. The Middle East and Africa also have rising incidences of diabetes. It is estimated that between 2010 and 2030 there will be a 69% increase in the number of adults with diabetes in developing countries compared with a 20% increase in developed countries.

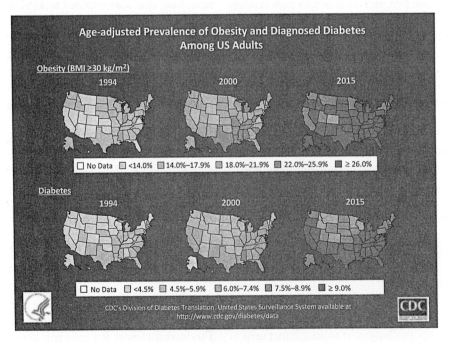

Fig. 1 Parallelism of diabetes and increased rates of obesity in the United States between 1994 and 2013

Furthermore, patients in developing countries tend to present at a younger age leading to a greater effect on their productivity [87].

Food insecurity, defined as an uncertain or limited availability of food owing to cost, is highly prevalent in the United States. Over 18% of the US population reported food insecurity between 2005 and 2014 [102]. The risk of developing type 2 diabetes is increased twofold in those who experience food insecurity [104]. Food insecurity has been associated with lower engagement in self-care behaviors and medication use, depression, distress, and worse glycemic management when compared with individuals who are food secure [103].

Along with global shifts in diabetes epidemiology, there has also been a rise in diabetes in younger populations. While type 1 diabetes is still the most common form of diabetes in young people in the United States, there has been a 30.5% increase in the overall prevalence of type 2 diabetes between 2001 and 2009. Similar to the pattern of type 2 diabetes in adults, the highest prevalence of type 2 diabetes is in Native Americans, Black, Hispanic, and Asian Pacific Islander youth, with the lowest prevalence in white youth. This is the opposite pattern of type 1 diabetes, which is more common in white youth and rare in Native Americans [21]. Prediabetes is also common among adolescents. Analysis of NHANES 2005–2006 showed an unadjusted prevalence of prediabetes of 16.1% among a diverse cross section of adolescents [58]. This increased population of young people diagnosed with diabetes will be at increased risk of complications given the long duration of the disease.

Pathophysiology

The pathophysiology of diabetes is a complex interplay between insulin resistance, beta-cell dysfunction, and other hormones that regulate metabolism. Normal glucose metabolism can be separated into fasting and fed states (Fig. 2). In the fasting state, the body relies on endogenous glucose production, mainly through hepatic glycogenolysis and gluconeogenesis. Hypoglycemia is prevented by maintaining a low insulin-to-glucose ratio in plasma. The brain is dependent on glucose so other tissues are provided with alternative sources of fuel such as fatty acids from adipose tissue lipolysis. This preserves glucose for use by the brain. In the fed state, blood glucose levels increase as a result of absorption of carbohydrates from the gut. This stimulates *insulin* production from islet β-cells and simultaneously suppresses glucagon secretion from α-cells. Insulin helps to lower blood sugar in multiple ways – it suppresses endogenous glucose production by the liver. Insulin also mediates glucose uptake by peripheral tissues through both oxidation to carbon dioxide and water and non-oxidative disposal through glycogen synthesis [73]. Insulin induces the *glucose transporter 4 (GLUT4)*, which catalyzes the uptake of glucose into adipose and muscle cells [93]. This effect is mediated through the nuclear receptor *peroxisome proliferator-activated receptor -Y (PPARγ)*. PPARγ is critical for adipocyte differentiation and glucose homeostasis, and humans with mutations in PPARγ have partial lipodystrophy and insulin resistance [4].

Extensive research has tried to elucidate the changes that lead from impaired fasting glucose to diabetes. Most of the initial research was based on cross-sectional studies of high-risk populations. The Pima Indians of Arizona have one of the highest documented rates of type 2 diabetes in the world [54]. However, there were environmental factors, such as the increased population of white settlers to the north, which led to the eventual diversion of the water that supported the Pimas Indian's way of life [55]. Their life changed from farming sustained though physical labor to one of food scarcity and little labor as they were forced to curtail their farming, which led to significant impacts on their food intake, physical activity, and their economy [83]. Research has also shown that there was a much lower prevalence of type 2 diabetes (6.9% in Mexican Pima Indians vs. 38% in US Pima Indians) and obesity in the Pima Indians in Mexico than in the USA, which indicates that even in populations genetically prone to these conditions, their development is determined mostly by environmental circumstances [84].

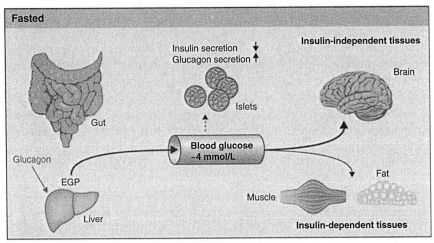

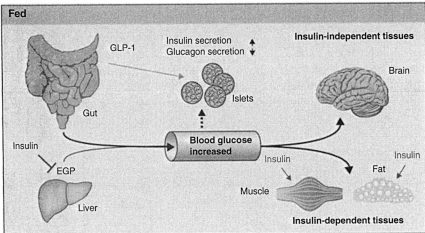

Fig. 2 Overview of normal glucose homeostasis. In the fasting state blood glucose concentration is determined by the balance between EGP production, mainly through hepatic glycogenolysis and gluconeogenesis, and use by insulin-independent tissues, such as the brain. EGP prevents hypoglycemia and is supported by a low insulin-to-glucagon ratio in plasma. The brain is dependent on glucose and, therefore, other tissues, such as heart and skeletal muscle, are mainly provided with nonglucose nutrients (e.g., nonesterified fatty acids from adipose tissue lipolysis). In the fed state (meal with carbohydrate), glucose concentrations in the blood rise because of absorption in the gut, which stimulates insulin secretion by islet β cells and suppresses glucagon secretion from α cells. EGP is suppressed (which helps to curtail total glucose input into blood) and uptake into insulin-sensitive peripheral tissues, such as the heart, skeletal muscle, and adipose tissue, is activated (which increases the rate of glucose disposal). Neurohormonal processes include the release of the incretin hormones, such as GLP-1, which increases glucose-stimulated insulin secretion and glucose-suppression of glucagon secretion. Adipose tissue lipolysis is suppressed and anabolic metabolism is promoted. Glucose concentrations become close to the fasting level within 2 h. *GLP-1* glucagon-like peptide 1, *EGP* endogenous glucose production

Longitudinal studies followed Pima Indians who progress from normal glucose tolerance (NGT) to impaired glucose tolerance (IGT) to determine the course of events. Subjects who progressed from NGT to IGT showed both a lower rate of insulin-stimulated glucose disposal and decreased insulin secretion in response to a glucose load. This suggests that both *insulin resistance* and decreased insulin secretion occur well before the development of overt diabetes. The decrease in glucose uptake in response to insulin was almost entirely due to decreased non-oxidative glucose disposal, suggesting that insulin resistance is primarily mediated by insulin's action on skeletal muscle glycogenesis [94]. Inappropriate endogenous glucose production by the liver appears to occur later in the development of diabetes.

When subjects in the longitudinal Pima Indian trial who progressed to diabetes were compared to subjects who retained normal glucose tolerance, both groups had impaired glucose disposal suggesting insulin resistance. However, the subjects who did not progress were able to compensate for this by increasing insulin secretion, maintaining normal glucose tolerance. The subjects who progressed to diabetes were not able to increase insulin secretion to compensate for decreased insulin action, suggesting that *beta-cell dysfunction* is key in the development of diabetes [94]. This hyperbolic relationship has been confirmed in healthy individuals as well – for any change in insulin sensitivity, there is a reciprocal change in beta-cell function to maintain euglycemia [49, 50]. Similar results were shown in the UKPDS, which showed that beta-cell function had already decreased by 50% at time of diagnosis of diabetes [33].

Primary cause of insulin resistance in type 2 diabetes appears to be a post-receptor defect, and the defect likely is an early step in the insulin signaling pathway. Possible candidates for the post-receptor defect are phosphatidylinositol-3-kinase, the insulin receptor substrates IRS-1 and IRS-2, and the glucose transporter Glut-4 [52].

The causes of beta-cell loss are multifactorial. *Glucolipotoxicity* is a term that refers to the toxic effect of hyperglycemia and elevated plasma fatty acid level, which occur early on in diabetes and may exert a destructive effect on beta-cells through increased oxidative stress [76]. In type 2 diabetes, islets show increased immune cell infiltration and cytokine release, which in turn directly impairs β-cell mass and function. *Amyloid* deposition in islet bodies is associated with decreased beta-cell area and increased beta-cell apoptosis, suggesting that islet amyloid deposition may play a role in beta-cell destruction [48]. Islet amyloid polypeptide secretion is increased in prediabetes because it is functionally coupled to the increased insulin demand. It activates and recruits additional immune cells to the islet by triggering chemokine release from β-cells

[79]. Compounding the problem of beta-cell loss is the fact that most studies suggest beta-cell mass is established early in life with limited ability to regenerate [19]. The reduction in beta-cell mass is not significant enough to explain the degree of impaired insulin release in type 2 diabetes, and further research is ongoing into the interplay between beta-cell mass and function [51].

While insulin resistance and beta-cell dysfunction are the foundation of our understanding of diabetes pathophysiology, there are numerous other hormones involved. *Glucagon* levels are inappropriately elevated in patients with type 2 diabetes. This elevation is thought to contribute to greater rates of glucose production by the liver and attenuated reduction after meals [20].

Incretin hormones play an important role in promoting glucose-stimulated insulin secretion. The incretin effect is the phenomenon in which oral glucose load elicits a greater endogenous insulin secretion as compared with intravenous glucose. This suggested that factors from the gut are involved in signaling insulin production. The two hormones responsible for the incretin effect are glucose-dependent insulinotropic hormone (GIP) and *glucagon-like peptide-1 (GLP-1)*. They are secreted after oral glucose loads and help increase insulin secretion. While GIP loses its effect on insulin secretion in diabetes, GLP-1 retains its stimulatory effect on insulin; however, its level is reduced in type 2 diabetes. This gave rise to GLP-1 as a target for type 2 diabetes [72].

While obesity is clearly associated with type 2 diabetes, the mechanism by which obesity leads to diabetes is still an area of active research. Adipose tissue secretes several proteins and cytokines, which are collectively termed *adipocytokines*, and it is thought that these may represent the link between obesity and diabetes. *Leptin* is produced by adipocytes and signals the hypothalamus regarding satiety and quantity of stored fat. Congenital leptin deficiency due to a mutation in the leptin gene leads to early-onset obesity, profound hyperphagia, and hyperinsulinemia with a dramatic response to treatment with leptin [31]. This condition is rare and typically seen in consanguineous marriages. In addition, leptin appears to act on the pancreas as well. In studies of pancreas-specific leptin receptor knockout mice (KO), when fed a standard diet, the KO mice had improved glucose tolerance as compared with controls. However, when the KO mice were challenged with a high-fat diet, they demonstrated poor compensatory islet growth and glucose intolerance when compared with controls [68].

Adiponectin is a hormone secreted by adipocytes that has anti-inflammatory and insulin-sensitizing properties. Adiponectin secretion is decreased in obesity, and higher adiponectin levels are associated with better glycemic control, more favorable lipid profile, and reduced inflammation in diabetic women [62].

Numerous other signaling molecules and pro-inflammatory cytokines have been studied, mainly in mouse models with some association studies in humans. *Tumor necrosis factor-alpha (TNFα)* released from adipose tissue may lead to impaired insulin action. Injection of TNFα into obese mice led to a two- to threefold increase in insulin-stimulated glucose utilization [40]. Plasminogen activator inhibitor 1 (PAI-1) is a pro-thrombotic factor released by adipocytes, which negatively regulates fibrinolysis by inhibiting tissue plasminogen activator. In a prospective study looking at incidence of type 2 diabetes, PAI-1 was an independent predictor of diabetes after controlling for other metabolic factors such as BMI and visceral fat [53]. Further research is needed to elucidate the relationship between obesity and diabetes with the goal of developing new therapeutic targets.

Diagnosis

The word diabetes was first coined by the ancient Greeks and literally means siphon, relating to the finding of frequent urination in those inflicted. The term mellitus, which is derived from the Latin word for sweet, was added by Englishman Thomas Willis in 1675 after noting the sweet taste of urine from patients with diabetes. In fact, sweet urine has been noted by physicians in ancient Egyptian, Persian, Indian, and Chinese societies. Today the most classic presenting symptoms of type 2 diabetes are polydipsia (frequent thirst), polyuria (frequent urination), blurry vision, and

unintentional weight loss. Typical physical exam findings include visceral adiposity and *acanthosis nigricans* – a velvety, hyperpigmented skin plaque often found on the neck and axilla. In more advanced cases of diabetes, one may see evidence of *diabetic retinopathy* on fundoscopic exam and decreased sensation in the feet.

The diagnosis of diabetes is mainly established through demonstrating hyperglycemia. If a patient has the above symptoms and a random blood glucose of 200 mg/dL (11.1 mmol/L), this establishes the diagnosis of diabetes. Asymptomatic individuals can be identified by any of the following criteria: fasting plasma glucose (FPG) value $\geq$126 mg/dL (7.0 mmol/L), 2-h post oral glucose 75 g tolerance test (OGTT) value of $\geq$200 mg/dL (11.1 mmol/L), and *glycated hemoglobin (A1C)* values $\geq$6.5% (48 mmol/mol) (Table 1). These criteria have been adopted by both the American Diabetes Association and the World Health Organization [7, 41]. While the ADA places less importance on the OGTT to diagnose diabetes citing its inconvenience, greater cost, and less reproducibility, the WHO encourages the use of the OGTT in diagnosing diabetes because of its greater sensitivity in diagnosing diabetes compared with FPG and evidence of worse health outcomes for patients diagnosed with diabetes by OGTT [42].

Glycated hemoglobin (A1c) is a product of hemoglobin's exposure to plasma glucose through nonenzymatic glycation and correlates to the average blood sugar for the prior 3 months. The ADA emphasizes using A1c because in some studies it is a stronger predictor of subsequent diabetes and cardiovascular events than fasting glucose [86]. Recent improvements in A1c assays have allowed its use for screening for diabetes. The National Glycohemoglobin Standardization Program (NGSP) has standardized the majority of the assays used in the United States to the Diabetes Control and Complications Trial (DCCT) standard. The A1c has many advantages including its convenience (fasting not required) and the stability of averaging blood sugars over a longer period of time. The disadvantages include greater cost, limited availability in certain regions, and factors that can alter A1c. Several studies report increased levels of HbA1c in nondiabetic elderly. Racial

Table 1 Diagnostic criteria for diabetes and prediabetes

	Diabetes ADA and WHO	
	mg/dL	mmol/L
Fasting plasma glucose OR	≥126	7.0
OGTT after 75 g oral glucose load OR	>200	11.1
Hemoglobin A1c	>6.5%	48 mmol/mol

	Prediabetes ADA		Prediabetes WHO	
	mg/dL	mmol/L	mg/dL	Mmol/L
IFG Fasting plasma glucose	100–125	5.6–6.9	110–125	6.1–6.9
IPG OGTT after 75 g oral glucose load	140–199	7.8–11.0	140–199 + FPG < 126	7.8–11.0 + FPG < 7.0
Prediabetes Hemoglobin A1c	5.7–6.4%	39–46 mmol/mol		

variations have been noted in A1c measurements as well. African Americans with and without diabetes have higher A1c levels than non-Hispanic whites when matched for fasting plasma glucose. Furthermore, conditions that alter hemoglobin such as hemoglobinopathies and anemia can cause variations in A1c measurements. The red blood cell (RBC) lifespan appears to be affected by several aging-associated changes compromising either RBC production or clearance ultimately influencing HbA1c measure in the elderly. Therefore, if there is a concern for diabetes in an elder patient with normal A1c consider doing an OGTT. The A1c test is also the least sensitive test, and it identifies one-third fewer cases of undiagnosed diabetes than a fasting glucose of ≥126 mg/dL (7.0 mmol/L) (ADA 2015). The disadvantage of lower sensitivity may be offset by the ease of testing, which facilitates screening larger numbers of people [75].

Patients can also be categorized as *prediabetic*, which confers an increased risk for diabetes. The ADA characterizes prediabetes as one of the following: impaired fasting glucose (IFG) defined as a FPG 100 mg/dL (5.6 mmol/L) to 125 mg/dL (6.9 mmol/L), impaired insulin glucose tolerance (IGT) defined as a 2-h plasma glucose in the 75-g OGTT of 140 mg/dL (7.8 mmol/L) to 199 mg/dL (11.0 mmol/L), or an A1c of 5.7–6.4%. This differs from the WHO, which defines IFG as a fasting glucose between 110 and 125 mg/dL (6.1–6.9 mmol/L) and defines IGT as both a

fasting glucose <126 (7.0 mmol/L) and a 2-h glucose ≥140 mg/dL (7.8 mmol/L) but <200 mg/dL (11.06 mmol/L). The WHO criteria use a higher threshold for defining IFG citing concerns that lowering the cut point would cause an overdiagnosis of IFG.

In general, *screening for diabetes* should be considered in overweight adults (defined as a BMI ≥25 kg/m^2 or 23 kg/m^2 in Asians) with additional risk factors including family history, hypertension, or a history of gestational diabetes. It is important to distinguish type 2 diabetes, which is the most common form, from other types of diabetes. The ADA classifies diabetes into four categories: (1) type 1 diabetes, (2) type 2 diabetes, (3) gestational, and (4) other. *Type 1 diabetes* is due to autoimmune destruction of pancreatic beta-cells resulting in absolute insulin deficiency. Patients often present with markedly elevated blood glucose and are prone to diabetic ketoacidosis, in contrast to *Type 2 diabetes*. Autoimmune markers are tested to confirm the diagnosis; these include islet cell autoantibodies, glutamic acid decarboxylase (GAD) antibodies, autoantibodies to insulin, autoantibodies to tyrosine phosphatases IA-2 and IA-2β, and autoantibodies to zinc transporter 8 (ZnT8). *Gestational diabetes (GDM)* is defined as diabetes diagnosed for the first time during pregnancy and as mentioned earlier is a risk factor for developing type 2 diabetes later in life.

Other less common forms of diabetes include monogenic diabetes syndrome, where a monogenic defect causes β-cell dysfunction. These include *maturity-onset diabetes of the young (MODY)*, which is characterized by impaired insulin secretion and is inherited in an autosomal dominant pattern with a wide range of clinical manifestations that require distinct treatment strategies. Currently, several MODY subtypes have been identified. The most common mutation is on chromosome 12 in hepatocyte nuclear factor (HNF)-1α. This mutation leads to reduced insulin secretion and often responds well to treatment with a sulfonylurea. Another common mutation is in the glucokinase gene on chromosome 7p. Glucokinase converts glucose to glucose-6-phosphate, which stimulates insulin secretion and acts as a glucose sensor. Mutations in this gene lead to a higher glucose threshold for insulin secretion with consequently higher baseline fasting blood glucose, which in most cases do not require treatment. Other forms of diabetes include cystic fibrosis-related diabetes (CFRD), which is due to insulin deficiency secondary to partial fibrotic destruction of islet mass. Diabetes can also be drug-induced and is commonly seen after treatment of HIV/AIDS and following immunosuppression for organ transplantation.

Treatment

The main goal of treating diabetes is lowering blood glucose to minimize the risk of both microvascular and macrovascular complications. *Microvascular complications* from diabetes include retinopathy, nephropathy, and neuropathy. *Macrovascular complications* in diabetes include coronary artery diseases, stroke, and peripheral vascular disease [8].

The cornerstone of diabetes treatment has been based on education on diet, exercise, and weight management. The Look AHEAD trial was designed to evaluate if intensive *lifestyle intervention for weight loss* would decrease cardiovascular morbidity and mortality in patients with type 2 diabetes. The clinical trial was ended after a median follow-up of 9.6 years when it was determined that despite a greater weight loss in the intervention group, there was no difference in the primary endpoints (i.e., death from cardiovascular causes, nonfatal myocardial infarction, nonfatal stroke, and later added hospitalization for angina) between the two groups (1.83 and 1.92 events per 100 person-years, in intervention and control groups, respectively; hazard ratio in the intervention group, 0.95; 95% confidence interval, 0.83–1.09; $p = 0.51$). However, the intensive lifestyle intervention group did have greater reductions in A1c, greater initial improvements in fitness, and greater reductions in all cardiovascular risk factors except for low-density-lipoprotein cholesterol levels [60]. Other clinical trials have shown lifestyle interventions in individuals with diabetes can provide other health benefits such as decreasing need for medications, improved well-being [97], and in some cases remission of diabetes [37]. Regular aerobic exercise was found to improve glycemic management in adults with type 2 diabetes, resulting in less daily time in hyperglycemia and ~ 0.6% reduction in HbA1c [24]. Given that most lifestyle modifications have few risks and some benefit, they remain the cornerstone of diabetes treatment.

In regard to medical therapy for glycemic control, the *Diabetes Control and Complications Trial (DCCT)* demonstrated that intensive therapy in type 1 diabetics delayed the onset and progression of microvascular complications such as diabetic retinopathy, nephropathy, and neuropathy [25]. Long-term follow-up of these patients showed a beneficial effect on the risk of cardiovascular disease as well [71]. For patients with type 2 diabetes, most, but not all, clinical trials showed a benefit of intensive treatment on preventing microvascular complications. The effect of intensive glucose control on macrovascular outcomes has proven more difficult to delineate.

The *United Kingdom Prospective Diabetes Study (UKPDS)* followed over 5000 newly diagnosed persons with type 2 diabetes and evaluated the effect of conventional versus intensive management on diabetes complications. The intensive therapy arm was treated with medication, while the conventional therapy arm was treated with diet alone with the addition of medications if their fasting blood glucose concentration was greater than 270 mg/dL (15 mmol/L). The average A1c was 7.0% in the intensive therapy group compared with 7.9% in the conventional therapy group. Over a 10-year period, the intensive treatment group had a 25% reduction in the risk of microvascular endpoints (7–40, $p = 0.0099$), most of which was due to reduced need for photocoagulation for diabetic retinopathy. However, the intensive therapy arm had more weight gain (4.0 kg for those receiving insulin and 1.7–2.7 kg for those receiving sulfonylurea) and increased incidence of hypoglycemia [90]. Other later studies showed reduction in microvascular endpoints such as nephropathy, while other studies did not show a reduction in microvascular endpoints [3, 28].

The major clinical trials investigating diabetes control and macrovascular complications are summarized in Table 2.

These trials were designed to evaluate the effect of intensive versus conventional therapy on cardiovascular outcomes in patients with long-standing diabetes (duration 8–12 years), and many who had already had one cardiovascular event. VADT and ADVANCE showed no difference in rates of macrovascular complications between intensive and conventional treatment arms [3, 28]. The *ACCORD trial* was ended early due to an increased mortality rate in the intensive glucose control group compared with conventional therapy [2]. The higher incidence of total and cardiovascular death in the intensive group versus standard persisted even after the intensive arm was transitioned to the standard therapy (HR for death from any cause 1.19, 95%

CI 1.03–1.38) [1]. While it was initially thought that the increased mortality rate may be due to hypoglycemia or the medications used, follow-up analysis has failed to demonstrate this conclusively [13].

Returning to the UKPDS trial discussed above, it continued with a post-trial monitoring phase in which all patients returned to community-based diabetes care with no attempt to maintain their previously randomized therapy. While initially the intensive group had a lower A1c, after 5 years, there was no significant difference in A1c between the two groups (A1c of around 7.8%). After a median follow-up of 17 years, there was still a significant reduction in microvascular complications with the intensive control group compared with the conventional treatment group (RR 0.76, 95% CI 0.64–0.89). Furthermore, while there was no significant difference in macrovascular outcome in the initial phase, a significant risk reduction for myocardial infarction (15%, $p = 0.01$) and death from any cause (13%, $p = 0.007$) emerged over time as more events occurred [39]. This gave rise to the term the "legacy effect" or "metabolic memory" suggesting that good glycemic control in the initial stages of diabetes can lower one's risk of both microvascular and macrovascular outcomes over a long period of time. This is in comparison to the initial phase of UKPDS and ADVANCE, which showed no benefit of good or near normal blood glucose control on macrovascular outcomes in the short term.

Based on these studies above, the ADA recommends an A1c target of 7% or less for most patients with diabetes, especially implemented

Table 2 Trial data for intensive glycemic control and macrovascular complications

	ACCORD	ADVANCE	VADT
N	10,251	11,140	1791
Mean duration T2DM	10 years	8 years	11.5 years
Known CVD	32%	35%	40%
A1c decrease	1.1% (6.4 vs. 7.5%)	0.7% (6.5 vs. 7.3%)	1.5% (6.9 vs. 8.4%)
Renal outcomes	−21%	−32%	−33%
CV outcomes	No effect*	No effect	No effect
NEJM publication	2008; 358: 2545	2008; 358: 2520	2009; 360: 129

ACCORD showed 22% increase in all-cause mortality

soon after diagnosis [8]. A more stringent goal of 6.5% or less can be considered if this can be achieved without significant hypoglycemia, especially in patients with a long life expectancy and little or no significant cardiovascular disease. Less stringent A1c goals such as 8% or less may be appropriate for patients with history of severe hypoglycemia and those patients who already have long-standing diabetes with complications or a decreased life expectancy.

The ADA emphasizes the importance of individualization based on key patient characteristics. Glycemic targets must be individualized in the context of shared decision-making to address individual needs and preferences and consider characteristics that influence risks and benefits of therapy. A1C targets should be reevaluated over time to balance the risks and benefits as patient factors change. This approach may optimize patient engagement and reduce the risks of polypharmacy and hypoglycemia.

Diabetes Management

Comprehensive care of the diabetic patient requires a multifaceted approach across multiple disciplines. Educating the patient about their disease and stressing modifiable risk factors for complications is the cornerstone of diabetes management. Patients should be informed of the benefit of weight loss, exercise, and dietary changes. While not one diet has proved itself superior in diabetics, it is reasonable to counsel patients to avoid trans-fat and highly refined carbohydrates that are often found in processed food in favor of increased fruits and vegetables, unprocessed meats, and omega-3 fatty acids. Emphasis should also be placed on smoking cessation, screening and treatment for depression, and routine immunizations.

Screening for diabetes complications should be done routinely and the ADA provides recommendations for standards of care for patients with diabetes. An annual dilated eye exam to look for *retinopathy* should be done at diagnosis. If there is no evidence of retinopathy for one or more annual eye exams and glycemia is well controlled,

then screening every 1–2 years may be considered. An annual foot exam should be performed to identify risk factors for ulcers and amputations. Urinary albumin and estimated glomerular filtration should be evaluated once a year in all patients with type 2 diabetes annually to screen for nephropathy. Treatment with an ACE inhibitor or angiotensin receptor blocker (ARB) is recommended for patients with elevated urinary albumin. In patients with type 2 diabetes and diabetic kidney disease, use of an SGLT-2 inhibitor in those with eGFR $\geq$20 mL/min/1.73 m^2 and UACR $\geq$200 mg/g creatinine is recommended to reduce chronic kidney disease progression and cardiovascular events.

For cardiovascular disease and risk management, the *blood pressure* should be measured at every visit. People with diabetes and hypertension qualify for antihypertensive drug therapy when the blood pressure is persistently elevated $\geq$130/80 mmHg. The on-treatment target blood pressure goal is <130/80 mmHg. A fasting *lipid profile* should be obtained at time of diagnosis and every 1–2 years afterwards. Statin therapy is recommended for most patients aged 40 or older, and can vary between moderate- and high-intensity statin therapy depending on age and risk factors. For people with diabetes aged 20–39 years, with additional atherosclerotic cardiovascular disease risk factors, such as a family history of premature ASCVD, it may be reasonable to initiate statin therapy in addition to lifestyle therapy.

Antiplatelet agents such as aspirin have been shown to be effective in reducing cardiovascular morbidity in high-risk patients with previous myocardial infarction or stroke (secondary prevention). Evidence for its use for primary prevention in diabetes is less clear, but it is reasonable to consider aspirin therapy for primary prevention in patients with increased cardiovascular risk (10-year risk >10%). Recommendations for using aspirin as primary prevention include both men and women aged $\geq$50 years with diabetes and at least one additional major risk factor (family history of premature ASCVD, hypertension, dyslipidemia, smoking, or CKD/albuminuria), who are not at increased risk of bleeding (older age, anemia, renal disease).

Medications commonly used for the treatment of type 2 diabetes are summarized in Table 3 [9].

There were several large cardiovascular outcomes trials in people with type 2 diabetes at high risk for cardiovascular disease or with existing cardiovascular disease such as EMPA-REG OUTCOME [BI 10773 (Empagliflozin) Cardiovascular Outcome Event Trial in Type 2 Diabetes Mellitus Patients], CANVAS (Canagliflozin Cardiovascular Assessment Study), and LEADER (Liraglutide Effect and Action in Diabetes: Evaluation of Cardiovascular Outcome Results). These large randomized controlled trials reported statistically significant reductions in major adverse cardiovascular events (MACE) for SGLT-2 inhibitors and GLP-1 receptor agonists. SGLT-2 inhibitors also reduce risk of heart failure hospitalization and progression of kidney disease in people with established ASCVD, multiple risk factors for ASCVD, or albuminuric kidney disease as these large cardiovascular outcome trials examined kidney effects as secondary outcomes [10].

In these cardiovascular outcome trials, SGLT-2 inhibitors and GLP-1 receptor agonists all had beneficial effects on indices of CKD. Some large clinical trials of SGLT-2 inhibitors have focused on people with advanced CKD. Some of the completed trials include the Dapagliflozin and Prevention of Adverse Outcomes in Chronic Kidney Disease (DAPA-CKD) and Canagliflozin and Renal Events in Diabetes with Established Nephropathy Clinical Evaluation (CREDENCE) study. Based on evidence from the CREDENCE and DAPA-CKD trials, as well as secondary

Table 3 Type 2 diabetes medications

Intervention	Action	Advantages	Disadvantages
Lifestyle	(+) Insulin sensitivity	Low cost Multiple benefits	Fails for most in first year
Metformin	Decreases gluconeogenesis	Low cost Weight neutral	Gastrointestinal (GI) side effects B12 deficiency Rare lactic acidosis
Sulfonylureas	Insulin secretagogue	Low cost	Hypoglycemia Weight gain
Thiazolidinediones	(+) Insulin sensitivity	No hypoglycemia Improved lipids Benefit in NASH	Weight gain Low cost Bone fracture Fluid retention
Alpha glucosidase Inhibitors	(−) Carb absorption	No hypoglycemia Weight neutral	GI side effects, frequent dosing
GLP-1 agonists	(+) Incretin effect	Benefit in ASCVD and DKD Weight loss No hypoglycemia	Injectable High cost GI side effects
GIP and GLP-1 agonists	(+) Incretin effect	Weight loss No hypoglycemia	Injectable High cost GI side effects
DPPIV-inhibitors	(+) Incretin effect	Weight neutral No hypoglycemia	High cost Lower potency
Glinides/meglitinides	Insulin secretagogue	Short acting	Frequent dosing Higher cost Weight gain Hypoglycemia
SGLT-2 inhibitors	Increases glycosuria	Benefit in HF, ASCVD, and DKD Weight loss	Genitourinary (GU) side effects High cost
Insulin	Increases insulin concentration	Efficacious	Injectable Can be high cost Weight gain

analyses of cardiovascular outcomes trials with SGLT-2 inhibitors, cardiovascular and renal events are reduced with SGLT-2 inhibitor use in patients with an eGFR of 20 mL/min/1.73 m^2 and higher independent of glucose-lowering effects [11].

Recent interest has focused on surgical treatments of type 2 diabetes through gastric bypass. Recent studies of gastric bypass in diabetic patients show that surgery often leads to improvements in diabetes control but at a cost of increased adverse events such as fracture and nutritional deficiency [29, 44]. Longer-term risks include vitamin and mineral deficiencies, anemia, osteoporosis, dumping syndrome, and severe hypoglycemia [106]. Post-bariatric hypoglycemia (PBH) can occur with RYGB, VSG, and other gastrointestinal procedures and may severely impact quality of life.

The Surgical Treatment and Medications Potentially Eradicate Diabetes Efficiently (STAMPEDE) trial, which randomized 150 participants with unmanaged diabetes to receive either metabolic surgery or medical treatment, found that 29% of those treated with Roux-en-Y gastric bypass (RYGB) and 23% treated with vertical sleeve gastrectomy (VSG) achieved A1C of 6.0% or lower after 5 years [105]. At least 35–50% of patients who initially achieve remission of diabetes eventually experience recurrence, however the majority of those who undergo surgery maintain substantial improvement of glycemia from baseline for at least 5–15 years.

Cross-References

▶ Adipokines and Metabolism
▶ Endocrine Disorders Associated with Obesity
▶ Genetics of Type 2 Diabetes
▶ Insulin Resistance in Obesity
▶ Linking Inflammation, Obesity, and Diabetes
▶ Non-alcoholic Fatty Liver Disease
▶ Overview of Metabolic Syndrome
▶ Pancreatic Islet Adaptation and Failure in Obesity

References

1. ACCORD Study Group, Gerstein HC, Miller ME, et al. Long-term effects of intensive glucose lowering on cardiovascular outcomes. N Engl J Med. 2011;364 (9):818–28.
2. Action to Control Cardiovascular Risk in Diabetes Study Group, Gerstein HC, Miller ME, et al. Effects of intensive glucose lowering in type 2 diabetes. N Engl J Med. 2008;358(24):2545–59.
3. ADVANCE Collaborative Group, Patel A, MacMahon S, et al. Intensive blood glucose control and vascular outcomes in patients with type 2 diabetes. N Engl J Med. 2008;358(24):2560–72.
4. Ahmadian M, Suh JM, Hah N, et al. PPARgamma signaling and metabolism: the good, the bad and the future. Nat Med. 2013;19(5):557–66.
5. Alonso-Magdalena P, Vieira E, Soriano S, et al. Bisphenol a exposure during pregnancy disrupts glucose homeostasis in mothers and adult male offspring. Environ Health Perspect. 2010;118(9):1243–50.
6. American Diabetes Association. Economic costs of diabetes in the U.S. in 2012. Diabetes Care. 2013;36 (4):1033–46.
7. American Diabetes Association. 2. Classification and diagnosis of diabetes: standards of care in diabetes – 2023. Diabetes Care. 2023a;46(Suppl 1):S19–40. https://doi.org/10.2337/dc23-S002.
8. American Diabetes Association. 6. Glycemic targets: standards of care in diabetes – 2023. Diabetes Care. 2023b;46(Suppl 1):S97–S110. https://doi.org/10.2337/dc23-S006.
9. American Diabetes Association. 9. Pharmacologic approaches to glycemic treatment: standards of care in diabetes – 2023. Diabetes Care. 2023c;46(Suppl 1):S140–57. https://doi.org/10.2337/dc23-S009.
10. American Diabetes Association. 10. Cardiovascular disease and risk management: standards of care in diabetes – 2023. Diabetes Care. 2023d;46(Suppl 1):S158–90. https://doi.org/10.2337/dc23-S010.
11. American Diabetes Association. 11. Chronic Kidney Disease and Risk Management: Standards of Care in Diabetes – 2023. Diabetes Care. 2023e;46(Suppl 1):S191–202. https://doi.org/10.2337/dc23-S011.
12. Barnett AH, Eff C, Leslie RDG, et al. Diabetes in identical twins. Diabetologia. 1981;20:87–93.
13. Bonds DE, Miller ME, Bergenstal RM, et al. The association between symptomatic, severe hypoglycaemia and mortality in type 2 diabetes: retrospective epidemiological analysis of the ACCORD study. BMJ. 2010;340:b4909.
14. Cappuccio FP, D'Elia L, Strazzullo P, et al. Quantity and quality of sleep and incidence of type 2 diabetes: a systematic review and meta-analysis. Diabetes Care. 2010;33(2):414–20.
15. Carlström M, Larsson SC. Coffee consumption and reduced risk of developing type 2 diabetes: a

systematic review with meta-analysis. Nutr Rev. 2018;76(6):395–417. https://doi.org/10.1093/nutrit/nuy014.

16. Centers for Disease Control and Prevention. National Diabetes Statistics Report: estimates of diabetes and its burden in the United States, 2014. Atlanta: U S Department of Health and Human Services; 2014.

17. Chan JM, Rimm EB, Colditz GA, et al. Obesity, fat distribution, and weight gain as risk factors for clinical diabetes in men. Diabetes Care. 1994;17(9): 961–9.

18. Chen L, Magliano DJ, Zimmet PZ. The worldwide epidemiology of type 2 diabetes mellitus – present and future perspectives. Nat Rev Endocrinol. 2011;8 (4):228–36.

19. Cobo-Vuilleumier N, Gauthier BR. To beta-e or not to beta-e replicating after 30: retrospective dating of human pancreatic islets. J Clin Endocrinol Metab. 2010;95(10):4552–4.

20. D'Alessio D. The role of dysregulated glucagon secretion in type 2 diabetes. Diabetes Res Clin Pract. 2011;13(s1):126–32.

21. Dabelea D, Mayer-Davis EJ, Saydah S, et al. Prevalence of type 1 and type 2 diabetes among children and adolescents from 2001 to 2009. JAMA. 2014;311 (17):1778–86.

22. Danaei G, Finucane MM, Lu Y, et al. National, regional, and global trends in fasting plasma glucose and diabetes prevalence since 1980: systematic analysis of health examination surveys and epidemiological studies with 370 country-years and 2.7 million participants. Lancet. 2011;378(9785):31–40.

23. Davies MJ, Aroda VR, Collins BS, et al. Management of hyperglycaemia in type 2 diabetes, 2022. A consensus report by the American Diabetes Association (ADA) and the European Association for the Study of Diabetes (EASD). Diabetologia. 2022;65(12):1925–66. https://doi.org/10.1007/s00125-022-05787-2.

24. Delevatti RS, Bracht CG, Lisboa SDC, et al. The role of aerobic training variables progression on glycemic control of patients with type 2 diabetes: a systematic review with meta-analysis. Sports Med Open. 2019;5: 22. https://doi.org/10.1186/s40798-019-0194-z.

25. Diabetes Control and Complications Trial Research Group. The effect of intensive treatment of diabetes on the development and progression of long-term complications in insulin-dependent diabetes mellitus. N Engl J Med. 1993;329(14):977–86.

26. Diabetes Prevention Program Research Group. 10-year follow-up of diabetes incidence and weight loss in the diabetes prevention program outcomes study. Lancet. 2009;374(9702):1677–86.

27. Drouin-Chartier JP, Zheng Y, Li Y, et al. Changes in consumption of sugary beverages and artificially sweetened beverages and subsequent risk of type 2 diabetes: results from three large prospective U.S. cohorts of women and men. Diabetes Care. 2019;42(12): 2181–9. https://doi.org/10.2337/dc19-0734.

28. Duckworth W, Abraira C, Moritz T, et al. Glucose control and vascular complications in veterans with type 2 diabetes. N Engl J Med. 2009;360(2):129–39.

29. ElSayed NA, Aleppo G, Aroda VR, et al. 8. Obesity and weight management for the prevention and treatment of type 2 diabetes: standards of care in diabetes – 2023. Diabetes Care. 2022;46(Suppl 1):S128–39. https://doi.org/10.2337/dc23-S008.

30. Estruch R, Ros E, Salas-Salvadó J, et al. Primary prevention of cardiovascular disease with a Mediterranean diet supplemented with extra-virgin olive oil or nuts. N Engl J Med. 2018;378(25):e34. https://doi.org/10.1056/NEJMoa1800389.

31. Farooqi IS, Matarese G, Lord GM, et al. Beneficial effects of leptin on obesity, T cell hyporesponsiveness, and neuroendocrine/metabolic dysfunction of human congenital leptin deficiency. J Clin Invest. 2002;110(8):1093.

32. Feig DS, Zinman BF, Wang X, et al. Risk of development of diabetes mellitus after diagnosis of gestational diabetes. CMAJ Can Med Assoc J. 2008;179 (3):229–39.

33. Festa A, Williams K, D'Agostino R Jr, et al. The natural course of beta-cell function in nondiabetic and diabetic individuals: the insulin resistance atherosclerosis study. Diabetes. 2006;55(4):1114–20.

34. Ford ES, Li CF, Sattar N. Metabolic syndrome and incident diabetes: current state of the evidence. Diabetes Care. 2008;31(9):1898–904.

35. Frati AC, Iniestra F, Ariza CR. Acute effect of cigarette smoking on glucose tolerance and other cardiovascular risk factors. Diabetes Care. 1996;19(2): 112–8.

36. Fung TT, Schulze M, Manson JE, et al. Dietary patterns, meat intake, and the risk of type 2 diabetes in women. Arch Intern Med. 2004;164(20):2235–40.

37. Gregg EW, Chen H, Wagenknecht LE, et al. Association of an intensive lifestyle intervention with remission of type 2 diabetes. JAMA. 2012;308(23): 2489–96.

38. Grøntved A, Hu FB. Television viewing and risk of type 2 diabetes, cardiovascular disease, and all-cause mortality: a meta-analysis. JAMA. 2011;305(23): 2448–55.

39. Holman RR, Paul SK, Bethel MA, et al. 10-year follow-up of intensive glucose control in type 2 diabetes. N Engl J Med. 2008;359(15):1577–89.

40. Hotamisligil GS, Shargill NS, Spiegelman BM. Adipose expression of tumor necrosis factor-alpha: direct role in obesity-linked insulin resistance. Science. 1993;259(5091):87–91.

41. http://www.idf.org/webdata/docs/WHO_IDF_definition_diagnosis_of_diabetes.pdf. Accessed 21 Apr 2015.

42. http://www.who.int/diabetes/publications/report-hba1c_2011.pdf. Accessed 21 Apr 2015.

43. Hu FB, Manson JE, Stampfer MJ, et al. Diet, lifestyle, and the risk of type 2 diabetes mellitus in women. N Engl J Med. 2001;345(11):790–7.

44. Ikramuddin S, Billington CJ, Lee WJ, et al. Roux-en-Y gastric bypass for diabetes (the diabetes surgery study): 2-year outcomes of a 5-year, randomised, controlled trial. Lancet Diabetes Endocrinol. 2015;3 (6):413–22.

45. InterAct Consortium, Scott RA, Langenberg C, et al. The link between family history and risk of type 2 diabetes is not explained by anthropometric, lifestyle or genetic risk factors: the EPIC-InterAct study. Diabetologia. 2013;56(1):60–9.

46. Jeon CY, Lokken RP, Hu FB, et al. Physical activity of moderate intensity and risk of type 2 diabetes: a systematic review. Diabetes Care. 2007;30(3): 744–52.

47. Jiang R, Manson JE, Stampfer MJ, et al. Nut and peanut butter consumption and risk of type 2 diabetes in women. JAMA. 2002;288(20):2554–60.

48. Jurgens CA, Toukatly MN, Fligner CL, et al. Beta-cell loss and beta-cell apoptosis in human type 2 diabetes are related to islet amyloid deposition. Am J Pathol. 2011;178(6):2632–40.

49. Kahn S. The relative contributions of insulin resistance and beta-cell dysfunction to the pathophysiology of type 2 diabetes. Diabetologia. 2003;46(1): 3–19.

50. Kahn SE, Prigeon RL, McCulloch DK, et al. Quantification of the relationship between insulin sensitivity and beta-cell function in human subjects. Evidence for a hyperbolic function. Diabetes. 1993;42(11): 1663–72.

51. Kahn SE, Cooper ME, Del Prato S. Pathophysiology and treatment of type 2 diabetes: perspectives on the past, present, and future. Lancet. 2014;383(9922): 1068–83.

52. Kalin MF, Goncalves M, John-Kalarickal J, Fonseca V. Pathogenesis of type 2 diabetes mellitus. In: Poretsky L, editor. Principles of diabetes mellitus. Cham: Springer International Publishing; 2017. p. 267–77. https://doi.org/10.1007/978-3-319-18741-9_13.

53. Kanaya AM, Wassel Fyr C, Vittinghoff E, et al. Adipocytokines and incident diabetes mellitus in older adults: the independent effect of plasminogen activator inhibitor 1. Arch Intern Med. 2006;166(3): 350–6.

54. Knowler WC, Pettitt DJ, Saad MF, et al. Diabetes mellitus in the pima indians: incidence, risk factors and pathogenesis. Diabetes Metab Rev. 1990;6(1): 1–27.

55. Knowler WC, Pettitt DJ, Saad MF, et al. Obesity in the Pima Indians: its magnitude and relationship with diabetes. Am J Clin Nutr. 1991;53(6 Suppl):1543S–51S. https://doi.org/10.1093/ajcn/53.6.1543S.

56. Knowler WC, Barrett-Connor E, Fowler SE, et al. Reduction in the incidence of type 2 diabetes with lifestyle intervention or metformin. N Engl J Med. 2002;346(6):393–403.

57. Lang IA, Galloway TS, Scarlett A, et al. Association of urinary bisphenol a concentration with medical disorders and laboratory abnormalities in adults. JAMA. 2008;300(11):1303–10.

58. Li C, Ford ES, Zhao G, et al. Prevalence of pre-diabetes and its association with clustering of cardiometabolic risk factors and hyperinsulinemia among U.S. adolescents: National Health and Nutrition Examination Survey 2005–2006. Diabetes Care. 2009;32(2):342–7.

59. Lo JC, Feigenbaum SL, Yang J, et al. Epidemiology and adverse cardiovascular risk profile of diagnosed polycystic ovary syndrome. J Clin Endocrinol Metab. 2006;91(4):1357–63.

60. Look AHEAD Research Group, Wing RR, Bolin P, et al. Cardiovascular effects of intensive lifestyle intervention in type 2 diabetes. N Engl J Med. 2013;369(2):145–54.

61. Malik VS, Popkin BM, Bray GA, Després JP, Willett WC, Hu FB. Sugar-sweetened beverages and risk of metabolic syndrome and type 2 diabetes. Diabetes Care. 2010;33(11):2477–83. https://doi.org/10.2337/dc10-1079.

62. Mantzoros CS, Li T, Manson JE, et al. Circulating adiponectin levels are associated with better glycemic control, more favorable lipid profile, and reduced inflammation in women with type 2 diabetes. J Clin Endocrinol Metab. 2005;90(8):4542–8.

63. McCarthy MI. Genomics, type 2 diabetes, and obesity. N Engl J Med. 2010;363(24):2339–50.

64. McMullan CJ, Schernhammer ES, Rimm EB, et al. Melatonin secretion and the incidence of type 2 diabetes. JAMA. 2013;309(13):1388–96.

65. Meigs JB, Cupples LA, Wilson PW. Parental transmission of type 2 diabetes: the Framingham offspring study. Diabetes. 2000;49(12):2201–7.

66. Melzer D, Rice NE, Lewis C, et al. Association of urinary bisphenol a concentration with heart disease: evidence from NHANES 2003/06. PLoS One. 2010;5 (1):e8673.

67. Micha RR, Wallace SB, Mozaffarian DM. Red and processed meat consumption and risk of incident coronary heart disease, stroke, and diabetes mellitus: a systematic review and meta-analysis. Circulation. 2010;121(21):2271–83.

68. Morioka T, Asilmaz E, Hu J, et al. Disruption of leptin receptor expression in the pancreas directly affects beta cell growth and function in mice. J Clin Invest. 2007;117(10):2860–8.

69. Mozaffarian D, Marfisi R, Levantesi G, et al. Incidence of new-onset diabetes and impaired fasting glucose in patients with recent myocardial infarction and the effect of clinical and lifestyle risk factors. Lancet. 2007;370(9588):667–75.

70. Narayan KMV, Boyle JP, Thompson TJ, et al. Effect of BMI on lifetime risk for diabetes in the U.-S. Diabetes Care. 2007;30(6):1562–6.

71. Nathan DM, Cleary PA, Backlund JY, et al. Intensive diabetes treatment and cardiovascular disease in patients with type 1 diabetes. N Engl J Med. 2005;353(25):2643–53.

72. Nauck MA, Baller B, Meier JJ. Gastric inhibitory polypeptide and glucagon-like peptide-1 in the pathogenesis of type 2 diabetes. Diabetes. 2004;53(Suppl 3):S190–6.

73. Nolan CJ, Damm P, Prentki M. Type 2 diabetes across generations: from pathophysiology to prevention and management. Lancet. 2011;378(9786):169–81.

74. Pan A, Sun Q, Bernstein AM, et al. Changes in red meat consumption and subsequent risk of type 2 diabetes mellitus: three cohorts of us men and women. JAMA Intern Med. 2013;173(14):1328–35.

75. Picon MJ, Murri M, Munoz A, et al. Hemoglobin A1c versus oral glucose tolerance test in postpartum diabetes screening. Diabetes Care. 2012;35(8):1648–53.

76. Poitout V, Robertson RP. Glucolipotoxicity: fuel excess and beta-cell dysfunction. Endocr Rev. 2008;29(3):351–66.

77. Ravelli AC, van der Meulen JH, Michels RP, et al. Glucose tolerance in adults after prenatal exposure to famine. Lancet. 1998;351(9097):173–7.

78. Rockette-Wagner B, Edelstein S, Venditti EM, et al. The impact of lifestyle intervention on sedentary time in individuals at high risk of diabetes. Diabetologia. 2015;58(6):1198–202.

79. Rohm TV, Meier DT, Olefsky JM, Donath MY. Inflammation in obesity, diabetes and related disorders. Immunity. 2022;55(1):31–55. https://doi.org/10.1016/j.immuni.2021.12.013.

80. Ruderman N, Chisholm D, Pi-Sunyer X, et al. The metabolically obese, normal-weight individual revisited. Diabetes. 1998;47(5):699–713.

81. Salas-Salvado J, Bullo M, Babio N, et al. Reduction in the incidence of type 2 diabetes with the mediterranean diet: results of the PREDIMED-Reus nutrition intervention randomized trial. Diabetes Care. 2011;34(1):14–9.

82. Salmerón J, Hu FB, Manson JE, et al. Dietary fat intake and risk of type 2 diabetes in women. Am J Clin Nutr. 2001;73(6):1019–26.

83. Schulz LO, Chaudhari LS. High-risk populations: the Pimas of Arizona and Mexico. Curr Obes Rep. 2015;4(1):92–8. https://doi.org/10.1007/s13679-014-0132-9.

84. Schulz LO, Bennett PH, Ravussin E, et al. Effects of traditional and western environments on prevalence of type 2 diabetes in Pima Indians in Mexico and the U.S. Diabetes Care. 2006;29(8):1866–71. https://doi.org/10.2337/dc06-0138.

85. Schulze M, Manson J, Ludwig D, et al. Sugar-sweetened beverages, weight gain, and incidence of type 2 diabetes in young and middle-aged women. JAMA. 2004;292(8):927–34.

86. Selvin E, Steffes MW, Zhu H, et al. Glycated hemoglobin, diabetes, and cardiovascular risk in non-diabetic adults. N Engl J Med. 2010;362(9):800–11.

87. Shaw JE, Sicree RA, Zimmet PZ. Global estimates of the prevalence of diabetes for 2010 and 2030. Diabetes Res Clin Pract. 2010;87(1):4–14.

88. Tinker LF, Bonds DE, Margolis KL, et al. Low-fat dietary pattern and risk of treated diabetes mellitus in postmenopausal women: the women's health initiative randomized controlled dietary modification trial. Arch Intern Med. 2008;168(14):1500–11.

89. Tuomilehto J, Lindstrom J, Eriksson JG, et al. Prevention of type 2 diabetes mellitus by changes in lifestyle among subjects with impaired glucose tolerance. N Engl J Med. 2001;344(18):1343–50.

90. UK Prospective Diabetes Study (UKPDS) Group. Intensive blood-glucose control with sulphonylureas or insulin compared with conventional treatment and risk of complications in patients with type 2 diabetes (UKPDS 33). Lancet. 1998;352(9131):837–53.

91. van Dam RM, Hu FB. Coffee consumption and risk of type 2 diabetes: a systematic review. JAMA. 2005;294(1):97–104.

92. van Dam RM, Willett WC, Stampfer MJ, et al. Dietary patterns and risk for type 2 diabetes mellitus in U.S. men. Ann Intern Med. 2002;136(3):201.

93. Watson RT, Kanzaki M, Pessin JE. Regulated membrane trafficking of the insulin-responsive glucose transporter 4 in adipocytes. Endocr Rev. 2004;25(2):177–204.

94. Weyer C, Bogardus C, Mott DM, et al. The natural history of insulin secretory dysfunction and insulin resistance in the pathogenesis of type 2 diabetes mellitus. J Clin Invest. 1999;104(6):787–94.

95. Whincup PH, Kaye SJ, Owen CG, et al. Birth weight and risk of type 2 diabetes: a systematic review. JAMA. 2008;300(24):2886–97.

96. Willi C, Bodenmann P, Ghali WA, et al. Active smoking and the risk of type 2 diabetes: a systematic review and meta-analysis. JAMA. 2007;298(22):2654–64.

97. Williamson DA, Rejeski J, Lang W, et al. Impact of a weight management program on health-related quality of life in overweight adults with type 2 diabetes. Arch Intern Med. 2009;169(2):163–71.

98. Yoon KH, Lee JH, Kim JW, et al. Epidemic obesity and type 2 diabetes in Asia. Lancet. 2006;368(9548):1681–8.

99. Zimmet P, Alberti KG, Shaw J. Global and societal implications of the diabetes epidemic. Nature. 2001;414(6865):782–7.

100. Zoeller RT, Brown TR, Doan LL, et al. Endocrine-disrupting chemicals and public health protection: a statement of principles from the endocrine society. Endocrinology. 2012;153(9):4097–110.

101. Schwingshackl L, Chaimani A, Hoffmann G, Schwedhelm C, Boeing H. A network meta-analysis on the comparative efficacy of different dietary approaches on glycaemic control in patients with type 2 diabetes mellitus. Eur J Epidemiol. 2018;33(2):157–170. https://doi.org/10.1007/s10654-017-0352-x

102. Walker RJ, Grusnick J, Garacci E, Mendez C, Egede LE. Trends in food insecurity in the USA for individuals with prediabetes, undiagnosed diabetes, and diagnosed diabetes. J Gen Intern Med. 2019;34(1):33–35. https://doi.org/10.1007/s11606-018-4651-z

103. Walker RJ, Garacci E, Ozieh M, Egede LE. Food insecurity and glycemic control in individuals with

diagnosed and undiagnosed diabetes in the United States. Prim Care Diabetes. 2021;15(5):813–818. https://doi.org/10.1016/j.pcd.2021.05.003

104. Hill JO, Galloway JM, Goley A, et al. Scientific statement: socioecological determinants of prediabetes and type 2 diabetes. Diabetes Care. 2013;36(8): 2430–2439. https://doi.org/10.2337/dc13-1161

105. Schauer PR, Bhatt DL, Kirwan JP, et al. Bariatric surgery versus intensive medical therapy for diabetes – 5-year outcomes. N Engl J Med. 2017;376(7): 641–651. https://doi.org/10.1056/NEJMoa1600869

106. Mechanick JI, Apovian C, Brethauer S, et al. Clinical practice guidelines for the perioperative nutrition, metabolic, and nonsurgical support of patients undergoing bariatric procedures – 2019 update: cosponsored by American association of clinical endocrinologists/ American college of endocrinology, the obesity society, American society for metabolic & bariatric surgery, obesity medicine association, and American society of anesthesiologists – executive summary. Endocr Pract. 2019;25(12):1346–1359. https://doi. org/10.4158/GL-2019-0406

Dyslipidemia in Metabolic Syndrome

28

Sue-Anne Toh and Michelle H. Lee

Contents

S.-A. Toh (✉)
Department of Medicine, Yong Loo Lin School of
Medicine, National University of Singapore, Singapore,
Singapore

NOVI Health, Singapore, Singapore

Regional Health System Office, National University
Health System, Singapore, Singapore
e-mail: mdcsates@nus.edu.sg

M. H. Lee
Department of Medicine, Yong Loo Lin School of
Medicine, National University of Singapore, Singapore,
Singapore

Abstract

Atherogenic dyslipidemia comprises the triad of elevated levels of small dense low-density lipoproteins (sdLDL) and triglycerides, coupled with lowered levels of cardioprotective high-density lipoproteins (HDL). This triad is a key component of the metabolic syndrome where its pathogenesis is driven by insulin resistance, and contributes to the development of atherosclerosis and cardiovascular disease (CVD). In the management of dyslipidemia, lowering LDL levels is the main strategy for reducing CVD risk. Clinical management includes dietary and

© Springer Nature Switzerland AG 2023
R. S. Ahima (ed.), *Metabolic Syndrome*,
https://doi.org/10.1007/978-3-031-40116-9_58

lifestyle interventions, coupled with drug treatment where needed, according to the individual's CVD risk. Statin is first-line therapy, followed by adding non-statin drug options as a combination therapy if statins alone do not sufficiently lower the LDL levels. Emerging non-statin therapies such as bempedoic acid and inclisiran are promising options to address the residual CVD risk following statin therapy and/or for those who are statin intolerant. Certain glucose-lowering drugs have additional benefits in lipid lowering with cardioprotective effects and can further reduce CVD risks in those with type 2 diabetes (T2D).

Keywords

Metabolic syndrome · Dyslipidemia · Insulin resistance · Atherosclerotic cardiovascular disease · Type 2 diabetes

Introduction

Metabolic syndrome (MetS) refers to a clustering of risk factors characterized by central obesity, hypertension, hyperglycemia, and atherogenic dyslipidemia [1]. MetS is associated with an increased risk of both type 2 diabetes (T2D) and cardiovascular disease (CVD), and has been shown to confer increased cardiovascular risk above and beyond the sum of each individual risk factor [2]. Insulin resistance is hypothesized to be the common factor responsible for the features of MetS, where it is defined as the pathophysiological condition of reduced insulin responsiveness in liver, muscle, and adipose tissue [3]. The characteristic lipid abnormalities in MetS are the atherogenic triad of elevated triglycerides, low levels of high-density lipoprotein (HDL) cholesterol, and an increase in small, dense low-density lipoprotein (LDL) particles [4]. It is estimated that 60–87% of individuals with MetS have at least one component of dyslipidemia [1]. In this chapter, we will discuss the role of insulin resistance in the pathogenesis of atherogenic dyslipidemia in metabolic syndrome, and how this relates to clinical management and frontiers for treatment.

Role of Insulin Resistance in the Development of Atherogenic Dyslipidemia

Insulin resistance, strongly associated with visceral adiposity [5], is a complex metabolic disorder that has several mechanisms [6]. In insulin-resistant states, three major events appear to underlie the development of atherogenic dyslipidemia: (i) overproduction of very low-density lipoproteins (VLDL), (ii) impaired catabolism of atherogenic (ApoB) lipoprotein remnants, and (iii) hypercatabolism of high-density lipoproteins (HDL). We will discuss each of these mechanisms.

VLDL Overproduction

Metabolic studies in humans have demonstrated that the insulin-resistant state is associated with an increased rate of hepatic production of VLDL triglycerides [7, 8] and is a hallmark of dyslipidemia in MetS [4]. As the role of VLDL is to transport excess energy, predominantly in the form of triglycerides (TG) out of the liver, it is not surprising that VLDL assembly and secretion is a substrate-dependent process that is highly regulated by the availability of TG [3]. It is well established that increased free fatty acid availability stimulates VLDL production and results in the incorporation of the newly derived TG [9, 10]. As shown in Fig. 1, a significant contribution of fatty acid flux to the liver for TG production comes from increased lipolysis of intra-abdominal adipose tissue [11], where in the insulin resistant state, insulin fails to suppress the hormone-sensitive lipase-mediated lipolysis of its TG stores [12]. Another major source of fatty acids results from de novo lipogenesis (DNL) in the liver, where it is increased in individuals with insulin resistance [11, 13]. Hyperglycemia associated with insulin resistance activates the glucose-mediated transcription factor carbohydrate responsive element-binding protein (ChREBP), where it induces the expression of various lipogenic enzymes involved in DNL [14]. In the insulin-resistant state, hepatic gluconeogenesis is enhanced through the failure of insulin to inhibit transcription factor Forkhead box protein

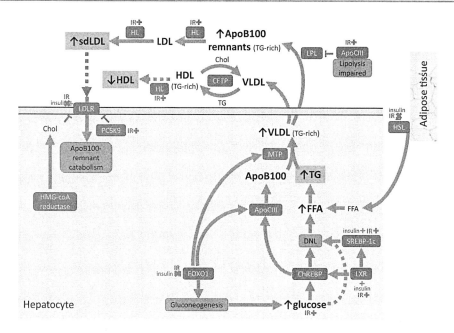

Fig. 1 Role of insulin resistance in the development of atherogenic dyslipidemia. CETP cholesteryl ester transfer protein, Chol cholesterol, ChREBP carbohydrate responsive element-binding protein, DNL de novo lipogenesis, FFA free fatty acid, FOXO1 Forkhead box protein O1, HDL high-density lipoproteins, HL hepatic lipase, HSL hormone sensitive lipase, LDL low-density lipoproteins, LDLR LDL receptor, LPL lipoprotein lipase, LXR liver X receptor, MTP microsomal triglyceride transfer protein, PCSK9 proprotein convertase subtilisin/kexin type 9, sdLDL small dense LDL, SREBP-1c sterol regulatory element binding protein 1c, TG triglycerides, VLDL very low-density lipoproteins

O1 (FOXO1), thereby further increasing hepatic hyperglycemia and eventually DNL, through the activation of ChREBP or other metabolic pathways such as uric acid synthesis [15]. Chronic hyperinsulinemia associated with obesity and T2D continues to stimulate insulin-mediated DNL in the liver despite the insulin resistance state [3]. Insulin, in part through stimulation of liver X receptor (LXR) [16], plays a central role in the upregulation of hepatic ChREBP expression and activity [17] as well as hepatic sterol regulatory element-binding protein 1c (SREBP-1c) expression [18] as shown in Fig. 1. SREBP-1c is a master regulator of the genes involved in DNL, including acetyl-CoA carboxylase, fatty acid synthase, long chain fatty acyl elongase and stearoyl CoA desaturase 1 (SCD1) [19]. Insulin also increases the proteolytic processing of SREBP-1c to its mature nuclear form via an LXR-independent mechanism [20].

The regulation of the assembly and secretion of VLDL from the liver is a major process affecting the production of VLDL. Microsomal triglyceride transfer protein (MTP), first described by Wetterau and Zilversmit in 1984 [21], resides principally in the endoplasmic reticulum of the liver and small intestine, although recent studies have also showed its presence in other organs [22]. Studies in patients with abetalipoproteinemia and mice show that MTP is essential for assembly and secretion of apoB-containing lipoproteins such as VLDL [23, 24], in part by catalyzing the transfer of neutral lipids to the apoB particle [25, 26]. Insulin negatively regulates MTP expression, possibly by inhibiting FOXO1 and preventing its translocation to the nucleus to activate the MTP promoter [27]. Hence, in the insulin resistant state, the failure of insulin to inhibit FOXO1 and hence MTP expression leads to an increase in VLDL assembly and secretion (Fig. 1). Insulin also negatively regulates ApoB secretion through other mechanisms [28] such as inhibiting the activity of Apo-CIII in the ApoB maturation process [29], and targeting the newly formed VLDL for lysosomal degradation [30].

These mechanisms are thought to be inhibited in insulin resistance [28].

Impaired Catabolism of ApoB-Lipoprotein Remnants

ApoB particles (e.g., VLDL, LDL, chylomicrons) are removed from the circulation primarily by the liver; this process is promoted by insulin [31] and impaired in insulin resistance and T2D [32]. Insulin stimulates the expression of the low-density lipoprotein receptor (LDLR) in the liver [33], which binds to ApoB100 and ApoE for the reuptake of these lipoprotein remnants into the liver cells from the circulation [34]. Proprotein convertase subtilisin/kexin type 9 (PCSK9), produced by the liver, binds to LDLR at the epidermal growth factor-binding site, initiating endocytosis and subsequent lysosomal degradation of the LDLR, thereby preventing recycling of the LDLR to the cell surface, which results in less efficient removal of LDL particles from the circulation [35]. As shown in Fig. 1, the adverse effects of insulin resistance on LDLR availability are two-fold – while hepatic insulin resistance impairs the insulin-stimulated LDLR production [32], PCSK9 levels increase with insulin resistance [36], leading to a net decrease of available LDLR on the cell surface for ApoB particle clearance [37].

Apolipoprotein CIII (apoC-III) is a glycoprotein produced mainly by the liver and is a protein constituent in HDL, as well as triglyceride-rich lipoproteins (VLDL and chylomicrons) [38]. ApoC-III negatively regulates the catabolism of circulating VLDL and chylomicrons by inhibiting the lipolytic activity of lipoprotein lipase [39]. ApoC-III also inhibits the LDLR-mediated hepatic clearance of triglyceride-rich remnants [40]. In the liver, apoC-III expression is inhibited by insulin through inhibiting FOXO1 [41] and stimulated by glucose in part via transcription factors HNF-4α and ChREBP [42]. Consequently, in people with insulin resistance and MetS, elevated plasma apoC-III concentrations were associated with increased plasma concentrations of atherogenic lipoprotein remnants [43] (Fig. 1).

Hepatic lipase (HL) is an enzyme that hydrolyzes TG from plasma lipoproteins and thus takes part in the metabolism of triglyceride-rich lipoprotein remnants and HDL [44]. Hepatic lipase, which is overactive in insulin resistance, remodels triglyceride-rich VLDL remnants, converts IDL to LDL particles, and mediates the hydrolysis of triglyceride-enriched LDL, promoting its conversion to small dense LDL (sdLDL) [44]. Insulin resistance is associated with an increased HL activity, resulting in the accelerated formation of sdLDL [45], although the basis for increased HL in the insulin resistance state remains unclear. The sdLDL particles are more intrinsically atherogenic owing to their enhanced susceptibility to oxidative modification and have reduced affinity for the LDL receptor, which results in them being less efficiently cleared from the circulation [46] (Fig. 1).

Hypercatabolism of HDL

The low levels of HDL in insulin-resistant states [47] can be attributed largely to accelerated HDL catabolism. One factor that accounts for this is activity of cholesteryl ester transfer protein (CETP), enhanced during the insulin resistance state [48], which mediates the transfer of cholesterol ester from HDL to apoB-containing lipoproteins in exchange for triglycerides. Increased levels of acceptor apoB-containing lipoprotein particles such as VLDL in insulin-resistant states may drive an increased rate [49] of CETP-mediated enrichment of triglycerides in HDL while depleting them from cholesteryl esters [50]. Such TG enrichment could render HDL particles more susceptible to hydrolysis by HL [51], overactive in insulin resistance, which further reduces their size even further [52]. These lipid-poor ApoA-I particles are more rapidly cleared from the kidney [53] (Fig. 1).

A relative of HL, endothelial lipase (EL), may also play an important role in contributing to reduced HDL levels in insulin resistance [54]. Endothelial lipase is secreted by endothelial cells and has a preferential affinity to hydrolyze phospholipids in HDL than other lipoproteins [55].

Experiments in mice show that overexpression of EL reduces HDL levels [56] by increasing the catabolism of HDL [57], whereas inhibition [58] or genetic deletion [56] of EL increases HDL levels by reducing the catabolic rate. In humans, loss-of-function variants of the EL gene are associated with the phenotype of high HDL [59]. There is evidence showing EL is regulated by insulin. Incubating human aortic endothelial cells with insulin showed a dose-dependent decrease in EL gene expression. Serum EL concentrations was also significantly decreased in diabetic patients after starting insulin therapy [60]. Hence, insulin-stimulated inhibition of EL expression may be impaired in the insulin resistance state, as EL levels are found to be significantly elevated in patients with MetS, highly correlated with the BMI, and inversely with HDL [54]. The effect of MetS and insulin resistance on EL activity warrants further research as the modulation of MetS on the association between EL and HDL may be more complex than just decreasing HDL levels [61].

Role of Atherogenic Dyslipidemia in Metabolic Syndrome in the Pathogenesis of CVD and T2D

Dyslipidemia is a major risk factor of CVD, mainly through the development of atherosclerosis [62]. The role of LDL in the pathogenesis of atherosclerosis has been evaluated extensively, with consistent evidence from multiple clinical and genetic studies establishing that LDL is a key player in the genesis of coronary artery disease [63]. Apolipoprotein B100-containing LDL binding to the negatively charged extracellular matrix proteoglycans leads to retention of LDL particles in the intima of the arterial wall, where they are susceptible to oxidation by reactive oxygen species or enzymes released from inflammatory cells. Oxidized LDL trigger further inflammation and immune cell infiltration, where macrophages phagocytose the trapped LDL and transform into foam cells [62]. Eventually fibroatheromatous plaques are formed, which are prone to rupture and cause thrombosis, leading

to obstruction of blood flow, and if it happens in the heart will lead to coronary heart disease [64]. Besides the concentration of LDL, the type of LDL particles also modulates the risk of CVD. sdLDL is the LDL subtype that is most atherogenic, as reported in the Prospective Framingham Offspring Study [65]. Possible mechanism explaining the enhanced atherogenic potential of sdLDL include: the exposure of apoB on the surface of sdLDL particles is reduced leading to their reduced affinity for LDLR and consequent prolonged plasma retention, their smaller size facilitates greater arterial entry and retention, and they are more vulnerable to oxidative modifications, as a consequence of their reduced antioxidant content [66].

Besides LDL, triglyceride-rich ApoB100 remnants (e.g., VLDL, chylomicrons, intermediate density lipoproteins) also contribute to the generation of foam cells and atherogenic plaques. Plasma triglycerides represent a marker for these remnants [67]. Non-fasting hypertriglyceridemia has been associated with increased myocardial infarction, ischemic heart disease, and death [68, 69]. The triglyceride component of these remnants does not appear to account for their atherogenicity – rather it is the cholesterol content of these lipoproteins that contribute to the intimal foam cells and plaques, and just like LDL can infiltrate the arterial intima [67]. In addition, the TG-rich ApoB100 remnants produce a greater inflammatory response than LDL [70], possibly due to their apolipoprotein CIII content [71].

HDL protects against atherosclerosis in several ways and, consequently, low plasma concentrations of HDL are associated with an increased risk of atherosclerotic cardiovascular disease [72]. The most established anti-atherogenic function of HDL is macrophage cholesterol efflux, where cholesterol from macrophage foam cells is removed through ATP-binding cassette transporter A1 (ABCA1) and taken up by HDL, thereby reducing the proinflammatory responses by arterial cholesterol-loaded macrophages [73]. Other beneficial effects of HDL include the promotion of endothelial synthesis of nitric oxide to mediate endothelial function, decreasing the expression of adhesion molecules on endothelial cells and thereby reducing inflammation, and anti-oxidant capability to reduce the oxidation of LDL [74]. Besides its cardioprotective effects, there is emerging evidence that HDL positively regulates glucose homeostasis [47]. Low levels of plasma HDL and its main protein component Apolipo-protein A-I are associated with T2D [75, 76]. In addition, reconstituted HDL infusion has been shown to reduce plasma glucose in T2D patients by increasing plasma insulin as well as activation of AMP-activated protein kinase (AMPK) in skel-etal muscle [77]. Recent findings indicate that HDL protects the pancreatic β-cells from cholesterol-induced toxicity, stress-induced apo-ptosis, and islet inflammation [78].

Management of Dyslipidemia

The treatment dyslipidemia is an essential part of CVD risk reduction, with LDL lowering being the primary target for reducing CVD risk. The inter-vention to reduce LDL should initially focus on lifestyle modifications including weight loss, die-tary modification and physical activity, and if necessary, pharmacologic therapies [79]. The 2019 European Society of Cardiology and European Atherosclerosis Society (ESC/EAS) guidelines for the management of dyslipidemias state that the LDL treatment targets depend on the individual's CVD risk: for those who have low or moderate CVD risk, the LDL goals are < 3.0 mmol/L (< 116 mg/dL) and < 2.6 mmol/L (< 100 mg/dL), respectively; for those who have high or very high CVD risk, the LDL goals are <1.8 mmol/L (< 70 mg/dL) and < 1.4 mmol/L (< 55 mg/dL), respectively, plus ≥ 50% reduc-tion in LDL levels from baseline [80]. Similarly, the American College of Cardiology (ACC) and American Heart Association (AHA) 2018 guide-lines also base LDL treatment goals on the strat-ification of CVD risk. However, unlike ESC/EAS, they do not specify an LDL target; instead, they state for intermediate or high CVD risk individ-uals, the goals are to reduce the LDL by 30–49% and ≥ 50%, respectively [81].

Dietary and Lifestyle Modification

Weight loss has been associated with regression in coronary arterial lesions and a reduction in CVD mortality [82], likely due to improvements in a number of CVD risk factors including insulin resistance and dyslipidemia [83]. A meta-analysis on 70 studies showed that weight loss from die-tary intervention resulted in significant decreases in plasma lipids and lipoproteins, where every 1 kg decrease in body weight resulted in 0.05 mmol/L, 0.02 mmol/L, and 0.0015 mmol/L decrease in total cholesterol, LDL, and TG, respectively [84]. Although weight loss is the most important goal for reducing cardiometabolic risk among overweight and obese individuals [85], maintaining the weight loss is challenging and many individuals regain weight [86].

Restriction of dietary saturated fatty acids (SFAs) has been a key guideline in the dietary management of CVD due to their positive associ-ation with LDL concentrations. SFAs can increase LDL by inhibiting LDL receptor activity and result in decreased clearance from the blood [87]. Dietary SFAs were originally linked to increased CVD risk in the Seven Countries Study [88]. However, recent meta-analyses showed mixed results on the influence of SFAs in increasing CVD risk, exposing the complex relationship between SFAs and CVD, with numer-ous factors influencing their relative contributions to CVD risk, including their chemical heteroge-neity, the type of replacement nutrient, interindividual variability in dietary response, and the dietary context in which SFAs are con-sumed [89]. While most epidemiological and clin-ical trial data support the replacement of SFAs with polyunsaturated fatty acids for reducing CVD risk, replacement of SFAs with dietary car-bohydrates has been associated with no improve-ment or even a worsening of CVD risk [90, 91, 92]. In insulin resistant, overweight, and obese individuals, a lower responsiveness to SFAs has been reported along with an increased sensitivity to carbohydrate [89], which can drive and exacerbate atherogenic dyslipidemia [93].

The effect of high carbohydrate intake on atherogenic dyslipidemia, and a recent study linking high sugar intake with increased CVD mortality [94] support the 2020 US Dietary Guidelines Advisory Committee to limit both added sugars and SFAs to a maximum of 10% each of total energy consumed [95]. There has been a shift from focusing on specific macronutrients in diets toward healthy dietary patterns in reducing CVD risk [85]. Diets such as the Mediterranean diet [96], the Dietary Approaches to Stop Hypertension (DASH) diet [97], and the Portfolio diet [98] have been shown to reduce dyslipidemia and CVD risk. Moreover, there is high evidence that the intake of certain food items such as soluble fiber psyllium, whole flaxseeds, tomatoes, and almonds can moderately reduce LDL concentrations. These findings warrant greater research and may aid future dietary guidelines for dyslipidemia [99].

Meta-analysis of studies in participants using aerobic exercise training alone consistently has shown increased HDL concentrations [100]. Aerobic exercise has minimal effect on LDL concentrations [101] unless there is a concomitant reduction in body weight [102]. Aerobic exercise training and dietary restriction have been proven to be very beneficial for individuals with MetS by improving blood pressure, body composition, blood triglycerides, and HDL concentrations [103]. Research studies regarding the benefits of resistance training on blood lipid and lipoprotein profiles have emerged in recent years. A meta-analysis of 29 studies showed that progressive resistance training significantly reduced total cholesterol, LDL, and triglyceride levels, but there was no change in HDL levels [104]. Exercise has a favorable effect on some of the CVD risk factors associated with the MetS [105]. Possible underlying mechanisms for reduction of blood lipid and lipoprotein levels and improvement of MetS characteristics likely include maintenance of skeletal muscle mass, higher resting metabolic rate, improved insulin sensitivity, and increased fat metabolism [103]. A recent meta-analysis suggests that combined exercise (aerobic + resistance) is the most effective choice in improving the metabolic syndrome and cardiovascular risk parameters [106]. According to the 2019 guidelines by the American Heart Association and the American College of Cardiology for treatment of elevated blood cholesterol levels, the amount of recommended physical activity is 150–300 min of moderate-intensity aerobic exercise and resistance exercise involving major muscle groups at least twice per week [107].

Current Drug Treatments

The priority of drug therapy is to reduce LDL levels to comply with the guideline-recommended treatment targets. When lifestyle interventions fail to reduce LDL levels, drug therapy should be considered next. For high risk individuals, drug therapy may be started concurrently with lifestyle interventions. Statin is recommended as the first line of therapy in most cases. The following section is based on a recent 2022 review [79], which provides an up-to-date account of the treatment strategies on dyslipidemia.

Statins
Statins are oral agents that inhibit HMG-coA reductase, an enzyme expressed in the liver, which catalyzes the conversion of HMG-coA to mevalonic acid, a cholesterol precursor [108]. As shown in Fig. 2, statin therapy depletes hepatic intracellular cholesterol and upregulates the LDL receptor, which in turn increases LDL particle catabolism and lowers circulating LDL levels [108]. Individuals on statin therapy can reduce their LDL cholesterol levels from 30% to over 50%, depending on the intensity of the regimen [80]. This in turn reduces exposure of the arterial wall to the atherogenic effects of LDL [64]. Meta-analysis of 27 randomized statin trials found that for each 1 mmol/L decrease in LDL cholesterol, there was a significant 9% reduction in all-cause mortality and a 24% reduction in risk of major coronary events [109]. Although statins are generally very well tolerated, they are associated with

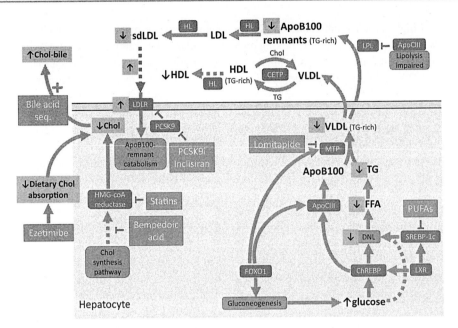

Fig. 2 Mode of action of various drugs to treat athero-genic dyslipidemia. Bile acid seq. Bile acid sequestrants, CETP cholesteryl ester transfer protein, Chol cholesterol, ChREBP carbohydrate responsive element-binding protein, DNL de novo lipogenesis, FFA free fatty acid, FOXO1 Forkhead box protein O1, HDL high-density lipoprotein, HL hepatic lipase, LDL low-density lipoprotein, LDLR LDL receptor, LPL lipoprotein lipase, LXR liver X receptor, MTP microsomal triglyceride transfer protein, PCSK9 proprotein convertase subtilisin/kexin type 9, PUFAs Omega-3 polyunsaturated fatty acids, sdLDL small dense LDL, SREBP-1c sterol regulatory element-binding protein 1c, TG triglycerides, VLDL very low-density lipoproteins

specific adverse effects such as statin-associated muscle aches and increased risk of new-onset diabetes and hemorrhagic stroke [80]. In patients who are unable to tolerate statins, or in some groups of patients such as those who are pregnant or planning for pregnancy, and patients at high risk for diabetes or stroke, there are other classes of lipid-lowering drugs that are commonly prescribed in combination with a statin.

Ezetimibe

Cholesterol absorption inhibitors reduce the absorption of dietary cholesterol or reabsorption of biliary cholesterol from the small intestine and liver, respectively, by inhibiting sterol transport protein Niemann-Pick C1-Like 1 (NPC1L1) [110] (Fig. 2). Currently, Ezetimibe is the only approved cholesterol absorption inhibitor for clinical use [79]. Ezetimibe, when used in combination with statin therapy, reduces LDL cholesterol levels on average by an additional 23% compared to statin monotherapy [111]. Moreover, in the

Improved Reduction of Outcomes: Vytorin Efficacy International Trial (IMPROVE-IT), which enrolled 18,144 patients with acute coronary syndrome, statin therapy combined with ezetimibe resulted in a significantly lower risk of CVD events than that with statin monotherapy, with a 2.0-percentage-point lower rate of CVD death, major coronary events, or nonfatal stroke [112]. In other randomized trials, ezetimibe was well tolerated and efficacious in reducing adverse CVD outcomes when used as monotherapy in patients 75 years and above [113] and in combination with a statin in patients with renal impairment [114]. Ezetimibe is recommended as a second-line therapy in combination with statins in clinical practice guidelines and is often prescribed to statin-intolerant patients [80].

PCSK9 Inhibitors

Circulating PCSK9 targets LDLR for lysosomal degradation, decreasing the liver's capacity to clear LDL particles from the blood [35].

Currently, PCSK9 inhibitors (Fig. 2) are not available orally and targeting strategies revolve around monoclonal antibodies or antisense RNA technology [35]. Two monoclonal antibodies have been approved for clinical use: evolocumab and alirocumab. These drugs are typically administered subcutaneously every 2 weeks [79]. Both drugs have been shown in large randomized trials such as the ODYSSEY OUTCOME and FOURIER trials to significantly reduce LDL cholesterol concentrations as well as adverse CVD events when used in combination with statin therapy compared to statin therapy alone [115]. These two drugs are generally well tolerated with occasional mild injection site reactions. Generation of auto-antibodies to the PCSK9 inhibitors are rare, but as the safety information is limited about 5 years, the safety of long-term use needs to be monitored [80, 116]. Due to the high cost of treatment, these drugs are likely to be considered cost-effective only in patients at very high-risk of ASCVD, and their use is recommended after response statin and ezetimibe is suboptimal [80].

Bile Acid Sequestrants

Bile acid sequestrants such as cholestyramine, colestipol, and colesevelam are nonabsorbable and indigestible positively charged polymeric resins. They bind to bile acids in the intestinal lumen, preventing their reabsorption into the enterohepatic circulation and resulting in their increased fecal excretion. This diverts hepatic cholesterol into bile synthesis and depletes intrahepatic cholesterol stores, resulting in the upregulation of LDLR activity and increased removal of LDL particles from the circulation [117] (Fig. 2). Meta-analysis of 15 studies found that bile acid sequestrants significantly lowered total cholesterol and LDL cholesterol levels, while increasing HDL cholesterol and triglyceride levels [118]. Another meta-analysis of nine studies showed that combining statin with bile acid sequestrant decreases LDL cholesterol by an average of 16.2% compared with statin use alone [119]. Despite evidence for reduction of ASCVD end points and a long safety record, their practical use is limited because of adverse gastrointestinal effects even at low doses. Moreover, as bile acid

sequestrants have major drug interactions due to the potential of these agents to bind to various drugs, timing of dosage needs to be considered while administrating these agents with other medications. Because bile acid sequestrants raise serum triglycerides, they must be avoided in individuals with hypertriglyceridemia [79, 80]. However, they are useful to treat certain patient groups where conventional statin therapy may not be recommended. Colesevelam has been shown to have glucose-lowering capabilities, possibly due to the increased activity of liver X receptors and increased secretion of incretins [120]. Colesevelam is also well tolerated as long-term therapy for T2D patients [121].

Lomitapide

As most currently available pharmaceutical options require the presence of at least partial LDL receptor function to mediate their effect, these treatments are often only partially effective for patients with Homozygous Familial Hypercholesterolemia (HoFH), as patients who suffer from this often have loss-of-function mutations in both copies of LDLR [122]. Microsomal triglyceride transfer protein (MTP) is essential for assembly and secretion of apoB-containing lipoproteins such as VLDL [23, 24], in part by catalyzing the transfer of neutral lipids to the apoB particle [25, 26] in the liver. Lomitapide is an MTP inhibitor, binding directly to MTP, which results in the reduction of VLDL production and its downstream product LDL [122] (Fig. 2). As a consequence of its mechanism of action, lomitapide has been associated with increased aminotransferase levels, which most likely reflects the increased fat in the liver, as well as poor gastro-intestinal tolerability [80]. Lomitapide is currently approved as a treatment option for HoFH patients. In a landmark 78-week open-label trial in 29 patients with HoFH, lomitapide, titrated to the maximal tolerable dose, decreased LDL cholesterol by 50% at the end of the efficacy phase (week 26) [123]. An extension trial where 17 of the patients participated in an additional 48-week extension further confirmed that lomitapide treatment added to other lipid-lowering therapies is highly effective in lowering LDL cholesterol levels with acceptable tolerability in HoFH patients [124].

Fibrates

Fibrates are agonists of transcription factor peroxisome proliferator-activated receptor-α (PPAR-α), which has pleiotropic effects on fatty acid and lipoprotein metabolism. As a consequence, fibrates can reduce triglyceride levels by 20–50% [125] although their LDL-lowering effect is modest [126]. However, clinical studies show little to no benefit of fibrates either as a monotherapy [127] or in combination with statin for ASCVD risk reduction in patients with mild to moderate hypertriglyceridemia such as the recent PROMINENT study with pemafibrate [128]. Fibrate use is mainly recommended for treatment of patients with severe hypertriglyceridemia to reduce risk of acute pancreatitis [80], or can also be considered as add-on therapy for patients with high ASCVD risk who may need a second agent due to elevated triglyceride levels [79].

Omega-3 Polyunsaturated Fatty Acids

Omega-3 polyunsaturated fatty acids (PUFAs) lower triglyceride levels by inhibiting DNL through the suppression of SREBP-1c expression (Fig. 2), and by increasing fatty acid oxidation through the activation of peroxisome proliferator activated receptor family members. Eicosapentaenoic acid (EPA) and docosahexaenoic acid (DHA) are among the most extensively studied omega-3 PUFAs for their potential clinical applications [129]. However, evidence for the reduction of ASCVD risk have been mixed. In the REDUCE-IT trial where 8179 patients who had elevated triglyceride levels and were on statin therapy, the risk of ischemic events, including cardiovascular death, was significantly lower among those who received 2 g of icosapent ethyl (purified EPA) twice daily than the placebo group [130]. A comparable study, the STRENGTH trial, showed that a combination of EPA and DHA had no significant reduction in major adverse CVD events in statin-treated patients [131], suggesting that purified EPA might have unique and pleiotropic effects to reduce ASCVD risk [79]. Current treatment guidelines recommend that for patients with triglyceride levels elevated at

1.5–5.6 mmol/L (135–499 mg/dL) despite statin treatment, icosapent ethyl at 2 × 2 g daily should be considered in combination with statin therapy [80].

Niacin

Niacin, also known as vitamin B3, is one of the few medications known to effectively raise HDL cholesterol levels, in addition to its triglyceride and LDL cholesterol-lowering effects. A 2 g dose of extended release niacin can lower LDL cholesterol and triglyceride levels by 16% and 32%, respectively, whereas HDL cholesterol levels are increased by 24% [132]. One of the large early clinical trials examining the long-term safety and efficacy of niacin as a monotherapy in the pre-statin era is the Coronary Drug Project from 1966 to 1975. With a mean follow-up of 15 years, nearly 9 years after termination of the trial, mortality from all causes in the niacin group was 11% lower than in the placebo group. This late benefit of niacin, occurring after discontinuation of the drug, may be a result of the early favorable effect of niacin in decreasing nonfatal reinfarction and its cholesterol-lowering effect [133]. However, with the advent of statins as a more superior therapy for reducing ASCVD, two pivotal clinical trials assessing the effect of adding niacin to statin therapy did not reduce ASCVD outcomes [134, 135]. Moreover, niacin is notorious for its side effects, which include flushing, worsened glucose tolerance, elevated liver enzymes, nausea, and vomiting [132]. Thus, its use has declined and niacin is no longer recommended in treatment guidelines [79].

Emerging Therapies

Since the approval of lovastatin in 1987, statins have revolutionized treatment for dyslipidemia and have become the mainstay therapy for the prevention of ASCVD [136]. However, certain patients may not achieve adequate reduction or are intolerant to statins, requiring additional non-statin therapies. This section highlights two emerging non-statin options that have potential in the near future to be viable options for dyslipidemia treatment.

Bempedoic Acid

Bempedoic acid is a synthetic fatty acid prodrug that, upon being metabolized by the liver, inhibits enzyme ATP-citrate lyase, which is part of the cholesterol biosynthetic pathway upstream of HMG-coA [137] (Fig. 2). Bempedoic acid when added to existing ezetimibe therapy in statin-intolerant patients reduced LDL cholesterol by 28.5% more than with placebo [138]. Bempedoic acid also significantly reduced LDL cholesterol by 18% when taken with statin therapy [139]. The recent CLEAR Outcomes clinical trial reported that in statin-intolerant patients, treatment with bempedoic acid was associated with a lower risk of major adverse cardiovascular events and was well tolerated [140]. Moreover, due to its specificity of action in the liver, the use of bempedoic acid may avoid the muscle-related adverse effects that is the primary cause of statin intolerance in patients [137]. Bempedoic acid is currently approved for clinical use both as monotherapy and in combination with ezetimibe [79], and its use is likely to be expanded following the favorable outcomes of recent clinical trials.

Inclisiran

Inclisiran is a new generation PCSK9 inhibitor, utilizing small interfering RNA (siRNA) technology to specifically inhibit synthesis of PCSK9 in the liver [141] (Fig. 2). Inclisiran is notable for its long duration of action, requiring subcutaneous administration once every 3–6 months as compared to once every 2–4 weeks with the monoclonal antibody inhibitors [79]. Meta-analysis of three randomized clinical trials comprising 3660 patients showed that inclisiran decreased LDL cholesterol levels by 51% and was associated with a 24% lower major adverse cardiovascular events rate [142]. A recent extended study of one of the clinical trials ORION-3 showed that twice-yearly administrations of inclisiran provided sustained reductions in LDL cholesterol and PCSK9 concentrations and was well tolerated over 4 years [143]. Inclisiran is approved in Europe and Canada for use in adults with primary hypercholesterolemia as an adjunct to diet [79]. Pending cost considerations and more evidence on its efficacy and safety in various patient populations, inclisiran will be likely useful in clinical situations as the PCSK9 inhibitor of choice.

New Indications for Dyslipidemia in Existing T2D Drug Treatments

Globally, CVD affects approximately 32.2% of all persons with T2D with coronary artery disease being one of the major contributors [144]. In addition to LDL-lowering drugs described in the previous section, at least two glucose-lowering drugs have added protective effects against CVD in T2D individuals.

Glucagon-Like Peptide 1 (GLP-1) Receptor Agonists

GLP-1 receptor agonists, are a class of that mimic the incretin hormone GLP-1 in activating the GLP-1 receptor. Besides its glucose-lowering ability as part of the T2D treatment, GLP-1 receptor agonists such as liraglutide and semaglutide have been shown in the recent LEADER and SUSTAIN-6 clinical trials to significantly reduce adverse CVD events in T2D patients, respectively [145, 146]. One possible mechanism is through the improvement in lipoprotein metabolism. Liraglutide reduces postprandial excursions of triglyceride and apolipoprotein B48 (a key component of chylomicrons) [147], fasting triglycerides and increases the catabolism of apoB100 remnants in T2D individuals [148]. Experiments in mice showed that liraglutide modifies the expression of genes involved in apoB100-containing lipoprotein catabolism, such as decreasing the mRNA expression of PSCK9 in the liver [148]. In addition to their effects on lipid metabolism, GLP-1 agonists also have been shown to reduce blood pressure, improve endothelial function, and reduce inflammation, all of which are important factors in the development of CVD [149].

Sodium-Glucose Cotransporter 2 (SGLT2) Inhibitors

SGLT2 inhibitors are a class of anti-diabetic drugs that inhibit the action of SGLT2 in the proximal tubules of the kidney, preventing renal glucose reabsorption and thus lowering blood glucose levels [150]. In the EMPA-REG OUTCOME clinical trial, T2D patients on SGLT2 inhibitor empagliflozin had 38% and 35% relative risk reduction of death from CVD causes and hospitalization for heart failure, respectively, as compared with the placebo group [151]. While SGLT2 inhibitors cause an increase in both LDL and HDL, sdLDL levels have been shown to decrease [152]. Besides their effects on lipid metabolism, SGLT2 inhibitors also have other pleiotropic effects on cardiovascular health such as improvement in ventricular loading, reduction of cardiac fibrosis [153], and fatty liver [154].

Conclusions

Atherogenic dyslipidemia, defined by elevated levels of triglycerides and sdLDL and low levels of HDL, is a key component of MetS. Insulin resistance, responsible for the pathogenesis of MetS, drives the development of dyslipidemia through the overproduction of VLDL, impaired catabolism of ApoB-lipoprotein remnants, and hypercatabolism of HDL. Dyslipidemia is a major risk factor of CVD, mainly through the development of atherosclerosis. sdLDL and triglyceride-rich ApoB100 remnants infiltrate the arterial intima, which in turn trigger inflammation and immune cell infiltration and cause the generation of macrophage foam cells and eventually the formation of fibro-atheromatous plaques. In contrast, HDL reverses atherogenesis where it functions to remove cholesterol from foam cells through ABCA1. In addition, HDL protects pancreatic β-cells from cholesterol-induced toxicity, thereby diminishing the progression of glucose dysregulation. Hence, the low levels of HDL in atherogenic dyslipidemia removes the cardioprotective and anti-hyperglycemia effects, increasing the risk of CVD and T2D, respectively.

Despite extensive evidence for each component of the dyslipidemic triad in its contribution to CVD, lowering LDL levels has proven the only effective strategy in reducing the risk for CVD. Reducing hypertriglyceridemia is only significant in preventing acute pancreatitis, while increasing HDL levels does not significantly reduce adverse CVD outcomes. Thus, in the management of dyslipidemia, LDL-lowering is the primary target for reducing CVD risk. Interventions should initially focus on lifestyle and dietary interventions, and then drug treatments, depending on the individual's CVD risk. Statins, which inhibit the production of LDL cholesterol through HMG-coA reductase, are the first-line therapy. However other drug options are available for those who are statin-intolerant, as well as in patients who require further reduction of LDL levels at the maximal tolerated statin doses. Research is now focused on developing more efficacious statin alternatives with good safety profiles to tackle the residual CVD risk following statin therapy, with bempedoic acid and inclisiran as promising candidates. In patients with T2D who are at high risk of developing CVD, glucose-lowering drugs such as GLP-1 receptor agonists and SGLT2 inhibitors have added cardioprotective effects in this population. Developing such drugs with multiple actions (lipid lowering, glucose lowering, weight reduction specifically with reduction in waist circumference) and demonstratable positive CVD outcomes could revolutionize treatment approaches, greatly reduce CVD mortality, and improve quality of life.

References

1. Pan WH, Yeh WT, Weng LC. Epidemiology of metabolic syndrome in Asia. Asia Pac J Clin Nutr. 2008;17(Suppl 1):37–42.
2. Lakka HM, Laaksonen DE, Lakka TA, Niskanen LK, Kumpusalo E, Tuomilehto J, et al. The metabolic syndrome and total and cardiovascular disease mortality in middle-aged men. JAMA. 2002;288:2709–16.
3. Choi SH, Ginsberg HN. Increased very low density lipoprotein (VLDL) secretion, hepatic steatosis, and insulin resistance. Trends Endocrinol Metab. 2011;22:353–63.
4. Adiels M, Olofsson SO, Taskinen MR, Boren J. Overproduction of very low-density lipoproteins is the hallmark of the dyslipidemia in the metabolic syndrome. Arterioscler Thromb Vasc Biol. 2008;28: 1225–36.
5. Bergman RN, Kim SP, Hsu IR, Catalano KJ, Chiu JD, Kabir M, et al. Abdominal obesity: role in the pathophysiology of metabolic disease and cardiovascular risk. Am J Med. 2007;120:S3–8; discussion S29-32
6. Samuel VT, Shulman GI. Mechanisms for insulin resistance: common threads and missing links. Cell. 2012;148:852–71.

7. Kissebah AH, Alfarsi S, Evans DJ, Adams PW. Integrated regulation of very low density lipoprotein triglyceride and apolipoprotein-B kinetics in non-insulin-dependent diabetes mellitus. Diabetes. 1982;31:217–25.

8. Duvillard L, Pont F, Florentin E, Galland-Jos C, Gambert P, Verges B. Metabolic abnormalities of apolipoprotein B-containing lipoproteins in non-insulin-dependent diabetes: a stable isotope kinetic study. Eur J Clin Investig. 2000;30:685–94.

9. Lewis GF, Uffelman KD, Szeto LW, Weller B, Steiner G. Interaction between free fatty acids and insulin in the acute control of very low density lipoprotein production in humans. J Clin Invest. 1995;95:158–66.

10. Boquist S, Hamsten A, Karpe F, Ruotolo G. Insulin and non-esterified fatty acid relations to alimentary lipaemia and plasma concentrations of postprandial triglyceride-rich lipoproteins in healthy middle-aged men. Diabetologia. 2000;43:185–93.

11. Fabbrini E, Mohammed BS, Magkos F, Korenblat KM, Patterson BW, Klein S. Alterations in adipose tissue and hepatic lipid kinetics in obese men and women with nonalcoholic fatty liver disease. Gastroenterology. 2008;134:424–31.

12. Costabile G, Annuzzi G, Di Marino L, De Natale C, Giacco R, Bozzetto L, et al. Fasting and post-prandial adipose tissue lipoprotein lipase and hormone-sensitive lipase in obesity and type 2 diabetes. J Endocrinol Investig. 2011;34:e110–4.

13. Diraison F, Moulin P, Beylot M. Contribution of hepatic de novo lipogenesis and reesterification of plasma non esterified fatty acids to plasma triglyceride synthesis during non-alcoholic fatty liver disease. Diabetes Metab. 2003;29:478–85.

14. Ameer F, Scandiuzzi L, Hasnain S, Kalbacher H, Zaidi N. De novo lipogenesis in health and disease. Metabolism. 2014;63:895–902.

15. Onyango AN. Excessive gluconeogenesis causes the hepatic insulin resistance paradox and its sequelae. Heliyon. 2022;8:e12294.

16. Tobin KA, Ulven SM, Schuster GU, Steineger HH, Andresen SM, Gustafsson JA, et al. Liver X receptors as insulin-mediating factors in fatty acid and cholesterol biosynthesis. J Biol Chem. 2002;277:10691–7.

17. Cha JY, Repa JJ. The liver X receptor (LXR) and hepatic lipogenesis. The carbohydrate-response element-binding protein is a target gene of LXR. J Biol Chem. 2007;282:743–51.

18. Higuchi N, Kato M, Shundo Y, Tajiri H, Tanaka M, Yamashita N, et al. Liver X receptor in cooperation with SREBP-1c is a major lipid synthesis regulator in nonalcoholic fatty liver disease. Hepatol Res. 2008;38:1122–9.

19. Horton JD, Goldstein JL, Brown MS. SREBPs: activators of the complete program of cholesterol and fatty acid synthesis in the liver. J Clin Invest. 2002;109:1125–31.

20. Hegarty BD, Bobard A, Hainault I, Ferre P, Bossard P, Foufelle F. Distinct roles of insulin and liver X receptor in the induction and cleavage of sterol regulatory element-binding protein-1c. Proc Natl Acad Sci U S A. 2005;102:791–6.

21. Wetterau JR, Zilversmit DB. A triglyceride and cholesteryl ester transfer protein associated with liver microsomes. J Biol Chem. 1984;259:10863–6.

22. Iqbal J, Jahangir Z, Al-Qarni AA. Microsomal triglyceride transfer protein: from lipid metabolism to metabolic diseases. Adv Exp Med Biol. 2020;1276:37–52.

23. Wetterau JR, Aggerbeck LP, Bouma ME, Eisenberg C, Munck A, Hermier M, et al. Absence of microsomal triglyceride transfer protein in individuals with abetalipoproteinemia. Science. 1992;258: 999–1001.

24. Raabe M, Veniant MM, Sullivan MA, Zlot CH, Bjorkegren J, Nielsen LB, et al. Analysis of the role of microsomal triglyceride transfer protein in the liver of tissue-specific knockout mice. J Clin Invest. 1999;103:1287–98.

25. Jamil H, Dickson JK Jr, Chu CH, Lago MW, Rinehart JK, Biller SA, et al. Microsomal triglyceride transfer protein. Specificity of lipid binding and transport. J Biol Chem. 1995;270:6549–54.

26. Patel SB, Grundy SM. Interactions between microsomal triglyceride transfer protein and apolipoprotein B within the endoplasmic reticulum in a heterologous expression system. J Biol Chem. 1996;271: 18686–94.

27. Kamagate A, Qu S, Perdomo G, Su D, Kim DH, Slusher S, et al. FoxO1 mediates insulin-dependent regulation of hepatic VLDL production in mice. J Clin Invest. 2008;118:2347–64.

28. Haas ME, Attie AD, Biddinger SB. The regulation of ApoB metabolism by insulin. Trends Endocrinol Metab. 2013;24:391–7.

29. Yao Z. Human apolipoprotein C-III - a new intrahepatic protein factor promoting assembly and secretion of very low density lipoproteins. Cardiovasc Hematol Disord Drug Targets. 2012;12:133–40.

30. Chamberlain JM, O'Dell C, Sparks CE, Sparks JD. Insulin suppression of apolipoprotein B in McArdle RH7777 cells involves increased sortilin 1 interaction and lysosomal targeting. Biochem Biophys Res Commun. 2013;430:66–71.

31. Mazzone T, Foster D, Chait A. In vivo stimulation of low-density lipoprotein degradation by insulin. Diabetes. 1984;33:333–8.

32. Howard BV, Abbott WG, Beltz WF, Harper IT, Fields RM, Grundy SM, et al. Integrated study of low density lipoprotein metabolism and very low density lipoprotein metabolism in non-insulin-dependent diabetes. Metabolism. 1987;36:870–7.

33. Wade DP, Knight BL, Soutar AK. Regulation of low-density-lipoprotein-receptor mRNA by insulin in human hepatoma Hep G2 cells. Eur J Biochem. 1989;181:727–31.

34. Go GW, Mani A. Low-density lipoprotein receptor (LDLR) family orchestrates cholesterol homeostasis. Yale J Biol Med. 2012;85:19–28.

35. Rakipovski G, Hovingh GK, Nyberg M. Proprotein convertase subtilisin/kexin type 9 inhibition as the next statin? Curr Opin Lipidol. 2020;31:340–6.

36. Lakoski SG, Lagace TA, Cohen JC, Horton JD, Hobbs HH. Genetic and metabolic determinants of plasma PCSK9 levels. J Clin Endocrinol Metab. 2009;94:2537–43.

37. Duvillard L, Florentin E, Lizard G, Petit JM, Galland F, Monier S, et al. Cell surface expression of LDL receptor is decreased in type 2 diabetic patients and is normalized by insulin therapy. Diabetes Care. 2003;26:1540–4.

38. Kohan AB. Apolipoprotein C-III: a potent modulator of hypertriglyceridemia and cardiovascular disease. Curr Opin Endocrinol Diabetes Obes. 2015;22:119–25.

39. Larsson M, Vorrsjo E, Talmud P, Lookene A, Olivecrona G. Apolipoproteins C-I and C-III inhibit lipoprotein lipase activity by displacement of the enzyme from lipid droplets. J Biol Chem. 2013;288: 33997–4008.

40. Sehayek E, Eisenberg S. Mechanisms of inhibition by apolipoprotein C of apolipoprotein E-dependent cellular metabolism of human triglyceride-rich lipoproteins through the low density lipoprotein receptor pathway. J Biol Chem. 1991;266:18259–67.

41. Altomonte J, Cong L, Harbaran S, Richter A, Xu J, Meseck M, et al. Foxo1 mediates insulin action on apoC-III and triglyceride metabolism. J Clin Invest. 2004;114:1493–503.

42. Caron S, Verrijken A, Mertens I, Samanez CH, Mautino G, Haas JT, et al. Transcriptional activation of apolipoprotein CIII expression by glucose may contribute to diabetic dyslipidemia. Arterioscler Thromb Vasc Biol. 2011;31:513–9.

43. Chan DC, Watts GF, Barrett PH, Mamo JC, Redgrave TG. Markers of triglyceride-rich lipoprotein remnant metabolism in visceral obesity. Clin Chem. 2002;48: 278–83.

44. Kobayashi J, Miyashita K, Nakajima K, Mabuchi H. Hepatic lipase: a comprehensive view of its role on plasma lipid and lipoprotein metabolism. J Atheroscler Thromb. 2015;22:1001–11.

45. Carr MC, Hokanson JE, Zambon A, Deeb SS, Barrett PH, Purnell JQ, et al. The contribution of intraabdominal fat to gender differences in hepatic lipase activity and low/high density lipoprotein heterogeneity. J Clin Endocrinol Metab. 2001;86: 2831–7.

46. Toth PP. Insulin resistance, small LDL particles, and risk for atherosclerotic disease. Curr Vasc Pharmacol. 2014;12:653–7.

47. Xepapadaki E, Nikdima I, Sagiadinou EC, Zvintzou E, Kypreos KE. HDL and type 2 diabetes: the chicken or the egg? Diabetologia. 2021;64: 1917–26.

48. Dullaart RP, Sluiter WJ, Dikkeschei LD, Hoogenberg K, Van Tol A. Effect of adiposity on plasma lipid transfer protein activities: a possible link between insulin resistance and high density

49. lipoprotein metabolism. Eur J Clin Investig. 1994;24:188–94.

49. Toh SA, Rader DJ. Dyslipidemia in insulin resistance: clinical challenges and adipocentric therapeutic frontiers. Expert Rev Cardiovasc Ther. 2008;6:1007–22.

50. von Eckardstein A, Nofer JR, Assmann G. High density lipoproteins and arteriosclerosis. Role of cholesterol efflux and reverse cholesterol transport. Arterioscler Thromb Vasc Biol. 2001;21:13–27.

51. Rashid S, Watanabe T, Sakaue T, Lewis GF. Mechanisms of HDL lowering in insulin resistant, hypertriglyceridemic states: the combined effect of HDL triglyceride enrichment and elevated hepatic lipase activity. Clin Biochem. 2003;36:421–9.

52. Thuren T. Hepatic lipase and HDL metabolism. Curr Opin Lipidol. 2000;11:277–83.

53. Horowitz BS, Goldberg IJ, Merab J, Vanni TM, Ramakrishnan R, Ginsberg HN. Increased plasma and renal clearance of an exchangeable pool of apolipoprotein A-I in subjects with low levels of high density lipoprotein cholesterol. J Clin Invest. 1993;91:1743–52.

54. Badellino KO, Wolfe ML, Reilly MP, Rader DJ. Endothelial lipase concentrations are increased in metabolic syndrome and associated with coronary atherosclerosis. PLoS Med. 2006;3:e22.

55. Knapp M, Gorski J. Endothelial lipase: regulation and biological function. J Physiol Pharmacol. 2022;73: 329–36.

56. Ishida T, Choi S, Kundu RK, Hirata K, Rubin EM, Cooper AD, et al. Endothelial lipase is a major determinant of HDL level. J Clin Invest. 2003;111:347–55.

57. Maugeais C, Tietge UJ, Broedl UC, Marchadier D, Cain W, McCoy MG, et al. Dose-dependent acceleration of high-density lipoprotein catabolism by endothelial lipase. Circulation. 2003;108:2121–6.

58. Jin W, Millar JS, Broedl U, Glick JM, Rader DJ. Inhibition of endothelial lipase causes increased HDL cholesterol levels in vivo. J Clin Invest. 2003;111:357–62.

59. Edmondson AC, Brown RJ, Kathiresan S, Cupples LA, Demissie S, Manning AK, et al. Loss-of-function variants in endothelial lipase are a cause of elevated HDL cholesterol in humans. J Clin Invest. 2009;119: 1042–50.

60. Shiu SW, Tan KC, Huang Y, Wong Y. Type 2 diabetes mellitus and endothelial lipase. Atherosclerosis. 2008;198:441–7.

61. Klobucar I, Stadler JT, Klobucar L, Lechleitner M, Trbusic M, Pregartner G, et al. Associations between endothelial lipase, high-density lipoprotein, and endothelial function differ in healthy volunteers and metabolic syndrome patients. Int J Mol Sci. 2023;24: 2073.

62. Weber C, Noels H. Atherosclerosis: current pathogenesis and therapeutic options. Nat Med. 2011;17: 1410–22.

63. Ference BA, Ginsberg HN, Graham I, Ray KK, Packard CJ, Bruckert E, et al. Low-density

lipoproteins cause atherosclerotic cardiovascular disease. 1. Evidence from genetic, epidemiologic, and clinical studies. A consensus statement from the European atherosclerosis society consensus panel. Eur Heart J. 2017;38:2459–72.

64. Bentzon JF, Otsuka F, Virmani R, Falk E. Mechanisms of plaque formation and rupture. Circ Res. 2014;114:1852–66.

65. Ikezaki H, Lim E, Cupples LA, Liu CT, Asztalos BF, Schaefer EJ. Small dense low-density lipoprotein cholesterol is the most atherogenic lipoprotein parameter in the prospective Framingham offspring study. J Am Heart Assoc. 2021;10:e019140.

66. Vekic J, Zeljkovic A, Cicero AFG, Janez A, Stoian AP, Sonmez A, et al. Atherosclerosis development and progression: the role of atherogenic small, dense LDL. Medicina (Kaunas). 2022;58:299.

67. Nordestgaard BG, Varbo A. Triglycerides and cardiovascular disease. Lancet. 2014;384:626–35.

68. Nordestgaard BG, Benn M, Schnohr P, Tybjaerg-Hansen A. Nonfasting triglycerides and risk of myocardial infarction, ischemic heart disease, and death in men and women. JAMA. 2007;298:299–308.

69. Bansal S, Buring JE, Rifai N, Mora S, Sacks FM, Ridker PM. Fasting compared with nonfasting triglycerides and risk of cardiovascular events in women. JAMA. 2007;298:309–16.

70. Varbo A, Benn M, Tybjaerg-Hansen A, Nordestgaard BG. Elevated remnant cholesterol causes both low-grade inflammation and ischemic heart disease, whereas elevated low-density lipoprotein cholesterol causes ischemic heart disease without inflammation. Circulation. 2013;128:1298–309.

71. Libby P. The changing landscape of atherosclerosis. Nature. 2021;592:524–33.

72. Gordon T, Castelli WP, Hjortland MC, Kannel WB, Dawber TR. High density lipoprotein as a protective factor against coronary heart disease. The Framingham Study. Am J Med. 1977;62:707–14.

73. Rosenson RS, Brewer HB Jr, Davidson WS, Fayad ZA, Fuster V, Goldstein J, et al. Cholesterol efflux and atheroprotection: advancing the concept of reverse cholesterol transport. Circulation. 2012;125:1905–19.

74. Rosenson RS, Brewer HB Jr, Ansell BJ, Barter P, Chapman MJ, Heinecke JW, et al. Dysfunctional HDL and atherosclerotic cardiovascular disease. Nat Rev Cardiol. 2016;13:48–60.

75. Wu X, Yu Z, Su W, Isquith DA, Neradilek MB, Lu N, et al. Low levels of ApoA1 improve risk prediction of type 2 diabetes mellitus. J Clin Lipidol. 2017;11:362–8.

76. Wu L, Parhofer KG. Diabetic dyslipidemia. Metabolism. 2014;63:1469–79.

77. Drew BG, Duffy SJ, Formosa MF, Natoli AK, Henstridge DC, Penfold SA, et al. High-density lipoprotein modulates glucose metabolism in patients with type 2 diabetes mellitus. Circulation. 2009;119:2103–11.

78. Kruit JK, Brunham LR, Verchere CB, Hayden MR. HDL and LDL cholesterol significantly influence beta-cell function in type 2 diabetes mellitus. Curr Opin Lipidol. 2010;21:178–85.

79. Berberich AJ, Hegele RA. A modern approach to dyslipidemia. Endocr Rev. 2022;43:611–53.

80. Authors/Task Force M, Guidelines ESCCfP, Societies ESCNC. ESC/EAS guidelines for the management of dyslipidaemias: lipid modification to reduce cardiovascular risk. Atherosclerosis. 2019;2019(290): 140–205.

81. Grundy SM, Stone NJ, Bailey AL, Beam C, Birtcher KK, Blumenthal RS, et al. 2018 AHA/ACC/AACVPR/AAPA/ABC/ACPM/ADA/AGS/APhA/ASPC/NLA/PCNA guideline on the Management of Blood Cholesterol: a report of the American College of Cardiology/American Heart Association Task Force on Clinical Practice Guidelines. Circulation. 2019;139:e1082–143.

82. Van Gaal LF, Wauters MA, De Leeuw IH. The beneficial effects of modest weight loss on cardiovascular risk factors. Int J Obes Relat Metab Disord. 1997;21 (Suppl 1):S5–9.

83. Chan DC, Barrett PH, Watts GF. The metabolic and pharmacologic bases for treating atherogenic dyslipidaemia. Best Pract Res Clin Endocrinol Metab. 2014;28:369–85.

84. Dattilo AM, Kris-Etherton PM. Effects of weight reduction on blood lipids and lipoproteins: a meta-analysis. Am J Clin Nutr. 1992;56:320–8.

85. Siri-Tarino PW, Krauss RM. Diet, lipids, and cardiovascular disease. Curr Opin Lipidol. 2016;27:323–8.

86. Greenway FL. Physiological adaptations to weight loss and factors favouring weight regain. Int J Obes. 2015;39:1188–96.

87. Dietschy JM. Dietary fatty acids and the regulation of plasma low density lipoprotein cholesterol concentrations. J Nutr. 1998;128:444S–8S.

88. Keys A, Aravanis C, Blackburn HW, Van Buchem FS, Buzina R, Djordjevic BD, et al. Epidemiological studies related to coronary heart disease: characteristics of men aged 40-59 in seven countries. Acta Med Scand Suppl. 1966;460:1–392.

89. Siri-Tarino PW, Chiu S, Bergeron N, Krauss RM. Saturated fats versus polyunsaturated fats versus carbohydrates for cardiovascular disease prevention and Treatment. Annu Rev Nutr. 2015;35:517–43.

90. Mensink RP, Katan MB. Effect of dietary fatty acids on serum lipids and lipoproteins. A meta-analysis of 27 trials. Arterioscler Thromb. 1992;12:911–9.

91. Jakobsen MU, Dethlofsen C, Joensen AM, Stegger J, Tjonneland A, Schmidt EB, et al. Intake of carbohydrates compared with intake of saturated fatty acids and risk of myocardial infarction: importance of the glycemic index. Am J Clin Nutr. 2010;91:1764–8.

92. Drouin-Chartier JP, Tremblay AJ, Lepine MC, Lemelin V, Lamarche B, Couture P. Substitution of dietary omega-6 polyunsaturated fatty acids for saturated fatty acids decreases LDL apolipoprotein B-100

production rate in men with dyslipidemia associated with insulin resistance: a randomized controlled trial. Am J Clin Nutr. 2018;107:26–34.

93. Te Morenga LA, Howatson AJ, Jones RM, Mann J. Dietary sugars and cardiometabolic risk: systematic review and meta-analyses of randomized controlled trials of the effects on blood pressure and lipids. Am J Clin Nutr. 2014;100:65–79.

94. Yang Q, Zhang Z, Gregg EW, Flanders WD, Merritt R, Hu FB. Added sugar intake and cardiovascular diseases mortality among US adults. JAMA Intern Med. 2014;174:516–24.

95. Snetselaar LG, de Jesus JM, DeSilva DM, Stoody EE. Dietary guidelines for Americans, 2020-2025: understanding the scientific process, guidelines, and key recommendations. Nutr Today. 2021;56:287–95.

96. Delgado-Lista J, Perez-Martinez P, Garcia-Rios A, Perez-Caballero AI, Perez-Jimenez F, Lopez-Miranda J. Mediterranean diet and cardiovascular risk: beyond traditional risk factors. Crit Rev Food Sci Nutr. 2016;56:788–801.

97. Chiu S, Bergeron N, Williams PT, Bray GA, Sutherland B, Krauss RM. Comparison of the DASH (dietary approaches to stop hypertension) diet and a higher-fat DASH diet on blood pressure and lipids and lipoproteins: a randomized controlled trial. Am J Clin Nutr. 2016;103:341–7.

98. Jenkins DJ, Chiavaroli L, Wong JM, Kendall C, Lewis GF, Vidgen E, et al. Adding monounsaturated fatty acids to a dietary portfolio of cholesterol-lowering foods in hypercholesterolemia. CMAJ. 2010;182:1961–7.

99. Schoeneck M, Iggman D. The effects of foods on LDL cholesterol levels: a systematic review of the accumulated evidence from systematic reviews and meta-analyses of randomized controlled trials. Nutr Metab Cardiovasc Dis. 2021;31:1325–38.

100. Kodama S, Tanaka S, Saito K, Shu M, Sone Y, Onitake F, et al. Effect of aerobic exercise training on serum levels of high-density lipoprotein cholesterol: a meta-analysis. Arch Intern Med. 2007;167:999–1008.

101. Kelley GA, Kelley KS, Vu TZ. Aerobic exercise, lipids and lipoproteins in overweight and obese adults: a meta-analysis of randomized controlled trials. Int J Obes. 2005;29:881–93.

102. Durstine JL, Grandjean PW, Cox CA, Thompson PD. Lipids, lipoproteins, and exercise. J Cardpulm Rehabil. 2002;22:385–98.

103. Gordon B, Chen S, Durstine JL. The effects of exercise training on the traditional lipid profile and beyond. Curr Sports Med Rep. 2014;13:253–9.

104. Kelley GA, Kelley KS. Impact of progressive resistance training on lipids and lipoproteins in adults: a meta-analysis of randomized controlled trials. Prev Med. 2009;48:9–19.

105. Pattyn N, Cornelissen VA, Eshghi SR, Vanhees L. The effect of exercise on the cardiovascular risk factors constituting the metabolic syndrome: a meta-analysis of controlled trials. Sports Med. 2013;43:121–33.

106. Liang M, Pan Y, Zhong T, Zeng Y, Cheng ASK. Effects of aerobic, resistance, and combined exercise on metabolic syndrome parameters and cardiovascular risk factors: a systematic review and network meta-analysis. Rev Cardiovasc Med. 2021;22:1523–33.

107. Barone Gibbs B, Hivert MF, Jerome GJ, Kraus WE, Rosenkranz SK, Schorr EN, et al. Physical activity as a critical component of first-line treatment for elevated blood pressure or cholesterol: who, what, and how?: a scientific statement from the American Heart Association. Hypertension. 2021;78:e26–37.

108. Stancu C, Sima A. Statins: mechanism of action and effects. J Cell Mol Med. 2001;5:378–87.

109. Cholesterol Treatment Trialists C, Fulcher J, O'Connell R, Voysey M, Emberson J, Blackwell L, et al. Efficacy and safety of LDL-lowering therapy among men and women: meta-analysis of individual data from 174,000 participants in 27 randomised trials. Lancet. 2015;385:1397–405.

110. Phan BA, Dayspring TD, Toth PP. Ezetimibe therapy: mechanism of action and clinical update. Vasc Health Risk Manag. 2012;8:415–27.

111. Morrone D, Weintraub WS, Toth PP, Hanson ME, Lowe RS, Lin J, et al. Lipid-altering efficacy of ezetimibe plus statin and statin monotherapy and identification of factors associated with treatment response: a pooled analysis of over 21,000 subjects from 27 clinical trials. Atherosclerosis. 2012;223:251–61.

112. Cannon CP, Blazing MA, Giugliano RP, McCagg A, White JA, Theroux P, et al. Ezetimibe added to statin therapy after acute coronary syndromes. N Engl J Med. 2015;372:2387–97.

113. Ouchi Y, Sasaki J, Arai H, Yokote K, Harada K, Katayama Y, et al. Ezetimibe lipid-lowering trial on prevention of atherosclerotic cardiovascular disease in 75 or older (EWTOPIA 75): a randomized, controlled trial. Circulation. 2019;140:992–1003.

114. Baigent C, Landray MJ, Reith C, Emberson J, Wheeler DC, Tomson C, et al. The effects of lowering LDL cholesterol with simvastatin plus ezetimibe in patients with chronic kidney disease (study of heart and renal protection): a randomised placebo-controlled trial. Lancet. 2011;377:2181–92.

115. Lee S, Cannon CP. Combination lipid-lowering therapies for the prevention of recurrent cardiovascular events. Curr Cardiol Rep. 2018;20:55.

116. Civeira F, Pedro-Botet J. Cost-effectiveness evaluation of the use of PCSK9 inhibitors. Endocrinol Diabetes Nutr (Engl Ed). 2021;68:369–71.

117. Islam MS, Sharif A, Kwan N, Tam KC. Bile acid sequestrants for hypercholesterolemia treatment using sustainable biopolymers: recent advances and future perspectives. Mol Pharm. 2022;19:1248–72.

118. Mazidi M, Rezaie P, Karimi E, Kengne AP. The effects of bile acid sequestrants on lipid profile and

blood glucose concentrations: a systematic review and meta-analysis of randomized controlled trials. Int J Cardiol. 2017;227:850–7.

119. Alder M, Bavishi A, Zumpf K, Peterson J, Stone NJ. A meta-analysis assessing additional LDL-C reduction from addition of a bile acid sequestrant to statin therapy. Am J Med. 2020;133:1322–7.

120. Aggarwal S, Loomba RS, Arora RR. Efficacy of colesevelam on lowering glycemia and lipids. J Cardiovasc Pharmacol. 2012;59:198–205.

121. Goldfine AB, Fonseca VA, Jones MR, Wang AC, Ford DM, Truitt KE. Long-term safety and tolerability of colesevelam HCl in subjects with type 2 diabetes. Horm Metab Res. 2010;42:23–30.

122. Berberich AJ, Hegele RA. Lomitapide for the treatment of hypercholesterolemia. Expert Opin Pharmacother. 2017;18:1261–8.

123. Cuchel M, Meagher EA, du Toit TH, Blom DJ, Marais AD, Hegele RA, et al. Efficacy and safety of a microsomal triglyceride transfer protein inhibitor in patients with homozygous familial hypercholesterolaemia: a single-arm, open-label, phase 3 study. Lancet. 2013;381:40–6.

124. Blom DJ, Averna MR, Meagher EA, du Toit TH, Sirtori CR, Hegele RA, et al. Long-term efficacy and safety of the microsomal triglyceride transfer protein inhibitor lomitapide in patients with homozygous familial hypercholesterolemia. Circulation. 2017;136:332–5.

125. Elisaf M. Effects of fibrates on serum metabolic parameters. Curr Med Res Opin. 2002;18:269–76.

126. Abourbih S, Filion KB, Joseph L, Schiffrin EL, Rinfret S, Poirier P, et al. Effect of fibrates on lipid profiles and cardiovascular outcomes: a systematic review. Am J Med. 2009;122(962):e961–8.

127. Saha SA, Kizhakepunnur LG, Bahekar A, Arora RR. The role of fibrates in the prevention of cardiovascular disease–a pooled meta-analysis of long-term randomized placebo-controlled clinical trials. Am Heart J. 2007;154:943–53.

128. Das Pradhan A, Glynn RJ, Fruchart JC, MacFadyen JG, Zaharris ES, Everett BM, et al. Triglyceride lowering with pemafibrate to reduce cardiovascular risk. N Engl J Med. 2022;387:1923–34.

129. Liu QK. Triglyceride-lowering and anti-inflammatory mechanisms of omega-3 polyunsaturated fatty acids for atherosclerotic cardiovascular risk reduction. J Clin Lipidol. 2021;15:556–68.

130. Bhatt DL, Steg PG, Miller M, Brinton EA, Jacobson TA, Ketchum SB, et al. Cardiovascular risk reduction with icosapent ethyl for hypertriglyceridemia. N Engl J Med. 2019;380:11–22.

131. Nicholls SJ, Lincoff AM, Garcia M, Bash D, Ballantyne CM, Barter PJ, et al. Effect of high-dose omega-3 fatty acids vs corn oil on major adverse cardiovascular events in patients at high cardiovascular risk: the STRENGTH randomized clinical trial. JAMA. 2020;324:2268–80.

132. Creider JC, Hegele RA, Joy TR. Niacin: another look at an underutilized lipid-lowering medication. Nat Rev Endocrinol. 2012;8:517–28.

133. Canner PL, Berge KG, Wenger NK, Stamler J, Friedman L, Prineas RJ, et al. Fifteen year mortality in coronary drug project patients: long-term benefit with niacin. J Am Coll Cardiol. 1986;8:1245–55.

134. Investigators A-H, Boden WE, Probstfield JL, Anderson T, Chaitman BR, Desvignes-Nickens P, et al. Niacin in patients with low HDL cholesterol levels receiving intensive statin therapy. N Engl J Med. 2011;365:2255–67.

135. Group HTC, Landray MJ, Haynes R, Hopewell JC, Parish S, Aung T, et al. Effects of extended-release niacin with laropiprant in high-risk patients. N Engl J Med. 2014;371:203–12.

136. Abdul-Rahman T, Bukhari SMA, Herrera EC, Awuah WA, Lawrence J, de Andrade H, et al. Lipid lowering therapy: an era beyond statins. Curr Probl Cardiol. 2022;47:101342.

137. Ruscica M, Sirtori CR, Carugo S, Banach M, Corsini A. Bempedoic acid: for whom and when. Curr Atheroscler Rep. 2022;24:791–801.

138. Ballantyne CM, Banach M, Mancini GBJ, Lepor NE, Hanselman JC, Zhao X, et al. Efficacy and safety of bempedoic acid added to ezetimibe in statin-intolerant patients with hypercholesterolemia: a randomized, placebo-controlled study. Atherosclerosis. 2018;277:195–203.

139. Banach M, Duell PB, Gotto AM Jr, Laufs U, Leiter LA, Mancini GBJ, et al. Association of Bempedoic Acid Administration with atherogenic lipid levels in phase 3 randomized clinical trials of patients with hypercholesterolemia. JAMA Cardiol. 2020;5:1124–35.

140. Nissen SE, Lincoff AM, Brennan D, Ray KK, Mason D, Kastelein JJP, et al. Bempedoic acid and cardiovascular outcomes in statin-intolerant patients. N Engl J Med. 2023;388(15):1353–64.

141. Frampton JE. Inclisiran: a review in hypercholesterolemia. Am J Cardiovasc Drugs. 2023;23:219–30.

142. Khan SA, Naz A, Qamar Masood M, Shah R. Meta-analysis of inclisiran for the treatment of hypercholesterolemia. Am J Cardiol. 2020;134:69–73.

143. Ray KK, Troquay RPT, Visseren FLJ, Leiter LA, Scott Wright R, Vikarunnessa S, et al. Long-term efficacy and safety of inclisiran in patients with high cardiovascular risk and elevated LDL cholesterol (ORION-3): results from the 4-year open-label extension of the ORION-1 trial. Lancet Diabetes Endocrinol. 2023;11:109–19.

144. Einarson TR, Acs A, Ludwig C, Panton UH. Prevalence of cardiovascular disease in type 2 diabetes: a systematic literature review of scientific evidence from across the world in 2007-2017. Cardiovasc Diabetol. 2018;17:83.

145. Marso SP, Daniels GH, Brown-Frandsen K, Kristensen P, Mann JF, Nauck MA, et al. Liraglutide

and cardiovascular outcomes in type 2 diabetes. N Engl J Med. 2016;375:311–22.

146. Marso SP, Bain SC, Consoli A, Eliaschewitz FG, Jodar E, Leiter LA, et al. Semaglutide and cardiovascular outcomes in patients with type 2 diabetes. N Engl J Med. 2016;375:1834–44.

147. Hermansen K, Baekdal TA, During M, Pietraszek A, Mortensen LS, Jorgensen H, et al. Liraglutide suppresses postprandial triglyceride and apolipoprotein B48 elevations after a fat-rich meal in patients with type 2 diabetes: a randomized, double-blind, placebo-controlled, cross-over trial. Diabetes Obes Metab. 2013;15:1040–8.

148. Verges B, Duvillard L, Pais de Barros JP, Bouillet B, Baillot-Rudoni S, Rouland A, et al. Liraglutide increases the catabolism of apolipoprotein B100-containing lipoproteins in patients with type 2 diabetes and reduces proprotein convertase subtilisin/kexin type 9 expression. Diabetes Care. 2021;44:1027–37.

149. Rizzo M, Nikolic D, Patti AM, Mannina C, Montalto G, McAdams BS, et al. GLP-1 receptor agonists and reduction of cardiometabolic risk: potential underlying mechanisms. Biochim Biophys Acta Mol basis Dis. 2018;1864:2814–21.

150. Fonseca-Correa JI, Correa-Rotter R. Sodium-glucose cotransporter 2 inhibitors mechanisms of action: a review. Front Med (Lausanne). 2021;8:777861.

151. Zinman B, Wanner C, Lachin JM, Fitchett D, Bluhmki E, Hantel S, et al. Empagliflozin, cardiovascular outcomes, and mortality in type 2 diabetes. N Engl J Med. 2015;373:2117–28.

152. Filippas-Ntekouan S, Tsimihodimos V, Filippatos T, Dimitriou T, Elisaf M. SGLT-2 inhibitors: pharmacokinetics characteristics and effects on lipids. Expert Opin Drug Metab Toxicol. 2018;14:1113–21.

153. Verma S, McMurray JJV. SGLT2 inhibitors and mechanisms of cardiovascular benefit: a state-of-the-art review. Diabetologia. 2018;61:2108–17.

154. Kahl S, Gancheva S, Strassburger K, Herder C, Machann J, Katsuyama H, et al. Empagliflozin effectively lowers liver fat content in well-controlled type 2 diabetes: a randomized, double-blind, phase 4, placebo-controlled trial. Diabetes Care. 2020;43:298–305.

Obesity and Cardiovascular Disease

29

Martin A. Alpert, Carl J. Lavie, and Natraj Katta

Contents

M. A. Alpert (✉)
Division of Cardiovascular Medicine, University of
Missouri School of Medicine, Columbia, MO, USA
e-mail: alpertm@health.missouri.edu

C. J. Lavie
John Ochsner Heart and Vascular Institute, New Orleans,
LA, USA

Ochsner Clinical School-The University of Queensland
School of Medicine, New Orleans, LA, USA
e-mail: clavie@ochsner.com

N. Katta
Bryan Heart, Lincoln, NE, USA
e-mail: natrajkatta24@gmail.com

Abstract

The metabolic syndrome comprises a variety of disorders that in aggregate potentiate the risk for cardiovascular disease (CVD) including coronary heart disease (CHD). The metabolic syndrome is characterized by the presence of three or more of the following five components: increased waist circumference ($\geq$ 102 cm in men and $\geq$ 88 cm in women), blood pressure $\geq$ 130/85 mmHg, serum triglyceride level $\geq$ 150 mg/dL, low high-density lipoprotein levels ($<$ 40 mg/dL in men and $<$ 50 mg/dL in women), and a serum glucose level $\geq$ 150 mg/ dL. Central obesity forms the nexus of the metabolic syndrome, interfacing with each of the other components. The metabolic syndrome is a potent risk factor for CVD, particularly CHD. Obesity is considered to be an independent risk factor for CVD due primarily to its association with established CVD risk factors. There is increasing evidence of an obesity paradox with regard to all-cause, CVD, and CHD mortality. Poor cardiorespiratory fitness facilitates CVD mortality. Limited data suggest that intentional (voluntary) weight loss may improve cardiovascular outcomes.

Keywords

Obesity · Overweight · Metabolic syndrome · Cardiovascular disease · Coronary artery disease · Coronary heart disease · Mortality · Obesity paradox

Introduction

In 1995, the 27th Bethesda Conference cited obesity as an independent risk factor for cardiovascular disease (CVD) [1]. They did so because of its strong association with known risk factors for CVD and due to accumulating epidemiologic evidence of an association between obesity and coronary artery disease (CAD) and its complications, commonly referred to as coronary heart disease (CHD) [2–20]. A relation between obesity and cerebrovascular disease exists, but is less robust than the relation between obesity and CAD/CHD [2, 4, 9, 20]. Studies of the relation between obesity and coronary artery pathology have produced mixed results. This chapter will review the epidemiologic evidence for an association between both overweight (OW) and obesity and CVD/CHD including the role of risk factors for CVD with special reference to the metabolic syndrome. In addition, it will explore the relation of OW and obesity to coronary artery pathology based on postmortem evaluation and coronary artery imaging studies, describe evidence for an obesity paradox with respect to CAD/CHD, and

discuss the effects of physical activity, cardiorespiratory fitness, and intentional (voluntary) weight loss on CVD and CHD outcomes in OW/obese patients.

Classifications and Definitions in Adults

The World Health Organization classification is the most commonly used classification of body weight with respect to OW and obesity [11]. This system classifies body weight in terms of body mass index (BMI), that is body weight in kilograms divided by height in meters and is expressed as kg/m^2. The World Health Organization body weight classification is as follows: underweight (<18.5 kg/m^2); normal weight (18.5–24.9 kg/m^2); OW (25–29.9 kg/m^2); class I obesity (30.0–34.9 kg/m^2); class II obesity (35–39.9 kg/m^2); and class III obesity also known as morbid or extreme obesity ($\geq$40 kg/m^2). In recent years, those with a BMI $\geq$ 50 kg/m^2 are described as having class IV obesity or super-obesity. Relative weight (%), also known as Metropolitan relative weight, assesses the relation of actual body weight to ideal body weight based on Metropolitan Life Insurance tables [6]. It is calculated by dividing actual body weight by ideal body weight, then multiplying the quotient by 100. Obesity is defined as a relative weight > 120%. Percent body fat is an important, but less commonly used method for classifying body weight [2, 8]. Obesity has also been classified based on the distribution of body fat including central (abdominal, visceral) and peripheral locations [2, 4, 6, 8, 9, 12, 13, 15, 20]. Distribution of body weight is most commonly based on measurements of waist-hip ratio and waist circumference. Normal waist-hip ratio is defined as <1.0 in men and < 0.8 in women. Normal waist circumference is defined as <102 cm in men and < 88 cm in women [2, 11, 12, 20]. The most common definition of the metabolic syndrome requires at least three of the five following components: waist circumference $\geq$ 102 cm in men and $\geq$ 88 cm in women; blood pressure $\geq$ 130/85 mmHg; serum triglyceride level ≥ 150 kg/dL; High-density lipo-protein (HDL) level < 40 mg/dL in men and < 50 mg/dL in women; and serum glucose level > 110 mg/dL [2, 9, 12, 17, 18, 20].

Risk Factors for CVD

There are a variety of genetic and pathophysiologic mechanisms that contribute to the development of atherosclerotic CVD including CHD. Many of these are associated with OW and obesity [2, 9, 10, 12–14, 20]. Traditional risk factors associated with OW and obesity include type 2 diabetes mellitus, systemic hypertension, and various dyslipidemias (elevated serum triglyceride levels, low serum levels of high-density lipoprotein, and increased serum levels of small dense low-density lipoprotein and apoprotein B). Nontraditional CVD risk factors associated with OW and obesity include insulin resistance with hyperinsulinemia, endothelial dysfunction, various inflammatory markers, adiponectin deficiency, and multiple pro-thrombotic factors. Central obesity is a key component of the metabolic syndrome which itself is considered an important risk factor for CVD [2, 9, 17, 18, 20]. An extensive discussion of the role of various CVD risk factors is beyond the scope of this chapter and is described in detail in multiple other chapters.

Epidemiology

Epidemiologic studies have provided extensive evidence of a relation between OW/obesity and CVD. Most of these studies have focused on CAD or CHD. Some have included risk assessment for cerebrovascular disease, primarily stroke. Peripheral arterial disease is rarely mentioned in these studies.

Relation of OW and Obesity to CVD and CHD: General Body Weight Indices

The Framingham Heart Study produced some of the earliest investigations of the relation between body weight indices or obesity and CVD in general and CHD in particular. Many of these studies were characterized by long-term follow-up. A study of 2818 women and 2252 men whose age ranged from 28 to 62 years and who were followed for 26 years showed that minimum relative weight was a risk factor for both CHD and stroke independent of traditional CVD risk factors [9, 20, 21]. In a study of 1126 women and 597 men whose age ranged from 55 to 65 years and who were followed for 23 years, there was a "U"-shaped mortality curve with the highest mortality at the extremes of BMI [9, 20, 22]. A trial of 2871 women and 2039 men whose age ranged from 35 to 70 years and who were followed for 24 years showed that the risk of CVD occurred in patients with abdominal obesity and general obesity in a linear fashion [9, 20, 23]. After 26 years of follow-up in this study, each standard deviation of relative weight gain predicted an increased risk of CHD and stroke of 22% in women and 15% in men. Optimal BMI to avoid CVD was 22.6 kg/m^2 [9, 20, 24]. Another study of women and men whose age ranged from 35 to 75 years and who were followed for 44 years showed that OW and obesity (based on BMI) were associated with an increased incidence of CVD including CHD [9, 20, 25].

The Nurse's Health Study also proved to be an important source of data related to the relation of body weight to CVD, in particular CHD. A study of 15,886 women whose age ranged from 30 to 56 years and who were followed for 8 years was assessed to determine if a relationship existed between obesity and CHD [9, 20, 26]. During follow-up, there were 605 coronary events including 306 myocardial infarctions, 83 deaths from CHD, and 206 cases of angina pectoris. A progressive increase in BMI (kg/m^2) showed a progressive increase in each manifestation of CHD with increasing BMI. After adjusting for age and cigarette smoking, relative risks were as follows; 1.0 for a BMI < 21 (referent); 1.3 for a BMI of 21 to <23; 1.3 for a BMI of 23 to <25; 1.8 for a BMI of 25 to <29; and 3.3 for a BMI of 29 to <32; ($p < 0.00001$ for the trend). An important determinant was weight gain after 18 years of age which substantially increased risk. The data were attenuated somewhat by the presence of hypercholesterolemia and diabetes mellitus. Thus, it would appear that even a modest rise in body weight early in adulthood increases the risk for CHD in middle age. A subsequent study by these investigators assessed the relation between BMI and all-cause mortality in women [9, 20, 27]. This study consisted of 115,195 women whose age ranged from 30 to 55 years who were followed for 10 years. There were 4726 deaths, 881 from CVD. Similar to the previous study, there was a progressive increase in the relative risk for all-cause mortality with increasing BMI, culminating in a relative risk for all-cause mortality of 2.1 for a BMI $\geq$ 32 kg/m^2. In this group, the relative risk for CVD was 4.1 (95%CI: 2.1–7.7). In both studies, the optimal weight for avoidance of the endpoints was 15% below the United States average at the time of the study. In a study of middle-aged women followed for 14 years, the highest BMI within the range of weight gain after 18 years predicted increased risk of CHD [9, 20, 28]. A study of 44,702 women nonsmokers whose BMI was 32 kg/m^2 or more showed that the relative risk of CVD mortality was 4.1 compared to women whose BMI was less than 19 kg/m^2 [9, 20, 29]. A study of 5897 women followed for 12 years showed that weight gain before the onset of diabetes mellitus was associated with increased risk of CHD after adjustment for selected CVD risk factors [9, 20, 30].

In the Health Professionals Follow-up Study which included 39,756 males whose age ranged from 40 to 75 years and who were followed for 10 years, the risk of CVD mortality rose progressively with increasing BMI in men <65 years old [9, 20, 31]. A previous iteration of this study showed no association between BMI and CVD mortality in men 65 years of age or older. A study that combined subgroups from Nurse's Health Study and the Health Professionals Follow-up Study consisting of 77,690 women and 40,060 men who were followed for 10 years showed that the risk of CHD and stroke rose in patients who were OW and with increasing severity of obesity [9, 20, 32].

The National Health and Nutrition Examination Survey (NHANES) has also provided important data concerning the relation between body weight indices or OW/obesity and CHD. The NHANES Epidemiologic Follow-up Study issued two reports concerning the relation of body weight to the risk of CHD. The first included 1259 women whose age ranged from 65 to 74 years and who were followed for 14 years [9, 20, 33]. This study showed that a BMI of $\geq$29 kg/m^2 was an independent risk factor for CHD. The second study included 960 women and 620 men whose mean age was 77 years and who were followed for 13 years [9, 20, 34]. This study showed that the presence of heavier weight in late-middle age was a risk factor for CHD later in life. Heavier weight during older age was a risk factor for CHD after adjusting for weight loss.

In a study of more than one million persons followed for 14 years, elevated BMI (26.5 kg/m^2 or more in men and more than 25 kg/m^2 in women) predicted CVD in men and women [9, 20, 35]. In subjects whose BMI was 40 kg/m^2 or more, the relative risks for CVD were 1.9 in women and 2.7 in men.

In a study of 22,025 Swedish men whose age ranged from 27 to 61 years and who were followed for 23 years, the cumulative mortality rate was 20% [9, 20, 36]. The relative risk for CHD events in patients who were OW was 1.26 (95%CI: 1.12–1.37) and was 1.76 (95%CI: 1.49–1.68) in obese subjects. CHD itself and CHD events were thought to be closely related to CVD risk factors.

A retrospective study of 866 African-American women and men who were followed for 7 years evaluated the relation of BMI to CAD confirmed by invasive coronary angiography showed that CAD occurred more frequently in OW subjects than in normal weight or obese patients [9, 20, 37].

In a study of 14 target populations which included 1974 women and men whose age ranged from 30 to 59 years and who were followed for 9 years, OW was found to be an independent predictor of CHD [9, 20, 38].

The Manitoba Heart Study included 3983 men whose mean age was 30.8 years at entry and who were followed for 26 years [9, 20, 39]. A total of 390 cases of CHD occurred during follow-up. Increased BMI was significantly associated with myocardial infarction, sudden death, and coronary insufficiency. These results did not become apparent until the sixteenth year of follow-up. After 20 years of follow-up, OW/obesity was the best predictor of myocardial infarction.

A meta-analysis of eight studies comprising 61,386 patients followed for more than 10 years was characterized by approximately 4000 adverse CVD events [9, 20, 40]. Obese subjects with the metabolic syndrome had a risk of CVD events 24% higher than normal weight participants without the metabolic syndrome. In the Copenhagen General Population Study, which included 71,527 adult subjects followed for a mean of 3.6 years, those with OW/obesity in association with the metabolic syndrome showed an increased risk of myocardial infarction relative to normal weight subjects [9, 20, 41]. Hazard ratios and 95%CI values for those with the metabolic syndrome were 1.37 (95%CI: 0.96–2.02) for normal weight subjects, 1.70 (1.35–2.15) for OW subjects, and 2.33 (1.81–3.00) for obese subjects. Hazard ratios for myocardial infarction for OW and obese subjects without the metabolic syndrome were substantially lower.

In a study of 16,113 women and men from Finland whose age ranged from 30 to 59 years and who were followed for 15 years, obesity proved to be an independent risk factor for CHD mortality in men, but was less predictive of CHD mortality in women [9, 20, 42]. The Chicago Western Electric Study consisted of 1701 men whose age ranged from 40 to 55 years who were followed for 22 years [9, 20, 43]. All indices of obesity studied except triceps skinfold thickness were significantly related to CHD mortality after 15 years of follow-up. Both BMI and fat patterning in African-American women followed for 25–38 years in the Charleston Heart Study failed to predict CHD mortality [9, 20, 44]. The Adventist Mortality Study included 12,576 women whose age ranged from 30 to 74 years and who were followed for 26 years [9, 20, 45]. It showed a "U"-shaped risk of mortality from CHD, hypertension, or stroke, especially during the fifth to seventh decades.

A prospective study of 7735 men whose age ranged from 40 and 59 years and who were followed for 14.8 years showed that subjects with a BMI of 22 kg/m^2 had the lowest CVD mortality risk. The Women's Health Australia Project included 13,431 women whose age ranged from 45 to 49 years and was designed to determine the relation between BMI and CVD risk [9, 20, 46]. A BMI range of 19–24 kg/m^2 conferred optimal minimization of CVD risk.

In a study of 2137 consecutive patients with CAD confirmed by coronary angiography (excluding coronary artery bypass graft surgery patients), multivariate analysis showed that higher BMI was associated with lower age at the onset of symptomatic CAD [47]. In patients whose BMI was 35–39 kg/m^2, the average age at onset of symptomatic CAD was 9.3 years younger than those with normal weight.

The results of a sub-study of the EPIC-CVD Study involving 520,00 patients followed for 2.2 years including 7637 with CHD showed that irrespective of BMI, metabolically unhealthy patients had higher CHD risk than metabolically healthy subjects [48]. Irrespective of metabolic health status, OW and obese patients had higher CHD risk than normal weight subjects.

In a study of 2129 patients whose age ranged from 20 to 59 years and who were followed up to 38 years, there were 389 CHD events [49]. Those who maintained stable OW or obese status throughout their adult life had increased CHD risk. In contrast, subjects who transitioned from normal weight to OW or obese status during adulthood did not have increased CHD risk.

A systematic review and meta-analysis derived from 95 cohorts involving 1.2 million participants showed that higher BMI had the same deleterious effect on CHD risk in females and males [50].

A study assessing the effect of obesity on long-term mortality in patients with acute myocardial infarction with and without diabetes mellitus showed that long-term mortality was increased in obese diabetics, but not in obese subjects without diabetes mellitus [51]. A study assessing the relation of BMI to mortality in patients with incident myocardial infarction, there was no mortality benefit in subjects who were OW or obese compared to normal weight patients [52].

In summary, studies using general body weight indices to assess the relation of body weight to CVD and CHD in the epidemiologic setting show that most, but not all support the existence of a relation between OW/obesity and both CVD and CHD morbidity and mortality.

Relation of Fat Distribution to CVD and CHD Risk

There is ample and increasing evidence that central obesity is superior to general body weight indices in predicting CVD and CHD morbidity and mortality. A study of 27,098 adults obtained from 52 countries reported that BMI was minimally associated with myocardial infarction after adjusting for other risk factors for CVD [9, 20, 53]. In this study, the odds ratio was 1.12 (95% CI was 1.03–1.22). In contrast, the odds ratios for waist-hip ratio in prediction of myocardial infarction were higher; 1.90 in the fourth and 2.50 in the fifth waist-hip ratio quintiles. The results of the INTERHEART Study showed that waist-hip ratio was the strongest predictor of myocardial infarction among body weight indices studied [9, 20, 54]. In this study, waist-hip ratio was a stronger predictor of myocardial infarction than BMI or other indices of central (abdominal) obesity. A review of relevant studies reported that high BMI and high waist-hip ratio were independent predictors of CHD mortality [9, 20, 55].

One study combined data from the Health Study of England with data from the Scottish Health Survey to determine the effect of lower metabolic risk on CVD risk [9, 20, 40]. There were 22,308 subjects whose mean age was 54 years. Lower metabolic risk was defined as waist circumference < 102 cm in men and < 88 cm in women, absence of hypertension and diabetes mellitus, normal C-reactive protein, and normal high-density lipoprotein cholesterol. Subjects with lower metabolic risk showed no increase in the risk of CVD compared to healthy normal weight patients.

A case-control study of women less than 70 years of age included 216 cases and 261 controls [9, 20, 56]. Increased mid-thigh girth and subcutaneous fat appeared to have a protective effect against CHD.

In a study of 44,702 women enrolled in the Nurse's Health Study, waist -hip ratio and waist circumference were both independently associated with the risk of CHD [9, 20, 57].

A study of 15,547 subjects (55% men, mean age 66 years) attempted to determine the relative associations of BMI and waist-hip ratio on 5-year survival [9, 20, 58]. There were 4699 deaths during a median follow-up period of 4.7 years. Subjects with a normal BMI and a high waist-hip ratio had a higher mortality rate than those with a normal BMI and normal waist-hip ratio, those who were OW with a normal waist-hip ratio, and those who were obese with a high waist-hip ratio ($p < 0.0001$ for all). In a study of 7057 patients with documented CAD who were > 65 years old and who were followed for a mean of 7.1 years, the highest mortality risk occurred in those with central obesity [59]. The hazard ratios were 1.29 (95%CI: 1.14–1.46) for high waist-hip ratio and 1.29 (95%CI: 1.12–1.50) for high waist circumference. High waist-hip ratio was predictive of overall mortality (hazard ratio 2.14, 95%CI: 1.93–2.38). High waist circumference was not predictive of overall mortality. This disparity may have occurred because high waist-hip ratio predicted mortality in both women and men, whereas high waist circumference predicted mortality only in men. Another study showed that the relative risk of CVD mortality rose progressively with increasing quintiles of waist circumference (1.00, 1.04, 1.04, 1.28, and 1.99) after adjustment for BMI and selected risk factors for CVD [9, 20, 60].

In a study of subjects 21 years of age or older, BMI, high waist-hip ratio, and weight gain were associated with increased risk of CAD [9, 20, 61]. In those 65 years of age or older, high waist-hip ratio was superior to BMI in predicting CAD. In the same study, high waist-hip ratio predicted increased CVD mortality in subjects ≥65 years old [9, 20, 31].

A study from Brazil involving 2396 patients assessed conicity index, body mass index, and waist circumference to determine if they were associated with CAD mortality [9, 20, 62]. None were found to be independent predictors of CAD mortality.

The Paris Prospective Study involved 6718 men whose age ranged from 42 to 53 years and who were followed for an averaged 6.6 years [9, 20, 63]. Thirteen upper and lower body skinfold thicknesses were measured. Higher ratios of truncal to mid-thigh skinfold thickness were highly predictive of CHD after adjusting for blood pressure, cholesterol, and diabetes mellitus.

In the Study of Men Born in 1913, 792 subjects were evaluated at 54 years of age with follow-up occurring 13 years later [9, 20, 64]. BMI, skinfold thickness, waist-hip ratio, and waist circumference were obtained. BMI, skinfold thickness, and waist circumference were not associated with ischemic heart disease, stroke or all-cause mortality. In contrast, increased waist-hip ratio was associated with ischemic heart disease and stroke ($p = 0.04$); however, adjustment for traditional CVD risk factors attenuated this association.

The relation between waist-hip ratio and four-year risk of fatal CAD was assessed in 32,858 women whose age ranged from 55 to 69 years [9, 20, 65]. In comparing the highest waist-hip tercile to the lowest tercile, the relative risk of death from CAD was 3.3 (95%CI:2.0–5.6). When the middle tercile was compared to the lowest tercile, there was a trend toward a significantly increased relative risk of death from CAD. High waist-hip ratio was an independent risk factor for CAD death; however, multiple other CVD risk factors were also identified for this endpoint.

In a study of 105,062 male veterans who were followed for 23 years, the relative risk of ischemic heart disease death per standard deviation of waist-hip ratio ranged from 1.10 to 1.17 and was higher in younger subjects [9, 20, 66]. BMI was not identified as a risk predictor for younger subjects, but was a significant risk predictor in those aged 21–30 years.

A study of 1462 Swedish women whose age ranged from 30 to 60 years and who were followed for more than 20 years showed that waist-hip ratio was an independent predictor of total mortality and death from myocardial infarction [9, 20, 67]. The relative risk was 1.67 (95% CI:1.18–2.36). A meta-analysis of 12 case-control studies showed that those with a high waist-hip ratio were at increased risk for myocardial infarction (odds ratio 2.62, 95% CI: 2.02–3.39) [68].

A study from Finland involving 1346 men with CVD whose age ranged from 42 to 60 years reported 123 acute CHD events during an average follow-up period of 10.6 years [9, 20, 69]. After adjustment for confounding variables, waist-hip ratio ($p < 0.009$), waist circumference ($p < 0.01$), and BMI ($p < 0.013$) cumulatively were associated with a nearly threefold risk of CHD events. Waist-hip ratio provided additional value over and above BMI. Those with central (abdominal) obesity who smoked cigarettes had a 5.5-fold increase in risk of CHD events compared to nonsmokers. Subjects with poor cardiorespiratory fitness had a 5.1-fold increase in risk of CHD events compared to those with normal cardiorespiratory fitness.

An Australian study of 9206 adults whose age ranged from 20 to 69 years showed that after adjustment for multiple CVD risk factors, waist-hip ratio was the dominant independent predictor of CVD and CHD mortality [9, 20, 70]. Waist-hip ratio was a better predictor of these endpoints than waist circumference which in turn was a better predictor of CVD and CHD death than BMI.

A Swedish study of 1462 women whose age ranged from 38 to 60 years assessed the relation of adipose tissue distribution to the risk of CVD and death [9, 20, 71]. Multivariate analysis showed that increased waist-hip ratio and waist circumference were associated with incidence of myocardial infarction independent of age, BMI, cigarette smoking, dyslipidemias, and systolic blood pressure.

A sub-study of the Honolulu Heart Study reported that in Japanese-American men, BMI, subscapular skinfold thickness, and centrality index predicted CHD after adjustment for selected risk factors for CVD [9, 20, 72].

In a study of 2512 men followed for 14 years, subscapular skinfold thickness significantly predicted ischemic heart disease after adjustment for age, cigarette smoking, and social status [9, 20, 73]. Other skinfold thickness measurements contributed marginally or not at all to prediction of ischemic heart disease relative to BMI.

In summary, High waist-hip ratio has contributed to CVD and CHD events most consistently among indices of central obesity. High waist circumference also appears to be a risk predictor of CVD and CHD events, but does so less consistently than high waist-hip ratio. High waist-hip ratio has proven to be superior to waist circumference and subscapular skinfold thickness as a predictor of CVD and CHD events in most direct comparisons. Markers of central obesity have been consistently superior to BMI as predictors of CVD and CHD events.

Pathology

Coronary artery pathology has been studied in OW and obese patients directly via postmortem evaluation and indirectly using invasive coronary angiography and computed tomographic (CT) techniques including coronary angiography and coronary artery calcium scoring.

Studies Derived from Postmortem Examination or Death Analysis

Postmortem studies have shown mixed results concerning the relation between OW/obesity and CAD/CHD. The International Atherosclerosis Project, which was active from 1960 to 1964, reported autopsy findings on 350 persons from six geographic regions [9, 20, 74]. Among those who died accidentally, there was no relation between the body weight indices measured and the extent of coronary atherosclerosis. In a Europe-based World Health Organization study, there was no significant difference in the prevalence of coronary stenoses or the extent of coronary atherosclerosis between normotensive nondiabetic obese subjects and those with normal body weight [9, 20, 75]. A study of 408 subjects whose age ranged from 15 to 89 years showed no significant difference in the extent of atherosclerosis between those who were underweight and OW subjects [9, 20, 76]. In a retrospective autopsy study of OW subjects and those who had "average" weight, the degree of coronary atherosclerosis between the two groups was similar [9, 20, 77]. A study of 237 men who died of

CHD and 297 men who suffered accidental death showed no significant difference in body weight between the two groups [9, 20, 78].

A study of 450 persons whose age range from 30 to 60 years and who died from acute myocardial infarction showed no significant difference in body weight between those who died and those with "average weight" in the age and gender-matched general population [9, 20, 79].

A retrospective analysis of the medical records of all nonelderly residents of Olmstead County, MN who died of nonnatural causes between 1981 and 2001 who had CAD on postmortem examination ($n = 595$) showed a nonlinear decrease in CAD over time which occurred concurrently with a decline in hypertension [9, 20, 80]. An end of the decline in CAD was attributed to a rise in obesity and diabetes mellitus.

Autopsy findings in a study of 37 Japanese-American men showed a positive correlation between CHD severity and relative weight of 116% or more [9, 20, 81]. Another study showed greater severity of CHD on postmortem examination and a higher incidence of catastrophic CHD events in normotensive men, but not in women [9, 20, 82].

In a study of 110 subjects from whom subcutaneous fat biopsies were obtained, the severity of coronary atherosclerosis correlated with the size, but not the number of fat cells [9, 20, 83].

Multiple postmortem studies of coronary atherosclerosis have shown an association with abdominal panniculus thickness. In an autopsy study of 1260 cases, advanced coronary atherosclerosis occurred twice as often in those with an abdominal panniculus thickness > 3 cm than in those with poor nutrition [9, 20, 84]. The Pathological Determinants of Atherosclerosis in Youth (PDAY) Study consisted of 3000 female and male subjects whose age ranged from 15 to 34 years [9, 20, 85]. This study reported the presence of fatty streaks in the right coronary artery and left anterior descending coronary artery in adolescents and young men with an increased BMI. Fatty streaks in the right coronary artery were greater in men with a thick abdominal panniculus. There was no association between BMI and extent of atherosclerosis in young women. A prior autopsy study by the same investigators of 1532 young persons who died of causes other than CHD showed that in males, the percentage of fatty streaks and raised right coronary lesions were two to four times more common in subjects whose abdominal panniculus was >17 mm than in those whose abdominal panniculus was less thick [9, 20, 86]. A postmortem study of 1108 males whose age range was 13–34 years who died from causes other than CHD showed a positive correlation between body weight-height indices and raised right coronary artery lesions in white men, but not in African-American men [9, 20, 87] In this study, the difference in abdominal panniculus thickness was small. A study of 672 postmortem cases whose age ranged from 25 to 64 years and in whom 70% suffered accidental death, there was a weak correlation between abdominal panniculus thickness and raised right coronary artery lesions in white men, but not in African-American men [9, 20, 88].

Studies Derived from Invasive Coronary Angiography

The Honolulu Heart Program studied 359 men drawn from 7591 subjects with established CHD [9, 20, 89]. Invasive coronary angiography was performed at the time of entry and was repeated during a 20-year follow-up period. The control group consisted of 35 men with <50% stenosis in any coronary artery. No significant difference was noted in BMI between the control group and those with greater degrees of coronary artery stenosis.

A study of 262 patients with established CAD confirmed by invasive coronary angiography was followed by repeat angiography 2–182 months after the initial study [9, 20, 90]. There was no significant difference in the progression of coronary atherosclerosis between subjects with a relative weight > 120% and those with lower relative weights.

Data derived from an invasive coronary angiography registry showed that even though black subjects had more CVD risk factors and were more commonly morbidly obese, they were less

likely to have clinically significant coronary artery stenosis on angiography [9, 20, 91].

These cross-sectional coronary angiographic studies and other similar studies have shown little or no relation between BMI and severity of CAD/CHD [9, 20, 92–97].

A study of 414 patients with suspected CAD who underwent invasive coronary angiography to determine the relation of both BMI and waist-hip ratio to severity of CAD was evaluated using the SYNTAX and Duke scoring systems [9, 20, 98]. The mean age was 61.2 years and 60.4% were male. There was a negative correlation between waist-hip ratio and both the SYNTAX and Duke scores ($p = 0.001$ for both). There was a positive correlation between waist-hip ratio and severity of CAD using the Duke scoring system ($p = 0.003$).

In a study of 7567 subjects hospitalized for chest pain who underwent invasive coronary angiography, there were 414 obese patients, 80% of whom had CAD [9, 20, 99]. Obese patients showed CAD at a younger age than nonobese patients (57 vs. 63 years of age). Of the 332 obese patients with CAD, 55.4% had obstructive CAD. Male gender and cigarette smoking favored obstructive CAD. Dyslipidemia favored nonobstructive CAD.

An invasive coronary angiographic study of 95 patients with acute myocardial infarction assessed the relation of obesity to SYNTAX score and coronary artery disease severity [9, 20, 100]. On univariate analysis, obesity was associated with a significantly lower SYNTAX score, fewer coronary artery stenoses >50%, and fewer proximal left anterior descending coronary artery stenoses. In contrast, age, cigarette smoking, and diabetes mellitus predicted more severe CAD. On multivariate analysis, obesity continued to be a significant predictor of less severe CAD characterized by lower SYNTAX score ($p = 0.04$), fewer coronary artery stenoses >50% (0.007), and fewer proximal left anterior descending coronary artery stenoses ($p = 0.03$). Age, cigarette smoking, and diabetes mellitus remained significant predictors of severe CAD.

A prospective study of 1299 consecutive patients who underwent invasive coronary angiography (69.7% male) utilized a variety of angiographic scores to quantify coronary atherosclerosis burden [9, 20, 93]. The study included 477 patients with normal weight, 567 patients who were overweight, and 255 who were obese. Compared to patients who were at normal weight on entry, those who were OW or obese had a higher prevalence of hypertension, hypercholesterolemia, and diabetes mellitus, but BMI was not associated with a greater extent of coronary atherosclerosis. Patients were followed for 24–82 months (mean: 40 months). At follow-up, obese and OW patients had a higher incidence of CHD events than normal weight patients (obese: 74.9%, OW: 67.7%, normal weight (53.2%)). The associated relative risks were as follows: obese versus OW (1.08, 95%CI: 1.02–1.23, $p < 0.05$), obese versus normal weight (1.17, 95%CI: 1.10–1.42, $p < 0.01$). Mortality from cardiac events was not significantly different among the groups studied. However, BMI was an independent predictor of acute coronary events ($p = 0.045$).

Studies Derived from CT Coronary Angiography, by Coronary Artery Calcium Scoring or Both

Assessment of the relation of obesity to CAD/CHD has been studied using CT coronary angiography, by coronary artery calcification scoring (Agaston score) or both.

A study of 13,874 patients with suspected CAD underwent CT coronary angiography [9, 20, 101]. Those with an elevated BMI showed a greater prevalence, extent, and severity of CAD that were not attributable solely to CVD risk factors. An independent association was present between BMI and myocardial infarction.

The Muscatine Heart Study consisted of 387 females and males who were 15 years old at entry and who were followed for 15 years [9, 20, 102]. Obesity, which was determined by BMI and triceps skinfold thickness, was associated with higher Agaston scores.

In the Dallas Heart Study, multiple indices of obesity were assessed [9, 20, 103]. Waist-hip ratio

was the only anthropomorphic measure of obesity associated with Agaston score.

A retrospective study of 6661 patients (mean age 57.1 years) evaluated the relation of Agaston score to indices of body weight including BMI and % body fat [9, 20, 104]. The study population included those who were underweight (0.1%), those with normal weight (21.3%), those who were OW (39.1%), and those who were obese (39.4%). There was an independent association between Agaston score and BMI (5 kg/m^2 increments, odds ratio 1.05, 95% CI:1.00–1.11, $p = 0.038$) and % body fat (odds ratio 2.38, 95% CI:1.05–5.40, $p = 0.038$). BMI and body surface area did not independently predict Agaston score. Percent body fat predicted Agaston score in men, but not in women.

The Coronary Artery Risk Development in Young Adults (CARDIA) Study consisted of 3275 patients whose age ranged from 18 to 30 years and who were followed up to 25 years [9, 20, 105]. Subjects were not initially obese. Assessment of CVD risk factors and CAD occurred at 5-year intervals. During follow-up, 40% of participants developed obesity which was either generalized or central (abdominal). In patients who were obese more than 20 years, Agaston score increased at a rate of 16/1000 patient-years compared to 11/1000 patient-years in nonobese subjects. Ten-year progression of Agaston score was seen in 25.2% of those with generalized obesity and in 27.2% of those with central obesity of more than 20 years duration.

A study of 1218 obese patients who were metabolically healthy determined the risk of developing the metabolic syndrome and progression of Agaston score during a median follow-up of 45 months [9, 20, 106]. Obese patients who were metabolically healthy were designated as class I if there was only one other component of the metabolic syndrome and class II if there was obesity and no other components of the metabolic syndrome. Metabolically healthy subjects without obesity served as the reference group. During follow-up, 32.2% of class I and 10.2% of class II obese patients developed the metabolic syndrome (hazard ratio 2.174, 95%CI: 1.513–3.127 for class I and 1.653, 95%CI: 0.434–3.129 for class II obese patients). Class I patients developed a significant increase in Agaston score during follow-up (hazard ratio 1.053, 95%CI: 1.144–2.390), whereas there was no significant change in Agaston score in class II patients. In class I patients who maintained metabolic health during follow-up, there was no significant change in Agaston score.

A study of 14,828 metabolically healthy patients (defined as no evidence of CVD or the metabolic syndrome and a normal homeostatic model assessment) assessed the effect of obesity versus absence of obesity on Agaston score [9, 20, 107]. Subjects who were metabolically healthy, but were obese had a higher prevalence of coronary artery calcium than in normal weight patients. The risk of developing coronary artery calcium in metabolically healthy obese patients was significantly higher than in metabolically healthy nonobese subjects (risk ratio 2.0, 95% CI: 1.48–3.43). Additional adjustment for metabolic risk factors below traditional levels weakened this association, negating the significant difference between groups.

In summary, postmortem studies and studies employing invasive or CT coronary angiography and/or coronary artery calcium scoring have produced mixed results regarding the association of OW and obesity to CAD. In most of these studies, obstructive CAD was not detected. This may relate to selection bias related to age at entry and entry criteria. Importantly, there does appear to be an association of OW/obesity to mild CAD, sometimes at an early age.

Obesity Paradox and CAD/CHD

The presence of an obesity paradox with regard to mortality is well established in patients with heart failure. There is an increasing body of evidence that an obesity paradox also exists for CAD and its complications, particularly for total (all-cause) and CHD mortality once CHD has been confirmed [9, 20, 108].

The largest study addressing this issue was a systematic review and meta-analysis involving 1,300,794 patients [20, 109]. Data were derived from 89 studies designed to assess the relation of

BMI to mortality and CV events in patients with established CAD during a mean follow-up of 3.2 years. Underweight status was associated with a significantly higher risk of short-term mortality compared to normal weight status (relative risk 2.24, 95%CI: 1.55–2.72) and long-term mortality (relative risk 1.70, 95%CI: 1.56–1.86). OW status was associated with significantly lower risk of short-term mortality (relative risk 0.69, 95% CI: 0.65–0.75) and long-term mortality (relative risk 0.79, 95%CI: 0.74–0.82) compared to normal weight status. Similarly, obesity was associated with significantly lower short-term mortality risk (relative risk 0.68, 95%CI: 0.61–0.75) and long-term mortality risk (relative risk 0.79, 95% CI: 0.73–0.85) compared to normal weight status. Long-term benefit of obesity attenuated over time and abated after 5 years. Class II and III obesities were associated with lower short-term mortality risk (relative risk 0.76, 95%CI: 0.62–0.92), but higher mortality risk after 5 years of follow-up (relative risk 1.25, 95% CI:1.14–1.38) compared to normal weight patients. The inverse relation between obesity and mortality became attenuated over a long period of follow-up.

A systematic review and meta-analysis of 40 studies involving more than 250,000 patients with documented CAD assessed total mortality risk in several CHD subgroups [9, 20, 110]. The referent group in this study had normal weight based on World Health Organization criteria. Underweight subjects (<19.0 kg/m^2) had the highest total mortality risk of the groups studied. Total mortality was lower in OW than in normal weight subjects. Total mortality in obese patients (BMI > 30 kg/m^2) was not significantly different from that of normal weight subjects. Total mortality in those whose BMI was ≥ 35 kg/m^2 was not significantly different than that of the referent group. Similar findings were noted in subgroups undergoing percutaneous coronary revascularization, coronary artery bypass grafting, and following acute myocardial infarction. CV mortality was somewhat lower in OW and obese subjects, but was higher than that of the referent group in those whose BMI was ≥ 35 kg/m^2.

A study of 15,828 patients drawn from the STABILITY Study database designed to assess the relation of BMI to cardiovascular outcomes in subjects with stable CAD assessed all-cause and CVD mortality risk [111]. The lowest all-cause and CVD mortality risks were noted in subjects whose BMI ranged from 25 to 35 kg/m^2. The highest all-cause and CVD risks were observed in subjects whose BMI was <20 kg/m^2 or $\geq$ 35 kg/m^2.

In a study of 50,149 patients with acute ST-segment myocardial infarction those with a BMI between 30 and 35 kg/m^2 had the lowest mortality rate of the groups studied [9, 20, 112]. Another study of patients with acute ST segment or non-ST segment myocardial infarction, adjusted mortality was lower in patients whose BMI was $\geq$40 kg/m^2 than in those whose BMI was <40 kg/m^2 [9, 20, 113]. A study drawn from the Nationwide Inpatient Sample assessing in-hospital mortality in patients with acute myocardial infarction showed that OW and obese subjects had lower in-hospital mortality than other BMI groups [114]. However, OW and obese patients were younger and had fewer comorbidities. In a study assessing the relation of BMI to mortality in patients with acute myocardial infarction, the mortality curve declined progressively in normal weight, OW, class I obese, and class II obese patients, but then increased in class III ($\geq$ 40 kg/m^2) patients [115]. A study drawn from the NCDR Registry assessing long-term outcomes in older adults (>65 years old) with ST segment myocardial infarction showed that class I obesity conferred the lowest mortality risk of the body weight groups studied including normal weight status [116]. Mortality rates in normal weight subjects and extremely obese patients were higher than in class I obese subject, thus forming a "U-shaped" mortality curve. Another study demonstrated that myocardial infarct size was smaller in obese subjects than in normal weight patient [20, 117].

A study of 1307 patients undergoing percutaneous coronary intervention was performed to determine the effect of OW and obesity on restenosis rates and multiple adverse cardiac events [9, 20, 118]. Patients received either a bare metal stent or a drug (paclitaxel)-eluting stent. The study population consisted of 17.8% with normal weight, 40.6% who were OW, and 41.5% who were obese. Patients assigned to the bare metal stent group experienced restenosis rates of 29.2% in OW subjects, 30.5% in those who were obese, and 9.3% in normal weight subjects ($p = 0.01$). Major adverse cardiac events in the bare metal stent group occurred in 20.8% of OW patients, 23.2% in obese subjects, and 11.3% of normal weight patients. Lower restenosis and multiple adverse cardiac event rates were noted in the drug-eluting stent group and there were no significant differences in either endpoint among normal weight, OW, and obese patients. Other studies of patients undergoing drug-eluting stent placement have reported successful deployment and lower target lesion restenosis and/or mortality rates in OW and/or obese patients compared to normal weight subjects [9, 20, 119–122]. In contrast, a German registry study did not show better outcomes with percutaneous coronary interventions in obese compared to nonobese patients [9, 20, 123]. Another study reported no difference in multiple adverse cardiac events between obese and normal weight patients after 1 year of follow-up; however, there was a lower mortality rate in obese than in normal weight subjects after 5 years of follow-up [9, 20, 124, 125].

Studies assessing the relation of OW and obesity to mortality and other outcomes in patients undergoing coronary artery bypass grafting have shown mixed results. In a study of 6068 patients undergoing coronary artery bypass grafting, 12-year mortality was similar in normal weight subjects and those with a 32–36 kg/m^2, but was significantly greater in those with a BMI $\geq$ 36 kg/m^2 [20, 126]. In a study of 4713 obese, 243 morbidly obese, and 1014 normal weight patients who underwent coronary artery bypass grafting, there were no significant differences in mortality, myocardial infarction, stroke, or reexploration of the thorax during short-term follow-up among the three body weight groups studied [20, 127]. A study of 1471 patients undergoing coronary artery bypass grafting at a single center showed that mortality rates at 30 days were 5% for normal weight patients, 1.3% for OW subjects, and 0% for those who were obese [128]. At 10 years, mortality rates were 13.2%

for normal weight patients, 7.8% for OW subjects, and 12.7% in those who were obese.

In a study derived from the APPROACH Registry involving 7560 patients undergoing coronary artery bypass grafting and 30,258 subjects undergoing percutaneous coronary intervention, all-cause mortality in class I obese patients was significantly lower than in normal weight subjects after 5 and 10 years of follow-up [20, 129]. Class III obese patients had higher all-cause mortality rates than normal weight subjects after 5 and 10 years of follow-up.

A study of 3269 normal weight, 6660 OW, 3821 obese, and 211 morbidly obese subjects studied the relation of BMI to early and late mortality after first-time coronary artery bypass surgery [9, 20, 130]. Using propensity scoring, early mortality was not affected by OW, obesity, or morbid obesity status regardless of risk factor profile. OW status was not protective against late death compared to normal weight subjects. Obesity was associated with a significant risk for late death (hazard ratio 1.22, 95% CI: 1.07–2.66, $p < 0.006$). and a somewhat less significant risk of late death with morbid obesity (hazard ratio 1.36, 95% CI: 0.24–2.49).

In a study of 31,621 patients with CHD who were followed for 46 months, medically treated patients who were OW or had class I obesity had significantly lower mortality risk than normal weight or underweight subjects [9, 20, 131]. In patients undergoing coronary artery bypass grafting, those with a BMI of 35–39.9 kg/m^2 had the lowest mortality rates among the body weight groups studied. Other studies have reported similar findings [9, 20, 132–135].

In a study of 519 patients with CHD before and after cardiac rehabilitation, subjects were followed for more than 3 years [9, 20, 136]. All-cause mortality was highest in the patients with a higher CRP level and lower BMI. Higher BMI was associated with lower mortality in higher and lower CRP subgroups. High body fat was associated with lower mortality in the higher CRP group, but not in the lower CRP group.

In summary, patients with CHD who are OW or have class I obesity tend to have mortality rates comparable to or lower than normal weight subjects. Mortality risk in class II and class III obesity is more variable, particularly in those who have undergone nonmedical interventions. This may be due in part to selection bias. Underweight subjects with CHD consistently have the highest mortality risk among body weight subgroups. Thus, there is credible evidence supporting the existence of an obesity paradox in patients with CHD.

Physical Activity and Cardiorespiratory Fitness: Relation to OW and Obese Patients

Evidence is accumulating to suggest that physical activity and cardiorespiratory fitness have great impact on the incidence of CVD, all-cause mortality, and CVD mortality in patients with and without established CHD [20, 137–140].

A study of 9563 men with CHD whose mean age was 33.4 years and who were matched for age and gender assessed the relation of cardiorespiratory fitness to all-cause mortality [20, 141]. Patients in the lowest tercile of cardiorespiratory fitness were classified as unfit, whereas those in the highest cardiorespiratory fitness tercile were classified as fit. During follow-up, fit patients had a good prognosis relating to all-cause and CVD mortality regardless of BMI, waist circumference, or percent body fat. In the unfit group, subjects with the lowest BMI, waist circumference, and percent body fat had a worse prognosis than those with greater degrees of adiposity. As previously noted, a study of 1356 men from Finland with abdominal obesity and no evidence of CVD at entry was shown to have a 5.1-fold increase in risk for CHD events if poor cardiorespiratory fitness was present [9, 20, 69].

A study from Norway comprising 6493 participants with CHD who were followed for a median of 12.5 years assessed the effect of physical activity and BMI on all-cause mortality [20, 142]. Patients who were OW or obese had lower all-cause and CVD mortality than did lower weight patients, thus supporting the presence of an obesity paradox. These findings however, were noted only in subjects who did not meet international physical activity guidelines. This suggests that physical activity was more important than BMI in predicting prognosis. A follow-up study of 3307 patients with CHD drawn from the same cohort was followed for a mean of 15.7 years [20, 143]. The purpose of the study was to assess the effects of changes in BMI and physical activity on all-cause and CVD mortality. Weight loss did not produce a significant reduction in all-cause or CVD mortality. There was a decrease in mortality associated with weight gain in those with a normal BMI at entry. Sustained or increased physical activity during follow-up was associated with a decrease in all-cause and CVD mortality. These findings make a compelling case for physical activity and cardiorespiratory fitness as prognostic markers in OW and obese patients. In contrast, a study of more than 88,000 patients showed that moderate physical activity did not decrease the risk of CVD in persistently OW and obese patients [144].

In summary, the preponderance of evidence suggests that low levels of physical activity and poor cardiorespiratory fitness adversely affect CVD and CHD mortality. Conversely, adequate levels of physical activity and preserved cardiorespiratory fitness are associated with a good prognosis with regard to CVD and CHD mortality. It is possible that cardiorespiratory fitness may be more important than BMI as a prognostic marker.

Effects of Intentional (Voluntary) Weight Loss

It is well established that intentional (voluntary) weight loss can favorably modify many CVD risk factors related to obesity including hypertension, atherogenic dyslipidemia, type 2 diabetes mellitus, insulin resistance with hyperinsulinemia, inflammation, and endothelial dysfunction. Intentional weight loss also reduces the incidence of the metabolic syndrome.

The Asia Pacific Cohort Collaboration investigators studied 33 cohorts comprising 310,000 patients [20, 145]. Each 2 kg/m^2 decrease in BMI was associated with a 14% decline in the risk of CHD. In the Australia/New Zealand cohort, the decrease was 10%.

A systematic review and meta-analysis involving 33,335 patients was performed to determine the importance of weight loss in those with CAD [20, 146]. The study endpoint was a composite of all-cause mortality, CVD mortality, and major adverse cardiac events. The average age of the study group was 64 years, 72% were males, and the average BMI was 30 kg/m^2. The average follow-up period was 3.2 years. Overall lack of weight loss was associated with increased risk of developing the composite endpoint (relative risk 1.30, 95% CI:1.00–1.69, $p = 0.05$). Intentional weight loss was associated with improvement of the composite endpoint (0.67, 95% CI:0.56–0.80, $p < 0.001$) In contrast, observational weight loss was associated with greater risk of the composite endpoint (relative risk 1.62, 95% CI:1.06–2.08, $p < 0.001$).

In summary, although data concerning the effect of intentional (voluntary) weight loss on CVD risk are sparse, these studies suggest that intentional weight reduction may improve prognosis in OW or obese patients with CVD. Further studies are needed to confirm and extend these results.

References

1. 27th Bethesda Conference. Matching the intensity of risk factor management with the hazard for coronary disease events. September 14–15, 1995. J Am Coll Cardiol. 1996;27:957.
2. Powell-Wiley TM, Poirier P, Burke LE, et al. Obesity and cardiovascular disease: a scientific statement from the American Heart Association. Circulation. 2021;143:e984–e1010.
3. Manoharan MP, Raja R, Jamil A, et al. Obesity and coronary artery disease. An updated systematic review. Cureus. 2022;14(9):e29490. https://doi.org/10.7759/cureus.29490. eCollection 2022 Sep.
4. Koliaki C, Liatis S, Kokkinos A. Obesity and cardiovascular disease: revisiting an old relationship. Metab Clin Exp. 2019;92:98–107.
5. Poirier P, Eckel RH. Obesity and cardiovascular disease. Curr Atheroscler Rep. 2002;4:448–53.
6. Alexander JK. Obesity and coronary heart disease. Am J Med Sci. 2001;321:215–24.
7. Barrett-Connor EL. Obesity, atherosclerosis and coronary heart disease. Ann Intern Med. 1985;103:1010–9.
8. Jahangir E, de Schutter A, Lavie CJ. The relation between obesity and coronary artery disease. Transl Res. 2014;164:336–44.

9. Alpert MA. Obesity and cardiac disease. In: Ahima RS, editor. Metabolic syndrome: a comprehensive textbook. New York: Springer Meteor; 2016. p. 619–36.
10. Mandviwala T, Khalid Y, Deswal A. Obesity and cardiovascular disease: risk factor or risk marker? Curr Atheroscler Rep. 2016;18(5):21. https://doi.org/10.1007/s11883-0575-4.
11. World Health Organization technical report 894. Obesity: Preventing and managing the global epidemic. Geneva: World Health Organization; 2000.
12. Bastien N, Poirier P, Lemieux I, Despres JP. Overview of epidemiology and contribution of obesity to cardiovascular disease. Prog Cardiovasc Dis. 2014;56: 369–81.
13. Nicklas B, Berman D, Penninx B, et al. Visceral adipose tissue cutoffs associated with metabolic risk factors for coronary heart disease in women. Diabetes Care. 2014;26:1413–20.
14. Berenson G, Wattigney W, Tracy R, et al. Atherosclerosis of the aorta and coronary arteries and cardiovascular risk factors in persons age 6 to 30 years and studied at necropsy (the Bogalusa heart study). Am J Cardiol. 1992;70:851–8.
15. Despres JP. Body fat distribution and risk of cardiovascular disease: an update. Circulation. 2012;126: 1301–13.
16. Wormser D, Kaptoge S, Di Angelantonio S, for the Emerging Risk Factors Collaboration, et al. Separate and combined associations of body-mass index and abdominal adiposity with cardiovascular disease: collaborative analysis of 58 prospective studies. Lancet. 2011;377:1085–95.
17. Lakka HM, Laaksonen D, Lakka T, et al. The metabolic syndrome and total and cardiovascular disease mortality in middle-age men. JAMA. 2002a;288: 2709–16.
18. Isomaa B, Almgren P, Tuomi T, et al. Cardiovascular morbidity and mortality associated with the metabolic syndrome. Diabetes Care. 2001;24:683–9.
19. Schulte H, Cullen P, Assmann G. Obesity mortality and cardiovascular disease in the Munster heart study (PROCAM). Atherosclerosis. 1999;144:199–209.
20. Katta N, Loethen T, Lavie CJ, Alpert MA. Obesity and coronary heart disease: epidemiology, pathology, and coronary artery imaging. Curr Probl Cardiol. 2021;46(3):100655. https://doi.org/10.1016/j.cpcardiol.2020.100655.
21. Hubert HB, Feinleib M, McNamara PM, Castelli WP. Obesity as an independent risk factor for cardiovascular disease: a 26-year follow-up of participants in the Framingham heart study. Circulation. 1983,67. 968–97.
22. Harris T, Cook F, Garrison R, et al. Body mass index and mortality among non- smoking older persons. The Framingham Heart Study. JAMA. 1998;259: 1520–4.
23. Kannel W, Cupples L, Ramaswami R, et al. Regional obesity and risk of cardiovascular disease: the Framingham study. J Clin Epidemiol. 1991;44:183–90.
24. Kannel W, D'Agostino R, Cobb J. Effect of weight on cardiovascular disease. Am J Clin Nutr. 1996;63: S419–21.
25. Wilson PW, D'Agostino RB, Sullivan L, Parise H, Kannel WB. Overweight and obesity as determinants of cardiovascular risk: the Framingham experience. Arch Intern Med. 2002;162:1867–72.
26. Manson JE, Colditz GA, Stampfer MJ, et al. A prospective study of obesity and risk of coronary heart disease in women. N Engl J Med. 1990;322:822–89.
27. Manson J, Willett W, Stampfer M, et al. Body weight and mortality among women. N Engl J Med. 1995;333:677–85.
28. Willett W, Manson J, Stampfer M, et al. Weight, weight change and coronary heart disease in women. JAMA. 1995;276:461–5.
29. Rexrode K, Hennekens C, Willett W, et al. A prospective study of body mass index, weight change, and risk of stroke in women. JAMA. 1995;277:1539–45.
30. Cho E, Colditz G, Manson J, et al. A prospective study of obesity and risk of coronary heart disease among diabetic women. Diabetes Care. 2002;35: 1142–8.
31. Baik I, Ascherio A, Rimm E, et al. Adiposity and mortality in men. Am J Epidemiol. 2000;152:264–71.
32. Field A, Coakley E, Must A, et al. Impact of overweight on the risk of developing common chronic diseases during a 10-year period. Arch Intern Med. 2001;161:1581–6.
33. Harris T, Ballard-Barbasch R, Madans J, et al. Overweight, weight loss and risk of coronary heart disease in older women. Am J Epidemiol. 1993;137:1318–27.
34. Harris T, Launer L, Madans J, et al. Cohort study of effect of being overweight and change in weight on risk of coronary heart disease in old age. Br Med J. 1997;314:1791–2.
35. Calle EE, Thun MJ, Petielli JM, et al. Body mass index and mortality in a prospective cohort of U.-S. adults. N Engl J Med. 1999;341:1097–105.
36. Jonsson S, Hedblad B, Engstrom G, Nilsson P, Bergland G, Janzon L. Influence of obesity on cardiovascular risk. Twenty-three-year follow-up of 22,025 men from an urban Swedish population. Int J Obes. 2002;26:1046–53.
37. Adams-Campbell K, Pensiton RL, Kim KS, Nensa E. Body mass index and coronary artery disease in African-Americans. Obes Res. 1995;3:215–9.
38. Zhou B, Wu Y, Li Y, et al. 2002. Overweight is an independent risk factor for cardiovascular disease in Chinese populations. Obes Rev. 2002;3:147–56.
39. Rabkin SW, Mathewson FA, Hsu PH. Relation of body weight of development of ischemic heart disease in a cohort of young north American men after a 26-year observation period: the Manitoba study. Am J Cardiol. 1977;39:452–8.
40. Kramer CK, Zinman B, Retnakaran R. Are metabolically healthy overweight and obesity benign conditions? A systematic review and meta-analysis. Ann Intern Med. 2013;159:758–69.

41. Thomsen M, Nordestgaard BG. Myocardial infarction and ischemic heart disease in overweight and obesity with and without metabolic syndrome. JAMA Intern Med. 2014;174:15–22.

42. Jousilahti P, Tumilehto J, Vartiainen E, et al. Body weight, cardiovascular risk factors, and coronary mortality. 15-year follow-up of middle-aged men and women in eastern Finland. Circulation. 1996;93:1372–9.

43. Spataro J, Dyer A, Stamler J, et al. Measures of adiposity and coronary heart disease mortality in the Chicago Western electric company study. J Clin Epidemiol. 1996;49:849–57.

44. Stevens J, Keil JE, Rust PF, et al. Body mass index and body girth as predictors of mortality in black and white women. Arch Intern Med. 1992;52:1557–62.

45. Singh P, Landsted K. Body mass and 26-year risk of mortality from specific diseases among women who never smoked. Epidemiology. 1998;52:1557–62.

46. Brown WJ, Dobson AJ, Mishra G. What is healthy weight for middle-aged women? Int J Obes Relat Metab Disord. 1998;22:520–8.

47. Atique SM, Shadbolt MP, Farshid A. Association between body mass index and age of presentation with symptomatic coronary artery disease. Clin Cardiol. 2016;39:653–7.

48. Lassale C, Tzoulaki I, Moons KG, et al. Separate and combined associations of obesity and metabolic health with coronary heart disease: a pan-European case-control study. Eur Heart J. 2018;39:397–406.

49. Calling S, Johansson SE, Nymberg VM, Sundquist J, Sundquist S. Trajectory of body mass index and risk for coronary heart disease. A 38-year follow-up study. PLoS One. 2021;16(10):e0258395. https://doi.org/10.1371/journal.pone.0258395.

50. Mongraw-Chapin ML, Peters SE, Huxley RR, Woodward M. The sex-specific relationship between body mass index and coronary heart disease: a systematic review of 95 cohorts with 1.2 million participants. Lancet Diabetes Endocrinol. 2015;3:437–9.

51. Colombo MG, Meisinger C, Amann U, et al. Association of obesity and long-term mortality in patients with acute myocardial infarction, with and without diabetes mellitus: results from the MONICA-KORA myocardial infarction registry. Cardiovasc Diabetol. 2015;14:24.

52. Al Shaar L, Li Y, Rimm EB, et al. Body mass index and mortality among adults with incident myocardial infarction. Am J Epidemiol. 2021;190:2019–28.

53. Yusuf S, Hawken S, Ounpuu S, et al. Obesity and the risk of myocardial infarction in 27,000 participants from 52 countries: a case-control study. Lancet. 2005;366:1640–52.

54. Yusuf S, Hawken S, Ounpuu S, et al. Effect of potentially modifiable risk factors associated with myocardial infarction in 52 countries (INTERHEART study): case-control study. Lancet. 2004;364:937–52.

55. Rao S, Donahue M, Pi-Sunyer F, et al. Obesity as a risk factor in coronary artery disease. Am Heart J. 2001;142:1102–7.

56. Kahn H, Austin H, Williamson D, et al. Simple anthropometric indices associated with ischemic heart disease. J Clin Epidemiol. 1996;49:1017–24.

57. Rexrode K, Carey V, Hennekens C, et al. Abdominal adiposity and coronary heart disease. JAMA. 1998;280:1843–8.

58. Coutinho T, Goel K, Correa de So D, et al. Combining body mass index with measures of central obesity in the assessment of mortality in subjects with coronary artery disease. Role of normal weight central obesity. J Am Coll Cardiol. 2013;61:553–60.

59. Sharma S, Batsis JA, Coutinho T, et al. Normal weight central obesity and mortality risk in older adults with coronary artery disease. Mayo Clin Proc. 2016;91:343–51.

60. Zhang C, Rexrode KM, van Dam RM, et al. Abdominal obesity the risk of all-cause, and cancer mortality: sixteen years of follow-up in U.S. women. Circulation. 2008;117:1658–67.

61. Rimm E, Stampfer M, Giovannucci E, et al. Body size and fat distribution as predictors of coronary heart disease among middle-aged and older U.S. men. Am J Epidemiol. 1995;141:1117–27.

62. Fontela PC, Winkelmann ER, Nazurio Viecili PR. Study of conicity index, body mass index and waist circumference as predictors of coronary artery disease. Rev Port Cardiol. 2017;36:357–64.

63. Dulcimetriere P, Richard JL, Combien F. The pattern of subcutaneous fat distribution in middle-aged men and risk of coronary heart disease. The Paris prospective study. Int J Obes. 1986;10:229–40.

64. Larsson K, Svardsudd L, Welin L, Wilhelm L, Bjorntrop P, Tibblen G. Abdominal adipose distribution, obesity, and risk of cardiovascular disease and death: 13-year follow-up of the study of men born in 1913. Br Med J. 1984;12:1401–4.

65. Prineas RJ, Folsom AR, Kay SA. Central obesity and increased risk of coronary heart disease mortality in older women. Am J Epidemiol. 1993;3:35–41.

66. Terry RB, Page WF, Haskell WC. Waist-hip ratio, body mass index and premature cardiovascular disease mortality in US Army veterans during a 23-year follow-up study. J Obes. 1992;16:417–28.

67. Bengtsson C, Bjorklund C, Lapidus L, Lissner L. Associations of severe lipid concentrations and obesity with mortality in women: 20-year follow-up of participants in prospective population study in Gothenburg, Sweden. BMJ. 1993;307:1395–89.

68. Cao Q, Yu S, Xiong W, et al. Waist-hip ratio as a predictor of myocardial infarction risk. Medicine. 2018;97(30):e11639. https://doi.org/10.1097/MD.000000000000.11639.

69. Lakka HM, Lakka TA, Toumilehto J, Salonen JT. Abdominal obesity is associated with increased risk of acute coronary events in men. Eur Heart J. 2002b;23:706–13.

70. Wellborn TA, Dhaliwal SS, Bennett SA. Waist-hip ratio is the dominant risk factor precipitation cardiovascular death in Australia. Med J Aust. 2003;179:580–5.

71. Lapidus L, Bengtsson C, Larrsson B, Pennert K, Rybo E, Sjostrum L. Distribution of adipose tissue and risk of cardiovascular disease and death: a 12-year follow-up of participants in the population study of women in Gothenburg, Sweden. BMJ. 1984;285:1257–61.
72. Curb JP, Marcus EB. Body fat, coronary heart disease, and stroke in Japanese men. Am J Clin Nutr. 1991;53: 1612s–5s.
73. Yarnell JW, Patterson CC, Thomas HF, Sweetnam PM. Central obesity: predictive value of skinfold measurements for subsequent ischemic heart disease at 14 years follow-up in the Caerphilly study. Int J Obes Relat Metab Disord. 2001;25:1546–9.
74. Montenegro MR, Salsberg LA. Obesity, body weight, body length and atherosclerosis. Lab Investig. 1968;18:594–603.
75. Sternby NH. Atherosclerosis and body build. Bull World Health Organ. 1976;53:601–4.
76. Giertsen JC. Atherosclerosis in an autopsy series. Acta Pathol Microbiol Scand. 1966;67:305–21.
77. Ackerman RF, Dry TJ, Edwards JE. Relationship of various factors to degree of coronary atherosclerosis in women. Circulation. 1950;1:1345–50.
78. Yater WM, Traum AH, Spring S, et al. Coronary artery disease in men 18-39 years of age. Am Heart J. 1948;36:334–72.
79. Lee KT, Thomas WA. Relationship of body weight to acute myocardial infarction. Am Heart J. 1956;52: 581–91.
80. Smith CY, Bailey KR, Emerson JA, et al. Contributions of increasing obesity and diabetes to slowing decline in subclinical coronary artery disease. J Am Heart Assoc. 2015;4(4):e001524. https://doi.org/10.1161/JAHA.114.001574.
81. Rhoads G, Kagan A. The relation of coronary disease, stroke and morality to weight in youth and in middle age. Lancet. 1983;16:492–5.
82. Wilkens RH, Roberts JC Jr, Moser C. Autopsy studies in atherosclerosis. Circulation. 1959;20:527–36.
83. Bjurulf P. Atherosclerosis and body build. Acta Med Scand. 1959;349(Suppl):1–99.
84. Wilens SL. Bearing of general nutritional state on atherosclerosis. Arch Intern Med. 1947;79:129–47.
85. McGill HC Jr, McMahon CA, Herderick EE, et al. Obesity accelerates the progression of coronary atherosclerosis in young men. Circulation. 2002;105: 2712–8.
86. McGill HC Jr, McMahan CA, Malcom GT, Oalmann MC, Strong JP. Relation of glycohemoglobin and adiposity to atherosclerosis in youth. Pathobiological determinates of atherosclerosis in youth. Arterioscler Thromb Vasc Biol. 1995;15:431–40.
87. Strong JP, Oalmann MC, Newman WP II, et al. Coronary heart disease in young black and white male coronary heart disease unity pathology study. Am Heart J. 1984;108(3 Pt 2):747–59.
88. Patel YC, Eggen DA, Strong JP. Obesity, smoking, and atherosclerosis. Atherosclerosis. 1980;36: 482–90.
89. Reed D, Yano K. Predictors of arteriographically defined coronary stenosis in the Honolulu heart program. Am J Epidemiol. 1991;134:111–22.
90. Cramer K, Paulin S, Werko L. Coronary angiographic findings in correlation with age, body weight, blood pressure, serum lipids, and smoking habits. Circulation. 1966;33:888–900.
91. Stalls CM, Triplette MA, Viera AJ, et al. The association between body mass index and coronary artery disease severity: a comparison of black and white patients. Am Heart J. 2014;167:514–20.
92. Flynn MA, Cogg MN, Gibney MJ, et al. Indices of obesity and body fat distribution in arteriographically defined coronary artery disease in men. Ir J Med Sci. 1993;162:503–9.
93. Rossi R, Iaccarino D, Nuzzo A, et al. Influence of body mass index on extent of coronary atherosclerosis and cardiac events in a cohort of patients at risk of coronary artery disease. Nutr Metab Cardiovasc Dis. 2011;21:86–93.
94. Morricone L, Ferrari M, Enrini R, et al. Angiographically determined coronary artery disease in relation to obesity and body fat distribution. Int J Obes. 1996;20(Suppl 4):109–14.
95. Hauner H, Stangl K, Schmatz C, et al. Body fat distribution in men with angiographically confirmed coronary artery disease. Atherosclerosis. 1990;85: 203–10.
96. Clark LT, Karve NM, Rones KT, et al. Obesity, distribution of body fat and coronary disease in black women. Am J Cardiol. 1994;73:895–6.
97. Zamboni M, Armellini F, Sheiban I, et al. Relation of body fat distribution in men and degree of coronary narrowing's in coronary artery disease. Am J Cardiol. 1992;70:1135–8.
98. Farhang A, Para Z, Jahanshahi B. Is the relationship of body mass index to severity of coronary artery disease different from that of waist-hip ratio and severity of coronary artery disease? Paradoxical findings. Cardiovasc J Afr. 2015;26:13–6.
99. Alkhawam H, Nguyen J, Sayanlar J, et al. Coronary artery disease in patients with body mass index $\geq$ 30 kg/m^2: a retrospective chart analysis. J Community Hosp Intern Med Perspect. 2016; https://doi.org/10.3402/chimp.v6.31483.eCollection.
100. Cepeda-Valery B, Chaudry K, Slipczuk L, et al. Association between obesity and severity of coronary artery disease at the time of acute myocardial infarction: another piece of the puzzle in the "obesity paradox". Int J Cardiol. 2014;176:247–9.
101. Labounty TM, Gomez MJ, Achenbach S, et al. Body mass index the prevalence severity and risk of coronary artery disease: an international study of 13,874 patients. Eur Heart J Cardiovasc Imaging. 2013;14: 456–63.
102. Mahoney L, Burns T, Stanford W, et al. Coronary risk factors measure in childhood and young adult life are associated with coronary artery calcification in young adults: the Muscatine study. J Am Coll Cardiol. 1996;27:277–84.

103. See R, Abdullah SM, McGuine DK, et al. The association of differing measures of overweight and obesity with prevalent atherosclerosis. The Dallas heart study. J Am Coll Cardiol. 2007;50:752–9.

104. Aljizeer A, Coutinho T. Pen, et al. obesity and coronary calcification. Can it explain the obesity paradox? Int J Cardiovasc Imaging. 2015;31:1063–70.

105. CARDIA Investigators. Duration of obesity linked with coronary artery calcification. BMJ. 2013;347 https://doi.org/10.1136/bmj.f4682.

106. Yoon JW, Jung MK, Park HE, et al. Influence of the definition of "metabolically health obesity" on progression of coronary artery calcification. PLoS One. 2017; https://doi.org/10.1371/journal.pone.0178741June2.

107. Chang Y, Kim BK, Yan KE, et al. Metabolically healthy obesity and coronary artery calcification. J Am Coll Cardiol. 2014;63:2679–86.

108. Lavie CJ, Milani RV, Ventura HO. Obesity and cardiovascular disease: risk factor, paradox, and impact of weight loss. J Am Coll Cardiol. 2009a;53:1925–32.

109. Wang ZJ, Zhou YJ, Galper BJ, Mauri FG. Association of body mass index with mortality and cardiovascular events: a systematic review and meta-analysis. BMJ. 2015;101:1631. https://doi.org/10.1136/heartjnl-2014-307119.

110. Romero-Corral A, Montori VM, Sommers VK, et al. Association of body weight with total mortality and with cardiovascular events in coronary artery disease: a systematic review of cohort studies. Lancet. 2006;68:666–78.

111. Held C, Hadziosmanovic N, Aylward PE, et al. Body mass index and association with cardiovascular outcomes in patients with stable coronary heart disease-A STABILITY sub-study. J Am Heart Assoc. 2022;1(3): e023667. https://doi.org/10.1161/JAHA.121.023667.

112. Das SR, Alexander KP, Chen AY, et al. Impact of body weight and extreme obesity on the presentation, treatment, and in-hospital outcomes of 50,149 patients with ST-segment elevation myocardial infarction results from the NCDR (National Cardiovascular Data Registry). J Am Coll Cardiol. 2011;58: 2642–50.

113. Kragelund C, Hassager C, Hildebrandt P, Torp-Pederssen C, Kober L. Impact of obesity on long-term prognosis following acute myocardial infarction. Int J Cardiol. 2005;98:121–31.

114. Pottlolla SH, Gurumurthy G, Sundaragiri PR, Cheungpositporn W, Vallabhajosyula S. Body mass index and in-hospital management and outcomes of acute myocardial infarction. Medicina. 2021;57(9): 926. https://doi.org/10.3390/medicina.57090926.

115. Bucholz EM, Rathone SS, Reid KJ, Jones PG, Chan PS, Rich MW. Body mass index and mortality in acute myocardial infarction. Am J Med. 2012;125: 796–803.

116. Neeland IJ, Das S, Simon DN, et al. The obesity paradox, extreme obesity and long-term outcomes in older adults with ST-segment myocardial infarction. Eur Heart J Qual Care Clin Outcomes. 2017;3: 183–91.

117. Pingitore A, Di BG, Lombardi M, et al. The obesity paradox and myocardial infarct size. J Cardiovasc Med. 2007;8:713–7.

118. Nikolsky E, Kosinski E, Mishkel GJ, et al. Impact of obesity on revascularization and restenosis rates after bare-mental and drug-eluting stent implantation (from the TAXUS-IV trial). Am J Cardiol. 2005;95:709–15.

119. Mehta L, Devlin W, McCullough PA, et al. Impact of body mass index on outcomes after percutaneous coronary intervention in patients with acute myocardial infarction. Am J Cardiol. 2007;99:906–10.

120. Gruberg L, Weissman NJ, Wakman R, et al. The impact of obesity on the short-term and long-term outcomes after percutaneous coronary intervention: the obesity paradox? J Am Coll Cardiol. 2002;39: 578–84.

121. Lancefield T, Clark DJ, Andrianopoulos N, et al. Is there an obesity paradox after percutaneous coronary intervention in the contemporary era? An analysis from a multicenter Australian registry. Cardiovasc Interv. 2010;3:660–8.

122. Wang ZJ, Zhou YJ, Zhao YX, et al. Effect of obesity on repeat revascularization in patients undergoing percutaneous coronary intervention with drug-eluting stents. Obesity. 2012;20:141–6.

123. Akin I, Tolg R, Hochadel M, et al. No evidence of "obesity paradox" after treatment with drug-eluting stents in a routine clinical practice: results from prospective multicenter German DES DE (German drug-eluting stent) registry. J Am Coll Cardiol Cardiovasc Interv. 2012;5:162–9.

124. Sarno G, Garg S, Onuma Y, et al. The impact of body mass index on the one-year outcomes of patients treated by percutaneous coronary intervention with Biolimus-and Sirolimus-eluting stents (from the LEADERS trial). Am J Cardiol. 2010;105:475–9.

125. Sarno G, Raber L, Onuma Y, et al. Impact of body mass index on the five-year outcome of patients having percutaneous coronary interventions with drug-eluting stents. Am J Cardiol. 2011;108:195–201.

126. Habib RH, Zacharius A, Schwann TA, Rioron CJ, Durham SJ, Shah A. Effects of obesity and small body size on operative and long-term outcomes of coronary artery bypass surgery: a propensity matched analysis. Ann Thorac Surg. 2005;79:1976–86.

127. Kuduvalli M, Grayson AD, Oo AY, Fabri BM, Abbas R. Eur J Cardiothorac Surg. 2002;22:787–93.

128. Lv M, Gao F, Liu B, et al. The effects of obesity following coronary artery bypass graft surgery. A retrospective study from a single center in China. Med Sci Monit PLoS Med. 2020;17(10):e1003351. https://doi.org/10.1371/journal.pmed.1003351.

129. Terada T, Forhan M, Norris CM, et al. Differences in short- and long-term mortality associated with body mass index following coronary revascularization. J Am Heart Assoc. 2017;33:882–9.

130. Shaper A, Wannamethee S, Walker M. Body weight: implications for coronary heart disease, stroke, and diabetes mellitus in a cohort of middle-aged men. British Med J. 1997;314:1311–7.

131. Oreopoulos A, Padwal R, Norris CM, Mullen JC, Pretorius V, Kalantar-Zadeh K. Effect of obesity on short-and long-term mortality postcoronary revascularization: a meta-analysis. Obesity. 2008;16:442–50.

132. Stamou SC, Nussbaum M, Stiegel RM, et al. Effect of body mass index on outcomes after cardiac surgery: is there an obesity paradox. Ann Thorac Surg. 2011;91:42–7.

133. Wagner BD, Grunwald GK, Rumsfeld JS, et al. Relationship of body mass index with outcomes after coronary artery bypass graft surgery. Ann Thorac Surg. 2007;84:10–6.

134. Koocheneski V, Amestejaru M, Salmanzadeh HR, Ardabili SS. The effect of obesity on mortality and morbidity after isolated coronary artery bypass graft surgery. Int Cardiovasc Res J. 2012;6:46–50.

135. Lavie CJ, Milani RV, Artham SM, Patel DA, Ventura HO. The obesity paradox and coronary disease. Am J Med. 2009b;122:1106–14.

136. de Schutter A, Kachur S, Lavie CJ, Boddepalli RS, Milani RV. The impact of inflammation on the obesity paradox in coronary heart disease. Int J Obes. 2016;40:1730–5.

137. Lavie CJ, Laddu D, Arena R, Ortega FB, Alpert MA, Kushner RF. Healthy weight and obesity prevention. J Am Coll Cardiol. 2018;72:1506–31.

138. Lavie CJ, Ozemek C, Carbone S, Katzmarzyk PT, Blair SN. Sedentary behavior, exercise and cardiovascular health. Circ Res. 2019;124:799–805.

139. Barry VW, Caputo JC, Kang M. The joint association of fitness and fatness on cardiovascular disease. Prog Cardiovasc Dis. 2018;61:136–41.

140. Lavie CJ, Blair SN. Fitness or fatness. Which is more important? JAMA. 2018;319:231–2.

141. McAuley PA, Artero EG, Sui X, et al. The obesity paradox, cardiorespiratory fitness, and coronary heart disease. Mayo Clin Proc. 2012;87:443–5.

142. Moholdt T, Lavie CJ, Nauman J. Interaction of physical activity and body mass index on mortality in coronary heart disease: data from the Nord-Trondelag health study. Am J Med. 2017;130:949–57.

143. Moholdt T, Lavie CJ, Nauman J. Sustained physical activity, not weight loss is associated with improved survival in coronary heart disease. J Am Coll Cardiol. 2018;71:1094–101.

144. Tian Q, Wang B, Chen S, Wu S. Moderate physical activity may not reduce the risk of cardiovascular disease. J Transl Med. 2022; https://doi.org/10.1186/s12967-021-03212-7.

145. Asia-Pacific Cohort Collaboration Investigators. Body mass index and cardiovascular disease in the Asia-Pacific region: an overview of 33 cohorts involving 310,000 participants. Int J Epidemiol. 2003;33:751–8.

146. Pack QR, Rodriguez-Escudero JP, Thomas R, et al. Importance of weight loss in coronary artery disease: a systematic review and meta-analysis. Mayo Clin Proc. 2016;89:1368–77.

Non-alcoholic Fatty Liver Disease

30

Sangwon F. Kim and Jang Hyun Choi

Contents

S. F. Kim (✉)
Division of Endocrinology, Diabetes, and Metabolism,
Johns Hopkins University School of Medicine, Baltimore,
MD, USA
e-mail: skim132@jhmi.edu

J. H. Choi (✉)
Department of Biological Sciences, Ulsan National
Institute of Science and Technology, Ulsan, Republic of
Korea
e-mail: janghchoi@unist.ac.kr

© Springer Nature Switzerland AG 2023
R. S. Ahima (ed.), *Metabolic Syndrome*,
https://doi.org/10.1007/978-3-031-40116-9_36

Abstract

Obesity is associated with nonalcoholic fatty liver disease (NAFLD), cardiovascular disease (CVD), and type 2 diabetes mellitus (T2DM). In recent years, NAFLD has emerged as the most common liver disease, affecting 25% of the global population. NAFLD is characterized by the accumulation of excessive lipids within hepatocytes, insulin resistance, abdominal fat distribution, dyslipidemia, and high blood pressure. NAFLD is highly prevalent in the United States, and represents abnormalities ranging from hepatic steatosis to more severe forms of nonalcoholic steatohepatitis, which can induce cirrhosis, fibrosis, and hepatocellular carcinoma. NAFLD involves a reprogrammed hepatic metabolic machinery that leads to excessive lipid accumulation and imbalances in lipid metabolism and lipid catabolism in the liver. Hepatic lipid homeostasis is well elucidated as a complex processes, including cellular signaling and transcriptional pathways and genes associated with fatty acid (FA) uptake and oxidation and lipogenesis. This chapter discusses the definition, risk factors, and diagnosis of NAFLD. We also describe animal models used to study the disease, i.e., dietary and genetic models. Lastly, we discuss the current therapies for NAFLD.

Keywords

Obesity · Nonalcoholic fatty liver disease (NAFLD) · Nonalcoholic steatohepatitis (NASH) · Cirrhosis · Fibrosis · Hepatocellular carcinoma (HCC) · Lipid accumulation · Insulin resistance · Fatty acid (FA) oxidation · Lipogenesis · FA uptake

Introduction

Obesity is a major health problem worldwide [1]. Obesity is attributed to imbalance between intake and expenditure, and the global prevalence has nearly tripled since 1975. In addition to excessive lipid stores in adipose tissues, obesity leads to ectopic lipid accumulation in the liver, skeletal muscle, heart and pancreas, which alters the function of these organs [2]. Studies have shown that obesity is caused by genetic, environmental, and lifestyle factors [3]. Obesity is preventable and yet it is difficult to maintain a healthy weight due to the busy lifestyle and energy-dense food in modern societies. The rising trends of obesity drives several diseases, including nonalcoholic fatty liver disease (NAFLD), cardiovascular disease

(CVD), type 2 diabetes mellitus (T2DM), and cancer [4]. In particular, obesity is strongly associated with a high incidence of NAFLD [5].

At present, NAFLD is the most common liver disease, affecting 25% of the global population, and is strongly associated with T2DM, dyslipidemia, and CVD [6]. The NAFLD spectrum includes hepatic steatosis, nonalcoholic steatohepatitis (NASH), fibrosis, cirrhosis, and hepatocellular carcinoma (HCC) [7]. Hepatic steatosis results from excessive hepatocellular triglyceride accumulation, and the rate of de novo lipogenesis (DNL) is greater than that of fatty acid (FA) oxidation and export of very low-density lipoprotein (VLDL). NASH is defined as the accumulation of excessive lipid content associated with oxidative injury of hepatocytes, inflammation, and fibrosis [8]. NASH may progress to cirrhosis, characterized by hepatocellular death from apoptosis, severe fibrosis, and distortion of liver architecture, and can lead to liver failure and HCC [9]. Recent reports suggest that over 40% of HCC patients have cirrhosis [10]. Although the pathogenesis of NAFLD has been widely elucidated for many years, our understanding of the molecular mechanisms is still evolving.

Definition of NAFLD

NAFLD is a disease that involves excessive lipid accumulation in the liver. Approximately 25% of the global population has NAFLD [5], which is projected to increase to 33.5% by 2030 [4]. NAFLD is distinguished from alcohol-associated liver disease a history of high alcohol intake. According to diagnostic criteria for NAFLD by the European Association for the Study of the Liver (EASL), National Institute for Health and Care Excellence (NICE), Italian Association for the Study of the Liver (AISF), and American Association for the Study of Liver Diseases, male patients with less than 30 g/day and female patients with less than 20 g/day of alcohol intake can be categorized as NAFLD patients [11]. In addition, the liver disease of NAFLD must be independent of other causes, such as viral hepatitis, autoimmune disease, and other systemic diseases. NAFLD can be divided into the nonalcoholic fatty liver (NAFL), which accumulates fat without inflammation or fibrosis, and nonalcoholic steatohepatitis (NASH), which involves hepatic steatosis with inflammation, ballooned hepatocytes, and fibrosis. Recently, a new definition was proposed to address the uncertain aspect of the current definition of NAFLD. Whether NAFLD is an appropriate name has been argued, as the term, "nonalcoholic" overemphasizes the absence of alcohol. Thus, the newly proposed name metabolic-associated fatty liver disease (MAFLD) was presented by an international panel of experts in 2020 to better define the pathogenesis of the disease owing to the connection between existing liver steatosis and evolving metabolic dysfunction, such as insulin resistance or impaired glucose metabolism [12]. MAFLD indicates a fatty liver disease associated with metabolic dysfunction, and does not exclude patients with alcohol intake, which is the most significant difference between MAFLD and NAFLD. Furthermore, the presence of metabolic disorders is necessary to diagnose MAFLD [13].

Epidemiology

Prevalence of NAFLD

The prevalence of NAFLD is increasing, affecting approximately 25% of the general population [7]. This number is expected to grow steadily to 33.5% by 2030 [4]. To understand the prevalence of NAFLD and select risk factors, several studies have reported the prevalence of NAFLD according to region and sex, among others. Patients with alcohol intake status and viral hepatitis were excluded according to the definition of NAFLD. There are various diagnostic criteria for NAFLD according to EASL, NICE, AISF, and AASLD. Typically, imaging and histology require >5% hepatic steatosis, and there should be no other cause for steatosis. According to medical guidelines, conventional liver biochemistry methods such as measurement of aspartate aminotransferase (AST) and alanine aminotransferase (ALT) levels and imaging such as ultrasound (US) or magnetic resonance imaging are initially used as noninvasive methods, followed by liver biopsy for accurate diagnosis. However, a biopsy is not recommended because it is invasive and increases risk of complications. Due to these criteria, the diagnosis of NAFLD has been the focus of various studies. In the USA, an extended 34-pooled prevalence study of 368,569 patients conducted from 2004 to 2016 found that NAFLD had a prevalence of 11.2% [14]. In addition, according to a cross-sectional analysis of the National Health and Nutrition Examination Survey from 2011 to 2014, the prevalence of NAFLD was 21.9% (30.7% in women and 15.3% in men). The prevalence according to age was 9.41% for those 40 years or younger, 24.65% for those >40–59 years, and 46.52% for those >60 years, which tended to increase with age [15].

In Asia, the prevalence of NAFLD is estimated at 31%, according to 195 pooled prevalence studies of 1,753,168 patients from 1989 to 2017 [16]. In a cohort study of 565 subjects performed in Hong Kong, the incidence of NAFLD was estimated to be 34 per 1000 persons per year [17]. A meta-analysis reported that the incidence of NAFLD in Asia was approximately 52 per 1000 persons per year, whereas in Israel, NAFLD incidence was 28 per 1000 person-years [7]. The same meta-analysis showed that the incidence of advanced fibrosis in patients with NASH was approximately 68 per 1000 person-years, whereas the incidence rate of HCC was estimated to be 5 per 1000 person-years [7]. In addition, in a Chinese cohort, the incidence of NAFLD increased with age. The incidence was 11.7% for those aged 20–34 years, 15.9% for those aged 35–49 years, 21.5% for those aged 50–64 years, and 22.8% for those aged 65 years or older [18].

In Europe, an observational cohort study in Poland diagnosed NAFLD using the NAFLD fibrosis score and showed prevalence of 37.2%. In addition, depending on the age group, the prevalence of NAFLD was 68.7% under the age of 80 and 36.3% over the age of 80 [19]. In other regions, the prevalence of NAFLD was as follows: 31.79% in the Middle East based on 1592 patients in three studies; 30.45% in South America based on 424 patients in three studies; and 13.48% in Africa in two studies with 250 patients

[7]. When summarizing the results of 32 studies from 2003 to 2018, the prevalence of NAFLD ranged from 11.2% to 37.2%, and the rate of NAFLD progression to biopsy-confirmed NASH ranged from 15.9% to 68.3% [20].

Clinical Impact of NAFLD

According to a review of 45 studies, the mortality rate was 15.4 per 1000 NAFLD patients and 25.6 per 1000 NASH patients [7]. The liver-related mortality was 0.77 per 1000 for NAFLD and 11.77 for NASH. In the United States, 10–20% of patients with HCC are diagnosed with NAFLD [21]. This shows 0.44 per 1000 people per year [7]. Furthermore, NASH is currently the fastest-growing cause of liver transplantation and was the second-highest reason for transplantation in men and the highest reason for transplantation in women in 2016 [22]. In addition to liver-related deaths, NAFLD is associated with clinical CVD. CVD is the most common cause of death in patients with NAFLD, and a meta-analysis of the association of NAFLD with diabetes and hypertension, which are risk factors for CVD, further supports this phenomenon [7].

Risk Factors of NAFLD

Genetic Factors

The difference in the prevalence of NAFLD between races shows that genetic factors are a risk factor for NAFLD. Genetic factors associated with NAFLD include triglyceride (TG) accumulation, hepatocellular dysfunction, chronic liver inflammation, and fibrosis. The incidence of NAFLD increases by up to 27% in the presence of specific mutations in or around *TM6SF2* and *PNPLA3*, which are associated with liver fat accumulation or elevated liver enzymes and are involved in TG and phospholipid metabolism [23]. Additionally, *MBOAT7*, *GCKR*, and *HMOX-1* are associated with NAFLD.

TM6SF2: TM6SF2 (transmembrane 6 superfamily member 2) is highly expressed in human and mouse liver, intestine, and kidney, and encodes proteins involved in liver TG secretion [24]. According to population genetic studies, the TM6SF2 E167K variant resulted in changes in liver TG, total cholesterol content, and ALT, confirming that TM6SF2 is a risk factor for NAFLD [25]. However, the TM6SF2 E167K variant has also been reported to have a cardioprotective effect with reduced CVD risk [26].

PNPLA3: PNPLA3 (patatin-like phospholipase domain-containing 3) is a highly expressed gene in the human liver that binds mainly to lipid droplets in mammalian cells and acts as a lipase [27]. The mutated variant of the PNPLA3 accumulates lipid droplets and disrupts lipid metabolism due to its altered lipase activity [28]. In addition, the I148M mutation in PNPLA3 indirectly affects the liver by triggering TG accumulation in brown adipocytes [29].

MBOAT7: MBOAT7 (membrane-bound O-acyltransferase domain-containing 7) is highly expressed in inflammatory cells and associated with acyltransferase activity. The resulting acyl chain remodeling of phospholipids improves susceptibility to steatosis. The rs641738C>T variant near the MBOAT7 locus is associated with fibrosis in liver diseases, including NAFLD and primary liver fibrosis [30]. Mboat7 deficiency in mice and humans indicates an inflammation-independent pathway of liver fibrosis that may be mediated by lipid signaling [31]. MBOAT7 is also involved in lipid droplet remodeling and steatosis [32].

GCKR: GCKR (glucokinase regulator) functions as a post-transcriptional regulator of glucokinase in the liver. Hepatic glucokinase stimulates glycogen accumulation and de novo lipogenesis DNL. The rs780094 and rs1260326 variants of GCKR are associated with metabolism of TG, VLDL, high-density lipoprotein, etc., which affect the pathogenesis of NAFLD [33]. Moreover, the rs780094 variant correlates with the progression of hepatic fibrosis [34].

MMOX1: HO-1 (heme oxygenase 1, encoded by *HMOX1*) is the main heme catabolic enzyme that degrades free heme to iron, carbon monoxide, and biliverdin [35]. Pediatric NAFLD patients with genetic polymorphisms in the HMOX1 promoter region showed increased serum ALT levels [36]. Inhibition of HO-1 can enhance lipogenesis and collagen production, which can induce liver fibrosis [37]. Canesin et al. demonstrated that deletion of HO-1 in myeloid cells promotes liver injury and fibrosis via a Notch-1-dependent pathway [38].

Obesity

Several studies have shown a connection between obesity and NAFLD. With liver biopsies in obese patients undergoing bariatric surgery in the USA, the NAFLD, and NASH prevalence were 41.9% and 30.4%, respectively [39]. In 2016, a literature review and meta-analysis of 368,569 high-risk patients from 34 studies showed a pooled NAFLD prevalence of 55.7%. In this study, 55.5% of White, 48.8% of Hispanic, and 47.6% of Black patients had NAFLD [14]. An analysis of obese adults referred for bariatric surgery conducted in 2007–2009 in France showed a 12.6% prevalence when NASH was measured using the NAFLD activity score [40]. Abdominal obesity significantly affects NAFLD, and visceral adipose tissue area is associated with an increased risk of NASH and fibrosis [41]. The risk of developing NAFLD has been reported to increase in response to a weight increase of 2 kg [42]. A recent systematic meta-analysis estimated the prevalence of NAFLD, NAFL, and NASH in obese patients. Among all overweight individuals, the estimated NAFLD prevalence was 59.7% in Asian and Middle Eastern countries or territories, and 75% in European countries and North and South America. These data strongly suggest that obesity is a major risk factor for NAFLD [43].

Type 2 Diabetes

Type 2 diabetes mellitus (T2DM) is also strongly associated with NAFLD. Insulin resistance, caused by T2DM, affects liver steatosis. Insulin resistance triggers lipolysis in adipose tissue, provides free fatty acids (FFAs) to the liver, and promotes DNL to increase fat accumulation [44, 45].

T2DM also alters macrophages and is related to leptin resistance and liver inflammation [46]. Systematic literature reviews and meta-analyses of 17 studies on adults with T2DM from 2005 to 2017 found that 54% of 10,897 T2DM patients had NAFLD [47]. In addition, in a study based on papers from 1989 to 2017, 65.3% of T2DM patients had NASH: 78% were in the Western Pacific region, 76% in Southeast Asia, and 59% in America [48]. In addition, an estimated 25% of the adult population in Western countries have NAFLD, but this prevalence increases to 60–80% in patients with obesity or T2DM and can reach 80–100% when both risk factors are present [5, 49]. Of these NAFLD cases, 20–30% progress to liver inflammation and fibrosis. The prevalence of NAFLD in patients with dysregulated glucose metabolism, such as insulin resistance, is increasing. It has been demonstrated that patients with NAFLD showed significantly impaired fasting glucose and impaired glucose tolerance [50]. Furthermore, patients with both T2DM and NAFLD have a higher risk of developing NASH, which can predispose to liver cancer. Collectively, these data suggest that the pathogenesis of NAFLD is tightly associated with impaired glucose metabolism and insulin resistance.

Circadian Rhythm

Circadian rhythms are tightly regulated by clock proteins and play an essential role in various physiological functions in the body including metabolic processes [51]. The dysregulation of the circadian clock contributes to NAFLD progression through lipid dysregulation, oxidative stress, and inflammation [52, 53]. Bmal1-deficient mice have metabolic defects, including high serum triglyceride (TG) and low circulating insulin levels [54, 55]. Specific disruption of the hepatic circadian rhythm via liver-specific Bmal1 deletion exacerbates hepatic steatosis, increases insulin resistance, and impairs hepatic gluconeogenesis in obese mice [53]. Furthermore, Clock mutant mice display impaired glucose tolerance, hyperinsulinemia, T2DM, and hepatic steatosis [55].

Studies have shown that poor sleep quality and sleep deprivation are associated with obesity and NAFLD [56]. Yang et al. reported that people with poor nighttime sleep and prolonged daytime napping have the highest risk of developing NAFLD [57]. Improvement in nighttime sleep quality resulted in a 29% reduction in NAFLD progression. The levels of inflammatory cytokines interleukin-6 (IL-6) and tumor necrosis factor-alpha (TNF-α) were increased with sleep deprivation, promoting hepatic steatosis and adipocyte lipolysis [58]. In population cohort studies, sleep deprivation is associated with NAFLD with an odd ratio of 1.28 for men and 1.71 for women [59].

Gut Microbiota

The gut microbiota plays important physiological roles in host digestion, immunity, and metabolism [60]. Increasing evidence has demonstrated a causal role of gut microbiota in NAFLD pathophysiology. Direct fecal microbiota transplantation from obese mice to germ-free recipients significantly increased NAFLD progression, including increased hepatic steatosis and dysregulation of gene expression in the lipid metabolism [61]. In addition, co-housing healthy wild-type mice with genetically modified mice prone to developing NASH resulted in a NAFLD phenotype with liver steatosis and inflammation in the healthy wild-type mice [62]. How does the gut microbiota regulate the progression of NAFLD and NASH? Gut microbes may increase intestinal permeability, which leads to the release of lipopolysaccharide (LPS, a major component of the gram-negative bacterial outer membrane) into the host's circulation. LPS can induce systemic inflammation and alter microbial metabolites, such as trimethylamine N-oxide, choline, and ethanol, affecting immune responses [63]. An imbalanced gut microbiota increases free fatty acid (FFA) absorption by increasing intestinal permeability and the release of inflammatory cytokines, such as IL-6 and TNF-α [64], leading to intestinal lipid accumulation and inflammation. Bacterial communities also produce short-chain

FAs, including butyrate, propionate, and acetate shown to mediate beneficial or anti-inflammatory effects that could prevent the progression of NAFLD and NASH [63].

Deconjugation of primary bile acids into secondary bile acids is another major function of gut microbiota. Primary and secondary bile acids perform critical functions through different receptors [65]. The gut microbiota regulates secondary bile acid metabolism and lipid synthesis in the liver by acting on the farnesoid X receptor (FXR) [66]. Dysregulated bile acid composition is significantly associated with metabolic diseases, such as insulin resistance and NAFLD [67]. In addition, intestinal microbial groups can cause NAFLD along with lipid accumulation in the intestine through FXR activation via changes in bile acid metabolism [68].

Diagnosis

Most individuals with NAFLD are asymptomatic and show elevated liver enzymes (usually less than five times the upper limit of the normal level) or evidence of steatosis in imaging studies [69, 70]. For the diagnosis of NAFLD, evidence of hepatic steatosis on imaging or histology is required, and liver disease or other causes of steatosis must be ruled out [71]. Unlike NAFLD, NASH is diagnosed based on the presence of steatohepatitis on the liver biopsy [72]. Currently, markers that can accurately and specifically diagnose NAFLD are lacking. The NAFLD liver fat score is calculated using the presence of metabolic syndrome, T2DM, insulin resistance, low albumin levels (less than 3.6 g per dL [36 g per L]), fasting serum insulin, fasting serum AST, and the AST/ALT ratio (AAR), as well as TG and cholesterol levels above the normal range [71, 72]. It is important to highlight that the degree of AST increase may not be proportional to the degree of hepatocellular injury associated with the NAFLD/NASH [73]. Gamma glutamyltransferase is often elevated in patients with NAFLD and associated with advanced fibrosis and increased mortality [70]. The AST to platelet (PLT) ratio index (APRI), fibrosis-4 (FIB-4) index = Age ([yr] ×

Table 1 Grading of NAFLD/NASH

Grade or stage	Brunt criteria	NASH Clinical Research Network
Fibrosis		
0	None	None
1	Zone 3 perisinusoidal fibrosis	Perisinusoidal or periportal fibrosis
2	Zone 3 perisinusoidal and periportal fibrosis	Perisinusoidal and periportal fibrosis
3	Bridging fibrosis	Bridging fibrosis
4	Cirrhosis	Cirrhosis
Hepatocyte ballooning		
0	None	None
1	Mild in zone 3	Few
2	Prominent in zone 3	Many
3	Marked in zone 3	
Lobular inflammation		
0	None	None
1	1–2 foci per 20X field	<2 foci per 20X field
2	2–4 foci per 20X field	2–4 foci per 20X field
3	>4 foci per 20X field	>4 foci per 20X field
Portal inflammation		
0	None	None
1	Mild	Mild
2	Moderate	Moderate
3	Severe	
Hepatocyte steatosis		
0	None	<5%
1	≤33%	5–33%
2	33–66%	33–67%
3	>66%	>67%

AST [U/L]/(PLT [10^9/L]) × (ALT [U/L])(1/2)), and FibroScan results are used for the evaluation of hepatic fibrosis. NAFLD/NASH can be diagnosed and staged through histological examination [74]; Table 1; Figs. 1 and 2.

Animal Models of NAFLD

Animal models show various aspects of the NAFLD spectrum, i.e., steatosis, hepatocyte injury, inflammation, and fibrosis (Table 2).

Dietary Models

Dietary models, including obesogenic and nutrient-deficient models, can effectively trigger the development of NAFLD and NASH.

High-Fat Diet: One of the simplest ways to induce hepatic steatosis is by disrupting lipid metabolism by feeding a high-fat diet (HFD; 60% fat, 20% protein, and 20% carbohydrate) to mice [75, 76]. With a HFD, the total caloric intake of animals is 45–75%, and HFD represents the most commonly used obesity model in rodents [77]. HFD mice develop hyperlipidemia, hyperinsulinemia, glucose intolerance, hepatic steatosis, increased liver TG levels, hepatocyte swelling, increased fasting glucose, and decreased adiponectin levels [78, 79]. Despite hepatic steatosis, no evidence of fibrosis was observed until 19 weeks of HFD intake [76]. After long-term (34–36 weeks) HFD feeding, significant increases in circulating liver enzyme levels, (e.g., ALT and AST) were observed; these mice showed only minor signs of inflammation and fibrosis [80], even after prolonged administration

Fig. 1 Liver histology from a patient with NASH. Hematoxylin and Eosin staining shows nodules of hepatocytes with steatosis. Reticulin staining highlights nodular liver architecture. Trichrome staining shows bands of fibrosis. (Image source: https://www.aasld.org/liver-fellow-network/core-series/pathology-pearls/liver-pathology-steatohepatitis)

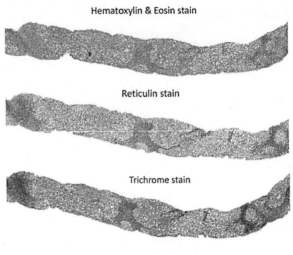

Fig. 2 NASH histology showing periportal hepatosteatosis, ballooning degeneration (enlarged hepatocytes with granular cytoplasm representing collapsed cytoskeleton), and Mallory hyaline bodies (representing clumps of eosinophilic misfolded and aggregated keratin filaments). (Image sources: https://commons.wikimedia.org/wiki/File:Periportal_hepatosteatosis_intermed_mag.jpg; https://www.aasld.org/liver-fellow-network/core-series/pathology-pearls/liver-pathology-steatohepatitis)

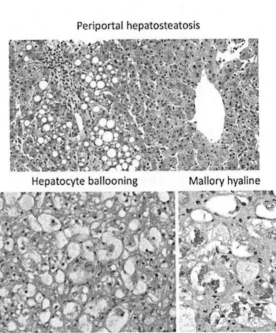

for up to 50 weeks [76]. Thus, HFD-fed animals mainly mimic the histopathology of human obesity, insulin resistance, hepatic steatosis, and hyperglycemia (Fig. 3).

High-Fat/High-Fructose/Sucrose: To increase hepatic fibrosis and steatosis, a high fat/high-fructose or high-sucrose (HF/HFr or HF/sucrose, respectively) consumption can be used [81, 82]. Administration of an alternative fast food-like diet based on HF/HFr (41%/30%) has also been shown to induce NASH [83]. Fructose metabolism differs from that of glucose. The hepatic metabolism of

fructose favors DNL and stimulates the synthesis of TG and FFAs. Fructose overconsumption is associated with obesity [84]. In addition, HFr consumption and increased fat intake have been reported as risk factors for developing NAFLD. Even in the absence of obesity, fructose consumption causes severe changes, such as dyslipidemia, insulin resistance, and NAFLD, with areas of inflammation. Compared to lean controls, male mice fed an HFr diet alone or combined with an HFD (HF/HFr) had increased plasma cholesterol and TG levels and insulin resistance.

Table 2 Animal models of NAFLD

Model	Obesity	Steatosis	NASH	Fibrosis
Dietary model				
HFD	++	++	+	–
HF/HFr	++	++	++	++
MCD	–	++	++	++
WD	++	++	+	–
Genetic model				
db/db	++	++	–	–
ob/ob	++	++	–	–
PPARα KO	–	++	++	++
SREBP1c Tg	–	++	++	++
CD36 Tg	–	+	–	–

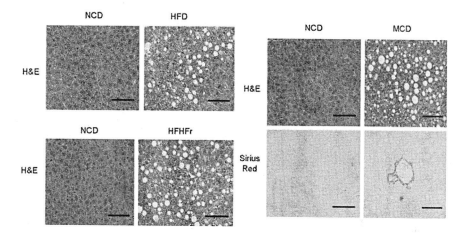

Fig. 3 Liver histology from mice fed with normal chow, high-fat diet (HFD), HFD with high-fructose/sucrose (HF/HFr), or methionine- and choline-deficient (MCD) diet. Hematoxylin and eosin (H&E) staining shows lipid droplet accumulation. Liver fibrosis was examined by Sirius Red staining. Scale bars, 100 μm

Methionine- and Choline-Deficient (MCD) Diet: Diets with low content or lacking certain nutrients can also be used to develop NAFLD/NASH features. MCD diets are generally high in sucrose (40%) and moderately rich in fat (10%) but lack methionine and choline, which are essential for hepatic β-oxidation and VLDL production [85]. Choline is a crucial nutrient mainly stored and metabolized in the liver. Animals deprived of only choline have impaired liver VLDL secretion, resulting in hepatic steatosis, oxidative stress, hepatocyte death, and altered cytokine and adipose cytokine levels, resulting in mild liver inflammation and fibrosis [86]. However, mice fed a diet deficient in both choline and methionine showed rapid NASH development with severe liver fibrosis within 4–10 weeks [87], most likely due to reduced VLDL synthesis and hepatic β-oxidation [79]. MCD has also been associated with hepatic microsomal lipid peroxidation. The liver showed macrosteatosis, inflammation, and perivenular and pericellular fibrosis [88]. The severity of NASH induced by the MCD diet differs among mouse strains. The MCD diet in C57BL/6 J mice primarily resulted in inflammation and necrosis and most closely approximated the histological features of the NASH [89]. The MCD diet better mimics the pathological features of severe NASH in humans. In addition, inflammation, fibrosis, and hepatocyte apoptosis occurred faster and more severely than in the HFD-fed mice. Therefore, this model is suitable for studying histologically advanced NASH and the mechanisms of inflammation and fibrosis [90].

Western Diet: Excessive food intake with high saturated fat, high carbohydrates, and cholesterol, known as the Western diet (WD), is a major reason for NAFLD development in humans and mice. In a mouse model, WD can induce hepatic steatosis, NASH, and hepatic fibrosis in a pathophysiological process similar to humans. Unlike the MCD diet, researchers can vary the composition of WD. Liver changes in mice fed a WD are highly variable, depending on the contents of the diet. Specifically, WD-fed male mice showed significantly impaired insulin sensitivity and increased hepatic steatosis by regulating lipid metabolism, such as downregulation of genes involved in FA oxidation and FA uptake and upregulation of genes associated with DNL [79]. However, WD barely induces hepatic fibrosis.

Genetic Models

db/db and ob/ob Mice: **Mice lacking functional leptin receptor**, *db/db*, are homozygous for the autosomal recessive diabetic gene (*db*). The *lepr* (*db*) gene encodes a point mutation in the leptin receptor, which leads to a defective leptin signaling [91]. Therefore, *db/db* mice have elevated leptin levels but are resistant to these effects. Leptin inhibits food inake [92], thus, *db/db* mice are hyperphagic, and develop early-onset obesity with severe insulin resistance, hyperglycemia, and neuroendocrine deficits [93]. *db/db* mice have macrovesicular hepatic steatosis but do not spontaneously develop steatohepatitis or fibrosis. Prolonged overfeeding (>1 month) leads to slightly aggravated hepatic inflammation [91]. Therefore, *db/db* mice are a good model for NAFLD but not NASH. Nevertheless, *db/db* mice fed an MCD diet showed increased inflammation and serum ALT levels compared to *db/db* mice and *ob/ob* mice fed a control diet. Moreover, *db/db* mice fed an MCD diet showed pericellular fibrosis [94].

ob/ob mice carry an autosomal recessive mutation in the leptin (*lep*) gene [95]. Unlike *db/db* mice, *ob/ob* mice have functional leptin receptors but truncated, nonfunctional leptin. These mice are hyperphagic and obese and prone to the development of steatosis, insulin resistance, hyperinsulinemia, hyperglycemia, severely reduced energy expenditure, and neuroendocrine deficits [96]. The advantage of *db/db* and *ob/ob* mice is they show characteristics of fatty liver and metabolic syndrome, rather than NASH or fibrosis, unlike the MCD dietary model [87].

Peroxisome Proliferator-Activated Receptor α (PPARα) Knockout (KO) Mice: PPARα is a ligand-activated nuclear receptor mainly expressed in the liver. PPARα acts as a nutritional regulator that controls the rates of FA catabolism and ketogenesis in response to fasting [97]. FA oxidation is regulated by PPARα, which provides an energy source for adenosine triphosphate (ATP) generation in mitochondria. PPARα controls the gene expression level of rate-limiting enzymes, including acyl-CoA oxidase 1, and FA uptake into the mitochondrial membrane is mediated by carnitine palmitoyltransferase-1 [98]. Knockout of PPARα in mice fed a HFD upregulated the markers of hepatic lipid metabolism, inflammation, and oxidative stress, resulting in hepatic steatosis [99]. Comparing wild-type and PPARα KO mice fed with MCD diet, the PPARα KO mice displayed more severe NASH progression, including hepatic TG accumulation and hepatocellular injury than wild-type mice [100]. Thus, PPARα plays a crucial role in the pathogenesis of NAFLD and NASH by regulating lipid metabolism and inflammation.

Sterol Regulatory Element-Binding Protein 1c (SREBP1c) Transgenic Mice: DNL is the process of synthesizing new fatty acids from acetyl-CoA produced in the mitochondria. Acetyl-CoA is transformed to malonyl-CoA by acetyl-CoA carboxylase (ACC) and then converted to FAs by fatty acid synthase (FASN) [101]. These FAs form TG, which is stored in hepatocytes and exported as VLDL vesicles to peripheral organs for energy consumption. Thus, excessive DNL significantly induces the development of NAFLD and NASH by increasing FA levels, causing severe inflammation and fibrosis [102]. The transcriptional regulation of DNL is controlled by SREBP1c, which is induced by carbohydrates, lipids, and insulin signaling. SREBP1c transgenic mice showed high levels of hepatic TG and expression of lipogenic genes. Also, elevated SREBP1c significantly increased the expression of downstream targets in DNL, including ACC and FASN, with excessive lipid accumulation in hepatocytes, which impairs FA oxidation and inflammation with lipotoxicity [103]. Thus, SREBP1c-mediated DNL is an important pathway in the development of NAFLD and NASH.

Cluster of Differentiation 36 (CD36) Transgenic Mice: Fatty acid (FA) uptake in the liver depends on FA transporters. CD36 regulates the transport of FAs regulated by PPARα and liver X receptor [104]. CD36 is important in NAFLD in that its expression is strongly correlated with the pathogenesis of the disease. Overexpression of hepatic Cd36 in mice results in a marked increase in hepatic FFA uptake and TG storage. The influx of massive amounts of FAs drives hepatic lipotoxicity via impairment of mitochondrial FA oxidation and inflammation. In contrast, hepatocyte-specific Cd36 KO mice were protected from HFD-induced liver steatosis and [105].

Current Therapies for NAFLD

NAFLD is a chronic liver disease associated with obesity and other metabolic disorders such as T2DM and insulin resistance. Currently, the primary treatment for NAFLD includes weight loss, as it can decrease fat accumulation in the liver and improve liver function. In addition, pharmacological treatment and bariatric surgery are also used for NAFLD treatment (Table 3).

Pharmacological Treatment

Although changes in lifestyle, such as exercise and dietary changes, help improve liver function, effective treatment of NAFLD remains challenging. More specifically, no drugs have been approved by the US Food and Drug Administration or the European Medicines Agency for NASH treatment; current drugs are off-label. In addition, pharmacological treatment is recommended only for patients with NASH, fibrosis, or NASH with high inflammatory activity [108, 115]. Insulin-sensitizing agents, such as pioglitazone and metformin, can improve insulin sensitivity and reduce liver fat accumulation. Lipid-lowering agents, such as statins, lower cholesterol levels and reduce the risk of CVD.

Pioglitazone: Pioglitazone is an insulin-sensitizing agent that ameliorates insulin resistance in patients with T2DM. As a PPARγ agonist, pioglitazone shows improved insulin sensitivity, reduced steatosis, and inflammation effects in

Table 3 Current therapies for NAFLD

Treatment	Mechanism of action	Clinical evidence	Reference
Pioglitazone	Activates PPARγ, improves insulin sensitivity	Promising results in several randomized controlled trials	[106, 107]
Vitamin E	Antioxidant properties, reduces oxidative stress	Mixed results in randomized controlled trials, potential for increased risk of prostate cancer	[107, 108]
Metformin	Improves insulin sensitivity, decreases gluconeogenesis	Mixed results in randomized controlled trials, potential for gastrointestinal side effects and lactic acidosis	[109, 110]
Statins	Reduce cholesterol synthesis, anti-inflammatory properties	Mixed results in randomized controlled trials, potential for liver toxicity	[111]
SGLT2 inhibitors	Inhibit glucose reabsorption in kidneys, increases urinary glucose excretion	Positive results in several randomized controlled trials, and increased risk of urinary tract infection	[112]
GLP-1 receptor agonists	Stimulate insulin secretion, reduces appetite and weight	Positive results in randomized controlled trials, potential for gastrointestinal symptoms	[113]
Bariatric surgery	Reduces caloric intake and weight, alters gut hormones and bile acid metabolism	Significant improvement in liver histology and resolution of NASH	[114]

patients with T2DM or NASH [116]. Although the EASL considers the use of pioglitazone only in patients with both NAFLD and diabetes, the NICE and AASLD allow the use of pioglitazone for patients with NAFLD alone [117], as studies showed improvements in NASH over placebo in patients without diabetes. In addition, positive outcomes have been reported from several clinical trials exploring the use of pioglitazone for NAFLD. In a randomized, double-blind, placebo-controlled trial involving 55 patients with NAFLD, pioglitazone improved liver steatosis and critical hepatic enzymes compared to the placebo after 6 months of administration [118]. However, side effects such as weight gain and bone fracture occurred; thus, the use of pioglitazone is limited [119, 120].

Vitamin E: Vitamin E is an antioxidant that reduces oxidative stress, and studies have shown that in NAFLD models, fibrotic genes such as TGF-β and MMP-2 are suppressed, and liver steatosis and inflammation are alleviated [121]. Clinical trials have shown that vitamin E can be effective in patients with NAFLD, particularly those with NASH, a more severe form of the disease. In a randomized, double-blind, placebo-controlled trial involving 247 patients with NASH, vitamin E improved liver histology compared with the placebo after 96 weeks of administration [107]. Although vitamin E is considered in the NICE and AASLD guidelines [108, 117], it is still important to note that a high dose of vitamin E is toxic and may increase the risk of bleeding, which can be a fatal factor in T2DM or CVD.

Metformin: Metformin is an oral antidiabetic medication that is commonly used to treat T2DM. Metformin is an AMP-activated protein kinase-activating agent that effectively improves liver function by reducing hepatic gluconeogenesis and improving insulin sensitivity; however, this is controversial. A clinical trial by Loomba et al. confirmed improved liver histology compared to the placebo after 12 months of treatment [109], but no improvement in the histological characteristics of NAFLD was observed in a study by Bugianesi et al. [122]). Therefore, metformin may not be beneficial in NAFLD.

Statins: Statins are used to treat dyslipidemia and are effective against cardiovascular disease

(CVD). Statins reduce cholesterol synthesis by acting as HMG-CoA reductase inhibitors. Due to the association between NAFLD and CVD, many patients with NAFLD receive statins. In practice, statins effectively relieve cardiovascular morbidity in patients with NAFLD [123]. Statin treatment is often safe and well tolerated by patients; however, in patients with decompensated cirrhosis, especially those with Child-Pugh class C cirrhosis, benefits are more limited, and risks are increased [124].

SGLT2 and GLP-1 Agonists: SGLT2 (sodium-glucose cotransporter 2) inhibitors and GLP-1 (glucagon-like peptide-1) receptor agonists are effective for treatment of T2DM and may also have beneficial effects on NAFLD. In a randomized controlled trial, an SGLT2 inhibitor improved hepatic enzymes and ameliorated hepatic steatosis in patients with NAFLD and T2DM [112, 125]. GLP-1 receptor agonists reduce weight and may improve NAFLD [113, 126].

Bariatric Surgery: For patients with severe obesity and other metabolic disorders, bariatric surgery is recommended. Gastric bypass is a type of bariatric surgery that reduces the size of the stomach and reroutes the small intestine to reduce the amount of food consumed and absorbed. It has been shown to improve liver function and reduce liver fat in patients with NAFLD [127]. Sleeve gastrectomy is another type of bariatric surgery that removes a portion of the stomach to reduce its size and limit the amount of food consumed. It has also been effective in reducing liver fat in patients with NAFLD [128]. Biliopancreatic diversion is a more complex type of bariatric surgery that reroutes the small intestine to limit the amount of food that can be absorbed and stimulate bile production. It improves liver function and reduces liver fat in patients with NAFLD [129].

Conclusions

With the increasing association of metabolic disorders associated with obesity, there is an increase in the burden of NAFLD. According to the WHO, NAFLD is currently the most common liver disease worldwide, associated with T2DM, dyslipidemia, and CVD. Despite growing evidence of NAFLD progression, there remains a lack of treatment strategies beyond lifestyle. Therefore, a better understanding of NAFLD pathophysiology is necessary for prevention and effective treatment.

Acknowledgments JHC is supported by NRF-2021R1I1A2041463 and KGM5392212, and SFK is supported by the American Heart Association 20SFRN35210662

References

1. Younossi Z, et al. Global burden of NAFLD and NASH: trends, predictions, risk factors and prevention. Nat Rev Gastroenterol Hepatol. 2018;15(1):11–20.
2. Kim D, et al. Changing trends in etiology-based annual mortality from chronic liver disease, from 2007 through 2016. Gastroenterology. 2018;155(4):1154–63.e3.
3. Fan JG, Kim SU, Wong VW. New trends on obesity and NAFLD in Asia. J Hepatol. 2017;67(4):862–73.
4. Estes C, et al. Modeling the epidemic of nonalcoholic fatty liver disease demonstrates an exponential increase in burden of disease. Hepatology. 2018;67(1):123–33.
5. Younossi Z, et al. Global perspectives on nonalcoholic fatty liver disease and nonalcoholic steatohepatitis. Hepatology. 2019;69(6):2672–82.
6. Anstee QM, Targher G, Day CP. Progression of NAFLD to diabetes mellitus, cardiovascular disease or cirrhosis. Nat Rev Gastroenterol Hepatol. 2013;10(6):330–44.
7. Younossi ZM, et al. Global epidemiology of nonalcoholic fatty liver disease-meta-analytic assessment of prevalence, incidence, and outcomes. Hepatology. 2016;64(1):73–84.
8. Feijo SG, et al. The spectrum of non alcoholic fatty liver disease in morbidly obese patients: prevalence and associate risk factors. Acta Cir Bras. 2013;28(11):788–93.
9. White DL, Kanwal F, El-Serag HB. Association between nonalcoholic fatty liver disease and risk for hepatocellular cancer, based on systematic review. Clin Gastroenterol Hepatol. 2012;10(12):1342.
10. Yang JD, et al. A global view of hepatocellular carcinoma: trends, risk, prevention and management. Nat Rev Gastroenterol Hepatol. 2019;16(10):589–604.
11. Yamamura S, et al. MAFLD identifies patients with significant hepatic fibrosis better than NAFLD. Liver Int. 2020;40(12):3018–30.
12. Eslam M, et al. A new definition for metabolic dysfunction-associated fatty liver disease: an

international expert consensus statement. J Hepatol. 2020;73(1):202–9.
13. Chalasani N, et al. The diagnosis and management of non-alcoholic fatty liver disease: practice guideline by the American Gastroenterological Association, American Association for the Study of Liver Diseases, and American College of Gastroenterology. Gastroenterology. 2012;142(7):1592–609.
14. Rich NE, et al. Racial and ethnic disparities in non-alcoholic fatty liver disease prevalence, severity, and outcomes in the United States: a systematic review and meta-analysis. Clin Gastroenterol Hepatol. 2018;16(2):198–210 e2.
15. Wong RJ, Liu B, Bhuket T. Significant burden of nonalcoholic fatty liver disease with advanced fibrosis in the US: a cross-sectional analysis of 2011-2014 National Health and Nutrition Examination Survey. Aliment Pharmacol Ther. 2017;46(10):974–80.
16. Li J, et al. Prevalence of non-alcoholic fatty liver disease(Nafld) in Asia: a systematic review and meta-analysis of 195 studies and 1,753,168 subjects from 15 countries and areas. Gastroenterology. 2018;154(6):S1165.
17. Wong VW, et al. Incidence of non-alcoholic fatty liver disease in Hong Kong: a population study with paired proton-magnetic resonance spectroscopy. J Hepatol. 2015;62(1):182–9.
18. Lin Y, et al. Age patterns of nonalcoholic fatty liver disease incidence: heterogeneous associations with metabolic changes. Diabetol Metab Syndr. 2022;14(1):181.
19. Hartleb M, et al. Non-alcoholic fatty liver and advanced fibrosis in the elderly: results from a community-based polish survey. Liver Int. 2017;37(11):1706–14.
20. Dufour J-F, et al. The global epidemiology of non-alcoholic steatohepatitis (NASH) and associated risk factors – a targeted literature review. Endocr Metabol Sci. 2021;3:100089.
21. Mantovani A, et al. Complications, morbidity and mortality of nonalcoholic fatty liver disease. Metabolism. 2020;111S:154170.
22. Noureddin M, et al. NASH leading cause of liver transplant in women: updated analysis of indications for liver transplant and ethnic and gender variances. Am J Gastroenterol. 2018;113(11):1649–59.
23. Rotman Y, et al. The association of genetic variability in patatin-like phospholipase domain-containing protein 3 (PNPLA3) with histological severity of nonalcoholic fatty liver disease. Hepatology. 2010;52(3):894–903.
24. Smagris E, et al. Inactivation of Tm6sf2, a gene defective in fatty liver disease, impairs lipidation but not secretion of very low density lipoproteins. J Biol Chem. 2016;291(20):10659–76.
25. Kozlitina J, et al. Exome-wide association study identifies a TM6SF2 variant that confers susceptibility to nonalcoholic fatty liver disease. Nat Genet. 2014;46(4):352–6.

26. Holmen OL, et al. Systematic evaluation of coding variation identifies a candidate causal variant in TM6SF2 influencing total cholesterol and myocardial infarction risk. Nat Genet. 2014;46(4):345–51.

27. Sookoian S, Pirola CJ. PNPLA3, the triacylglycerol synthesis/hydrolysis/storage dilemma, and non-alcoholic fatty liver disease. World J Gastroenterol. 2012;18(42):6018–26.

28. BasuRay S, et al. The PNPLA3 variant associated with fatty liver disease (I148M) accumulates on lipid droplets by evading ubiquitylation. Hepatology. 2017;66(4):1111–24.

29. Yang A, et al. Dynamic interactions of ABHD5 with PNPLA3 regulate triacylglycerol metabolism in brown adipocytes. Nat Metab. 2019;1(5):560–9.

30. Teo K, et al. rs641738C>T near MBOAT7 is associated with liver fat, ALT and fibrosis in NAFLD: a meta-analysis. J Hepatol. 2021;74(1):20–30.

31. Thangapandi VR, et al. Loss of hepatic Mboat7 leads to liver fibrosis. Gut. 2021;70(5):940–50.

32. Meroni M, et al. Mboat7 down-regulation by hyper-insulinemia induces fat accumulation in hepatocytes. EBioMedicine. 2020;52:102658.

33. Stancakova A, et al. Effects of 34 risk loci for type 2 diabetes or hyperglycemia on lipoprotein subclasses and their composition in 6,580 nondiabetic Finnish men. Diabetes. 2011;60(5):1608–16.

34. Petta S, et al. Glucokinase regulatory protein gene polymorphism affects liver fibrosis in non-alcoholic fatty liver disease. PLoS One. 2014;9(2):e87523.

35. Canesin G, et al. Heme-derived metabolic signals dictate immune responses. Front Immunol. 2020;11:66.

36. Chang PF, et al. Heme oxygenase-1 gene promoter polymorphism and the risk of pediatric nonalcoholic fatty liver disease. Int J Obes. 2015;39(8):1236–40.

37. Raffaele M, et al. Inhibition of Heme oxygenase antioxidant activity exacerbates hepatic steatosis and fibrosis in vitro. Antioxidants (Basel). 2019;8(8):277.

38. Canesin G, et al. Heme oxygenase-1 mitigates liver injury and fibrosis via modulation of LNX1/Notch1 pathway in myeloid cells. iScience. 2022;25(9):104983.

39. Mehta R, et al. The role of mitochondrial genomics in patients with non-alcoholic steatohepatitis (NASH). BMC Med Genet. 2016;17(1):63.

40. Anty R, et al. A new composite model including metabolic syndrome, alanine aminotransferase and cytokeratin-18 for the diagnosis of non-alcoholic steatohepatitis in morbidly obese patients. Aliment Pharmacol Ther. 2010;32(11–12):1315–22.

41. Yu SJ, et al. Visceral obesity predicts significant fibrosis in patients with nonalcoholic fatty liver disease. Medicine (Baltimore). 2015;94(48):e2159.

42. Chang Y, et al. Weight gain within the normal weight range predicts ultrasonographically detected fatty liver in healthy Korean men. Gut. 2009;58(10):1419–25.

43. Quek J, et al. Global prevalence of non-alcoholic fatty liver disease and non-alcoholic steatohepatitis in the overweight and obese population: a systematic review and meta-analysis. Lancet Gastroenterol Hepatol. 2023;8(1):20–30.

44. Polyzos SA, Kountouras J, Zavos C. Nonalcoholic fatty liver disease: the pathogenetic roles of insulin resistance and adipocytokines. Curr Mol Med. 2009;9(3):299–314.

45. Bugianesi E, et al. Insulin resistance in nonalcoholic fatty liver disease. Curr Pharm Des. 2010;16(17):1941–51.

46. Polyzos SA, et al. The potential adverse role of leptin resistance in nonalcoholic fatty liver disease a hypothesis based on critical review of the literature. J Clin Gastroenterol. 2011;45(1):50–4.

47. Amiri Dash Atan N, et al. Type 2 diabetes mellitus and non-alcoholic fatty liver disease: a systematic review and meta-analysis. Gastroenterol Hepatol Bed Bench. 2017;10(Suppl1):S1–7.

48. Golabi P, et al. The worldwide prevalence of non-alcoholic steatohepatitis (NASH) in patients with type 2 diabetes mellitus (DM). J Hepatol. 2018;68:S841.

49. Powell EE, Wong VW, Rinella M. Non-alcoholic fatty liver disease. Lancet. 2021;397(10290):2212–24.

50. Ortiz-Lopez C, et al. Prevalence of prediabetes and diabetes and metabolic profile of patients with non-alcoholic fatty liver disease (NAFLD). Diabetes Care. 2012;35(4):873–8.

51. Serin Y, Acar Tek N. Effect of circadian rhythm on metabolic processes and the regulation of energy balance. Ann Nutr Metab. 2019;74(4):322–30.

52. Adamovich Y, et al. Circadian clocks and feeding time regulate the oscillations and levels of hepatic triglycerides. Cell Metab. 2014;19(2):319–30.

53. Jacobi D, et al. Hepatic Bmal1 regulates rhythmic mitochondrial dynamics and promotes metabolic fitness. Cell Metab. 2015;22(4):709–20.

54. Rudic RD, et al. BMAL1 and CLOCK, two essential components of the circadian clock, are involved in glucose homeostasis. PLoS Biol. 2004;2(11):e377.

55. Marcheva B, et al. Disruption of the CLOCK components CLOCK and BMAL1 leads to hypoinsulinaemia and diabetes. Nature. 2010;466(7306):627–31.

56. Perumpail BJ, et al. Clinical epidemiology and disease burden of nonalcoholic fatty liver disease. World J Gastroenterol. 2017;23(47):8263–76.

57. Yang J, et al. Sleep factors in relation to metabolic dysfunction-associated fatty liver disease in middle-aged and elderly Chinese. J Clin Endocrinol Metab. 2022;107(10):2874–82.

58. Langin D, Arner P. Importance of TNFalpha and neutral lipases in human adipose tissue lipolysis. Trends Endocrinol Metab. 2006;17(8):314–20.

59. Kim CW, et al. Sleep duration and quality in relation to non-alcoholic fatty liver disease in middle-aged workers and their spouses. J Hepatol. 2013;59(2):351–7.

60. Fouhy F, et al. Composition of the early intestinal microbiota: knowledge, knowledge gaps and the use of high-throughput sequencing to address these gaps. Gut Microbes. 2012;3(3):203–20.

61. Le Roy T, et al. Intestinal microbiota determines development of non-alcoholic fatty liver disease in mice. Gut. 2013;62(12):1787–94.

62. Henao-Mejia J, et al. Inflammasome-mediated dysbiosis regulates progression of NAFLD and obesity. Nature. 2012;482(7384):179–85.

63. Leung C, et al. The role of the gut microbiota in NAFLD. Nat Rev Gastroenterol Hepatol. 2016;13(7):412–25.

64. Kirpich IA, Marsano LS, McClain CJ. Gut-liver axis, nutrition, and non-alcoholic fatty liver disease. Clin Biochem. 2015;48(13–14):923–30.

65. Wahlstrom A, et al. Intestinal crosstalk between bile acids and microbiota and its impact on host metabolism. Cell Metab. 2016;24(1):41–50.

66. Sayin SI, et al. Gut microbiota regulates bile acid metabolism by reducing the levels of Tauro-beta-muricholic acid, a naturally occurring FXR antagonist. Cell Metab. 2013;17(2):225–35.

67. Staley C, Khoruts A, Sadowsky MJ. Contemporary applications of fecal microbiota transplantation to treat intestinal diseases in humans. Arch Med Res. 2017;48(8):766–73.

68. Arab JP, et al. Bile acids and nonalcoholic fatty liver disease: molecular insights and therapeutic perspectives. Hepatology. 2017;65(1):350–62.

69. Jennifer Gallacher SM. Practical diagnosis and staging of nonalcoholic fatty liver disease: a narrative review. Hepatology. 2018;3:108. https://doi.org/10.33590/emj/10314271.

70. Tahan V, et al. Serum gamma-glutamyltranspeptidase distinguishes non-alcoholic fatty liver disease at high risk. Hepato-Gastroenterology. 2008;55(85):1433–8.

71. Dyson JK, Anstee QM, McPherson S. Non-alcoholic fatty liver disease: a practical approach to diagnosis and staging. Frontline Gastroenterol. 2014;5(3):211–8.

72. Borrelli A, et al. Role of gut microbiota and oxidative stress in the progression of non-alcoholic fatty liver disease to hepatocarcinoma: current and innovative therapeutic approaches. Redox Biol. 2018;15:467–79.

73. Giboney PT. Mildly elevated liver transaminase levels in the asymptomatic patient. Am Fam Physician. 2005;71(6):1105–10.

74. Brunt EM, et al. Nonalcoholic fatty liver disease (NAFLD) activity score and the histopathologic diagnosis in NAFLD: distinct clinicopathologic meanings. Hepatology. 2011;53(3):810–20.

75. Jacobs A, et al. An overview of mouse models of nonalcoholic steatohepatitis: from past to present. Curr Protoc Mouse Biol. 2016;6(2):185–200.

76. Ito M, et al. Longitudinal analysis of murine steatohepatitis model induced by chronic exposure to high-fat diet. Hepatol Res. 2007;37(1):50–7.

77. Speakman JR. Use of high-fat diets to study rodent obesity as a model of human obesity. Int J Obes. 2019;43(8):1491–2.

78. Fakhoury-Sayegh N, et al. Characteristics of non-alcoholic fatty liver disease induced in Wistar rats following four different diets. Nutr Res Pract. 2015;9(4):350–7.

79. Chen K, et al. Advancing the understanding of NAFLD to hepatocellular carcinoma development: from experimental models to humans. Biochim Biophys Acta Rev Cancer. 2019;1871(1):117–25.

80. Vonghia L, et al. CD4+ROR gamma t++ and Tregs in a mouse model of diet-induced nonalcoholic steatohepatitis. Mediat Inflamm. 2015;2015:239623.

81. Lustig RH, Schmidt LA, Brindis CD. The toxic truth about sugar. Nature. 2012;482(7383):27–9.

82. Nomura K, Yamanouchi T. The role of fructose-enriched diets in mechanisms of nonalcoholic fatty liver disease. J Nutr Biochem. 2012;23(3):203–8.

83. Abe N, et al. Longitudinal characterization of diet-induced genetic murine models of non-alcoholic steatohepatitis with metabolic, histological, and transcriptomic hallmarks of human patients. Biol Open. 2019;8(5):bio041251.

84. Bray GA, Nielsen SJ, Popkin BM. Consumption of high-fructose corn syrup in beverages may play a role in the epidemic of obesity. Am J Clin Nutr. 2004;79(4):537–43.

85. Korinkova L, et al. Pathophysiology of NAFLD and NASH in experimental models: the role of food intake regulating peptides. Front Endocrinol (Lausanne). 2020;11:597583.

86. Corbin KD, Zeisel SH. Choline metabolism provides novel insights into nonalcoholic fatty liver disease and its progression. Curr Opin Gastroenterol. 2012;28(2):159–65.

87. Lau JK, Zhang X, Yu J. Animal models of non-alcoholic fatty liver disease: current perspectives and recent advances. J Pathol. 2017;241(1):36–44.

88. Leclercq IA, et al. CYP2E1 and CYP4A as microsomal catalysts of lipid peroxides in murine non-alcoholic steatohepatitis. J Clin Invest. 2000;105(8):1067–75.

89. Kirsch R, et al. Rodent nutritional model of non-alcoholic steatohepatitis: species, strain and sex difference studies. J Gastroenterol Hepatol. 2003;18(11):1272–82.

90. Machado MV, et al. Mouse models of diet-induced nonalcoholic steatohepatitis reproduce the heterogeneity of the human disease. PLoS One. 2015;10(5):e0127991.

91. Trak-Smayra V, et al. Pathology of the liver in obese and diabetic ob/ob and db/db mice fed a standard or high-calorie diet. Int J Exp Pathol. 2011;92(6):413–21.

92. Yang SQ, et al. Obesity increases sensitivity to endotoxin liver injury: implications for the pathogenesis of steatohepatitis. Proc Natl Acad Sci U S A. 1997;94(6):2557–62.

93. Campfield LA, Smith FJ, Burn P. The OB protein (leptin) pathway – a link between adipose tissue mass and central neural networks. Horm Metab Res. 1996;28(12):619–32.

94. Sahai A, et al. Obese and diabetic db/db mice develop marked liver fibrosis in a model of nonalcoholic steatohepatitis: role of short-form leptin receptors and osteopontin. Am J Physiol Gastrointest Liver Physiol. 2004;287(5):G1035–43.

95. Pelleymounter MA, et al. Effects of the obese gene product on body weight regulation in ob/ob mice. Science. 1995;269(5223):540–3.

96. Wang B, Chandrasekera PC, Pippin JJ. Leptin- and leptin receptor-deficient rodent models: relevance for human type 2 diabetes. Curr Diabetes Rev. 2014;10(2):131–45.

97. Pawlak M, Lefebvre P, Staels B. Molecular mechanism of PPAR alpha action and its impact on lipid metabolism, inflammation and fibrosis in non-alcoholic fatty liver disease. J Hepatol. 2015;62(3):720–33.

98. Liss KHH, Finck BN. PPARs and nonalcoholic fatty liver disease. Biochimie. 2017;136:65–74.

99. Gao Q, et al. PPAR alpha-deficient Ob/Ob obese mice become more obese and manifest severe hepatic steatosis due to decreased fatty acid oxidation. Am J Pathol. 2015;185(5):1396–408.

100. Stec DE, et al. Loss of hepatic PPAR alpha promotes inflammation and serum hyperlipidemia in diet-induced obesity. Am J Phys Regul Integr Comp Phys. 2019;317(5):R733–45.

101. Ipsen DH, Lykkesfeldt J, Tveden-Nyborg P. Molecular mechanisms of hepatic lipid accumulation in non-alcoholic fatty liver disease. Cell Mol Life Sci. 2018;75(18):3313–27.

102. Pei K, et al. An overview of lipid metabolism and nonalcoholic fatty liver disease. Biomed Res Int. 2020;2020:1.

103. Bence KK, Birnbaum MJ. Metabolic drivers of non-alcoholic fatty liver disease. Mol Metabol. 2020;50:50.

104. Rada P, et al. Understanding lipotoxicity in NAFLD pathogenesis: is CD36 a key driver? Cell Death Dis. 2020;11(9):802.

105. Wilson CG, et al. Hepatocyte-specific disruption of CD36 attenuates fatty liver and improves insulin sensitivity in HFD-fed mice. Endocrinology. 2016;157(2): 570–85.

106. Cusi K, et al. Long-term pioglitazone treatment for patients with nonalcoholic steatohepatitis and prediabetes or type 2 diabetes mellitus: a randomized trial. Ann Intern Med. 2016;165(5):305–15.

107. Sanyal AJ, et al. Pioglitazone, vitamin E, or placebo for nonalcoholic steatohepatitis. N Engl J Med. 2010;362(18):1675–85.

108. Chalasani N, et al. The diagnosis and management of nonalcoholic fatty liver disease: practice guidance from the American Association for the Study of Liver Diseases. Hepatology. 2018;67(1):328–57.

109. Loomba R, et al. Clinical trial: pilot study of metformin for the treatment of non-alcoholic steatohepatitis. Aliment Pharmacol Ther. 2009;29(2):172–82.

110. Uygun A, et al. Metformin in the treatment of patients with non-alcoholic steatohepatitis. Aliment Pharmacol Ther. 2004;19(5):537–44.

111. Athyros VG, et al. Safety and efficacy of long-term statin treatment for cardiovascular events in patients with coronary heart disease and abnormal liver tests in the Greek Atorvastatin and Coronary Heart Disease Evaluation (GREACE) study: a post-hoc analysis. Lancet. 2010;376(9756): 1916–22.

112. Kuchay MS, et al. Effect of Empagliflozin on liver fat in patients with type 2 diabetes and nonalcoholic fatty liver disease: a randomized controlled trial (E-LIFT trial). Diabetes Care. 2018;41(8):1801–8.

113. Armstrong MJ, et al. Liraglutide safety and efficacy in patients with non-alcoholic steatohepatitis (LEAN): a multicentre, double-blind, randomised, placebo-controlled phase 2 study. Lancet. 2016;387(10019): 679–90.

114. Schauer PR, et al. Bariatric surgery versus intensive medical therapy in obese patients with diabetes. N Engl J Med. 2012;366(17):1567–76.

115. Sanyal AJ, et al. Challenges and opportunities in drug and biomarker development for nonalcoholic steatohepatitis: findings and recommendations from an American Association for the Study of Liver Diseases-U.S. Food and Drug Administration Joint Workshop. Hepatology. 2015;61(4): 1392–405.

116. Belfort R, et al. A placebo-controlled trial of pioglitazone in subjects with nonalcoholic steatohepatitis. N Engl J Med. 2006;355(22):2297–307.

117. National Institute for Health and Care Excellence. Non-alcoholic fatty liver disease: assessment and management. National Institute for Health and Care Excellence (NICE), London, UK: 2016.

118. Promrat K, et al. Randomized controlled trial testing the effects of weight loss on nonalcoholic steatohepatitis. Hepatology. 2010;51(1):121–9.

119. Lincoff AM, et al. Pioglitazone and risk of cardiovascular events in patients with type 2 diabetes mellitus – a meta-analysis of randomized trials. JAMA. 2007;298(10):1180–8.

120. Loke YK, Singh S, Furberg CD. Long-term use of thiazolidinediones and fractures in type 2 diabetes: a meta-analysis. Can Med Assoc J. 2009;180(1): 32–9.

121. Karimian G, et al. Vitamin E attenuates the progression of non-alcoholic fatty liver disease caused by partial hepatectomy in mice. PLoS One. 2015;10(11):e0143121.

122. Bugianesi E, et al. A randomized controlled trial of metformin versus vitamin E or prescriptive diet in nonalcoholic fatty liver disease. Am J Gastroenterol. 2005;100(5):1082–90.

123. Cohen DE, Anania FA, Chalasani N. An assessment of statin safety by hepatologists. Am J Cardiol. 2006;97(8a):77c–81c.

124. Abraldes JG, et al. Addition of simvastatin to standard therapy for the prevention of variceal rebleeding does not reduce rebleeding but increases survival in patients with cirrhosis. Gastroenterology. 2016;150(5):1160–1170 e3.

125. Armstrong MJ, et al. Glucagon-like peptide 1 decreases lipotoxicity in non-alcoholic steatohepatitis. J Hepatol. 2016;64(2):399–408.

126. Ito D, et al. Comparison of Ipragliflozin and pioglitazone effects on nonalcoholic fatty liver disease in patients with type 2 diabetes: a randomized, 24-week, open-label, active-controlled trial. Diabetes Care. 2017;40(10):1364–72.

127. Fakhry TK, et al. Bariatric surgery improves non-alcoholic fatty liver disease: a contemporary systematic review and meta-analysis. Surg Obes Relat Dis. 2019;15(3):502–11.

128. Esquivel CM, et al. Laparoscopic sleeve gastrectomy resolves NAFLD: another formal indication for bariatric surgery? Obes Surg. 2018;28(12):4022–33.

129. Aller R, et al. Effect on liver enzymes of biliopancreatic diversion: 4 years of follow-up. Ann Nutr Metab. 2015;66(2–3):132–6.

Sarcopenic Obesity

31

Danae C. Gross, Ray Cheever, and John A. Batsis

Contents

D. C. Gross · R. Cheever
Department of Nutrition, Gillings School of Global Public Health, University of North Carolina, Chapel Hill, NC, USA

J. A. Batsis (✉)
Department of Nutrition, Gillings School of Global Public Health, University of North Carolina, Chapel Hill, NC, USA

Division of Geriatric Medicine, School of Medicine, University of North Carolina, Chapel Hill, NC, USA

Center for Aging and Health, University of North Carolina, Chapel Hill, NC, USA
e-mail: john.batsis@unc.edu

Abstract

An aging population in conjunction with a worsening obesity epidemic worldwide is leading to a public health epidemic of older adults with considerable mobility and functional limitations. Sarcopenia is the age-related progression of decreased muscle mass, strength, and function. Though sarcopenia naturally occurs as part of the aging process, it can be exacerbated when coupled with obesity. Older adults with sarcopenic obesity are thought to have a synergistic risk of adverse outcomes compared to those with either sarcopenia or obesity alone. Consensus groups continue their efforts in creating standardized terms and definitions for identifying those at risk for sarcopenic obesity. The standardization of definitions is critically important in developing clinical trials for sarcopenic obesity that will lead to improvement in body composition and physical function. Multicomponent management strategies consisting of physical exercise and dietary modifications are safely recommended to mitigate worsening sarcopenia, preserve muscle strength, and promote weight loss. Promising, novel therapies have the potential to improve body composition and muscle physiology in this subgroup of patients.

Keywords

Sarcopenia · Obesity · Health promotion

Abbreviations

BMI	Body mass index
EASO	European Association for the Study of Obesity
ESPEN	European Society for Clinical Nutrition and Metabolism
EWGSOP	European Working Group for the Study of Sarcopenia in Older People
FNIH	Foundation for the National Institutes for Health
GLIS	Global Leadership Initiative in Sarcopenia
NHANES	National Health and Nutrition Examination Survey
SarcO	Sarcopenic Obesity
SDOC	Sarcopenic Definitions Outcome Consortium

Introduction: An Aging Population

The population in the United States and other countries globally continues to increase. Older adults, those aged 65 years and older, are a rapidly growing demographic group [1]. In 2022, older adults made up 10% of the global population – this number is projected to increase to 16% in 2050 [1]. It is estimated that by the year 2050, the number of older adults worldwide are projected to be more than twice the number of children under age 5 [1]. Two known major reasons contribute to these trends: first, the baby boom cohort, those who turned 65 years old in 2011, will continue to fuel the growing population of older adults [1]; second, the lower mortality and increased survival from improved medical care. Furthermore, the age distribution has shifted upward as a result of an ongoing drop in fertility levels [1]. A combination of all these factors have led to the rapid expansion of older adults aged ≥65 years across the world and in the United States.

Aging is the primary driver of the development of chronic diseases. Alterations in the underlying hallmarks of aging (e.g., altered metabolism, chronic inflammation, epigenetic changes, senescence) accumulate over time, leading to an increase in the number of chronic medical conditions. In one study of Medicare beneficiaries, 82% had more than one chronic medical condition and 65% had multiple problems [2]. As such, an aging older adult with multimorbidity is at increased risk for incident disability resulting from the accumulation of medical comorbidities [3]. Additionally, impaired physical function is strongly associated with an increased risk of frailty [4] and death [5]. Such impaired physical function may result in loss of independence and increased healthcare utilization. Table 1 lists activities of daily living used to measure functional status [3, 6]. Patient-specific secondary outcome measures include quality of life, which has been shown to decrease with higher rates of comorbidity [7] and disability [8]. As the total number of older adults increase, so will the impact of accumulated comorbidity and

Table 1 Functional status – activities of daily living [6, 99]

Basic	Instrumental
Bathing	Shopping
Dressing	Housekeeping
Transferring from bed to chair	Preparing meals
Toileting	Taking medications
Eating	Finances
Walking	Using transportation
	Making phone calls

disability, further impacting health and healthcare utilization significant to society.

Obesity

Obesity in both adult and pediatric populations continues to be a public health epidemic that has drawn considerable attention as a result of its impact on patients and society. Recent epidemiologic surveys found the prevalence rate of adults with obesity measured using body mass index (BMI) increased to 41.9% in 2017–2020 from 30.5% in 1999–2000 [9]. As a result, more than 65% of the United States population is classified as having obesity or overweight (BMI 25–29.9 kg/m^2). The rapid expansion of the population aged 65 years and older will lead to larger numbers of persons with obesity. Rates are continuing to rise [9]. Even in older adults, the rates of obesity remain high. The most recent National Health and Nutrition Examination Survey (NHANES) found that 41.5% of adults 60 years of age and older, were classified as having a BMI of 30 kg/m^2 or more. Despite similar prevalence rates to those of the general population, the impact of obesity in older adults has been given little attention despite the growing epidemic.

Body mass index (BMI) is often used as a representation of body fat as it is simple and inexpensive to measure and calculate (using height and weight). Clinically, this is a quality measure in the United States and is universally measured and available in electronic health records [9]. BMI is calculated by dividing an individual's weight (in kilograms) by the individual's height (in meters) squared. "Obesity" occurs when an individual's body fat and fat distribution exceed what is considered healthy and increases the risk for disease. In adult populations, a BMI of 30 kg/m^2 or greater would be considered a diagnosis and a weight classification of having obesity. However, changes in body composition occur as a normal manifestation of aging [10]. Muscle mass and its strength peak in the third decade of life, and then start progressively declining, with a rate

increasing after the age of 60 years. Additionally, body fat gradually increases with age, reaching a peak between 60 and 75 years old [11]. Changes in adipose tissue, due to the aging process, involve redistribution of deposits and composition and are exacerbated by excessive energy intake and inactivity. Progressive loss of skeletal muscle mass, coupled with increases in visceral adiposity, makes use of a BMI measurement in older adults, a relatively inaccurate index [12]. Other assessment measures of obesity and body fat composition can be considered, including waist circumference and body fat.

It has been hypothesized that there are likely subtypes of obesity, including those with and without metabolic abnormalities [13]. There likely is a component of genetic predisposition to surviving, and further research is needed to better identify patients at lower risk. Both duration of obesity during the lifespan [14], and obesity at the age of 65 years are associated with increased risk of physical impairments, disability [14], and nursing home placement [15]. Using seven-year follow-up data from the Health, Aging, and Body Composition Study, of 2845 community-dwelling US adults, men and women who were classified as overweight or having obesity at all three designated time points (25 years old, 50 years, and at the time of study (70–709 years old)) had increased risk of mobility limitations compared to a normal BMI (HR 1.61 [1.25–2.06] and 2.85 [2.15–3.78], respectively) [14]. Whether functional impairment is due to increased load on joints or metabolic changes due to coexistent underlying inflammation is currently under study of investigation.

Researchers and clinicians have long debated the manner in diagnosing obesity, whether by anthropometric measures (and which ones) or by radiological means. Irrespective of its assessment, it is well accepted that obesity is detrimental to overall function in older adults [16]. A recent systematic review by Schaap et al. noted a risk ratio of 1.60 [1.43, 1.80] of impaired function in those with a BMI $\geq$ 30 kg/m^2 [16]. In addition, body fat assessed by bioelectrical impedance has been associated with a risk of impaired function [17]. Epidemiological studies have demonstrated a robust relationship between obesity and hypertension, hyperlipidemia, diabetes, sleep apnea [18], and other disorders, including osteoarthritis [19] and cancer [20]. Obesity, particularly if developed in mid-life, has been strongly also associated with cognitive dysfunction [21]. These relationships exist in older adults as well. The risk of obesity-related cardiovascular disease has been shown to be higher in older adults [22]. Yet, people who are classified as overweight or having obesity often die prematurely. In one study, having excess weight was associated with approximately 500,000 excess death in the United States [23] suggesting a critical need to develop effective therapies to mitigate this epidemic.

Many studies routinely use BMI for weight and obesity classifications. While this anthropometric measure is practical and easy to measure clinically, it does have several limitations. First, adults tend to decrease in height as they age [24]. Second, changes in body composition can lead to changes in weight [25]. Third, a BMI cutoff of 30 kg/m^2 to classify obesity was based on older epidemiological studies [26]. For instance in older adults age >65 years, a BMI between 26 and 27 kg/m^2 may be associated with the lowest mortality rates [27]. Additionally, BMI accounts for both fat mass and muscle mass, and may poorly reflect specific differences in body composition. For instance, a 25-year-old male who is a body builder has very little fat mass with a considerable proportion of dense muscle mass; however, this individual may inadvertently be classified as having obesity. As will be discussed below, BMI fails to account for the changes in muscle mass and muscle quality with aging. While a discussion on these measures is outside the scope of this chapter, sole use of BMI can be problematic since there is a subset of persons with elevated central adiposity who are at higher risk of disability [17] and mortality [28], both in cross-sectional and longitudinal studies [29]. In fact, one study conducted by our group using NHANES data, we demonstrate that while specificity was high, sensitivity was low, particularly as age increased [30].

Sarcopenia

Sarcopenia is an under-recognized and under-characterized syndrome in clinical medicine. A term initially coined in 1989 by Rosenberg, sarcopenia is characterized by the natural reduction of muscle mass with aging. The word sarcopenia is derived from the Greek word, "sarcos" meaning flesh, and "penia" meaning lack of. The syndrome of sarcopenia is located on the spectrum of frailty and disability [30]. While sarcopenia is primarily a disease of older adults, it may be associated with other chronic health conditions seen in younger patients, including disuse, cancer, malnutrition, and cachexia [31]. Muscle mass increases with age up until the third or fourth decade of life (30–40 years old), then starts decreasing in the fourth decade of life (Fig. 1). However, the trajectory of muscle loss is also known to be altered with physical exercise and/or environmental changes. Once an individual reaches and drops below a given threshold of muscle loss, it is believed they may be at risk for a higher risk of incident disability [32]. This age-related decline in muscle, parallels that observed with bone mass [33]. For instance, once bone mass reaches a critical level, one's risk of a fracture is increased [34]. Emerging studies suggest that future definitions may parallel that using bone density, that is, using t-scores to evaluate those at intermediate or high risk.

The definition of sarcopenia has evolved considerably over the years and has led to considerable debate in identifying the natural history and advancing the science of this syndrome. In the past, definitions of sarcopenia were primarily based on muscle mass. Such definitions accounted for total body skeletal muscle mass and appendicular skeletal muscle mass, often adjusted for height in meters squared. Many of these threshold definitions were based on epidemiological studies, using two standard deviations below the population mean of a healthier population. Alternatively, they were based on the bottom two quintiles of a given target population [35]. Basing threshold definitions on mathematical definitions and distributions and not proven clinical

Fig. 1 Muscle mass, strength, and function during the life cycle. Muscle mass, strength, and function increase in early in life, peaks in the third and fourth decades, and then decreases in later life. (Adapted from Sayer et al. [32])

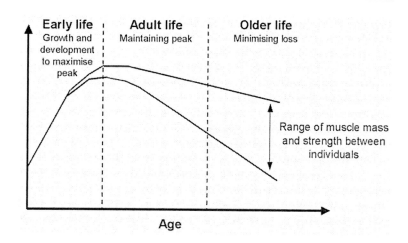

outcomes led in part to such disparate definitions. Many advocated the need to create thresholds and cutoffs that corresponded to validated clinical outcomes such as disability, mortality, and institutionalization [30]. These shortcomings led to two groups, one in Europe, and the other in the United States to address these issues.

The European Working Group for the Study of Sarcopenia in Older People (EWGSOP) [30] developed a clinical algorithm to identify those with sarcopenia and outlined key outcomes (Table 3). This consensus group included muscle quality and strength in their definition of sarcopenia. They also recommended incorporating muscle mass and function (strength or performance) into the definition of sarcopenia for its diagnosis. While their initial definition was published in 2010, an updated consensus definition in 2019 uses reduced muscle strength as a key characteristic for sarcopenia rather than low muscle mass. This updated consensus guideline recommended using gait speed as a measure to assess severity of sarcopenia, not diagnostic criterion, since gait speed has unclear associations with determining sarcopenia [36]. The EWGSOP recommends use of grip strength or a chair stand measure, with specific cutoff points for each test, to assess for sarcopenia [36]. For research studies, other methods to measure strength, such as knee flexion and extension, were suggested as potential recommendations for use [36].

In the United States, the Foundation for the National Institutes for Health (FNIH) initiated the Sarcopenia project [37]. This consensus group develops clinically appropriate threshold measures to predict incident disability and adverse outcomes [37]. At the 2014 consensus meeting, the group determined that the diagnosis of sarcopenia was most sensitive to low lean muscle mass adjusted for body mass index and grip strength [37]. Based on epidemiological studies [38–40], muscle strength was more predictive of impaired physical function compared to muscle mass alone. Muscle mass was believed to indirectly impact function. In community-dwelling older adults, low muscle mass has been associated with weakness or "dynapenia," both of which have been associated with reduced physical function. Importantly, low muscle mass was found to be less likely to be associated with impaired physical function [16]. Hence, the causal pathway between muscle mass to strength to function is now being challenged. In fact, there are likely two patient phenotypes: those with weakness but with preserved muscle mass; and those with low muscle mass leading to weakness. This consortium identified a number of large-scale epidemiological studies to ascertain these relationships and selected mobility impairment as a primary outcome (gait speed <0.8 m/s) as such a measure predicts mortality and disability [41].

To validate and build upon the findings of the Sarcopenia Project, The Sarcopenic Definitions Outcome Consortium (SDOC) includes clinical trials of older adults and clinical datasets from

Table 2 Cut points for weakness using grip strength

Cut point	Males	Females
Grip strength	<35.5 kg	<20 kg
Grip strength over body mass index	<1.05	<0.79
Grip strength over total body fat	<1.66	<0.65
Grip strength over arm lean mass	<6.1	<3.26
Grip strength over body weight	<0.45	<0.34

Table adapted from the Sarcopenia Definition and Outcomes Consortium [44]
Grip strength measured using a dynamometer
Abbreviations: *BMI*, body mass index

epidemiologic studies. Published in 2020, the panel agreed that both weakness, defined by low grip strength, and slowness, defined by low usual gait speed, should be included in the definition of sarcopenia [42]. It was identified that sex-specific cut points for low grip strength, either absolute or normalized for body size were an important discriminator of slowness [42]. Low grip strength, with or without normalization to weight or BMI, was a predictor of adverse health outcomes such as falls, self-reported mobility limitation, hip fracture, and mortality in older adults [42]. Table 2 outlines the current thresholds and cut points that have been proposed for use by clinicians and researchers. A recent analysis noted that the prevalence of sarcopenia and sarcopenia with obesity varied markedly depending on the definition used [35]. One author conservatively estimated that sarcopenia may affect more than 50 million persons today; this potentially can increase to 200 million within the next 40 years [43]. The estimated direct health costs of $18.5 billion in the year 2000 are not insignificant [44].

To provide a clear, standardized framework for discussing sarcopenia-related terms in both research and clinical settings, the Global Leadership Initiative in Sarcopenia (GLIS) assembled a glossary of terms commonly encountered in the sarcopenia literature with corresponding proposed definitions [45]. Because different researchers may attribute widely varying meanings to the same sarcopenia-related terms, the GLIS glossary of terms and definitions is needed to avoid confusion about the meanings of common sarcopenia-related terms and prevent

Table 3 Proposed outcomes from the European working group for the study of sarcopenia in older adults [30]

Primary outcome domains	Physical performance
	Muscle strength
	Muscle mass
Secondary outcome domains	Activities of daily living
	Quality of life
	Metabolic & biochemical markers
	Markers of inflammation
	Global impression of change by subject or physician
	Falls
	Admission to the hospital or nursing home
	Social support
	Mortality

obfuscation of research on similar sarcopenia-related outcome [45]. By adhering to the standardized GLIS glossary of terms in sarcopenia research, it will become easier to draw concise conclusions from disparate research studies on sarcopenia that investigate similar variables such as muscle strength and muscle quality. The GLIS has provided definitions for a sizable list of terms common in the sarcopenia literature such as muscle strength, muscle power, lean mass, fat-free mass, muscle quality, and muscle density [45]. While enumerating the GLIS-proposed definitions for all these terms is beyond the scope of the present chapter, we advise that researchers studying sarcopenia refer to the GLIS glossary of sarcopenia-related terms to ensure the transferability of their research findings to other similar studies.

Sarcopenic Obesity

Sarcopenic obesity (SarcO) is believed to impact more than one in ten older adults around the world [11]. While both obesity and sarcopenia have been evaluated separately, individuals present with definitions and clinical features of both. Thus, SarcO is characterized by the combination of obesity and sarcopenia. Co-occurrence of sarcopenia and obesity was found to lead to a synergistically higher risk for metabolic disease and functional impairment compared to those caused by the cumulative risk of each condition separately [46]. This distinction is of critical importance is that in clinical practice, identifying those at synergistic risk of complications may permit targeted interventions in the future.

In numerous epidemiology-based studies, the prevalence of SarcO has been shown to be higher in older adults [35, 39, 48–55]. The result of age-related changes observed in body composition [46] and risk factors that accelerate the onset of sarcopenia in individuals with obesity may be key reasons for this observation. Some examples include systemic and muscle oxidative stress, inflammation, and insulin resistance. These may be exacerbated in the presence of other metabolic complications and comorbidities [47–49]. Yet, it is important to note that SarcO is not exclusively a condition limited to older adults as it has been observed in middle-aged and younger individuals with obesity, oftentimes due to acute and chronic diseases, and as a result of rapid changes in weight [46]. A recent systematic review found that mean age of the studied population was below 65 years in a third of the studies reviewed [46]. In another study conducted by Poggiogalle et al., of a sample of 727 persons with obesity, the rate of SarcO was 34.8% in males and 50.1% in females but their mean age was 45.6 ± 13.5 years and 45.8 ± 13.6 years, respectively [48].

Common Underlying Mechanisms + Theoretical Framework

While the underlying pathophysiology and mechanisms to explain the development of SarcO have previously been unclear, emerging evidence suggests that common inflammatory pathways that link sarcopenia and obesity. When physical inactivity is coupled with sarcopenic obesity, there are negative alterations in myokines and adipokines. These changes lead to decreases in interleukin-10 (IL-10), interleukin-15 (IL-15), insulin-like growth factor hormone (IGF-1), irisin, leukemia inhibitory factor (LIF), fibroblast growth factor-21 (FGF-21), adiponectin, and apelin [51]. In contrast, there are increases in myostatin, leptin, interleukin-6 (IL-6), interleukin-8 (IL-8), and resistin [50]. Changes in these myokines and adipokines can lead increased inflammatory factors and fat mass, degradation of muscle proteins, and decreased muscle tissue, all of which exacerbate SarcO [50]. Figure 2 highlights the interplay between fat and muscle signaling that are contributing factors to SarcO.

Studies have revealed that changes in body composition in those with SarcO are likely due to fat infiltration of muscle. Such fat infiltration, or myosteatosis, contributes to lower muscle quality and reduced work performance [51]. Fat and muscle are known to be both metabolically active. As noted in Fig. 2, they can impact each other. For instance, excess energy intake, decreased physical inactivity, low-grade inflammation, and insulin resistance from losses of skeletal muscle, result in changes of hormonal homeostasis in the development of SarcO [43]. Adipokines and pro-inflammatory cytokines (IL-6, TNF-a) produced by adipocytes or by infiltrating macrophages in adipose tissue, can potentially induce C-reactive protein in the liver. These mechanisms can explain the robust association of C-reactive protein with low handgrip strength and high body fat suggesting that underlying inflammation is a causative factor [52]. Leptin and low adiponectin concentrations negatively impact muscle mass leading to reductions in muscle quality [53]. In fact, leptin resistance is hypothesized as an underlying mechanism linking atherosclerosis and metabolic syndrome [54], and in one study has shown that it is negatively related to appendicular skeletal muscle mass adjusted for fat mass [55]. Further data from the INChianti study have demonstrated that global and central obesity negatively affects

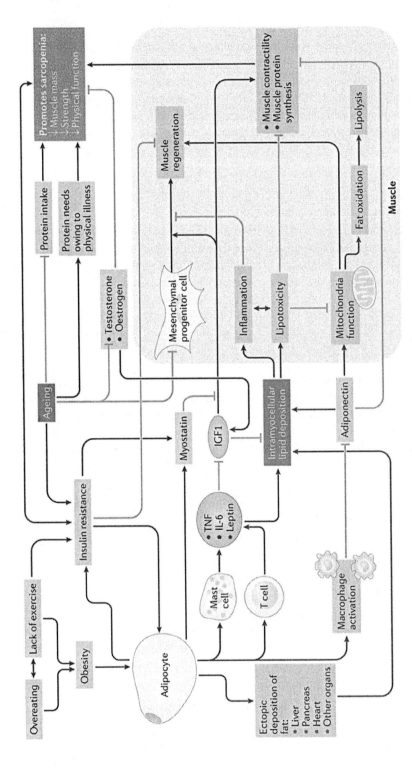

Fig. 2 A proposed model of mechanisms leading to sarcopenic obesity The proposed interplay between adipose and muscle tissue, which is believed to contribute to the development of sarcopenic obesity, is shown. The black lines are stimulatory, while red lines with flat ends indicate inhibition. IGF1, insulin-like growth factor 1; TNF, tumor necrosis factor. Myostatin A transforming growth factor-related protein that is synthesized and secreted in skeletal muscle and negatively regulates muscle mass and function. An excess of fatty acids in the organism leads to apoptosis of pancreatic β-cells and consequently to reduce secretion of insulin. This results in deregulation of the muscular PKB/Akt pathway and a decreased translocation of GLUT4 transporters leading to insulin insensitivity. Moreover, protein turnover is altered due to changes in S6K1 activity. Secretion of IL-15, a paracrine anabolic myokine, is suppressed by adipose tissue. Hence, TNFα induces muscle atrophy by stimulation of apoptosis as well as by upregulation of the proteasomal decay of filament proteins. Satellite cells dedifferentiate to an adipocyte-like phenotype stunting regeneration of muscle fibers.

muscle strength leading to the development and progression of sarcopenic obesity [56].

These findings suggest that there may be a higher risk of cardiovascular disease in those patients with SarcO. Additionally, high levels of circulating free fatty acids appear to play a role in the development of SarcO [52]. The pathogenesis is complex which was summarized by Kob et al. [57] in (Fig. 2). With aging, increases in fat and progressive loss of muscle mass, may exacerbate excess fatty acids deposit in extra-adipose tissues, which could lead to lipotoxicity and eventual insulin resistance. Deposition of fat into muscle alters their morphology, size, and function, and protein turnover occurs. Future research needs to leverage the use of epidemiology-based datasets to answer some of these important questions.

Screening, Diagnosis, and Evaluation

The European Society for Clinical Nutrition and Metabolism (ESPEN) and the European Association for the Study of Obesity (EASO) launched an initiative to reach expert consensus on a definition and diagnostic criteria for SarcO [46]. This international expert panel proposed a standardized definition of SarcO that defined this syndrome as the co-existence of excess fat mass and low skeletal muscle mass or function [46]. The group strongly recommended that a diagnosis of SarcO should be considered in clinical practice, particularly in at-risk individuals who together have an elevated BMI or waist circumference, representative of obesity, but also in those with markers of low skeletal muscle mass or physical function [46]. ESPEN/EASO recommended a two-stage approach. First, screening in the primary care setting. Second, that diagnostic procedures should include an assessment of skeletal muscle function, followed by assessment of body composition. This coexistent presence of excess adiposity and low skeletal muscle mass (or related body compartments) would confirm the diagnosis of SarcO [46]. More will be discussed about screening, diagnosis, and staging later in this chapter.

This consortium was clear to suggest that SarcO should be considered a unique clinical condition. Their rationale was as a result of: (1) the interaction between body fat mass accumulation and the loss of skeletal muscle mass and function; and (2) the negative clinical interactions between obesity and sarcopenia [46].

Among the leading guidelines for diagnosing sarcopenic obesity are the recent diagnostic criteria proposed by Donini and colleagues [46]. In their proposed framework put forth by the Sarcopenic Obesity Global Leadership Initiative (Fig. 3), the diagnosis of SarcO entails a consecutive, two-step process to determine both skeletal muscle functional parameters and body composition. According to Donini et al., the determination of skeletal muscle functional parameters depends on tests of skeletal muscle strength such as handgrip strength, knee extensor strength, or chair stand test with results of these tests adjusted for patient-specific variables such as sex, ethnicity, and age [47]. If subjects meet diagnostic criteria for sarcopenia based on these tests of skeletal muscle function, then researchers and clinicians should proceed to assess body composition via dual-energy X-ray absorptiometry (DXA) or bioelectrical impedance analysis (BIA), with DXA being the preferred option [47]. Furthermore, as many have suggested, the classification of sarcopenic obesity may require consideration of the pathophysiology of the condition: namely, whether the sarcopenic obesity has occurred because of long-standing adiposity-mediated inflammation or the presence of an acute trigger in a prior nonsarcopenic individual with obesity. However, diagnostic criteria for sarcopenic obesity do not differ between these two potentially distinct phenotypes [47]. In addition to merely determining the presence of sarcopenic obesity, Donini et al. stress the need to stage sarcopenic obesity based on certain associated complications, with stage one sarcopenic obesity entailing no complications related to altered body composition and skeletal muscle function, and stage two sarcopenic obesity entailing one or more such complications, including metabolic disease, disability secondary to high fat mass or low muscle mass, or cardiorespiratory disease [47].

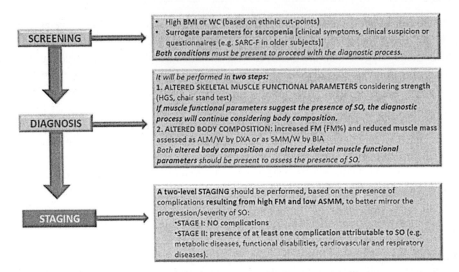

Fig. 3 Diagnostic procedure for the assessment of sarcopenic obesity. Abbreviations: ALM/W, appendicular lean mass adjusted to body weight; ASMM, absolute skeletal muscle mass; BIA, bioelectrical impedance analysis; BMI, body mass index; DXA, dual X-ray absorptiometry; FM, fat mass; HGS, handgrip strength; SMM/W, total skeletal muscle mass adjusted by weight; SarcO, sarcopenic obesity; WC, waist circumference; SARC-F, strength, assistance with walking, rising from a chair, climbing stairs and falls. (Donini Lorenzo et al. [46])

Consequences and Implications on Function in Older Adults

Moving beyond the challenges of a concrete definition of SarcO, most past studies used a combination of muscle mass and BMI to define this entity. The impact of sarcopenia, obesity, and physical performance has increasingly been a topic of increased study. Using bioelectrical impedance, subjects with SarcO in a Taiwanese cohort were found to have worse physical performance than those without [58]. Early epidemiologic studies, however, demonstrated inconsistent results on impairment of function [59, 60]. For instance, SarcO is related to subjective impairment in physical performance [61], including falls [62]. Baumgartner et al. used the New Mexico Aging Process Health Study and noted that the risk of incident disability was a HR 2.63 [1.19,5.85] over the course of an eight-year follow-up [63]. The EPIDOS study in Europe noted that SarcO had 2.60 higher odds of having difficulty climbing stairs and 2.35 higher odds of difficulty going downstairs than those without any of these entities [64]. A study using the Quebec Longitudinal Study (Nutrition as a Determinant of Successful Aging)

compared four groups of high/low muscle mass and high/low obesity. Their outcomes examined their characteristics of physical function [59]. Their results did not demonstrate that SarcO had lower physical capacity as compared to non-sarcopenic/obese individuals in this cohort. A clear outcome from this study was the impact of obesity on function. Inflammatory markers, including C-reactive protein, homeostasis model assessment (IR_{HOMA}) were higher in subjects with SarcO in NHANES 1999–2004 [65] and also in the INChianti study [56], suggesting that pro-inflammatory cytokines may be critical in both the development and progression of SarcO. Certain studies have demonstrated important associations between SarcO and important functional measures. For instance, using a sample from a community-based cohort of 1655 older adults suggested that fat mass negative impacting domains of physical performance and overall functioning and that its inter-relation with lean mass importantly impacts these estimates [66].

The Korean National Health and Nutrition Examination Survey (KNHANES) had considerable data on older adults. These authors observed, in a cross-sectional analysis, that SarcO was associated with radiographic knee osteoarthritis (OR 3.51 [2.15–5.75]) in contrast to those with sarcopenia and obesity (OR 2.38 [1.80–3.15]) [67]. A specific SarcO study performed in South Korea has been instrumental in better characterizing the associations between this entity and important geriatric outcomes. While inherent ethnic differences in body composition exist, this population focused predominantly on a population of Asian descent and ethnicity. Applying the National Cholesterol Education Program-Adult Treatment Panel III guidelines to the Korean NHANES cohort, persons with SarcO had a higher risk for dyslipidemia (OR 2.82 [1.76–4.51]) than the other groups [68]. The risk of metabolic syndrome was also elevated in those with SarcO (OR 3.24 [1.21,8.66]) in both females and 5.13 [0.90–29.30] in males [69]. This was confirmed in a longitudinal study noting that SarcO was at higher risk for metabolic syndrome (OR 8.28 [4.45–15.40]) than either obesity or sarcopenia alone [70]. This same cohort demonstrated that over a period of 28 months, visceral fat was associated with future loss of skeletal muscle mass in Korean adults [71].

Mortality

The relationship between mortality and sarcopenia and obesity suggests that SarcO is likely to be strongly associated with an increased risk of death. In one prospective Cardiovascular Health Study of 3336 community-dwelling older adults without cardiovascular disease at baseline, persons were classified as having SarcO based on measures of muscle mass or strength, and waist circumference [72]. After a mean follow-up of 8 years, persons classified as having SarcO had a 23% increased risk of death (95% CI: 0.99–1.54) [72]. Another epidemiological study using data from the NHANES III epidemiological study defined SarcO using body fat and total skeletal muscle mass adjusted for height^2 cutoffs and had a higher mortality risk in females (HR 1.35 [1.05–1.74]) than in males (HR 0.98 [0.77–1.25]) [73]. Additionally, in the British Regional Heart Study, a community-based study

of 4107 men aged 60–79 years, the risk of all-cause mortality was increased in persons with SarcO [74]. Individuals with a high waist circumference (>102 cm) and the lowest quartile of mid-arm muscle circumference had a 55% increase in mortality risk compared with non-sarcopenic, nonobese individuals during the six-year follow-up period [74]. The same study population was reexamined 11 years later and the risk of mortality increased by 41% in the sarcopenic group and 21% the obese group [76]. The highest risk of death was found in males with sarcopenic obesity with a 72% increase, compared with the nonsarcopenic, nonobese group, after adjusting for lifestyle and cardiovascular risk factors [75]. This study also included fat-free mass index and fat mass index when defining SarcO but found no significant relationships using these measures [75]. Further evaluation with recent recommended thresholds and cut points is needed, and sex-specific analyses would be helpful in identifying whether differences exist between these demographic groups.

Management of Sarcopenic Obesity

Despite recent and emerging findings, formal guidelines for the management of SarcO have not been well established. Disparities in defining SarcO and the small number of primary outcomes to evaluate have contributed to the limited number of clinical trials that investigate possible interventions in reducing fat and preserving muscle.

Role of Nutrition and Exercise

Physical activity (including exercise) and proper nutritional habits are effective ways to prevent or slow down the development of SarcO. Weight loss is the cornerstone of management in older adults with SarcO yet providers remain cautious about recommending it in clinical practice as caloric restriction can lead to the loss in muscle mass and worsen sarcopenia [51]. Importantly, a limited number of clinical trials focus exclusively on sarcopenic obesity. Yet, recent studies with older adults have shown positive effects of intentional weight loss on morbidity and physical function [76–78]. Following a meta-analysis of randomized trials of adults with obesity aged ≥55 years, which had follow-up times of 4 years or more, researchers reported a 16% reduction in mortality (95% CI 0.71–0.99) [79]. As with any lifestyle modification program, the foundation of management includes dietary (caloric) restriction, behavioral counseling, and increased physical activity through aerobic or resistance exercise. Weight reduction of 5–10% can lead to improvement or resolution of comorbidities. A recent benefit available to Medicare Beneficiaries has led to reimbursable models for primary care clinicians to counsel older adults with obesity [80].

Combining physical exercise (specifically resistance exercises) with nutrition interventions such as calorie restriction and protein supplementation have shown promise as potential therapies for sarcopenic obesity. In older adults, exercise has been known to affect hormonal balance, reduce oxidative stress, improve muscle oxidative capacity, and increase muscle protein synthesis despite age-related decreases in anabolic signaling [81]. In patients with sarcopenia and obesity, combined weight loss with exercise improved physical function and was found to ameliorate frailty compared to each intervention alone [78]. Furthermore, resistance exercise has been shown to have the greatest improvements in muscle strength [81]. To address the potential downregulation of protein synthesis and loss of lean muscle mass during acute calorie restriction, early pilot studies have shown preservation of appendicular lean mass during weight loss [82]. Protein intake of 1.0–1.2 g/kg/day of body weight is essential to compensate for the anabolic resistance commonly found in this group [82, 83]. However, caution is advised in prescribing higher protein diets to prevent renal dysfunction for older adults.

While vitamin D levels decline with age, and deficiencies may be associated with reduced muscle strength, statin myopathy, reduced function, falls, and fractures [84, 85], its D replacement is associated with reduced mortality [86] and can be considered as part of the multimodal approach to treatment and care. In addition, recent studies revealed the effect of vitamin D on muscle physiology to regulate calcium signaling which is associated with the contractile force in muscle fibers [87]. Vitamin D doses of 50,000 units can be considered in older adults in the form of Vitamin D2 or Vitamin D3 [88]. Additionally, calcium should be supplemented with vitamin D therapy to mitigate the potential risks of unopposed supplementation [81].

Emerging Pharmacotherapy Revise

A number of Food and Drug Administration and experimental therapies are being currently tested. In the phase I trials and in rodent models, therapies that have been trialed in the past but have been unsuccessful or fraught with challenges when translated to human studies. Emerging pharmacological interventions studied include testosterone supplementation, selective androgen receptor modulators, myostatin inhibitors, and antiobesity drugs. To the reader, we emphasize that there are no approved drugs for the treatment of SarcO in older adults.

As testosterone concentrations drop with age, they parallel the changes observed in body composition observed as well. While hypogonadal males appear to have some benefit with therapy [89]; however, disparate results have been observed with healthy older males [90]. For instance, testosterone therapy with exercise altered body composition favorably by reducing fat mass and increasing skeletal muscle but did not alter physical performance. Other studies have observed similar findings. In one multicenter trial of 75 obese males, testosterone therapy was associated with a significant decrease in whole body and appendicular fat mass, whereas the placebo group revealed a significant increase in both measures [91]. Additionally, the testosterone group had a higher increase in their lean body mass compared to the placebo group [91]. Despite these promising findings, the Food and Drug Administration has placed a warning on supplementation with testosterone. Adverse events [92] include erythrocytosis, prostate cancer, blood clots, stroke, myocardial infarction, and heart failure [93].

A potential contributing factor to the development of SarcO has been a decline in growth hormone and IGF-1 synthesis, and elevated levels of myostatin. While supplementation of these compounds appears physiologically plausible, clinical studies have again been fraught with disappointment and adverse events [94]. Emerging analogs are being studied that potentially can alter body composition, and future studies should examine their effects on physical function. Myostatin inhibitors reduce the expression of myostatin in both aerobic and resistance exercises and may have promising benefits in treating SarcO [81]. Also, a recent systematic review of DHEA therapy demonstrated changes in body composition [95], but future studies are needed to determine whether it impacts physical function.

Recently, Metformin, has been considered a promising antiaging drug through regulation of bone, muscle, and joint functions, and slowing the progression of sarcopenia. In regard to aging, metformin is known to regulate intracellular signaling pathways by way of AMPK activation and other pathways which have protective anti-inflammatory effects [96]. Despite these promising findings, there are limited studies on metformin and the aging adult, and most of them are conducted in rodent studies. More clinical trials are needed to evaluate the antiaging effect of Metformin in sarcopenic obesity. Targeting Aging with Metformin (TAME) is a proposed clinical trial in which researchers will investigate metformin and the molecular aging pathways to slow the incidence of age-related multimorbidity and decline in functional status [97]. The blood-based biomarkers under investigation include IL-6, TNF-alpha receptor I or II, C-reactive protein (CRP), GDF-15, insulin, IGF-1, cystatin-C, NT-proBNP, and hemoglobin A1c [97].

Glucagon-like peptide-1 (GLP-1) receptor agonist is an emerging treatment for overweight and obese adults. The GLP-1 receptor analog, liraglutide, shows promise in preservation of muscle mass [98]. Perna et al. evaluated the use of liraglutide in overweight and obese older adults with type 2 diabetes mellitus [98]. After 6 months of weeks of treatment, reduction of body weight was mostly due to the decrease of fat [98].

Liraglutide was found to preserve the stability of skeletal muscle and prevent the degradation of muscle protein and none of the participants developed sarcopenia [98]. More studies are needed to investigate the effectiveness and safety of GLP-1 receptor agonists in fat loss and musculoskeletal health, specifically to prevent sarcopenia in older adults.

Future Directions and Conclusion

The phenotype of sarcopenic obesity is gaining increased recognition from both the research and clinical perspectives. With a burgeoning aging population expecting to increase from 10% in 2022 to 16% by the year 2050, there will be a concomitant growth of cases of sarcopenic obesity. Older adults with obesity are at risk of developing sarcopenia and incident frailty, leading to an increased risk for adverse events and healthcare utilization. Ongoing standardization of definitions related to outcomes for both sarcopenia and obesity is being worked on and an important next step. Gaining an understanding of the basic biological mechanisms of sarcopenic obesity will permit us to fully understand the possible mechanisms that could inform drug development and its targets in the future. As practitioners identify patients with sarcopenic obesity, they could prescribe lifestyle modifications that include combined weight loss and aerobic and resistance exercise that will favorably alter body composition by loss of fat and preservation or improvement of muscle mass and quality. Clinical trials are critically needed to test both known and experimental interventions that could potentially prevent or reverse functional decline in patients with sarcopenic obesity.

References

1. Roberts AW, Ogunwole SU, Blakeslee L, Rabe MA. The population 65 years and older in the United States: 2016. American Community Survey Reports. Vol ACS-38. United States Census Bureau 2018.
2. Wolff JL, Starfield B, Anderson G. Prevalence, expenditures, and complications of multiple chronic conditions in the elderly. Arch Intern Med. 2002;162(20): 2269–76.

3. Dunlop DD, Hughes SL, Manheim LM. Disability in activities of daily living: patterns of change and a hierarchy of disability. Am J Public Health. 1997;87 (3):378–83.

4. Fried LP, Tangen CM, Walston J, Newman AB, Hirsch C, Gottdiener J, Seeman T, Tracy R, Kop WJ, Burke G, McBurnie MA. Cardiovascular health study collaborative research G. Frailty in older adults: evidence for a phenotype. J Gerontol A Biol Sci Med Sci. 2001;56(3):M146–56.

5. Guiding principles for the care of older adults with multimorbidity: an approach for clinicians. Guiding principles for the care of older adults with multimorbidity: an approach for clinicians: American geriatrics society expert panel on the care of older adults with multimorbidity. J Am Geriatr Soc. 2012;60(10): E1–E25.

6. Lawton MP, Brody EM. Assessment of older people: self-maintaining and instrumental activities of daily living. The Gerontologist. 1969;9(3):179–86.

7. Chambers BA, Guo SS, Siervogel R, Hall G, Chumlea WC. Cumulative effects of cardiovascular disease risk factors on quality of life. J Nutr Health Aging. 2002;6 (3):179–84.

8. Rosemann T, Grol R, Herman K, Wensing M, Szecsenyi J. Association between obesity, quality of life, physical activity and health service utilization in primary care patients with osteoarthritis. Int J Behav Nutr Phys Act. 2008;5:4.

9. Health TfAs. State of obesity 2022. Better policies for a healthy America 2022.

10. Baumgartner RN. Body composition in healthy aging. Ann N Y Acad Sci. 2000;904:437–48.

11. Gao Q, Mei F, Shang Y, Hu K, Chen F, Zhao L, Ma B. Global prevalence of sarcopenic obesity in older adults: a systematic review and meta-analysis. Clin Nutr. 2021;40(7):4633–41.

12. Okorodudu DO, Jumean MF, Montori VM, Romero-Corral A, Somers VK, Erwin PJ, Lopez-Jimenez F. Diagnostic performance of body mass index to identify obesity as defined by body adiposity: a systematic review and meta-analysis. Int J Obes. 2010;34(5): 791–9.

13. Kramer CK, Zinman B, Retnakaran R. Are metabolically healthy overweight and obesity benign conditions?: a systematic review and meta-analysis. Ann Intern Med. 2013;159(11):758–69.

14. Houston DK, Ding J, Nicklas BJ, Harris TB, Lee JS, Nevitt MC, Rubin SM, Tylavsky FA, Kritchevsky SB, Health ABCS. Overweight and obesity over the adult life course and incident mobility limitation in older adults: the health, aging and body composition study. Am J Epidemiol. 2009;169(8):927–36.

15. Zizza CA, Herring A, Stevens J, Popkin BM. Obesity affects nursing-care facility admission among whites but not blacks. Obes Res. 2002;10(8):816–23.

16. Schaap LA, Koster A, Visser M. Adiposity, muscle mass, and muscle strength in relation to functional decline in older persons. Epidemiologic reviews. 2012;35:51.

17. Batsis JA, Sahakyan KR, Rodriguez-Escudero JP, Bartels SJ, Lopez-Jimenez F. Normal weight obesity and functional outcomes in older adults. Eur J Intern Med. 2014;25(6):517–22.

18. Gregg EW, Cheng YJ, Cadwell BL, Imperatore G, Williams DE, Flegal KM, Narayan KM, Williamson DF. Secular trends in cardiovascular disease risk factors according to body mass index in US adults. JAMA. 2005;293(15):1868–74.

19. Ambrose NL, Keogan F, O'Callaghan JP, O'Connell PG. Obesity and disability in the symptomatic Irish knee osteoarthritis population. Ir J Med Sci. 2010;179 (2):265–8.

20. Reeves GK, Pirie K, Beral V, Green J, Spencer E, Bull D, Million Women Study C. Cancer incidence and mortality in relation to body mass index in the Million Women Study: cohort study. BMJ (Clin Res ed). 2007;335(7630):1134.

21. Hassing LB, Dahl AK, Thorvaldsson V, Berg S, Gatz M, Pedersen NL, Johansson B. Overweight in midlife and risk of dementia: a 40-year follow-up study. Int J Obes. 2009;33(8):893–8.

22. Lopez-Jimenez F, Batsis JA, Roger VL, Brekke L, Ting HH, Somers VK. Trends in 10-year predicted risk of cardiovascular disease in the United States, 1976 to 2004. Circ Cardiovasc Qual Outcomes. 2009;2(5): 443–50.

23. Ward ZJ, Willett WC, Hu FB, Pacheco LS, Long MW, Gortmaker SL. Excess mortality associated with elevated body weight in the USA by state and demographic subgroup: a modelling study. eClinicalMedicine. 2022;48:101429.

24. Sorkin JD, Muller DC, Andres R. Longitudinal change in height of men and women: implications for interpretation of the body mass index: the Baltimore longitudinal study of aging. Am J Epidemiol. 1999;150(9): 969–77.

25. Williamson DF. Descriptive epidemiology of body weight and weight change in U.S. adults. Ann Intern Med. 1993;119(7 Pt 2):646–9.

26. Physical status: the use and interpretation of anthropometry. Report of a WHO expert committee. World Health Organ Tech Rep Ser. 1995;854.: World Health Organization:1–452.

27. Kuk JL, Ardern CI. Influence of age on the association between various measures of obesity and all-cause mortality. J Am Geriatr Soc. 2009;57(11):2077–84.

28. Batsis JA, Sahakyan KR, Rodriguez-Escudero JP, Bartels SJ, Somers VK, Lopez-Jimenez F. Normal weight obesity and mortality in United States subjects >/=60 years of age (from the third National Health and nutrition examination survey). Am J Cardiol. 2013;112 (10):1592–8.

29. Batsis JA, Zhbelik AJ, Scherer E, Barre LK, Bartels S. Normal weight central obesity, physical activity, and functional decline: data from the osteoarthritis

initiative. Journal of the American Geriatrics Society. 2015;63(8):1552–60.

30. Cruz-Jentoft AJ, Baeyens JP, Bauer JM, Boirie Y, Cederholm T, Landi F, Martin FC, Michel JP, Rolland Y, Schneider SM, Topinkova E, Vandewoude M, Zamboni M. Sarcopenia: European consensus on definition and diagnosis. Age Ageing. 2010;39(4):412–23.

31. Morley JE, Anker SD, Evans WJ. Cachexia and aging: an update based on the fourth international cachexia meeting. J Nutr Health Aging. 2009;13(1):47–55.

32. Sayer AA, Syddall H, Martin H, Patel H, Baylis D, Cooper C. The developmental origins of sarcopenia. J Nutr Health Aging. 2008;12(7):427–32.

33. Warming L, Hassager C, Christiansen C. Changes in bone mineral density with age in men and women: a longitudinal study. Osteoporos Int. 2002;13(2): 105–12.

34. Kanis JA, Johnell O, Oden A, Johansson H, McCloskey E. FRAX and the assessment of fracture probability in men and women from the UK. Osteoporos Int. 2008;19(4):385–97.

35. Batsis JA, Barre LK, Mackenzie TA, Pratt SI, Lopez-Jimenez F, Bartels SJ. Variation in the prevalence of sarcopenia and sarcopenic obesity in older adults associated with different research definitions: dual-energy X-ray absorptiometry data from the National Health and nutrition examination survey 1999-2004. J Am Geriatr Soc. 2013;61(6):974–80.

36. Cruz-Jentoft AJ, Bahat G, Bauer J, Boirie Y, Bruyère O, Cederholm T, Cooper C, Landi F, Rolland Y, Sayer AA, Schneider SM, Sieber CC, Topinkova E, Vandewoude M, Visser M, Zamboni M. Sarcopenia: revised European consensus on definition and diagnosis. Age Ageing. 2019;48(1):16–31.

37. Studenski SA, Peters KW, Alley DE, Cawthon PM, McLean RR, Harris TB, Ferrucci L, Guralnik JM, Fragala MS, Kenny AM, Kiel DP, Kritchevsky SB, Shardell MD, Dam TT, Vassileva MT. The FNIH sarcopenia project: rationale, study description, conference recommendations, and final estimates. J Gerontol A Biol Sci Med Sci. 2014;69(5):547–58.

38. RR ML, Shardell MD, Alley DE, Cawthon PM, Fragala MS, Harris TB, Kenny AM, Peters KW, Ferrucci L, Guralnik JM, Kritchevsky SB, Kiel DP, Vassileva MT, Xue QL, Perera S, Studenski SA, Dam TT. Criteria for clinically relevant weakness and low lean mass and their longitudinal association with incident mobility impairment and mortality: the foundation for the National Institutes of Health (FNIH) sarcopenia project. J Gerontol A Biol Sci Med Sci. 2014;69(5): 576–83.

39. Dam TT, Peters KW, Fragala M, Cawthon PM, Harris TB, McLean R, Shardell M, Alley DE, Kenny A, Ferrucci L, Guralnik J, Kiel DP, Kritchevsky S, Vassileva MT, Studenski S. An evidence-based comparison of operational criteria for the presence of sarcopenia. J Gerontol A Biol Sci Med Sci. 2014;69 (5):584–90.

40. Cawthon PM, Peters KW, Shardell MD, McLean RR, Dam TT, Kenny AM, Fragala MS, Harris TB, Kiel DP, Guralnik JM, Ferrucci L, Kritchevsky SB, Vassileva MT, Studenski SA, Alley DE. Cutpoints for low appendicular lean mass that identify older adults with clinically significant weakness. J Gerontol A Biol Sci Med Sci. 2014;69(5):567–75.

41. Studenski S, Perera S, Patel K, Rosano C, Faulkner K, Inzitari M, Brach J, Chandler J, Cawthon P, Connor EB, Nevitt M, Visser M, Kritchevsky S, Badinelli S, Harris T, Newman AB, Cauley J, Ferrucci L, Guralnik J. Gait speed and survival in older adults. JAMA. 2011;305(1):50–8.

42. Bhasin S, Travison TG, Manini TM, Patel S, Pencina KM, Fielding RA, Magaziner JM, Newman AB, Kiel DP, Cooper C, Guralnik JM, Cauley JA, Arai H, Clark BC, Landi F, Schaap LA, Pereira SL, Rooks D, Woo J, Woodhouse LJ, Binder E, Brown T, Shardell M, Xue QL, D'Agostino RB, Orwig D, Gorsicki G, Correa-De-Araujo R, Cawthon PM. Sarcopenia definition: the position statements of the sarcopenia definition and outcomes consortium. J Am Geriatr Soc. 2020;68(7): 1410–8.

43. Santilli V, Bernetti A, Mangone M, Paoloni M. Clinical definition of sarcopenia. Clin Cases Miner Bone Metab. 2014;11(3):177–80.

44. Janssen I, Shepard DS, Katzmarzyk PT, Roubenoff R. The healthcare costs of sarcopenia in the United States. J Am Geriatr Soc. 2004;52(1):80–5.

45. Cawthon PM, Visser M, Arai H, Ávila-Funes JA, Barazzoni R, Bhasin S, Binder E, Bruyère O, Cederholm T, Chen L-K, Cooper C, Duque G, Fielding RA, Guralnik J, Kiel DP, Kirk B, Landi F, Sayer AA, Von Haehling S, Woo J, Cruz-Jentoft AJ. Defining terms commonly used in sarcopenia research: a glossary proposed by the global leadership in sarcopenia (GLIS) steering committee. Eur Geriat Med. 2022;13 (6):1239–44.

46. Donini LM, Busetto L, Bischoff SC, Cederholm T, Ballesteros-Pomar MD, Batsis JA, Bauer JM, Boirie Y, Cruz-Jentoft AJ, Dicker D, Frara S, Frühbeck G, Genton L, Gepner Y, Giustina A, Gonzalez MC, Han HS, Heymsfield SB, Higashiguchi T, Laviano A, Lenzi A, Nyulasi I, Parrinello E, Poggiogalle E, Prado CM, Salvador J, Rolland Y, Santini F, Serlie MJ, Shi H, Sieber CC, Siervo M, Vettor R, Villareal DT, Volkert D, Yu J, Zamboni M, Barazzoni R. Definition and diagnostic criteria for sarcopenic obesity: ESPEN and EASO consensus statement. Clin Nutr. 2022;41(4):990–1000.

47. Donini M, Lorenzo BL, Bischoff C, Stephan CT, Ballesteros-Pomar D, Maria BA, John BM, Juergen BY, Cruz-Jentoft J, Alfonso DD, Frara S, Frühbeck G, Genton L, Gepner Y, Giustina A, Gonzalez C, Maria HH-S, Heymsfield B, Steven HT, Laviano A, Lenzi A, Nyulasi I, Parrinello E, Poggiogalle E, Prado M, Carla SJ, Rolland Y, Santini F, Serlie J, Mireille SH, Sieber C, Cornel SM, Vettor R, Villareal T, Dennis VD, Yu J, Zamboni M,

Barazzoni R. Definition and diagnostic criteria for sarcopenic obesity: ESPEN and EASO consensus statement. Obesity Facts. 2022;15(3):321–35.

48. Poggiogalle E, Lubrano C, Sergi G, Coin A, Gnessi L, Mariani S, Lenzi A, Donini LM. Sarcopenic obesity and metabolic syndrome in adult Caucasian subjects. J Nutr Health Aging. 2016;20(9):958–63.

49. Poggiogalle E, Lubrano C, Gnessi L, Mariani S, Di Martino M, Catalano C, Lenzi A, Donini LM. The decline in muscle strength and muscle quality in relation to metabolic derangements in adult women with obesity. Clin Nutr. 2019;38(5):2430–5.

50. Alizadeh PH. Exercise therapy for people with sarcopenic obesity: myokines and adipokines as effective actors. Front Endocrinol (Lausanne). 2022;13: 811751.

51. Villareal DT, Banks M, Siener C, Sinacore DR, Klein S. Physical frailty and body composition in obese elderly men and women. Obes Res. 2004;12(6): 913–20.

52. Stenholm S, Harris TB, Rantanen T, Visser M, Kritchevsky SB, Ferrucci L. Sarcopenic obesity: definition, cause and consequences. Curr Opin Clin Nutr Metab Care. 2008;11(6):693–700.

53. Hamrick MW, Herberg S, Arounleut P, He HZ, Shiver A, Qi RQ, Zhou L, Isales CM, Mi QS. The adipokine leptin increases skeletal muscle mass and significantly alters skeletal muscle miRNA expression profile in aged mice. Biochem Biophys Res Commun. 2010;400(3):379–83.

54. Sweeney G. Cardiovascular effects of leptin. Nat Rev Cardiol. 2010;7(1):22–9.

55. Waters DL, Qualls CR, Dorin RI, Veldhuis JD, Baumgartner RN. Altered growth hormone, cortisol, and leptin secretion in healthy elderly persons with sarcopenia and mixed body composition phenotypes. J Gerontol A Biol Sci Med Sci. 2008;63(5):536–41.

56. Schrager MA, Metter EJ, Simonsick E, Ble A, Bandinelli S, Lauretani F, Ferrucci L. Sarcopenic obesity and inflammation in the InCHIANTI study. J Appl Physiol (Bethesda, MD : 1985). 2007;102(3):919–25.

57. Kob R, Bollheimer LC, Bertsch T, Fellner C, Djukic M, Sieber CC, Fischer BE. Sarcopenic obesity: molecular clues to a better understanding of its pathogenesis? Biogerontology. 2015;16(1):15–29.

58. Chang CI, Huang KC, Chan DC, Wu CH, Lin CC, Hsiung CA, Hsu CC, Chen CY. The impacts of sarcopenia and obesity on physical performance in the elderly. Obes Res Clin Pract. 2014;9:256–65.

59. Bouchard DR, Dionne IJ, Brochu M. Sarcopenic/obesity and physical capacity in older men and women: data from the nutrition as a determinant of successful aging (NuAge)-the Quebec longitudinal study. Obesity. 2009;17(11):2082–8.

60. Davison KK, Ford ES, Cogswell ME, Dietz WH. Percentage of body fat and body mass index are associated with mobility limitations in people aged 70 and older from NHANES III. J Am Geriatr Soc. 2002;50(11):1802–9.

61. Auyeung TW, Lee JS, Leung J, Kwok T, Woo J. Adiposity to muscle ratio predicts incident physical limitation in a cohort of 3,153 older adults – an alternative measurement of sarcopenia and sarcopenic obesity. Age (Dordr). 2013;35(4):1377–85.

62. Baumgartner RN, Koehler KM, Gallagher D, Romero L, Heymsfield SB, Ross RR, Garry PJ, Lindeman RD. Epidemiology of sarcopenia among the elderly in New Mexico. Am J Epidemiol. 1998;147(8):755–63.

63. Baumgartner RN, Wayne SJ, Waters DL, Janssen I, Gallagher D, Morley JE. Sarcopenic obesity predicts instrumental activities of daily living disability in the elderly. Obes Res. 2004;12(12):1995–2004.

64. Rolland Y, Lauwers-Cances V, Cristini C, Abellan van Kan G, Janssen I, Morley JE, Vellas B. Difficulties with physical function associated with obesity, sarcopenia, and sarcopenic-obesity in community-dwelling elderly women: the EPIDOS (EPIDemiologie de l'OSteoporose) study. Am J Clin Nutr. 2009;89(6):1895–900.

65. Levine ME, Crimmins EM. The impact of insulin resistance and inflammation on the association between sarcopenic obesity and physical functioning. Obesity (Silver Spring, MD). 2012;20(10):2101–6.

66. Sternfeld B, Ngo L, Satariano WA, Tager IB. Associations of body composition with physical performance and self-reported functional limitation in elderly men and women. Am J Epidemiol. 2002;156 (2):110–21.

67. Lee S, Kim TN, Kim SH. Sarcopenic obesity is more closely associated with knee osteoarthritis than is non-sarcopenic obesity: a cross-sectional study. Arthritis Rheum. 2012;64(12):3947–54.

68. Baek SJ, Nam GE, Han KD, Choi SW, Jung SW, Bok AR, Kim YH, Lee KS, Han BD, Kim DH. Sarcopenia and sarcopenic obesity and their association with dyslipidemia in Korean elderly men: the 2008-2010 Korea National Health and nutrition examination survey. J Endocrinol Investig. 2014;37(3):247–60.

69. Kim TN, Yang SJ, Yoo HJ, Lim KI, Kang HJ, Song W, Seo JA, Kim SG, Kim NH, Baik SH, Choi DS, Choi KM. Prevalence of sarcopenia and sarcopenic obesity in Korean adults: the Korean sarcopenic obesity study. Int J Obes. 2009;33(8):885–92.

70. Lim S, Kim JH, Yoon JW, Kang SM, Choi SH, Park YJ, Kim KW, Lim JY, Park KS, Jang HC. Sarcopenic obesity: prevalence and association with metabolic syndrome in the Korean longitudinal study on Health and aging (KLoSHA). Diabetes Care. 2010;33(7): 1652–4.

71. Kim TN, Park MS, Ryu JY, Choi HY, Hong HC, Yoo HJ, Kang HJ, Song W, Park SW, Baik SH, Newman AB, Choi KM. Impact of visceral fat on skeletal muscle mass and vice versa in a prospective cohort study: the Korean Sarcopenic obesity study (KSOS). PLoS One. 2014;9(12):e115407.

72. Stephen WC, Janssen I. Sarcopenic-obesity and cardiovascular disease risk in the elderly. J Nutr Health Aging. 2009;13(5):460–6.

73. Batsis JA, Mackenzie TA, Barre LK, Lopez-Jimenez F, Bartels SJ. Sarcopenia, sarcopenic obesity and mortality in older adults: results from the National Health and nutrition examination survey III. Eur J Clin Nutr. 2014;68(9):1001–7.

74. Atkins JL, Wannamathee SG. Sarcopenic obesity in ageing: cardiovascular outcomes and mortality. Br J Nutr. 2020;124(10):1102–13.

75. Atkins JL, Whincup PH, Morris RW, Lennon LT, Papacosta O, Wannamethee SG. Sarcopenic obesity and risk of cardiovascular disease and mortality: a population-based cohort study of older men. J Am Geriatr Soc. 2014;62(2):253–60.

76. Beavers KM, Beavers DP, Nesbit BA, Ambrosius WT, Marsh AP, Nicklas BJ, Rejeski WJ. Effect of an 18-month physical activity and weight loss intervention on body composition in overweight and obese older adults. Obesity (Silver Spring, MD). 2014;22(2):325–31.

77. Shea MK, Houston DK, Nicklas BJ, Messier SP, Davis CC, Miller ME, Harris TB, Kitzman DW, Kennedy K, Kritchevsky SB. The effect of randomization to weight loss on total mortality in older overweight and obese adults: the ADAPT study. J Gerontol A Biol Sci Med Sci. 2010;65(5):519–25.

78. Villareal DT, Chode S, Parimi N, Sinacore DR, Hilton T, Armamento-Villareal R, Napoli N, Qualls C, Shah K. Weight loss, exercise, or both and physical function in obese older adults. N Engl J Med. 2011;364(13):1218–29.

79. Kritchevsky SB, Beavers KM, Miller ME, Shea MK, Houston DK, Kitzman DW, Nicklas BJ. Intentional weight loss and all-cause mortality: a meta-analysis of randomized clinical trials. PLoS One. 2015;10(3):e0121993.

80. Batsis JA, Huyck KL, Bartels SJ. Challenges with the medicare obesity benefit: practical concerns & proposed solutions. J Gen Intern Med. 2014;30:118.

81. Batsis JA, Villareal DT. Sarcopenic obesity in older adults: aetiology, epidemiology and treatment strategies. Nat Rev Endocrinol. 2018;14(9):513–37.

82. Verreijen AM, Engberink MF, Memelink RG, Van Der Plas SE, Visser M, Weijs PJM. Effect of a high protein diet and/or resistance exercise on the preservation of fat free mass during weight loss in overweight and obese older adults: a randomized controlled trial. Nutr J. 2017;16(1)

83. Trouwborst I, Verreijen A, Memelink R, Massanet P, Boirie Y, Weijs P, Tieland M. Exercise and nutrition strategies to counteract Sarcopenic obesity. Nutrients. 2018;10(5):605.

84. Holick MF, Binkley NC, Bischoff-Ferrari HA, Gordon CM, Hanley DA, Heaney RP, Murad MH, Weaver CM, Endocrine S. Evaluation, treatment, and prevention of vitamin D deficiency: an Endocrine Society clinical practice guideline. J Clin Endocrinol Metab. 2011;96(7):1911–30.

85. Wicherts IS, van Schoor NM, Boeke AJ, Visser M, Deeg DJ, Smit J, Knol DL, Lips P. Vitamin D status predicts physical performance and its decline in older persons. J Clin Endocrinol Metab. 2007;92(6):2058–65.

86. Zittermann A, Iodice S, Pilz S, Grant WB, Bagnardi V, Gandini S. Vitamin D deficiency and mortality risk in the general population: a meta-analysis of prospective cohort studies. Am J Clin Nutr. 2012;95(1):91–100.

87. Poggiogalle E, Parrinello E, Barazzoni R, Busetto L, Donini LM. Therapeutic strategies for sarcopenic obesity: a systematic review. Curr Opin Clin Nutr Metab Care. 2021;24(1):33–41.

88. American Geriatrics Society Workgroup on Vitamin DSfOA. Recommendations abstracted from the American Geriatrics Society consensus statement on vitamin D for prevention of falls and their consequences. J Am Geriatr Soc. 2014;62(1):147–52.

89. Behre HM, Tammela TL, Arver S, Tolra JR, Bonifacio V, Lamche M, Kelly J, Hiemeyer F, European Testogel Study T, Giltay EJ, Gooren LJ. A randomized, double-blind, placebo-controlled trial of testosterone gel on body composition and health-related quality-of-life in men with hypogonadal to low-normal levels of serum testosterone and symptoms of androgen deficiency over 6 months with 12 months open-label follow-up. Aging Male. 2012;15(4):198–207.

90. Emmelot-Vonk MH, Verhaar HJ, Nakhai Pour HR, Aleman A, Lock TM, Bosch JL, Grobbee DE, van der Schouw YT. Effect of testosterone supplementation on functional mobility, cognition, and other parameters in older men: a randomized controlled trial. JAMA. 2008;299(1):39–52.

91. Bhasin S, Parker RA, Sattler F, Haubrich R, Alston B, Umbleja T, Shikuma CM, Team ACTGPAS. Effects of testosterone supplementation on whole body and regional fat mass and distribution in human immunodeficiency virus-infected men with abdominal obesity. J Clin Endocrinol Metab. 2007;92(3):1049–57.

92. Fernandez-Balsells MM, Murad MH, Lane M, Lampropulos JF, Albuquerque F, Mullan RJ, Agrwal N, Elamin MB, Gallegos-Orozco JF, Wang AT, Erwin PJ, Bhasin S, Montori VM. Clinical review 1: adverse effects of testosterone therapy in adult men: a systematic review and meta-analysis. J Clin Endocrinol Metab. 2010;95(6):2560–75.

93. Xu L, Freeman G, Cowling BJ, Schooling CM. Testosterone therapy and cardiovascular events among men: a systematic review and meta-analysis of placebo-controlled randomized trials. BMC Med. 2013;11:108.

94. Nair KS, Rizza RA, O'Brien P, Dhatariya K, Short KR, Nehra A, Vittone JL, Klee GG, Basu A, Basu R, Cobelli C, Toffolo G, Dalla Man C, Tindall DJ, Melton LJ 3rd, Smith GE, Khosla S, Jensen MD. DHEA in elderly women and DHEA or testosterone in elderly men. N Engl J Med. 2006;355(16):1647–59.

95. Baker WL, Karan S, Kenny AM. Effect of dehydroepiandrosterone on muscle strength and physical function in older adults: a systematic review. J Am Geriatr Soc. 2011;59(6):997–1002.

96. Konopka AR, Laurin JL, Schoenberg HM, Reid JJ, Castor WM, Wolff CA, Musci RV, Safairad OD, Linden MA, Biela LM, Bailey SM, Hamilton KL, Miller BF. Metformin inhibits mitochondrial adaptations to aerobic exercise training in older adults. Aging Cell. 2019;18(1):e12880.

97. Justice JN, Ferrucci L, Newman AB, Aroda VR, Bahnson JL, Divers J, Espeland MA, Marcovina S, Pollak MN, Kritchevsky SB, Barzilai N, Kuchel GA. A framework for selection of blood-based biomarkers for geroscience-guided clinical trials: report from the TAME biomarkers workgroup. Geroscience. 2018;40(5–6):419–36.

98. Perna S, Guido D, Bologna C, Solerte SB, Guerriero F, Isu A, Rondanelli M. Liraglutide and obesity in elderly: efficacy in fat loss and safety in order to prevent sarcopenia. A perspective case series study. Aging Clin Exp Res. 2016;28(6):1251–7.

99. Katz S, Ford AB, Moskowitz RW, Jackson BA, Jaffe MW. Studies of illness in the aged. The index of ADL: a standardized measure of biological and psychosocial function. JAMA. 1963;185:914–9.

Linking Obesity, Metabolism, and Cancer

32

Ivana Vucenik, Laundette P. Jones, and John C. McLenithan

Contents

I. Vucenik (✉)
Department of Medical and Research Technology,
University of Maryland School of Medicine, Baltimore,
MD, USA

Department of Pathology, University of Maryland School
of Medicine, Baltimore, MD, USA
e-mail: ivucenik@som.umaryland.edu

L. P. Jones
Department(s) of Pharmacology & Epidemiology and
Public Health, University of Maryland School of
Medicine, Baltimore, MD, USA
e-mail: LPJones@som.umaryland.edu

J. C. McLenithan
Department of Medicine, University of Maryland School
of Medicine, Baltimore, MD, USA
e-mail: jmcle001@umaryland.edu;
jmclenithan@som.umaryland.edu

© Springer Nature Switzerland AG 2023
R. S. Ahima (ed.), *Metabolic Syndrome*,
https://doi.org/10.1007/978-3-031-40116-9_50

Abstract

The pandemics of obesity and cancer are major health challenges worldwide. In addition to diabetes and cardiovascular disease, epidemiological evidence shows that people who are overweight or obese are at increased risk of developing some types of cancer. Obesity may also affect tumor progression for many cancers, and obesity presents an obstacle in cancer treatment. In this chapter we discuss potential mechanisms linking obesity to cancer development, progression, and mortality, including energy imbalance, insulin resistance, and altered hormone signaling. We especially focus on chronic inflammation, and its local and systemic effects. Understanding the mechanisms involved in obesity–cancer link is important not only to prevent both cancer and obesity, but also for developing potential therapeutics.

Keywords

Obesity · Cancer · Metabolism · Mechanisms · Inflammation · Prevention · Interventions

Key Points

1. Excess body weight and adiposity pose significant health risk for cardiovascular disease, type 2 diabetes, and various types of cancer, but are modifiable risk factors
2. Heterogeneity of obesity affects pathophysiology at cellular and systemic levels
3. Obesity is characterized by an increase in body fat, increased macrophage infiltration of white adipose tissue, and abnormal adipokine and cytokine production, contributing to a low-grade chronic inflammation

4. Inflammation provides an important link between obesity, insulin resistance, and cancer, but there are significant differences in the inflammatory profile of distinct abdominal fat depots

Introduction

Obesity rates have been steadily increasing over recent decades, reaching pandemic proportions with significant implications for public health. Obesity rates continue to rise, and by 2030 it is predicted that the number of people with obesity globally will have doubled since 2010. The World Obesity Federation's 2023 atlas predicts that 51% of the world, or more than 4 billion people, will be obese or overweight within the next 12 years. Rates of obesity are rising particularly among children and in lower-income countries [1]. It is projected that by 2030, about 50% of the adult population in the USA will be obese [2].

There are multiple health consequences of overweight and obesity. Obesity is a risk factor for cardiovascular disease, type 2 diabetes, hypertension, dyslipidemia, musculoskeletal disorders, some cancers, dementia, psychosocial problems, and increased mortality [3]. In addition to its serious health consequences, health-care expenditure for obesity-related diseases is increasing and it is predicted that the global economic impact of overweight and obesity will reach $4.32 trillion annually if prevention and treatment measures do not improve [1].

Obesity is defined as abnormal or excessive accumulation of body fat. Definitions for classifying and reporting healthy weight, overweight, and obesity in populations have historically been based on measures of weight and height rather than clinical measures of adiposity. By far the most widely used weight-for-height measure is the body mass index (BMI), which is defined as weight (in kilograms) divided by height (in meters squared); BMI of 18.8–24.0 kg/m^2 indicates healthy weight, 25.0–29.9 overweight, and BMI of 30 kg/m^2 or higher obesity [4]. Although BMI is the same for both sexes and for all ages of adults, it should be considered as a rough guide, because it may not correspond to the same degree of adiposity in different individuals. Additionally, heritability of obesity and variability of BMI related to the race, ethnicity, and culture indicate that the obesity standards may need to be reevaluated. There are other methods to evaluate body fat and body fat distribution, such as waist circumference (WC), body shape index (ABSI), and estimating the visceral adipose tissue (VAT) and abdominal subcutaneous adipose tissue (SAT) by ultrasound, computed tomography, and magnetic resonance imaging. The heterogeneity of obesity is shown by existence of distinct subsets of obese individuals, a subgroup who have reduced cardiometabolic risk despite being obese, as opposed to lean individuals with a high risk for cardiometabolic complications [5–8]. These phenotypically distinct subgroups have been recognized in early 1980s and are known as metabolically healthy obese (MHO) and metabolically unhealthy normal weight (MUNW). The prevalence of MHO varies from 20% to 30% among obese individuals. Compared to regular obese individuals, MHO subjects have high levels of insulin sensitivity and the absence of diabetes, dyslipidemia, or hypertension. MHO phenotype is characterized by a more favorable inflammatory profile, smaller adipocyte cell size, less visceral fat, and less infiltration of macrophages into adipose tissue [7].

The Association of Obesity and Cancer

The worldwide burden of cancer continues to grow. Cancer is the second leading cause of death worldwide and exposure to risk factors plays an important role in the biology and burden of many cancer types. Therefore, understanding the magnitude of cancer burden attributable to potentially modifiable risk factors is crucial for development of effective prevention strategies, and guiding policy makers and researchers [9]. New research strategies and infrastructure that combine population-based and laboratory research at a global level are needed to enhance cancer prevention [10].

Excess adiposity is associated with the risk of developing several types of cancer. To date, over 500 observational epidemiologic studies have examined the associations between obesity, physical activity, and cancer incidence [11]. Many of the global concerns regarding the links between environmental factors and diet, nutrition, obesity, and cancer are addressed by the World Cancer Research Fund (WCRF) and American Institute for Cancer Research (AICR) [12] and their various publications [13]. The WCRF and AICR conducted a comprehensive and systemic evaluation of the available literature on diet, physical activity, weight, and cancer prevention, considering epidemiologic, clinical, and experimental data, and concluded that body fatness was an established risk factor for several cancers, e.g., breast, endometrium, colon, esophagus, gall bladder, pancreas, kidney, prostate, and liver [12]. Furthermore, the WCRF/AICR has estimated that about 21% of cancer in the USA can be attributed to obesity, 17% in Great Britain, 13% in Brazil, and 11% in China [12, 13]. In addition to WCRF/AICR, this evidence has been evaluated and summarized for the Physical Activity Guidelines for Americans (PAGA) 2018 Report as part of their recommendations on physical activity for cancer risk reduction [11–14]. These reviews of the evidence, as well as multiple systematic reviews and meta-analyses on the topic concluded that there is strong evidence that physical activity reduces the risk of bladder, breast, colon, endometrial, esophageal adenocarcinoma, and gastric cancers [11]. There is moderate evidence for an association between higher levels of physical activity with lower occurrence of renal, ovarian, pancreatic, and lung cancers [11].

Adiposity Patterns and Heterogeneity

Adiposity pattern and fat topography, in particular the upper (central, android) and lower (peripheral, gynoid) types of obesity, are also related to pathogenesis of cancer. Studies have demonstrated that expansion of visceral adipose tissue (VAT) rather than subcutaneous adipose tissue (SAT) is critical for the development of obesity-associated insulin resistance [15], and at least in overweight/obese subjects, expansion of SAT depots may be protective. However, absolute quantification of VAT and SAT may not reflect the relative distribution of body fat, and recent data suggest that a high VAT/SAT ratio, a measure of relative body fat distribution between VAT and SAT depots, is a unique risk marker independent of overall adiposity. Less is known regarding associations between adipose depots and cancer risk. A study by Murphy et al. [16] provides insight into relationships between specific fat depots and cancer risk and suggest differential relationships among men and women. The total fat mass and VAT were positively associated with cancer risk among women but there was no association with cancer risk among men. Visceral abdominal fat was recently associated with an increased risk of colorectal adenoma; the findings of the study implicate abdominal VAT in the development and progression of colorectal adenoma, and it was better indicator of obesity for colorectal adenoma than the BMI in both sexes [17]. There is a growing appreciation of a pathogenic role of ectopic fat, supported by findings that the visceral adiposity is associated with incident cardiovascular disease and cancer [18], renal cell carcinoma [19], and gastrointestinal cancers [20]. In terms of the body shape, it was shown that body shape is not a risk for breast cancer and that being "apple-shaped" (android adiposity) does not significantly increase breast cancer risk than being "pear-shaped" (gynoid adiposity) [21].

It seems that molecular and metabolic characteristics of white adipose tissue, immune cellular infiltration, and adipokine production are associated with MHO and MUNW phenotype, and that biological pathways and processes such as oxidative phosphorylation, branched-chain amino acid catabolism, and fatty acid beta-oxidation differ between these phenotypes [8]. The potential role of genetic predisposition, and also lifestyle factors such as diet, needs to be clarified in MHO [7]. However, only few studies have addressed the relationship of MHO and MUNW phenotype with cancer. One of those studies was a 15-year prospective study conducted in Cremona, Italy, where the prevalence of MHO was relatively low, only 11% [5, 22]. These subjects had normal insulin sensitivity, and their all-cause cardiovascular disease and cancer mortality, adjusted for age and sex, was lower than in obese insulin-resistant people [22]. Although the prevalence of MUNW is higher in Asian populations, its association with cancer has not been studied.

Adipose tissue is heterogeneous at the cellular level, with morphological and functional diversity. White adipose tissue (WAT) mainly stores energy as triglyceride, whereas brown adipose tissue (BAT) is rich in mitochondria and highly thermogenic [23]. WAT and BAT distributions vary depending on sex, age, and cancer microenvironment, but their specific functions in onset or progression of cancer are unknown.

Potential Mechanisms Linking Obesity and Cancer

Understanding the link between being overweight or obese, and a wide variety of cancers, as well as the biological mechanisms involved, remains an evolving and currently very active area of research. The complex physiological changes that occur with obesity include alterations in the adipose tissue production of growth factors, hormones, and reactive oxygen species (ROS) that can impact the development of cancer [24, 25]. Underlying the comorbid disease states that are associated with obesity including many cancers is a state of chronic low level inflammation [24, 25]. Inflammation has been implicated in every stage of cancer development including transformation, survival, proliferation, invasion, angiogenesis, and metastasis [26]. We will briefly discuss mechanisms linking obesity and cancer as well as the role of inflammatory pathways.

The Role of Inflammation

Inflammation is a complex biological response that can result in both local tissue and systemic physiological changes. Acute inflammation is a rapid high-grade response to tissue damage or pathogen invasion. The cascade of chemokines, cytokines, immune cell infiltration into a damaged, necrotic, or infected tissue is initiated by cells of the innate immune system consisting of macrophages, mast cells, and other stromal-vascular cell types. Chemokines produced by resident cells recruit circulating neutrophils from the microvasculature into the damaged tissue. Activated neutrophils then release anti-microbial peptides and ROS to kill invading pathogens. At this point either the wound healing response will continue or assistance from the adaptive immune system (B and T cell-mediated) will be initiated. The wound healing process involves tissue remodeling including cellular hyperplasia and angiogenesis triggered by cytokines and growth factors released into the local environment [27].

Obesity is the result of a hypertrophic and hyperplastic response of adipocytes within adipose tissue to caloric intake in excess of the requirement for metabolic homeostasis. This is usually the result of chronic positive energy balance, decreased energy expenditure, or both. Obesity is also characterized by a state of chronic low-grade inflammation in contrast to the acute inflammatory response to microbial invasion or tissue damage described previously. In obesity, adipocyte hypertrophy can result in endoplasmic reticulum stress and inadequate microcirculation leading to tissue hypoxia. These stressors can induce modified tissue damage or wound healing response in adipose tissue characterized by the release of pro-inflammatory cytokines, such as tumor necrosis factor-α (TNF-α) and chemokines, such as monocyte chemoattractant protein-1 (MCP 1). MCP-1 recruits monocytes into the adipose tissue that differentiate into pro-inflammatory M1 macrophages that release additional cytokines, such as interleukin-1 (IL-1) and interleukin-6 (IL-6) and chemokines, such as interleukin-8 (IL-8) and macrophage inflammatory protein-1α (MIP-1α). Additionally, chemokine and cytokine gradients attract neutrophils and more monocytes that further exacerbate the inflammatory state in a feed-forward regulation [28]. Secreted pro-inflammatory cytokines contribute to systemic inflammation but have important localized paracrine effects promoting adipocyte insulin resistance leading to elevated lipolysis and the increased release of free fatty acids (FFAs) that can further provoke local and systemic inflammation and lipotoxicity [28].

Comorbidities of obesity include type 2 diabetes, dyslipidemia, hypertension, endothelial dysfunction, and hepatic steatosis leading to increased incidence of cardiovascular disease, renal failure, and several types of cancer. These comorbidities can be attributed directly or indirectly to a chronic inflammatory state [28]. Although these pathophysiological states are associated with increased BMI, they are most highly associated with increases in visceral obesity. It is important to recognize that chronic inflammation is a common characteristic of all adipose tissue depots in the obese state, however, the level and the contribution of a particular adipose tissue depot to local and systemic inflammation can vary dramatically [15, 28]. Adipose tissue is a highly vascularized complex tissue containing multiple cell types in addition to adipocytes including endothelial cells, preadipocytes, multipotent stem cells, fibroblasts, macrophages, monocytes, neutrophils, mast cells, natural killer (NK) cells, T-cells, dendritic cells [23], and mesothelial cells (only visceral adipose tissue) [29]. It is the secretory factors or secretome of the combined cell types within an adipose depot that contribute to its systemic endocrine and local paracrine effects on metabolism and disease susceptibility. Visceral adipose tissue has a greater pro-inflammatory cytokine, plasminogen activator inhibitor-1 (PAI-1), vascular endothelial growth factor (VEGF), and free fatty acid (FFA) secretory profile than subcutaneous adipose tissue by nature of its location in the visceral cavity, higher nutrient and endotoxin exposure from the portal circulation, and its differing cellular composition [15]. Therefore, it is no surprise that increased visceral adipose tissue (VAT) is highly associated with inflammation-dependent disease states such as type 2 diabetes, cardiovascular disease, and cancer as discussed previously [15]. The prominent link between inflammation and obesity has been further highlighted by finding that the inflammasomes may contribute to the pathology [30].

Hyperinsulinemia and Growth Factors

Insulin and insulin-like growth factors (IGFs) have been implicated in a wide range of cancers due to their antiapoptotic and growth promoting properties [24, 25, 30]. Obesity is associated with inflammation-dependent increases in insulin resistance resulting in hyperglycemia and compensatory hyperinsulinemia, and eventually type 2 diabetes [24, 25]. High levels of insulin promote insulin-like growth factor-1 (IGF-1) production. Therefore, patients with obesity and type 2 diabetes have increased cancer mortality, perhaps due to hyperinsulinemia, and/or elevated IGF-1, which leads to increased cancer cell growth, proliferation, and survival. Although insulin target tissues affecting glucose metabolism exhibit insulin resistance in prediabetes or type 2 diabetes, cancer cells maintain sensitivity toward insulin, thus allowing additional growth promotion in the hyperinsulinemic state [23, 25, 30]. In contrast, patients with low circulating insulin and IGFs appear to be protected from cancer development. Patients with type 2 diabetes, receiving insulin therapy or drugs to stimulate insulin secretion have a significantly higher incidence of cancer than those treated with metformin, an insulin-sensitizing anti-diabetic drug that reduces insulin requirement [31]. Epidemiological studies have consistently associated metformin use with decreased cancer incidence and cancer-related mortality; thus, metformin is emerging as a potential anticancer agent [31], underscoring the importance of insulin sensitivity and energy metabolism in cancer biology. Additionally, metformin can activate 5'AMP-activated protein kinase (AMPK), a central regulator of energy metabolism and promoter of fatty acid oxidation [32]. Caloric restriction, which increases insulin sensitivity and reduces circulating insulin and IGF-1 levels, is a potent suppressor of carcinogenesis [33–35]. In several animal models, the effect of caloric restriction on carcinogenesis reduces the PI3K/Akt/mTOR pathway activation via AMPK activation [34, 35], and can be abrogated by restoration of IGF-1 levels [33]. Tumors with mutations activating the PI3K/Akt/mTOR signaling pathway are resistant to caloric restriction [36]. The PI3K/Akt/mTOR and Ras/Raf/MAPK axes are common effector pathways for many growth factors including insulin, IGF, and leptin, regulating tumor survival, growth, and proliferation [37]. Accordingly, PI3K/Akt/mTOR inhibition has been an active target to reduce carcinogenesis and tumor incidence.

Dysregulation of the Adipose Tissue Secretome

Adipose tissue synthesizes and secretes bioactive peptides, adipokines, which include leptin, adiponectin, and numerous others including cytokines and chemokines as well as bioactive lipids and steroid hormones [28].

Leptin acts in the brain to inhibit feeding, and regulate energy metabolism and neuroendocrine axis. Leptin also acts directly on the immune system by stimulating monocytes and lymphocytes to produce pro-inflammatory cytokines [24, 25, 30, 38]. Plasma leptin is increased in proportion to body fat. In obesity, the rise in leptin is unable to prevent weight gain, hence the concept of "leptin resistance." Signaling of leptin through its receptor activates numerous cascades, including the JAK-STAT, IRS-1/2, MAPK, and Akt/PI3K, and decreases the activity of 5'AMP-activated protein kinase (AMPK), a master regulator of cellular energy homeostasis [39, 40]. Despite the leptin resistance observed in obesity, elevated leptin levels can promote tumor growth, and thus, has been viewed as a major mediator of obesity-related cancers [30, 41, 42].

Adiponectin is the most abundant adipokine and circulates in multimeric forms. Adiponectin has potent insulin-sensitizing and anti-inflammatory actions and promotes fatty acid oxidation [40]. In contrast to leptin, adiponectin decreases with increasing adiposity [30, 43, 44], inhibits proliferation of colon, prostate, endometrial, and breast cancer cells and is associated with decreased risk of cancers of the uterus, colon, and breast in epidemiological studies [23, 25, 45]. The anticancer activity of adiponectin [44] may result from modulation of energy balance by decreasing insulin/IGF-1 and mTOR signaling via activation of AMPK and by exerting anti-inflammatory actions via the inhibition of pro-inflammatory signaling [43]. The association between the adiponectin-to-leptin ratio has been suggested as an important risk marker of cancer [46, 47].

Omentin-1 is a 34 kDa adipokine that is highly expressed in visceral adipose tissue (VAT), has both insulin-sensitizing and anti-inflammatory activities, and exerts anti-oxidative and anti-apoptotic roles and regulates endothelial dysfunction [48, 49]. Omentin-1 also has protective effects against cancer, atherosclerosis, type 2 diabetes, and metabolic bone disease [49]. Omentin-1 is decreased with increasing adiposity, and it has been shown to promote apoptosis via p53 deacetylation [48].

Visfatin (Nicotinamide phosphoribosyltransferase, or pre-B-cell colony-enhancing factor) is secreted by adipocytes, macrophages, and endothelial; has pro-inflammatory properties [28]; and may be related to obesity-induced insulin resistance and cancer [50]. Visfatin regulates cancer cell proliferation, angiogenesis, metastasis, and drug resistance.

Vaspin (Visceral adipose tissue-derived serine protease inhibitor) is a 50 kDa adipokine discovered in visceral white adipose tissue of Otsuka Long-Evans Tokushima rat, a model of obesity and type 2 diabetes. Studies have suggested that changes in vaspin levels may be linked with metabolic syndrome, obesity, and impaired insulin sensitivity [51]. High circulating levels of vaspin, omentin-1, and visfatin were shown in patients with colorectal cancer, suggesting a potential role in obesity-dependent cancer [52].

Vascular endothelial growth factor VEGF is a 40–45 kDa homodimeric protein secreted by many cell types. VEGF-A modulates cell migration, endothelial cell sprouting, mitogenesis, vasodilation, and vascular permeability. VEGF-B regulates angiogenesis and mediate metastasis. VEGF-C and VEGF-D regulate lymphangiogenesis, and PlGF regulates vasculogenesis, inflammation, and cancer cell survival. Locally increased levels of VEGF contribute to tumor neovascularization and metastasis [15, 53].

Pro-inflammatory cytokines such as IL-1, IL-6, and TNF-α, are highly elevated in adipose tissue from obese individuals and contribute to chronic localized as well as systemic inflammation. In addition to creating an insulin resistant state in adipose tissue, these factors play a crucial role in tumor growth and invasiveness [54]. IL-1 and TNF-α activate nuclear factor κB (NF-κB)-dependent increases in pro-inflammatory cytokines, angiogenic factors (VEGF and IL-8), matrix metalloproteinases (MMPs) for remodeling and invasion, chemokines and inflammatory enzymes, prostaglandin-endoperoxide synthase 2 (PGHS-2 or COX-2), and 5-lipoxygenase (5-LOX). IL-6 promotes growth and antiapoptotic pathways through IL-6R/JAK activation of STAT3-dependent transcription [26].

Chemokines are soluble chemotactic cytokines that are grouped into four classes based on the positions of key cysteine residues: C, CC, CXC, and CX3C. Several studies have reported the involvement of chemokines and chemokine receptors in cell proliferation, migration, invasion, and metastasis of different types of tumors [55, 56]. They are produced in large amounts from inflamed obese adipose tissue, such as MCP-1 (CCL2), and with IL-8 further exacerbate the inflammatory state by increasing monocyte and neutrophil infiltration of the tissue. IL-8, acting as a chemokine and a pro-angiogenic factor, has been linked with progression, metastasis, and poor prognosis for cancers of the colon, liver, prostate, lung, ovary, and melanoma [53, 55]. Expression of CXCR4, the chemokine receptor that binds stromal cell-derived factor-1 (SDF-1), has been associated with metastasis and poor prognosis in a variety of cancers [53, 55]. Although, the chemokine receptor CXCR4 is expressed on adipocytes and macrophages in adipose tissue, its role in this tissue remains unclear [57].

A list of various interleukins (ILs) and chemokines associated with cancer initiation and promotion, and a role of COX-2, 5-LOX, and

MMPs in cancer are briefly summarized in Table 1 [24, 26–28, 55, 57]. The table also estimates the preventable fractions for selected cancers in the USA attributed to excess adiposity [12, 13, 58].

Steroid hormones, i.e., estrogen, progesterone, androgens, and glucocorticoids are involved in obesity-dependent cancers [60, 61]. Adipose tissue can produce significant amounts of estrogens via aromatase-catalyzed conversion of gonadal and adrenal androgens to estrogen in men and postmenopausal women [61]. In obesity, the elevated pro-inflammatory environment induces elevated expression of aromatase in adipose tissue, thereby contributing to higher local and systemic levels of estrogen [54]. Estrogen and estrogen receptor-α (ER-α) have been implicated in the pathogenesis of postmenopausal breast and endometrial cancers by inducing cellular proliferation, VEGF expression and angiogenesis, and inhibiting apoptosis, and targeting estrogen as a preventive intervention has been demonstrated by clinical data [62]. Selectively reducing aromatase expression and excessive estrogen production has been targeted to reduce ER-dependent obesity-associated cancer [63]. Treatment with exemestane, an aromatase inhibitor, decreased the risk of invasive breast cancer by 65% [64, 65]. Although androgens levels are not consistently associated with prostate cancer risk in men, obesity has been associated with poor prognosis and more aggressive prostate tumors. It is possible that androgen-independent activation of androgen receptor by elevated IL-6 and IGF-1 may be a mediator of aggressive prostate cancer

Table 1 Linking obesity to risk for selected cancers: Proposed mechanisms and a role of inflammation

Cancer	Associated with increased BMI and preventable[a] (%)	Proposed mechanism(s)	Inflammation-driven cancers and inflammatory mediators most likely involved	References
Breast (postmenopausal)	17	Systemic or local estrogen and inflammatory factors	COX-2; CXCR4 and CCR7 in metastasis	[12, 13, 55, 56, 58]
Endometrial	50	Endogenous circulating estrogen from adipose tissue	Circulating and local tissue cytokines might be involved	[12, 13, 58]
Ovarian	5	Systemic and local tissue inflammation	CXCR4, SDF-1, CXCL12, and IL-8 in invasion and growth	[12, 13, 53, 55, 58]
Colorectal	16	Systemic inflammation, cytokines, leptin, IGF-1	IL-6, COX-2, and 5-LOX in increased risk	[12, 13, 26, 28, 55, 58]
Esophageal	35	Acid reflux causing local inflammation	COX-2 in increased risk, invasion, and angiogenesis	[12, 13, 55, 58]
Gallbladder	21	Gall stones causing local inflammation	MMP-9 in aggressiveness and poor prognosis; VEGF, TNF-α, and NF-κB in the lymphangiogenesis	[12, 13, 55, 58, 59]
Pancreatic	19	Systemic inflammation and other circulating factors	IL-1, COX-2, MMP-9 in metastasis and cell invasion	[12, 13, 28, 55, 58]
Liver	27	Fatty infiltration with chronic local inflammation	Oxidative stress and ROS, IL-6 and other inflammatory mediators in liver carcinogenesis	[12, 13, 23, 24, 27, 53, 55, 58]
Kidney	14	Systemic inflammation and growth-stimulating factors	5-LOX in tumor progression	[12, 13, 55, 58]
Prostate	11	Systemic inflammation, other circulating factors, such as IGF-1	IL-6, IL-8, and COX-2 in angiogenesis and clinically more aggressive form of prostate cancer	[12, 13, 55, 56, 58]

[a] The World Cancer Research Fund/American Institute for Cancer Research (WCRF/AICR) estimated the preventable fraction for selected cancers in the USA attributed to excess adiposity. (Refs. [12, 13, 58])

in obesity [54]. Glucocorticoid production from adipose tissue is elevated in obesity, associated with local and systemic insulin resistance, increased lipolysis and elevated FFA levels, and may contribute to pathophysiology of cancer [28, 54, 66].

Bioactive lipids mediate a wide range of biological functions. In the obese insulin resistant state, adipocytes, particularly visceral adipocytes, are highly lipolytic. Free fatty acids (FFAs) released in elevated amounts lead to ectopic deposition in non-adipose tissues such as liver, muscle pancreas causing lipotoxicity, worsening insulin resistance, and pancreatic beta cell dysfunction [28, 54]. FFAs released into the tumor microenvironment can promote tumor growth by supplying metabolic fuels for energy metabolism and generation of pro-tumorigenic signaling lipids [24]. In addition to ectopic tissue accumulation, saturated FFAs can initiate pro-inflammatory signaling to NF-κB through binding and activation of toll-like receptor 4 (TLR4) [28]. Pro-inflammatory signaling by FFAs or cytokines triggers NF-κB-dependent transcription of several genes promoting tumor formation and development including cyclooxygenase-2 (PGHS-2 or COX-2) and 5-lipoxygenase (5-LOX) that produce bioactive pro-inflammatory and tumorigenic lipids, prostaglandin E_2 (PGE$_2$) and leukotrienes, respectively [55, 66].

Some Emerging Mechanisms and New Concepts in Obesity and Cancer Link

Interactions with the Tumor Microenvironment

The tumor microenvironment is a complex interplay of cellular, extracellular matrix (ECM), secretory factor, and metabolite interactions that promote all stages of tumorigenesis. In its simplest form, this environment is composed of tumor cells, the surrounding normal tissue or stromal cells, tumor-associated inflammatory cells, the secretome unique to this environment, as well as systemic factors that may impact tumor growth such as elevated insulin, IGF-1, or

systemic inflammation in type 2 diabetes. In obesity-related cancers such as colon, renal, breast, liver, endometrial, prostate, and pancreatic, the proximal location of dysfunctional adipose tissue in the microenvironment greatly enhances the tumorigenic nature of these complex interactions. Obese adipose tissue and tumors both resemble tissues that are wounded and are undergoing remodeling and repair processes [54]. At these sites hypoxic conditions induce hypoxia-inducible factor 1α (HIF-1α)-dependent increases in several genes, such as *VEGF*, vascular endothelial growth factor receptor (*VEGFR*), cytokine-inducible nitric oxide synthase (*iNOS*), *COX-2*, erythropoietin (*EPO*) that promote angiogenesis/neovascularization, cell proliferation, and inflammation. Even under normoxic conditions elevated IL-1β and TNF-α have been shown to maintain HIF-1α activity. Elevated HIF1-α is associated with increased metastasis and poor prognosis for many cancers [55]. Tissue remodeling in obese adipose tissue is indicated by the presence of crown-like structures (CLS), i.e., dead adipocytes surrounded by macrophages [15]. As discussed earlier, these stresses induce an ever-escalating cascade of prostaglandin E_2 (PGE$_2$), chemokines, cytokines, and immune cell infiltration that create the state of chronic inflammation. As part of the chronic inflammatory and wound healing environment, elevated remodeling enzymes such as matrix metalloproteinase (MMP)-2, -7, -9 and urokinase plasminogen activator (u-PA) promote cancer cell invasion and metastasis [26]. Additionally, elevated ROS (reactive oxygen species) released by infiltrating myeloid cells increase oxidative stress in the microenvironment contributing to DNA damage, mutagenesis, and further activation of pro-inflammatory signaling to NF-κB [55]. Although the emphasis has been on adipose tissue contribution of adipokines, cytokines, chemokines, and bioactive lipids to tumorigenesis, activation of central transcriptional pathways such as HIF-1, signal transducer, and activator of transcription 3 (STAT3) and NF-κB are important in the tumor as well as the dysfunctional adipose tissue. STAT3 and NF-κB-dependent transcription synergizes to increase tumor inflammation, decrease antitumor responses, and promote tumor growth and metastasis. These synergistic interactions within the tumor and between obese adipose tissue and the tumor underscore the overwhelming contribution of inflammation, particularly NF-κB activation in the tumor microenvironment [26] (Fig. 1). Thus, critical targets such as NF-κB and COX-2 may become important targets for cancer prevention.

Activity of Natural Killer (NK) Cells

Adiposity is known to be related to the impaired immune competence and these alterations in the immune system could play a role for cancer risk in obese patients. Patients with obesity exhibit lower activity of NK cells [67], and consequently lower cytotoxic activity against precancerous and cancer cells. A weight loss of 26% after 6 months, as a result of gastric bypass surgery, led to an increase in NK cell cytotoxic activity [67]. Furthermore, it is known that an important cause of obesity-induced insulin resistance is chronic systemic inflammation originating in VAT, and that VAT inflammation is associated with accumulation of pro-inflammatory macrophages in adipose tissue, but the immunological signals that trigger their accumulation remain unknown. Recently it was found that a phenotypically distinct population of tissue-resident NK cells might represent a crucial link between obesity-induced adipose stress and VAT inflammation [68]. Obesity was associated with upregulation of ligands of the NK cell-activating receptor NCR1 on adipocytes; this stimulated NK cell proliferation and interferon-γ (IFN-γ) production, which in turn triggered the differentiation of pro-inflammatory macrophages and promoted insulin resistance. Deficiency of NK cells, NCR1, or IFN-γ prevented the accumulation of pro-inflammatory macrophages in VAT and greatly ameliorated insulin sensitivity. Thus,

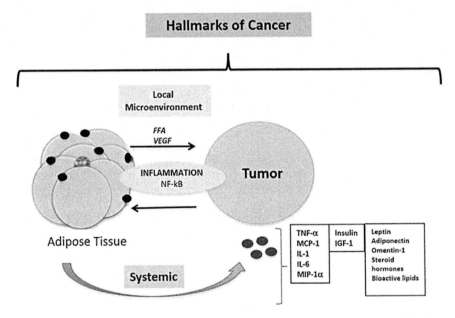

Fig. 1 Obesity alters adipose tissue's production of cytokines/adipokines, growth factors, and steroid hormones that can impact tumor development. A few examples are provided: FFA, free fatty acids; IL-1, interleukin 1; IL-6, interleukin 6; IGF-1, insulin-like growth factor 1; MCP-1, monocyte chemoattractant protein-1; MIP-1a, macrophage inflammatory protein 1a; NF-kB, nuclear factor kappa-light-chain-enhancer of activated B cells; VEGF, vascular endothelial growth factor. Additionally, the "Hallmarks of Cancer" (e.g., sustained proliferative signaling, evasion of growth suppressors, resistance to cell death, enabling replicative immortality, induction of angiogenesis, activation of metastasis, reprogrammed energy metabolism, avoidance of immune destruction, promotion of inflammation) provides an overarching framework to further consider how obesity might influence the carcinogenic hallmarks in somatic cells [78]

NK cells are key regulators of macrophage polarization and insulin resistance in response to obesity-induced adipocyte stress [68]. Because NK functions are dysregulated in obesity and obesity-associated cancer, NK therapies may potentially be used to overcome immune dysfunction in obesity-associated cancer [69].

Role of the Microbiome

The role of gut microbiota in metabolic disorders is increasingly gaining importance. Gut microbiota has been indicated as a critical player in the development of both obesity and diabetes [70, 71]. The involvement of gut microbiota in the generation of obesity-associated low-grade inflammation and diabetes [72] has been discussed, and maintenance of gut microbiota homeostasis is important. Metabolites from the gut microbes contribute to the gut barrier integrity, and a compromised barrier may lead to leakage of inflammatory mediators into systemic circulation and to increase of insulin resistance [73]. Emerging evidence suggests that the complex interplay relating microbiota both to neoplastic and metabolic diseases could aid strategies for cancer treatment and outcomes [74].

Role of Epigenetics

Another factor connecting obesity and cancer is the role of epigenetics; the interaction of epigenome with the environment, including nutrition, can alter patterns of gene expression. Micro RNAS (miRNAs) are small noncoding RNAs that regulate gene expression at the post-transcription level and thus biological processes in different tissues. A major function of miRNAs in adipose tissue is to regulate the differentiation of adipocytes, and consequently metabolic and endocrine function. Although numerous miRNAs are present in human adipose tissue, the expression of only few is altered in individuals with obesity and diabetes [75]. Furthermore, studies have revealed that miRNAs play crucial roles in regulating brown adipocyte differentiation [76], important in obesity and related metabolic disorders,

indicating new strategies for the treatment of these diseases. Epigenetic changes in DNA and associated chromatin proteins are increasingly being considered as important mediators of the linkage between obesity and cancer, and multiple agents, targeted at epigenetic changes, are being tested for cancer therapy [77].

Kynurenines

The kynurenine pathway represents the dominant pathway of tryptophan catabolism, accounting for the disposal of around 95% of the tryptophan not used for protein synthesis [30]. The kynurenine pathway is also driven physiologically by eating, and obesity may involve the effects of kynurenines in the central control of adipose metabolism by the modulation of neuronal glutamate receptors [30].

Summarizing mechanisms that link obesity and cancer, the framework of "hallmarks of cancer" (seminal work by Hanahan and Weinberg) was used to delineate how obesity might influence the carcinogenic hallmarks in somatic cells [78]. The effects of obesity on sustaining proliferative signaling, on evading growth suppressors, on resisting cell death, on enabling replicative immortality, on inducing angiogenesis, on activating invasion and metastasis, reprogramming energy metabolism, on avoiding immune destruction, together with its effects on genome instability and tumor-promoting inflammation was discussed [78]. This interesting approach is important, because clarifying how these cancer hallmarks are affected by obesity may lead to novel prevention and treatment strategies in this pandemic of obesity and cancer.

Prevention and Interventions

Prevention

Obesity is mostly preventable. Throughout history, various methods addressing obesity have been documented and many of these methods actually mirror strategies seen today. Ancient Egyptians practiced binging and purging,

Pythagoras (570–490 BC) recommended eating in moderation, while Iccus and Herodicus (500–400 BC) combined exercise with diet for optimal health [3]. Hippocrates of Kos (460–370 BC), "father of medicine," was among the first to realize the danger of obesity, and Tobias Venner (1577–1660), an English physician and medical writer, was recognized as the first to use a term "obesity." Interestingly, one of the earliest images of the body, the Venus of Willendorf, suggests that features of fatness and fertility would have been highly desirable for people who lived in a harsh ice-age environment.

Based on the available evidence, the WCRF/AICR developed guidelines and personal recommendations for individuals, as well as goals for the population as whole, made by world experts, including those from the International Obesity Task Force, to prevent both obesity and cancer [12, 13]. Although setting these targets was a vital first step, equally important has been understanding how to achieve them. This is a reason why WCRF/AICR published an evidence-based Policy and Action for Cancer Prevention report that provides evidence-based recommendations to key groups in society on how to help people make healthier choices to reduce their chances of developing cancer [13]. Similar recommendations and guidelines on nutrition and physical activity for cancer prevention were given by the American Cancer Society (ACS) [79] and by the Physical Activity Advisory Committee [14].

Obesity is an indicator of an unhealthy lifestyle. Strategies, such as healthy diet, change in lifestyle, or even pharmacological, that disrupt the obesity–cancer axis may be useful for reducing the rise of cancer or its progression.

Some phytochemicals, such as resveratrol, curcumin, and quercetin have been shown to be potent in breaking the obesity–cancer link by interacting with inflammatory and growth factor signals that underlie this link [80]. Also, naturally appearing and widely distributed in animal and plant tissues, inositol phosphates (if water soluble) [81, 82] or inositide (if lipid-bound) [83] have shown implications in obesity, diabetes, and cancer. Mediterranean Diet has been shown to be beneficial for cardiovascular diseases and to

have a preventive role on cancer [84]. The combination of polyphenols contained in fruits, vegetables, grains, legumes, and olive oil have been recognized for their antioxidant and anti-inflammatory properties contributing to antitumor and antiatherogenic abilities. Polyphenols control and reduce inflammation through a series of pathways preventing cancer and other age-related diseases with an inflammatory pathogenesis. Moreover, resveratrol, quercetin, and other polyphenols exert their anticancer and chemopreventive action through mechanisms that mimic caloric restriction (sirtuin and mTOR pathways) [84]. However, the mechanism behind these effects of phytochemicals on cancer is very complex and still unclear because these compounds certainly do much more than just disrupt the obesity–cancer axis.

Obesity–Cancer Intervention

The number of cancer survivors is steadily increasing. Although obesity has been an established factor for cancer incidence, accumulating evidence suggest that obesity is predictive of poor cancer prognosis among cancer survivors [62]. There are several challenges and various modalities of cancer treatment in obese patients, related to dosage, pharmacokinetics, and resistance to chemotherapy [85]. There is a gap in our knowledge of the role of obesity in cancer survival and recurrence, and we need to identify new targets and strategies for improved cancer outcomes in obese patients [85].

Results from diet and weight loss studies show that cancer survivors are motivated and able to make dietary and lifestyle modifications. The Women's Intervention Nutrition Study (WINS) [86] and the Women's Healthy Eating and Lifestyle (WHEL) [87] trials, conducted among early-stage breast cancer survivors, tested the effects of dietary interventions on cancer recurrence and survival. By promoting a low-fat diet through individualized counseling provided by registered dietitian in WINS trial, there were significantly lower rates of recurrence observed in intervention arm at 5 years [86, 88]. In contrast, the WHEL intervention used telephone-based dietary counseling to promote a daily intake of vegetable, fruits, and fiber, and although intake of fruits and vegetable were increased, and intake of fat was decreased, there were no differences in weight change between arms. Additionally, after a median follow-up of 7.3 years, there were no between-arm differences in recurrence [87, 88]. The FRESH START trial conducted on newly diagnosed breast and prostate cancer survivors resulted in a modest but significant weight loss because of lower fat, high fruit, and vegetable diets [88, 89]. However, only a few interventions have pursued weight loss as a specific arm [88]. The Healthy Weight Management (HWM) [90] and the Survivors Health And Physical Exercise (SHAPE) [91] interventions in breast cancer survivors tested the impact of a cognitive behavioral weight loss program plus telephone counseling against a wait-list control, and both interventions resulted in significant improvements in physical activity and weight loss. Although few physical activity trials have focused on survival, they have shown improvements in many health outcomes in cancer survivors, including health-related fitness, fatigue, depression, and quality of life [88]. A multinational trial in Canada and Australia, the Colon Health and Life-Long Exercise Change (CHALLENGE) trial, is currently open to accrual and incorporates intervention approaches shown effective [92]. The Exercise and Nutrition to Enhance Recovery and Good Health for You (ENERGY) trial is designed as a vanguard component of a fully powered trial of at least 2500 women with breast cancer recurrence endpoints [93]. With a goal to reduce breast cancer recurrence, this study has a high potential to have a major impact on clinical management and outcomes after a breast cancer diagnosis. This trial initiates the effort to establish weight loss support for overweight or obese breast cancer survivors as a new standard of clinical care. However, while weight loss may be a good cancer prevention strategy, it could actually be harmful in patients who have already succumbed to disease. During weight loss, white adipose tissue (WAT) undergoes remodeling, and it remains to be seen how tumor cells respond to this change in

systemic and local environment. While awaiting definitive evidence from ongoing randomized trials, breast cancer patients can reasonably be counseled to avoid weight gain and reduce body weight if overweight or obese and increase or maintain a moderate level of physical activity [94]. While lifestyle interventions for weight loss are efficacious, sometimes their long-term durability is limited. Therefore, in addition to these nutrition interventions, several pharmacological interventions may also prove to be useful in targeting obesity cancer risk. These interventions may include FDA-approved weight-loss drugs, although these drugs might be associated with side effects that may not be acceptable to patients [95, 96]. And the cost of Medicare covering new obesity medications, such as semaglutide (Wegovy), could be financially devastating, health economists are warning [97]. Another agent that targets obesity-associated physiology and signaling pathways is metformin, previously discussed [31, 32, 95].

Bariatric surgery is very effective for weight loss, reversal of type 2 diabetes, and reduces the risk of cancer. For example, in the SPLENDID (Surgical Procedures and Long-term Effectiveness in Neoplastic Disease Incidence and Death) matched cohort study, patients with a BMI of 35 or greater who underwent bariatric surgery at a US health system were matched 1:5 to patients who did not undergo surgery for their obesity, resulting in a total of 30,318 patients, bariatric surgery ($n = 5053$), including Roux-en-Y gastric bypass and sleeve gastrectomy, versus non-surgical care ($n = 25,265$). During follow-up, 96 patients in the bariatric surgery group and 780 patients in the nonsurgical control group had an incident obesity-associated cancer, incidence rate of 3.0 events versus 4.6 events, respectively, per 1000 person-years. The cumulative incidence of the primary end point at 10 years was 2.9% in the bariatric surgery group and 4.9% in the nonsurgical control group (absolute risk difference, 2.0% [95% CI, 1.2–2.7%]; adjusted hazard ratio, 0.68 [95% CI, 0.53–0.87], $P = 0.002$). The cumulative incidence of cancer-related mortality at 10 years was 0.8% in the bariatric surgery group and 1.4% in the nonsurgical control group (absolute risk difference, 0.6% [95% CI, 0.1–1.0%]; adjusted hazard ratio, 0.52 [95% CI, 0.31–0.88], $P = 0.01$). Thus, bariatric surgery was associated with a significantly lower incidence of obesity-associated cancer and cancer-related mortality.

Some traditional medicines and dietary supplements claim weight loss but may be controversial [96]. A recent review highlights and addresses current recommendations and feasible interventions that clinicians may consider to further reduce the incidence and recurrence of cancer in patients with obesity [98]. The ongoing NIH clinical trial is investigating fiber-rich foods to treat obesity and prevent colon cancer, and testing whether a high-legume, high-fiber diet will simultaneously increase weight loss and suppress intestinal biomarkers of cancer risk compared to a control diet [99]. Interestingly, inositol and inositol phosphates, particularly phytic acid (inositol hexaphosphate) are fiber-rich components with ability to fight both cancer and obesity through their metabolites and pathways [81, 82, 100].

Historically, white adipose tissue (WAT) has been the primary focus of obesity research. However, based on research in mice, there has been interest in activating brown adipose tissue (BAT) as a target to reduce obesity [23, 101, 102]. In contrast to WAT that stores energy, BAT dissipates energy and produces heat [23, 101]. This process is mediated by the mitochondrial uncoupling protein 1 (UCP1). Notably, the amount of BAT is inversely correlated with obesity and BMI [101]. Morphological and imaging studies demonstrate that BAT is functional, leading to an explosion of research that seeks to pharmacologically convert white to brown fat, in order to burn off excess calories and combat human obesity [103–109]. Beige/brite cells reside within anatomical sites of classical WAT throughout the body and are highly activated in response to thermogenic stimuli, including beta-3 adrenergic agonists and thyroid hormone. While the evidence for the benefits of activating brown fat in mice is clear, the therapeutic potential of activating brown fat in humans is uncertain [110]. However, the stimulation of brown fat in white fat depots poses a potential problem since this process is associated with increases in vascularity and secretion of angiogenic and growth factors [111]. Indeed, it is known that these characteristics are essential steps for breast cancer progression and dissemination [5]. Particularly, recent emphasis has been made on the association of browning of adipose tissue with mutated tumor suppressor genes, such as *PTEN* [111] and *BRCA1* [112]. A few PET/CT studies in humans have shown that BAT activity is greater in patients with active cancer compared to age-, sex-, and BMI-matched BAT-positive patients without active cancer [113–116]. However, additional studies are needed to further define the role of BAT in cancer development and progression.

Conclusion

Interventions, either diet, lifestyle, or pharmacological, that disrupt the obesity–cancer connection may be useful for reducing the rise of cancer or its progression. Identification of key molecules that can serve as biological markers, targets, and modulators are critical to break the association of obesity and cancer. Inflammation is a major link between obesity and cancer, and inflammation-associated molecules can be activated by several environmental and lifestyle-related factors. More than half of the cancers occurring today are preventable by applying knowledge that we already have, because tobacco, obesity, and physical inactivity are all modifiable causes of cancer that generate the most diseases [117]. The obstacles are complex and are driven and perpetuated by interrelated factors at multiple levels including personal (i.e., biological, psychological), organizational/institutional, environmental (i.e., both social and physical), and policy levels [118]. These factors, known as social determinants of health (SDH), influence people's health at every stage of life and inequalities in these factors lead to widespread and persistent inequalities in life expectancy and time spent in good health [118]. Given the SDH that lie outside the realm of the individual and medical care, to achieve maximal possible cancer prevention, we need better ways to implement what we know, and use public health models that seek health equity for all, including those facing the greatest social obstacles.

The obesity epidemic is driven by excess consumption of energy-dense processed food and sedentary lifestyle. In the USA, obesity prevalence is highest in lower socioeconomic groups, and will likely trigger rapid increase in obesity-related cancers [119]. There is an urgent need to understand the pathophysiology, develop biomarkers for screening, and implement preventive and therapeutic strategies to reverse this trend.

References

1. https://www.worldobesity.org/resources/resource-library/world-obesity-atlas-2023/. Accessed 25 Mar 2023.
2. Ward ZJ, Bleich SN, Cradock AL, Barrett JL, Giles CM, Flax C, et al. Projected U.S. State-level prevalence of adult obesity and severe obesity. N Engl J Med. 2019;381:2440–50.
3. Rossen LM, Rossen EA. Obesity 101. New York: Springer Publishing Co., LLC; 2012.
4. https://www.cdc.gov/obesity/basics/adult-defining.html/. Assessed 26 Mar 2023.
5. Bernstein LM. Cancer and heterogeneity of obesity: a potential contribution of brown fat. Future Oncol. 2012;8:1537–48.
6. Boonchaya-anant P, Apovian M. Metabolically healthy obesity – does it exist? Curr Atheroscler Rep. 2014;16:441.
7. Navarro E, Funtikova AN, Fito M, Schröder H. Can metabolically healthy obesity be explained by diet, genetics, and inflammation? Mol Nutr Food Res. 2015;59:75–93.
8. Badoud F, Perreault ZMA, Mutch DM. Molecular insights into the role of white adipose tissue in metabolically unhealthy normal weight and metabolically healthy obese individuals. FASEB J. 2015;29:748–58.
9. GBD. Cancer Risk Factors Collaborators/The global burden of cancer attributable to risk factors, 2010–19: a systematic analysis for the Global Burden of Disease Study 2019. Lancet. 2019;2022(400):563–91.
10. Brennan P, Davey-Smith G. Identifying novel causes of cancers to enhance cancer prevention: new strategies are needed. J Natl Cancer Inst. 2022;114:353–60.
11. Friedenreich CM, Ryder-Burbidge C, McNeil J. Physical activity, obesity and sedentary behavior in cancer etiology: epidemiologic evidence and biological mechanisms. Mol Oncol. 2021;15:790–800.
12. World Cancer Research Fund/American Institute for Cancer Research. Food, nutrition, physical activity, and the prevention of cancer: a global perspective. Washington, DC: AICR; 2007.
13. https://www.wcrf.org/policy/our-publications/. Assessed 27 Mar 2023.
14. 2018 Physical Activity Guidelines Advisory Committee. 2018 Physical Activity Guidelines Advisory Committee Scientific report. Washington, DC: Department of Health and Human Services; 2018.
15. Lee M-J, Wu Y, Fried SK. Adipose tissue heterogeneity: implications of depot differences in adipose tissue for obesity complications. Mol Asp Med. 2013;34:1–11.
16. Murphy RA, Bureyko TF, Miljkovic I, Cauley JA, Satterfield S, Hue TF, et al. Association of total and computed tomographic measures of regional adiposity with incident cancer risk: a prospective population-based study of older adults. Appl Physiol Nutr Metab. 2014;39:687–92.
17. Nagata N, Sakamoto K, Arai T, Niikura R, Shimbo R, Shinozaki M, et al. Visceral abdominal fat measured by computed tomography is associated with an increased risk of colorectal adenoma. Int J Cancer. 2014;135:2273–81.
18. Britton KA, Massaro JM, Murabito JM, Kreger BE, Hoffmann U, Fox CS. Body fat distribution, incident cardiovascular disease, cancer, and all-cause mortality. J Am Coll Cardiol. 2013;62:921–5.
19. Zhu Y, Wang H-K, Zhang H-L, Yao X-D, Zhang S-L, Dai B, et al. Visceral obesity and risk of high grade disease in clinical T1a renal cell carcinoma. J Urol. 2013;189:447–53.
20. Harada K, Baba Y, Ishimoto T, Kosumi K, Tokunaga R, Izumi D et al. Low visceral fat content is associated with poor prognosis in a database of 507 upper gastrointestinal cancers. Ann Surg Oncol. 2015 Feb 25 [Epub ahead of print].
21. Kabat GC, Xue X, Kamensky V, Lane D, Bea JW, Chen C, et al. Risk of breast, endometrial, colorectal, and renal cancers in postmenopausal women in association with a body shape index and other anthropometric measures. Cancer Causes Control. 2015;26:219–29.
22. Calori G, Lattuada G, Piemonti L, Garancini MP, Ragogna F, Villa M, et al. Prevalence, metabolic features, and prognosis of metabolically healthy obese Italian individuals: the Cremona study. Diabetes Care. 2011;34:210–5.
23. Ràfols ME. Adipose tissue: cell heterogeneity and functional diversity. Endocrinol Nutr. 2014;61:100–12.
24. Louie SM, Roberts LS, Nomura DK. Mechanisms linking obesity and cancer. BBA. 1831;2013:1499–508.
25. Ungefroren H, Gieseler F, Fliedner S, Leh H. Adiposopathy in cancer and (cardio)metabolic diseases: an endocrine approach. Horm Mol Clin Invest. 2015;21:17–41.
26. Multhoff G, Molls M, Radons J. Chronic inflammation in cancer development. Front Immunol. 2012;2:98.
27. Headland SE, Norling LV. The resolution of inflammation: principles and challenges. Semin Immunol. 2015;27:149–60.

28. Maury E, Brichard SM. Adipokine dysregulation, adipose tissue inflammation and metabolic syndrome. Mol Cell Endocrinol. 2010;314:1–16.

29. Darimont C, Avanti O, Blancher F, Wagniere S, Mansourian R, Zbinden I, et al. Contribution of mesothelial cells in the expression of inflammatory-related factors in omental adipose tissue of obese subjects. Int J Obes. 2008;32:112–1120.

30. Stone TW, McPherson M, Darlington LG. Obesity and cancer: existing and new hypotheses for a causal connection. EBioMedicine. 2018;30:14–28.

31. Dowling RJ, Niraula S, Stambolic V, Goodwin PJ. Metformin in cancer: translational challenges. J Mol Endocrinol. 2012;2012(48):R31–43.

32. Salani B, Del Rio A, Sambuceti G, Cordera R, Maggi D. Metformin, cancer and glucose metabolism. Endocr Relat Cancer. 2014;21:R461–71.

33. Hursting SD, Smith SM, Lashinger LM, Harvey AE, Perkins. Calories and carcinogenesis: lessons learned from 30 years of calorie restriction research. Carcinogenesis. 2010;31:83–9.

34. Moore T, Beltran L, Carbajal S, Strom S, Traag J, Hursting SD, et al. Dietary energy balance modulates signaling through the Akt/Mammalian Target of Rapamycin pathways in multiple epithelial tissues. Cancer Prev Res. 2008;1:65–76.

35. Jiang W, Zhu Z, Thompson HJ. Dietary energy restriction modulates the activity of Akt and mTOR in mammary carcinomas, mammary gland, and liver. Cancer Res. 2008;68:5492–9.

36. Kalaany NY, Sabatini DM. Tumours with PI3K activation are resistant to dietary restriction. Nature. 2009;458:725–31.

37. Dunn SE, Kari FW, French J, Leininger JR, Travlos G, Wilson R, et al. Dietary restriction reduces insulin-like growth factor I levels, which modulates apoptosis, cell proliferation, and tumor progression in p53-deficient mice. Cancer Res. 1997;57:4667–72.

38. Ottero M, Lago R, Gomez R, Dieguez C, Lago C, Gómez-Reino GO. Rheumatology. 2006;45:944–50.

39. Münzberg H, Myers MG Jr. Molecular and anatomical determinants of central leptin resistance. Nat Neurosci. 2005;8:566–70.

40. Yadav A, Kataria MA, Saini V, Yadav A. Role of leptin and adiponectin in insulin resistance. Clin Chim Acta. 2013;417:80–4.

41. Friedman JM, Mantzoros CS. 20 years of leptin: from the discovery of leptin gene to leptin in our therapeutic armamentarium. Metabolism. 2015;64:1–4.

42. Park H-K, Ahima RS. Physiology of leptin: energy homeostasis, neuroendocrine function and metabolism. Metabolism. 2015;64:24–34.

43. Dalamaga M, Diakopoulos KN, Mantzoros CS. The role of adiponectin in cancer: a review of current evidence. Endocr Rev. 2012;33:547–94.

44. Perrier S, Jardé T. Adiponectin, an anti-carcinogenic hormone? A systematic review on breast, colorectal, liver and prostate cancer. Curr Med Chem. 2012;19: 5501–12.

45. Khan S, Shukla S, Sinha S, Meeran SM. Role of adipokines and cytokines in obesity-associated breast cancer: therapeutic targets. Cytokines Growth Factor Rev. 2013;24:503–13.

46. Hursting SD, Hursting MJ. Growth signals, inflammation, and vascular perturbation: mechanistic links between obesity, metabolic syndrome, and cancer. Arterioscler Thromb Vasc Biol. 2012;32:1766–70.

47. Cleary MP, Ray A, Rogozina OP, Dogan S, Grossmann ME. Targeting the adiponectin: leptin ratio for postmenopausal breast cancer prevention. Front Biosci. 2009;1:329–57.

48. Zhang YY, Zhou LM. Omentin-1, a new adipokine, promotes apoptosis through regulating Sirt1-dependent p53 deacetylation in hepatocellular carcinoma cells. Eur J Pharmacol. 2013;698:137–44.

49. Zhao A, Xiao H, Zhu Y, Liu S, Zhang S, Yang Z, et al. Omentin-1: a newly discovered warrior against metabolic related diseases. Expert Opin Ther Targets. 2022;26:275–89.

50. Abdalla MMI. Role of visfatin in obesity-induced insulin resistance. World J Clin Cases. 2022;10: 10840–51.

51. Pilarski L, Pelczyńska M, Koperska A, Seraszek-Jaros A, Szulińska M, Bogdański P. Association of serum vaspin concentration with metabolic disorders in obese individuals. Biomol Ther. 2023;13:508.

52. Fazeli MS, Dashti H, Akbarzadeh S, Assadi M, Aminian A, Keramati MR, et al. Circulating levels of novel adipocytokines in patients with colorectal cancer. Cytokine. 2013;62:81–5.

53. Aggarwal BB, Gehlot P. Inflammation and cancer: how friendly is the relationship for cancer patients? Curr Opin Pharmacol. 2009;9:351–69.

54. Iyengar NM, Hudis CA, Dannenberg AJ. Obesity and cancer: local and systemic mechanisms. Ann Rev Med. 2015;66:297–309.

55. Sethi G, Shanmugam MK, Ramachandran L, Kuman AP, Tergaonkar V. Multifaceted link between cancer and inflammation. Biosci Rep. 2012;32:1–15.

56. Muller A, Homey B, Soto H, Ge N, Catron D, Buchanan ME, et al. Involvement of chemokine receptors in breast cancer metastasis. Nature. 2001;410:50–6.

57. Yao L, Heuser-Baker J, Herlea-Pana O, Zhang N, Szweda LI, Griffin TM, et al. Deficiency in adipocyte chemokine receptor CXCR4 exacerbates obesity and compromises thermoregulatory responses of brown adipose tissue in a mouse model of diet-induced obesity. FASEB J. 2014;28:4534–50.

58. Byers T, Sedjo RL. Body fatness as a cause of cancer: epidemiological clues to biologic mechanisms. Endocr Relat Cancer. 2015;22:R125–34.

59. Du Q, Jiang L, Wang X, Wang M, She F, Chen Y. Tumor necrosis factor-α promotes lymphangiogenesis of gallbladder carcinoma through nuclear factor-κB-mediated upregulation upregulation of vascular endothelial growth factor-C. Cancer Sci. 2014;105: 1261–71.

60. Hursting SD, Lashinger LM, Wheatley KW, Rogers CJ, Colbert LH, Nunez NP, et al. Reducing the weight of cancer: mechanistic targets for breaking the obesity-carcinogenesis link. Best Pract Res Endocrinol Metab. 2008;22:659–69.

61. Kaaks R, Lukanova A, Kurzer MS. Obesity, endogenous hormones, and endometrial cancer risk: a synthetic review. Cancer Epidemiol Biomark Prev. 2001;11:1531–43.

62. Institute of Medicine. The role of obesity in cancer survival and recurrence: workshop summary. Washington, DC: The National Academic Press; 2012.

63. Bulun SE, Chen D, Moy I, Brooks DC, Zhao H. Aromatase, breast cancer and obesity: a complex interaction. Trends Endocrinol Metab. 2012;23:83–9.

64. Hursting SD, DiGiovanni J, Dannenberg AJ, Azrad M, Leroith D, Demark-Wahnefried W, et al. Obesity, energy balance and cancer: new opportunities for prevention. Cancer Prev Res. 2012;5:1260–72.

65. Goss PE, Ingle JN, Ales-Martinez JE, Cheung AM, Cheung AM, Chlebowski RT, Wactawski-Wende J, et al. Exemestane for breast-cancer prevention in postmenopausal women. N Engl J Med. 2011;364:2381–91.

66. Nakanishi M, Rosenberg DW. Multifaceted role of PGE_2 in inflammation and cancer. Semin Immunopathol. 2013;35:123–37.

67. Moulin CM, Rizzo LV, Halpern A. Effect of surgery-induced weight loss on immune function. Expert Rev Gastroenterol Hepatol. 2008;2:617–9.

68. Wensveen FM, Jelenčić V, Valentić S, Šestan M, Wensveen TT, et al. NK cells link obesity-induced adipose stress to inflammation and insulin resistance. Nat Immunol. 2015;16:376–85.

69. Mylod E, Lysaght J, Conroy MJ. Natural killer cell therapy: a new frontier for obesity-associated cancer. Cancer Lett. 2022;535:215620.

70. van Olden C, Groen AK, Nieuwdorp M. Role of intestinal microbiome in lipid and glucose metabolism in Diabetes Mellitus. Clin Ther. 2015 Apr 24 [Epub ahead of print].

71. Tai N, Wong FS, Wen L. The role of gut microbiota in the development of type 1, type 2 diabetes mellitus and obesity. Rev Endocr Metab Disord. 2015;16:55–65.

72. Cani PD, Osto M, Geurtis L, Everard A. Involvement of gut microbiota in the development of low-grade inflammation and type 2 diabetes associated with obesity. Gut Microbes. 2012;3:279–88.

73. Upadhyaya S, Banerjee G. Type 2 diabetes and gut microbiome: at the intersection of known and unknown. Gut Microbes. 2015;6:85–92.

74. Marzullo P, Bettini S, Menafra D, Aprano S, Muscogiuri G, Barrea L, et al. Spot-light on microbiota in obesity and cancer. Int J Obes. 2021;45:2291–9.

75. Arner P, Kulyté A. MicroRNA regulatory networks in human adipose tissue and obesity. Nat Rev Endocrinol. 2015;11:276–88.

76. Yuntao G, Xiangyang M. MicroRNAs in the regulation of brown adipocyte differentiation. Yi Chuan. 2015;37:240–9.

77. Berger NA, Scacheri PC. Targeting epigenetics to prevent obesity promoted cancers. Cancer Prev Res. 2018;11:125–8.

78. Harris BHL, Macaulay VM, Harris DA, Klenerman P, Karpe F, Lord SR, et al. Obesity: a perfect storm for carcinogenesis. Cancer Metastasis Rev. 2022;41:491–515.

79. Rock CL, Thomson C, Gansler T, Gapstur SM, McCullough ML, Patel AV, et al. American Cancer Society guideline for diet and physical activity for cancer prevention. CA Cancer J Clin. 2020;70:245–71.

80. Ford NA, Lashinger LM, Allott EH, Hursting SD. Mechanistic targets and phytochemical strategies for breaking the obesity-cancer link. Front Oncol. 2013;3:209.

81. Vucenik I, Stains JP. Obesity and cancer risk: evidence, mechanisms, and recommendations. Ann N Y Acad Sci. 2012;1271:37–43.

82. Kim JN, Han SN, Kim HK. Phytic acid and myo-inositol support adipocyte differentiation and improve insulin sensitivity in 3T3-L1 cells. Nutr Res. 2014;34:723–31.

83. Manna P, Jain SK. Phosphatidylinositol-3,4,5-triphosphate and cellular signaling: implications for obesity and diabetes. Cell Physiol Biochem. 2015;35:1253–75.

84. Ostan R, Lanzarini C, Pini E, Scruti M, Vianello D, Bertarelli C, et al. Inflammaging and cancer: a challenge for the Mediterranean Diet. Nutrients. 2015;7:2589–621.

85. Lashinger LM, Rossi EL, Hursting SD. Obesity and resistance to cancer therapy: interacting roles of inflammation and metabolic dysregulation. Clin Pharmacol Ther. 2014;96:458–63.

86. Chlebowski RT, Blackburn GL, Thompson CA, Nixon DW, Shapiro A, Hoy MK, et al. Dietary fat reduction and breast cancer outcome: interim efficacy results from the Woman's Intervention Nutrition Study. J Natl Cancer Inst. 2006;98:1767–76.

87. Pierce JP, Natarajan L, Caan BJ, Parker BA, Greenberg ER, Flatt SW, et al. Influence of a diet very high in vegetables, fruit, and fiber and low in fat on prognosis following treatment for breast cancer: the Women's Healthy Eating and Living (WHEL) randomized trial. JAMA. 2007;298:289–98.

88. Demark-Wahnefried W, Platz EA, Ligibel JA, Blair CK, Courneya KS, Meyerhardt JA, et al. The role of obesity in cancer survival and recurrence. Cancer Epidemiol Biomark Prev. 2012;21:1244–59.

89. Demark-Wahnefried W, Clipp EC, Lipkus IM, Lobach D, Snyder DC, Sloane R, et al. Main outcomes of the FRESH START trial: a sequentially tailored, diet and exercise mailed print intervention among breast and prostate cancer survivors. J Clin Oncol. 2007;25:2709–18.

90. Mefferd K, Nichols JF, Pakiz B, Rock CL. A cognitive behavioral therapy intervention to promote

weight loss improves body composition and blood lipid profiles among overweight survivors. Breast Cancer Res Treat. 2007;104:145–52.

91. Taylor DL, Nichols JF, Pakiz B, Bardwell WA, Flatt SW, Rock CL. Relationships between cardiorespiratory fitness, physical activity, and psychosocial variables in overweight and obese breast cancer survivors. Int J Behav Med. 2010;17:264–70.

92. Courneya KS, Booth CM, Gill S, O'Brien P, Vardy J, Friedenreich CM, et al. The colon health and life-long exercise change trial: a randomized trial of the National Institute of Canada Clinical Trials Group. Curr Oncol. 2008;15:279–85.

93. Rock CL, Byers TE, Colditz GA, Demark-Wahnefried W, Ganz PA, Wolin KY, et al. Reducing breast cancer recurrence with weight loss, a vanguard trial: the Exercise and Nutrition to Enhance Recovery and Good Health for You (ENERGY) trial. Contemp Clin Trials. 2013;34:282–95.

94. Chlebowski RT. Nutrition and physical activity influence on breast cancer incidence and outcome. Breast. 2013;22:S30–7.

95. Goodwin P, Stambolic V. Impact of obesity epidemic on cancer. Annu Rev Med. 2015;66:281–96.

96. Mordes JP, Liu C, Xu S. Medications for weight loss. Curr Opin Endocrinol Diabetes Obes. 2015;22:91–7.

97. Baig K, Dusetzina SB, Kim DD, Leech AA. Medicare Part D coverage of antiobesity medication – challenges and uncertainty ahead. N Engl J Med. 2023;388:961–3.

98. Bhardwaj NJ, Chae K, Sheng JY, Yeh H-C. Clinical interventions to break the obesity and cancer link: a narrative review. Cancer Metastasis Rev. 2022;41:719–35.

99. https://clinicaltrials.gov/ct2/show/NCT04780477

100. Chatree S, Thongmaen N, Tantivejkul K, Sitticharoon C, Vucenik I. Role of inositol and inositol phosphates in energy metabolism. Molecules. 2020;25(21):5079.

101. Sidossis L, Kajimura S. Brown and beige fat in humans: thermogenic adipocytes that control energy and glucose homeostasis. J Clin Invest. 2015;125:478–86.

102. Banks MA. Brown fat holds promise for addressing obesity and a host related ills. Proc Natl Acad Sci U S A. 2022;119(43):e2216435119.

103. Zafir B. Brown adipose tissue: research milestones of a potential player in human energy balance and obesity. Horm Metab Res. 2013;45:774–85.

104. Gunawardana SC, Piston DW. Reversal of type 1 diabetes in mice by brown adipose tissue transplant. Diabetes. 2012;61:674–82.

105. Stanford KI, Middelbeek RJ, Townsend KL, An D, Nygaard EB, Hitchcox KM, et al. Brown adipose

tissue regulates glucose homeostasis and insulin sensitivity. J Clin Invest. 2013;123:215–23.

106. Villarroya J, Cereijo R, Villaroya F. An endocrine role for brown adipose tissue? Am J Physiol Endocrinol Metab. 2013;305:E567–72.

107. Cypess AM, Kahn CR. Brown fat as a therapy for obesity and diabetes. Curr Opin Endocrinol Diabetes Obes. 2010;2:143–9.

108. Frühbeck G, Becerril S, Sáinz N, Garrastachu P, García-Velloso MJ. BAT: a new target for human obesity? Trends Pharmacol Sci. 2009;30:387–96.

109. Tseng Y-H, Cypess AM, Kahn CR. Cellular bioenergetics as a target for obesity therapy. Nat Rev Drug Discov. 2010;9:465–82.

110. Yoneshiro T, Wang Q, Tajima K, Matsushita M, Maki H, Igarashi K, et al. BCAA catabolism in brown fat controls energy homeostasis through CLC25A44. Nature. 2019;572:614–9.

111. Ortega-Molina A, Efeyan A, Lopez-Guadamillas E, Muñoz-Martin M, Gómez-López G, Cañamero M, et al. Pten positively regulates brown adipose function, energy expenditure, and longevity. Cell Metab. 2012;15:382–94.

112. Jones LP, Buelto D, Tago E, Owusu-Boaltey KE. Abnormal mammary adipose tissue environment of Brca 1 mutant mice show a persistent deposition of highly vascularized multilocular adipocytes. J Cancer Sci Ther. 2011;S2:1–6.

113. Cao Q, Hersl J, La A, Smith M, Jenkins J, Goloubeva O, et al. A pilot study of FDG PET/CT detects a link between brown adipose tissue and breast cancer. BMC Cancer. 2014;14:126.

114. Bos SA, Gill CM, Martinez-Salazar EL, Torriani M, Bredella MA. Preliminary investigation of brown adipose tissue assessed by PET/CT and cancer activity. Skelet Radiol. 2019;48:413–9.

115. Yin X, Chen Y, Ruze R, Xu R, Song J, Wang C, et al. The evolving view of thermogenic fat and its implications in cancer and metabolic diseases. Signal Transduct Target Ther. 2022;7:324.

116. Pace L, Nicolai E, Basso L, Garbino N, Soricelli A, Salvatore M. Brown adipose tissue in breast cancer evaluated by [18F] FDG-PET/CT. Mol Imaging Biol. 2020;4:1111–5.

117. Colditz GA, Wolin KY, Gehlert S. Applying what we know to accelerate cancer prevention. Sci Transl Med. 2012;4:4127rv4.

118. Braveman P, Gottlieb L. The social determinants of health: it's time to consider the causes of the causes. Public Health Rep. 2014;129(Suppl 2):19–31.

119. Żukiewicz-Sobczak W, Wróblewska P, Zwoliński J, Chmielewska-Badora J, Adamczuk P, Krasowska E, et al. Obesity and poverty paradox in developed countries. Ann Agric Environ Med. 2014;21:590–4.

Endocrine Disorders Associated with Obesity

33

Hyeong-Kyu Park and Rexford S. Ahima

Contents

Abstract

Several endocrine disorders, including diabetes, insulinoma, Cushing syndrome, hypothyroidism, polycystic ovary syndrome (PCOS), and growth hormone deficiency (GHD) are associated with obesity. The mechanisms for the development of obesity vary according to the abnormalities of endocrine function. The primary actions of insulin, glucocorticoids, thyroid hormone, and growth hormone are associated with energy metabolism in liver, muscle, and adipose and other tissues. This chapter describes the pathogenesis of obesity and metabolic dysfunction associated with excess insulin or glucocorticoids, and deficiency of thyroid hormone or growth hormone.

H.K.P and R.S.A co-wrote the review article.

H.-K. Park
Department of Internal Medicine, Soonchunhyang
University College of Medicine, Seoul, South Korea
e-mail: hkpark@schmc.ac.kr

R. S. Ahima (✉)
Department of Medicine, Division of Endocrinology,
Diabetes and Metabolism, Johns Hopkins University
School of Medicine, Baltimore, MD, USA
e-mail: ahima@jhmi.edu

© Springer Nature Switzerland AG 2023
R. S. Ahima (ed.), *Metabolic Syndrome*,
https://doi.org/10.1007/978-3-031-40116-9_42

Keywords

Cushing syndrome · Growth hormone
deficiency · Hyperinsulinism ·
Hypothyroidism · Obesity · Type 2 diabetes

Introduction

Hyperinsulinemia, hypercortisolism, hypothyroidism, and growth hormone deficiency are
often associated with obesity. Insulin is a potent
anabolic hormone, and treatment with insulin or
some antidiabetic drugs results in weight gain
through direct effects on adipogenesis and lipid
storage. Insulinoma is a rare cause of hyperinsulinism associated with hypoglycemia, hunger, and
rapid weight gain. Excessive glucocorticoid exposure in Cushing syndrome results in central obesity, sarcopenia, osteoporosis, hypertension, and
dyslipidemia. The local production of active glucocorticoids in adipose tissue by 11β (beta)-
hydroxysteroid dehydrogenase type 1 has been
implicated in obesity, insulin resistance, and
hypertension. Hypothyroidism increases body
weight by decreasing thermogenesis and increasing fluid retention and interstitial accumulation of
glycosaminoglycans. Hypothyroidism also
increases cholesterol synthesis and impairs insulin
sensitivity. Growth hormone deficiency in adults
decreases lean tissue mass and increases fat. The
focus of this chapter will be on putative mechanisms linking obesity to excessive exposure to
insulin and glucocorticoids, and thyroid and
growth hormone deficiencies.

Insulin

Insulin is secreted by the pancreatic β (beta) cells
of the islets of Langerhans in response to elevated
blood glucose levels during the postprandial
period, potentiated by the effects of amino acids
and fatty acids and incretin hormones produced in
the gastrointestinal tract [1]. Insulin is a key anabolic hormone responsible for promoting glycogen storage in the liver and skeletal muscle, and
triglyceride storage in adipose tissue and liver.

Following secretion, insulin binds to insulin
receptor, which consists of two α (alpha) subunits
and two β (beta) subunits that form a hetero-
tetrameric complex. Insulin binds to the extracellular (alpha) subunits, transmitting a signal across
the plasma membrane that activates the intracellular tyrosine kinase domain of the β (beta) subunit. Insulin binding to the external component of
its receptor results in activation of receptor tyrosine kinase [2]. Once activated, the insulin receptor (IR) can phosphorylate a number of substrate
proteins that initiate downstream signaling pathways. Intracellular substrates of IR tyrosine
kinase include IRS (IR substrate) proteins, Shc,
Cbl, APS, Gab-1 (Grb2-associated binder-1). The
core cellular processes downstream of the insulin
signaling network involves the phosphatidylinositol 3-kinase (PI3-kinase) and the mitogen-
activated protein kinase (MAPK) pathways [3].

While a pathway leading to activation of
MAPK promotes cell division, protein synthesis,
and cell growth by phosphorylating transcription
factors leading to activation of gene expression,
the regulatory roles of insulin in energy metabolism are largely mediated by the PI3-kinase pathway [4, 5]. The major metabolic pathways
stimulated by insulin are glycolysis, glycogen
synthesis, lipogenesis, and protein synthesis. In
contrast, insulin inhibits gluconeogenesis, glycogenolysis, lipolysis, fatty acid oxidation, and protein degradation. The PI3-kinase pathway also
regulates glucose uptake through the translocation
of glucose transporter GLUT4 to the membrane of
muscle and fat cells [6]. Insulin stimulates glycogen synthesis, while it downregulates glucose
production by suppressing gluconeogenesis and
glycogenolysis in liver. Insulin increases the rate
of glycolysis by increasing glucose transport and
the activities of hexokinase and
6-phosphofructokinase in muscle. Glycogen synthase, the key regulating enzyme for glycogen
synthesis, is activated by insulin. During fasting,
the fall in insulin and increase in
counter-regulatory hormones, such as glucagon,
epinephrine, glucocorticoids, and growth hormone, stimulate glycogenolysis and gluconeogenesis in the liver, leading to glucose release to
ensure adequate fuel supply to the brain and

other vital organs. Insulin also plays an important role in lipid metabolism. Insulin decreases lipolysis in adipose tissue by inhibiting hormone-sensitive lipase activity, thereby lowering plasma fatty acid level [7]. Insulin resistance attenuates lipolysis, especially of upper body or visceral fat, in obesity. Thus, individuals with obesity with a predominance of intra-abdominal fat have higher rates of fatty acid mobilization and greater resistance to the anti-lipolytic effects of insulin when compared with individuals with excess lower body fat [8, 9]. Insulin also stimulates de novo lipogenesis from glucose in the liver and adipose tissue. Insulin is a strong activator of lipogenesis through increased expression of lipogenic enzymes such as fatty acid synthase (FAS) and acetyl-CoA carboxylase (ACC). Insulin stimulates the re-esterification of fatty acids in adipose tissue and liver in the form of triglyceride (TG). Insulin also increases lean and muscle mass, by suppressing proteolysis and enhancing protein synthesis [10].

Hyperinsulinism and Obesity

Obesity and diabetes are closely linked and increasing worldwide. Because most patients with type 2 diabetes (T2D) are overweight or obese at the time of diagnosis, iatrogenic weight gain is an important clinical issue that can become a barrier to successful management. Unfortunately, insulin and several oral antidiabetic drugs increase body weight. For example, after 1 year of treatment, a study showed that patients on thiazolidinedione (TZD) treatment gained 5.0 kg, in comparison with 3.3 kg in those using insulin, and 1.8 kg in those treated with sulfonylureas (SUs). In contrast, patients on metformin lost 2.4 kg [11]. In the United Kingdom Prospective Diabetes Study (UKPDS), an increase in body weight was associated with intensified treatment and improved glycemic control. The patients on intensive treatment gained 3 kg more than conventionally treated patients during the 10-year follow-up period, with most of the weight increase occurring within the first 12 months. Weight gain was seen with all drugs used for intensive intervention, with the exception of metformin. Weight gain was highest among the insulin-treated patients, who gained a mean of 6.5 kg [12, 13].

Weight gain in type 1 diabetes is often perceived as desirable; however, overweight or obesity in type 1 diabetes can become a problem with intensive insulin therapy. The Diabetes Control and Complications Trial (DCCT) showed that insulin-associated weight gain was greater in patients receiving intensive treatment compared to conventional treatment (5.1 vs. 3.7 kg, during the first 12 months of therapy), but the mean weight of both groups increased to values beyond ideal. After 12 months of therapy, the intensively treated group had a weight that was 10% above ideal. After 8 years, body weight continued to increase every year in both groups – more so in the intensively treated cohort. After about 6 years of follow-up, the patients in the intensively treated group gained nearly 5 kg more than their conventionally treated counterparts [14–16].

How does chronically elevated insulin or improvement in glycemic control in diabetes result in weight gain? A possible explanation is a defensive or unconscious increase in food intake caused by the fear or experience of hypoglycemia. Insulin significantly increases the risk of hypoglycemia. In fact, some patients increase their intake of carbohydrates episodically or chronically to counteract a threat or experience of hypoglycemia. Increased insulin level in response to increased caloric intake promotes adipogenesis and lipid storage. Weight gain in treated diabetes may also result from the resolution of glycosuria. If the food intake is not reduced to compensate for improved glycemic control, the reduction in glycosuria will result in a net gain in weight. Combining sodium glucose co-transporter 2 (SGLT2) inhibitors, which induce glycosuria with insulin not only improves hyperglycemia but also lessens insulin-associated weight gain [17]. Subcutaneous administration of insulin may also contribute to weight gain in diabetes. When insulin is given subcutaneously, the absorbed insulin first circulates systemically, so muscle and adipose tissues are over-insulinized while the liver is under-insulinized. It is possible that systemically elevated insulin levels promote fat accumulation, which in turn increases in the therapeutic insulin requirements [16]. Novel long-acting basal insulin analogs have been shown to have less day-to-day variability of action and thus less weight gain [18].

Weight management through diet and exercise is essential for all patients with diabetes. Weight reduction in patients with T2D can decrease diabetes-related complications and improve cardiovascular risk factors. Recent studies have shown a strong relationship between the magnitude of weight loss and likelihood of diabetes remission [19]. Anti-hyperglycemic agents have significant effects on body weight. Metformin is the most commonly used first-line therapy for T2D, and often induces weight loss or is generally considered weight neutral (Table 1). Among other antidiabetic drugs, dipeptidyl peptidase-IV (DPP-IV) inhibitors are weight neutral. In contrast, insulin, SUs, and TZDs are associated with weight gain. However, the SGLT2 inhibitors, amylin analogs, glucagon-like peptide-1 (GLP-1) receptor agonists, and dual glucose-dependent insulinotropic polypeptide (GIP)/GLP-1 receptor co-agonist promote significant weight loss [20, 21]. Thus, adjunctive treatment with metformin, SGLT2 inhibitors, DPP-IV inhibitors, GLP-1 receptor agonists, and GIP/GLP-1 receptor co-agonist should be encouraged to reduce insulin doses and avoid weight gain in patients with T2D. Moreover, practitioners should consider weight-neutral alternatives of medications for hypertension, depression, and other diseases when treating patients with diabetes (Table 1).

Insulinoma, the most common functioning islet cell tumor of the pancreas, is a rare cause of rapid weight gain. Patients with insulinoma present with symptoms of hypoglycemia secondary to excessive and uncontrolled secretion of insulin. Common symptoms range from intense hunger, tremor, palpitations, and sweating to severe neuroglycopenic manifestations, such as anxiety, confusion, behavioral changes, and coma. Symptoms often occur in the morning after an overnight fast and may be precipitated by exercise. The symptoms are episodic due to the intermittent secretion of insulin by insulinoma. Patients with insulinoma learn to avoid these symptoms by eating frequent meals, often high sugar snacks, which promotes weight gain. The diagnosis of insulinoma is established with the determination of fasting hyperinsulinemia (plasma insulin >6 µIU/ml), and symptomatic hypoglycemia (fasting plasma glucose <45 mg/dl). Increased levels of C-peptide and proinsulin distinguish insulinoma from factitious insulin therapy [22]. Several options are available for imaging and localizing insulinoma tumors, including ultrasonography, computed tomography, and intra-arterial calcium stimulation with venous sampling [23]. Surgical resection is the treatment of choice and offers the only chance of cure of insulinoma [24, 25]. Malignant insulinoma is extremely rare. Aggressive surgical and medical approaches including administration of octreotide are recommended in patients with malignant insulinoma to control hypoglycemia [26]. Continuous glucose monitoring can help to detect and prevent hypoglycemic episodes and monitor responses to therapy in patients with insulinoma [27].

Glucocorticoids

Cortisol is the main active glucocorticoid (GC) in humans, and an important regulator of many physiological pathways, particularly during stress or illness [28]. GCs are involved in several physiological processes, including metabolism, immune response, growth and development, and reproduction. Secretion of GCs by the adrenal cortex is normally regulated by the hypothalamo-pituitary-adrenal (HPA) axis (Fig. 1). Activation of the HPA axis starts with the secretion of hypothalamic corticotropin-releasing hormone (CRH), stimulation of pituitary pro-opiomelanocortin (POMC) gene transcription, secretion of the POMC-encoded adrenocorticotropic hormone (ACTH), and stimulation of adrenal GC synthesis and secretion (Fig. 2). GCs, in turn, inhibit CRH gene expression and secretion at the hypothalamic level, and POMC transcription and ACTH-secretion in the anterior pituitary, thereby

Table 1 Hormones and drugs associated with weight gain

Drug class	Drugs that may cause weight gain	Alternatives that cause less weight gain, weight loss, or are weight neutral
Diabetes treatment	Insulin, sulfonylureas, thiazolidinediones	Metformin, DPP-IV inhibitors, SGLT2 inhibitors, GLP-1 receptor agonists, GIP/GLP-1 receptor co-agonist, amylin analogs, acarbose
Steroid hormones	Corticosteroids, progestational steroids	NSAIDs
Oral contraceptives	Progestational steroids, hormonal contraceptives	Barrier methods, IUDs
Endometriosis treatment	Depot leuprolide acetate	Surgical methods
Antihistamines/anticholinergics	Diphenhydramine, doxepin, cyproheptadine	Decongestants, steroid inhalers
Antihypertensives	α-blocker, β-blocker	ACE inhibitors, calcium channel blockers
Antipsychotic	Risperidone, olanzapine, clozapine	Ziprasidone, aripiprazole
Antidepressants and mood stabilizers	TCAs, paroxetine, mirtazapine, citalopram, venlafaxine, MAOIs	Bupropion, nefazodone
Anticonvulsants	Carbamazepine, gabapentin, valproate	Lamotrigine, topiramate, zonisamide

ACE, angiotensin converting enzyme; DPP-IV, dipeptidyl peptidase-IV; GIP, glucose-dependent insulinotropic polypeptide; GLP-1, glucagon-like peptide-1; IUD, intrauterine device; MAOI, monoamine oxidase inhibitor; NSAID, nonsteroidal anti-inflammatory drug; TCA, tricyclic antidepressant; SGLT2, sodium glucose co-transporter 2

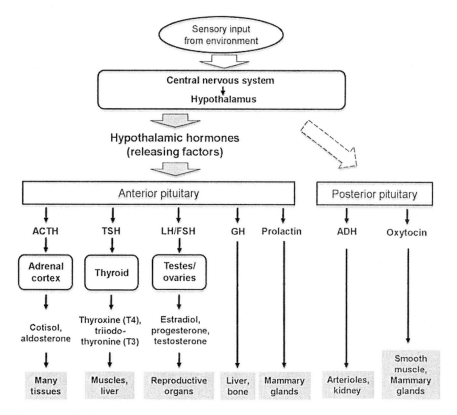

Fig. 1 Major neuroendocrine systems

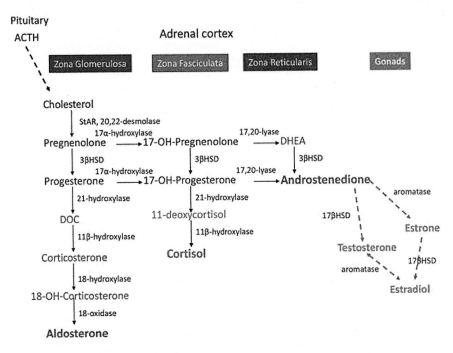

Fig. 2 Steroid hormone biosynthesis in adrenal cortex

establishing a regulatory feedback loop [29, 30]. The activity of HPA axis can further be increased in response to physiological and emotional stress. Once secreted, circulating GCs are bound to and transported by plasma proteins such as corticosteroid-binding globulin and albumin [31]. GCs mediate their physiologic effects by binding to an intracellular receptor, the GC receptor, the nuclear receptor superfamily of transcription factors. Upon GC binding in the cytosol, the GC receptor translocates into the nucleus where it serves as a DNA sequence-specific transcriptional regulator of distinct GC-responsive target genes. The main biological functions of GC include the suppression of inflammation and control of energy homeostasis. Excessive GC from exogenous treatment, e.g., for asthma and inflammatory conditions, or from endogenous overproduction due to pituitary adenoma, ectopic ACTH-producing tumors, or adrenal tumors, results in central obesity, sarcopenia, hyperglycemia, insulin resistance, dyslipidemia, fatty liver, hypertension, and immunodeficiency (Table 1). Some of these complications of GC excess (Cushing syndrome) resemble the metabolic syndrome associated with common forms of obesity [32].

Cushing Syndrome

Cushing syndrome is a rare condition that results from prolonged exposure to high circulating cortisol levels. Cushing syndrome can be divided into (i) ACTH-dependent Cushing syndrome, in which inappropriately high plasma ACTH concentrations stimulate the adrenal cortex to produce excessive amounts of cortisol, and (ii) ACTH-independent Cushing syndrome, in which excessive production of cortisol by abnormal adrenocortical tissue causes the syndrome and suppresses the secretion of both CRH and ACTH. ACTH-dependent Cushing syndrome accounts for about 80% of cases of endogenous hypercortisolism. Most cases of Cushing syndrome are caused by ACTH-secreting pituitary adenoma, often benign adenomas. The incidence of pituitary-dependent Cushing disease and adrenal adenomas in women is three to four times that of men [33].

The clinical features of Cushing syndrome may vary depending on the extent and duration of cortisol excess exposure. The typical symptoms and signs include a rapid increase in body weight, central obesity, mooning and plethora of the face, dorsocervical fat pad (buffalo hump) and supraclavicular fat pad, oligomenorrhea or amenorrhea, decreased libido in men, spontaneous ecchymoses, proximal muscle wasting and weakness, and the development of multiple wide purplish striae on the abdomen or proximal extremities. Depression and insomnia are common in Cushing syndrome. Patients may have mild hirsutism and acne, but severe androgenization, especially hirsutism and virilization, strongly suggests adrenal carcinoma. Cutaneous hyperpigmentation occurs in patients with ectopic ACTH syndrome in whom plasma ACTH concentrations are markedly elevated. Cushing syndrome shares similar clinical features with metabolic syndrome, characterized by central obesity, insulin resistance, glucose intolerance, hypertension, and dyslipidemia [34, 35].

The key biochemical features of Cushing syndrome consist of excessive endogenous secretion of cortisol, loss of the normal feedback of the HPA axis, and disturbance of the normal circadian rhythm of cortisol secretion. Recent guidelines on the diagnosis of Cushing syndrome recommend using at least two of the screening tests. Screening tests include 24-h urine free cortisol (UFC), late-night salivary cortisol, or low-dose dexamethasone suppression (1 mg overnight or 2 mg over 48 h) test. The determination of 24-h excretion of cortisol in urine is a reliable measure of cortisol secretion. UFC integrates the plasma-free cortisol concentrations during the entire day, with a raised level being consistent with Cushing syndrome. In a patient thought to have Cushing syndrome, cortisol should be measured in two or three consecutive 24-h urine specimens. Occasionally, cyclic, or episodic hypercortisolism requires several UFC determinations over a period of 3–6 months to establish a firm diagnosis [36]. A UFC test may show false-positive elevation in an individual drinking more than 5 liters of fluid daily or false-negative result in a patient with moderate to severe renal impairment. The loss of circadian rhythm with absence of a late-night

cortisol nadir in patients with Cushing syndrome provides the basis for measurement of a late-night salivary cortisol. Using different assays and various diagnostic criteria, investigators have reported that late-night salivary cortisol levels on two separate evenings yield a 92–100% sensitivity and a 93–100% specificity for the diagnosis of Cushing syndrome [37, 38]. The late-night salivary cortisol test, which measures free fraction, is appropriate for women taking estrogens. However, this test may be abnormal in shift-workers. An overnight 1 mg dexamethasone suppression test (DST) is a simple screening test for endogenous hypercortisolism. The test involves the oral administration of 1 mg dexamethasone between 11 pm and midnight, after which a plasma cortisol sample is obtained between 8 and 9 a.m. the next morning. A cortisol concentration of 1.8 or 3.6 μg/dL or less achieves high sensitivity; however, up to 30% of false-positive may occur as a result of primary obesity, chronic illness, psychiatric disorders, and even in normal individuals [37]. The 2-day, low-dose DST (0.5 mg every 6 h for 2 days) identifies patients with Cushing syndrome. The DST tests may be abnormal in women taking oral estrogens or patients on drugs that alter dexamethasone metabolism, e.g., phenytoin, rifampicin, or itraconazole.

The next challenge after establishing high cortisol levels is to identify the source of excess cortisol. The mainstay of differential diagnosis is the measurement of morning ACTH level. Plasma ACTH levels <5–10 pg/mL suggest an adrenal source of cortisol. Normal or elevated ACTH concentration suggests a pituitary or an ectopic source of ACTH. The standard 2-day, high-dose DST (2 mg every 6 h for 2 days), distinguishes Cushing disease, in which there is only relative resistance to GC negative feedback, from ectopic ACTH syndrome, in which there is usually complete resistance. The high-dose DST is performed on 24 h collections of urine for the measurement of UFC, and the degree of suppression is calculated from day 1 to day 3 after the administration of oral dexamethasone. Suppression of UFC by 90% has 100% specificity and 83% sensitivity for the diagnosis of pituitary disease [39]. As an alternative, a single 8-mg dose of dexamethasone is given orally at 11 pm, and plasma cortisol is measured at 8 am before and after dexamethasone administration. This test has a sensitivity ranging from 57% to 92% and a specificity ranging from 57% to 100% [40]. The most direct way to demonstrate pituitary hypersecretion of ACTH is to document a central-to-peripheral-venous gradient in blood draining the tumor [41].

Pseudo-Cushing Syndrome

Patients with certain non-endocrine disorders may exhibit some of the clinical or biochemical features of Cushing syndrome. As many as 80% of patients with major depressive disorder have increased HPA axis activity. Their hormonal abnormalities presumably result from hyperactivity of the HPA axis that disappears with remission of depression. Chronic alcoholism can mimic Cushing syndrome. These clinical features often disappear with abstinence from alcohol. The mechanism of hypercortisolism in chronic alcoholism may involve either increased CRH secretion or impaired hepatic metabolism of cortisol. Patients with chronic kidney disease have a disrupted circadian rhythm and abnormal dexamethasone-induced cortisol suppression. Hypercortisolism in chronic kidney disease seems to be associated with activation of the HPA axis [42].

The dexamethasone-CRH and desmopressin stimulation test has been used to distinguish patients with pseudo-Cushing syndrome from those with Cushing syndrome. The test is performed with low-dose DST followed by CRH (1 µg/kg body weight) stimulation and cortisol measurements. In patients with pseudo-Cushing syndrome, the pituitary corticotroph is appropriately suppressed by GCs and does not respond to CRH, while in Cushing syndrome the corticotroph tumor is resistant to dexamethasone and responds to CRH. Therefore, a serum cortisol level greater than 1.4 µg/dL in response to CRH after dexamethasone suppression supports the diagnosis of Cushing syndrome, whereas lower cortisol values are seen in normal individuals and those with pseudo-Cushing syndrome. The desmopressin stimulation test is performed in the morning measuring circulating ACTH and cortisol levels before and after desmopressin (10 µg) administration. Despite many limitations, these tests may provide valuable diagnostic information to distinguish between Cushing syndrome and pseudo-Cushing syndrome. Measurements of late-night salivary or midnight serum cortisol can also be used to differentiate patients with Cushing syndrome from those with pseudo-Cushing syndrome. The circadian rhythm of cortisol is preserved in pseudo-Cushing syndrome but disrupted in Cushing syndrome [43]. While true hypercortisolism will persist and the symptoms worsen over time in Cushing syndrome, hypercortisolism associated with pseudo-Cushing syndrome typically resolves spontaneously, or following definitive treatment, e.g., antidepressant treatment or abstinence from alcohol [36].

Linking Cortisol Metabolism and Obesity

Although there is a striking resemblance between some of the physical and biochemical features of Cushing syndrome and the metabolic syndrome associated with primary obesity, the plasma cortisol levels tend to be normal or reduced in the latter. This paradox was explained by the discovery that intracellular GC reactivation occurs in adipose tissue and liver of obese rodents and humans. Circulating free GCs can diffuse through the cell membrane to exert their function due to their lipophilic nature. However, the bioavailable GC levels in the cytoplasm are regulated by 11β (beta)-hydroxysteroid dehydrogenase enzymes as well as HPA axis activity. 11β (beta)-hydroxysteroid dehydrogenase type 1 (11β-HSD1) is the enzyme that mediates the conversion of inactive cortisone to active cortisol in humans (Fig. 3), and deoxycorticosterone to corticosterone in rodents. 11β-HSD1 is located within the endoplasmic reticulum and it is highly expressed in liver and adipose tissue. Tissue-specific dysregulation of cortisol metabolism due to increased adipose mass and decreased hepatic 11β-HSD1 activity has been shown in individuals with obesity [44].

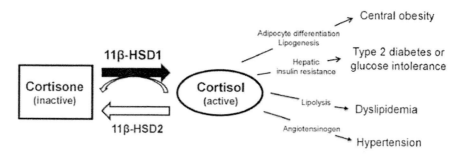

Fig. 3 Role of 11β (beta)-hydroxysteroid dehydrogenase type 1 (11β-HSD1) in the metabolic syndrome. 11β-HSD1, highly expressed in liver and adipose tissue, generates active cortisol from inactive cortisone. In contrast, 11β-HSD2 is mainly expressed in kidney and colon, and converts cortisol to cortisone. Enhanced activity of 11β-HSD1 in adipose tissue has been implicated in central obesity, insulin resistance, type 2 diabetes, dyslipidemia, and atherogenic cardiovascular diseases. Inhibition of 11β-HSD1 might be a promising target for treating metabolic syndrome

Transgenic mice overexpressing 11β-HSD1 in liver produced mild insulin resistance, fatty liver, hyperlipidemia, and hypertension, but not obesity or glucose intolerance. Targeted overexpression of 11β-HSD1 in adipose tissue exhibited a similar profile with visceral obesity, and dyslipidemia. In contrast, 11β-HSD1 knock-out (11β-HSD1−/−) mice had improved glucose tolerance, improved lipid profile, and reduced weight and visceral fat when fed a high-fat diet [45]. Pharmacologic inhibition of 11β-HSD1 in obese rodent models also improved lipid profile and glucose tolerance [46, 47].

Studies in individuals with obesity have demonstrated increased 11β-HSD1 expression and activity in subcutaneous and omental adipose tissue, with positive correlations with body mass index (BMI), body fat, and insulin resistance [48]. However, the role of 11β-HSD1 in individuals with metabolic syndrome and T2D has not been consistent. In a case report of Cushing disease that failed to present with a classical Cushingoid phenotype, a partial functional defect of 11β-HSD1 activity was identified, suggesting that intracellular 11β-HSD1 activity may significantly affect clinical manifestations in Cushing syndrome. Pharmacologic inhibition of 11β-HSD1 may offer therapeutic strategy for obesity-related metabolic disorders. However, selective 11β-HSD1 inhibitor treatment in obesity, metabolic syndrome, and T2D has shown overall disappointing results in clinical trials [49].

Thyroid Hormone

Thyroid hormone is essential for normal growth and development and metabolic regulation in mammals. Thyroid hormone plays a key role during embryogenesis and early life, and has profound effects in adult life, including the regulation of energy homeostasis, thermogenesis, and nutrient metabolism. The synthesis and secretion of thyroid hormone are regulated by a feedback system, the hypothalamo-pituitary-thyroid (HPT) axis. Thyrotropin-releasing hormone (TRH) is synthesized in the paraventricular nucleus of the hypothalamus, and transported via axons to the median eminence, where it is released into the portal capillary plexus and stimulates TSH synthesis and secretion of thyroxine (T4) and tri-iodothyronine (T3) [50]. T4 is more abundant in the circulation and is peripherally converted into more biologically active triiodothyronine (T3). The majority of thyroid hormones circulate in the bloodstream bound to specific carrier proteins, including thyroxine-binding globulin (TBG), transthyretin, and albumin. Protein-bound thyroid hormones cannot enter cells and thus are considered to be biologically inert. Only less than 1% of serum thyroid hormone is free hormone available for uptake by target tissues [51]. Circulating free thyroid hormone is transported across the plasma membrane via specific transporters, including monocarboxylate transporter (MCT)8, MCT10, and organic anion-transporting polypeptide 1C1. Plasma and cellular T3 levels are mainly derived from T4 conversion via type 1 (D1) and type 2 (D2) iodothyronine deiodinases. The type 3 (D3) iodothyronine deiodinase deactivates T4 and T3. Deiodinases are differentially expressed in various tissues. Local activation of T3 from T4 appears to be an important mechanism of regulation of thyroid hormone action at the tissue level [52]. Free thyroid hormone enters target cells and acts mainly through its nuclear receptors, thyroid hormone receptor (TR) α (alpha) and β (beta). TR forms a heterodimeric complex, with retinoid X receptor (RXR), which binds to a thyroid hormone response element (TRE) to regulate the expression of genes involved in metabolism of lipids, carbohydrates, bile acids, and other processes. In the absence of T3, TR recruits a corepressor to mediate transcriptional repression. The binding of T3 to TR leads to dismissal of the corepressor complex and recruitment of coactivators to stimulate gene expression. While the hypothalamic-pituitary-thyroid (HPT) axis modulates to keep thyroid hormone levels stable,

intracellular availability of thyroid hormone is strongly regulated by deiodinases, transporters, TR, and nuclear receptor coregulators in target cells [53].

Thyroid hormone plays a major role in regulating energy balance and metabolism. Thyroid hormone increases the basal metabolic rate via Na/K-ATPase, and also interacts with the adrenergic nervous system to produce heat in response to cold exposure. This process, termed adaptive thermogenesis, occurs in rodent brown adipose tissue (BAT), requires both TRα (alpha) and TRβ (beta), and involves uncoupling protein (UCP)-1 expression. Deiodinase 2 (D2) is expressed in BAT, white fat, and skeletal muscle, and is required for adaptive thermogenesis. During cold exposure, the adrenergic system induces D2 expression in BAT, thereby stimulating thermogenesis [54]. Thyroid hormone also stimulates lipolysis in adipose tissue. While thyroid hormone stimulates lipogenesis in the liver, there is a net reduction in total triglycerides through increased mobilization, degradation, and fatty acid oxidation (Fig. 4). Thyroid hormone reduces serum

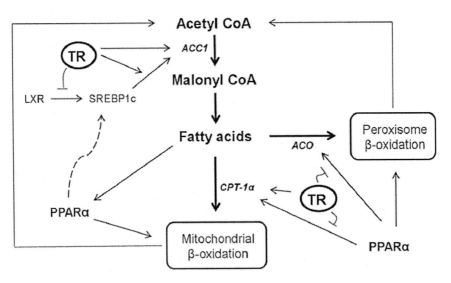

Fig. 4 Effects of thyroid hormone on fatty acid metabolism in liver. The ACC1 promoter contains a thyroid hormone receptor response element (TRE) and sterol regulating element-binding protein response element (SRE). Thyroid hormone directly stimulates the synthesis of ACC1, which catalyzes the formation of fatty acids. Thyroid hormone increases fatty acid oxidation by upregulating expression of CPT-1α (alpha). Unliganded thyroid hormone receptor (TR) blocks stimulation of CPT-1α (alpha) and ACO by PPARα (alpha). ACC, acetyl-CoA carboxylase; ACO, acetyl-CoA oxidase; CPT, carnitine palmitoyl-transferase; PPAR, peroxisome proliferator-activated receptor

cholesterol levels by increasing hepatic expression of low-density lipoprotein receptor and converting cholesterol into bile acids in liver [55]. Glucose metabolism is also modulated by thyroid hormone. Excess thyroid hormone stimulates hepatic gluconeogenesis and glucose production, increases GLUT4 in skeletal muscle, and impairs glucose-stimulated insulin release [54].

Clinical Features of Hypothyroidism

Weight gain is a common complaint in hypothyroid patients. The commonest cause of hypothyroidism in developed countries is chronic autoimmune thyroiditis. High levels of anti-thyroid antibodies are present in patients with autoimmune thyroiditis. Radioiodine ablation or surgical thyroidectomy as treatment for hyperthyroidism or thyroid cancer can also lead to hypothyroidism if thyroxine replacement is inadequate. Hypothyroidism may be drug-induced (e.g., lithium, amiodarone), or result from disorders of the pituitary (secondary) or hypothalamus (tertiary). The prevalence of hypothyroidism in the general population varies between 3% and 5% in the United States and Europe, depending on the definition used. Anti-thyroid peroxidase (TPO) antibodies are associated with hypothyroidism, and this is more common in women and with aging [56]. The clinical manifestations of hypothyroidism may be severe or mild, ranging from myxedema coma to nonspecific symptoms. Common symptoms of hypothyroidism include fatigue, depression, cold intolerance, constipation, dryness of the skin, and menstrual irregularities. As the disorder becomes fully established, the classic features of non-pitting edema (myxedema) of the skin, periorbital edema, hoarseness, sinus bradycardia, hypothermia, and delayed relaxation of the deep tendon reflexes appear [57, 58].

The serum TSH is the most sensitive test for detecting early thyroid failure. An increase in TSH precedes a decline of serum free T4 by several months and sometimes years. Serum T3 concentrations are often normal. Adults presenting with symptomatic hypothyroidism often have a TSH level >10 mU/L, and reductions in the serum free or total T4 concentrations. The early stage of hypothyroidism occurs when a serum TSH level is elevated (between 5 and 10 mU/L) while circulating levels of thyroid hormone are normal. This is termed "subclinical hypothyroidism," and in many patients represents a state of compensated or mild thyroid failure [57]. Anti-thyroid antibodies can be detected in 80% of patients with subclinical hypothyroidism, and 80% of patients with subclinical hypothyroidism have a serum TSH less than 10 mU/L. Patients with subclinical hypothyroidism have a high rate of progression to clinically overt hypothyroidism, ~2.6% per year, if TPO antibodies are absent, and 4.3% if TPO is present. A TSH level greater than 10 mIU/L predicts a higher rate of progression of hypothyroidism [59]. Laboratory investigation of hypothyroidism may reveal mild anemia, increased creatine phosphokinase concentrations indicating myopathy, and abnormal lipid profile with increased total and low-density lipoprotein cholesterol and decreased high-density lipoprotein cholesterol concentrations [60].

Central hypothyroidism is rare and affects both sexes equally. Central hypothyroidism is characterized by a defect of thyroid hormone production due to insufficient stimulation by TSH of a normal thyroid gland. Central hypothyroidism can be congenital or acquired in the case of lesions affecting either the pituitary (secondary hypothyroidism) or the hypothalamus (tertiary hypothyroidism). The diagnosis is based on biochemical tests showing a low serum free T4 level and inappropriately low-to-normal TSH level. TRH testing may help in the differential diagnosis between tertiary (hypothalamic) and secondary (pituitary) hypothyroidism. In the latter, the TSH response may be absent or impaired, whereas tertiary hypothyroidism is characterized by normal, exaggerated, or delayed TSH response to TRH injection [61].

Hypothyroidism and Obesity

Individuals with overt hypothyroidism have variable degrees of weight gain. An increase in body weight associated with hypothyroidism may arise from body fat accumulation, water retention, and increased deposition of glycoaminoglycans [62]. Thyroid hormone modulates the basal metabolic rate, and stimulates resting energy expenditure (REE) by increasing ATP production in muscle. Thyroid status is known to be associated with changes in weight and REE. Studies have demonstrated a positive cross-sectional association between serum TSH levels and the BMI. Increased serum TSH levels within the normal reference range are strongly and linearly associated with weight gain [54].

Hypothyroidism is also associated with structural and functional cardiac abnormalities, e.g., cardiac wall stiffness, bradycardia, and depressed myocardial contractility, which account for reduced cardiac output [63]. A low cardiac output and a decrease in renal blood flow and glomerular filtration rate lead to impaired renal water excretion, which contributes to edema and weight gain [64]. Hypothyroidism also causes generalized interstitial deposition of glycosaminoglycans, which in turn leads to fluid and sodium retention. Hyaluronan, an abundant non-sulfated glycosaminoglycan, accumulates in many tissues including the skin, myocardium, kidney, and vasculature in severe, long-standing hypothyroidism due to a reduced clearance rate and increased synthetic rate. Hyaluronan exhibits a remarkable avidity for water, thus causing the tissues to expand greatly [65, 66]. Restoration of euthyroidism by T4 treatment increases REE and decreases body weight, mainly by decreasing the lean mass. Thyroxine treatment normalizes the tissue composition and increases water excretion [67].

Thyroid hormone plays a pivotal role in controlling whole body metabolism, fat metabolism, and cardiovascular function. TRβ, the prevalent thyroid receptor isoform in liver, is responsible for regulating serum cholesterol levels, whereas TRα isoform is predominant in heart and bone. Several thyroid hormone analogs, which have beneficial effects on body weight and serum cholesterol levels without deleterious effects on heart, muscle, and bone by targeting selectively TRβ have been developed and evaluated [68, 69]. In spite of disappointing results in early clinical trials, recent novel TRβ-selective, liver-selective analogs showed encouraging results for the treatment of non-alcoholic steatohepatitis (NAFLD) [70, 71]. Moreover, thyroid hormone metabolites also gained significant attention, since early studies with these metabolites revealed beneficial metabolic effects without adverse side effects in obese rodent models [72]. Recent clinical trials of synthetic thyroid hormone analogs have shown improvements in glycemic control, lipids and blood pressure, supporting the therapeutic potential of thyromimetics in obesity-related metabolic disorders [73, 74].

Growth Hormone

Growth hormone (GH) is secreted by the anterior pituitary somatotrophs. GH secretion is stimulated by GH-releasing hormone (GHRH) and ghrelin, and inhibited by somatostatin. GH secretion is inhibited by insulin, glucose, and fatty acids, while arginine stimulates GH secretion [75]. GH pulses occur mainly at night. Fasting increases and food consumption inhibits GH secretion during the day. Ghrelin, secreted mainly from the stomach, stimulates GH release in a synergistic manner with GHRH [76]. GH secretion increases during puberty under the influence of sex steroids and declines gradually thereafter throughout life. Obesity is associated with decreased GH secretion. GH receptor is expressed on multiple tissues, including liver, cartilage, muscle, and adipose tissue. The binding of GH to GH receptor dimers triggers intracellular signal transduction to regulate target genes. Several of the proteins phosphorylated and activated by the GH receptor through JAK2 serve as adapters, linking GH signaling to a variety of signal transduction pathways [77]. GH is the main regulator of insulin-like growth factor (IGF)-1. Liver is a major target tissue of GH action and produces IGF-1 and IGF-binding protein-3 (IGFBP-3) in response to GH. IGFBP-3 prolongs the half-life of IGF-I. Unbound IGF-1 mediates a negative feedback control of GH secretion by acting directly on the somatotroph and on hypothalamic GHRH and somatostatin neurons [75]. A number of studies have demonstrated that both GH and IGF-1 play key roles in the normal growth of bone and muscle. GH also modulates metabolism and energy homeostasis in various tissues, including liver, adipose tissue, and pancreas. GH stimulates hepatic glucose production, and plays an important role in triglyceride secretion from liver. The main effect of GH in adipose tissue is the stimulation of lipolysis. GH may also regulate tissue glucocorticoid action by inhibiting 11β-HSD1, leading to less cortisol production in adipose tissue. GH appears to exert direct effects on pancreatic β-cells, affecting insulin synthesis and secretion [78]. In addition, GH has a significant effect on maintaining the structure and function of heart and vascular system. Both GH and IGF-1 may have a regulatory role for peripheral vascular resistance and myocardial contractility [79].

Cardiometabolic Complications of GH Deficiency

Growth hormone deficiency (GHD) may be isolated or occur as part of multiple hormone deficiencies. GHD often results from damage to the pituitary gland or hypothalamus, caused by a tumor, traumatic brain injury, or following surgical resection or radiotherapy. In adults, GHD is associated with adverse cardiometabolic risk profile and increased fracture risk, and reduced quality of life. Individuals with GHD typically have central obesity, decreased lean mass and bone mineral density, reduced exercise capacity, and elevated levels of total and low-density lipoprotein cholesterol and triglyceride. Accumulation of visceral fat in GHD may be linked to decreased lipolysis and increased local cortisol production by enhanced 11β-HSD1 activity in adipose tissue. Whereas GH antagonizes insulin action, GHD is characterized by central obesity, associated with insulin resistance and increased prevalence of metabolic syndrome and type 2 diabetes (T2D). In addition to the traditional cardiovascular risk factors, endothelial dysfunction, pro-inflammatory state, increased oxidative stress, and impaired adipokine levels may also contribute to the development of premature atherosclerosis in GHD [80]. Several retrospective studies have demonstrated an increased risk of cardiovascular morbidity and mortality in patients with GHD [81, 82].

GH secretion is pulsatile and GH has a short half-life. Because GH levels may be undetectable between secretory spikes in healthy adults, random GH measurement is unreliable in the evaluation of GHD. Low serum IGF-1 levels do not always establish the diagnosis of GHD. Moreover, reduced IGF-1 levels are seen in several conditions, e.g., starvation, chronic liver and kidney diseases, hypothyroidism, and diabetes. However, low IGF-1 in patients with multiple pituitary hormone deficiencies may indicate GHD. The diagnosis of GHD generally relies on the measurements of GH secretory reserve in response to GH stimulation tests. Among the tests, insulin tolerance test (ITT), considered the gold standard test of GHD, is accurate if the plasma nadir glucose level is less than 40 mg/dL. GHD is diagnosed if a peak GH level is less than 5 μg/L. The ITT is labor-intensive, contraindicated in the elderly and pregnant women, and in adults with cardiovascular disease or seizure disorder. The combined administration of GHRH and arginine represents a dual stimulus to GH secretion. GH response to GHRH-arginine is inversely associated with central adiposity. Accordingly, BMI-dependent values of GH are recommended for this test. Glucagon stimulation test is also accurate and widely used in the evaluation of GHD. However, it requires an intramuscular injection and can cause side effects in older people. BMI-appropriate peak GH values for the diagnosis of GHD are recommended during this test. Macimorelin is an orally active ghrelin-mimetic, which stimulates endogenous GH secretion. Macimorelin stimulation test was reported to have good sensitivity and specificity compared with the ITT. Oral macimorelin, 0.5 mg/kg after fasting for at least 8 h, is a simple, well-tolerated, reproducible diagnostic test without serious adverse effects. Importantly, some concurrent drugs may interact with macimorelin and cause prolongation of QT interval, i.e., antipsychotic medication (e.g., chlorpromazine, haloperidol, thioridazone, ziprasidone), antibiotics (e.g., moxiloxacin), class 1A antiarrhythmics (e.g., quinidine, procainamide), and class III antiarrhythmics (e.g., amiodarone, sotalol). CYP3A4 inducers (e.g., carbamazepine, enzalutamide, mitotane, phenytoin, rifampin, St. John's wort, bosentan, efavirenz, etravirine, modafinil, armodafinil, rufinamide), and GH therapy should be discontinued before macimorelin administration [83, 84].

Adequate GH replacement in GHD has been shown to exert favorable effects in body composition, bone metabolism, lipid profile, exercise capacity, quality of life, and several cardiovascular risk factors. However, GH replacement does not ameliorate all cardiometabolic abnormalities observed in patients with GHD. Several studies demonstrated an increased mortality in patients with hypopituitarism including GHD. Excess mortality in these patients seems to be multifactorial, including unreplaced GHD, inadequate replacement of other hormones, and comorbidities. Whether treatment with GH definitely reduces mortality in patients with GHD remains inconclusive [82, 85]. GH replacement can increase blood glucose, since GH has an anti-insulin effect. Therefore, periodic monitoring of glycemic status is advisable in individuals with obesity or a family history of T2D. The combined effects of GH/IGF-1 action that include pro-proliferative and antiapoptotic properties have raised some concerns regarding the safety of GH replacement. Recent studies have shown no association between GH replacement and the development of new neoplasm. Nevertheless, GH should not be given to patients with active malignancy or avoided in those with a history of cancer [86]. GH replacement may have several side effects, including edema, arthralgia, carpal tunnel syndrome, and paresthesia, especially in older, heavier, and female patients with GHD. To avoid adverse effects, GH replacement should be initiated with a low dose and titrated based on clinical response and serum IGF-1 levels [87]. Recently, long-acting GH preparations that allow for decreased injection frequency are developed. The long-acting GH analogs have different pharmacokinetic and pharmacodynamic properties, compared with daily recombinant GH products. Therefore, long-term implications of prolonged elevation of GH levels after an injection of a long-acting GH analog that may cause metabolic aberrations need to be addressed [88].

Conclusion

Obesity can be a manifestation of hyperinsulinism, hypercortisolism, hypothyroidism, or growth hormone deficiency. It is well established that obesity is strongly associated with glucose intolerance or diabetes, atherogenic dyslipidemia, hypertension, and an increased risk of atherosclerotic cardiovascular diseases. In contrast to primary obesity, obesity resulting from abnormal regulation of insulin, glucocorticoids, thyroid hormone, or growth hormone tends to have a rapid onset and progression, and to be associated with unique symptoms and signs of the underlying diseases. Understanding the pathogenesis, clinical features, and hormonal evaluation of endocrinopathies can provide practitioners specific treatment strategies.

Practice Points

- Insulinoma is the most common functioning islet cell tumor of the pancreas and a rare cause of rapid weight gain.
- Excessive glucocorticoid from endogenous production or exogenous treatment results in central obesity, sarcopenia, hyperglycemia, hypertension, and dyslipidemia.
- Weight gain associated with hypothyroidism results from decreased thermogenesis and increased fluid retention and interstitial accumulation of glycosaminoglycans.
- Growth hormone deficiency is associated with central obesity and adverse cardiometabolic risk profile.

Research Agenda

- Selective inhibition of 11β (beta)-hydroxysteroid dehydrogenase for obesity-related metabolic disorders
- Synthetic thyroid hormone analogs or metabolites for obesity-related metabolic disorders

- Long-term surveillance data of long-acting growth hormone analogs on safety, efficacy, and cost-effectiveness

References

1. Campbell JE, Newgard CB. Mechanisms controlling pancreatic islet cell function in insulin secretion. Nat Rev Mol Cell Biol. 2021;22:142–58.
2. Newsholme P, Cruzat V, Arfuso F, Keane K. Nutrient regulation of insulin secretion and action. J Endocrinol. 2014;221:R105–20.
3. Rahman MS, Hossain KS, Das S, Kundu S, Adegoke EO, Rahman MA, et al. Role of insulin in health and disease: an update. Int J Mol Sci. 2021;22:6403.
4. Avruch J, Khokhlatchev A, Kyriakis JM, Luo Z, Tzivion G, Vavvas D, et al. Ras activation of the Raf kinase: tyrosine kinase recruitment of the MAP kinase cascade. Recent Prog Horm Res. 2001;56:127–55.
5. Khan AH, Pessin JE. Insulin regulation of glucose uptake: a complex interplay of intracellular signalling pathways. Diabetologia. 2002;45:1475–83.
6. Saltiel AR. Insulin signaling in health and disease. J Clin Invest. 2021;131:e142241.
7. Dimitriadis G, Mitrou P, Lambadiari V, Maratou E, Raptis SA. Insulin effects in muscle and adipose tissue. Diabetes Res Clin Pract. 2011;93(Suppl 1):S52–9.
8. Guo Z, Hensrud DD, Johnson CM, Jensen MD. Regional postprandial fatty acid metabolism in different obesity phenotypes. Diabetes. 1999;48:1586–92.
9. Savage DB, Semple RK. Recent insights into fatty liver, metabolic dyslipidaemia and their links to insulin resistance. Curr Opin Lipidol. 2010;21:329–36.
10. Capeau J. Insulin resistance and steatosis in humans. Diabetes Metab. 2008;34:649–57.
11. Nichols GA, Gomez-Caminero A. Weight changes following the initiation of new anti-hyperglycaemic therapies. Diabetes Obes Metab. 2007;9:96–102.
12. Intensive blood-glucose control with sulphonylureas or insulin compared with conventional treatment and risk of complications in patients with type 2 diabetes (UKPDS 33). UK Prospective Diabetes Study (UKPDS) Group. Lancet. 1998;352:837–53.
13. Effect of intensive blood-glucose control with metformin on complications in overweight patients with type 2 diabetes (UKPDS 34). UK Prospective Diabetes Study (UKPDS) Group. Lancet. 1998;352:854–65.
14. Weight gain associated with intensive therapy in the diabetes control and complications trial. The DCCT Research Group. Diabetes Care. 1988;11:567–73.
15. Influence of intensive diabetes treatment on body weight and composition of adults with type 1 diabetes in the Diabetes Control and Complications Trial. Diabetes Care. 2001;24:1711–21.
16. Russell-Jones D, Khan R. Insulin-associated weight gain in diabetes – causes, effects and coping strategies. Diabetes Obes Metab. 2007;9:799–812.
17. Carver C. Insulin treatment and the problem of weight gain in type 2 diabetes. Diabetes Educ. 2006;32:910–7.
18. Brown A, Guess N, Dornhorst A, Taheri S, Frost G. Insulin-associated weight gain in obese type 2 diabetes mellitus patients: what can be done? Diabetes Obes Metab. 2017;19:1655–68.
19. Lingvay I, Sumithran P, Cohen RV, le Roux CW. Obesity management as a primary treatment goal for type 2 diabetes: time to reframe the conversation. Lancet. 2022;399:394–405.
20. Apovian CM, Okemah J, O'Neil PM. Body weight considerations in the management of type 2 diabetes. Adv Ther. 2019;36:44–58.
21. Nauck MA, D'Alessio DA. Tirzepatide, a dual GIP/GLP-1 receptor co-agonist for the treatment of type 2 diabetes with unmatched effectiveness regrading glycaemic control and body weight reduction. Cardiovasc Diabetol. 2022;21:169.
22. Vaidakis D, Karoubalis J, Pappa T, Piaditis G, Zografos GN. Pancreatic insulinoma: current issues and trends. Hepatobiliary Pancreat Dis Int. 2010;9:234–41.
23. Guettier JM, Kam A, Chang R, Skarulis MC, Cochran C, Alexander HR, et al. Localization of insulinomas to regions of the pancreas by intraarterial calcium stimulation: the NIH experience. J Clin Endocrinol Metab. 2009;94:1074–80.
24. Tucker ON, Crotty PL, Conlon KC. The management of insulinoma. Br J Surg. 2006;93:264–75.
25. Grant CS. Insulinoma. Best Pract Res Clin Gastroenterol. 2005;19:783–98.
26. Oberg K, Kvols L, Caplin M, Delle Fave G, de Herder W, Rindi G, et al. Consensus report on the use of somatostatin analogs for the management of neuroendocrine tumors of the gastroenteropancreatic system. Ann Oncol. 2004;15:966–73.
27. Okabayashi T, Shima Y, Sumiyoshi T, Kozuki A, Ito S, Ogawa Y, et al. Diagnosis and management of insulinoma. World J Gastroenterol. 2013;19:829–37.
28. Sacta MA, Chinenov Y, Rogatsky I. Glucocorticoid signaling: an update from a genomic perspective. Annu Rev Physiol. 2016;78:155–80.
29. Malkoski SP, Dorin RI. Composite glucocorticoid regulation at a functionally defined negative glucocorticoid response element of the human corticotropin-releasing hormone gene. Mol Endocrinol. 1999;13:1629–44.
30. Watts AG. Glucocorticoid regulation of peptide genes in neuroendocrine CRH neurons: a complexity beyond negative feedback. Front Neuroendocrinol. 2005;26:109–30.
31. Timmermans S, Souffriau J, Libert C. A general introduction to glucocorticoid biology. Front Immunol. 2019;10:1545.
32. Vegiopoulos A, Herzig S. Glucocorticoids, metabolism and metabolic diseases. Mol Cell Endocrinol. 2007;275:43–61.
33. Barbot M, Zilio M, Scaroni C. Cushing's syndrome: overview of clinical presentation, diagnostic tools and complications. Best Pract Res Clin Endocrinol Metab. 2020;34:101380.

34. Nieman LK. Cushing's syndrome: update on signs, symptoms and biochemical screening. Eur J Endocrinol. 2015;173:M33–8.

35. Ferriere A, Tabarin A. Cushing's syndrome: treatment and new therapeutic approaches. Best Pract Res Clin Endocrinol Metab. 2020;34:101381.

36. Tsigos C, Chrousos GP. Differential diagnosis and management of Cushing's syndrome. Annu Rev Med. 1996;47:443–61.

37. Nieman LK, Biller BM, Findling JW, Newell-Price J, Savage MO, Stewart PM, et al. The diagnosis of Cushing's syndrome: an Endocrine Society Clinical Practice guideline. J Clin Endocrinol Metab. 2008;93:1526–40.

38. Raff H. Update on late-night salivary cortisol for the diagnosis of Cushing's syndrome: methodological considerations. Endocrine. 2013;44:346–9.

39. Flack MR, Oldfield EH, Cutler GB Jr, Zweig MH, Malley JD, Chrousos GP, et al. Urine free cortisol in the high-dose dexamethasone suppression test for the differential diagnosis of the Cushing syndrome. Ann Intern Med. 1992;116:211–7.

40. Newell-Price J, Trainer P, Besser M, Grossman A. The diagnosis and differential diagnosis of Cushing's syndrome and pseudo-Cushing's states. Endocr Rev. 1998;19:647–72.

41. Orth DN. Cushing's syndrome. N Engl J Med. 1995;332:791–803.

42. Findling JW, Raff H. Diagnosis of endocrine disease: differentiation of pathologic/neoplastic hypercortisolism (Cushing's syndrome) from physiologic/non-neoplastic hypercortisolism (formerly known as pseudo-Cushing's syndrome). Eur J Endocrinol. 2017;176:R205–r16.

43. Nieman LK. Diagnosis of Cushing's syndrome in the modern era. Endocrinol Metab Clin N Am. 2018;47:259–73.

44. Stomby A, Andrew R, Walker BR, Olsson T. Tissue-specific dysregulation of cortisol regeneration by 11betaHSD1 in obesity: has it promised too much? Diabetologia. 2014;57:1100–10.

45. Gomez-Sanchez EP, Gomez-Sanchez CE. 11-β-hydroxysteroid dehydrogenases: a growing multitasking family. Mol Cell Endocrinol. 2021;526:111210.

46. Berthiaume M, Laplante M, Festuccia W, Gélinas Y, Poulin S, Lalonde J, et al. Depot-specific modulation of rat intraabdominal adipose tissue lipid metabolism by pharmacological inhibition of 11beta-hydroxysteroid dehydrogenase type 1. Endocrinology. 2007;148:2391–7.

47. Taylor A, Irwin N, McKillop AM, Flatt PR, Gault VA. Sub-chronic administration of the 11beta-HSD1 inhibitor, carbenoxolone, improves glucose tolerance and insulin sensitivity in mice with diet-induced obesity. Biol Chem. 2008;389:441–5.

48. Li X, Wang J, Yang Q, Shao S. 11β-hydroxysteroid dehydrogenase type 1 in obese subjects with type 2 diabetes mellitus. Am J Med Sci. 2017;354:408–14.

49. Gregory S, Hill D, Grey B, Ketelbey W, Miller T, Muniz-Terrera G, et al. 11β-hydroxysteroid dehydrogenase type 1 inhibitor use in human disease-a systematic review and narrative synthesis. Metabolism. 2020;108:154246.

50. Shupnik MA, Ridgway EC, Chin WW. Molecular biology of thyrotropin. Endocr Rev. 1989;10:459–75.

51. van der Spek AH, Fliers E, Boelen A. The classic pathways of thyroid hormone metabolism. Mol Cell Endocrinol. 2017;458:29–38.

52. Brent GA. Mechanisms of thyroid hormone action. J Clin Invest. 2012;122:3035–43.

53. Mendoza A, Hollenberg AN. New insights into thyroid hormone action. Pharmacol Ther. 2017;173:135–45.

54. Mullur R, Liu YY, Brent GA. Thyroid hormone regulation of metabolism. Physiol Rev. 2014;94:355–82.

55. Sinha RA, Singh BK, Yen PM. Direct effects of thyroid hormones on hepatic lipid metabolism. Nat Rev Endocrinol. 2018;14:259–69.

56. Hollowell JG, Staehling NW, Flanders WD, Hannon WH, Gunter EW, Spencer CA, et al. Serum TSH, T(4), and thyroid antibodies in the United States population (1988 to 1994): National Health and Nutrition Examination Survey (NHANES III). J Clin Endocrinol Metab. 2002;87:489–99.

57. Vaidya B, Pearce SH. Management of hypothyroidism in adults. BMJ. 2008;337:a801.

58. Chaker L, Bianco AC, Jonklaas J, Peeters RP. Hypothyroidism. Lancet. 2017;390:1550–62.

59. Fatourechi V. Subclinical hypothyroidism: an update for primary care physicians. Mayo Clin Proc. 2009;84:65–71.

60. Woeber KA. Update on the management of hyperthyroidism and hypothyroidism. Arch Intern Med. 2000;160:1067–71.

61. Lania A, Persani L, Beck-Peccoz P. Central hypothyroidism. Pituitary. 2008;11:181–6.

62. Santini F, Marzullo P, Rotondi M, Ceccarini G, Pagano L, Ippolito S, et al. Mechanisms in endocrinology: the crosstalk between thyroid gland and adipose tissue: signal integration in health and disease. Eur J Endocrinol. 2014;171:R137–52.

63. Fazio S, Palmieri EA, Lombardi G, Biondi B. Effects of thyroid hormone on the cardiovascular system. Recent Prog Horm Res. 2004;59:31–50.

64. Montenegro J, Gonzalez O, Saracho R, Aguirre R, Gonzalez O, Martinez I. Changes in renal function in primary hypothyroidism. Am J Kidney Dis. 1996;27:195–8.

65. Smith TJ, Murata Y, Horwitz AL, Philipson L, Refetoff S. Regulation of glycosaminoglycan synthesis by thyroid hormone in vitro. J Clin Invest. 1982;70:1066–73.

66. Gianoukakis AG, Jennings TA, King CS, Sheehan CE, Hoa N, Heldin P, et al. Hyaluronan accumulation in thyroid tissue: evidence for contributions from epithelial cells and fibroblasts. Endocrinology. 2007;148:54–62.

67. Laurberg P, Knudsen N, Andersen S, Carle A, Pedersen IB, Karmisholt J. Thyroid function and obesity. Eur Thyroid J. 2012;1:159–67.

68. Mondal S, Mugesh G. Novel thyroid hormone analogues, enzyme inhibitors and mimetics, and their action. Mol Cell Endocrinol. 2017;458:91–104.
69. Kowalik MA, Columbano A, Perra A. Thyroid hormones, thyromimetics and their metabolites in the treatment of liver disease. Front Endocrinol (Lausanne). 2018;9:382.
70. Saponaro F, Sestito S, Runfola M, Rapposelli S, Chiellini G. Selective thyroid hormone receptor-beta (TRβ) agonists: new perspectives for the treatment of metabolic and neurodegenerative disorders. Front Med (Lausanne). 2020;7:331.
71. Zucchi R. Thyroid hormone analogues: an update. Thyroid. 2020;30:1099–105.
72. Senese R, Cioffi F, Petito G, Goglia F, Lanni A. Thyroid hormone metabolites and analogues. Endocrine. 2019;66:105–14.
73. Sane R, Wirth EK, Köhrle J. 3,5-T2-an endogenous thyroid hormone metabolite as promising lead substance in anti-steatotic drug development? Metabolites. 2022;12:582.
74. Joshi D, Gj P, Ghosh S, Mohanan A, Joshi S, Mohan V, et al. TRC150094, a novel mitochondrial modulator, reduces cardio-metabolic risk as an add-on treatment: a phase-2, 24-week, multi-center, randomized, double-blind, clinical trial. Diabetes Metab Syndr Obes. 2022;15:615–31.
75. Meinhardt UJ, Ho KK. Modulation of growth hormone action by sex steroids. Clin Endocrinol. 2006;65:413–22.
76. Tritos NA, Biller BMK. Current concepts of the diagnosis of adult growth hormone deficiency. Rev Endocr Metab Disord. 2021;22:109–16.
77. Melmed S. Pathogenesis and diagnosis of growth hormone deficiency in adults. N Engl J Med. 2019;380: 2551–62.
78. Vijayakumar A, Yakar S, Leroith D. The intricate role of growth hormone in metabolism. Front Endocrinol (Lausanne). 2011;2:32.
79. Isgaard J, Arcopinto M, Karason K, Cittadini A. GH and the cardiovascular system: an update on a topic at heart. Endocrine. 2015;48:25–35.
80. Ratku B, Sebestyén V, Erdei A, Nagy EV, Szabó Z, Somodi S. Effects of adult growth hormone deficiency and replacement therapy on the cardiometabolic risk profile. Pituitary. 2022;25:211–28.
81. Gazzaruso C, Gola M, Karamouzis I, Giubbini R, Giustina A. Cardiovascular risk in adult patients with growth hormone (GH) deficiency and following substitution with GH – an update. J Clin Endocrinol Metab. 2014;99:18–29.
82. van Bunderen CC, Olsson DS. Growth hormone deficiency and replacement therapy in adults: impact on survival. Rev Endocr Metab Disord. 2021;22: 125–33.
83. Yuen KCJ, Biller BMK, Radovick S, Carmichael JD, Jasim S, Pantalone KM, et al. American Association of Clinical Endocrinologists and American College of Endocrinology guidelines for management of growth hormone deficiency in adults and patients transitioning from pediatric to adult care. Endocr Pract. 2019;25: 1191–232.
84. Garcia JM, Biller BMK, Korbonits M, Popovic V, Luger A, Strasburger CJ, et al. Macimorelin as a diagnostic test for adult GH deficiency. J Clin Endocrinol Metab. 2018;103:3083–93.
85. Díez JJ, Sangiao-Alvarellos S, Cordido F. Treatment with growth hormone for adults with growth hormone deficiency syndrome: benefits and risks. Int J Mol Sci. 2018;19:893.
86. Boguszewski MCS, Boguszewski CL, Chemaitilly W, Cohen LE, Gebauer J, Higham C, et al. Safety of growth hormone replacement in survivors of cancer and intracranial and pituitary tumours: a consensus statement. Eur J Endocrinol. 2022;186:35–52.
87. Johannsson G, Ragnarsson O. Growth hormone deficiency in adults with hypopituitarism-what are the risks and can they be eliminated by therapy? J Intern Med. 2021;290:1180–93.
88. Yuen KCJ, Miller BS, Boguszewski CL, Hoffman AR. Usefulness and potential pitfalls of long-acting growth hormone analogs. Front Endocrinol (Lausanne). 2021;12:637209.

Obesity, Metabolic Syndrome, and Sleep Disorders

34

Daisy Duan and Jonathan C. Jun

Contents

D. Duan
Department of Medicine, Division of Endocrinology,
Diabetes and Metabolism, Johns Hopkins University
School of Medicine, Baltimore, MD, USA
e-mail: dduan5@jhmi.edu

J. C. Jun (✉)
Division of Pulmonary and Critical Care, Department of
Medicine, Johns Hopkins University School of Medicine,
Baltimore, MD, USA
e-mail: jjun2@jhmi.edu

Abstract

This chapter will focus on two sleep-related breathing disorders associated with metabolic syndrome, obstructive sleep apnea (OSA), and obesity hypoventilation syndrome (OHS). OSA is characterized by obstructive apneas, hypopneas, and/or respiratory effort-related arousals caused by repetitive collapse of the upper airways during sleep. OSA commonly coexists with metabolic syndrome. While obesity contributes towards the pathogenesis of OSA, some studies suggest that OSA is an independent risk factor for metabolic dysfunction. Intermittent

© Springer Nature Switzerland AG 2023
R. S. Ahima (ed.), *Metabolic Syndrome*,
https://doi.org/10.1007/978-3-031-40116-9_53

hypoxia and sleep fragmentation are hall-marks of OSA pathophysiology that could mediate the metabolic dysfunction seen in OSA. Effective weight loss improves but does not usually lead to complete resolution of OSA. The primary modality for OSA treatment is continuous positive airway pressure (CPAP), although CPAP is associated with modest weight gain. However, combining a lifestyle intervention for weight loss and CPAP can be synergistic and more impactful in improving OSA and metabolic outcomes. Studies on the impact of CPAP therapy on glycemic outcomes show conflicting results, which may be explained by differences in CPAP adherence, sex differences, and stages of diabetes. OHS describes the triad of obesity, hypercapnia not adequately explained by other causes, and sleep-disordered breathing. The majority of subjects with OHS have concomitant OSA. Obesity is necessary but not sufficient for the development of OHS. While OHS shares risk factors with OSA, it remains unknown why some patients develop OHS while others with a similar BMI or fat distribution do not. Treatment of OHS includes CPAP with non-invasive ventilation, supplemental oxygen to correct hypoxemia, and weight loss that is often challenging to achieve.

Keywords

Sleep apnea · Hypoventilation · Obesity · Metabolic syndrome · Diabetes

Introduction

Sleep-disordered breathing (SDB) is a common comorbidity associated with the metabolic syndrome. SDB includes several forms of respiratory dysfunction during sleep such as snoring, obstructive sleep apnea (OSA), central sleep apnea, and hypoventilation. This review will focus on two forms of SDB: OSA, and obesity hypoventilation syndrome (OHS), with an emphasis on their associations with obesity and metabolic syndrome and the impact of treatment of SDB on metabolic outcomes.

Overview of Obstructive Sleep Apnea

Definition and Epidemiology

Obstructive sleep apnea (OSA) is characterized by obstructive apneas, hypopneas, and/or respiratory effort-related arousals caused by repetitive collapse of the upper airways during sleep. OSA is the most common sleep-related breathing disorder. The severity of OSA is based on the apnea-hypopnea index (AHI), defined as the number of apneas (pauses in breathing lasting ≥ 10 s) plus hypopneas (episodes of shallow breathing lasting ≥ 10 s accompanied by a desaturation or sleep arousal) per hour of sleep. Mild OSA is defined by AHI 5–14.9 events/h of sleep, moderate OSA is defined by AHI 15–29.9 events/h of sleep, and severe OSA is defined by AHI ≥ 30 events/h. The estimated prevalence of OSA in the USA is 26.6% in men and 8.7% in women among individuals aged 30–49 years, and 43.2% in men and 27.8% in women among individuals aged 50 to 70 years [1]. Risk factors for OSA include older age, male sex, obesity, enlarged upper airway soft tissues, and craniofacial abnormalities [2]. There are racial and ethnic differences in the prevalence of OSA, with a higher prevalence of OSA (53.6%) among African Americans aged 50–80 years seen in the Jackson Heart Sleep Study [3]. Additionally, in the Multi-Ethnic Study of Atherosclerosis, the prevalence of moderate-to-severe OSA appears higher in adults aged 54–93 with Hispanic ethnicity (38.2%), participants of Chinese descent (39.4%), and African Americans (32.4%), compared to white individuals (30.3%) [4].

Symptoms and Diagnosis

The common symptoms of OSA are excessive sleepiness, fatigue, or unrefreshing sleep, present in 73–90% of patients. Witnessed breathing pauses, choking, or gasping are the most specific symptoms for OSA. Other common symptoms include snoring, nocturnal gastroesophageal reflux (GERD), nocturia, and morning headaches [2]. Diagnostic testing for OSA is recommended for any patient with unexplained excessive sleepiness, fatigue, or unrefreshing sleep. Testing should be considered in patients with unexplained nocturia, nocturnal GERD, morning headache, or frequent nocturnal awakenings, particularly in the setting of snoring, witnessed nocturnal apneas, or overweight body habitus. Historically, OSA is diagnosed by laboratory-based polysomnography, which monitors both sleep and respiratory parameters. Over the last 10 to 20 years, portable technologies have been developed that can monitor airflow, respiratory effort, and oxygen saturation in the home environment. Home sleep apnea testing (HSAT) has become a convenient and common method for OSA diagnosis with a relatively high sensitivity (79%) and specificity (79%) in patients with a high pretest probability of disease. However, HSATs may not be appropriate for complex medical patients with cardiopulmonary comorbidities. In addition, some patients with high suspicion for OSA and a negative HSAT warrant laboratory-based polysomnography since HSATs may not detect certain features of OSA such as sleep fragmentation [2].

Treatment

Behavioral interventions for OSA include weight loss, regular aerobic exercise, abstinence from alcohol, and avoiding supine sleep position. Weight loss via any modality (lifestyle intervention, bariatric surgery, or pharmacotherapy) is associated with improvement in OSA severity, in a dose-dependent manner [5–7]. Exercise may improve OSA via weight-independent effects in small randomized clinical trials of patients with moderate-to-severe OSA [8]. The primary therapy for symptomatic OSA is positive airway pressure (PAP), which can normalize AHI in >90% of patients while wearing the device [9]. However, the benefit of PAP therapy depends on adherence. Alternative treatment options include oral appliances (mandibular repositioning devices) for those with mild to moderate OSA, and surgical

procedures such as uvulopalatopharyngoplasty and hypoglossal nerve stimulation. There are currently no approved pharmacologic therapies for OSA, although some drugs are in development that target upper airway neuromuscular tone or that control of breathing [10].

OSA and Metabolic Syndrome

The prevalence of OSA in metabolic syndrome and vice versa is high. While obesity is a major contributor of this link, metabolic syndrome is nine times more likely to be present in OSA even after adjusting for BMI [11]. Intermittent hypoxia and sleep fragmentation are both hallmarks of OSA pathophysiology that could mediate the metabolic dysfunction seen in OSA via several proposed mechanisms, including increased activation of the sympathetic nervous system and hypoathalamic-pituitary-adrenal axis, and increased oxidative stress and inflammation [12]. While treatment of OSA with continuous positive airway pressure (CPAP) is associated with improvements in some parameters related to the proposed pathogenic pathways, CPAP therapy has not been definitively proven to improve metabolic syndrome components in patients with OSA.

Obstructive Sleep Apnea and Obesity

Contribution of Obesity to the Pathogenesis of Obstructive Sleep Apnea

The role of obesity in the pathogenesis of OSA is well established. Population studies in the USA, Europe, Asia, and Australia have demonstrated a graded increase in the prevalence of OSA with various measures of adiposity (i.e., BMI, neck circumference, waist-to-hip ratio) [13]. OSA is twice as common in individuals who are overweight and four times as common in individuals with obesity compared to individuals with normal weight [1]. Among individuals in the USA with BMI 30–39.9 kg/m^2, the prevalence of OSA is 44.6% in men and 13.5% in women

[1]. Longitudinal studies have found significant associations between changes in weight and changes in AHI. Peppard et al. found that a 10% increase in weight over 4 years predicted about 32% increase in AHI and a sixfold increase in the odds of developing moderate-to-severe OSA [14]. In the Sleep Heart Healthy Study with >2000 community-dwelling participants, the effect of weight loss on decreases in AHI was less pronounced compared to the effect of weight gain on increases in AHI. For example, men who gained at least 10 kg over 5 years had 5.21 times the odds of having a large (>15 events/h) increase in AHI while men who had lost at least 10 kg had 2.9-fold lower odds of a large (>15 events/h) decrease in AHI [15]. A reason for the inconsistent relationship of AHI and body weight may be that the AHI reflects the frequency of events, which is a function of respiratory *stability* whereas the changes in body weight affect airway *collapsibility*. The respiratory stability and airway collapsibility represent related as well as independent features of OSA pathogenesis.

Obesity promotes OSA because upper body fat can contribute to airway obstruction through structural changes in the tongue, neck, and lung size [16]. For example, the cross-sectional area of abdominal visceral fat obtained from CT images was highly correlated with AHI [17]. Similarly, patients with obesity and OSA had a significantly greater amount of abdominal visceral fat than patients with obesity but without OSA [18]. Thus, OSA often reflects increased visceral fat content which in turn is an independent risk factor for increased mortality [19]. On the other hand, body mass index (BMI) lacks quantification of fat distribution or function. Not surprisingly, BMI was not well correlated with AHI as compared with visceral adiposity [18].

Contribution of Obstructive Sleep Apnea to the Pathogenesis of Obesity

One possible explanation for the OSA-adiposity association is that OSA causes weight gain. OSA can result in insufficient and/or disrupted sleep, which may promote behavioral, metabolic, and hormonal changes that induce weight gain.

Insufficient sleep, often studied in sleep deprivation protocols in healthy adults without OSA, induces positive energy balance with resultant weight gain due to increased energy intake that far exceeds the additional energy expenditure of nocturnal wakefulness [20]. In adults with OSA, resting metabolic rate appears to be elevated compared to controls, but leptin resistance and high ghrelin levels seen in OSA could drive energy intake [21]. However, studies that measure food intake in OSA patients have not consistently demonstrated an increase in caloric intake. One study that examined OSA patients enrolled in a randomized controlled study of CPAP vs sham found no changes in diet behavior (measured by food frequency questionnaire) after 4 months of treatment [22]. A study of patients in middle to late childhood with obesity and OSA found that AHI was significantly associated with total calories consumed at dinner and more severe OSA was associated with an increased preference for calorie-dense foods that are high in fat and carbohydrates [23]. Furthermore, in the Swedish Obese Subjects Cohort, participants with high likelihood of OSA (self-reported loud snoring and observed breathing pauses) reported higher energy intake than weight-matched controls without OSA symptoms [24]. Additionally, OSA has been found to reduce physical activity, which may be the result of increased sleepiness, and could contribute to obesity [21]. However, treatment of OSA with CPAP does not consistently show improvement in physical activity [22, 25]. Hence, there are limited data showing that OSA actually causes obesity.

Impact of Weight Loss on Obstructive Sleep Apnea

Effective weight loss with any modality is known to improve but rarely cures OSA. A meta-analysis of 15 studies in patients who underwent bariatric surgery found a pooled mean reduction of AHI from 39 to 12.5 events/h with a mean reduction in BMI by 13.2 kg/m^2 and weight loss of 35.4 kg [26]. However, 70–90% of patients continued to have residual OSA following both behavioral and surgical weight loss approaches [27]. Currently, there are only a few studies examining the effects of US FDA-approved weight loss medications on OSA outcomes. A randomized, double-blind, placebo-controlled trial in 45 patients with obesity and moderate-to-severe OSA who could not tolerate PAP and without cardiac disease found that treatment with phentermine/topiramate extended-release in addition to lifestyle counseling achieved greater weight loss(-6.5 kg) and improvement in AHI by 15 events/h compared to lifestyle counseling alone after 28 weeks [28]. Liraglutide 3.0 mg dose has also been studied in a randomized, double-blinded study in 359 patients with obesity and moderate-or-severe OSA but without diabetes and found to induce 4.2% more weight loss and reduction in AHI by 6.1 events/h than placebo after 32 weeks [7]. In both studies, the improvement in AHI was thought to be related to the degree of weight loss. More recently, long-acting incretin therapies with semaglutide (GLP-1 receptor agonist) and tirzepatide (GLP-1/GIP dual receptor agonist) have achieved a mean weight loss of 15–20% in patients with obesity without diabetes [29, 30]. There is currently an ongoing trial evaluating the efficacy of tirzepatide for the treatment of OSA (SURMOUNT-OSA; NCT05412004). In particular, as GLP-1 receptor agonists have been shown to have cardiometabolic benefits in patients with type 2 diabetes, it would be interesting to evaluate cardiometabolic benefits of these medications in patients with OSA.

Impact of CPAP on Body Weight

Studies have consistently demonstrated that treatment of OSA with CPAP is associated with modest but significant weight gain. A meta-analysis of >3000 patients from 25 randomized controlled trials reported that CPAP use significantly increased body weight by 0.42 kg on average, compared to control conditions without CPAP use [31]. The proposed mechanism for weight gain with CPAP therapy is a decrease in energy expenditure. In adults with OSA, resting metabolic rate is elevated compared to controls, likely related to increased sympathetic nerve activity or increased work of breathing during the sleep

period [21]. CPAP is associated with a small reduction in energy expenditure, effectively normalizing the modestly elevated basal metabolic rate seen in untreated OSA [32–34]. Tachikawa et al. found that in patients with newly diagnosed OSA, CPAP therapy reduced the basal metabolic rate by about 5% (75 kcal/day) from baseline, and the reduction in basal metabolic rate was associated with reduced sympathetic nerve activity (measured by reduced urine norepinephrine) [34]. Furthermore, the basal metabolic rate decreased more in those with higher CPAP adherence. In this study, the patients who gained weight had greater food intake despite similar reductions in metabolic rate, and unchanged physical activity compared to patients without weight gain, suggesting a contribution of increased energy intake rather than expenditure. On the other hand, long-term data showed that CPAP use in patients with moderate-to-severe OSA after an average of 3.8 years did not cause weight change [35]. These results suggest that weight gain may not be cumulative or related to acute effects of CPAP. One hypothesis is that weight gain may be the result of fluid accumulation with positive pressure ventilation or reversal of OSA-associated nocturia [36]. In support of this hypothesis, 24 highly CPAP-adherent patients were studied during CPAP or after 1 week of CPAP withdrawal using a randomized crossover design. CPAP treatment caused higher weight gain by 0.37 kg, and a trend towards higher extracellular body water and lower 24-h urine volume [37].

Despite the modest weight gain associated with CPAP, studies show that CPAP does not hinder weight loss efficacy in the context of intensive lifestyle modification. In a retrospective study of patients with obesity who started an intensive weight management program, those who had OSA achieved similar weight loss at 12 months as those without OSA, regardless of CPAP use [38]. In fact, the addition of lifestyle or behavioral intervention for weight loss to CPAP therapy can be synergistic for improving AHI and metabolic outcomes. In patients with severe OSA and obesity undergoing CPAP treatment for OSA, a randomized control trial involving a 48-week intensive weight loss program resulted in about 8 kg weight loss vs 0.1 kg in the control group at 12 months, and a greater reduction in AHI at 3 months despite similar CPAP adherence [39]. At 12 months, although the AHI reduction was no longer significantly different between the groups, intensive weight loss resulted in significant reductions in C-reactive protein (CRP) and glycated hemoglobin (HbA1c), and an increase in HDL cholesterol. A parallel-arm, open-label, randomized clinical trial in 89 men with CPAP-treated moderate-to-severe OSA and overweight/obesity were randomized to usual care or an 8-week lifestyle intervention. The lifestyle intervention group had a greater decrease in AHI than the control group (mean between-group difference of 23.8 events/h), along with greater reduction in body weight (mean between-group difference of −5.7 kg) at 6 months [40]. There were also significant differences in systolic and blood pressure reductions, improvement in insulin resistance, and improvement in lipid profile with lower LDL cholesterol and triglycerides in the lifestyle intervention group compared to usual care. One limitation is that the study did not report CPAP adherence data and did not specify CPAP adherence rates as an inclusion criteria in order to increase the generalizability of results. Thus, it is unknown if there were differences in CPAP adherence during the study. A randomized controlled trial in patients with overweight and moderate-to-severe OSA who received CPAP only vs CPAP plus a behavioral sleep medicine intervention targeting physical activity and eating behavior found that 6 months of CPAP therapy plus behavioral intervention resulted in more a pronounced improvement in OSA, with a reduction in AHI by 9.9 events/h vs 1.9 events/h in the CPAP-only group, which was not explained by CPAP adherence in a multivariate regression analysis [41]. Notably, there were no metabolic or weight outcomes reported in this study. Overall, the CPAP therapy combined with behavioral weight loss may be more effective in improving sleep and breathing parameters along with metabolic outcomes.

Obstructive Sleep Apnea and Insulin Resistance

Contribution of Obstructive Sleep Apnea to the Pathogenesis of Insulin Resistance

Studies in patients without preexisting type 2 diabetes have shown that OSA is associated with insulin resistance independent of obesity. A study in 270 participants without diabetes and with OSA found that AHI was an independent determinant of insulin resistance such that each additional apnea or hypopnea per sleep hour increased fasting insulin level and homeostatic model assessment for insulin resistance (HOMA-IR) by 0.5% [42]. In the Sleep Heart Health Study, participants with mild SDB and moderate-to-severe SDB had an adjusted odds ratio of 1.27 and 1.46, respectively, for fasting glucose intolerance [43]. In the Multi-Ethnic Study of Atherosclerosis, moderate-to-severe OSA was significantly associated with abnormal fasting glucose in African Americans (odds ratio 2.14) and white participants (odds ratio 2.85), but not among Chinese or Hispanic participants, after adjusting for site, age, sex, waist circumference, and sleep duration [44]. A hyperinsulinemic-euglycemic clamp study revealed that in patients with obesity and OSA, there was an increase in insulin resistance and adipose tissue lipolysis, and reduced glucose uptake into adipose tissue and skeletal muscle compared to patients with obesity but without OSA [45].

Longitudinal studies demonstrate an increased risk for incident diabetes in patients with moderate-to-severe OSA. One study found a 4.4-fold risk of developing type 2 diabetes after 11 years of follow-up after adjusting for BMI and interval weight gain [46]. A meta-analysis reported a 63% increased risk for developing diabetes in OSA patients [47]. Once patients develop type 2 diabetes, the prevalence of OSA ranges 58–86% depending on presence of obesity and age [48, 49]. In patients with type 2 diabetes, increasing OSA severity is associated with higher HbA1c levels independent of BMI, age, sex, and diabetes-related factors [50].

Proposed Mechanisms Linking OSA and Metabolic Dysfunction

Intermittent hypoxia and sleep fragmentation are both hallmarks of OSA pathophysiology that could mediate the metabolic dysfunction seen in OSA. Intermittent hypoxia (IH) describes the cyclical pattern of hypoxia and reoxygenation during sleep. Animal models of IH have shown that IH could induce hyperglycemia through increased insulin resistance [51–53], increased adipose tissue inflammation [54], and increased pancreatic β-cell apoptosis in a polygenic rodent model of type 2 diabetes [55]. Cross-sectional and intervention studies support the association between IH and hyperglycemia. In the Sleep Heart Health Study, sleep-related hypoxemia was associated with glucose intolerance that was independent of age, BMI, and waist circumference [43]. A cross-sectional study of patients with uncontrolled type 2 diabetes found that patients with intermittent hypoxia (defined by 4% oxyhemoglobin desaturation index ≥15) had higher HbA1c than those without intermittent hypoxia after adjusting for obesity, age at onset and duration of diabetes, insulin requirement, sleep quality, and depressed mood [56]. A randomized crossover study of 13 healthy volunteers exposed to 5 h of intermittent hypoxia or normoxia during wakefulness found decreased insulin sensitivity (measured by intravenous glucose tolerance test) after IH, related to increased sympathetic nervous system (SNS) activity [57]. Sleep fragmentation is another hallmark of OSA, referring to the interruption of sleep by frequent, brief arousals that follow obstructive respiratory events. One clinical study demonstrated that sleep fragmentation using auditory stimuli induced aberrant glucose homeostasis in healthy volunteers [58, 59].

Proposed mechanisms for how IH or sleep fragmentation may lead to insulin resistance include (i) increased sympathetic activity; (ii) altered activity of the hypothalamic-pituitary-adrenal (HPA) axis; (iii) increased oxidative stress with increased formation of reactive oxygen species; and (iv) increased inflammation [12].

Patients with OSA have increased SNS activity during both sleep and wakefulness, which

decreases with CPAP therapy [34, 60]. IH stimulates chemoreflexes in the carotid body which then can activate the SNS [61]. In fact, carotid body denervation in mice prevented IH-stimulated hepatic glucose output and liver expression of phosphoenolpyruvate carboxykinase, a rate-limiting hepatic enzyme of gluconeogenesis [62]. Additionally, OSA can cause arousals from sleep and hypercapnia, which may synergistically enhance SNS activity [63]. In animal studies, alpha-adrenergic blockade (phentolamine) or adrenal medullectomy abolished IH-induced glucose intolerance [53]. Acute hypoxia-induced insulin resistance was attenuated by sympathetic inhibition with clonidine in healthy men [64]. Lastly, patients with OSA have elevated plasma free fatty acid levels, which may be mediated by SNS-induced lipolysis [65, 66]. During CPAP withdrawal, nocturnal glucose increased dynamically with heart rate elevation, suggesting autonomic influence [67].

Increased stress response with overactivation of the HPA axis has also been observed in patients with OSA. Several studies have demonstrated elevated cortisol levels in patients with OSA compared to controls, and a reduction in cortisol levels with CPAP therapy [68–71]. Elevated cortisol levels are also seen during acute CPAP withdrawal [67]. Excess cortisol is known to impair insulin secretion and insulin action resulting in hyperglycemia, which could contribute to impaired glucose homeostasis observed in OSA.

Studies have demonstrated that patients with OSA exhibit elevated markers of oxidative stress such as lipid peroxidation, isoprostane concentrations, and markers of DNA oxidation. IH is postulated to promote the formation of reactive oxygen species (ROS) and induce oxidative stress in a pattern similarly seen in ischemia-reperfusion injury [72]. Consequently, increased oxidative stress is implicated in the pathogenesis of insulin resistance and pancreactic β-cell dysfunction [73]. Several clinical studies have demonstrated reduction in markers of oxidative stress in patients with OSA after CPAP treatment [74–76]. Furthermore, small clinical studies of antioxidant treatments in patients with OSA, such as vitamin C, allopurinol, and N-acetylcysteine, have found improvement in oxidative stress markers, improved endothelial function (measured by flow-mediated dilation of the brachial artery), and even improvement in OSA parameters [12]. However, the specific role in oxidative stress in mediating metabolic dysfunction in OSA remains unclear.

In vitro and in vivo models have demonstrated that IH activates transcription factor nuclear factor-kappa B (NF-κB), a key player in inflammatory and innate immune responses. NF-κB are upregulated in patients with OSA when compared to matched controls, and are reduced by CPAP treatment [77]. Similarly, tumor necrosis factor α (TNF-α), an inflammatory cytokine activated by NF-κB, is also elevated in patients with OSA compared to matched controls and were lowered by CPAP therapy. Notably, IH (as defined by oxygen desaturation index) was the strongest predictor of TNF-α levels [78]. One study in mice found that IH exposure induced insulin resistance and proinflammatory M1 macrophage polarization in visceral adipose tissue. The authors of this study also showed that, in a clinical cohort of 186 patients, OSA severity was significantly associated with M1 macrophage inflammatory marker sCD163 independent of anthropometric and demographic factors [54].

Impact of CPAP on Glycemic Outcomes

Studies on the impact of CPAP therapy on glycemic outcomes show conflicting results. Important considerations for interpreting the studies include variability in CPAP adherence, duration of follow-up, and glycemic status of the study population. In general, short-term, in-laboratory studies where CPAP adherence was directly observed tended to reveal a beneficial effect of CPAP on glycemic outcomes. Conversely, longer-term, outpatient clinical trials may have null effects but often with low rate of CPAP adherence. Additionally, sex differences in OSA and metabolic outcomes are increasingly recognized although most clinical studies recruited predominantly male patients, given the higher prevalence of OSA in men. Moreover, the optimal timing of CPAP treatment in the disease progression of type 2 diabetes is

unknown but studies generally support improvement in blood glucose with CPAP therapy in patients with prediabetes rather than type 2 diabetes.

CPAP may improve glucose tolerance and diabetes risk in OSA patients without preexisting diabetes. A retrospective cohort study from Hong Kong found that untreated moderate-to-severe OSA patients had a higher risk of developing diabetes with a hazard ratio of 2.01 and 2.62, respectively, within a median follow-up of 7.3 years, which was reduced with regular CPAP use [79]. A meta-analysis of nine randomized controlled trials in patients with OSA but without diabetes found that CPAP therapy improved insulin resistance but without changes in fasting glucose [80]. A randomized controlled trial of 80 patients with severe obesity and severe OSA without diabetes who were randomized to CPAP vs conservative treatment for 12 weeks found that CPAP group had more improvement in 2-h plasma glucose during an oral glucose tolerance test without between-group differences in weight loss [81]. However, in a landmark trial where 146 patients with obesity and OSA were randomized to (1) weight loss, (2) CPAP only, or (3) weight loss + CPAP, 6-months follow-up results revealed more reductions in CRP levels, insulin resistance, and serum triglyceride levels in the weight loss only and weight loss plus CPAP groups compared to the CPAP group [82]. This result suggests that the effect of CPAP treatment on metabolic outcomes is likely less than that of weight loss.

Laboratory studies in which CPAP adherence was ensured found beneficial effects of CPAP on glycemic outcomes in patients with prediabetes and diabetes. Mokhlesi et al. found that 1 week of effective in-laboratory CPAP therapy reduced the 24-h mean glucose level by 13.5 mg/dL without changes in insulin levels in 12 patients with type 2 diabetes and OSA [83]. Specifically, CPAP reduced the "dawn phenomenon" triggered by nocturnal hypoglycemia and reduced the fasting glucose level. Similarly, in patients with OSA and prediabetes randomly assigned to 8-h nightly CPAP vs placebo, 2 weeks of directly observed OSA adherence reduced the area under the curve for glucose during a 2-h oral glucose tolerance test, improved insulin sensitivity, and reduced norepinephrine levels and 24-h blood pressure [84]. Conversely, acute CPAP withdrawal in 31 patients with moderate-to-severe OSA who were habitual CPAP users induced nocturnal hyperglycemia, especially in patients with type 2 diabetes [67].

A recent meta-analysis of seven randomized controlled trials of CPAP vs sham in patients with type 2 diabetes and OSA found that CPAP significantly improved HbA1c, fasting glucose, HOMA-IR, systolic and diastolic blood pressure [85]. Interestingly, a post-hoc analysis of one study revealed that patients on oral hypoglycemic medications only, but not insulin therapy, had improvement in glycemic control [86]. This suggests that CPAP may have limited benefit in those with more advanced diabetes. A recent randomized controlled trial of 100 patients with metabolic syndrome and moderate-or-severe OSA randomized to CPAP or nasal dilator strips for 6 months found that the rate of metabolic syndrome reversibility was higher after CPAP (18% in CPAP group vs 4% in control). Individual metabolic syndrome components that were significantly improved include a significant reduction in waist circumferences by 1.2 cm, systolic blood pressure by 7.5 mmHg, and diastolic blood pressure by 5 mmHg. Notably, there was no changes in fasting glucose levels. Non-metabolic syndrome components that improved included a change in total cholesterol by −9.0 mg/dL, non-HDL cholesterol by −7.5 mg/dL, and VLDL cholesterol by −3.0 mg/dL. However, most patients retained their metabolic syndrome diagnosis despite improvement in sleep parameters [87]. Notably, there was no significant weight loss in either treatment arm and as demonstrated by another trial [82], CPAP therapy likely needs to be combined with a weight loss intervention to induce clinically meaningful metabolic benefits.

Several randomized controlled trials in patients with type 2 diabetes and OSA did not show any differences in glycemic outcomes after CPAP [88–90]. In one study, there was a trend towards better glycemic indices in the subgroup with high CPAP adherence [88]. However, in another study, there were no between-group differences in HbA1c, even in analyses stratified by baseline glycemic control, sleep apnea severity, or CPAP adherence [89]. A substudy of the Sleep Apnea and cardiovascular Endpoints (SAVE) study of ~900 patients with preexisting diabetes, prediabetes, or new diagnoses of diabetes found no difference in serum glucose or HbA1c when randomized to CPAP vs usual care after a median follow-up of 4.3 years [90]. Furthermore, CPAP adherence showed no relationship with glycemic outcomes. However, the authors found a sex and CPAP interaction such that women with diabetes had worsening glycemic control (measured by glucose only, not HbA1c) in the usual care group while women in the CPAP group had stable glycemic status. Another open-label randomized control trial of 3 months of PAP therapy + lifestyle counseling vs lifestyle counseling alone in 184 adults with type 2 diabetes and newly diagnosed moderate-to-severe OSA found that CPAP therapy did not have an effect on glucose variability (measured by continuous glucose monitor [CGM]-derived standard deviation of glucose values), mean glucose, or HbA1c [91]. Adherence was quite high at 77%. In women (49% of the cohort), CPAP reduced glycemic variability compared to control, with a mean difference of 3.5 mg/dL in within-person standard deviation of interstitial glucose. CPAP also reduced mean glucose by 0.5 mg/dL in women, while the control condition caused an increase in mean glucose by 14 mg/dL in women after 3 months. Lastly, a study with the longest follow-up period found that 47 patients with type 2 diabetes and OSA using CPAP (58% adherence rate) had stable HbA1c and fasting plasma glucose levels at 56 weeks [92]. Notably, the study was non-randomized and the participants had more advanced type 2 diabetes as shown by higher baseline HbA1c, and nearly a third of participants were on insulin therapy. Taken together, CPAP therapy may have a modest and heterogeneous impact on glycemic outcomes, with more significant effects in women and in patients in the early stages of type 2 diabetes or prediabetes.

Obesity Hypoventilation Syndrome

Definition and Diagnosis

The Posthumous Papers of the Pickwick Club published in 1837 by Charles Dickens contained a character named Joe "The Fat Boy," described as severely obese, voraciously hungry, and prone to fall asleep with loud snoring while running errands. Burwell later published a case report of a patient who resembled this character who sought medical treatment for falling asleep during Poker [93]. This case report popularized the term "Pickwickian syndrome," which is now referred to as *obesity hypoventilation syndrome* (OHS). Currently, OHS is defined as obesity (BMI ≥ 30 kg/m^2) and arterial hypercapnia (partial pressure of carbon dioxide [PaCO$_2$] >45 mmHg) not adequately explained by causes such as pulmonary dysfunction, airway disorders, or neuromuscular disease. The majority of subjects with OHS have concomitant OSA, while about 10% have sleep-related hypoventilation without upper airway obstruction [94]. Thus, OHS is a triad of obesity, hypercapnia, and sleep-disordered breathing. The sleep-disordered breathing could take the form of OSA or sleep-induced hypoventilation (in adults, defined as PaCO$_2$ level >55 mmHg for ≥ 10 min, PaCO$_2$ increase by ≥ 10 mmHg compared to awake supine level up to a level of >50 mmHg for ≥ 10 min [95]).

A formal diagnosis of OHS requires an arterial blood gas (ABG) showing an elevated partial pressure of carbon dioxide. However, blood gases are not commonly performed in ambulatory settings. Therefore, surrogates of PaCO$_2$ are often used in clinical practice to suggest the diagnosis. Increased serum bicarbonate, reflecting metabolic compensation for hypercapnia, can serve as a relatively sensitive marker of hypoventilation. In an American Thoracic Society guideline [96], several studies [97–99] were pooled to assess diagnostic accuracy of elevated bicarbonate (>27 mmol/L) for OHS, yielding a sensitivity of 0.86 and specificity of 0.77. The guideline further applied this threshold to hypothetical cohorts differing in OHS prevalence, based on the degree of obesity. Bicarbonate would be expected to have the highest negative predictive value in low pre-test probability settings (e.g., BMI 30–35 kg/m^2) and the highest positive predictive value in populations with an expected prevalence of $>20\%$ OHS, such as among those with BMI >40 kg/m^2.

The majority of patients with OHS have OSA; the more severe the OSA, the higher the likelihood of daytime hypercapnia. For example, 79 of 522 patients referred to a sleep clinic were found to have OSA and elevated bicarbonate level (>27 mmol/L). Within this subset, 76% of patients with an AHI ≥ 100 events/h had hypercapnia, whereas 36% with an AHI <100 events/h had hypercapnia. Patients with OHS may also have low arterial oxygen saturation, due to shunt (low functional residual capacity) as well as alveolar hypoventilation. In a 2009 meta-analysis of 15 studies that examined determinants of hypercapnia among patients with obesity and OSA, the authors reported that the overnight average oxygen saturation was ~5% lower (85.5 vs 90.3%) in hypercapnic patients. The percentage of sleep time spent with oxygen saturation (SpO$_2$) $<90\%$ was also 56% in hypercapnic patients, but 19% in those without hypercapnia [100]. Supine positioning, especially in obese patients, causes a fall in functional residual capacity and can elicit modest decreases in oxygen saturation even while awake. Chung et al. leveraged this physiology to examine supine SpO$_2$ as a marker of OHS [101]. Among patients with a BMI of >50 kg/m^2, supine oxygen saturation prior to sleep (during the first 90s of data collection) was used to predict the presence of daytime hypercapnia. SpO$_2$ $<91.2\%$ had 34.8% sensitivity and 96.6% specificity while a cutoff of SpO$_2$ $<96.7\%$ had 87.0% sensitivity and 20.7% specificity for daytime hypercapnia.

Prevalence and Risk Factors

OHS is estimated to affect 10–20% of patients with OSA, 0.6% of the general population [102] and a large proportion of bariatric surgery referrals [103]. The prevalence increases with the degree of obesity as well as severity of concomitant OSA. With dramatic increases in the rates of worldwide obesity [104], the prevalence of OHS is likely to increase. Among hospitalized adults with severe obesity (BMI >35 kg/m^2), the prevalence of OHS can be as high as 31% [105]. Other than obesity, risk factors for OHS are unclear. Some studies suggest a higher risk of OHS in post-menopausal women than in men [106]. Since hypercapnia can occur in several other conditions, Bulbul et al. examined predictors of OHS among patients admitted to the hospital who underwent ABG [107]. In multivariate logistic regression of the patients with chronic hypoventilation by ABG (n = 118), BMI >35 kg/m^2, arterial oxygen saturation <91.4% and ratio of PaCO$_2$/BMI <1.5 were significantly related to OHS. The PaCO$_2$/BMI <1.5 ratio criterion suggests that OHS is characterized by less pronounced hypercapnia with morbid obesity, while other conditions (e.g. COPD) typically involve marked hypercapnia and thinner body habitus. In a retrospective analysis of 577 patients presenting to a bariatric surgery center in China, the authors investigated variables associated with OHS, which was present in 17.9% [108]. They identified BMI, neck circumference, type 2 diabetes, serum bicarbonate, and CRP levels as independent risk factors for OHS and incorporated these 5 variables into a normogram with a robust C-index of 0.830. This model indicates that diabetes and inflammation are associated with OHS, but whether these factors are causes, consequences, or parallel comorbidities with OHS is unclear.

Clinical Manifestations

Since the majority of patients with OHS have concomitant OSA, clinical manifestations are similar including snoring, daytime sleepiness, hypertension, and nocturnal episodes of choking or gasping. However, many patients with OHS present in acute hypercapnic respiratory failure [109]. When matched with obese controls, patients with OHS had twofold rates of hospitalization, 2.5-fold health care costs, and fivefold risks of hospitalization [110]. OHS patients matched to OSA patients of similar age, sex, and duration of PAP usage had a twofold increase in

the risk of mortality and double the risk of cardiovascular events [111]. Marik et al. reported that 8% of their critical care unit admissions met criteria for OHS, of which 18% died in hospital [112]. At another academic medical center, mortality of OHS patients at 3 years post-discharge was 31% [113].

Chronically reduced oxygen levels in OHS also places patients at risk for pulmonary hypertension, with a prevalence of about 50%, when pulmonary hypertension was defined as echocardiographic evidence of pulmonary artery systolic pressure ≥40 mmHg. Masa et al. examined factors associated with pulmonary hypertension in patients with untreated OHS enrolled in the Pickwick trial (described below) with echocardiographic data [114]. In a multivariable model, they found that partial pressure of oxygen (PaO$_2$) (OR = 0.96) and high BMI (OR = 1.07) were independently associated pulmonary hypertension risk. These findings suggest that obesity per se (even when adjusting for oxygen level) could promote pulmonary hypertension through mechanisms such as increased cardiac output, higher pulmonary vascular resistance (due to reduced lung volume), and perivascular fat accumulation (leading to mechanical resistance and to secretion of inflammatory mediators and vasoactive peptides such as endothelin-1) [115].

Treatment

Mainstays of OHS treatment are positive airway pressure during sleep, correction of hypoxemia, and weight loss. Less well studied therapies related to OHS pathogenesis will be described in section "Pathophysiology."

Positive airway pressure (PAP): CPAP provides a pneumatic splint to maintain the airway during sleep, and effectively treats OSA as well as many cases of OHS [96]. Non-invasive ventilation (NIV) refers to devices that enhance breathing often by providing inspiratory pressure alternating with positive end-expiratory pressure (PEEP). Theoretically, NIV augments tidal volume and may be more effective in reversing OHS-associated hypercapnia. NIV stabilizes breathing in OHS during acute respiratory failure [116] and improve mortality after hospital discharge [117]. On the other hand, CPAP may offer similar benefits as NIV in longitudinal outpatient settings. Piper et al randomized patients with OHS to 3 months of CPAP or NIV and reported about 7 mmHg reductions in $PaCO_2$ regardless of PAP modality [118]. The Spanish multi-center "Pickwick study" compared efficacy of NIV, CPAP, and lifestyle modification for patients with stable OHS including subgroups with or without severe OSA [119, 120]. In the combined OHS + OSA subgroup (n = 221), NIV and CPAP were equivalent and both were superior to lifestyle in terms of gas exchange and functional outcomes at 2 months [119] as well as after 3 years [121]. In the OHS subgroup without severe OSA (AHI <30 events/h), the authors compared NIV versus lifestyle modification [122]. NIV improved gas exchange compared to lifestyle modification but did not alter rates of hospitalization. On the other hand, PAP may not fully correct hypoventilation and hypoxemia in part due to non-obstructive physiology [123] and due to suboptimal PAP adherence [118, 124, 125]. A recent observational study (n = 143) examined factors associated with persistent hypercapnia in OHS patients treated with NIV for a mean of 4.6 years of follow up [126]. About half of the patients in this cohort exhibited $PaCO_2$ >45 mmHg. In multivariable regression, the authors reported that higher baseline $PaCO_2$ (OR = 1.05), lung capacity (OR = 0.96), female sex (male OR = 0.25), and lower BMI (OR = 0.92) were independent predictors of persistent hypercapnia. The surprising finding that BMI was "protective" illustrates that other factors that more directly affect lung mechanics are important for OHS pathogenesis. Thus, CPAP and/or NIV mitigates upper airway contributions to hypoventilation, but does not consistently address other causes of hypoventilation. In retrospective studies, PAP-related reduction in $PaCO_2$ is associated with improved survival in the 10 years following initiation of therapy. Higher mortality was related to reduced baseline PaO_2, or elevated CRP, pH, or leukocytes [127].

Supplemental oxygen: Many patients with OHS require supplemental oxygen, with similar prescription criteria as that of other chronic pulmonary diseases such as COPD. While it is reasonable to correct hypoxemia to address chronic right heart failure, the actual effects of oxygen on long-term OHS outcomes is unknown. In some short-term studies, supplemental O_2 further increased CO_2 [128, 129]. In a post-hoc analysis of patients enrolled in the Pickwick study, investigators compared outcomes among patients who were on supplemental oxygen versus no oxygen treatment (irrespective of assignment to NIV, CPAP, or lifestyle groups) 2 months post-enrollment [130]. They found no differences in functional status, symptoms, or hospital resource utilization, but indirect markers of worsening hypoventilation during sleep such as trends towards morning confusion and headache with oxygen use.

Weight loss: In the previously mentioned "Pickwick Study," subjects in the lifestyle modification group were encouraged to consume <1000 calories per day but only lost <2 kg during the 2-month trial. Mandal et al randomized newly diagnosed OHS patients to either (A) a 3-month nutrition and exercise rehabilitation ("NERO") program with initiation of NIV, or (B) NIV-only, and examined weight loss after 12 months [131]. The NERO intervention facilitated weight loss at 3 months(−3 kg in control, −10 kg in NERO), but provided no additional CO_2-lowering effect beyond that of NIV. In a bariatric cohort [132], Sugerman et al followed 38 patients with OHS for 6 years post-surgery [132]. Patients lost 30% body weight (163 to 115 kg), PaO_2 increased from 54 to 68 mmHg, and $PaCO_2$ decreased from 53 to 47 mmHg [96]. In a meta-analysis of weight loss surgeries, BMI decreased from 55 to 38 kg/m^2 but 62% had residual sleep apnea (AHI >15 events/h) [27]. After 10 years of follow up, most patients with OSA or OHS who underwent laparoscopic banding still required NIV [133]. Thus, weight loss of sufficient magnitude to reverse OHS is difficult to achieve.

Pathophysiology

Obesity is necessary but not sufficient for the development of OHS, as evidenced by a lack of a linear increase in serum bicarbonate levels with BMI in a large health system database [134]. Clues to additional pathogenic factors have been gleaned from studies comparing eucapnic to hypercapnic patients with obesity. Generally, those with hypercapnia have higher BMI and/or body surface area, more severe OSA, and lower lung volumes [100]. Excessive accumulation of adipose tissue restricts the thoracic cage and increases work of breathing [135]. On pulmonary function testing, patients with severe obesity may exhibit reduced lung volumes including the total lung capacity, functional residual capacity (the air remaining in the lungs after a normal exhalation). Overall minute ventilation (VE) is equivalent in those with hypercapnia, but inappropriately so; VE is low after adjustment for body mass [136] suggesting a mismatch between respiratory output and ventilatory requirements. In a recent study, patients with OHS patients with BMI 30–40 kg/m^2 had their respiratory muscle endurance tested against patients with OHS and BMI >40 kg/m^2, as well as patient controls with BMI 30–40 kg/m^2 and low likelihood of OSA/OHS (by STOP-BANG screen). Respiratory muscle endurance was tested with an incremental loading test involving inhaling maximally through a resistance system. Those with OHS (in both weight categories) had reduced respiratory muscle endurance compared to controls. Interestingly, those using chronic PAP had higher endurance, suggesting that NIV may relieve work of breathing during sleep [137].

The leading theory of OHS contends that OSA is the "first hit" on the pathway to OHS. Some people have longer apneas and brief inter-apnea respiratory arousals [138] and do not appropriately compensate for this ventilatory load. This leads to CO_2 retention during sleep, which persists during waking hours, perhaps via bicarbonate retention [139]. According to the European Respiratory Society Task Force, patients with obesity and OSA are considered to be at risk ("Stage 0") for OHS [140]. "Stage I" patients develop sleep-related hypoventilation but normalize ventilation upon awakening and have normal bicarbonate levels. As hypoventilation progresses, serum bicarbonate levels increase ("Stage II" OHS), foreshadowing the development of sustained hypercapnia ("Stage III" OHS). When accompanied by cardio-metabolic comorbidities, "Stage IV" OHS is established [139].

While the sequence above is logical, it remains a mystery why some patients develop OHS while others with a similar BMI or fat distribution do not [141]. Leptin, an anorexigenic hormone secreted from adipose tissue, was discovered in 1994 [142] and may be involved in OHS pathogenesis. Leptin suppresses appetite while stimulating energy expenditure through targets in the hypothalamus. Leptin levels are elevated in common forms of obesity, indicative of leptin resistance [143]. Leptin resistance may result from impairment of transport across the blood-brain barrier (BBB) or leptin receptor signaling defects. Some studies support saturation of BBB transport capacity at low levels of circulating leptin [144], and low ratios of cerebrospinal fluid:serum leptin in humans with obesity, supporting the BBB transport hypothesis [145]. On the other hand, other studies contradict the BBB as the main culprit in leptin resistance [146, 147].

Whichever the underlying mechanisms of leptin resistance, the absence of leptin signaling in the hypothalamus has respiratory consequences. *ob/ob* mice lacking leptin and *db/db* mice with leptin receptor defect are not only hyperphagic and obese [148], but they also have elevated $PaCO_2$. The metabolic and respiratory defects in *ob/ob* mice are corrected by leptin infusion [149]. In addition, diet-induced obese mice exhibit high circulating leptin levels (leptin resistance), flow-limited breathing during sleep, and hypercapnia [150], which are improved after administration of intranasal (but not intravenous) leptin [151]. The precise neural targets of leptin leading to changes in ventilation are still under investigation [152].

Conclusion

OSA and OHS are manifestations of sleep-disordered breathing and commonly occur with obesity and metabolic syndrome. There is likely a bidirectional relationship between OSA and metabolic dysfunction. Intermittent hypoxia and sleep fragmentation have been investigated to mediate metabolic dysfunction seen in OSA via several proposed mechanisms. Effective weight loss can significantly improve OSA but may be difficult to achieve and sustain. Conversely, treatment of OSA with CPAP can result in modest weight gain. Furthermore, benefits of CPAP on glycemic outcomes are not consistently shown but may be present in select patient populations such as those with prediabetes or early stages of type 2 diabetes. Limited studies suggest a possible sex difference with more metabolic benefits of CPAP in women but this warrants further investigation. Studies on the cardiovascular effects of incretin-based pharmacotherapy are needed in patients are at high risk for cardiometabolic diseases. Future research is needed to better understand the mechanisms connecting OSA, OHS, and metabolic syndrome, and potential targets for the development of specific and effective therapies for this complex interplay of disorders.

References

1. Peppard PE, Young T, Barnet JH, Palta M, Hagen EW, Hla KM. Increased prevalence of sleep-disordered breathing in adults. Am J Epidemiol. 2013;177(9):1006–14.
2. Gottlieb DJ, Punjabi NM. Diagnosis and management of obstructive sleep apnea: a review. JAMA. 2020;323(14):1389–400.
3. Johnson DA, Guo N, Rueschman M, Wang R, Wilson JG, Redline S. Prevalence of correlates of obstructive sleep apnea among African Americans: the Jackson Heart Sleep Study. Sleep. 2018;41:zsy154.
4. Chen X, Wang R, Zee P, Lutsey PL, Javaheri S, Alcántara C, et al. Racial/ethnic differences in sleep disturbances: the multi-ethnic study of atherosclerosis (MESA). Sleep. 2015;38(6):877–88.
5. Foster GD, Borradaile KE, Sanders MH, Millman R, Zammit G, Newman AB, et al. A randomized study on the effect of weight loss on obstructive sleep apnea among obese patients with type 2 diabetes: the sleep

AHEAD study. Arch Intern Med. 2009;169(17):1619–26.
6. Dixon JB, Schachter LM, O'Brien PE, Jones K, Grima M, Lambert G, et al. Surgical vs conventional therapy for weight loss treatment of obstructive sleep apnea: a randomized controlled trial. JAMA. 2012;308(11):1142–9.
7. Blackman A, Foster GD, Zammit G, Rosenberg R, Aronne L, Wadden T, et al. Effect of liraglutide 3.0 mg in individuals with obesity and moderate or severe obstructive sleep apnea: the SCALE Sleep Apnea randomized clinical trial. Int J Obes (Lond). 2016;40(8):1310–9.
8. Iftikhar IH, Bittencourt L, Youngstedt SD, Ayas N, Cistulli P, Schwab R, et al. Comparative efficacy of CPAP, MADs, exercise-training, and dietary weight loss for sleep apnea: a network meta-analysis. Sleep Med. 2017;30:7–14.
9. Patil Susheel P, Ayappa Indu A, Caples Sean M, John KR, Patel Sanjay R, Harrod Christopher G. Treatment of adult obstructive sleep apnea with positive airway pressure: an American Academy of sleep medicine systematic review, meta-analysis, and GRADE assessment. J Clin Sleep Med. 2019;15(2):301–34.
10. Schütz SG, Dunn A, Braley TJ, Pitt B, Shelgikar AV. New frontiers in pharmacologic obstructive sleep apnea treatment: a narrative review. Sleep Med Rev. 2021;57. https://pubmed.ncbi.nlm.nih.gov/33853035/
11. Coughlin SR, Mawdsley L, Mugarza JA, Calverley PMA, Wilding JPH. Obstructive sleep apnoea is independently associated with an increased prevalence of metabolic syndrome. Eur Heart J. 2004;25(9):735–41.
12. Mesarwi OA, Sharma EV, Jun JC, Polotsky VY. Metabolic dysfunction in obstructive sleep apnea: a critical examination of underlying mechanisms. Sleep Biol Rhythms. 2015;13(1):2–17.
13. Young T, Peppard PE, Taheri S. Excess weight and sleep-disordered breathing. J Appl Physiol. 2005;99(4):1592–9.
14. Peppard PE, Young T, Palta M, Dempsey J, Skatrud J. Longitudinal study of moderate weight change and sleep-disordered breathing. JAMA. 2000;284(23):3015–21.
15. Newman AB, Foster G, Givelber R, Nieto FJ, Redline S, Young T. Progression and regression of sleep-disordered breathing with changes in weight: the Sleep Heart Health Study. Arch Intern Med. 2005;165(20):2408–13.
16. Kim AM, Keenan BT, Jackson N, Chan EL, Staley B, Poptani H, et al. Tongue fat and its relationship to obstructive sleep apnea. Sleep. 2014;37(10):1639–48.
17. Öğretmenoğlu O, Süslü AE, Yücel ÖT, Önerci TM, Şahin A. Body fat composition: a predictive factor for obstructive sleep apnea. Laryngoscope. 2005;115(8):1493–8.
18. Vgontzas AN, Papanicolaou DA, Bixler EO, Hopper K, Lotsikas A, Lin HM, et al. Sleep apnea and daytime sleepiness and fatigue: relation to

visceral obesity, insulin resistance, and hypercytokinemia. J. Clin. Endocrinol. Metabol. 2000;85(3):1151–8.

19. Lee SW, Son JY, Kim JM, Hwang SS, Han JS, Heo NJ. Body fat distribution is more predictive of all-cause mortality than overall adiposity. Diabetes Obes Metab. 2018;20(1):141–7.

20. Duan D, Kim LJ, Jun JC, Polotsky VY. Connecting insufficient sleep and insomnia with metabolic dysfunction. Ann N Y Acad Sci. 2022. https://doi.org/10.1111/nyas.14926.

21. Shechter A. Obstructive sleep apnea and energy balance regulation: a systematic review. Sleep Med Rev. 2017;34:59–69.

22. Batool-Anwar S, Goodwin JL, Drescher AA, Baldwin CM, Simon RD, Smith TW, et al. Impact of CPAP on activity patterns and diet in patients with obstructive sleep apnea (OSA). J Clin Sleep Med. 2014;10(5):465–72.

23. Beebe DW, Miller N, Kirk S, Daniels SR, Amin R. The association between obstructive sleep apnea and dietary choices among obese individuals during middle to late childhood. Sleep Med. 2011;12(8):797–9.

24. Grunstein RR, Stenlof K, Hedner J, Sjostrom L. Impact of obstructive sleep apnea and sleepiness on metabolic and cardiovascular risk factors in the Swedish Obese Subjects (SOS) study. Int J Obes Relat Metab Disord. 1995;19(6):410–8.

25. Jean RE, Duttuluri M, Gibson CD, Mir S, Fuhrmann K, Eden E, et al. Improvement in physical activity in persons with obstructive sleep apnea treated with continuous positive airway pressure. J Phys Act Health. 2017;14(3):176–82.

26. Wong AM, Barnes HN, Joosten SA, Landry SA, Dabscheck E, Mansfield DR, et al. The effect of surgical weight loss on obstructive sleep apnoea: a systematic review and meta-analysis. Sleep Med Rev. 2018;42:85–99.

27. Greenburg DL, Lettieri CJ, Eliasson AH. Effects of surgical weight loss on measures of obstructive sleep apnea: a meta-analysis. Am J Med. 2009;122(6):535–42.

28. Winslow DH, Bowden CH, Didonato KP, McCullough PA. A randomized, double-blind, placebo-controlled study of an oral, extended-release formulation of phentermine/topiramate for the treatment of obstructive sleep apnea in obese adults. Sleep. 2012;35(11):1529–39.

29. Wilding JPH, Batterham RL, Calanna S, Davies M, Van Gaal LF, Lingvay I, et al. Once-weekly semaglutide in adults with overweight or obesity. N Engl J Med. 2021;384(11):989–1002.

30. Jastreboff AM, Aronne LJ, Ahmad NN, Wharton S, Connery L, Alves B, et al. Tirzepatide once weekly for the treatment of obesity. N Engl J Med. 2022;387(3):205–16.

31. Drager LF, Brunoni AR, Jenner R, Lorenzi-Filho G, Bensenor IM, Lotufo PA. Effects of CPAP on body weight in patients with obstructive sleep apnoea: a meta-analysis of randomised trials. Thorax. 2015;70 (1468–3296):258–64.

32. Stenlof K, Grunstein R, Hedner J, Sjostrom L. Energy expenditure in obstructive sleep apnea: effects of treatment with continuous positive airway pressure. Am J Physiol. 1996;271(6 Pt 1):E1036–43.

33. Bamberga M, Rizzi M, Gadaleta F, Grechi A, Baiardini R, Fanfulla F. Relationship between energy expenditure, physical activity and weight loss during CPAP treatment in obese OSA subjects. Respir Med. 2015;109(4):540–5.

34. Tachikawa R, Ikeda K, Minami T, Matsumoto T, Hamada S, Murase K, et al. Changes in energy metabolism after continuous positive airway pressure for obstructive sleep apnea. Am J Respir Crit Care Med. 2016;194(6):729–38.

35. Ou Q, Chen B, Loffler KA, Luo Y, Zhang X, Chen R, et al. The effects of long-term CPAP on weight change in patients with comorbid OSA and cardiovascular disease. Chest. 2019;155(4):720–9.

36. Miyazato M, Tohyama K, Touyama M, Nakamura H, Oshiro T, Ueda S, et al. Effect of continuous positive airway pressure on nocturnal urine production in patients with obstructive sleep apnea syndrome. Neurourol Urodyn. 2017;36(2):376–9.

37. Herculano S, Grad GF, Drager LF, de Albuquerque ALP, Melo CM, Lorenzi-Filho G, et al. Weight gain induced by continuous positive airway pressure in patients with obstructive sleep apnea is mediated by fluid accumulation: a randomized crossover controlled trial. Am J Respir Crit Care Med. 2021;203 (1):134–6.

38. Kobuch S, Tsang F, Chimoriya R, Gossayn D, O'Brien S, Jamal J, et al. Obstructive sleep apnoea and 12-month weight loss in adults with class 3 obesity attending a multidisciplinary weight management program. BMC Endocr Disord. 2021;21(1). https://pubmed.ncbi.nlm.nih.gov/34774056/

39. López-Padrós C, Salord N, Alves C, Vilarrasa N, Gasa M, Planas R, et al. Effectiveness of an intensive weight-loss program for severe OSA in patients undergoing CPAP treatment: a randomized controlled trial. J Clin Sleep Med. 2020;16(4):503–14.

40. Carneiro-Barrera A, Amaro-Gahete FJ, Guillén-Riquelme A, Jurado-Fasoli L, Sáez-Roca G, Martín-Carrasco C, et al. Effect of an interdisciplinary weight loss and lifestyle intervention on obstructive sleep apnea severity: the INTERAPNEA Randomized Clinical Trial. JAMA Netw Open. 2022;5(4):E228212.

41. Igelström H, Åsenlöf P, Emtner M, Lindberg E. Improvement in obstructive sleep apnea after a tailored behavioural sleep medicine intervention targeting healthy eating and physical activity: a randomised controlled trial. Sleep Breath Schlaf Atmung. 2018;22(3):653–61.

42. Ip MS, Lam B, Ng MM, Lam WK, Tsang KW, Lam KS. Obstructive sleep apnea is independently

associated with insulin resistance. Am J Respir Crit Care Med. 2002;165(5):670–6.

43. Punjabi NM, Shahar E, Redline S, Gottlieb DJ, Givelber R, Resnick HE. Sleep-disordered breathing, glucose intolerance, and insulin resistance: the sleep heart health study. Am J Epidemiol. 2004;160(6): 521–30.

44. Bakker JP, Weng J, Wang R, Redline S, Punjabi NM, Patel SR. Associations between obstructive sleep apnea, sleep duration, and abnormal fasting glucose. The multi-ethnic study of atherosclerosis. Am J Respir Crit Care Med. 2015;192(6):745–53.

45. Koh HCE, van Vliet S, Cao C, Patterson BW, Reeds DN, Laforest R, et al. Effect of obstructive sleep apnea on glucose metabolism. Eur J Endocrinol. 2022;186(4):457–67.

46. Lindberg E, Theorell-Haglow J, Svensson M, Gislason T, Berne C, Janson C. Sleep apnea and glucose metabolism: a long-term follow-up in a community-based sample. Chest. 2012;142(4): 935–42.

47. Wang X, Bi Y, Zhang Q, Pan F. Obstructive sleep apnoea and the risk of type 2 diabetes: a meta-analysis of prospective cohort studies. Respirology. 2013;18 (1):140–6.

48. Resnick HE, Redline S, Shahar E, Gilpin A, Newman A, Walter R, et al. Diabetes and sleep disturbances: findings from the Sleep Heart Health Study. Diabetes Care. 2003;26:702–9.

49. Foster GD, Sanders MH, Millman R, Zammit G, Borradaile KE, Newman AB, et al. Obstructive sleep apnea among obese patients with type 2 diabetes. Diabetes Care. 2009;32(6):1017–9.

50. Aronsohn RS, Whitmore H, Van Cauter E, Tasali E. Impact of untreated obstructive sleep apnea on glucose control in type 2 diabetes. Am J Respir Crit Care Med. 2010;181(5):507–13.

51. Iiyori N, Alonso LC, Li J, Sanders MH, Garcia-Ocana A, O'Doherty RM, et al. Intermittent hypoxia causes insulin resistance in lean mice independent of autonomic activity. Am J Respir Crit Care Med. 2007;175(8):851–7.

52. Polak J, Shimoda LA, Drager LF, Undem C, McHugh H, Polotsky VY, et al. Intermittent hypoxia impairs glucose homeostasis in C57BL6/J mice: partial improvement with cessation of the exposure. Sleep. 2013;36(10):1483–90.

53. Jun JC, Shin MK, Devera R, Yao Q, Mesarwi O, Bevans-Fonti S, et al. Intermittent hypoxia-induced glucose intolerance is abolished by α-adrenergic blockade or adrenal medullectomy. Am J Physiol Endocrinol Metab. 2014;307(11):E1073–83.

54. Murphy AM, Thomas A, Crinion SJ, Kent BD, Tambuwala MM, Fabre A, et al. Intermittent hypoxia in obstructive sleep apnoea mediates insulin resistance through adipose tissue inflammation. Eur Respir J. 2017;49(4). https://pubmed.ncbi.nlm.nih.gov/28424360/

55. Sherwani SI, Aldana C, Usmani S, Adin C, Kotha S, Khan M, et al. Intermittent hypoxia exacerbates pancreatic β-cell dysfunction in a mouse model of diabetes mellitus. Sleep. 2013;36(12):1849–58.

56. Torrella M, Castells I, Gimenez-Perez G, Recasens A, Miquel M, Simó O, et al. Intermittent hypoxia is an independent marker of poorer glycaemic control in patients with uncontrolled type 2 diabetes. Diabetes Metab. 2015;41(4):312–8.

57. Louis M, Punjabi NM. Effects of acute intermittent hypoxia on glucose metabolism in awake healthy volunteers. J Appl Physiol. 2009;106(5):1538–44.

58. Stamatakis KA, Punjabi NM. Effects of sleep fragmentation on glucose metabolism in normal subjects. Chest. 2010;137(1):95–101.

59. Tasali E, Ip MS. Obstructive sleep apnea and metabolic syndrome: alterations in glucose metabolism and inflammation. Proc Am Thorac Soc. 2008;5(2): 207–17.

60. Somers VK, Dyken ME, Clary MP, Abboud FM. Sympathetic neural mechanisms in obstructive sleep apnea. J Clin Invest. 1995;96(4):1897–904.

61. Gonzalez-Martin MC, Vega-Agapito MV, Conde SV, Castaneda J, Bustamante R, Olea E, et al. Carotid body function and ventilatory responses in intermittent hypoxia. Evidence for anomalous brainstem integration of arterial chemoreceptor input. J Cell Physiol. 2011;226:1961–9.

62. Shin MK, Yao Q, Jun JC, Bevans-Fonti S, Yoo DY, Han W, et al. Carotid body denervation prevents fasting hyperglycemia during chronic intermittent hypoxia. J Appl Physiol. 2014;117(7):765–76.

63. Somers VK, Mark AL, Abboud FM. Sympathetic activation by hypoxia and hypercapnia – implications for sleep apnea. Clin Exp Hypertens. 1988;10(Suppl 1):413–22.

64. Peltonen GL, Scalzo RL, Schweder MM, Larson DG, Lucksasen GJ, Irwin D, et al. Sympathetic inhibition attenuates hypoxia induced insulin resistance in healthy adult humans. J Physiol. 2012;590(11): 2801–9.

65. Jun JC, Drager LF, Najjar SS, Gottlieb SS, Brown CD, Smith PL, et al. Effects of sleep apnea on nocturnal free fatty acids in subjects with heart failure. Sleep. 2011;34(9):1207–13.

66. Barcelo A, Pierola J, de la Pena M, Esquinas C, Fuster A, Sanchez-de-la-Torre M, et al. Free fatty acids and the metabolic syndrome in patients with obstructive sleep apnoea. Eur Respir J. 2011;37: 1418–23.

67. Chopra S, Rathore A, Younas H, Pham LV, Gu C, Beselman A, et al. Obstructive sleep apnea dynamically increases nocturnal plasma free fatty acids, glucose, and cortisol during sleep. J Clin Endocrinol Metab. 2017;102(9):3172–81.

68. Kritikou I, Basta M, Vgontzas AN, Pejovic S, Fernandez-Mendoza J, Liao D, et al. Sleep apnea and the hypothalamic-pituitary-adrenal axis in men

and women: effects of continuous positive airway pressure. Eur Respir J. 2016;47(2):531–40.

69. Vgontzas AN, Pejovic S, Zoumakis E, Lin HM, Bentley CM, Bixler EO, et al. Hypothalamic-pituitary-adrenal axis activity in obese men with and without sleep apnea: effects of continuous positive airway pressure therapy. J Clin Endocrinol Metab. 2007;92: 4199–207.

70. Henley DE, Russell GM, Douthwaite JA, Wood SA, Buchanan F, Gibson R, et al. Hypothalamic-pituitary-adrenal axis activation in obstructive sleep apnea: the effect of continuous positive airway pressure therapy. J Clin Endocrinol Metab. 2009;94(11):4234–42.

71. Carneiro G, Togeiro SM, Hayashi LF, Ribeiro-Filho FF, Ribeiro AB, Tufik S, et al. Effect of continuous positive airway pressure therapy on hypothalamic-pituitary-adrenal axis function and 24-h blood pressure profile in obese men with obstructive sleep apnea syndrome. Am J Physiol Endocrinol Metab. 2008;295:E380–4.

72. Lavie L, Lavie P. Molecular mechanisms of cardiovascular disease in OSAHS: the oxidative stress link. Eur Respir J. 2009;33(6):1467–84.

73. Pitocco D, Tesauro M, Alessandro R, Ghirlanda G, Cardillo C. Oxidative stress in diabetes: implications for vascular and other complications. Int J Mol Sci. 2013;14(11):21525–50.

74. Schulz R, Mahmoudi S, Hattar K, Sibelius U, Olschewski H, Mayer K, et al. Enhanced release of superoxide from polymorphonuclear neutrophils in obstructive sleep apnea. Impact of continuous positive airway pressure therapy. Am J Respir Crit Care Med. 2000;162(2 Pt 1):566–70.

75. Carpagnano GE, Kharitonov SA, Resta O, Foschino-Barbaro MP, Gramiccioni E, Barnes PJ. 8-Isoprostane, a marker of oxidative stress, is increased in exhaled breath condensate of patients with obstructive sleep apnea after night and is reduced by continuous positive airway pressure therapy. Chest. 2003;124(4): 1386–92.

76. Celec P, Hodosy J, Behuliak M, Pálffy R, Gardlík R, Halčák L, et al. Oxidative and carbonyl stress in patients with obstructive sleep apnea treated with continuous positive airway pressure. Sleep Breath. 2012;16(2):393–8.

77. Ryan S, Taylor CT, McNicholas WT. Selective activation of inflammatory pathways by intermittent hypoxia in obstructive sleep apnea syndrome. Circulation. 2005;112(17):2660–7.

78. Ryan S, Taylor CT, McNicholas WT. Predictors of elevated nuclear factor-kappaB-dependent genes in obstructive sleep apnea syndrome. Am J Respir Crit Care Med. 2006;174:824–30.

79. Xu PH, Hui CKM, Lui MMS, Lam DCL, Fong DYT, Ip MSM. Incident type 2 diabetes in OSA and effect of CPAP treatment: a retrospective clinic cohort study. Chest. 2019;156(4):743–53.

80. Abud R, Salgueiro M, Drake L, Reyes T, Jorquera J, Labarca G. Efficacy of continuous positive airway pressure (CPAP) preventing type 2 diabetes mellitus in patients with obstructive sleep apnea hypopnea syndrome (OSAHS) and insulin resistance: a systematic review and meta-analysis. Sleep Med. 2019;62: 14–21.

81. Salord N, Fortuna AM, Monasterio C, Gasa M, Pérez A, Bonsignore MR, et al. A randomized controlled trial of continuous positive airway pressure on glucose tolerance in obese patients with obstructive sleep apnea. Sleep. 2016;39(1):35–41.

82. Chirinos JA, Gurubhagavatula I, Teff K, Rader DJ, Wadden TA, Townsend R, et al. CPAP, weight loss, or both for obstructive sleep apnea. N Engl J Med. 2014;370(24):2265–75.

83. Mokhlesi B, Grimaldi D, Beccuti G, Van Cauter E. Effect of one week of CPAP treatment of obstructive sleep apnoea on 24-hour profiles of glucose, insulin and counter-regulatory hormones in type 2 diabetes. Diabetes Obes Metab. 2017;19(3):452–6.

84. Pamidi S, Wroblewski K, Stepien M, Sharif-Sidi K, Kilkus J, Whitmore H, et al. Eight hours of nightly continuous positive airway pressure treatment of obstructive sleep apnea improves glucose metabolism in patients with prediabetes. A randomized controlled trial. Am J Respir Crit Care Med. 2015;192 (1):96–105.

85. Shang W, Zhang Y, Wang G, Han D. Benefits of continuous positive airway pressure on glycaemic control and insulin resistance in patients with type 2 diabetes and obstructive sleep apnoea: a meta-analysis. Diabetes Obes Metab. 2021;23(2):540–8.

86. Martinez-Ceron E, Barquiel B, Bezos AM, Casitas R, Galera R, Garcia-Benito C, et al. Effect of continuous positive airway pressure on glycemic control in patients with obstructive sleep apnea and type 2 diabetes a randomized clinical trial. Am J Respir Crit Care Med. 2016;194(4):476–85.

87. Giampá SQC, Furlan SF, Freitas LS, Macedo TA, Lebkuchen A, Cardozo KHM, et al. Effects of CPAP on metabolic syndrome in patients with OSA: a randomized trial. Chest. 2022;161(5):1370–81.

88. Banghøj AM, Krogager C, Kristensen PL, Hansen KW, Laugesen E, Fleischer J, et al. Effect of 12-week continuous positive airway pressure therapy on glucose levels assessed by continuous glucose monitoring in people with type 2 diabetes and obstructive sleep apnoea; a randomized controlled trial. Endocrinol Diabet Metabol. 2021;4(2). https:// onlinelibrary.wiley.com/doi/10.1002/edm2.148

89. Shaw JE, Punjabi NM, Naughton MT, Willes L, Bergenstal RM, Cistulli PA, et al. The effect of treatment of obstructive sleep apnea on glycemic control in type 2 diabetes. Am J Respir Crit Care Med. 2016. http://www.ncbi.nlm.nih.gov/pubmed/26926656

90. Loffler KA, Heeley E, Freed R, Meng R, Bittencourt LR, Gonzaga Carvalho CC, et al. Continuous positive airway pressure treatment, glycemia, and diabetes risk in obstructive sleep apnea and comorbid cardiovascular disease. Diabetes Care. 2020;43(8):1859–67.

91. Aurora RN, Rooney MR, Wang D, Selvin E, Punjabi NM. Effects of positive airway pressure therapy on glycemic variability in patients with type 2 diabetes and OSA: a randomized controlled trial. Chest. 2023. https://www.sciencedirect.com/science/article/pii/S0012369223005147

92. Torrella M, Castells I, Gimenez-Perez G, Recasens A, Miquel M, Simó O, et al. Continuous positive airway pressure improves sleep quality, but not glycaemic control, in patients with poorly controlled long-standing type 2 diabetes. Diabetes Metab. 2017;43(6):547–9.

93. Burwell R, Whaley B. Exteme obesity associated with alveolar hypoventilation – a Pickwickian Syndrome. Am J Med. 1956;21:811–8.

94. Mokhlesi B. Obesity hypoventilation syndrome: a state-of-the-art review. Respir Care. 2010;55(10):1347–62; discussion 1363–5

95. Böing S, Randerath WJ. Chronic hypoventilation syndromes and sleep-related hypoventilation. J Thorac Dis. 2015;7(8):1273–85.

96. Mokhlesi B, Masa JF, Brozek JL, Gurubhagavatula I, Murphy PB, Piper AJ, et al. Evaluation and management of obesity hypoventilation syndrome. An official American Thoracic Society Clinical Practice guideline. Am J Respir Crit Care Med. 2019;200(3):e6–24.

97. Mokhlesi B, Tulaimat A, Faibussowitsch I, Wang Y, Evans AT. Obesity hypoventilation syndrome: prevalence and predictors in patients with obstructive sleep apnea. Sleep Breath. 2007;11(2):117–24.

98. Bingol Z, Pıhtılı A, Cagatay P, Okumus G, Kıyan E. Clinical predictors of obesity hypoventilation syndrome in obese subjects with obstructive sleep apnea. Respir Care. 2015;60(5):666–72.

99. Macavei VM, Spurling KJ, Loft J, Makker HK. Diagnostic predictors of obesity-hypoventilation syndrome in patients suspected of having sleep disordered breathing. J Clin Sleep Med. 2013;9(9):879–84.

100. Kaw R, Hernandez AV, Walker E, Aboussouan L, Mokhlesi B. Determinants of hypercapnia in obese patients with obstructive sleep apnea: a systematic review and metaanalysis of cohort studies. Chest. 2009;136(3):787–96.

101. Chung Y, Garden FL, Jee AS, Srikantha S, Gupta S, Buchanan PR, et al. Supine awake oximetry as a screening tool for daytime hypercapnia in super-obese patients. Intern Med J. 2017;47(10):1136–41.

102. Masa JF, Pépin JL, Borel JC, Mokhlesi B, Murphy PB, Sánchez-Quiroga MÁ. Obesity hypoventilation syndrome. Eur Respir Rev. 2019;28(151):180097.

103. Tran K, Wang L, Gharaibeh S, Kempke N, Rao Kashyap S, Cetin D, et al. Elucidating predictors of obesity hypoventilation syndrome in a large bariatric surgery cohort. Ann Am Thorac Soc. 2020;17(10):1279–88.

104. Ng M, Fleming T, Robinson M, Thomson B, Graetz N, Margono C, et al. Global, regional, and national prevalence of overweight and obesity in children and adults during 1980–2013: a systematic analysis for the Global Burden of Disease Study 2013. Lancet. 2014;384(9945):766–81.

105. Nowbar S, Burkart KM, Gonzales R, Fedorowicz A, Gozansky WS, Gaudio JC, et al. Obesity-associated hypoventilation in hospitalized patients: prevalence, effects, and outcome. Am J Med. 2004;116(1):1–7.

106. BaHammam AS, Almeneessier AS. Is obesity hypoventilation syndrome a postmenopausal disorder? Open Respir Med J. 2019;13(1):51–4.

107. Bülbül Y, Ayik S, Ozlu T, Orem A. Frequency and predictors of obesity hypoventilation in hospitalized patients at a tertiary health care institution. Ann Thorac Med. 2014;9(2):87–91.

108. Chen W, Feng J, Dong S, Guo J, Liang Y, Hu R, et al. A novel nomogram and online calculator for predicting the risk of obesity hypoventilation syndrome in bariatric surgery candidates. Obes Surg. 2023;33(1):68–77.

109. Lee WY, Mokhlesi B. Diagnosis and management of obesity hypoventilation syndrome in the ICU. Crit Care Clin. 2008;24(3):533–49. vii

110. Berg G, Delaive K, Manfreda J, Walld R, Kryger MH. The use of health-care resources in obesity-hypoventilation syndrome. Chest. 2001;120(2):377–83.

111. Castro-Añón O, Pérez de Llano LA, De la Fuente Sánchez S, Golpe R, Méndez Marote L, Castro-Castro J, et al. Obesity-hypoventilation syndrome: increased risk of death over sleep apnea syndrome. PLoS One. 2015;10(2):e0117808.

112. Marik PE, Desai H. Characteristics of patients with the "malignant obesity hypoventilation syndrome" admitted to an ICU. J Intensive Care Med. 2013;28(2):124–30.

113. Marik PE, Chen C. The clinical characteristics and hospital and post-hospital survival of patients with the obesity hypoventilation syndrome: analysis of a large cohort. Obes Sci Pract. 2016;2(1):40–7.

114. Masa JF, Benítez ID, Javaheri S, Mogollon MV, de Sánchez-Quiroga MÁ, Terreros F, Corral J, et al. Risk factors associated with pulmonary hypertension in obesity hypoventilation syndrome. J Clin Sleep Med. 2022;18(4):983–92.

115. Virdis A, Duranti E, Rossi C, Dell'Agnello U, Santini E, Anselmino M, et al. Tumour necrosis factor-alpha participates on the endothelin-1/nitric oxide imbalance in small arteries from obese patients: role of perivascular adipose tissue. Eur Heart J. 2015;36(13):784–94.

116. Carrillo A, Ferrer M, Gonzalez-Diaz G, Lopez-Martinez A, Llamas N, Alcazar M, et al. Noninvasive ventilation in acute hypercapnic respiratory failure caused by obesity hypoventilation syndrome and chronic obstructive pulmonary disease. Am J Respir Crit Care Med. 2012;186(12):1279–85.

117. Mokhlesi B, Masa JF, Afshar M, Almadana Pacheco V, Berlowitz DJ, Borel JC, et al. The effect of hospital discharge with empiric noninvasive

ventilation on mortality in hospitalized patients with obesity hypoventilation syndrome: an individual patient data meta-analysis. Ann ATS. 2020. https://www.atsjournals.org/doi/abs/10.1513/AnnalsATS.201912-887OC

118. Piper AJ, Wang D, Yee BJ, Barnes DJ, Grunstein RR. Randomised trial of CPAP vs bilevel support in the treatment of obesity hypoventilation syndrome without severe nocturnal desaturation. Thorax. 2008;63(5):395–401.

119. Masa JF, Corral J, Alonso ML, Ordax E, Troncoso MF, Gonzalez M, et al. Efficacy of different treatment alternatives for obesity hypoventilation syndrome. Pickwick study. Am J Respir Crit Care Med. 2015;192(1):86–95.

120. López-Jiménez MJ, Masa JF, Corral J, Terán J, Ordaz E, Troncoso MF, et al. Mid- and long-term efficacy of non-invasive ventilation in obesity hypoventilation syndrome: the Pickwick's study. Arch Bronconeumol. 2016;52(3):158–65.

121. Masa JF, Mokhlesi B, Benítez I, Gomez de Terreros FJ, Sánchez-Quiroga MÁ, Romero A, et al. Long-term clinical effectiveness of continuous positive airway pressure therapy versus non-invasive ventilation therapy in patients with obesity hypoventilation syndrome: a multicentre, open-label, randomised controlled trial. Lancet. 2019;393(10182):1721–32.

122. Masa JF, Benítez I, Sánchez-Quiroga MÁ, Gomez de Terreros FJ, Corral J, Romero A, et al. Long-term noninvasive ventilation in obesity hypoventilation syndrome without severe OSA: the Pickwick randomized controlled trial. Chest. 2020;158(3):1176–86.

123. Rapoport DM, Garay SM, Epstein H, Goldring RM. Hypercapnia in the obstructive sleep apnea syndrome. A reevaluation of the "Pickwickian syndrome". Chest. 1986;89(5):627–35.

124. Mokhlesi B, Tulaimat A, Evans AT, Wang Y, Itani A, Hassebella HA, et al. Impact of adherence with positive airway pressure therapy on hypercapnia in obstructive sleep apnea. J Clin Sleep Med. 2006;2(1):57–62.

125. Borel JC, Tamisier R, Gonzalez-Bermejo J, Baguet JP, Monneret D, Arnol N, et al. Noninvasive ventilation in mild obesity hypoventilation syndrome: a randomized controlled trial. Chest. 2012;141(3):692–702.

126. Agossou M, Barzu R, Awanou B, Bellegarde-Joachim J, Arnal JM, Dramé M. Factors associated with the efficiency of home non-invasive ventilation in patients with obesity-hypoventilation syndrome in Martinique. J Clin Med. 2023;12(10):3381.

127. Budweiser S, Riedl SG, Jorres RA, Heinemann F, Pfeifer M. Mortality and prognostic factors in patients with obesity-hypoventilation syndrome undergoing noninvasive ventilation. J Intern Med. 2007;261(4):375–83.

128. Hollier CA, Harmer AR, Maxwell LJ, Menadue C, Willson GN, Unger G, et al. Moderate concentrations of supplemental oxygen worsen hypercapnia in obesity hypoventilation syndrome: a randomised crossover study. Thorax. 2014;69(4):346–53.

129. Wijesinghe M, Williams M, Perrin K, Weatherall M, Beasley R. The effect of supplemental oxygen on hypercapnia in subjects with obesity-associated hypoventilation: a randomized, crossover, clinical study. Chest. 2011;139(5):1018–24.

130. Masa JF, Corral J, Romero A, Caballero C, Terán SJ, Alonso-Álvarez Maria L, et al. The effect of supplemental oxygen in obesity hypoventilation syndrome. J Clin Sleep Med. 2016;12(10):1379–88.

131. Mandal S, Suh ES, Harding R, Vaughan-France A, Ramsay M, Connolly B, et al. Nutrition and exercise rehabilitation in obesity hypoventilation syndrome (NERO): a pilot randomised controlled trial. Thorax. 2018;73(1):62–9.

132. Sugerman HJ, Fairman RP, Sood RK, Engle K, Wolfe L, Kellum JM. Long-term effects of gastric surgery for treating respiratory insufficiency of obesity. Am J Clin Nutr. 1992;55(2 Suppl):597S–601S.

133. Feigel-Guiller B, Drui D, Dimet J, Zair Y, Le Bras M, Fuertes-Zamorano N, et al. Laparoscopic gastric banding in obese patients with sleep apnea: a 3-year controlled study and follow-up after 10 years. Obes Surg. 2015;25(10):1886–92.

134. Duan D, Perin J, Osman A, Sgambati F, Kim LJ, Pham LV, et al. Effects of sex, age, and body mass index on serum bicarbonate. Front Sleep. 2023;2:1195823.

135. Lee MY, Lin CC, Shen SY, Chiu CH, Liaw SF. Work of breathing in eucapnic and hypercapnic sleep apnea syndrome. Respiration. 2009;77(2):146–53.

136. Javaheri S, Simbartl LA. Respiratory determinants of diurnal hypercapnia in obesity hypoventilation syndrome. What does weight have to do with it? Ann ATS. 2014;11(6):945–50.

137. Dusgun ES, Aslan GK, Abanoz ES, Kiyan E. Respiratory muscle endurance in obesity hypoventilation syndrome. Respir Care. 2022;67(5):526–33.

138. Berger KI, Ayappa I, Sorkin IB, Norman RG, Rapoport DM, Goldring RM. Postevent ventilation as a function of CO(2) load during respiratory events in obstructive sleep apnea. J Appl Physiol. 2002;93(3):917–24.

139. Manuel AR, Hart N, Stradling JR. Is a raised bicarbonate, without hypercapnia, part of the physiologic spectrum of obesity-related hypoventilation? Chest. 2015;147:362–8.

140. Randerath W, Verbraecken J, Andreas S, Arzt M, Bloch KE, Brack T, et al. Definition, discrimination, diagnosis and treatment of central breathing disturbances during sleep. Eur Respir J. 2017;49(1):1600959.

141. Turnbull CD, Wang SH, Manuel AR, Keenan BT, McIntyre AG, Schwab RJ, et al. Relationships between MRI fat distributions and sleep apnea and

obesity hypoventilation syndrome in very obese patients. Sleep Breath. 2018;22(3):673–81.

142. Zhang Y, Proenca R, Maffei M, Barone M, Leopold L, Friedman JM. Positional cloning of the mouse obese gene and its human homologue. Nature. 1994;372 (6505):425–32.

143. Considine RV, Sinha MK, Heiman ML, Kriauciunas A, Stephens TW, Nyce MR, et al. Serum immunoreactive-leptin concentrations in normal-weight and obese humans [see comments]. N Engl J Med. 1996;334(5):292–5.

144. Banks WA, Clever CM, Farrell CL. Partial saturation and regional variation in the blood-to-brain transport of leptin in normal weight mice. Am J Physiol Endocrinol Metab. 2000;278(6):E1158–65.

145. Schwartz MW, Peskind E, Raskind M, Boyko EJ, Porte D Jr. Cerebrospinal fluid leptin levels: relationship to plasma levels and to adiposity in humans. Nat Med. 1996;2(5):589–93.

146. Izquierdo AG, Crujeiras AB, Casanueva FF, Carreira MC. Leptin, obesity, and leptin resistance: where are we 25 years later? Nutrients. 2019;11(11):2704.

147. Harrison L, Schriever SC, Feuchtinger A, Kyriakou E, Baumann P, Pfuhlmann K, et al. Fluorescent blood–brain barrier tracing shows intact leptin transport in obese mice. Int J Obes. 2019;43(6):1305–18.

148. Lindström P. The physiology of obese-hyperglycemic mice [ob/ob mice]. ScientificWorldJournal. 2007;7: 666–85.

149. O'Donnell CP, Tankersley CG, Polotsky VY, Schwartz AR, Smith PL. Leptin, obesity, and respiratory function. Respir Physiol. 2000;119:163–70.

150. Fleury Curado T, Pho H, Berger S, Caballero-Eraso C, Shin MK, Sennes LU, et al. Sleep-disordered breathing in C57BL/6J mice with diet-induced obesity. Sleep. 2018;41(8):zsy089.

151. Berger S, Pho H, Fleury-Curado T, Bevans-Fonti S, Younas H, Shin MK, et al. Intranasal leptin relieves sleep-disordered breathing in mice with diet-induced obesity. Am J Respir Crit Care Med. 2018;199(6): 773–83.

152. Amorim MR, Aung O, Mokhlesi B, Polotsky VY. Leptin-mediated neural targets in obesity hypoventilation syndrome. Sleep. 2022;45(9):zsac153.

Connecting Obesity and Reproductive Disorders

35

Rexford S. Ahima and Jenny Pena Dias

Contents

Abstract

Obesity predisposes to reproductive disorders in both women and men. Polycystic ovary syndrome (PCOS) is a common endocrine disorder in women of reproductive age. PCOS prevalence is higher in women with obesity, associated with insulin resistance, glucose intolerance, sleep apnea, increased risk of cardiovascular diseases, and the commonest cause

R. S. Ahima (✉) · J. P. Dias
Department of Medicine, Division of Endocrinology, Diabetes and Metabolism, Johns Hopkins University School of Medicine, Baltimore, MD, USA
e-mail: ahima@jhmi.edu

© Springer Nature Switzerland AG 2023
R. S. Ahima (ed.), *Metabolic Syndrome*,
https://doi.org/10.1007/978-3-031-40116-9_54

of anovulatory infertility. Obesity in men is linked to secondary hypogonadism and impaired semen quality and infertility. In addition, men with testosterone deficiency are prone to developing increased adiposity and reduced muscle mass, indicating a bidirectional relationship between obesity and hypogonadism. This review will focus on pathophysiology of PCOS and male obesity-associated hypogonadism, diagnostic approaches, and current therapies.

Keywords

Obesity · Polycystic ovary disease · Sex hormone · Hypogonadism · Fertility

Introduction

Adequate nutrition and integration of metabolic signals from energy stores with the hypothalamic-pituitary-gonadal (HPG) axis are essential for reproduction. Gonadotropin releasing hormone (GnRH) neurons located in the preoptic area, septum, and anterior hypothalamus in rodents, or periventricular area and mediobasal hypothalamus in primates respond to sex steroids and metabolic signals, and secrete GnRH in a pulsatile manner into the hypophyseal portal circulation in the median eminence. GnRH acts on gonadotropes in the anterior pituitary to regulate the synthesis and secretion of luteinizing hormone (LH) and follicle-stimulating hormone (FSH). LH and FSH regulate steroidogenesis and gametogenesis in the gonads, and the sex steroids in turn act via feedback mechanisms in the hypothalamus [1].

Extremes of body weight and adiposity have disruptive effects on the HPG axis [1–3]. Malnutrition or limited adipose tissue, e.g., in starvation or lipodystrophy, causes delayed puberty, menstrual disruption, and infertility [3–5]. This is characterized by reduced levels of LH and sex steroids, implying a central regulation of HPG axis by metabolic signals. Obesity in women is linked to early onset of puberty, menstrual irregularities, infertility, and pregnancy complications [6–8]. Men with obesity are prone to secondary

hypogonadism, characterized by reduced levels of LH and testosterone, and infertility [9, 10].

Over the past four decades, obesity has become a global epidemic affecting about 650 million adults, representing 13% of the world's adult population [11]. The worldwide obesity rate has tripled since 1975. The World Obesity Federation predicts that by 2030, 1 in 5 women and 1 in 7 men will have obesity [12]. The obesity prevalence in the USA increased from 30.5% in 1999–2000 to 41.9% in 2017–2020, and the prevalence of severe obesity increased from 4.7–9.2% during that period [13]. Obesity-related diseases, including type 2 diabetes, heart disease, stroke, and certain types of cancer, are among the leading causes of morbidity and mortality. Obesity also has adverse effects on reproduction, including ovulatory and menstrual functions, fertility, and pregnancy outcomes.

This chapter focuses on the commonest reproductive disorders associated with obesity: polycystic ovary syndrome (PCOS) in women and secondary hypogonadism in men. We discuss the current pathophysiology, diagnosis, and management.

Polycystic Ovary Syndrome

Polycystic ovary syndrome (PCOS) is the most common endocrine disorder affecting 5–20% of reproductive-age women, depending on the disease definition and population [14]. PCOS typically develops during adolescence and clinical features of hyperandrogenism (acne, hirsutism, and male-pattern baldness) and reproductive dysfunction (oligo-amenorrhea and associated subfertility). Although metabolic dysfunction is not required for the definition of PCOS, studies show a high prevalence of obesity (especially central obesity), type 2 diabetes, and cardiovascular disease in patients with PCOS [14, 15]. In large epidemiological studies, 38–88% of women with PCOS are either overweight or obese [16, 17]. Women with obesity have an odds ratio of 2.7 for the development of PCOS compared to nonobese women [18]. Genome-wide studies also show a shared genetic architecture between PCOS, obesity, and various metabolic traits and PCOS [19, 20].

Pathophysiology of PCOS

Hyperandrogenism is a key feature of PCOS, and the main source of testosterone in PCOS is ovarian androgen hypersecretion [6] (Fig. 1). Women with PCOS have high GnRH pulse frequency resulting in hypersecretion of LH and androgen production by ovarian theca cells. Low or normal FSH level in PCOS suppresses the growth and maturation of ovarian follicles, resulting in follicular arrest and the formation of multiple ovarian cysts, and oligo-ovulation or anovulation. As the number of pre-antral and antral follicles increases, anti-Mullerian hormone synthesis and secretion increases, and this stimulates the activity of GnRH neurons and GnRH-dependent secretion of LH, which further stimulates ovarian androgen production. Insulin resistance in PCOS results in hyperinsulinemia, which also stimulates GnRH secretion and ovarian theca cell androgen production as well as suppresses sex hormone binding globulin (SHBG) synthesis in the liver, resulting in high levels of free testosterone in the circulation that mediates the clinical symptoms of hyperandrogenism.

The etiology of PCOS is complex, several phenotypes constitute the syndrome, and the factors mediating heterogeneity of ovarian abnormalites, elevated androgen levels, and metabolic dysfunction vary among diverse populations. PCOS is influenced by genetic and environmental factors [21]. Hyperandrogenemia in PCOS has an estimated heritability of 70%, and 20 susceptibility loci and rare genetic variants, e.g., in *AMH2* and *DENND1*, have been identified [21]. GWAS has also determined a shared genetic link between PCOS and obesity, type 2 diabetes, and cardiovascular risk [22]. Women with PCOS have increased weight gain and higher levels of androgens and AMH during pregnancy [23]. Daughters of women with PCOS have elevated androgen and AMH levels [24] as well as PCOS-like ovarian morphology before the onset of puberty, suggesting in utero programming plays an important role in the pathogenesis of PCOS [25]. Transgenerational studies indicate that female as well as male relatives of women with PCOS have increased risk of insulin resistance and metabolic syndrome [22, 26]. A combination of the maternal hormonal milieu and intrauterine environment may influence the function of fetal HPG axis and contribute to the transgenerational transmission of PCOS [22, 27].

Despite the high prevalence of PCOS, the underlying mechanisms are not well understood. Animal models have provided insight to the pathogenesis of PCOS [28–30] (Table 1). Administration of sex steroids and their modulators is the most widely used method to induce PCOS-like phenotypes in rodents (Table 1). Pre- or postnatal administration of testosterone in female rats induces abnormal estrus cycles and changes in sex hormones and ovaries. DHEA is produced mainly in the adrenal gland, and women with PCOS have high DHEA levels. Female rats treated with DHEA develop irregular cycles accompanied by increased number of cystic follicles, elevated testosterone levels, and higher LH/FSH ratio. Dihydrotestosterone (DHT) has potent androgenic activity and is not converted into E2 by aromatase. Female rats and mice prenatally exposed to DHT develop irregular cycles, elevated levels of LH and E2, increased number of antral and atretic follicles. Aromatase converts testosterone and androstenedione into E2 and estrone. Letrozole, a nonsteroidal aromatase inhibitor, blocks the conversion of androgens to estrogen. Female rats treated with letrozole are acyclic, have elevated LH, FSH, and testosterone levels, and increased ovary weight, atretic antral follicles, and follicular cysts, as well as increased body weight and inguinal adipose tissue, and insulin resistance. Mifepristone (RU486), a progesterone receptor antagonist, suppresses ovulation and formation of corpus luteum. Female rats treated with RU486 develop persistent estrus, elevated testosterone, LH, and prolactin levels, and increased numbers of preantral and antral follicles and atretic follicles. Female rats treated with estradiol valerate, a long-acting estrogen, have prolonged estrus or proestrus, elevated testosterone and E2 levels, and large cyst-like ovarian follicles.

Rodent models with spontaneous or engineered gene mutations linked to obesity and abnormal lipid and glucose metabolism often develop hyperinsulinemia, abnormal estrus cycles, ovarian cysts, and impaired fertility [29, 30]. Female mice fed a

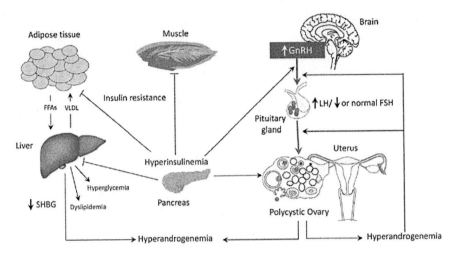

Fig. 1 Pathophysiology of PCOS. PCOS is characterized by hyperactivity of GnRH neurons, hypersecretion of GnRH and LH, and ovarian theca cell androgen over-production. Insulin resistance induces hyperinsulinemia, stimulation of HPG axis, reduction in SHBG, and increase in free (active) testosterone. Abbreviations: *FFAs* free fatty acids, *VLDL* very low density lipoprotein

high fat/high sucrose diet or exposed to endocrine disruptors or environmental perturbation may develop reproductive abnormalities. These models are useful but do not display the full spectrum of PCOS disorders [28–30].

Diagnosis of PCOS

The diagnostic criteria for PCOS evolved from the original National Institutes of Health criteria [31], i.e., clinical or biochemical evidence of hyperandrogenism and amenorrhea/oligomenorrhea, excluding other disorders. The most widely used criteria for PCOS, the Rotterdam criteria, require 2 out of 3 criteria, i.e., hyperandrogenism, oligomenorrhea or amenorrhea, or polycystic ovarian morphology [31]. Biochemical evidence of hyperandrogenism is based on the total testosterone, free calculated testosterone, or free testosterone measured preferably by liquid chromatography–mass spectrometry. As discussed earlier, AMH drives androgen production in PCOS. Serum AMH concentrations may be elevated or within the upper range of normal in women with PCOS. However, AMH measurement is not currently part of the laboratory evaluation of PCOS.

It is important to exclude conditions that may alter the measurement of sex hormones. For example, patients seen for evaluation of PCOS may be taking oral contraceptives, resulting in suppression of gonadotropins and ovarian androgens. Metformin and spironolactone also affect androgen levels. These medications should be stopped at least four to 6 weeks before evaluation of PCOS. In any reproductive-age woman presenting with amenorrhea or oligomenorrhea, other causes of irregular menses, e.g., pregnancy, hyperprolactinemia, thyroid disorders, and ovarian failure, should be investigated. The laboratory testing should include human chorionic gonadotropin (hCG), prolactin, and thyroid-stimulating hormone (TSH), and FSH. Of note, it is not essential to measure serum LH, since an elevated LH:FSH ratio is not a critical criterion for diagnosis of PCOS.

Nonclassic congenital adrenal hyperplasia (NCAH) is rare but may have a similar presentation as PCOS, i.e., hyperandrogenism, oligomenorrhea, and polycystic ovaries. NCAH, P450c21 (21-hydroxylase) deficiency, is an autosomal recessive disorder due to mutations in the *CYP21A2* gene. As with PCOS, NCAH may be associated with obesity and metabolic dysfunction. The prevalence of NCAH ranges from

Table 1 Animal models of PCOS

Model	Estrous cycle/Ovarian morphology	Sex hormones	Body weight/ Adiposity	Metabolic dysfunction
Rat; prenatal testosterone	Longer and irregular estrous cycles; increased antral follicles; and reduced corpus luteum	Increased T, LH, and LH/FSH; normal E2	Increased body weight	Increased blood glucose
Rat; postnatal DHEA	Irregular, mainly estrous; reduced corpus luteum	Increased T and LH/FSH; normal E2	No change in body weight	Increased blood glucose
Rat; prenatal DHT	Irregular estrous cycles; increased atretic cysts	Increased or normal T and E2; increased LH	No change in body weight; increased parametrial fat	Steatosis
Mouse: prenatal DHT	Irregular estrous cycles	Increased or normal T	No change in body weight; increased parametrial fat	Steatosis
Rat: postnatal DHT	Acyclic (diestrus); reduced antral follicles and corpus luteum	Normal T, E2, and LH	Increased body weight and fat	Insulin resistance
Mouse; postnatal; DHT	Acyclic (diestrus); atretic cysts	Normal T, E2, and LH	Increased body weight and fat	Insulin resistance; reduced adiponectin; and increased cholesterol
Rat; postnatal/adult letrozole	Acyclic (diestrus); cystic follicles	Increased, reduced E2, increased LH and FSH	Increased body weight and fat	Insulin resistance
Rat; adult mifepristone	Persistent estrous; increased antral follicles	Increased T, LH, and PRL	No change in body weight	No significant change in insulin sensitivity
Rat; postnatal/adult; estradiol valerate	Persistent estrous; large follicular cysts; increased atresia	Increased T, E2, and LH	No change in weight; increased inguinal fat	No significant change in insulin sensitivity
Mouse; aromatase knockout	Acyclic; ovarian cysts (hemorrhagic)	Increased T and LH	Not reported	Not reported
Mouse; transgenic LH β-CTP	Prolonged estrous; ovarian cysts	Increased T and LH	Not reported	Not reported
Mouse; transgenic expression of nerve growth factor driven by 17α-hydroxylase/C_{17-20}lyase promoter (17NF mice)	Prolonged estrous	Increased T	Increased body weight and fat	Increased insulin; glucose intolerance
Mouse; theca-specific (CYP17) ERα KO	Irregular cycles; ovarian cysts (hemorrhagic)	Increased T and reduced LH	Not reported	Not reported

0.6–9%, with higher prevalence among Ashkenazi Jews, Mediterranean, Middle Eastern, Indian, and Hispanic populations. The reduction in P450c21 activity impairs the conversion of 17-hydroxyprogesterone (17-OHP) to 11-deoxycortisol, and progesterone (P4) to deoxycorticosterone, resulting in elevation of serum levels of 17-OHP, P4, and androstenedione. To screen for NCAH, a morning serum 17-OHP level is measured in the early follicular phase in women who have spontaneous menstrual cycles, or on a random day in women without cycles. A value less than 200 ng/dL (6 nmol/L) in the early follicular phase makes the diagnosis of NCAH unlikely. A value greater than 200 ng/dL in the early follicular phase strongly suggests the diagnosis, and it may be confirmed by a (250 mcg) corticotropin ($ACTH_{1-24}$) stimulation test. The response to cosyntropin in most NCAH patients exceeds 1500 ng/dL (43 nmol/L). Genetic testing is important in patients with NCAH considering pregnancy, and it can also identify compound heterozygote individuals carrying an allele encoding a severe defect in *CYP21A2*.

Androgen-secreting ovarian or adrenal tumors or ovarian hyperthecosis often occur in postmenopausal women, but may occasionally occur in premenopausal women. These conditions are characterized by rapid onset of hirsutism, rapidly worsening hirsutism, and virilization (e.g. frontal balding, severe acne, and clitoromegaly). Serum testosterone concentrations are greater than 150 ng/dL (5.2 nmol/L), and patients with adrenal tumors have serum dehydroepiandrosterone sulfate (DHEAS) concentrations higher than 800 mcg/dL (21.6 micromol/L).

Clinical Features of Hyperandrogenism

Clinical signs of hyperandrogenism include acne, hirsutism, and male-pattern baldness. The Ferriman-Gallwey score is used to assess the degree of hirsutism; however, there are limitations to this method among different racial groups. Mediterranean, South Asian, and Middle Eastern women have greater amounts of body hair, White and Black women have intermediate amount of body hair, and East Asian and Native American women have less body hair. Patients with virilization or rapid-onset hirsutism should be evaluated for other causes of hyperandrogenism, e.g., ovarian and adrenal androgen-secreting tumors.

Women with PCOS can present with a wide range of reproductive abnormalities including irregular menses, anovulation, infertility, and

pregnancy complications. PCOS is the primary cause of anovulatory infertility. A study in women with PCOS showed a 15-fold increased risk of infertility. Among these patients, 72% reported anovulatory infertility and higher rates of ovulation induction compared to women without PCOS. PCOS is associated with two- to three-fold increased risk for gestational diabetes, pregnancy-induced hypertension, preeclampsia, and premature birth [32, 33]. The rates of pregnancy loss and stillbirth, induction of labor, and caeserean section are all higher in PCOS [34, 35]. Women with PCOS may have more difficulty with lactation [36].

Although metabolic abnormalities are not required criteria for the diagnosis of PCOS, obesity, glucose intolerance, type 2 diabetes, dyslipidemia, and nonalcoholic fatty liver disease (NAFLD) are common in PCOS. Type 2 diabetes has an earlier age of onset in patients with PCOS, with a fourfold higher incidence compared to those without PCOS. A study of women with PCOS showed the incidence of type 2 diabetes was 3·21/1000/year in the normal weight group, 4·67/1000/year in the overweight goup, and 8·80/1000/year in the obese group [36, 37]. Dyslipidemia with PCOS is characterized by higher concentrations of triglycerides and LDL cholesterol, and reduced HDL cholesterol [38]. Women with PCOS have higher prevalence of hypertension [33]. In comparison with a control population matched by age and BMI, and site of clinical care, patients with PCOS showed a higher incidence of major cardiovascular events [33].

Depending on the diagnostic criteria, the prevalence of NAFLD in PCOS is more than twofold higher than in healthy women without PCOS [39]. Increased androgen levels in PCOS are associated with visceral adiposity, insulin resistance, hyperinsulinemia, hypoadiponectinemia, increase lipolysis, and de novo hepatic lipogenesis, resulting in hepatic steatosis. PCOS increases the risk of NAFLD even in the absence of obesity [40–42]. NAFLD increases the risk of developing type 2 diabetes [43].

Studies have also evaluated the role of genes linked to the development of PCOS and metabolic dysfunction [21, 31]. Polygenic risk scores linked to PCOS phenotypes show similar associations with hyperandrogenism and metabolic dysfunction in both women and men, suggesting similar pathways for these abnormalities [21, 31].

Transvaginal Ultrasound of Ovary

Transvaginal ultrasound (TVUS) is used to assess polycystic ovarian morphology (PCOM). However, it is important to point out that a patient presenting with oligomenorrhea and evidence of hyperandrogenism, excluding other causes, does not need an ultrasound to make a diagnosis of PCOS. TVUS or abdominal ovarian ultrasound is useful to determine PCOM in a patient who has regular menses and hyperandrogenism. PCOM is defined by the number and size of ovarian follicles, and not cysts. The Rotterdam criteria for PCOM is based on the presence of 12 or more follicles in either ovary, measuring 2–9 mm in diameter and/or increased ovarian volume (>10 mL). TVUS is also used in women with anovulatory infertility undergoing ovulation induction to monitor the growth and number of ovarian follicles.

Management of PCOS

Reproductive Disorders

Management of menstrual cycle abnormalities and hyperandrogenism are the primary goals for patients with PCOS. Reversal of anovulation or oligo-ovulation in PCOS avoids prolonged progesterone exposure which increases the risk of endometrial hyperplasia and cancer. Women with PCOS not trying to become pregnant are treated with combined oral contraceptive pills (COCP). The combined oral contraceptive exerts antiandrogenic action by increasing the levels of SHBG and reducing circulating androgens. General guidelines should be followed when prescribing COCP in PCOS, because there is no consensus regarding specific types or doses of estrogens and progestins. The contraindications and side effects of COCP should be discussed with the patient. If estrogen in contraindicated, cyclical progestogens, e.g., medroxyprogesterone acetate, can be used to regulate menses in PCOS patients with amenorrhea or oligomenorrhea.

Metformin improves insulin resistance and may enhance ovulation and regulate the menses; however, metformin does not reduce hyperandrogenism or prevent pregnancy. Extended-release preparation is preferred, starting at a low dose, with 500 mg increments weekly, to a maximum of 2.5 g in adults and 2 g in adolescents, to reduce side effects and improve compliance. Metfomin use is associated with vitamin B12 deficiency, especially in patients with diabetes, post-bariatric surgery, pernicious anemia, or on vegan diet. Patients should be monitored and treated accordingly. Metformin in combination with the COCP may be beneficial in PCOS patients with a BMI >30 kg/m^2, impaired glucose tolerance, or diabetes.

Anovulatory infertility is common in patients with PCOS. Intermenstrual intervals longer than 35 days are considered *oligo-ovulatory* and may require ovulation induction agents for pregnancy. In normally cycling women, the serum progesterone is measured on day 21 to determine whether ovulation has occurred. In women with PCOS and long intermenstrual intervals, serum progesterone is measured 7–10 days before the next anticipated menses. The timing of ovulation can be challenging, hence ultrasound may also be used to document ovulation. Fertility evaluation can be postponed until the patient is ready to pursue pregnancy. In PCOS patients with overweight or obesity, weight loss improves the likelihood of ovulation, conception, and pregnancy outcomes. Diet, exercise, and lifestyle interventions are essential during fertility treatment. Letrozole should be the first-line drug therapy for anovulatory infertility in women with PCOS, if there are no other infertility factors [44]. Letrozole use is off-label in some countries; where it is not allowed, clomiphene citrate is an alternative. Clomifene citrate causes a higher multiple pregnancy rate than letrozole, therefore patients should be monitored for multiple follicular development. If unsuccessful, the second-line therapy for anovulatory infertility is gonadotropins.

In vitro fertilization is recommended as third-line therapy, considering the use of invasive procedures and high costs involved. PCOS is associated with higher number of complications in pregnancy, intrapartum, delivery, and postpartum, due to obesity and diabetes. This requires screening and management of diabetes and hypertension, avoidance of multiple pregnancy, and weight control.

Dermatological Abnormalities

Hyperandrogenism in PCOS is characterized by hirsutism, acne, and male-pattern alopecia. The first-line treatment of hirsutism and acne in patents not seeking pregnancy is COCP. The estrogen in COCP stimulates hepatic production of SHBG, which then reduces the free (bioactive) circulating androgens. Progestins in COCP also inhibit androgen biosynthesis and impair androgen receptor binding.

Antiandrogens could be considered for the treatment of hirsutism in women with PCOS, if there is a suboptimal response after 6 months of COCP. Antiandrogens include androgen receptor blockers, e.g., spironolactone, flutamide and cyproterone acetate, and 5α-reductase inhibitor, e.g., finasteride. Patients must be counseled regarding the teratogenic potential of anti-androgen therapy, i.e., risk of feminization of male fetus. To avoid this, patients should use effective contraception, e.g., intrauterine device or COCP, while taking antiandrogen medication. Spironolactone at doses of 25–100 mg/day appears to be safe, finasteride increases the risk of hepatotoxicity, cyproterone acetate >10 mg/day increases meningioma risk, and flutamide and bicalutamide have an increased risk of severe hepatotoxicity.

Localized facial hirsutism may be treated with a topical solution of eflornithine hydrochloride, an irreversible inhibitor of ornithine decarboxylase, in the hair follicle. Hormonal therapy for hirsutism can be combined with cosmetic treatment, e.g., shaving, depilation, laser therapy, and electrolysis. Topical antibiotics, and topical or oral retinoids may be used for the treatment of acne, and minoxidil for hair transplantation and treatment of alopecia.

Other Disorders Associated with PCOS

Patients with PCOS have higher prevalence of obesity, glucose intolerance, diabetes, hypertension, obstructive sleep apnea, and mood and eating disorders [30, 40, 45, 46]. Table 2 is a summary of management recommendations.

Male Obesity and Reproductive Disorders

Secondary Hypogonadism

The most common abnormality associated with obesity in men is secondary hypogonadism (male-associated secondary hypogonadism, MOSH). Overall, obesity suppresses the hypothalamic-pituitary-testicular (HPT) axis, but results in population studies may be influenced by degree of adiposity, age, as well as comorbid conditions, e.g., diabetes and sleep apnea, infections and pro-inflammatory states, and drugs, e.g., opioids and glucocorticoids [47, 48]. Men with severe obesity have decreased total and free testosterone levels as well as reduced inhibin-B and LH pulse amplitude and secretion [48, 49]. These changes are mediated via peripheral factors, i.e., hyper-leptinemia, leptin resistance, hyperinsulinemia, insulin resistance, and increased peripheral conversion of testosterone to estrogen and a chronic inflammatory state, interacting with kisspeptin and other CNS pathways to disrupt the HPT axis [47, 48].

In young and middle-aged men with class I obesity (BMI 30 to <35 kg/m^2) and class II obesity (BMI 35 to <40 kg/m^2), the total testosterone is low, free testosterone is normal, gonadotrophins are not elevated, and dynamic testing with GnRH, clomiphene, or human chorionic gonadotrophin

Table 2 Management of disorders associated with PCOS

Disorder	Recommendation
Obesity: Patients with PCOS have high prevalence of obesity	• Lifestyle intervention: healthy diet, exercise, and behavioral strategies • Behavioral strategies: set realistic goals, self-monitoring, problem-solving, reinforcement, emotional wellbeing, and maintenance of healthy lifestyle • Prevention of further weight gain, and long-term weight maintenance • In overweight or obese patients, the energy deficit target for weight loss should be individualized • Good diet quality, allowing for a flexible, individualized dietary approach to achieve healthy weight (5–10% less), and avoid unhealthy (nutritionally unbalanced/fad) diets • Physical activity in all forms • Limit sedentary time (sitting and screen time) and increase light, moderate high intensity activities (walking, housework, and exercise) • Minimum of 250 min/week of moderate intensity activities, or 150 min/week of high intensity activities. Strength exercises on 2 days per week
Glucose intolerance: Patients with PCOS have increased risk of impaired fasting glucose, glucose intolerance, and type 2 diabetes regardless of age and BMI	• Assess glycemic status at the time of diagnosis • Assess glycemic status every 1–3 years, based on individual risk factors • Assess glycemic status using the 75 g oral glucose tolerance test (OGTT) • Measure fasting plasma glucose and/or glycated HbA1c if OGTT cannot be done • OGTT should be done when planning pregnancy • If not performed preconception, OGTT can be done at the first prenatal visit, and should be done at 24–28 weeks of gestation • Combination of COCP and metformin is beneficial in patients with BMI >30 kg/m^2, impaired glucose tolerance, or type 2 diabetes • GLP-1 receptor agonists should be considered for obesity treatment • Bariatric surgery could be considered for weight loss
Cardiovascular disease: Patients with PCOS have an increased risk of cardiovascular disease, though the overall risk of cardiovascular disease is low in premenopausal women	• Assess plasma lipid profile (total cholesterol, LDL cholesterol, HDL cholesterol, and triglyceride) at diagnosis of PCOS, and thereafter based on the extent of hyperlipidemia and other cardiovascular risk factors • Measure blood pressure annually and when planning pregnancy or seeking fertility treatment
Obstructive sleep apnea: Patients with PCOS have higher prevalence of obstructive sleep apnea, independent of BMI	• Assess for symptoms of obstructive sleep apnea (snoring, daytime sleepiness or fatigue, and apneic episodes), screen with validated questionnaire, and refer to a sleep specialist, if necessary
Eating disorders: Eating disorders and disordered eating should be assessed in PCOS, regardless of BMI	• If eating disorder is detected, refer patient to qualified practitioners for further assessment and management
Anxiety and depression: PCOS is associated with high prevalence of anxiety and/or depressive symptoms	• Screen for anxiety and depression using validated tools • If anxiety or depressive symptoms are detected, refer patient to qualified practitioners or further assessment and management

shows normal pituitary and testicular functions [50, 51]. The low total testosterone concentration is caused by a reduction in sex hormone binding globulin (SHBG) that binds to testosterone in the circulation. Typically, there is no clinical evidence of androgen deficiency associated with hypogonadism in mild obesity [50, 51]. In contrast, in more severe obesity, i.e., class III obesity (BMI $\geq$ 40 kg/m^2), the total testosterone is low, free testosterone and gonadotropins may be reduced, and LH pulse amplitude and secretion are diminished [47, 48, 52].

A meta-analysis of 18 studies with a total of 4546 men with obesity found a high prevalence of low testosterone (50–80%) [53]. Although advanced age is a major contributor to HPT axis suppression, several studies show that obesity independently leads to low testosterone levels. Obesity is associated with reduced testosterone levels even in young men aged 24–41 years [54]. The Coronary Artery Risk Development in Young Adults (CARDIA) study showed a close association of obesity, especially central obesity, and low testosterone in young men aged 18–30 years [46, 54]. Among men with obesity aged 33–45 years in a primary care setting, up to 75% have low testosterone, and this high prevalence is similar to that seen in older men with obesity [55, 56]. In the MMAS, an increase in BMI of 4–5 kg/m^2 was associated with reduced testosterone levels [57]. In the European Male Aging Study (EMAS) comprising of 3369 men aged 40–79 years, men with BMI $\geq$30 kg/m^2 had 30% lower testosterone levels, and 13-fold increase in prevalence of low testosterone compared to men with normal weight [58]. Moreover, the prospective EMAS data showed that after 4 years of follow-up, 10% weight gain was associated with 2.4 nmol/L reduction in testosterone, while 10% reduction in weight was associated with 2.9 nmol/L increase in testosterone [59].

MOSH is associated with sexual dysfunction, impaired fertility, osteopenia, reduction in muscle mass and physical performance, and increased body fat [60, 61]. In the EMAS, obesity was associated with low testosterone levels and sexual dysfunction [62]. In the T trials comprising of men with low testosterone and clinical evidence of androgen deficiency, 63% of participants were obese [63]. Low testosterone levels associated with obesity and comorbid conditions such as diabetes and sleep apnea contribute to subfertility or infertility, erectile dysfunction, and abnormal semen quality [50, 64].

Metabolic and Reproductive Effects of Low Testosterone

There is also evidence for a reverse effect of low testosterone levels on the development of obesity. A study of 3351 men showed that low testosterone level is associated with higher BMI, waist size, and risk of metabolic syndrome [65]. Low testosterone is a strong predictor of visceral fat accumulation [66]. Induction of hypogonadism in men with prostate cancer increases total body fat as well as visceral fat [67]. Conversely, testosterone treatment reduces BMI, waist circumference, waist-to-height ratio, total body fat mass, and visceral fat [68–70]. In a study of 115 men receiving testosterone undecanoate injections for 10 years, body weight decreased by 18.5%, and waist circumference decreased by 12% [71].

The effect of testosterone treatment was studied in 823 men, 474 (57.6%) obese, 286 (34.8%) overweight, and 63 (7.7%) normal weight [72]. Testosterone undecanoate injections were administered every 12 weeks for up to 11 years in 281 men with obesity, 121 men with overweight, and 26 men with normal weight, and the remaining 395 men served as controls. Testosterone treatment reduced body weight by 4.8% in the normal weight group while the control group gained 8% in weight. In the overweight group, testosterone treatment resulted in 9.6% weight loss in men, while the control group gained 6.9% in weight. In the obese group, testosterone treatment resulted in 20.6% weight loss, while the control group gained 5.1% in weight. Similar changes were seen in the waist circumference and were accompanied by corresponding changes in glucose and lipids [72].

In 316 men with prediabetes and low testosterone, testosterone treatment led to significant improvement in fasting blood glucose and HbA$_{1c}$, whereas the untreated group worsened over time [73]. Testosterone treatment decreased body weight by 8%, while the control group gained 9% in weight [73]. Another study of 356 men with type 2 diabetes and low testosterone showed significant reduction in body weight and waist circumference and improvement in glycemic parameters [74]. Testosterone-treated men had a reduction in insulin dose requirement compared with the untreated group, 46.6% of the testosterone-treated group achieved normal glucose control, whereas no reduction in glucose or HbA$_{1c}$ levels was observed in the untreated group [74]. Thus, testosterone treatment improves beta cell function in patients with obesity and diabetes and low testosterone.

Men with obesity and moderate-to-severe erectile dysfunction or lower urinary tract symptoms may benefit from testosterone treatment [72, 75]. Testosterone undecanoate injections for up to 12 years significantly reduced body weight, waist circumference, and BMI, and improved erectile dysfunction [72].

Testosterone Therapy

The diagnosis of secondary hypogonadism in men with obesity should be comprehensive and guided by each patient's symptoms of androgen deficiency, potential benefits, and risks (Table 3). Testosterone deficiency should be evaluated using reliable assays, and testosterone replacement therapy recommended only for conditions that are likely to improve, and avoided in conditions that could be adversely impacted, such as prostate cancer, heart failure, hypercoagulation, or erythrocytosis. The benefits of testosterone therapy, i.e., body composition (body fat and muscle mass), muscle strength, sexual function, HbA$_{1c}$, lipids, and quality of life require long-term treatment.

Table 3 Testosterone therapy for hypogonadism in men with obesity

Parameter	Recommendation
Diagnosis	• Diagnosis of hypogonadism in men with clinical symptoms and signs consistent with testosterone deficiency, and repeated serum testosterone concentrations measured using accurate assays for total and free testosterone on fasting morning serum samples • Distinguish between primary and secondary hypogonadism by measuring serum LH and FSH levels
Testosterone therapy	• Primary treatment of obesity, diabetes, and sleep apnea • Testosterone therapy can be used to improve symptoms of testosterone deficiency • Discuss potential benefits and risks • Assess prostate cancer risk before starting testosterone treatment, 3–12 months after starting testosterone, and plan long-term monitoring
Contraindication	• Testosterone therapy should not be routinely prescribed to older men (≥ 65 years) or patients with type 2 diabetes with low testosterone levels • Men planning fertility • Breast cancer, prostate cancer, palpable prostate nodule or induration, and prostate-specific antigen (PSA) >4 ng/mL, PSA >3 ng/mL with high prostate cancer risk (without further evaluation) • Elevated hematocrit • Severe untreated obstructive sleep apnea • Severe untreated lower urinary tract symptoms • Heart failure, myocardial infarction, or stroke within the last 6 months
Monitoring	• Evaluate symptoms and signs of androgen deficiency, compliance, and adverse effects • Urological evaluation during the first 12 months of testosterone therapy if PSA >1.4 ng/mL above baseline, or PSA >4.0 ng/mL, or prostate abnormality is detected on digital rectal examination • After 1 year, if there is no abnormality, prostate monitoring should be based on standard guidelines according to and race of the patient

Obesity, Weight Loss, and Fertility

Epidemiological studies have described conflicting associations between obesity and sperm parameters [76, 77]. There is a J-curve relationship between BMI and sperm quality: An optimal sperm concentration is associated with normal BMI, and a reduction in sperm concentration is associated with lower BMI <20 or a higher BMI >25. After adjusting the data for age, ethnicity, smoking, alcohol, and medication use, being overweight was associated with reduction in ejaculate volume and sperm motility [78]. A meta-analysis of 13,077 overweight or obese men showed higher odds of having oligospermia or azoospermia [77]. Some studies have reported a decline in semen volume, total sperm count, or sperm concentration, without changes in sperm motility, and others have not found a significant association between adiposity and semen parameters [78–80]. Mechanisms proposed to explain adverse effects of obesity on spermatogenesis include low serum testosterone, increased scrotal temperature, and oxidative stress.

Obesity in men is also associated with worse pregnancy outcomes [81–83]. Men with obesity are more likely to experience infertility during treatment, and the live birth per cycle of in vitro fertilization may be reduced [82, 83]. However, studies are often low quality or have multiple confounding factors. Paternal obesity may have a negative impact on offspring health via epigenetic and transgenerational mechanisms [84].

Weight loss in men with obesity increases serum testosterone levels and may have positive effects on sexual function and semen parameters [85, 86]. A study of 32 overweight and 86 obese men on a weight loss regimen found an increase in total and free testosterone levels during the weight loss and maintenance phases [86]. Hakonsen et al. [87] studied 43 men with severe obesity over 14 weeks of weight loss and found an increased levels of testosterone, SHBG, AMH, total sperm count, and semen volume.

Studies have also examined the impact of bariatric surgery on sex hormones in men with obesity [88]. A retrospective cohort study of patients undergoing laparoscopic sleeve gastrectomy or Roux-en-Y gastric bypass investigated sexual function using the International Index of Erectile Function (IIEF) questionnaire. Sex hormones were measured before and at least one-year post-surgery. BMI and waist circumference were negatively correlated with testosterone levels, and BMI was a predictor of severity of erectile dysfunction. Both types of bariatric surgery led to improvement in sexual function [89]. A prospective study showed a positive impact of sleeve gastrectomy on increasing testosterone levels and improving semen parameters at 12 months [90]. The serum testosterone levels significantly increased after surgical weight loss, and the sperm concentration increased significantly in azoospermic and oligospermic groups compared to the normospermic group [90]. Other studies have reported significant improvement in FSH, LH, total and free testosterone, SHBG, semen volume, total sperm count, sperm viability, and DNA fragmentation rate [88].

Conclusion

Obesity and metabolic syndrome are closely associated with adverse effects on reproduction. PCOS is associated with infertility, adverse pregnancy outcomes, metabolic dysfunction, and increased cardiovascular risk. MOSH is associated with infertility, metabolic dysfunction, and increased cardiovascular risk. Although progress has been made over the past decades, current diagnostic and management approaches are based on component diseases instead of specific pathways linking the HPG axis to metabolism and regulation of various systems. In this review, we provide an update on the pathophysiology, diagnosis, clinical features, and treatment of PCOS and MOSH, including lifestyle and medical treatment. We discuss evidence-based guidelines for management. Knowledge gaps include genetic and environmental etiology, whether PCOS is primarily initiated by CNS and/or peripheral mechanisms, the role of adipose tissue as an energy storage site as well as a source of adipokines and other secreted factors connecting energy homeostasis and regulation of HPG axis,

the effects of obesity-related inflammation on metabolism and reproduction, the mechanisms connecting PCOS and MOSH to metabolic syndrome, obstructive sleep apnea, and mental health disorders, and the long-term health benefits of reversal of PCOS and MOSH.

Cross-References

▷ Adipokines and Metabolism
▷ Bariatric Surgery
▷ Diet and Obesity
▷ Diet, Exercise, and Behavior Therapy
▷ Endocrine Disorders Associated with Obesity
▷ Overview of Metabolic Syndrome
▷ Principles of Energy Homeostasis

Acknowledgments RSA is supported by Bloomberg Distinguished Professorship. JPD is supported by National Institutes of Health grant K01-AG079680.

References

1. Hill JW, Elias CF. Neuroanatomical framework of the metabolic control of reproduction. Physiol Rev. 2018;98(4):2349–80.
2. Ahima RS. Body fat, leptin, and hypothalamic amenorrhea. N Engl J Med. 2004;351(10):959–62.
3. Frisch RE. Body fat, menarche, fitness and fertility. Hum Reprod. 1987;2(6):521–33.
4. Akinci B, Meral R, Oral EA. Phenotypic and genetic characteristics of lipodystrophy: pathophysiology, metabolic abnormalities, and comorbidities. Curr Diab Rep. 2018;18(12):143–9.
5. Boutari C, Pappas PD, Mintziori G, et al. The effect of underweight on female and male reproduction. Metabolism. 2020;107:154229.
6. Witchel SF, Azziz R, Oberfield SE. History of polycystic ovary syndrome, premature adrenarche, and hyperandrogenism in pediatric endocrinology. Horm Res Paediatr. 2022;95(6):557–67.
7. Vatier C, Christin-Maitre S, Vigouroux C. Role of insulin resistance on fertility – focus on polycystic ovary syndrome. Ann Endocrinol (Paris). 2022;83(3): 199–202.
8. Practice Committee of the American Society for Reproductive Medicine. American Society for Reproductive Medicine position statement on qualifications for providing ultrasound procedures in reproductive medicine. Fertil Steril. 2022;118(4):668–70.
9. Ahmed B, Konje JC. The epidemiology of obesity in reproduction. Best Pract Res Clin Obstet Gynaecol. 2023;89:102342.
10. Ameratunga D, Gebeh A, Amoako A. Obesity and male infertility. Best Pract Res Clin Obstet Gynaecol. 2023;90:102393.
11. WHO. https://www.who.int/news-room/fact-sheets/detail/obesity-and-overweight Website.
12. World obesity. https://www.worldobesity.org/resources/resource-library/world-obesity-atlas-2023 Website.
13. CDC. https://www.cdc.gov/nchs/fastats/obesity-overweight.htm Website.
14. Escobar-Morreale HF. Polycystic ovary syndrome: definition, aetiology, diagnosis and treatment. Nat Rev Endocrinol. 2018;14(5):270–84.
15. Gambineri A, Patton L, Altieri P, et al. Polycystic ovary syndrome is a risk factor for type 2 diabetes: results from a long-term prospective study. Diabetes. 2012;61(9): 2369–74.
16. Gibson-Helm M, Teede H, Dunaif A, Dokras A. Delayed diagnosis and a lack of information associated with dissatisfaction in women with polycystic ovary syndrome. J Clin Endocrinol Metab. 2017;102(2):604–12.
17. Dokras A, Saini S, Gibson-Helm M, Schulkin J, Cooney L, Teede H. Gaps in knowledge among physicians regarding diagnostic criteria and management of polycystic ovary syndrome. Fertil Steril. 2017;107(6): 1380–1386.e1.
18. Al Wattar BH, Bueno A, Martin MG, et al. Harmonizing research outcomes for polycystic ovary syndrome (HARP), a marathon not a sprint: current challenges and future research need. Hum Reprod. 2021;36(3): 523–8.
19. Gorsic LK, Dapas M, Legro RS, Hayes MG, Urbanek M. Functional genetic variation in the anti-Mullerian hormone pathway in women with polycystic ovary syndrome. J Clin Endocrinol Metab. 2019;104(7): 2855–74.
20. Brower MA, Hai Y, Jones MR, et al. Bidirectional Mendelian randomization to explore the causal relationships between body mass index and polycystic ovary syndrome. Hum Reprod. 2019;34(1):127–36.
21. Shrivastava S, Conigliaro RL. Polycystic ovarian syndrome. Med Clin North Am. 2023;107(2):227–34.
22. Risal S, Pei Y, Lu H, et al. Prenatal androgen exposure and transgenerational susceptibility to polycystic ovary syndrome. Nat Med. 2019;25(12):1894–904.
23. Ruth KS, Day FR, Tyrrell J, et al. Using human genetics to understand the disease impacts of testosterone in men and women. Nat Med. 2020;26(2):252–8.
24. Teede H, Misso M, Tassone EC, et al. Anti-Mullerian hormone in PCOS: a review informing international guidelines. Trends Endocrinol Metab. 2019;30(7): 467–78.
25. Tay CT, Hart RJ, Hickey M, et al. Updated adolescent diagnostic criteria for polycystic ovary syndrome: impact on prevalence and longitudinal body mass

index trajectories from birth to adulthood. BMC Med. 2020;18(1):389.

26. Risal S, Li C, Luo Q, et al. Transgenerational transmission of reproductive and metabolic dysfunction in the male progeny of polycystic ovary syndrome. Cell Rep Med. 2023;4(5):101035.

27. Lim SS, Norman RJ, Davies MJ, Moran LJ. The effect of obesity on polycystic ovary syndrome: a systematic review and meta-analysis. Obes Rev. 2013;14(2):95–109.

28. Paixao L, Ramos RB, Lavarda A, Morsh DM, Spritzer PM. Animal models of hyperandrogenism and ovarian morphology changes as features of polycystic ovary syndrome: a systematic review. Reprod Biol Endocrinol. 2017;15(1):12.

29. Indran IR, Lee BH, Yong E. Cellular and animal studies: insights into pathophysiology and therapy of PCOS. Best Pract Res Clin Obstet Gynaecol. 2016;37:12–24.

30. Roland AV, Moenter SM. Reproductive neuroendocrine dysfunction in polycystic ovary syndrome: insight from animal models. Front Neuroendocrinol. 2014;35(4):494–511.

31. Rosenfield RL, Ehrmann DA. The pathogenesis of Polycystic Ovary Syndrome (PCOS): the hypothesis of PCOS as functional ovarian Hyperandrogenism revisited. Endocr Rev. 2016;37(5):467–520.

32. Wekker V, van Dammen L, Koning A, et al. Long-term cardiometabolic disease risk in women with PCOS: a systematic review and meta-analysis. Hum Reprod Update. 2020;26(6):942–60.

33. Berni TR, Morgan CL, Rees DA. Women with polycystic ovary syndrome have an increased risk of major cardiovascular events: a population study. J Clin Endocrinol Metab. 2021;106(9):e3369–80.

34. Bahri Khomami M, Joham AE, Boyle JA, et al. Increased maternal pregnancy complications in polycystic ovary syndrome appear to be independent of obesity-a systematic review, meta-analysis, and meta-regression. Obes Rev. 2019;20(5):659–74.

35. Valgeirsdottir H, Kunovac Kallak T, Sundstrom Poromaa I, et al. Polycystic ovary syndrome and risk of stillbirth: a nationwide register-based study. BJOG. 2021;128(13):2073–82.

36. Joham AE, Nanayakkara N, Ranasinha S, et al. Obesity, polycystic ovary syndrome and breastfeeding: an observational study. Acta Obstet Gynecol Scand. 2016;95(4):458–66.

37. Kakoly NS, Earnest A, Teede HJ, Moran LJ, Joham AE. The impact of obesity on the incidence of type 2 diabetes among women with polycystic ovary syndrome. Diabetes Care. 2019;42(4):560–7.

38. Ramezani Tehrani F, Montazeri SA, Hosseinpanah F, et al. Trend of cardio-metabolic risk factors in polycystic ovary syndrome: a population-based prospective cohort study. PLoS One. 2015;10(9):e0137609.

39. Paschou SA, Polyzos SA, Anagnostis P, et al. Non-alcoholic fatty liver disease in women with polycystic ovary syndrome. Endocrine. 2020;67(1):1–8.

40. Rocha ALL, Faria LC, Guimaraes TCM, et al. Non-alcoholic fatty liver disease in women with polycystic ovary syndrome: systematic review and meta-analysis. J Endocrinol Investig. 2017;40(12):1279–88.

41. Asfari MM, Sarmini MT, Baidoun F, et al. Association of non-alcoholic fatty liver disease and polycystic ovarian syndrome. BMJ Open Gastroenterol. 2020;7(1): e000352. https://doi.org/10.1136/bmjgast-000352.

42. Mantovani A, Petracca G, Csermely A, et al. Non-alcoholic fatty liver disease and risk of new-onset heart failure: an updated meta-analysis of about 11 million individuals. Gut. 2022.

43. Gastaldelli A, Cusi K. From NASH to diabetes and from diabetes to NASH: mechanisms and treatment options. JHEP Rep. 2019;1(4):312–28.

44. Wang R, Kim BV, van Wely M, et al. Treatment strategies for women with WHO group II anovulation: systematic review and network meta-analysis. BMJ. 2017;356:j138.

45. Teede HJ, Tay CT, Laven JJE, et al. Recommendations from the 2023 international evidence-based guideline for the assessment and management of polycystic ovary syndrome. J Clin Endocrinol Metab. 2023.

46. Gapstur SM, Kopp P, Gann PH, Chiu BC, Colangelo LA, Liu K. Changes in BMI modulate age-associated changes in sex hormone binding globulin and total testosterone, but not bioavailable testosterone in young adult men: the CARDIA male hormone study. Int J Obes. 2007;31(4):685–91.

47. Giagulli VA, Kaufman JM, Vermeulen A. Pathogenesis of the decreased androgen levels in obese men. J Clin Endocrinol Metab. 1994;79(4):997–1000.

48. Veldhuis J, Yang R, Roelfsema F, Takahashi P. Proinflammatory cytokine infusion attenuates LH's feedforward on testosterone secretion: modulation by age. J Clin Endocrinol Metab. 2016;101(2):539–49.

49. Vermeulen A, Kaufman JM, Deslypere JP, Thomas G. Attenuated luteinizing hormone (LH) pulse amplitude but normal LH pulse frequency, and its relation to plasma androgens in hypogonadism of obese men. J Clin Endocrinol Metab. 1993;76(5):1140–6.

50. Glass AR, Swerdloff RS, Bray GA, Dahms WT, Atkinson RL. Low serum testosterone and sex-hormone-binding-globulin in massively obese men. J Clin Endocrinol Metab. 1977;45(6):1211–9.

51. Schneider G, Kirschner MA, Berkowitz R, Ertel NH. Increased estrogen production in obese men. J Clin Endocrinol Metab. 1979;48(4):633–8.

52. Dias JP, Veldhuis JD, Carlson O, et al. Effects of transdermal testosterone gel or an aromatase inhibitor on serum concentration and pulsatility of growth hormone in older men with age-related low testosterone. Metabolism. 2017;69:143–7.

53. van Hulsteijn LT, Pasquali R, Casanueva F, et al. Prevalence of endocrine disorders in obese patients: systematic review and meta-analysis. Eur J Endocrinol. 2020;182(1):11–21.

54. Gapstur SM, Gann PH, Kopp P, Colangelo L, Longcope C, Liu K. Serum androgen concentrations

in young men: a longitudinal analysis of associations with age, obesity, and race. The CARDIA male hormone study. Cancer Epidemiol Biomark Prev. 2002;11 (10 Pt 1):1041–7.

55. Molina-Vega M, Asenjo-Plaza M, Garcia-Ruiz MC, et al. Cross-sectional, primary care-based study of the prevalence of hypoandrogenemia in nondiabetic young men with obesity. Obesity (Silver Spring). 2019;27(10): 1584–90.

56. Calderon B, Gomez-Martin JM, Vega-Pinero B, et al. Prevalence of male secondary hypogonadism in moderate to severe obesity and its relationship with insulin resistance and excess body weight. Andrology. 2016;4 (1):62–7.

57. Travison TG, Araujo AB, Esche GR, McKinlay JB. The relationship between body composition and bone mineral content: threshold effects in a racially and ethnically diverse group of men. Osteoporos Int. 2008;19(1):29–38.

58. Wu FCW, Tajar A, Pye SR, et al. Hypothalamic-pituitary-testicular axis disruptions in older men are differentially linked to age and modifiable risk factors: the European Male Aging Study. J Clin Endocrinol Metab. 2008;93(7):2737–45.

59. Camacho EM, Huhtaniemi IT, O'Neill TW, et al. Age-associated changes in hypothalamic-pituitary-testicular function in middle-aged and older men are modified by weight change and lifestyle factors: longitudinal results from the European Male Ageing Study. Eur J Endocrinol. 2013;168(3):445–55.

60. Tajar A, Huhtaniemi IT, O'Neill TW, et al. Characteristics of androgen deficiency in late-onset hypogonadism: results from the European Male Aging Study (EMAS). J Clin Endocrinol Metab. 2012;97(5): 1508–16.

61. Krasnoff JB, Basaria S, Pencina MJ, et al. Free testosterone levels are associated with mobility limitation and physical performance in community-dwelling men: the Framingham Offspring Study. J Clin Endocrinol Metab. 2010;95(6):2790–9.

62. Wu FCW, Tajar A, Beynon JM, et al. Identification of late-onset hypogonadism in middle-aged and elderly men. N Engl J Med. 2010;363(2):123–35.

63. Snyder PJ, Bhasin S, Cunningham GR, et al. Effects of testosterone treatment in older men. N Engl J Med. 2016;374(7):611–24.

64. Kley HK, Deselaers T, Peerenboom H. Evidence for hypogonadism in massively obese males due to decreased free testosterone. Horm Metab Res. 1981;13(11):639–41.

65. Chasland LC, Knuiman MW, Divitini ML, et al. Higher circulating androgens and higher physical activity levels are associated with less central adiposity and lower risk of cardiovascular death in older men. Clin Endocrinol. 2019;90(2):375–83.

66. Tsai EC, Boyko EJ, Leonetti DL, Fujimoto WY. Low serum testosterone level as a predictor of increased visceral fat in Japanese-American men. Int J Obes Relat Metab Disord. 2000;24(4):485–91.

67. Hamilton EJ, Gianatti E, Strauss BJ, et al. Increase in visceral and subcutaneous abdominal fat in men with prostate cancer treated with androgen deprivation therapy. Clin Endocrinol. 2011;74(3):377–83.

68. Snyder PJ, Peachey H, Hannoush P, et al. Effect of testosterone treatment on body composition and muscle strength in men over 65 years of age. J Clin Endocrinol Metab. 1999;84(8):2647–53.

69. Marin P, Holmang S, Jonsson L, et al. The effects of testosterone treatment on body composition and metabolism in middle-aged obese men. Int J Obes Relat Metab Disord. 1992;16(12):991–7.

70. Dias JP, Melvin D, Simonsick EM, et al. Effects of aromatase inhibition vs. testosterone in older men with low testosterone: randomized-controlled trial. Andrology. 2016;4(1):33–40.

71. Yassin AA, Nettleship J, Almehmadi Y, Salman M, Saad F. Effects of continuous long-term testosterone therapy (TTh) on anthropometric, endocrine and metabolic parameters for up to 10 years in 115 hypogonadal elderly men: real-life experience from an observational registry study. Andrologia. 2016;48(7):793–9.

72. Saad F, Caliber M, Doros G, Haider KS, Haider A. Long-term treatment with testosterone undecanoate injections in men with hypogonadism alleviates erectile dysfunction and reduces risk of major adverse cardiovascular events, prostate cancer, and mortality. Aging Male. 2020;23(1):81–92.

73. Yassin A, Haider A, Haider KS, et al. Testosterone therapy in men with hypogonadism prevents progression from prediabetes to type 2 diabetes: eight-year data from a registry study. Diabetes Care. 2019;42(6): 1104–11.

74. Haider KS, Haider A, Saad F, et al. Remission of type 2 diabetes following long-term treatment with injectable testosterone undecanoate in patients with hypogonadism and type 2 diabetes: 11-year data from a real-world registry study. Diabetes Obes Metab. 2020;22 (11):2055–68.

75. Saad F, Doros G, Haider KS, Haider A. Hypogonadal men with moderate-to-severe lower urinary tract symptoms have a more severe cardiometabolic risk profile and benefit more from testosterone therapy than men with mild lower urinary tract symptoms. Investig Clin Urol. 2018;59(6):399–409.

76. Macdonald AA, Stewart AW, Farquhar CM. Body mass index in relation to semen quality and reproductive hormones in New Zealand men: a cross-sectional study in fertility clinics. Hum Reprod. 2013;28(12): 3178–87.

77. Sermondade N, Faure C, Fezeu L, et al. BMI in relation to sperm count: an updated systematic review and collaborative meta-analysis. Hum Reprod Update. 2013;19(3):221–31.

78. Hammiche F, Laven JSE, Twigt JM, Boellaard WPA, Steegers EAP, Steegers-Theunissen RP. Body mass index and central adiposity are associated with sperm quality in men of subfertile couples. Hum Reprod. 2012;27(8):2365–72.

79. Guo D, Wu W, Tang Q, et al. The impact of BMI on sperm parameters and the metabolite changes of seminal plasma concomitantly. Oncotarget. 2017;8(30):48619–34.

80. Eisenberg ML, Kim S, Chen Z, Sundaram R, Schisterman EF, Louis GMB. The relationship between male BMI and waist circumference on semen quality: data from the LIFE study. Hum Reprod. 2015;30(2):493–4.

81. Bakos HW, Mitchell M, Setchell BP, Lane M. The effect of paternal diet-induced obesity on sperm function and fertilization in a mouse model. Int J Androl. 2011;34(5 Pt 1):402–10.

82. Campbell JM, Lane M, Owens JA, Bakos HW. Paternal obesity negatively affects male fertility and assisted reproduction outcomes: a systematic review and meta-analysis. Reprod Biomed Online. 2015;31(5):593–604.

83. Merhi ZO, Keltz J, Zapantis A, et al. Male adiposity impairs clinical pregnancy rate by in vitro fertilization without affecting day 3 embryo quality. Obesity (Silver Spring). 2013;21(8):1608–12.

84. Houfflyn S, Matthys C, Soubry A. Male obesity: epigenetic origin and effects in sperm and offspring. Curr Mol Biol Rep. 2017;3(4):288–96.

85. Andersen E, Juhl CR, Kjoller ET, et al. Sperm count is increased by diet-induced weight loss and maintained by exercise or GLP-1 analogue treatment: a randomized controlled trial. Hum Reprod. 2022;37(7):1414–22.

86. Collins CE, Jensen ME, Young MD, Callister R, Plotnikoff RC, Morgan PJ. Improvement in erectile function following weight loss in obese men: the SHED-IT randomized controlled trial. Obes Res Clin Pract. 2013;7(6):450.

87. Hakonsen LB, Thulstrup AM, Aggerholm AS, et al. Does weight loss improve semen quality and reproductive hormones? Results from a cohort of severely obese men. Reprod Health. 2011;8:24.

88. Di Vincenzo A, Busetto L, Vettor R, Rossato M. Obesity, male reproductive function and bariatric surgery. Front Endocrinol (Lausanne). 2018;9:769.

89. Chen G, Sun L, Jiang S, et al. Effects of bariatric surgery on testosterone level and sexual function in men with obesity: a retrospective study. Front Endocrinol (Lausanne). 2023;13:1036243.

90. El Bardisi H, Majzoub A, Arafa M, et al. Effect of bariatric surgery on semen parameters and sex hormone concentrations: a prospective study. Reprod Biomed Online. 2016;33(5):606–11.

Metabolic Syndrome and Kidney Diseases

Vincent Boima, Alexander B. Agyekum, and Augustus K. Eduafo

Contents

V. Boima
Department of Medicine and Therapeutics, University of Ghana Medical School, College of Health Sciences, University of Ghana, Accra, Ghana
e-mail: vboima@ug.edu.gh

A. B. Agyekum
National Cardiothoracic Center, Korle Bu Teaching Hospital, Accra, Ghana

A. K. Eduafo (✉)
Wright State University Boonshoft School of Medicine, Transplant Nephrology, Dayton, OH, USA
e-mail: augustus.eduafo@wright.edu

Abstract

The metabolic syndrome (MetS) affects 20–25% of people worldwide and increases the risk of cardiovascular disease (CVD). MetS is associated with kidney abnormalities, including activation of the renin-angiotensin-aldosterone system (RAAS), glomerular hyperfiltration, podocyte injury, albuminuria, and fibrosis. This chapter describes the epidemiology and pathogenesis of chronic kidney disease (CKD) in MetS, including the roles of

© Springer Nature Switzerland AG 2023
R. S. Ahima (ed.), *Metabolic Syndrome*,
https://doi.org/10.1007/978-3-031-40116-9_57

obesity, insulin resistance, diabetes, adipokines, oxidative stress, inflammation, and endothelial dysfunction, and the current and future strategies for prevention and treatment of CKD.

Keywords

Obesity · Diabetes · Hypertension · Kidney disease · Inflammation · Albuminuria

Abbreviations

ACE-I	Angiotensin-Converting Enzyme Inhibitor
ANG II	Angiotensin II
ARB	Angiotensin Receptor Blocker
BMI	Body mass index
CHD	Congenital Heart Disease
CKD	Chronic Kidney Disease
DMT2	Diabetes Mellitus type 2
DPP-4	Dipeptidyl Peptidase 4
ESRD	End-stage kidney disease
FBS	Fasting Blood Sugar
GBM	Glomerular Basement Membrane
GDF	Growth Differentiation Factor
GFR	Glomerular Filtration Rate
GI	Gastrointestinal
HDL	High Density Lipoprotein
IR	Insulin Resistance
KDIGO	Kidney Disease Improving Global Outcomes
LDL	Low-Density Lipoprotein
MetS	Metabolic Syndrome
RAAS	Renin-Angiotensin-Aldosterone System
ROS	Reactive Oxygen Species
SGLT2	Sodium-glucose Cotransporter-2
TG	Triglycerides
VLDL	Very Low-Density Lipoprotein
WC	Waist circumference

Introduction

Chronic kidney disease (CKD) is one of the leading causes of morbidity and mortality worldwide. The risk factors for the rising incidence of CKD include obesity, hypertension, diabetes, and dyslipidemia. It is estimated that 843.6 million individuals are affected by CKD globally. Low- and middle-income countries are the most burdened by CKD due to their limited resources. In the United States, one in seven adults have CKD, and nine in ten with CKD are unaware of their disease. Approximately two in five adults with severe CKD have no knowledge that they have CKD [1–6]. CKD is more common in people aged 65 years or older (38%) compared to those aged 45–64 years (12%) or 18–44 years (6%), although, CKD patients in LMIC are mostly young. Women have a slightly higher prevalence (14%) compared to men (12%). Non-Hispanic Black adults have a higher prevalence (16%) compared to non-Hispanic White (13%), Asian (13%) or Hispanic (14%) [5, 7]. Metabolic syndrome (MetS) has adverse effects on kidney function, including glomerular hyperfiltration, RAAS activation, microalbuminuria, profibrotic factors, and podocyte injury [8].

Metabolic Syndrome

The MetS is a cluster of cardiovascular disease (CVD) risk factors [9–16]. Reaven was the first to propose the idea of "syndrome X," which he later called "MetS," speculating that it was a key factor in the development of coronary artery disease and type 2 diabetes [17]. There is no universal diagnostic standard criteria for MetS, and various studies have used different criteria proposed by the World Health Organization (WHO, 1998), National Cholesterol Education/Adult Treatment Panel III (NCEPATPIII, 2001), Modified NCEP-ATP III, 2010, American Heart Association (AHA, 2005), International Diabetes Federation (IDF, 2005), or the Chinese Diabetes Society (CDS, 2020). Central obesity, impaired glucose tolerance, waist circumference (WC), blood pressure, high density lipoprotein (HDL) cholesterol, triglycerides (TG), and glucose are often included in the diagnostic criteria. According to the WHO, diabetes or impaired glucose metabolism are the main criteria for diagnosing MetS, whereas the IDF based its diagnosis of MetS on central obesity. The prevalence of MetS varies according to different diagnostic criteria. In order to standardize the definition of MetS, the IDF, American Heart Association and the National Heart, Lung, and Blood Institute (AHA/NHLBI) issued a Joint Interim Statement (JIS). The following criteria are included in the JIS definition of MetS: (1) increased fasting blood glucose (FBG) or the use of hypoglycemic medications; (2) raised blood pressure or the use of blood pressure medications; (3) increased plasma TG or the use of lipid lowering medications; (4) a decreased HDL cholesterol; and (5) the Chinese definition of central/visceral obesity, i.e., a waist circumference of >85 cm for men and > 80 cm for women. If three or more of the aforementioned criteria were satisfied, MetS is diagnosed. The JIS and NCEP-ATPIII criteria are consistent with the China Diabetes Association and Chinese Medical Association definitions of MetS [8] (Table 1).

MetS is rising along with the obesity epidemic. In the United States, more than one-fourth of the population met the diagnostic criteria for metabolic syndrome in 2008, with over two-third of the population being overweight or obese [9]. The prevalence of MetS varies among countries, with an estimated 20–25% of the world's population having the condition. The differences in MetS prevalence are affected by gender, age, race, diet, physical activity, socioeconomic, and cultural factors. From 1980 to 2012, the prevalence of MetS in the United States rose to 35%. The National Health and Nutrition Examination (NHANES) data from 2020 revealed that the incidence rate of MetS was 24% in males and 22% in women [8]. The MetS prevalence is high in African Americans, especially women, due to the increased rates of obesity, hypertension, and diabetes. A 1988–1994 survey indicated that Mexican Americans had the greatest age-adjusted prevalence of metabolic syndrome in the United States, affecting 31.9% compared to 27% in the general population [9].

The specific causes of metabolic syndrome are unknown. Family history, poor diet, and insufficient exercise are all recognized risk factors for MetS. The growing availability and consumption of high-calorie, low-fiber fast food as well as the decline in physical activity brought on by sedentary lifestyle and mechanized transportation are major factors. At the molecular level, insulin resistance and dysfunctional adipose tissue play significant roles in the pathophysiology of MetS. Excessive accumulation of fat in adipose tissues and ectopically in the liver and skeletal muscles results in insulin resistance. The release of pro-inflammatory cytokines occurs as a result of both adipose cell enlargement and the infiltration of macrophages into adipose tissue, promoting insulin resistance. Adipose tissue's function in metabolic syndrome is influenced by how it is distributed. Subcutaneous fat does not correlate with inflammation, whereas visceral or intra-abdominal fat does. Adipokines, e.g., leptin, adiponectin, resistin, and plasminogen activator inhibitor, have been linked to abnormal glucose and lipid metabolism, oxidative stress, and vascular injury in MetS. Psychosocial stress is associated with a higher risk of MetS [9, 19–24]. In a study of 28,209 patients, those with MetS who had normoglycemia or mild hyperglycemia had annual conversion rates to diabetes of 0.6%, but those with intermediate hyperglycemia (6.1–7.0 mmol/L) had a higher diabetes conversion rate of 2.5%, putting them at high risk for CVD [25].

The Relationship Between CKD and Metabolic Syndrome

Despite the imprecise definition of MetS, it has been demonstrated to be linked to histopathological signs of CKD, such as tubular atrophy and interstitial fibrosis, and CKD markers [26]. Single or multiple components of MetS have been linked to CKD, posing a major threat to health, financial burden, and a lower quality of life [27]. Xie et al. found significant associations between CKD and MetS components, including hypertension, high triglycerides (TG), elevated fasting blood sugar (FBS), and elevated waist circumference [16]. Microalbuminuria is twice as common in MetS patients with one or two components compared to those without MetS, and 130% more common in those with more than three MetS features [25]. In patients with type 2 diabetes, MetS accurately predicted new onset CKD [25].

Table 1 Diagnosis of metabolic syndrome

	WHO, 1998	IDF, 2005	NCEP ATP III, 2004	Modified NCEP ATP III, 2010	AHA, 2005	CDS, 2020
Serum glucose	Presence of impaired glucose tolerance with any 2 of the following criteria	Presence of central adiposity with 2 or more of the following criteria	Presence of 3 or more of the following criteria			
	Plasma glucose at 2 h after glucose load ≥7.8 mmol/L	FPG ≥100 mg/dL (5.6 mmol/L) or previously diagnosed type 2 diabetes	FPG ≥ 110 mg/dL (6.1 mmol/L)	FPG ≥ 100 mg/dL (5.6 mmol/L)	FPG ≥100 mg/dL (5.6 mmol/L)	FPG ≥6.1 mmol/L or plasma glucose at 2 h after glucose load ≥7.8 mmol/L
WC	–	M: > 90 cm; F: > 80 cm	M: >102 cm; F: >88 cm	M: >102 cm; F: >88 cm (Asian origin, M: >90 cm and F: >80 cm)	M: >102 cm; F: >88 cm	M: ≥ 90 cm; F: ≥ 85 cm
BMI	>30 kg/m2					
WHR	M > 0.90; F > 0.85					
Hypertension	≥140/≥90 mmHg	≥130/≥85 mmHg	≥130/≥85 mmHg	≥130/≥85 mmHg or current use of antihypertensive drugs	≥130/≥85 mmHg	≥130/≥85 mmHg
HDL cholesterol	M: < 35 mg/dL (0.9 mmol/L); F: < 39 mg/dL (1 mmol/L)	M: < 40 mg/L (1.03 mmol/L); F: < 50 mg/L (1.29 mmol/L) or receiving treatment	M: <40 mg/dL (1.03 mmol/L); F: <50 mg/dL (1.29 mmol/L)	M: <40 mg/dL (1.03 mmol/L); F: <50 mg/dL (1.29 mmol/L)	M: <40 mg/dL (1.03 mmol/L); F: <50 mg/dL (1.29 mmol/L)	<40 mg/dL (1.04 mmol/L)
Triglycerides	≥150 mg/dL (1.7 mmol/L)	≥150 mg/dL (1.7 mmol/L) or receiving treatment	≥150 mg/dL (1.7 mmol/L)			

The MetS is an independent risk factor for the development of CKD, even after adjusting for diabetes and hypertension. Compared to those without MetS, nephrectomy patients with MetS had a higher prevalence of CKD-related signs, such as loss of kidney function and global and segmental glomerulosclerosis. Additionally, research suggests that having MetS before a kidney transplant increases the risk of developing new-onset diabetes after the procedure, and that having MetS afterward has a negative impact on allograft survival and mortality. Thus, MetS is a catalyst for kidney injury in CKD and amplifies the adverse effects of diabetes and other metabolic dysfunction [25, 28–34]. Enhanced pro-inflammatory cytokine production, insulin resistance, oxidative stress, profibrotic factor production, connective tissue expansion, increased microvascular injury, and kidney ischemia are some of the potential mechanisms of kidney damage in MetS [26].

Pathogenesis of Renal Damage from METS

Insulin resistance appears to play an important role in MetS-related CKD (Fig. 1). Insulin resistance and chronic hyperglycemia in type 2 diabetes are associated with oxidative stress, inflammation, and kidney insufficiency. Hyperinsulinemia increases the synthesis of insulin-like growth factor 1 (IGF-1), which promotes connective tissue growth and fibrosis. Obesity increases the release of leptin, interleukin-6, and tumor necrosis factor-alpha (TNF-α). Glomerulosclerosis may result from leptin-induced intrarenal expression of transforming growth factor-beta (TGF-β). The synthesis of type IV collagen may also be promoted. Reactive oxygen species (ROS) may be produced as a result of TNF-α, and ROS can then result in dysfunction of kidney endothelial cell, mesangial enlargement, and fibrosis. Adiponectin is reduced in

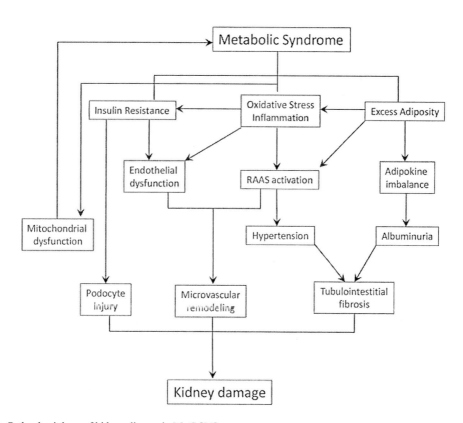

Fig. 1 Pathophysiology of kidney disease in MetS [25]

obesity and associated with insulin resistance and kidney pathology. Vascular intima thickening and proliferation of smooth muscle cells are linked to adiponectin insufficiency. Obesity results in an expanded glomerular volume, podocyte hypertrophy, and mesangial matrix growth, which precede the pathogenesis of CKD. Angiotensin II induces ROS formation in conjunction with another MetS component, hypertension, resulting in a reduction in nitric oxide synthase production and kidney microvascular injury, ischemia, and tubulointerstitial damage [26, 35–39].

Renal Microvascular Remodeling

MetS causes kidney parenchymal abnormalities like tubular atrophy and interstitial fibrosis in humans and animals. Microvascular remodeling has also been seen in kidney lesions in patients with MetS, manifesting as arterial and arteriolar sclerosis. Animal studies have provided evidence of effects of MetS on microvessels. A 6-week MetS diet containing 60% fructose in rats led to wall thickening in outer cortical and juxtamedullary afferent arterioles, simulating human arteriolar sclerosis. After 16 weeks, it was shown that the renin-angiotensin-aldosterone system (RAAS) was activated in MetS, which led to dysregulated angiogenesis, increased tissue fibrosis, and elevated levels of Ang II. Numerous cytokines that are abundant in adipose tissue, such as tumor necrosis factor (TNF)-α and interleukin-6 (IL-6), may cause neovascularization as a result of visceral adipose tissue accumulation and fat infiltration of the kidney. MetS enhanced kidney microvascular proliferation in its early stages. An increase in vascular endothelial growth factor expression likely induced by oxidative stress is seen in MetS and linked to the increase in microvascular density. The small microvessels may help to maintain kidney perfusion and explain the higher kidney blood flow and glomerular filtration rate (GFR) that defines the early stage of MetS. It is possible that in a later stage of MetS, the intrarenal vessels may be defective and unstable because those newly created vessels frequently have an unorganized architecture.

Furthermore, continuous mechanical stress brought on by hyperfiltration on glomerular capillaries increases the likelihood of microvascular loss [25, 39–47].

Inflammation, Insulin Resistance, and Kidney Disease

The kidney has been identified as a target organ frequently engaged in the inflammatory response in animal models of MetS. Pigs fed a 16-week MetS diet had higher levels of circulating oxidized low-density lipoprotein and soluble E-selectin, which attracts inflammatory cells and pro-inflammatory macrophage infiltration in the kidney, leading to the development of glomerulosclerosis. Zucker fatty diabetic rats exhibit widespread fibrosis and neutrophil infiltration in peritubular capillaries as well as macrophage infiltration in the tubular-interstitium. Inflammation may therefore have a role in MetS kidney fibrosis and glomerulosclerosis progression [25, 48, 49].

Fasting hyperinsulinemia has historically been used to identify insulin resistance. Postprandial hyperinsulinemia, however, already exists before fasting hyperinsulinemia develops. Hyper-insulinemia promotes the absorption of glucose by muscle and inhibits the liver's endogenous glucose synthesis. Insulin's capacity to increase glucose absorption and reduce hepatic glucose synthesis is compromised in insulin-resistant states. As a result, hyperglycemia is sustained, which drives postprandial insulin secretion. High insulin concentrations may overstimulate the arterial wall cells in the skeletal muscle. Typically, when insulin binds to the insulin receptor, the receptor's tyrosine kinase activity is activated. Tyrosine residues on substrate proteins are phosphorylated by the insulin receptor when it is activated, starting a signaling cascade. Phosphatidylinositol-3 kinase (PI-3K) and mitogen-activated protein (MAP) kinase pathways are the two main routes for insulin signaling. Tyrosine phosphorylation of a member of the insulin receptor substrate family, which is connected to the p85 regulatory subunit, starts the PI-3K pathway and activates the enzyme.

Phosphatidylinositol 3,4,5-phosphate (PIP3) is formed as a result of PI-3 K. As a result, Akt and other effector molecules that mediate the metabolic response to insulin are activated. This includes the membrane translocation of the glucose transporter type 4 (GLUT4). The insulin receptor substrate is phosphorylated to bind Grb2 and activate Ras, which starts the MAP kinase cascade. Ras then attaches to Raf inhibiting it and, activating MEK1 kinase. Extracellular signal-regulated kinases ERK1 and ERK2 are activated by MEK1. The mitogenic and pro-inflammatory effects of insulin signaling are mediated by the ERKs. The routes that activate PI-3K are disrupted in MetS and type 2 diabetes. Even in the presence of insulin resistance, the activation of the ERK-MAPK pathway promotes the development and proliferation of smooth muscle cells, thereby enhancing atherogenesis. Another important characteristic of MetS is that insulin resistance promotes an increase in adipose lipolysis and release of free fatty acids. The development of insulin resistance in muscle and other target tissues is significantly influenced by higher plasma free fatty acid level, which inhibits, PI-3K signaling, decreases nitric oxide, and promotes vascular endothelial dysfunction [15, 50, 51]. Reduced endothelial nitric oxide generation and increased oxidative stress are linked to insulin resistance and hyperinsulinemia, and the development of diabetic nephropathy [15, 52].

Obesity and Kidney Disease

Body mass index (BMI), measurements of central obesity (such as waist circumference and waist-to-hip ratio), and assessments of body composition are used to define obesity. The most practical method to assess the severity of obesity is BMI [53]. The WHO's classifications of obesity based on BMI are the most extensively used: underweight – BMI of <18.5 kg/m2, normal weight 18.5–24.9, overweight 25.0–29.9, Grade 1 obesity 30.0–34.9, Grade 2 obesity 35.0–39.9, Grade 3 or severe obesity ≥40.0.

Indicators of central (visceral) adiposity, which is connected to insulin resistance, dyslipidemia,

and an elevated risk of CVD, include the waist circumference and waist-to-hip ratio. When combined with BMI categories, these measurements have been demonstrated to guide the risk assessment and outcomes of CVD. Central obesity is defined as follows: Waist circumference: men >102 cm (40 in), women >88 cm (35 in), waist-to-hip ratio: men ≥0.90; women ≥0.85.

There is a need for accurate body composition assessment because the BMI is unable to distinguish between fat-free mass and fat mass. However, accurate technologies for measuring body composition, such as dual-energy X-ray absorptiometry, MRI, and CT scan are expensive, and used in research and not clinical settings [53–55].

Obesity prevalence has increased, and it is now a serious global health issue that affects both adults and children [56]. The abdominal fat surrounding the mesentery and omentum is known as visceral adipose tissue. The portal circulation receives the free fatty acids that are released from the visceral fat. In addition to adipokines, cytokines, and chemokines, adipocytes secrete angiotensinogen that regulates the synthesis of aldosterone. Aldosterone levels are elevated in MetS and linked to hypertension through renal tubular reabsorption of sodium, causing water retention [15, 57–61]. In patients with obesity, activated RAAS induces hemodynamic alterations such as increased GFR and renal plasma flow (RPF), which results in compensatory glomerulomegaly, glomerular hyperfiltration, and segmental sclerosis [8, 62–66]. Elevated aldosterone is linked to activation of transforming growth factor 1, reactive oxygen species (ROS), and plasminogen activator inhibitor-1, promoting fibrosis and kidney failure. Aldosterone also enhances the loss of podocytes, which results in a reduction in the integrity of the slit-pore membrane and consequent proteinuria. Additionally, aldosterone enhances renal tubular and interstitial oxidative stress and inflammation, which aggravate salt-induced tubulo-glomerular damage [15, 67–70]. The most prevalent morphological kidney abnormalities seen in kidney biopsies from patients with obesity are glomerulomegaly, and focal and segmental glomerulosclerosis [15, 71] (Fig. 2).

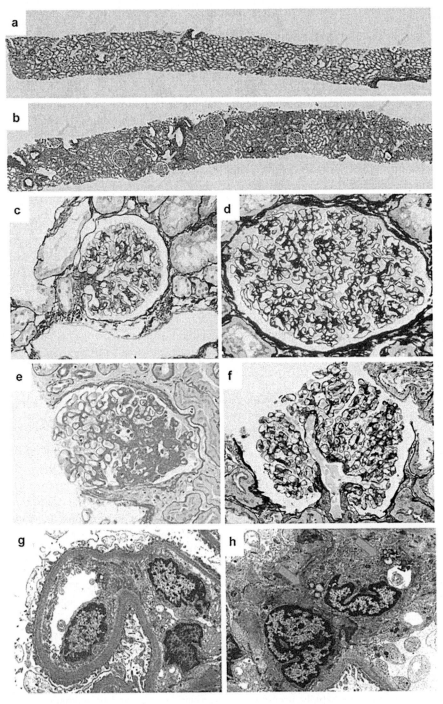

Fig. 2 Histopathology of obesity-related glomerulopathy. Kidney biopsy from (**a**) nonobese kidney transplantation donor showing normal glomerular density, and (**b**) a patient with obesity-related glomerulopathy showing reduced glomerular density. Arrows point to non-sclerotic (glomeruli stained with periodic acid-methenamine silver staining, original magnification ×25). (**c**) Glomerulus from a nonobese patient showing minimal change nephrotic syndrome. (**d**) hypertrophied glomerulus from a patient with obesity (magnification ×400). (**e**) Segmental glomerular sclerosis is often seen in relation to the vascular pole. (**f**) Dilated glomerular afferent arterioles in a patient with obesity-related glomerulopathy. (**g**) Electron micrograph showing mild thickening of the glomerular basement

Dyslipidemia and Kidney Disease

Increased small LDL particles, low HDL cholesterol, and raised triglycerides (TG) are the hallmarks of this MetS. A higher level of total apo-B, which is typically seen with atherogenic dyslipidemia, is caused by an increase in the amount of VLDL and LDL particles. Small and dense LDL particles are frequently linked to atherogenic dyslipidemia and MetS. Smaller LDL particles may enter the artery wall more readily and be more susceptible to atherogenic alteration. Atherosclerosis risk is also predicted by low HDL cholesterol levels. The dyslipidemia seen in MetS leads to increased oxidative stress and endothelial damage, both of which contribute to atherosclerosis and CKD. Low HDL cholesterol and high TG are independent risk factors for the onset of CKD [15, 73–79].

Hypertension and CKD

An important component of MetS is high blood pressure [13]. Although the prevalence of both hypertension and MetS is largely age-dependent, type 2 diabetes and the obesity epidemic have dramatically increased blood pressure (BP) levels in children [14]. Compared to lean people, obese people have a higher prevalence of high blood pressure. Hypertension is a well-known risk factor for coronary artery disease, heart failure, stroke, and CKD [15]. Insulin resistance and hyperinsulinemia affect blood pressure [12, 15]. When administered intravenously to lean individuals, insulin has a vasodilatory effect and increases renal sodium reabsorption. In people with obesity, the renal effect on sodium reabsorption can be sustained in the presence of insulin resistance while the vasodilatory effects of insulin can be lost. Salt-sensitive hypertension is also related to MetS. Hyperinsulinemia may promote salt reabsorption as a result of the increased insulin resistance in CKD [15, 80, 81]. Plasma aldosterone levels and sympathetic nerve activity both have a strong correlation with hypertension in MetS. Angiotensinogen is secreted by visceral adipocytes and activates the RAAS. Furthermore, the perinephric fat increases in people with MetS, compressing the renal parenchymal cells, leading to pressure natriuresis. Other adipokines altered in MetS patients, e.g., elevated leptin levels and low adiponectin levels, result in increased sympathetic nerve activity, which exacerbates hypertension. Ischemia from hypertension primarily damages the kidneys. Renal tubular, renal vascular, and glomerular damage are the most common effects of ischemia. Angiotensin II, which can further constrict blood vessels and cause the growth of renal parenchymal cells, is also produced and secreted more often during ischemia, which can damage the kidney through both hemodynamic and non-hemodynamic effects [8, 82–89].

Diagnosis of MetS-Related Kidney Disease

Glomerular hyperfiltration, eGFR $<60/\text{mL/min}$ per 1.73 m^2, proteinuria and/or microalbuminuria, renal tubular dysfunction, abnormalities on ultrasound (e.g., increased intrarenal resistive indices), and histopathological abnormalities are all features of MetS-related kidney disease. MetS-related renal disease is different from CKD in a patient with MetS. Glomerulomegaly, podocytopathy, mesangial cell and matrix proliferation, Glomerular basement membrane (GBM) thickening, global sclerosis, segmental sclerosis, tubular atrophy, interstitial fibrosis, and renal vascular injuries (arterial sclerosis and hyalinosis) are among the pathological features seen in MetS patients. Studies have shown that

Fig. 2 (continued) membrane, mild podocyte foot process effacement, and widening of the subendothelial space in a patient with obesity-related glomerulopathy (magnification ×5000). (**h**) Arrows point to intracytoplasmic lipid vacuoles in glomerular mesangial cells in a patient with obesity-related glomerulopathy (magnification ×5000). (This figure was reproduced from an open access article under the Creative Commons license. Tsuboi et al. [72])

some biomarkers, e.g., growth differentiation factor-11 (GDF-11), are altered in the blood and urine of MetS patients. GDF-11 has a negative correlation with BMI and WC in MetS. Growth differentiation factor 15 (GDF-15) has been independently linked to MetS and considerably higher in elderly patients with MetS [8].

Management of Kidney Disease in Metabolic Syndrome

The most crucial first measures in treating MetS are lifestyle modification and weight loss. Westernized diets are substantially linked to an increased risk of MetS, according to studies comparing ethnically similar people exposed to various dietary environments [9].

Lifestyle Modification

The use of lifestyle interventions, such as dietary changes, with a focus on a diet high in vegetables, fruits, whole grains, medium-chain fatty acids, and short-chain fatty acids, aerobic exercise, adequate sleep, quitting smoking, improve the outcome of MetS [8]. The DASH diet, high in low-fat dairy foods, fruits and vegetables, has positive benefits on blood pressure and lipids. Fruit and vegetable fiber and other phytonutrients may provide protection by reducing cholesterol or inflammation [15, 90, 91].

First-line treatments to halt the course of MetS kidney damage include weight management and exercise. The Coronary Artery Risk Development in Young Adults (CARDIA) study serves as an example of the importance of weight control in reducing the progression of MetS. When compared to young individuals who maintained stable body mass index (BMI) across the research period, regardless of the baseline BMI, increasing the BMI over 15 years was related with unfavorable progression of MetS components in this observational analysis of 5115 young adults, ages 18–30 years. A multimodal strategy to weight loss, involving food, exercise, and medications, is most effective [92–95]. In addition to helping people lose weight, exercise may also

help them lose abdominal fat more specifically, at least in females. Guidelines for physical activity recommend practical, consistent, and moderate exercise routines. A daily minimum of 30 min of moderate-intensity physical activity, including brisk walking, is the typical exercise prescription. The positive effect on metabolic health appears to be further enhanced by increasing physical activity levels [90, 95, 96]. Studies have shown that food restriction, especially when paired with aerobic activity, lowers serum creatinine and albuminuria, raises the GFR, improves renal hemodynamics, and lowers the risk of kidney stone formation [8].

Antihypertensive Medications

Patients with MetS and hypertension are at a higher risk of developing heart and renal problems [15]. First, hypertensive patients should follow a salt-restricted diet. Antihypertensive medication administration is the second intervention. In order to regulate hypertension in MetS, it is advised to utilize angiotensin-converting enzyme inhibitors (ACEI) and angiotensin receptor antagonists (ARB). Doing so helps to lower RAAS activation, relieve glomerular hyperfiltration, and decrease proteinuria. Exercise training and RAAS blockers work together to more effectively lower the hypertension, urine albumin-to-creatinine ratio, and serum creatinine of MetS patients. Losartan can effectively lower blood pressure while preserving the circadian rhythm of blood pressure and protecting the kidneys [97, 98].

Oral Hypoglycemics

Patients with MetS have been treated with various diabetes drugs, including metformin, pioglitazone, dipeptidyl peptidase-4 (DPP-4) inhibitors, glucagon-like peptide-1 (GLP-1) receptor agonists, and sodium-glucose cotransporter 2 (SGLT2) inhibitors. Metformin is generally safe and improves insulin sensitivity. Pioglitazone improves insulin resistance and glycemic control, and decreases inflammation, and may protect endothelial cell function. GLP-1 receptor agonists have the benefits of reducing body weight and improving glycemia. SGLT2 inhibitors reduce blood glucose, promote weight loss, and reduce blood pressure [99–104]. SGLT2 inhibitors reduces onset of heart failure and CKD patients with type 2 diabetes and improves outcomes of heart failure and CKD in patients with and without type 2 diabetes [105, 106]. For patients with heart failure pioglitazone is contraindicated [107].

Lipid-Lowering Medications

It is well known that statins are effective at significantly lowering LDL cholesterol [15]. Statins are the first-line medication for hyperlipidemia in MetS patients because of their potent ability to manage hyperlipidemia, stabilize atherosclerosis, and lower the risk of cardiovascular disease. Statins can also lessen proteinuria in individuals with MetS and slow the progression of kidney disease due to their anti-inflammatory, antioxidant, antithrombotic, anti-fibrotic effects, and improvement in endothelial function. Statin therapy in patients with MetS increased the eGFR by 13.7 ml/min/1.73 m². Statins are safe for treatment of hyperlipidemia in MetS patients with CKD [108–111].

For secondary prevention in type 2 diabetes, ATP III suggested a goal of serum low-density lipoprotein (LDL) cholesterol of less than 100 mg/dL (2.6 mmol/L), but other studies have suggested a more aggressive goal of less than 80 mg/dL (2.1 mmol/L) with a regimen that includes taking a statin [95]. Simvastatin (20–40 mg) was administered to participants in the 4S study who met the lipid criteria for MetS. They had different LDL cholesterol reduction of 37.5%, TG reduction of 24.1%, and HDL cholesterol increase of 10.3%. Rosuvastatin at a dose of 10 mg lowered TG by 23%, apolipoprotein B by 37%, and LDL cholesterol by 47%, while raising

Table 2 Therapeutic options for MetS

MetS criterion	Treatment	Effects
Obesity	Diet	Reduction in weight; improve glycemia and albuminuria
	Physical activity	Beneficial when combined with diet and/or weight loss medication
	Weight loss medication	Role in slowing CKD progression is unclear; moderate weight loss may improve GFR and albuminuria
	Bariatric surgery	Reduces weight, and improves hypertension, diabetes, dyslipidemia, and slows CKD
Dyslipidemia	Statins	Improves cardiovascular risk, but current data regarding CKD progression are conflicting
	Ezetimibe	Often combined with statins, and well tolerated in CKD
	Niacin	Triglyceride reduction and positive effects on phosphate metabolism; limited by side effect profile
	Omega-3 polyunsaturated fatty acids	Reduction in albuminuria; no effect on GFR
Hypertension	ACEI/ARB	Recommended for MetS patients
	Thiazide diuretics	May worsen glycemia; need to watch for hyperuricemia and hypokalemia, which can lead to worsening CKD
Diabetes mellitus	Thiazolidinedione (Pioglitazone)	Reduction in albuminuria; improve glycemia
	Dipeptidyl peptidase-4 (DPP-4) inhibitors	Improve glycemia
	Glucagon-like peptide-1 (GLP-1) receptor agonists	Improve glycemia; weight loss
	Sodium-glucose transporter-2 (SGLT-2) inhibitors	Improve glycemia; weight loss; reno-protection

Adapted from Ref. [116]

HDL cholesterol by 10% [15]. The rate of major cardiovascular events at 5 years was reduced when individuals with established coronary artery disease and MetS were treated with atorvastatin 80 mg versus 10 mg [95].

Bariatric Surgery

In the prospective clinical trial by Lee et al., 52.2% of the morbidly obese participants had MetS. Significant weight loss 1 year after gastric bypass surgery improved every element of MetS [15, 112]. Bariatric surgery is an effective treatment for achieving sustained weight loss, and improves blood pressure and glycemia, including remission of diabetes. Bariatric surgery may diminish the decline in kidney function in MetS. There are also risks in bariatric surgery, e.g., acute kidney injury and nephrolithiasis.

Other Treatment Approaches for MetS

Probiotics may have some benefits for MetS patients by reducing blood sugar and homocysteine levels, improving the inflammatory status and protecting against MetS-related kidney impairment [113]. Patients with MetS may have lower plasma glycine levels than healthy people. A number of clinical signs of MetS, including impaired glucose metabolism, hypertension, and hyperlipidemia, may be alleviated by glycine supplementation. A daily supplementation of glycine (15 g/day) in patients with MetS reduced oxidative stress, including superoxide dismutase-specific activity and thiobarbituric acid reactive chemicals, and improvement in hypertension [114, 115] (Table 2).

References

1. Arora P. Chronic Kidney Disease (CKD): practice essentials, pathophysiology, etiology. Medscape. 2021. Available from https://emedicine.medscape.com/article/238798-overview
2. Dehghani A, Alishavandi S, Nourimajalan N, Fallahzadeh H, Rahmanian V. Prevalence of chronic kidney diseases and its determinants among Iranian adults: results of the first phase of Shahedieh cohort study. BMC Nephrol. 2022;23(1):1–11. Available from https://bmcnephrol.biomedcentral.com/articles/10.1186/s12882-022-02832-5
3. CDC. Chronic Kidney Disease in the United States, 2021. Centers for Disease Control and Prevention. 2021. Available from https://www.cdc.gov/kidneydisease/publications-resources/ckd-national-facts.html
4. Kovesdy CP. Epidemiology of chronic kidney disease: an update 2022. Kidney Int Suppl (2011). 2022;12(1):7. Available from /pmc/articles/PMC9073222/
5. Obrador GT, Curhan GC, Tonelli M, Taylor EN. Epidemiology of chronic kidney disease – UpToDate. UpToDate. 2022. Available from https://www.uptodate.com/contents/epidemiology-of-chronic-kidney-disease
6. Sundström J, Bodegard J, Bollmann A, Vervloet MG, Mark PB, Karasik A, et al. Prevalence, outcomes, and cost of chronic kidney disease in a contemporary population of 24 million patients from 11 countries: The CaReMe CKD study. Lancet Reg Health Eur. 2022;20:100438. Available from http://www.thelancet.com/article/S2666776222001326/fulltext
7. Rosenberg M, Curhan GC, Tonelli M, Forman JP. Overview of the management of chronic kidney disease in adults – UpToDate. UpToDate. 2022. Available from https://www.uptodate.com/contents/overview-of-the-management-of-chronic-kidney-disease-in-adults?search=chronic%20kidney%20disease&source=search_result&selectedTitle=1~150&usage_type=default&display_rank=1
8. Lin L, Tan W, Pan X, Tian E, Wu Z, Yang J. Metabolic syndrome-related kidney injury: a review and update, Frontiers in endocrinology, vol. 13. Frontiers Media S.A.; 2022.
9. Wang SS. Metabolic syndrome: practice essentials, background, pathophysiology. Medscape. 2020. Available from https://emedicine.medscape.com/article/165124-overview
10. Agyemang-Yeboah F, Eghan BAJ, Annani-Akollor ME, Togbe E, Donkor S, Oppong AB. Evaluation of metabolic syndrome and its associated risk factors in type 2 diabetes: a Descriptive Cross-Sectional Study at the Komfo Anokye Teaching Hospital, Kumasi. Ghana. Biomed Res Int. 2019;2019.
11. Shin JA, Lee JH, Lim SY, Ha HS, Kwon HS, Park YM, et al. Metabolic syndrome as a predictor of type 2 diabetes, and its clinical interpretations and usefulness. J Diab Invest. 2013;4(4):334. Available from /pmc/articles/PMC4020225/
12. Mendizábal Y, Llorens S, Nava E. Hypertension in metabolic syndrome: vascular pathophysiology. Int J Hypertens. 2013;2013.
13. Yanai H, Tomono Y, Ito K, Furutani N, Yoshida H, Tada N. The underlying mechanisms for development of hypertension in the metabolic syndrome. Nutr J. 2008;7(1):10. Available from /pmc/articles/PMC2335113/

14. Franklin SS. Hypertension in the metabolic syndrome. Metab Syndr Relat Disord. 2006;4(4):287–98. Available from https://pubmed.ncbi.nlm.nih.gov/18370747/

15. Laguardia HA, Hamm LL, Chen J. The metabolic syndrome and risk of chronic kidney disease: Pathophysiology and intervention strategies. J Nutr Metab. 2012:2012.

16. Xie K, Bao L, Jiang X, Ye Z, Bing J, Dong Y, et al. The association of metabolic syndrome components and chronic kidney disease in patients with hypertension. Lipids Health Dis. 2019;18(1):1–6. Available from https://lipidworld.biomedcentral.com/articles/10.1186/s12944-019-1121-5

17. Kassi E, Pervanidou P, Kaltsas G, Chrousos G. Metabolic syndrome: definitions and controversies. BMC Med. 2011;9(1):1–13. Available from https://link.springer.com/articles/10.1186/1741-7015-9-48

18. Lin L, Tan W, Pan X, Tian E, Wu Z, Yang J. Metabolic syndrome related kidney injury: a review and update. Front Endocrinol (Lausanne). 2022;13:904001. https://doi.org/10.3389/fendo.2022.904001. eCollection 2022. PMID: 35813613

19. Goldbacher EM, Matthews KA. Are psychological characteristics related to risk of the metabolic syndrome? A review of the literature. Ann Behav Med. 2007;34(3):240–52. Available from https://pubmed.ncbi.nlm.nih.gov/18020934/

20. Després JP, Lemieux I, Bergeron J, Pibarot P, Mathieu P, Larose E, et al. Abdominal obesity and the metabolic syndrome: contribution to global cardiometabolic risk. Arterioscler Thromb Vasc Biol. 2008;28(6):1039–49. Available from https://pubmed.ncbi.nlm.nih.gov/18356555/

21. Gustafson B, Hammarstedt A, Andersson CX, Smith U. Inflamed adipose tissue: a culprit underlying the metabolic syndrome and atherosclerosis. Arterioscler Thromb Vasc Biol. 2007;27(11):2276–83. Available from https://pubmed.ncbi.nlm.nih.gov/17823366/

22. Lann D, LeRoith D. Insulin resistance as the underlying cause for the metabolic syndrome. Med Clin North Am. 2007;91(6):1063–77. Available from https://pubmed.ncbi.nlm.nih.gov/17964909/

23. Goossens GH. The role of adipose tissue dysfunction in the pathogenesis of obesity-related insulin resistance. Physiol Behav. 2008;94(2):206–18. Available from https://pubmed.ncbi.nlm.nih.gov/18037457/

24. Ogden CL, D Carroll M, Fryar CD, Flegal KM. Prevalence of obesity among adults and youth: United States, 2011–2014 – PubMed. PubMed. 2015. Available from https://pubmed.ncbi.nlm.nih.gov/26633046/

25. Zhang X, Lerman LO. The metabolic syndrome and chronic kidney disease. Transl Res. 2017;183:14–25.

26. Prasad GVR. Metabolic syndrome and chronic kidney disease: current status and future directions. World J Nephrol. 2014;3(4):210. Available from /pmc/articles/PMC4220353/

27. Xiao H, Shao X, Gao P, Zou H, Zhang X. Metabolic syndrome components and chronic kidney disease in a community population aged 40 years and older in Southern China: a cross-sectional study. Diab Metab Syndr Obes. 2022; 15:839–48. Available from https://www.dovepress.com/metabolic-syndrome-components-and-chronic-kidney-disease-in-a-communit-peer-reviewed-fulltext-article-DMSO

28. de Vries APJ, Bakker SJL, van Son WJ, van der Heide JJH, Ploeg RJ, The HT, et al. Metabolic syndrome is associated with impaired long-term renal allograft function; not all component criteria contribute equally. Am J Transplant. 2004;4(10):1675–83. Available from https://pubmed.ncbi.nlm.nih.gov/15367224/

29. Porrini E, Delgado P, Bigo C, Alvarez A, Cobo M, Checa MD, et al. Impact of metabolic syndrome on graft function and survival after cadaveric renal transplantation. Am J Kidney Dis. 2006;48(1):134–42. Available from https://pubmed.ncbi.nlm.nih.gov/16797396/

30. DeFina LF, Vega GL, Leonard D, Grundy SM. Fasting glucose, obesity, and metabolic syndrome as predictors of type 2 diabetes: the Cooper Center Longitudinal Study. J Invest Med. 2012;60(8):1164–8. Available from https://pubmed.ncbi.nlm.nih.gov/23111652/

31. Luk AOY, So WY, Ma RCW, Kong APS, Ozaki R, Ng VSW, et al. Metabolic syndrome predicts new onset of chronic kidney disease in 5829 patients with type 2 diabetes: a 5-year prospective analysis of the Hong Kong Diabetes Registry. Diab Care. 2008;31(12):2357–61. Available from https://pubmed.ncbi.nlm.nih.gov/18835954/

32. Hoehner CM, Greenlund KJ, Rith-Najarian S, Casper ML, McClellan WM. Association of the insulin resistance syndrome and microalbuminuria among non-diabetic native Americans. The Inter-Tribal Heart Project. J Am Soc Nephrol. 2002;13(6):1626–34. Available from https://pubmed.ncbi.nlm.nih.gov/12039992/

33. Alexander MP, Patel T, Farag YMK, Florez A, Rennke HG, Singh AK. Kidney pathological changes in metabolic syndrome: a cross-sectional study. Am J Kidney Dis. 2009;53(5):751–9. Available from https://pubmed.ncbi.nlm.nih.gov/19339092/

34. Chen J, Muntner P, Hamm LL, Jones DW, Batuman V, Fonseca V, et al. The metabolic syndrome and chronic kidney disease in U.S. adults. Ann Intern Med. 2004;140(3). Available from https://pubmed.ncbi.nlm.nih.gov/14757614/

35. Wahba IM, Mak RH. Obesity and obesity-initiated metabolic syndrome: mechanistic links to chronic kidney disease. Clin J Am Soc Nephrol. 2007;2(3):550–62. Available from https://pubmed.ncbi.nlm.nih.gov/17699463/

36. Wolf G, Chen S, Han DC, Ziyadeh FN. Leptin and renal disease. Am J Kidney Dis. 2002;39(1):1–11.

Available from https://pubmed.ncbi.nlm.nih.gov/11774095/

37. Wisse BE. The inflammatory syndrome: the role of adipose tissue cytokines in metabolic disorders linked to obesity. J Am Soc Nephrol. 2004;15(11):2792–800. Available from https://pubmed.ncbi.nlm.nih.gov/15504932/

38. Wang S, DeNichilo M, Brubaker C, Hirschberg R. Connective tissue growth factor in tubulointerstitial injury of diabetic nephropathy. Kidney Int. 2001;60(1):96–105. Available from https://pubmed.ncbi.nlm.nih.gov/11422741/

39. Locatelli F, Pozzoni P, del Vecchio L. Renal manifestations in the metabolic syndrome. J Am Soc Nephrol. 2006;17(4 Suppl 2). Available from https://pubmed.ncbi.nlm.nih.gov/16565254/

40. Hale LJ, Hurcombe J, Lay A, Santamaría B, Valverde AM, Saleem MA, et al. Insulin directly stimulates VEGF-A production in the glomerular podocyte. Am J Physiol Renal Physiol. 2013;305(2). Available from https://pubmed.ncbi.nlm.nih.gov/23698113/

41. Kim YW, Byzova T. Oxidative stress in angiogenesis and vascular disease. Blood. 2014;123(5):625–631. Available from https://pubmed.ncbi.nlm.nih.gov/24300855/

42. Li ZL, Woollard JR, Ebrahimi B, Crane JA, Jordan KL, Lerman A, et al. Transition from obesity to metabolic syndrome is associated with altered myocardial autophagy and apoptosis. Arterioscler Thromb Vasc Biol. 2012;32(5):1132–41. Available from https://pubmed.ncbi.nlm.nih.gov/22383702/

43. Li Z, Woollard JR, Wang S, Korsmo MJ, Ebrahimi B, Grande JP, et al. Increased glomerular filtration rate in early metabolic syndrome is associated with renal adiposity and microvascular proliferation. Am J Physiol Renal Physiol. 2011;301(5). Available from https://pubmed.ncbi.nlm.nih.gov/21775485/

44. Chade AR, Hall JE. Role of the renal microcirculation in progression of chronic kidney injury in obesity. Am J Nephrol. 2016;44(5):354–67. Available from https://pubmed.ncbi.nlm.nih.gov/27771702/

45. Buscemi S, Verga S, Batsis JA, Cottone S, Mattina A, Re A, et al. Intra-renal hemodynamics and carotid intima-media thickness in the metabolic syndrome. Diab Res Clin Pract. 2009;86(3):177–85. Available from https://pubmed.ncbi.nlm.nih.gov/19815301/

46. Zhang X, Li ZL, Woollard JR, Eirin A, Ebrahimi B, Crane JA, et al. Obesity-metabolic derangement preserves hemodynamics but promotes intrarenal adiposity and macrophage infiltration in swine renovascular disease. Am J Physiol Renal Physiol. 2013;305(3). Available from https://pubmed.ncbi.nlm.nih.gov/23657852/

47. Lerman LO, Lerman A. The metabolic syndrome and early kidney disease: another link in the chain? Rev Esp Cardiol. 2011;64(5):358. Available from /pmc/articles/PMC3107983/

48. Hotamisligil GS. Inflammation and metabolic disorders. Nature. 2006;444(7121):860–7. Available from https://pubmed.ncbi.nlm.nih.gov/17167474/

49. Dominguez JH, Wu P, Packer CS, Temm C, Kelly KJ. Lipotoxic and inflammatory phenotypes in rats with uncontrolled metabolic syndrome and nephropathy. Am J Physiol Renal Physiol 2007;293(3). Available from https://pubmed.ncbi.nlm.nih.gov/17596532/

50. le Roith D, Zick Y. Recent advances in our understanding of insulin action and insulin resistance. Diab Care. 2001;24(3):588–97. Available from https://diabetesjournals.org/care/article/24/3/588/22922/Recent-Advances-in-Our-Understanding-of-Insulin

51. Mathew A, Okada S, Sharma K. Obesity related kidney disease. Curr Diab Rev. 2011;7(1):41–9.

52. Sarafidis PA, Ruilope LM. Insulin resistance, hyperinsulinemia, and renal injury: mechanisms and implications. Am J Nephrol. 2006;26(3):232–244. Available from https://www.karger.com/Article/FullText/93632

53. Medina-Inojosa JR, Lavie CJ. Obesity: association with cardiovascular disease – UpToDate. UpToDate. 2023. Available from https://www.uptodate.com/contents/obesity-association-with-cardiovascular-disease?search=abdominal%20obesity&source=search_result&selectedTitle=1~150&usage_type=default&display_rank=1

54. Sahakyan KR, Somers VK, Rodriguez-Escudero JP, Hodge DO, Carter RE, Sochor O, et al. Normal weight central obesity: implications for total and cardiovascular mortality. Ann Intern Med. 2015;163(11):827. Available from /pmc/articles/PMC4995595/

55. WHO. Waist circumference and waist–hip ratio. WHO Expert. 2011;64(1):2–5. Available from http://www.nature.com/doifinder/10.1038/ejcn.2009.139

56. Engin A. The definition and prevalence of obesity and metabolic syndrome. Adv Exp Med Biol. 2017; 960: 1–17. Available from https://pubmed.ncbi.nlm.nih.gov/28585193/

57. Sowers JR, Whaley-Connell A, Epstein M. Narrative review: the emerging clinical implications of the role of aldosterone in the metabolic syndrome and resistant hypertension. Ann Intern Med. 2009;150(11):776–83.

58. Goodfriend TL, Ball DL, Egan BM, Campbell WB, Nithipatikom K. Epoxy-Keto derivative of linoleic acid stimulates aldosterone secretion. Hypertension. 2004;43(2):358–63. Available from https://www.ahajournals.org/doi/abs/10.1161/01.HYP.0000113294.06704.64

59. Lamounier-Zepter V, Ehrhart-Bornstein M. Fat tissue metabolism and adrenal steroid secretion. Curr Hypertens Rep. 2006;8(1):30–4. Available from https://link.springer.com/article/10.1007/s11906-006-0038-3

60. Aubert H, Frère C, Aillaud MF, Morange PE, Juhan-Vague I, Alessi MC. Weak and non-independent

association between plasma TAFI antigen levels and the insulin resistance syndrome. J Thromb Haemost. 2003;1(4):791–7. Available from https://onlinelibrary.wiley.com/doi/full/10.1046/j.1538-7836.2003.00147.x

61. Bosello O, Zamboni M. Visceral obesity and metabolic syndrome. Obes Rev. 2000;1(1):47–56. Available from https://onlinelibrary.wiley.com/doi/full/10.1046/j.1467-789x.2000.00008.x

62. Sharma I, Liao Y, Zheng X, Kanwar YS. New pandemic: obesity and associated nephropathy. Front Med (Lausanne). 2021; 8:673556. Available from /pmc/articles/PMC8275856/

63. Remuzzi G, Perico N, Macia M, Ruggenenti P. The role of renin-angiotensin-aldosterone system in the progression of chronic kidney disease. Kidney Int. 2005;68 (SUPPL 99):S57–65. Available from http://www.kidney-international.org/article/S0085253815512805/fulltext

64. Helal I, Fick-Brosnahan GM, Reed-Gitomer B, Schrier RW. Glomerular hyperfiltration: definitions, mechanisms and clinical implications. Nat Rev Nephrol. 2012;8(5):293–300. Available from https://pubmed.ncbi.nlm.nih.gov/22349487/

65. Muñoz-Durango N, Fuentes CA, Castillo AE, González-Gómez LM, Vecchiola A, Fardella CE, et al. Role of the Renin-Angiotensin-Aldosterone system beyond blood pressure regulation: molecular and cellular mechanisms involved in end-organ damage during arterial hypertension. Int J Mol Sci. 2016;17 (7). Available from https://pubmed.ncbi.nlm.nih.gov/27347925/

66. Min SH, Kim SH, Jeong IK, Cho HC, Jeong JO, Lee JH, et al. Independent association of serum aldosterone level with metabolic syndrome and insulin resistance in Korean adults. Korean Circ J. 2018;48(3):198–208. Available from https://pubmed.ncbi.nlm.nih.gov/29557106/

67. Bomback AS, Klemmer PJ. Renal injury in extreme obesity: the important role of aldosterone. Kidney Int. 2008;74(9):1216. Available from http://www.kidney-international.org/article/S0085253815535035/fulltext

68. Sowers JR. Hypertension, angiotensin II, and oxidative stress. https://doi.org/101056/NEJMe020054. 2002;346(25):1999–2001. Available from. https://www.nejm.org/doi/full/10.1056/NEJMe020054

69. Cooper SA, Whaley-Connell A, Habibi J, Wei Y, Lastra G, Manrique C, et al. Renin-angiotensin-aldosterone system and oxidative stress in cardiovascular insulin resistance. Am J Physiol Heart Circ Physiol. 2007;293(4).2009–23. Available from https://journals.physiology.org/doi/10.1152/ajpheart.00522.2007

70. Whaley-Connell A, Habibi J, Wei Y, Gutweiler A, Jellison J, Wiedmeyer CE, et al. Mineralocorticoid receptor antagonism attenuates glomerular filtration barrier remodeling in the transgenic Ren2 rat. Am J Physiol Renal Physiol. 2009;296(5):1013–22. Available from https://journals.physiology.org/doi/10.1152/ajprenal.90646.2008

71. Kambham N, Markowitz GS, Valeri AM, Lin J, D'Agati VD. Obesity-related glomerulopathy: an emerging epidemic. Kidney Int. 2001;59(4):1498–509. Available from http://www.kidney-international.org/article/S0085253815476264/fulltext

72. Tsuboi N, Okabayashi Y, Shimizu A, Yokoo T. The renal pathology of obesity. Kidney Int Rep. 2017;2(2): 251–60. https://doi.org/10.1016/j.ekir.2017.01.007).

73. Fried LF, Orchard TJ, Kasiske BL. Effect of lipid reduction on the progression of renal disease: a meta-analysis. Kidney Int. 2001;59(1):260–9. Available from http://www.kidney-international.org/article/S0085253815474617/fulltext

74. Muntner P, Coresh J, Smith JC, Eckfeldt J, Klag MJ. Plasma lipids and risk of developing renal dysfunction: The atherosclerosis risk in communities' study. Kidney Int. 2000;58(1):293–301. Available from http://www.kidney-international.org/article/S008525381547098X/fulltext

75. Mänttäri M, Tiula E, Alikoski T, Manninen V. Effects of hypertension and dyslipidemia on the decline in renal function. Hypertension. 1995;26(4):670–5.

76. Ou HC, Chou FP, Lin TM, Yang CH, Sheu WHH. Protective effects of honokiol against oxidized LDL-induced cytotoxicity and adhesion molecule expression in endothelial cells. Chem Biol Interact. 2006;161(1):1–13.

77. Ou HC, Lee WJ, da Lee S, Huang CY, Chiu TH, Tsai KL, et al. Ellagic acid protects endothelial cells from oxidized low-density lipoprotein-induced apoptosis by modulating the PI3K/Akt/eNOS pathway. Toxicol Appl Pharmacol. 2010;248(2):134–43.

78. Krauss RM. Dense low-density lipoproteins and coronary artery disease. Am J Cardiol. 1995;75(6): 53B–7B.

79. Krauss RM. Atherogenicity of triglyceride-rich lipoproteins. Am J Cardiol. 1998;81(4 A):13B–17B. Available from http://www.ajconline.org/article/S0002914998000320/fulltext

80. Steinberg HO, Brechtel G, Johnson A, Fineberg N, Baron AD. Insulin-mediated skeletal muscle vasodilation is nitric oxide dependent. A novel action of insulin to increase nitric oxide release. J Clin Invest. 1994;94(3):1172–9.

81. Tooke JE, Hannemann MM. Adverse endothelial function and the insulin resistance syndrome. J Intern Med. 2000;247(4):425–31. Available from https://onlinelibrary.wiley.com/doi/full/10.1046/j.1365-2796.2000.00671.x

82. Ferrara D, Montecucco F, Dallegri F, Carbone F. Impact of different ectopic fat depots on cardiovascular and metabolic diseases. J Cell Physiol. 2019;234(12):21630–41. Available from https://pubmed.ncbi.nlm.nih.gov/31106419/

83. Katsimardou A, Imprialos K, Stavropoulos K, Sachinidis A, Doumas M, Athyros V. Hypertension in metabolic syndrome: novel insights. Curr Hypertens Rev. 2020;16(1):12–8. Available from https://pubmed.ncbi.nlm.nih.gov/30987573/

84. da Silva AA, do Carmo JM, Li X, Wang Z, Mouton AJ, Hall JE. Role of hyperinsulinemia and insulin resistance in hypertension: metabolic syndrome revisited. Can J Cardiol. 2020;36(5):671–82. Available from https://pubmed.ncbi.nlm.nih.gov/32389340/

85. Hosseini A, Razavi BM, Banach M, Hosseinzadeh H. Quercetin and metabolic syndrome: a review. Phytother Res. 2021;35(10):5352–64. Available from https://pubmed.ncbi.nlm.nih.gov/34101925/

86. Mair KM, Gaw R, MacLean MR. Obesity, estrogens and adipose tissue dysfunction – implications for pulmonary arterial hypertension. Pulm Circ. 2020;10(3). Available from https://pubmed.ncbi.nlm.nih.gov/32999709/

87. Hall ME, do Carmo JM, da Silva AA, Juncos LA, Wang Z, Hall JE. Obesity, hypertension, and chronic kidney disease. Int J Nephrol Renovasc Dis. 2014;7: 75–88. Available from https://pubmed.ncbi.nlm.nih.gov/24600241/

88. Kang SH, Cho KH, Park JW, Yoon KW, Do JY. Association of visceral fat area with chronic kidney disease and metabolic syndrome risk in the general population: analysis using multi-frequency bioimpedance. Kidney Blood Press Res. 2015;40(3): 223–30. Available from https://pubmed.ncbi.nlm.nih.gov/25966816/

89. Escasany E, Izquierdo-Lahuerta A, Medina-Gomez G. Underlying mechanisms of renal lipotoxicity in obesity. Nephron. 2019;143(1):28–32. Available from https://pubmed.ncbi.nlm.nih.gov/30625473/

90. Xu H, Barnes GT, Yang Q, Tan G, Yang D, Chou CJ, et al. Chronic inflammation in fat plays a crucial role in the development of obesity-related insulin resistance. J Clin Invest. 2003;112(12):1821–30. Available from http://www.jci.org/cgi/content/full/

91. Azadbakht L, Mirmiran P, Esmaillzadeh A, Azizi T, Azizi F. Beneficial effects of a dietary approaches to stop hypertension eating plan on features of the metabolic syndrome. Diab Care. 2005;28(12):2823–31. Available from https://diabetesjournals.org/care/article/28/12/2823/22802/Beneficial-Effects-of-a-Dietary-Approaches-to-Stop

92. Heymsfield SB, Segal KR, Hauptman J, Lucas CP, Boldrin MN, Rissanen A, et al. Effects of weight loss with orlistat on glucose tolerance and progression to type 2 diabetes in obese adults. Arch Intern Med. 2000;160(9):1321–6. Available from https://pubmed.ncbi.nlm.nih.gov/10809036/

93. Lloyd-Jones DM, Liu K, Colangelo LA, Yan LL, Klein L, Loria CM, et al. Consistently stable or decreased body mass index in young adulthood and longitudinal changes in metabolic syndrome components: the Coronary Artery Risk Development in Young Adults Study. Circulation. 2007;115(8): 1004–11. Available from https://pubmed.ncbi.nlm.nih.gov/17283263/

94. Reaven G, Segal K, Hauptman J, Boldrin M, Lucas C. Effect of orlistat-assisted weight loss in decreasing coronary heart disease risk in patients with syndrome X. Am J Cardiol. 2001;87(7):827–31. Available from https://pubmed.ncbi.nlm.nih.gov/11274935/

95. Meigs JB, Nathan DM, Wolfsdorf JI, Givens J. Metabolic syndrome (insulin resistance syndrome or syndrome X) – UpToDate. UpToDate. 2022. Available from https://www.uptodate.com/contents/metabolic-syndrome-insulin-resistance-syndrome-or-syndrome-x?search=metabolic%20syndrome&source=search_result&selectedTitle=1~150&usage_type=default&display_rank=1

96. Thompson PD, Buchner D, Piña IL, Balady GJ, Williams MA, Marcus BH, et al. Exercise and physical activity in the prevention and treatment of atherosclerotic cardiovascular disease: a statement from the Council on Clinical Cardiology (Subcommittee on Exercise, Rehabilitation, and Prevention) and the Council on Nutrition, Physical Activity, and Metabolism (Subcommittee on Physical Activity). Circulation. 2003;107(24):3109–16. Available from https://pubmed.ncbi.nlm.nih.gov/12821592/

97. Stuard S, Belcaro G, Cesarone MR, Ricci A, Dugall AM, Pellegrini L, et al. Kidney function in metabolic syndrome may be improved with Pycnogenol® – PubMed. PubMed. 2010. Available from https://pubmed.ncbi.nlm.nih.gov/20657531/

98. Masajtis-Zagajewska A, Majer J, Nowicki M. Losartan and Eprosartan induce a similar effect on the acute rise in serum uric acid concentration after an oral fructose load in patients with metabolic syndrome. J Renin Angiotensin Aldosterone Syst 2021;2021:2214978. Available from https://pubmed.ncbi.nlm.nih.gov/34527078/

99. Ishii M, Shibata R, Kondo K, Kambara T, Shimizu Y, Tanigawa T, et al. Vildagliptin Stimulates Endothelial Cell Network Formation and Ischemia-induced Revascularization via an Endothelial Nitric-oxide Synthase-dependent Mechanism. J Biol Chem. 2014;289(39): 27235. Available from /pmc/articles/PMC4175356/

100. Salybekov AA, Masuda H, Miyazaki K, Sheng Y, Sato A, Shizuno T, et al. Dipeptidyl dipeptidase-4 inhibitor recovered ischemia through an increase in vasculogenic endothelial progenitor cells and regeneration-associated cells in diet-induced obese mice. PLoS One. 2019;14(3). Available from /pmc/articles/PMC6424405/

101. Ng HY, Leung FF, Kuo WH, Lee WC, Lee Cte. Dapagliflozin and xanthine oxidase inhibitors improve insulin resistance and modulate renal glucose and urate transport in metabolic syndrome. Clin Exp Pharmacol Physiol. 2021;48(12):1603–12. Available from https://pubmed.ncbi.nlm.nih.gov/34407232/

102. Nauck MA, Quast DR, Wefers J, Meier JJ. GLP-1 receptor agonists in the treatment of type 2 diabetes – state-of-the-art. Mol Metab. 2021;46. Available from https://pubmed.ncbi.nlm.nih.gov/33068776/

103. Rizzo M, Nikolic D, Patti AM, Mannina C, Montalto G, McAdams BS, et al. GLP-1 receptor agonists and reduction of cardiometabolic risk:

potential underlying mechanisms. Biochim Biophys Acta Mol Basis Dis. 2018;1864(9 Pt B):2814–21. Available from https://pubmed.ncbi.nlm.nih.gov/29778663/

104. Prakash S, Rai U, Kosuru R, Tiwari V, Singh S. Amelioration of diet-induced metabolic syndrome and fatty liver with sitagliptin via regulation of adipose tissue inflammation and hepatic Adiponectin/AMPK levels in mice. Biochimie. 2020; 168:198–209. Available from https://pubmed.ncbi.nlm.nih.gov/31715215/

105. Chan JC, Malik V, Jia W, Kadowaki T, Yajnik CS, Yoon KH, Hu FB. Diabetes in Asia: epidemiology, risk factors, and pathophysiology. JAMA. 2009;301(20):2129–40. https://doi.org/10.1001/jama.2009.726. PMID: 19470990.

106. Arnold SV, Kosiborod M, Wang J, Fenici P, Gannedahl G, LoCasale RJ. Burden of cardio-renal-metabolic conditions in adults with type 2 diabetes within the Diabetes Collaborative Registry. Diabetes Obes Metab. 2018;20(8):2000–2003. https://doi.org/10.1111/dom.13303. Epub 2018 Apr 19. PMID: 29577540.

107. Thomas MC, Cooper ME, Zimmet P. Changing epidemiology of type 2 diabetes mellitus and associated chronic kidney disease. Nat Rev Nephrol. 2016;12(2):73–81. https://doi.org/10.1038/nrneph.2015.173. Epub 2015 Nov 10. PMID: 26553517.

108. Athyros VG, Mikhailidis DP, Liberopoulos EN, Kakafika AI, Karagiannis A, Papageorgiou AA, et al. Effect of statin treatment on renal function and serum uric acid levels and their relation to vascular events in patients with coronary heart disease and metabolic syndrome: a subgroup analysis of the GREek Atorvastatin and Coronary heart disease Evaluation (GREACE) Study. Nephrol Dial Transplant. 2007;22(1):118–27. Available from https://pubmed.ncbi.nlm.nih.gov/16998214/

109. Velarde GP, Choudhary N, Bravo-Jaimes K, Smotherman C, Sherazi S, Kraemer DF. Effect of atorvastatin on lipogenic, inflammatory and thrombogenic markers in women with the metabolic syndrome. Nutr Metab Cardiovasc Dis. 2021;31(2):634–40. Available from https://pubmed.ncbi.nlm.nih.gov/33485731/

110. Malur P, Menezes A, DiNicolantonio JJ, O'Keefe JH, Lavie CJ. The microvascular and macrovascular benefits of fibrates in diabetes and the metabolic syndrome: a review. Mo Med. 2017;114(6):464. Available from /pmc/articles/PMC6139978/

111. Agrawal V, Shah A, Rice C, Franklin BA, McCullough PA. Impact of treating the metabolic syndrome on chronic kidney disease. Nat Rev Nephrol. 2009;5(9):520–8. Available from https://pubmed.ncbi.nlm.nih.gov/19636332/

112. Lee WJ, Huang MT, Wang W, Lin CM, Chen TC, Lai IR. Effects of obesity surgery on the metabolic syndrome. Arch Surg. 2004;139(10):1088–1092. Available from https://jamanetwork.com/journals/jamasurgery/fullarticle/770299

113. Bernini LJ, Simão ANC, Alfieri DF, Lozovoy MAB, Mari NL, de Souza CHB, et al. Beneficial effects of Bifidobacterium lactis on lipid profile and cytokines in patients with metabolic syndrome: A randomized trial. Effects of probiotics on metabolic syndrome. Nutrition. 2016;32(6):716–9. Available from https://pubmed.ncbi.nlm.nih.gov/27126957/

114. Díaz-Flores M, Cruz M, Duran-Reyes G, Munguia-Miranda C, Loza-Rodríguez H, Pulido-Casas E, et al. Oral supplementation with glycine reduces oxidative stress in patients with metabolic syndrome, improving their systolic blood pressure. Can J Physiol Pharmacol. 2013;91(10):855–60. Available from https://pubmed.ncbi.nlm.nih.gov/24144057/

115. Imenshahidi M, Hossenzadeh H. Effects of glycine on metabolic syndrome components: a review. J Endocrinol Invest. 2022;45(5):927–39. Available from https://pubmed.ncbi.nlm.nih.gov/35013990/

116. Ahima RS. Metabolic syndrome a comprehensive textbook. Cham: Springer; 2016.

Part VI

Prevention and Treatment

Diet, Exercise, and Behavior Therapy

37

Leah M. Schumacher, David B. Sarwer, and Kelly C. Allison

Contents

L. M. Schumacher
Department of Kinesiology and Center for Obesity
Research and Education, College of Public Health, Temple
University, Philadelphia, PA, USA
e-mail: leah.schumacher@temple.edu

D. B. Sarwer
Department of Social and Behavioral Sciences and Center
for Obesity Research and Education, College of Public
Health, Temple University, Philadelphia, PA, USA
e-mail: dsarwer@temple.edu

K. C. Allison (✉)
Department of Psychiatry, Perelman School of Medicine,
University of Pennsylvania, Philadelphia, PA, USA
e-mail: kca@pennmedicine.upenn.edu

© Springer Nature Switzerland AG 2023
R. S. Ahima (ed.), *Metabolic Syndrome*,
https://doi.org/10.1007/978-3-031-40116-9_43

Abstract

Diet composition, physical activity, and behavior change play an essential role in weight management. These three pillars of weight management are complementary, and when used in combination, yield clinically meaningfully weight loss and improvements in many aspects of physical and mental health. Specific approaches and techniques for modifying diet, physical activity, and weight-related behaviors are reviewed in this chapter. Considerations regarding treatment modality, delivery of lifestyle modification alone or in combination with other treatment approaches, and weight stigma are also discussed. Consistent with the World Health Organization's definition of obesity as a chronic progressive relapsing disease, weight loss maintenance remains challenging. Improvements in metabolic functioning and other aspects of health worsen when weight is regained. Research is thus needed to help match individuals to weight management approaches that may increase adherence and long-term maintenance of weight loss and health benefits.

Keywords

Lifestyle modification · Caloric restriction · Physical activity · Behavioral modification · Telemedicine · Weight maintenance · Dietary interventions

Introduction

Obesity is a complex, chronic progressive relapsing disease resulting from genetic, physiological, behavioral, environmental, and sociocultural factors [1]. As understanding of obesity has advanced over the years, it has become clear that simply instructing individuals to eat less and move more is insufficient to address obesity at the population level. A multidisciplinary, multilevel approach that includes but also extends beyond individual-level behavior is needed. That said, individuals' health behaviors, including their dietary behaviors and physical activity, strongly impact weight and metabolic health. Modifications to diet and physical activity can lead to clinically significant weight loss, typically defined as weight loss of 5–10% of initial body weight. Weight loss of this magnitude yields significant improvements in health, including a reduction in the incidence of diabetes [2, 3].

Typically, lifestyle modification interventions consist of three complementary elements: caloric restriction, increased physical activity, and behavior modification counseling. Dietary interventions may explicitly focus on creating an energy deficit through use of a daily calorie goal; they also may focus on aspects of eating such as macronutrient content and consumption or avoidance of certain types of foods. Physical activity intervention typically involves providing a weekly exercise goal focused on minutes of moderate-to-vigorous physical activity (MVPA). Lifestyle changes to increase light physical activity and decrease sedentary time are also encouraged. Behavior modification strategies rooted in cognitive-behavioral approaches seek to promote adherence to dietary and physical activity prescriptions and to equip individuals with skills to establish and maintain healthy lifestyles long term. Key strategies include self-monitoring, goal setting, stimulus control, and problem-solving, as well as strategies for dealing with unhelpful thought patterns.

Lifestyle modification intervention can be delivered in various modalities and settings. Although lifestyle modification is often delivered as a standalone intervention, it can also be delivered in conjunction with pharmacotherapy and, with some modifications, to patients who undergo bariatric surgery. Regardless of the format in which treatment is delivered, it is imperative to deliver care in a patient-centered manner that avoids perpetuating weight stigma – a widely prevalent form of bias that can have devastating impacts. Given the deleterious influence of weight stigma on health and well-being, research is underway to explore avenues for reducing weight stigma and lessening its negative effects among individuals seeking weight management intervention.

Dietary Approaches

The amount and types of foods that individuals eat has a profound impact on weight and metabolic health. Dietary change is thus a key component of lifestyle modification strategies. There are multiple evidence-based approaches for reducing energy intake and promoting cardiometabolic health. These include approaches that emphasize macronutrient composition, overall dietary patterns, specific types of food, and the timing of eating. These can be found in self-help books, on dedicated web pages, and imbedded in commercial weight loss programs.

There is considerable interest in the field and among the general public about whether one dietary approach is superior to others in promoting weight loss or metabolic health. While some approaches outperform others over short periods of time, such as 6 months, most large, systematic comparisons of different dietary approaches have found minimal differences in average weight loss when individuals are followed for a year or more [4]. This is especially true when overall energy intake is comparable [5]. Differences in metabolic biomarkers are also often small, although some diets may be preferred for individuals with certain health issues, such as cardiometabolic risk factors [2]. Consistent with the broader movement toward personalized or precision medicine within healthcare, there has been interest in whether individuals can be matched to an optimal dietary approach based on factors such as their genotype pattern or insulin secretion [6]. To date, these studies have had relatively limited success.

The most important takeaway from decades of research is that dietary changes that result in an energy deficit, regardless of macronutrient content, will result in weight loss for most individuals. Current clinical practice guidelines for the management of obesity recommend prescription of a daily calorie goal to achieve a 500–750 kcal/day energy deficit. Prescription of an evidence-based diet that restricts certain food types and thus also indirectly produces an energy deficit sufficient for weight loss may be of use for selected individuals [2, 7]. Individuals' taste and lifestyle preferences, their perceived ability to implement a particular dietary approach over the long-term, and their medical comorbidities should be considered when selecting a dietary approach. Fad diets, though popular, are typically unsustainable and have not been shown to improve health long term. These diets should be avoided.

Brief descriptions of several popular evidence-based dietary approaches are outlined. Detailed descriptions of these strategies and the current evidence state for each are available in several excellent consensus reports from health professional societies [2, 8].

Low Fat, Low Calorie

One of the most popular and widely used dietary approaches for obesity is a low-fat, low-calorie approach. This approach involves prescribing a daily intake goal based on an individual's current weight, with 1200–1500 kcal/day prescribed for individuals weighing <250 lbs. and 1500–1800 kcal/day prescribed for individuals weighing >250 lbs. These intake goals are designed to produce a calorie deficit resulting in 1–2 lbs. of weight loss per week and overall weight losses of ≥5–10%. Macronutrient goals of a low-fat diet include consuming <30% of intake from fats, 45–60% from carbohydrates, and 15–20% from proteins.

The rationale behind a low-fat diet for obesity relates to calorie density and food volume. Fat is more calorically dense (9 kcals per gram) than protein or carbohydrate (each 4 kcals per gram). When eating a low-fat diet, an individual can thus consume a higher volume of food than they would be able to consume on a higher-fat diet for the same number of calories. Because food volume is a powerful signal for satiety [9], eating a higher volume of foods can help manage hunger while adhering to a reduced daily intake goal. Eating low-fat, higher-volume foods also allows individuals to eat for a longer duration at a given meal. A low-fat approach particularly focused on decreasing saturated and trans fats may be useful for individuals with diabetes mellitus (T2DM) and/or cardiovascular disease (CVD) since these types of fat are known to increase risk for cardiovascular events and impair insulin sensitivity [10].

A low-fat, low-calorie approach has been used by many successful weight loss interventions, such as the Diabetes Prevention Program (DPP), Look AHEAD, and POWER Trials [11–14]. The Look AHEAD study, for example, was a multiyear investigation that randomized 5145 older Americans with overweight or obesity and T2DM to Intensive Lifestyle Intervention (ILI; including a low-fat diet and ongoing group and individual weight management counseling) or to a Diabetes Support and Education group (DSE; yearly support meetings). The ILI group showed greater weight loss throughout the study as compared to the DSE group (8.6% vs. 0.7% at 1 year; 6.0% vs. 3.5% at the 4 year final assessment) [12] and exhibited greater improvements than ILI in many other aspects of health, such as HbA1c levels [15], sleep apnea [16], quality of life [17], and mobility [18]. However, the rate of cardiovascular events was not different [19]. As this was the primary outcome measure, the results, when considered against the intensity of the intervention, raised concerns about the broad implementation of this dietary approach.

A low-fat, low-calorie approach is encouraged in clinical guidelines for healthy eating and weight loss developed by several professional societies; it is one approach encouraged by the American Diabetes Association [7, 20]. This is also the approach used by the commercial program WW (formerly known as Weight Watchers), although WW users track assigned point values versus calories and macronutrient percentages. It is also worth noting that the healthy eating guidelines provided by the US Departments of Agriculture and Health and Human Services, while not focused on weight loss, have consistently been based on a low-fat approach.

Low Carbohydrate

Several popular dietary approaches place primary emphasis on limiting carbohydrate intake and replacing carbohydrates with fat and/or protein. These approaches, including the Atkins and South Beach diets [21], encourage cutting carbohydrate and eating a diet of primarily fat and protein, and ketogenic diets, which advocate dramatically cutting carbohydrate to put the body into a metabolic state called ketosis [22]. When in ketosis, the body burns fat for energy instead of glucose. While there is no single definition of a low carbohydrate diet, this approach typically involves restricting carbohydrate to 26–45% of intake or less [8]. As a reference, national guidelines currently recommend 45–65% of energy intake from carbohydrates. Low carbohydrate diets often do not explicitly encourage calorie counting or restriction. However, carbohydrates need to be tracked.

The American Diabetes Association includes a low-carbohydrate diet among those appropriate for individuals with prediabetes or diabetes [8]. Several meta-analyses comparing low-carbohydrate to higher carbohydrate eating patterns indicate that a low-carbohydrate approach yields greater improvements in A1c, triglycerides, HDL-C, and blood pressure over the short term (i.e., 6 months) [23, 24]. Weight loss may also be slightly greater in the short term [25]. However, differences between low-carbohydrate and other approaches are minimal when examined over longer periods of time [23, 24, 26]. This may result from difficulties adhering to low carbohydrate approaches over time [25]. There are also potential risks and side effects associated with following a low carbohydrate approach, especially a very low carbohydrate plan, such as diuresis and halitosis.

High Protein

Another well-known and widely tested approach is the high protein diet. A high protein diet is defined as a diet in which 1.2–1.6 g protein/kg/day is consumed. This translates to about 25–30% of daily intake [27]. Approximately 30% of calories are from fat and 40–45% are from carbohydrates. In comparison, data from the National Health and

Nutrition Examination Survey show that Americans typically consume 14–16% of daily energy intake from protein [28]. Reduced energy intake is not inherent to a high protein diet, but patients should aim for energy deficit if weight loss is a goal.

A high protein diet is thought to be helpful for weight loss for a few reasons [29]. First, protein has been shown to promote satiety as compared to other macronutrients [27]. Eating a high protein diet can help individuals to reduce their overall energy intake while managing hunger. Second, protein has a higher thermic effect than carbohydrates or fat and therefore impacts energy balance. Third, protein may help maintain lean muscle mass. As lean muscle mass uses more energy than fat mass, this may allow individuals to consume more calories while losing weight or maintaining weight loss. This approach is intuitively appealing to many individuals and anecdotally is often appealing to men.

Several meta-analyses have examined the effects of a high protein diet for both weight loss and cardiovascular improvements [30, 31]. While these studies have shown some short-term advantages of high protein versus lower protein diets, such as greater body fat loss and lower fasting triglycerides, these differences disappear over time [30, 31]. As with other approaches, one's ability to adhere to a specific dietary approach is vital to its benefits for weight and metabolic health. Gastrointestinal side effects may occur with a high protein diet [32]. Recommendations from several health societies to limit intake of red meat is also a factor to consider against pursuing a high protein dietary approach.

Mediterranean Diet

A Mediterranean Diet focuses on overall dietary composition rather than specific macronutrient patterns. A Mediterranean approach emphasizes plant-based foods that include nuts, legumes, fruits, vegetables, seeds, and whole grains, and olive oil as the main source of added fat. Fish and seafood are included in moderation, while dairy and red meat are limited. Moderate consumption of red wine is sometimes encouraged [8]. A Mediterranean Diet does not inherently

limit caloric intake and instead focuses primarily on the types of foods eaten. Individuals seeking weight loss who wish to practice a Mediterranean style of eating will be most successful in meeting weight loss goals if they ensure an energy deficit.

Interest in the Mediterranean Diet stemmed from epidemiological data showing that individuals in countries that border the Mediterranean Sea, e.g., Italy and Greece, had lower rates of cardiovascular diseases (CVD) than individuals in the United States. A Mediterranean diet is hypothesized to be beneficial through mechanisms including reducing inflammation, blood sugar, and body weight. In head-to-head comparisons among diets, recent evidence is perhaps most supportive of a Mediterranean approach. Compared to other dietary approaches such as a low-fat diet, a Mediterranean diet appears to lead to greater improvements in cardiovascular risk factors and inflammatory markers [33, 34]. Lower intake of saturated fats coupled with higher intake of polyunsaturated and monounsaturated fat – like olive oil – is also associated with lower rates of CVD and of other major causes of death [35]. As such, the Mediterranean Diet is among those advocated in the American Heart Association's dietary guidelines to improve cardiovascular health [36]. It is also recommended by the American Diabetes Association as one of the dietary styles appropriate for individuals with prediabetes or T2D [7], and aligns with aspects of US national dietary guidelines.

Low Glycemic Index

Glycemic index (GI) refers to the degree to which foods containing carbohydrates affect the release of blood glucose after the food is consumed [37]. A low GI diet focuses on minimizing swings in blood sugar through attention to the types of carbohydrates eaten. Foods are ranked on a 0–100 scale, with glucose and white bread being the standard for comparison at a GI of 100. Foods with lower GI values are preferred when following a GI diet. The GI of foods is affected by many factors, such as processing, cooking, and storage [38]. GI values are not always intuitive. For example, low GI snack foods include nuts and "hummus" (spread of chickpeas, tahini, lemon, and spices) but also foods like Nutella and Snickers bars. Thus, it can be a complicated approach to follow.

A low GI diet aims to reduce spikes in blood glucose that results from consuming high levels of simple carbohydrates, which are broken down more quickly and release glucose into the bloodstream more rapidly than complex carbohydrates. Reducing blood glucose levels is hypothesized to reduce insulin levels and increases in body fat and weight. Energy intake levels are not reduced just by eating a low GI diet. Therefore, calorie restriction must be combined with a low GI approach for weight loss. While there is continued interest in the GI approach, especially in patients with T2D or polycystic ovary syndrome, the data on its efficacy has been mixed. Two recent systematic reviews showed no significant impact on A1c and mixed effects on fasting glucose [39, 40]. Limiting foods high in GI aligns with broader guidelines provided by some health societies [20].

Newer Dietary Approaches

Two dietary approaches that have received increased attention from researchers and the general public alike in recent years are intermittent fasting and plant-based diets.

Intermittent fasting, also called intermittent energy restriction or time restricted eating, refers to a variety of regimens in which the primary focus is on "when" rather than "what" individuals eat. This includes approaches such as alternative day fasting, the 5:2 diet, and time restricted eating [41]. In alternate day fasting, individuals alternate days of eating ad libitum with days of no eating or significantly reduced calories (e.g., 20–30% of normal intake). The 5:2 diet similarly involves 5 days of eating ad libitum and 2 days per week of fasting or reduced calorie intake. Time restricted eating involves limiting feeding to a certain time window each day (e.g., 8–10 h) and fasting the remainder of the 24-h period.

Intermittent fasting may be beneficial for several reasons. Small studies have shown that the calorie deficit created during the fast is not completely compensated for during the days of ad libitum eating, thus producing weight loss. Prolonged periods of fasting also increase utilization of fat stores for energy [42]. Intermittent fasting may be simpler to follow than some other dietary approaches given that it does not involve tracking calories or macronutrients, and there may be beneficial cellular processes triggered by fasting. Time restricted eating windows that restrict energy consumption to the biological day, which is when the body evolved to metabolize food, may help to promote circadian alignment and optimal health.

Meta-analyses of current data indicate that intermittent fasting is a viable alternative to continuous energy restriction achieved through adherence to a daily calorie goal or a diet that restricts intake of certain macronutrients, as described above [41, 43]. While some research suggests weight loss from intermittent fasting is greater than that achieved via other approaches [44], research controlling energy intake reveals similar weight outcomes [45]. Intermittent fasting also appears to have beneficial effects for several cardiometabolic outcomes, although studies with longer follow-up periods are needed [43].

Plant-based diets refer to both vegetarian and vegan diets. As with the Mediterranean diet, these diets emphasize general patterns of eating rather than specific macronutrient intake. A lacto-ovo-vegetarian diet excludes red meat, poultry, and fish but includes eggs and dairy, while a vegan diet excludes all animal-based products. The nutritional composition and quality of plant-based diets can vary widely depending on the types of foods consumed. A vegetarian diet composed primarily of fresh fruits and vegetables, whole grains, legumes, and nuts is much more healthy than a vegetarian diet consisting of many processed foods high in calories, fat, sodium, and sugar. Plant-based diets have long been touted for their health benefits but have only more recently been of interest as a specific dietary approach for weight loss. While data support several health benefits of a healthy vegetarian diet [46], well-controlled trials evaluating its efficacy for weight loss relative to other evidence-based approaches are limited. A healthy vegetarian or vegan diet is among those cited as beneficial by the American

Heart Association for cardiovascular health [36]. A vegan diet predisposes to deficiency of nutrients predominantly found in animal products, e.g., protein, vitamin B12, vitamin D, iron, omega-3 fats, calcium, and zinc. Thus, persons following a vegan diet require monitoring and nutrient supplementation.

Physical Activity

Although exercise is a popular strategy for trying to lose weight, many well-controlled trials have shown that exercise alone has a variable effect on body weight, with individuals on average experiencing minimal weight loss [47]. However, exercise combined with dietary change leads to more sustained weight loss than dietary change alone and individuals who engage in higher levels of moderate to vigorous physical activity (MVPA) tend to have better weight loss maintenance [48, 49]. For these reasons, as well as the many well-known health benefits of regular physical activity independent of weight change, exercise remains a pillar of lifestyle modification interventions.

Lifestyle modification programs typically focus primarily on increasing structured exercise – that is, purposeful activity undertaken for the purpose of improving health. Many also encourage increasing overall lifestyle activity and some encourage decreasing sedentary time. The US Department of Health and Human Services recommends that all adults engage in strength training on at least 2 days per week for overall health [50]. Strength training is typically not a major focus of lifestyle modification interventions given its modest impact on energy expenditure. However, strength training increases or preserves lean muscle mass and thus provides benefit for weight management in conjunction with aerobic activity [51].

Structured Exercise

Guidelines from the American College of Sports Medicine and The Obesity Society recommend that adults engage in at least 150 min of MVPA per week to prevent weight gain and 200–300 min or more per week to prevent weight regain after intentional weight loss [52]. This is equivalent to approximately 1200 kcals and 2000 kcals burned per week on average, respectively. These recommendations are based primarily on observations showing that individuals who engage in these high levels of MVPA are more successful with long-term weight maintenance. Some experimental work also supports the importance of regular exercise for weight management, although adherence to high levels of exercise can be challenging in randomized trials [49].

Exercise intensity is often measured in metabolic equivalents (METs). METs are a ratio of one's working metabolic rate relative to their resting metabolic rate, with one MET defined as the amount of oxygen required and the number of calories one burns at rest. Intensity can also be measured in terms of age-adjusted estimated maximum heart rate, which can be approximated by subtracting one's age in years from 220. Moderate intensity activity is defined as activity equivalent to 3–5.9 METs or approximately 65–75% of estimated maximum heart rate, while vigorous activity is any activity of 6 or greater METs or more than 75% of estimated maximum heart rate [53]. Examples of activities that often achieve at least a moderate intensity of activity include walking at 3–4 miles per hour, swimming, cycling (stationary or outdoors), aerobics classes, and use of cardiovascular workout machines like an elliptical or stair stepper. As exercise intensity is dependent on a particular individual's fitness level, the types of activities and intensity required to achieve a moderate-to-vigorous intensity level is highly variable. As such, lifestyle modification programs typically teach individuals strategies for gauging exercise intensity, such as manually taking their pulse, tracking heart rate with a smartwatch or other tracker, or using subjective measures like the "talk test," in which moderate-intensity exercise is equivalent to activity where an individual can talk but not sing.

Many individuals initiating weight management interventions are quite sedentary and may have low cardiorespiratory fitness. Exercise prescriptions are therefore typically progressive. For example, individuals may first be encouraged to exercise 3 days per week for 15 min per day, with the number of exercise days and minutes gradually increasing until 150–300 min/week is reached. Historically, individuals have been instructed to perform exercise in sessions, or "bouts," at least 10 min in duration. More recent data suggest that this minimum duration is not necessary to yield desired health benefits from exercise [54]. Accordingly, the 2018 Physical Activity Guidelines for Americans departed from previous versions by removing the 10-min bout requirement.

In the context of obesity treatment, it may still be helpful to emphasize exercise in bouts – unless individuals are implementing interval training, as discussed below – to facilitate exercise goal setting and self-monitoring. Additionally, multiple exercise days per week are usually encouraged to help individuals establish an exercise routine and make activity part of their lifestyle. Condensing exercise minutes into just a couple of days, sometimes referred to as a "weekend warrior" pattern, may work well for some. While additional research is needed on this exercise pattern, results from a large population-based study found that all-cause mortality was lower among active adults – including "weekend warriors" – relative to inactive adults [55].

Continuous Versus Interval Training

High-intensity internal training (HIIT) consists of exercise performed at intensities >80% maximal capacity for multiple, brief bursts, each of which is typically less than 1 min. These intervals are separated by periods of lower intensity active recovery. Interval training has become increasingly popular due to its time-effectiveness and its potential benefits for increasing cardiovascular fitness and strength. Data on the effects of HIIT relative to continuous exercise training are equivocal. Several recent meta-analyses among a variety of populations have found that HIIT produces greater improvements on maximal oxygen consumption, fat mass, and other metabolic outcomes compared to traditional moderate-intensity

continuous training [56, 57]. A meta-analysis specific to populations with obesity that compared HITT to continuous training similarly found superior improvements for HIIT on cardiorespiratory fitness and percent fat mass, although BMI did not differ [58]. However, the expert committee that drafted the most recent national physical activity guidelines concluded that HIIT produces benefits on par with continuous training [54]. The committee did note that individuals with obesity are more likely than those of healthy weight to derive benefit from HIIT. While not often explicitly prescribed in lifestyle modification interventions, varying one's intensity of activity to include HIIT may provide benefits. One downside of HIIT is that the higher intensity of exercise can cause it to be perceived as unpleasant. This may be especially true for individuals with obesity [59]. Adherence to higher intensity exercise regimens can thus be less consistent, especially earlier in the adaptation of the approach [59].

Minute Versus Step Goals

National physical activity guidelines and exercise recommendations provided in lifestyle modification interventions have historically emphasized MVPA minute goals. However, the proliferation of wrist-worn and smartphone-based step counters over the past decade has led to increased interest in the value of step goals for improving health and facilitating weight management. Research on the health benefits provided from steps alone, with no regard for whether those steps were accrued through light activity or MVPA, remains limited [54]. While some research suggests an inverse dose–response relationship of daily steps with health outcomes including cardiovascular events, T2D, and all-cause mortality, additional studies are needed to determine whether a step goal alone is sufficient for improved health [60, 61]. At present, primary focus continues to be on minutes of MVPA to maximize health gains. Individuals who want to count steps can first determine how many steps they take when engaging in MVPA, set an MVPA time goal, and to then use step counts to track progress toward that goal. For example, a patient could see how many steps they take during a 10-min brisk walk and then determine how many steps would be required for the equivalent of 20 min of MVPA.

Lifestyle Activity and Sedentary Time

Light intensity exercise, often referred to as lifestyle activity, refers to activities that require <3.0 METs. Examples include leisurely walking and light household activities. Lifestyle activity is most often measured through step counts. Lifestyle activity has some benefit for weight management. Although it has much less of an effect on energy expenditure than MVPA, lifestyle activity does contribute to energy expenditure and, in conjunction with dietary change and MVPA, can help create an energy deficit [52]. As noted above, steps may also relate to improvements in other health outcomes. Patients are therefore usually encouraged to increase their lifestyle activity in addition to increasing structured exercise.

Several studies have explored the associations of step counts with weight change. For every increase in 2100 steps per day, BMI is reduced by 0.4 kg/m^2 (holding energy intake equal) [62]. As a point of reference, 2000 steps is about a mile. One recent study found that individuals in a weight loss intervention who achieved at least a 10% weight loss at 18 months were engaging in 10,000 steps per day, with approximately 3500 of these steps being accrued through bouted MVPA [63]. A daily goal of 10,000 steps has gained popularity in the general public and is being adopted in some countries as a public health goal [64]. However, no specific step goal has been identified for US guidelines, although benefits appear to accrue as steps increase toward and meet the 10,000 mark [60].

Sedentary behavior refers to any waking behavior characterized by low levels of energy expenditure (<1.5 METSs) while sitting, reclining, or lying. Many weight management programs do not place strong emphasis on reducing sedentary behavior and instead focus on increasing MVPA and lifestyle activity (which indirectly displace sedentary time). However, some programs have begun directly targeting sedentary time given its negative effects on cardiovascular health. Greater time spent in sedentary behavior strongly relates to risk of CVD and all-cause mortality in adults [60]. Risk also depends on amount of MVPA. Among individuals with high levels of MVPA, the negative effects of high amounts of sedentary time are reduced. Among individuals with low levels of MVPA, the risk of all-cause mortality increases as time spent sitting increases [60]. For inactive adults, displacing sedentary time with physical activity, including lifestyle activity, is one way to reduce risk of all-cause mortality. Even greater reductions can be achieved through also increasing MVPA. There is currently debate about how much the patterning of sedentary behavior matters, namely, whether prolonged periods of sedentary time are more detrimental to health than sedentary behavior accrued across briefer periods. While more research is needed, many experts agree that frequent postural shifts are likely beneficial [65].

Effects of Exercise on Metabolic Parameters

Although the effect of physical activity on weight loss is not as large as many individuals seeking treatment would prefer, exercise can improve cardiovascular and metabolic parameters and reduce mortality risk independent of weight loss. It is likely beneficial to emphasizing these important outcomes when encouraging patients to increase exercise to manage expectations about exercise's effect on weight.

The importance of "fitness" versus "fatness" is a hot topic among both researchers in the field and the general public [66]. Teasing out the impact of fitness versus fatness on health is a difficult task, and findings on the independent and combined effects of fitness and fatness on health and mortality vary based on the population being studied and the design used. However, overall, it appears that high cardiorespiratory fitness buffers against many, but not all, of the health risks associated with excess weight [67, 68]. As an example of one study that highlights the profound benefits of high cardiorespiratory fitness, Arem and colleagues conducted a pooled analysis of over 660,000 participants across studies of the National Cancer Institute Cohort Consortium examining the 2008 physical activity guidelines and their effect on mortality risk [69]. They reported that engagement in any moderate or vigorous activity reduced risk by 20% as compared to those engaging in no activity. Those who engaged in one to two times the recommended amount of activity per week – 7.5 metabolic equivalent hours per week – decreased their mortality risk by 31%. This protective effect was found across BMI categories. One limitation of studies in this area is that most do not examine the potential differential effect of degree of obesity on outcomes, often collapsing individuals with BMIs >30 or > 35 kg.m^2 into a single group for analyses [66, 70]. Additionally, because some research suggests excess adiposity still confers risk for CVD outcomes and mortality independently of exercise, encouraging both exercise and weight management likely yields the greatest health benefits.

Behavioral Modification

Behavioral modification is a critical aspect of obesity treatment that enables individuals to establish healthy behaviors and lays the groundwork for long-term success. Interventions can be delivered through different modalities and in individual or group formats. Key behavioral modification skills common to most lifestyle interventions for obesity are discussed below. Other skills not reviewed here, such as stress management, are present in some approaches.

Self-Monitoring and Goal Setting

Consistent self-monitoring is one of the most reliable and strongest predictors of both short- and long-term weight loss [71–73]. Self-monitoring encourages behavior modification and promotes weight loss by providing individuals with regular feedback on their behaviors in relation to their goals – namely, how they are doing with meeting eating, activity, and weight loss goals. This regular feedback provides opportunities for patients to modify their behaviors appropriately and can provide a sense of accomplishment and reward when behaviors are on track [74].

Patients are typically instructed to keep daily records of their food intake, to track their exercise each week, and to weigh themselves regularly. There has been debate about the optimal self-weighing frequency. At least weekly self-weighing is recommended when patients are seeking both to lose weight and to maintain weight loss. Daily weighing is recommended for maintenance and may be more helpful than less frequent weighing for weight loss [75].

Paper and pencil logs were historically used for self-monitoring. A subset of patients still opts for this approach. However, most individuals now use websites and smartphone apps to monitor their food intake. There are a variety of commercial apps available for self-monitoring, including apps that are free of charge. Some of these apps include features like barcode scanners that automatically load nutritional information from pre-packaged foods into one's record. Additional forms of technology-based self-monitoring include food photography and bite counters. Many individuals now also use wearable physical activity trackers, like smartwatches and commercial wrist-worn activity trackers, to monitor their exercise and lifestyle activity. Wi-fi equipped smart scales that sync with apps or websites and automatically depict weight trends can also be useful for monitoring body weight. Many of these scales also measure metrics like body fat, although accuracy is of concern. Due to cost, smart scales are still often the exception rather than the norm in clinical practice.

These more automated forms of self-monitoring can reduce patient burden and save time, thus improving self-monitoring adherence [76]. However, these benefits may come with the trade-off of reduced accuracy. For example, photography-based food monitoring appears less effective than more traditional self-monitoring focused on tracking calories [77]. While some research shows that app-based monitoring of calorie intake is similar in accuracy to paper-and-pencil methods

[78], the increased self-monitoring adherence achieved through use of technology has typically not resulted in greater weight losses [76]. This raises the possibility that accuracy is a challenge for some. An additional benefit of automated self-monitoring besides reduced burden is that data can be easily shared with clinicians or other individuals to provide enhanced support and accountability. Several studies have examined the utility of data sharing in improving care with promising outcomes [79]. Patients may find it somewhat distressing to self-monitor when they are having difficulty meeting their goals or are gaining weight, leading to short-term breaks, or "lapses," in self-monitoring [80, 81]. While this difficulty is understandable, consistent self-monitoring relates to better long-term outcomes. Programs therefore encourage patients to continue self-monitoring even if, and perhaps especially if, experiencing difficulties meeting their goals.

Goal setting is another key behavioral modification strategy that complements self-monitoring. Patients' dietary and physical activity goals are typically set by their clinician or their selected weight loss program/approach, and patients use self-monitoring to assess their progress toward these goals day-to-day and week-to-week. During live treatment sessions, clinicians typically check in on goal progress at the outset of sessions and set new goals at the end of sessions. In automated programs, algorithms can be used to determine progress toward goals based on self-monitoring data and to provide automatic, tailored feedback. Tailoring appears to be especially important for patient success in programs that use digital technology [82]. Patients are taught to set specific, measurable, actionable behavioral targets to modify aspects of their lifestyle to meet their eating, physical activity, and weight loss goals. For example, if a patient is struggling to meet their calorie goal, they may target a behavior focused on reducing the frequency of restaurant eating or preparing more fruits and vegetables for snacks. Goal setting is essential for facilitating behavior change. Figure 1 shows an example of a weekly goal setting worksheet.

Stimulus Control and Problem Solving

Environmental and social cues play a major role in shaping behavior [83]. As such, patients are taught to modify cues in their immediate environment – such as their home and workplace – to both reduce cues that trigger unhealthy eating and inactivity and to increase cues for healthy eating and physical activity. The idea behind stimulus control is to reduce the need for individuals to rely on self-regulation to override cues for unhealthy behavior, and to create an environment where healthy

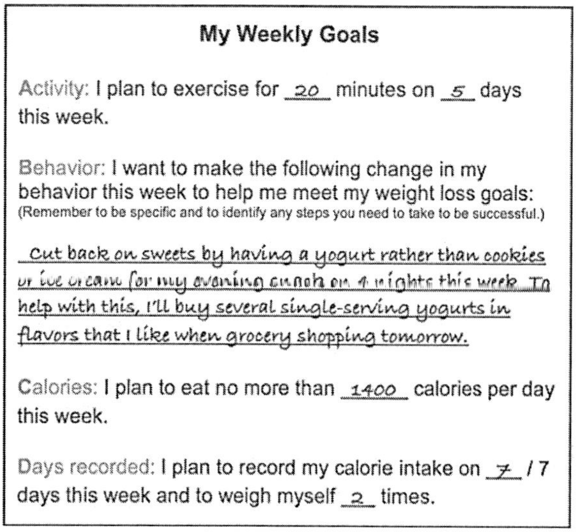

Fig. 1 Worksheets like the one shown here can assist patients in setting specific goals for key weight-related behaviors

My Weekly Goals

Activity: I plan to exercise for _20_ minutes on _5_ days this week.

Behavior: I want to make the following change in my behavior this week to help me meet my weight loss goals: (Remember to be specific and to identify any steps you need to take to be successful.)

Cut back on sweets by having a yogurt rather than cookies or ice cream for my evening snack on 4 nights this week. To help with this, I'll buy several single-serving yogurts in flavors that I like when grocery shopping tomorrow.

Calories: I plan to eat no more than _1400_ calories per day this week.

Days recorded: I plan to record my calorie intake on _7_ / 7 days this week and to weigh myself _2_ times.

behaviors are more of an automatic, default choice. This focus on automating healthy choices as much as possible aligns with theories of behavior change emphasizing the important role that less-conscious processes, like habit, play in health behavior [84]. Stimulus control can focus on reducing exposure to particularly tempting high-calorie foods, increasing the availability and visibility of healthy food, and creating cues for physical activity. Patients are also encouraged to modify social cues to create a social environment that helps, rather than hinders, their success. This can focus on asking for support for healthy behaviors from loved ones, modifying social patterns that do not serve health goals, and creating new social habits that center around physical activity and healthy eating.

Problem solving is another core behavioral skill. Patients identify a problem in detail, identify potential solutions to the problem, consider the pros and cons of each option, choose a solution, develop a plan to implement it, and evaluate the effectiveness of the chosen solution once the behavior has been implemented [73]. Making these plans as specific as possible and checking in with patients regarding their intentions to try to enact the plan during the coming week are necessary for adherence.

Managing Thoughts and Maintaining Motivation

Patients must maintain healthy patterns of eating and physical activity over time to maintain their weight loss and sustain improvements in health. A pressing issue is thus how to maintain motivation. Thought patterns affect both initial success in modifying behavior and maintenance of behavior changes. Strategies from cognitive behavioral therapies, including acceptance-based behavior therapy (ABBT), are often used in interventions to address thinking patterns and motivational issues.

Programs like the Diabetes Prevention Program (DPP) teach the skill of cognitive restructuring to deal with unhelpful thinking patterns [85]. This skill focuses on identifying thoughts that do not promote healthy behaviors, assessing their accuracy and helpfulness, and modifying these thoughts to make them more realistic and helpful. For example, a patient might think, "I have to have pizza on Friday nights with my friends. It's pizza night." The provider would help the patient explore how this thought impacts behavior and health goals. Alternative ways of viewing and responding to the situation could then be explored. For example, the patient may identify that they do not need to have pizza and that this is largely a learned habit. They could explore the pros and cons of eating pizza each Friday and emotions related to eating and not eating pizza in this context. Different behavioral options could be identified, such as alternating menu items for Friday nights to include healthier options, using portion control to have a smaller amount of pizza, or experimenting with new, healthier pizza recipes to improve the nutritional quality and decrease the caloric content of the pizza consumed. Socratic questioning can be used to help the patient generate their own solutions to weight loss barriers. This exercise also increases the patient's ability to identify triggers to overeating and automatic thoughts that lead to undesirable outcomes, allowing the individual to stop in the moment and respond in a manner more consistent with his or her weight loss or weight maintenance goals. Motivational barriers are often addressed through use of small rewards, regular reflections on benefits gained from lifestyle change, and incorporating novel foods and activities into one's healthy lifestyle to prevent behavioral drift due to boredom.

Acceptance-based behavior therapy (ABBT) is a variation of traditional cognitive behavioral therapy and has been shown to be an effective alternative approach for promoting long-term weight loss. ABBT focuses on changing one's response to thoughts and feelings, rather than the experiences themselves. It also emphasizes the importance of personal values for long-term motivation [86]. This approach posits that uncomfortable thoughts and feelings are at times inevitable when seeking to practice healthy behaviors. This is especially true given that we live in a society where unhealthy eating cues are ubiquitous, inactivity is increasingly the default, and our biology often works against long-term weight maintenance. Patients are taught mindfulness- and acceptance-based skills that focus on noticing and accepting that these thoughts and feelings are present, while at the same time choosing to engage in the healthy behaviors. Values, or the life domains or roles that patients care most deeply about, are used to foster motivation to engage in healthy behaviors in the face of challenging internal experiences.

As an example, patients who value being an involved parent might identify that healthy eating and regular physical activity gives them more energy and enhances their mobility, thus helping them to better "live out" their parenting values. As another example, patients who highly value community involvement might identify ways in which lifestyle modification allows them to serve as a positive role model for others in their community. Connections between healthy behaviors and values serve as motivation to sustain long-term behavior change. ABBT has been shown to be efficacious for weight loss when delivered in groups over multiple months, in-person workshops, and in remote formats [87, 88].

Other Treatment Considerations

The treatment components described above can be implemented in a variety of formats. The importance of both avoiding stigmatizing individuals for their weight and considering weight stigma when conceptualizing treatment is also discussed.

Intervention Settings and Modalities

Lifestyle modification interventions can be delivered through individual counseling sessions with a nutritionist, psychologist, physician, or other ancillary medical staff. The Centers for Medicare and Medicaid Services covers intensive lifestyle modification delivered by select providers in individual sessions in primary care. Excellent

resources exist to facilitate effective treatment delivery in this setting [89]. Because individual intervention is time-intensive and expensive, group interventions are often employed. Not only are groups more cost-effective than individual treatment, they also provide social support and can help participants be more engaged and feel more accountable for their efforts. Whether delivered in individual or group-based formats, it is recommended that patients receive high-intensity comprehensive intervention – defined as 14 or more sessions in 6 months with a trained interventionist – to achieve 5–10% weight loss [2].

Landmark programs like the DPP and Look AHEAD were delivered face-to-face in-person. In-person treatment continues to be a common treatment modality, including in medical settings, specialty weight management clinics, community-based settings (e.g., YMCAs), and commercial programs. Interventions are also frequently delivered via telephone and videoconferencing, either solely through these modalities or in hybrid remote/in-person models. More recently, researchers have explored the potential of delivering treatment through social media platforms, apps, and fully automated online programs. This line of inquiry was accelerated during the COVID-19 pandemic when many forms of health care delivery quickly pivoted to the use of technology to deliver care. The efficacy of these approaches varies, with weight losses achieved often less than those seen in in-person programs. However, some programs demonstrate impressive outcomes on par with many in-person treatments. For example, a fully automated 12-week program developed by Thomas and colleagues produced 5% weight loss at 12 weeks in several trials, including a pragmatic trial in primary care [90].

Combining Lifestyle Modification with Other Treatment Approaches

Lifestyle modification is a first-line treatment for obesity and is often used as a standalone treatment approach [2]. However, it can also be combined with pharmacotherapy, also referred to as anti-obesity medications. The FDA has approved several anti-obesity medications, including the newer glucagon-like peptide-1 (GLP-1) agents, semaglutide and liraglutide, with several others in development. These medications have shown great promise for increasing weight losses, as described in detail elsewhere in the book. For example, in one 68-week long randomized trial among adults with obesity without T2D, once weekly semaglutide resulted in −14.9% weight loss as compared with −2.4% with placebo [91]. Anti-obesity medications are most effective when combined with behavioral weight management [92]. Many components of lifestyle modification can also be used to enhance outcomes from bariatric surgery, although specific dietary practices must be implemented to ensure adequate nutrition and prevent complications [93, 94].

Weight Stigma

Weight stigma refers to social devaluation of people because of their body weight [95]. Weight stigma can lead to negative weight-based stereotypes, weight-based discrimination, and internalized weight bias, in which individuals with obesity apply negative stereotypes to themselves. An overwhelming body of literature clearly shows the many detrimental effects of weight stigma and internalized bias [95]. This includes negative effects on physical health, mental health, social functioning, and even domains like employment. Ironically – and contrary to the belief held by some that stigma will motivate individuals to lose weight – weight stigma and internalized bias contribute to obesity and its comorbidities through both behavioral and physiological pathways [95]. Unfortunately, patients frequently report experiencing weight stigma and discrimination in healthcare settings, including from obesity providers [96]. Stigma and discrimination from providers may owe in part to the low priority of obesity education among medical schools [97]. A lack of comprehensive education on the complex etiology of obesity, its conceptualization as a chronic disease, and evidence-based treatments for obesity leaves many providers unprepared to manage obesity among their patients.

Given the adverse effects of weight stigma, there have been calls to action to increase research on this topic and to take steps to reduce stigma and internalized bias. This includes reducing stigma in healthcare settings. Excellent discussions of strategies to reduce weight stigma in healthcare settings can be found elsewhere but include measures such as policy changes, increased education, provision of appropriate seating and equipment for larger bodies, and increased involvement of persons with obesity in the development of obesity-related policies and care [98, 99]. Identifying strategies for decreasing the negative effect of weight stigma on health behaviors and outcomes, including skills to reduce internalization of these biases in individuals, can be incorporated into conventional weight management programs or used as stand-alone interventions. This is a developing priority in this area [100].

Disordered Eating

A subset of persons with obesity may engage in disordered eating behaviors. These may predate behavioral weight management attempts, or they may begin after the start of such a program. Clinicians should monitor for meal-skipping, which can lead to episodes of loss of control over eating, which can include binge episodes. Others may engage in inappropriate compensatory behaviors, such as vomiting, laxative use, or compulsive exercise to counteract food intake. Still others may engage in night-eating, including waking to eat. Individuals in all BMI categories can engage in disordered eating behaviors, so it is important to monitor for their presence. Staples of these treatments, such as tracking one's caloric intake and daily weighing may be triggering in persons with disordered eating. Clinicians should use their judgment to pause weight loss goals until these eating disordered thoughts and behaviors are addressed, and consider if and when it would be better to pursue weight management goals. Stabilization of weight or weight maintenance should be the revised goal in the presence of active disordered eating attitudes and behaviors.

Conclusions

Lifestyle modification plays a key role in weight management efforts. Its components include choosing a specific dietary plan, promoting MVPA, and using behavioral modification strategies. Different dietary approaches produce weight loss successfully, typically between a 5% and 10% loss of initial body weight, which is related to improvements in cardiovascular and metabolic health. As better long-term dietary adherence relates to better outcomes, individuals' preferences and perceived ability to adhere to a certain diet is of utmost importance when selecting a dietary approach. Supplementing dietary change with physical activity generally increases weight loss, predicts longer-term weight loss maintenance, and improves overall health. The use of behavioral modification techniques helps improve adherence to a diet and exercise plan through specific action plans and accountability. These techniques can also help sustain long-term motivation.

Future research in this area likely will focus on matching lifestyle modification strategies to individuals based on factors like genetics, taste, and behavioral preferences. More research is also needed to understand how individual-level change can be bolstered through larger, community- and systems-based changes, how to best combine behavioral intervention with other treatment approaches, and how to decrease stigma and its negative effects. Until then, providing ample support to those seeking weight loss, encouraging self-monitoring, targeting specific calorie or other macronutrient goals, and providing specific plans for increasing physical activity should be a part of any prescribed weight management program.

References

1. Bray G, Kim K, Wilding J, Federation WO. Obesity: a chronic relapsing progressive disease process. A position statement of the world obesity Federation. Obes Rev. 2017;18(7):715–23.
2. Jensen MD, Ryan DH, Apovian CM, et al. 2013 AHA/ACC/TOS guideline for the management of overweight and obesity in adults: a report of the American College of Cardiology/American Heart Association Task Force on Practice Guidelines and The Obesity Society. J Am Coll Cardiol. 2014;63(25): 2985–3023.
3. Curry SJ, Krist AH, Owens DK, et al. Behavioral weight loss interventions to prevent obesity-related morbidity and mortality in adults: US preventive services task force recommendation statement. JAMA. 2018;320(11):1163–71.
4. Tobias DK, Chen M, Manson JE, Ludwig DS, Willett W, Hu FB. Effect of low-fat diet interventions versus other diet interventions on long-term weight change in adults: a systematic review and meta-analysis. Lancet Diabetes Endocrinol. 2015;3(12): 968–79.
5. Sacks FM, Bray GA, Carey VJ, et al. Comparison of weight-loss diets with different compositions of fat, protein, and carbohydrates. N Engl J Med. 2009;360 (9):859–73.
6. Gardner CD, Trepanowski JF, Del Gobbo LC, et al. Effect of low-fat vs low-carbohydrate diet on 12-month weight loss in overweight adults and the association with genotype pattern or insulin secretion: the DIETFITS randomized clinical trial. JAMA. 2018;319(7):667–79.
7. Committee ADAPP, Committee: ADAPP. 8. Obesity and weight management for the prevention and treatment of type 2 diabetes: standards of medical care in diabetes – 2022. Diabetes Care. 2022;45(Supp 1): S113–24.
8. Evert AB, Dennison M, Gardner CD, et al. Nutrition therapy for adults with diabetes or prediabetes: a consensus report. Diabetes Care. 2019;42(5):731–54.
9. Rolls BJ. The relationship between dietary energy density and energy intake. Physiol Behav. 2009;97 (5):609–15.
10. Kim Y, Je Y, Giovannucci EL. Association between dietary fat intake and mortality from all-causes, cardiovascular disease, and cancer: a systematic review and meta-analysis of prospective cohort studies. Clin Nutr. 2021;40(3):1060–70.
11. Group DPPR. Reduction in the incidence of type 2 diabetes with lifestyle intervention or metformin. N Engl J Med. 2002;346(6):393–403.
12. Group LAR. Long-term effects of a lifestyle intervention on weight and cardiovascular risk factors in individuals with type 2 diabetes mellitus: four-year results of the look AHEAD trial. Arch Intern Med. 2010;170 (17):1566–75.
13. Appel LJ, Clark JM, Yeh H-C, et al. Comparative effectiveness of weight-loss interventions in clinical practice. N Engl J Med. 2011;365(21):1959–68.
14. Wadden TA, Volger S, Sarwer DB, et al. A two-year randomized trial of obesity treatment in primary care practice. N Engl J Med. 2011;365(21):1969–79.
15. Group LAR. Reduction in weight and cardiovascular disease risk factors in individuals with type 2 diabetes: one-year results of the look AHEAD trial. Diabetes Care. 2007;30(6):1374–83.

16. Foster GD, Borradaile KE, Sanders MH, et al. A randomized study on the effect of weight loss on obstructive sleep apnea among obese patients with type 2 diabetes: the sleep AHEAD study. Arch Intern Med. 2009;169(17):1619–26.

17. Williamson DA, Rejeski J, Lang W, et al. Impact of a weight management program on health-related quality of life in overweight adults with type 2 diabetes. Arch Intern Med. 2009;169(2):163–71.

18. Rejeski WJ, Ip EH, Bertoni AG, et al. Lifestyle change and mobility in obese adults with type 2 diabetes. N Engl J Med. 2012;366(13):1209–17.

19. Group LAR. Cardiovascular effects of intensive lifestyle intervention in type 2 diabetes. N Engl J Med. 2013;369(2):145–54.

20. Gonzalez-Campoy JM, Castorino K, Ebrahim A, et al. Clinical practice guidelines for healthy eating for the prevention and treatment of metabolic and endocrine diseases in adults: cosponsored by the American Association of Clinical Endocrinologists/the American College of Endocrinology and the Obesity Society. Endocr Pract. 2013;19: 1–82.

21. Astrup A, Larsen TM, Harper A. Atkins and other low-carbohydrate diets: hoax or an effective tool for weight loss? Lancet. 2004;364(9437):897–9.

22. Yancy WS, Mitchell NS, Westman EC. Ketogenic diet for obesity and diabetes. JAMA Intern Med. 2019;179(12):1734–5.

23. van Zuuren EJ, Fedorowicz Z, Kuijpers T, Pijl H. Effects of low-carbohydrate-compared with low-fat-diet interventions on metabolic control in people with type 2 diabetes: a systematic review including GRADE assessments. Am J Clin Nutr. 2018;108(2): 300–31.

24. Sainsbury E, Kizirian NV, Partridge SR, Gill T, Colagiuri S, Gibson AA. Effect of dietary carbohydrate restriction on glycemic control in adults with diabetes: a systematic review and meta-analysis. Diabetes Res Clin Pract. 2018;139:239–52.

25. Bueno NB, de Melo ISV, de Oliveira SL, da Rocha AT. Very-low-carbohydrate ketogenic diet v. low-fat diet for long-term weight loss: a meta-analysis of randomised controlled trials. Br J Nutr. 2013;110(7): 1178–87.

26. Apekey TA, Maynard MJ, Kittana M, Kunutsor SK. Comparison of the effectiveness of low carbohydrate versus low fat diets in type 2 diabetes: systematic review and meta-analysis of randomized controlled trials. Nutrients. 2022;14(20):4391.

27. Leidy HJ, Clifton PM, Astrup A, et al. The role of protein in weight loss and maintenance. Am J Clin Nutr. 2015;101(6):1320S–9S.

28. Phillips SM, Fulgoni VL III, Heaney RP, Nicklas TA, Slavin JL, Weaver CM. Commonly consumed protein foods contribute to nutrient intake, diet quality, and nutrient adequacy. Am J Clin Nutr. 2015;101(6): 1346S–52S.

29. Pesta DH, Samuel VT. A high-protein diet for reducing body fat: mechanisms and possible caveats. Nutr Metab (Lond). 2014;11(1):1–8.

30. Yu Z, Nan F, Wang LY, Jiang H, Chen W, Jiang Y. Effects of high-protein diet on glycemic control, insulin resistance and blood pressure in type 2 diabetes: a systematic review and meta-analysis of randomized controlled trials. Clin Nutr. 2020;39(6):1724–34.

31. Wycherley TP, Moran LJ, Clifton PM, Noakes M, Brinkworth GD. Effects of energy-restricted high-protein, low-fat compared with standard-protein, low-fat diets: a meta-analysis of randomized controlled trials. Am J Clin Nutr. 2012;96(6):1281–98.

32. Santesso N, Akl E, Bianchi M, et al. Effects of higher- versus lower-protein diets on health outcomes: a systematic review and meta-analysis. Eur J Clin Nutr. 2012;66(7):780–8.

33. Nordmann AJ, Suter-Zimmermann K, Bucher HC, et al. Meta-analysis comparing Mediterranean to low-fat diets for modification of cardiovascular risk factors. Am J Med. 2011;124(9):841–51. e842

34. Dinu M, Pagliai G, Angelino D, et al. Effects of popular diets on anthropometric and cardiometabolic parameters: an umbrella review of meta-analyses of randomized controlled trials. Adv Nutr. 2020;11(4): 815–33.

35. Sacks FM, Lichtenstein AH, Wu JH, et al. Dietary fats and cardiovascular disease: a presidential advisory from the American Heart Association. Circulation. 2017;136(3):e1–e23.

36. Lichtenstein AH, Appel LJ, Vadiveloo M, et al. 2021 dietary guidance to improve cardiovascular health: a scientific statement from the American Heart Association. Circulation. 2021;144(23):e472–87.

37. Jenkins DJ, Wolever T, Taylor RH, et al. Glycemic index of foods: a physiological basis for carbohydrate exchange. Am J Clin Nutr. 1981;34(3):362–6.

38. Makris A, Foster GD. Dietary approaches to the treatment of obesity. Psychiatr Clin. 2011;34(4):813–27.

39. Franz MJ, MacLeod J, Evert A, et al. Academy of nutrition and dietetics nutrition practice guideline for type 1 and type 2 diabetes in adults: systematic review of evidence for medical nutrition therapy effectiveness and recommendations for integration into the nutrition care process. J Acad Nutr Diet. 2017;117 (10):1659–79.

40. Vega-López S, Venn BJ, Slavin JL. Relevance of the glycemic index and glycemic load for body weight, diabetes, and cardiovascular disease. Nutrients. 2018;10(10):1361.

41. Elortegui Pascual P, Rolands MR, Eldridge AL, et al. A meta-analysis comparing the effectiveness of alternate day fasting, the 5: 2 diet, and time-restricted eating for weight loss. Obesity. 2022;31:9.

42. De Cabo R, Mattson MP. Effects of intermittent fasting on health, aging, and disease. N Engl J Med. 2019;381(26):2541–51.

43. Patikorn C, Roubal K, Veettil SK, et al. Intermittent fasting and obesity-related health outcomes: an umbrella review of meta-analyses of randomized clinical trials. JAMA Netw Open. 2021;4(12):e2139558–8.

44. Borgundvaag E, Mak J, Kramer CK. Metabolic impact of intermittent fasting in patients with type 2 diabetes mellitus: a systematic review and meta-

analysis of interventional studies. J Clin Endocrinol Metab. 2021;106(3):902–11.

45. Liu D, Huang Y, Huang C, et al. Calorie restriction with or without time-restricted eating in weight loss. N Engl J Med. 2022;386(16):1495–504.

46. Viguiliouk E, Kendall CW, Kahleová H, et al. Effect of vegetarian dietary patterns on cardiometabolic risk factors in diabetes: a systematic review and meta-analysis of randomized controlled trials. Clin Nutr. 2019;38(3):1133–45.

47. Swift DL, McGee JE, Earnest CP, Carlisle E, Nygard M, Johannsen NM. The effects of exercise and physical activity on weight loss and maintenance. Prog Cardiovasc Dis. 2018;61(2):206–13.

48. Johns DJ, Hartmann-Boyce J, Jebb SA, Aveyard P. Diet or exercise interventions vs combined behavioral weight management programs: a systematic review and meta-analysis of direct comparisons. J Acad Nutr Diet. 2014;114(10):1557–68.

49. Jakicic JM, Rogers RJ, Sherman SA, Kovacs SJ. Physical activity and weight management. In: Wadden TA, Bray GA, editors. Handbook of obesity treatment. 2nd ed. New York: The Guillford Press; 2018. p. 322–35.

50. Piercy KL, Troiano RP, Ballard RM, et al. The physical activity guidelines for Americans. JAMA. 2018;320(19):2020–8.

51. Jm O, Bellicha A, van Baak MA, et al. Exercise training in the management of overweight and obesity in adults: synthesis of the evidence and recommendations from the European Association for the Study of obesity physical activity working group. Obes Rev. 2021;22:e13273.

52. Donnelly JE, Blair SN, Jakicic JM, Manore MM, Rankin JW, Smith BK. American College of Sports Medicine Position Stand. Appropriate physical activity intervention strategies for weight loss and prevention of weight regain for adults. Med Sci Sports Exerc. 2009;41(2):459–71.

53. American College of Sports Medicine. ACSM's guidelines for exercise testing and prescription. Philadelphia: Lippincott Williams & Wilkins; 2020.

54. 2018 Physical ACtivity Guidelines Advisory Committee. 2018 physical activity guidelines advisory committee scientific report. Washington, DC: U.S. Department of Health and Human Services; 2018.

55. O'Donovan G, Lee I-M, Hamer M, Stamatakis E. Association of "weekend warrior" and other leisure time physical activity patterns with risks for all-cause, cardiovascular disease, and cancer mortality. JAMA Intern Med. 2017;177(3):335–42.

56. Milanović Z, Sporiš G, Weston M. Effectiveness of high-intensity interval training (HIT) and continuous endurance training for VO2max improvements: a systematic review and meta-analysis of controlled trials. Sports Med. 2015;45(10):1469–81.

57. Costa EC, Hay JL, Kehler DS, et al. Effects of high-intensity interval training versus moderate-intensity continuous training on blood pressure in adults with pre-to established hypertension: a systematic review

and meta-analysis of randomized trials. Sports Med. 2018;48(9):2127–42.

58. Türk Y, Theel W, Kasteleyn M, et al. High intensity training in obesity: a meta-analysis. Obes Sci Pract. 2017;3(3):258–71.

59. Ekkekakis P, Vazou S, Bixby WR, Georgiadis E. The mysterious case of the public health guideline that is (almost) entirely ignored: call for a research agenda on the causes of the extreme avoidance of physical activity in obesity. Obes Rev. 2016;17(4):313–29.

60. Kraus WE, Janz KF, Powell KE, et al. Daily step counts for measuring physical activity exposure and its relation to health. Med Sci Sports Exerc. 2019;51 (6):1206.

61. Paluch AE, Bajpai S, Bassett DR, et al. Daily steps and all-cause mortality: a meta-analysis of 15 international cohorts. Lancet Public Health. 2022;7(3): e219–28.

62. Bravata DM, Smith-Spangler C, Sundaram V, et al. Using pedometers to increase physical activity and improve health: a systematic review. JAMA. 2007;298(19):2296–304.

63. Creasy SA, Lang W, Tate DF, Davis KK, Jakicic JM. Pattern of daily steps is associated with weight loss: secondary analysis from the step-up randomized trial. Obesity. 2018;26(6):977–84.

64. Duncan MJ, Brown WJ, Mummery WK, Vandelanotte C. 10,000 steps Australia: a community-wide eHealth physical activity promotion programme. Br J Sports Med. 2018;52(14):885–6.

65. Biddle SJ, Bennie JA, De Cocker K, et al. Controversies in the science of sedentary behaviour and health: insights, perspectives and future directions from the 2018 Queensland sedentary behaviour think tank. Int J Environ Res Public Health. 2019;16(23):4762.

66. Kennedy AB, Lavie CJ, Blair SN. Fitness or fatness: which is more important? JAMA. 2018;319(3):231–2.

67. Barry VW, Caputo JL, Kang M. The joint association of fitness and fatness on cardiovascular disease mortality: a meta-analysis. Prog Cardiovasc Dis. 2018;61 (2):136–41.

68. Fogelholm M. Physical activity, fitness and fatness: relations to mortality, morbidity and disease risk factors: a systematic review. Obes Rev. 2010;11(3): 202–21.

69. Arem H, Moore SC, Patel A, et al. Leisure time physical activity and mortality: a detailed pooled analysis of the dose-response relationship. JAMA Intern Med. 2015;175(6):959–67.

70. Willey JZ, Moon YP, Sherzai A, Cheung YK, Sacco RL, Elkind MS. Leisure-time physical activity and mortality in a multiethnic prospective cohort study: the northern Manhattan study. Ann Epidemiol. 2015;25(7):475–9. e472

71. Burke LE, Wang J, Sevick MA. Self-monitoring in weight loss: a systematic review of the literature. J Am Diet Assoc. 2011;111(1):92–102.

72. Dombrowski SU, Sniehotta FF, Avenell A, Johnston M, MacLennan G, Araújo-Soares V. Identifying active ingredients in complex behavioural interventions for obese adults with

obesity-related co-morbidities or additional risk factors for co-morbidities: a systematic review. Health Psychol Rev. 2012;6(1):7–32.

73. Sarwer DB, Butryn ML, Forman E, Bradley LE. Lifestyle modification for the treatment of obesity. In: Still C, Sarwer DB, Blankenship J, editors. The ASMBS textbook of bariatric surgery. Volume 2: integrative health. New York: Springer; 2014. p. 147–55.

74. Carver CS, Scheier MF. Control theory: a useful conceptual framework for personality–social, clinical, and health psychology. Psychol Bull. 1982;92(1):111.

75. Steinberg DM, Bennett GG, Askew S, Tate DF. Weighing every day matters: daily weighing improves weight loss and adoption of weight control behaviors. J Acad Nutr Diet. 2015;115(4):511–8.

76. Spring B, Pellegrini CA, Pfammatter A, et al. Effects of an abbreviated obesity intervention supported by mobile technology: the ENGAGED randomized clinical trial. Obesity. 2017;25(7):1191–8.

77. Dunn CG, Turner-McGrievy GM, Wilcox S, Hutto B. Dietary self-monitoring through calorie tracking but not through a digital photography app is associated with significant weight loss: the 2SMART pilot study – a 6-month randomized trial. J Acad Nutr Diet. 2019;119(9):1525–32.

78. Hutcheson MJ, Rollo ME, Callister R, Collins CE. Self-monitoring of dietary intake by young women: online food records completed on computer or smartphone are as accurate as paper-based food records but more acceptable. J Acad Nutr Diet. 2015;115(1):87–94.

79. Butryn ML, Martinelli MK, Crane NT, et al. Counselor surveillance of digital self-monitoring data: a pilot randomized controlled trial. Obesity. 2020;28(12):2339–46.

80. Schumacher LM, Martinelli MK, Convertino AD, Forman EM, Butryn ML. Weight-related information avoidance prospectively predicts poorer self-monitoring and engagement in a behavioral weight loss intervention. Ann Behav Med. 2021;55(2):103–11.

81. Chang BP, Webb TL, Benn Y. Why do people act like the proverbial ostrich? Investigating the reasons that people provide for not monitoring their goal progress. Front Psychol. 2017;8:152.

82. Berry R, Kassavou A, Sutton S. Does self-monitoring diet and physical activity behaviors using digital technology support adults with obesity or overweight to lose weight? A systematic literature review with meta-analysis. Obes Rev. 2021;22(10):e13306.

83. Belfort-DeAguiar R, Seo D. Food cues and obesity: overpowering hormones and energy balance regulation. Curr Obes Rep. 2018;7(2):122–9.

84. Hagger MS. Non-conscious processes and dual-process theories in health psychology. Health Psychol Rev. 2016;10(4):375–80.

85. Group DPPR. The diabetes prevention program (DPP): description of lifestyle intervention. Diabetes Care. 2002;25(12):2165–71.

86. Butryn ML, Schumacher LM, Forman EM. Alternative behavioral weight loss approaches:

acceptance and commitment therapy and motivational interviewing. In: Wadden TA, Bray GA, editors. Handbook of obesity treatment. 2nd ed. New York: The Guillford Press; 2018. p. 508–21.

87. Forman EM, Butryn ML, Manasse SM, et al. Acceptance-based versus standard behavioral treatment for obesity: results from the mind your health randomized controlled trial. Obesity. 2016;24(10):2050–6.

88. Lillis J, Niemeier HM, Thomas JG, et al. A randomized trial of an acceptance-based behavioral intervention for weight loss in people with high internal disinhibition. Obesity. 2016;24(12):2509–14.

89. Wadden TA, Tsai AG, Tronieri JS. A protocol to deliver intensive behavioral therapy (IBT) for obesity in primary care settings: the MODEL-IBT program. Obesity. 2019;27(10):1562–6.

90. Thomas JG, Panza E, Espel-Huynh HM, et al. Pragmatic implementation of a fully automated online obesity treatment in primary care. Obesity. 2022;30(8):1621–8.

91. Wilding JP, Batterham RL, Calanna S, et al. Once-weekly semaglutide in adults with overweight or obesity. N Engl J Med. 2021;384:989.

92. Apovian CM, Aronne LJ, Bessesen DH, et al. Pharmacological management of obesity: an endocrine society clinical practice guideline. J Clin Endocr. 2015;100(2):342–62.

93. Mechanick JI, Youdim A, Jones DB, et al. Clinical practice guidelines for the perioperative nutritional, metabolic, and nonsurgical support of the bariatric surgery patient – 2013 update: cosponsored by American Association of Clinical Endocrinologists, the Obesity Society, and American Society for Metabolic & bariatric surgery. Obesity. 2013;21(S1):S1–S27.

94. Sarwer DB, Heinberg LJ. A review of the psychosocial aspects of clinically severe obesity and bariatric surgery. Am Psychol. 2020;75(2):252.

95. Puhl RM, Himmelstein MS, Pearl RL. Weight stigma as a psychosocial contributor to obesity. Am Psychol. 2020;75(2):274.

96. Puhl RM, Lessard LM, Himmelstein MS, Foster GD. The roles of experienced and internalized weight stigma in healthcare experiences: perspectives of adults engaged in weight management across six countries. PLoS One. 2021;16(6):e0251566.

97. Butsch WS, Kushner RF, Alford S, Smolarz BG. Low priority of obesity education leads to lack of medical students' preparedness to effectively treat patients with obesity: results from the US medical school obesity education curriculum benchmark study. BMC Med Educ. 2020;20(1):1–6.

98. Flint SW. Time to end weight stigma in healthcare. EClinicalMedicine. 2021;34:34.

99. Talumaa B, Brown A, Batterham RL, Kalea AZ. Effective strategies in ending weight stigma in healthcare. Obes Rev. 2022;23:e13494.

100. Pearl RL, Wadden TA, Bach C, et al. Effects of a cognitive-behavioral intervention targeting weight stigma: a randomized controlled trial. J Consult Clin Psychol. 2020;88(5):470.

Pharmacotherapy of Obesity and Metabolic Syndrome

38

Daisy Duan and Rexford S. Ahima

Contents

D. Duan · R. S. Ahima (✉)
Department of Medicine, Division of Endocrinology,
Diabetes and Metabolism, Johns Hopkins University
School of Medicine, Baltimore, MD, USA
e-mail: dduan5@jhmi.edu; ahima@jhmi.edu

Abstract

The management of metabolic syndrome requires a healthy low-calorie diet, increased physical activity, and other behaviors that promote optimal loss weight loss, maintenance of weight loss, and control of glycemia, blood pressure, and lipids. Medications for obesity, diabetes, hypertension, and dyslipidemia may be necessary for the treatment of components of metabolic syndrome and to reduce the risk of cardiovascular disease. This chapter describes current medications available for treatment of obesity and metabolic syndrome.

Keywords

Obesity · Metabolic syndrome · Diabetes · Hypertension · Lipid · Cardiovascular

Introduction

The prevalence of metabolic syndrome has increased worldwide mainly due to the obesity epidemic [70]. Weight loss and long-term maintenance of weight loss have been shown to improve comorbid diseases associated with metabolic syndrome (Table 1). Diet and increased physical activity are essential for weight management. Medications or bariatric surgery may be needed to achieve and maintain a healthy weight [2, 25, 26, 42, 62, 63, 66, 84, 96, 99, 133, 136, 144, 146, 150, 156]. For weight management to be successful, it is crucial for patients to be actively involved in their care and be monitored frequently for weight loss, comorbid disease outcomes, and adverse effects of treatment.

Weight Loss Medications

Medications for weight loss are indicated as adjunctive therapies to lifestyle modifications in patients with BMI $\geq 30 \, kg/m^2$ or BMI $\geq 27 \, kg/m^2$ with at least one weight-related comorbid condition, such as type 2 diabetes, hypertension,

Table 1 Weight reduction improves clinical outcomes of obesity-related diseases

Disease	References
Type 2 diabetes	[26, 99, 133]
Hypertension	[66, 156]
Dyslipidemia	[66, 156]
Cardiovascular disease	[150]
Nonalcoholic fatty liver diseases (NAFLD)	[63, 144]
Sleep apnea	[84]
Osteoarthritis	[25, 42, 62, 96, 146]
Cancer	[2, 136]

dyslipidemia, or obstructive sleep apnea (OSA) [9]. Currently, medications approved by the United States Food and Drug Administration (FDA) for long-term treatment of obesity include orlistat, phentermine combined with topiramate, naltrexone combined with bupropion, liraglutide, and semaglutide. Notably, clinical trials evaluating medications for chronic weight management have implemented lifestyle interventions concurrently in both placebo and treatment arms. A weight loss medication is typically deemed effective if it results in weight loss $\geq 5\%$ of body weight in 12–16 weeks. However, the recidivism rate for weight loss is very high, and weight regain after discontinuation of pharmacotherapy is common. Long-term use of obesity medications can help to sustain weight loss maintenance. In general, medications that are ineffective after 12 weeks of treatment or have adverse effects or safety concerns should be discontinued and alternative therapies considered. Table 2 summarizes pharmacotherapies for obesity and their effects on the components of metabolic syndrome. Weight loss efficacy of FDA-approved medications for chronic management of obesity is summarized in Fig. 1.

Glucagon-Like Peptide 1 Receptor Agonists

Liraglutide is an acylated glucagon-like peptide 1 (GLP-1) analogue that shares 97% amino acid sequence homology to endogenous GLP-1 (7–37). Liraglutide, which is derived from the addition of an albumin-binding C16 fatty acid side chain, has a prolonged plasma half-life compared with endogenous GLP-1 (13 h vs. 2 min) [82]. Liraglutide activates the GLP-1 receptor and triggers several responses, including glucose-dependent insulin secretion, inhibition of pancreatic glucagon secretion, delay in gastric emptying, and reduction of appetite and weight through brainstem and hypothalamic neuronal pathways [105]. Liraglutide is administered once daily via subcutaneous injection and was initially approved for the treatment of type 2 diabetes in 2010, with a maximum dose of 1.8 mg daily (Victoza). Liraglutide at the higher dose of 3 mg (Saxenda) was approved for weight

Table 2 Summary of pharmacotherapy of obesity medications and their effects on components of metabolic syndrome

Medication	Mechanism of action	Weight loss efficacy[a]	Adverse effects and contraindications	Glycemic outcomes	BP	Lipids	Cardiovascular outcomes
Orlistat (Xenical) 120 mg TID Approved in 1999	Pancreatic lipase inhibitor; reduces intestinal digestion of fat	−2.9% at 1 year [129]	Abdominal discomfort, flatulence, and oily and loose stools Contraindications: pregnancy, cholestasis, chronic malabsorption syndrome, and hypersensitivity	↓ Risk of diabetes incidence by 37% after 4 years in patients without diabetes [141]; ↓ Hb_{A1c} by an additional 0.43% (placebo-subtracted) in T2D after 6–12 months [67]	↓ Systolic BP by 1.7 mmHg and diastolic BP by 1.6 mmHg [76]	↓ LDL by 8.7 mg/dL; ↓ HDL by 1.1 mg/dL [76]	Not studied
Phentermine/ topiramate (Qsymia) 15 mg/92 mg Approved in 2012	Phentermine stimulates norepinephrine levels in the hypothalamus ↑ appetite suppression Topiramate stimulates GABA receptor activity, but it is unclear if this is directly involved in appetite suppression and weight loss	−8.6% at 1 year [46]	Paresthesia, dizziness, altered taste sensation, dry mouth, insomnia, and constipation Contraindications: pregnancy, glaucoma, hyperthyroidism, MAOI therapy within 14 days, and hypersensitivity	↓ Hb_{A1c} by 0.2% after 1 year ([76]; [46]); ↓ Hb_{A1c} by 0.3% in T2D after 1 year [46]	↓ Systolic BP by 3.7 mmHg and diastolic BP by 1.4 mmHg [76]	↓ LDL by 4.2 mg/dL; increased ↑ HDL by 2.2 mg/dL [76]	Not studied
Naltrexone/ bupropion (Contrave) 16 mg/ 180 mg BID Approved in 2014	Bupropion stimulates POMC neurons in the hypothalamus to reduce food intake Naltrexone is an opioid receptor antagonist that suppresses the inhibitory opioid feedback on the POMC neurons, to facilitate greater weight loss	−4.8% at 1 year [54]	Nausea, constipation, headache, vomiting, dizziness, insomnia, dry mouth, and diarrhea Contraindications: pregnancy, uncontrolled hypertension, seizure disorder, eating disorder, use of other bupropion-containing products, chronic opioid use, severe hepatic dysfunction, and use	↓ Hb_{A1c} by an additional 0.5% (placebo-subtracted) in T2D after 1 year [60]	No significant changes in systolic or diastolic BP [76]	No significant changes in LDL; ↑ HDL by 2.5 mg/dL [76]	Inconclusive due to early termination of the trial [109]

(continued)

Table 2 (continued)

Medication	Mechanism of action	Weight loss efficacy[a]	Adverse effects and contraindications	Glycemic outcomes	BP	Lipids	Cardiovascular outcomes
Liraglutide (Saxenda) 3 mg Approved in 2014	GLP-1 receptor agonist; enhances glucose-dependent insulin release, inhibits glucagon secretion, delays gastric emptying, and reduces food intake via reducing appetite	−5.4% at 1 year [115]	Nausea, diarrhea, constipation, and vomiting; increased HR; acute pancreatitis, acute cholecystitis Contraindication: pregnancy; hypersensitivity, personal or family history of MTC, or in patients with MEN2 within 14 days of taking MAOIs	↓ Hb$_{A1c}$ by 0.80% (on metformin background therapy) and 1.45% (drug naïve) in T2D [142]	↓ systolic BP by 2.85 mmHg and diastolic BP by 0.66 mmHg [100]	↓ LDL by 2.9 mg/dL [100]	↓ MACE (composite outcome) and death from CV causes and all-cause mortality in patients with T2D at high cardiovascular risk with liraglutide 1.2–1.8 mg doses [92]; no excess cardiovascular risk in patients with overweight/obesity (97% without diabetes) on liraglutide 3.0 mg dose [31]
Semaglutide (Wegovy) 2.4 mg Approved in 2021	GLP-1 receptor agonist; enhances glucose-dependent insulin release, inhibits glucagon secretion, delays gastric emptying, and reduces food intake via reducing appetite	−12.4% at 1 year [153]	Nausea, diarrhea, constipation, and vomiting; increased HR; acute pancreatitis, acute cholecystitis; and diabetic retinopathy (in T2D) Contraindications: hypersensitivity, personal or family history of MTC or in patients with MEN2	↓ Hb$_{A1c}$ by 1.33% (on metformin background therapy) and by 1.48% (drug naïve) in T2D [142]	↓ Systolic BP by 5.1 mmHg and diastolic BP by 2.4 mmHg [153]	↓ LDL by 4%; ↓ non-HDL by 6%; ↓ and triglycerides by 16% [83]	↓ MACE (composite outcome) in patients with T2D at high cardiovascular risk with semaglutide 0.5–1.0 mg doses [93]; CV outcome study with semaglutide 2.4 mg dose in people with obesity and cardiovascular disease without diabetes is ongoing (SELECT)

| Tirzepatide (Mounjaro) 15 mg Pending approval (fast track designation in 2022) | Dual GIP and GLP-1 receptor agonist; enhances glucose-dependent insulin release, reduces glucagon levels, delays gastric emptying, and reduces food intake via reducing appetite | −17.8% at 1 year [69] | Nausea, diarrhea, decreased appetite, vomiting, and constipation; increased HR; and hypoglycemia (in T2D), acute gallbladder disease, and acute pancreatitis Contraindications: hypersensitivity, personal or family history of MTC, or in patients with MEN2 | ↓ Hb_{A1c} by 2.06% in T2D [73] | ↓ Systolic BP by 6.1 mmHg and diastolic BP by 4.0 mmHg [69] | ↓ LDL by 4.2%, ↓ triglycerides by 20.3%, and ↑ HDL by 8.8% [69] | Ongoing study comparing tirzepatide versus dulaglutide in patients with T2D on cardiovascular outcomes will be completed by 2024 [98] |

[a]Percent weight losses are expressed as placebo-subtracted values. Abbreviations: BID, twice a day; BP, blood pressure; CV, cardiovascular; GABA, gamma-aminobutyric acid; GLP-1, glucagon-like peptide-1; GIP, gastric inhibitory polypeptide; Hb_{A1c}, hemoglobin A1c; HR, heart rate; MACE, major adverse cardiovascular events; MAOI, monoamine oxidase inhibitors; MEN2, multiple endocrine neoplasia type 2; MTC, medullary thyroid carcinoma; POMC, pro-opiomelanocortin; TID, three times a day; and T2D, type 2 diabetes mellitus

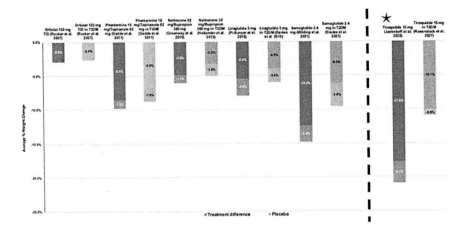

Fig. 1 Summary of weight loss efficacy of FDA-approved medications for obesity treatment

management in 2014. The recommended starting dose of liraglutide is 0.6 mg daily, with up-titration by 0.6 mg weekly until 3.0 mg target dose is achieved. The safety and efficacy of Saxenda have been evaluated in several clinical trials in adults with overweight or obesity with or without comorbid diseases [10, 30, 115, 148]. In a 56-week study, 3731 patients with obesity or overweight with ≥1 weight-related comorbidities and without diabetes were randomized to liraglutide 3.0 mg versus placebo while also receiving lifestyle counseling [115]. The liraglutide group lost 8.0% of their body weight, compared to 2.6% in the placebo group. Notably, 63.2% of the liraglutide-treated group lost ≥5% of their body weight, compared to 27.1% of the placebo group. Saxenda treatment also leads to improvement in systolic and diastolic blood pressure and reduction in LDL cholesterol [100]. Among patients with type 2 diabetes on oral hypoglycemic agents only and with overweight/ or obesity, Saxenda treatment resulted in an average weight loss of 6.0% from baseline compared to placebo as an adjunct to hypocaloric diet and increased physical activity at 56 weeks with an estimated treatment difference of −4.0%. Notably, 54.3% of patients treated with Saxenda lost at least 5% of their body weight compared to 21.4% of patients treated with placebo [30]. In patients with type 2 diabetes and high cardiovascular risk, treatment with higher dose liraglutide (Victoza) 1.2–1.8 mg doses resulted in significant reduction of major adverse cardiovascular events (LEADER Trial, [92]). In patients with

overweight/obesity (97% without diabetes), liraglutide (Saxenda) 3.0 mg dose did not show excess cardiovascular risk [31].

Semaglutide is a long-acting GLP-1 analogue that shares 94% sequence homology to human GLP-1. Through albumin binding facilitated by modification of position 26 lysine with a hydrophilic spacer and a C18 fatty diacid addition, along with an amino acid replacement in position 8 which prevents dipeptidyl peptidase 4 (DPP-4) degradation, semaglutide has a half-life of 165 hours, compared to liraglutide's half-life of 13–15 hours). This allows semaglutide injection to be dosed once weekly instead of daily. Semaglutide comes in both injection and oral preparations. Semaglutide injection up to 2 mg weekly (Ozempic) was approved for the treatment of type 2 diabetes in 2017, while semaglutide injection up to 2.4 mg weekly (Wegovy) was approved for chronic treatment of obesity in 2022. The starting dose of Wegovy is 0.25 mg weekly, with up-titration to the next dose (0.5 mg, 1.0 mg, 1.7 mg, and maximum of 2.4 mg) every 4 weeks as tolerated. The safety and efficacy of Wegovy 2.4 mg has been evaluated in a series of clinical trials called the Semaglutide Treatment Effect for People with obesity (STEP) program. STEP 1 and STEP 3 trials evaluated adults with obesity or overweight with ≥1 weight-related comorbidities and without diabetes [149, 153]. At 68 weeks, STEP 1 Trial found that in 1900 adults, lifestyle intervention alone, which involved monthly individual counseling on hypocaloric diet and increased physical activity, resulted in 2.4% average weight loss compared to 14.9% receiving lifestyle intervention and semaglutide 2.4 mg, with a treatment difference of 12.4% [153]. Additionally, 86.4% of patients in the semaglutide group attained weight reduction of 5% or more, compared to 31.5% in the placebo group. STEP 3 Trial similarly found that in 600 adults, intensive behavioral therapy with an initial 8-week low-calorie diet provided as meal replacements resulted in 5.7% weight reduction, compared to 16% weight reduction when semaglutide 2.4 mg was added, with a treatment difference of 10.3% [149]. In 1200 participants with type 2 diabetes on oral hypoglycemic agents and overweight/obesity, semaglutide 2.4 mg versus semaglutide 1.0 mg versus placebo as an adjunct to lifestyle intervention for 68 weeks resulted in an average weight loss of 9.6%, 7.0%, and 3.4%, respectively [32]. Notably, 68.8% of patients on semaglutide 2.4 mg achieved weight reduction of at least 5% compared to 28.5% in the placebo group. In the longest study with semaglutide where 304 patients with overweight or obesity without diabetes were randomized to receive placebo versus semaglutide 2.4 mg for 2 years. The semaglutide group lost 15.2% of their body weight, compared to 2.6% in the placebo group, with an estimated treatment difference of 12.6% [48]. Wegovy treatment also decreased blood pressure and improved cholesterol levels [83, 153]. In patients with type 2 diabetes at high cardiovascular risk, treatment with semaglutide (Ozempic) 0.5–1.0 mg doses resulted in significant reduction in cardiovascular events (SUSTAIN-6, [93]). Cardiovascular outcomes with Wegovy 2.4 mg dose in patients with obesity and cardiovascular disease without diabetes are being studied in the ongoing SELECT trial, expected to be completed by 2023 (NCT03574597). In 2023, Wegovy received FDA approval for the treatment of obesity in pediatric patients aged 12 years and older, after a double-blind randomized placebo-controlled trial in 201 adolescents (age 12 to <18 years) with obesity or overweight and at least 1 weight-related coexisting condition found a mean change in BMI of −16.1% with semaglutide 2.4 mg compared to 0.6% with placebo after 68 weeks of treatment [152].

The most common side effects for GLP-1 receptor agonists are nausea, diarrhea, constipation, and vomiting. Nausea may be due to transient delayed gastric emptying, with the frequency of nausea waning as treatment is continued. Overall, gastrointestinal adverse reactions led to discontinuation of therapy in 4.3% of patients treated with Wegovy versus 0.7% placebo-treated patients and 6.2% of patients treated with Saxenda versus 0.8% of placebo-treated patients. GLP-1 receptor agonists caused dose-dependent and treatment-duration-dependent increase in the incidence of thyroid C-cell tumors in rodents, but it is unknown whether the drug causes thyroid C-cell tumors, including medullary thyroid carcinoma (MTC), in humans. Wegovy and Saxenda are contraindicated in patients with a personal or family history of MTC or in patients with MEN2. Serious but rare adverse effects of GLP-1 receptor agonists include acute cholecystitis, acute pancreatitis, renal impairment (majority of events occurred in patients who had experienced dehydration due to gastrointestinal side effects), and suicidal thoughts. Both Wegovy and Saxenda can increase the resting heart rate (mean increase of 1–4 beats per minute) and should be discontinued in patients who experience a sustained increase in resting heart rate. Unique to semaglutide, in patients with type 2 diabetes, diabetic retinopathy was reported by 4.0% of Wegovy-treated patients versus 2.7% placebo-treated patients with the absolute risk increase for diabetic retinopathy larger among patients with a history of diabetic retinopathy at baseline. The association with worsening of diabetic retinopathy is thought to be due to rapid improvement in glucose control although the effect of long-term glycemic control with semaglutide on diabetic retinopathy has not been studied. Additionally, there is an increased risk for hypoglycemia in patients with type 2 diabetes when GLP-1 receptor agonists were used concurrently with a sulfonylurea. There is currently a pregnancy exposure registry set up to monitor pregnancy outcomes in women exposed to semaglutide during pregnancy. Saxenda is contraindicated in pregnancy. Saxenda has not been studied and is not approved for use in pediatric patients younger than 18 years. Safety and efficacy of Wegovy have not been established in pediatric patients younger than age 12. In the clinical trials for both Saxenda and Wegovy, only a small number of participants were of older age (6.9–8.8% were 65 years and over, and 0.5–0.9% were 75 years or older), but no overall differences in safety or effectiveness were observed in older versus younger patients.

A head-to-head study compared semaglutide 2.4 mg versus liraglutide 3.0 mg versus placebo added to counseling for diet and physical activity in 338 patients with overweight or obesity and without diabetes over 68 weeks [127]. Weight loss was superior with semaglutide, with a mean weight loss of 15.8% compared to 6.4% with liraglutide and 1.9% with placebo. Adverse events were similar between semaglutide and liraglutide groups, with 84.1% of semaglutide-treated patients and 82.7% of liraglutide-treated patients reporting gastrointestinal disorders (compared to 55.3% of placebo-treated patients). Reports of gastrointestinal adverse effects were most frequent during and shortly after dose escalation. The rate of permanent treatment discontinuation due to adverse effects was higher in liraglutide (12.6%) compared to semaglutide (3.2%). Currently, the exact mechanisms underlying the differences in weight loss efficacy between semaglutide and liraglutide are unknown and under investigation. Both semaglutide and liraglutide induce weight loss through caloric reduction though this effect is more potent with semaglutide (35% energy reduction compared to placebo) than liraglutide (16% energy reduction compared to placebo) [45].

Naltrexone/Bupropion

Bupropion is a dopamine and norepinephrine reuptake inhibitor used in the treatment of depression and smoking cessation. Bupropion can stimulate the pro-opiomelanocortin (POMC) neurons in the arcuate nucleus of the hypothalamus to decrease food intake. However, POMC stimulation results in compensatory autoinhibitory feedback, which is regulated by endogenous opioids. Naltrexone is an opioid receptor antagonist approved for the treatment of alcohol or opioid dependence. Naltrexone has minimal effect on body weight if given alone;

however, when used in conjunction with bupropion (POMC stimulator), naltrexone suppresses the inhibitory opioid feedback on the POMC neurons, to facilitate greater weight loss via inhibition of food intake [53]. Contrave is a combination of naltrexone and bupropion administered as an extended-release formulation that was approved by the FDA in 2014. The effectiveness of Contrave has been evaluated in randomized clinical trials involving about 4500 participants with obesity or overweight and significant weight-related conditions treated for 1 year [8, 54, 60, 147]. All participants received lifestyle modification consisting of a reduced calorie diet and regular physical activity. The results showed a mean weight loss of 4.8% with Contrave over placebo treatment at 1 year [54]. About 48% of participants treated with Contrave lost at least 5% of their body weight compared to 16% to placebo-treated patients. In participants with overweight/obesity and type 2 diabetes on oral medications, Contrave resulted in an average weight loss of 3% better than placebo treatment at 1 year and an additional 0.5% reduction in hemoglobin A1c (HbA$_{1c}$) [60]. About 44% of patients treated with Contrave lost at least 5% of their body weight compared to 19% in the placebo-treated group. A meta-analysis found no significant changes in blood pressure or LDL levels with Contrave treatment [76].

Patients on maintenance doses of Contrave should be evaluated after 12 weeks, and the drug should be discontinued if they have not lost at least 5% of baseline body weight. The most common adverse effects of Contrave include nausea, constipation, headache, vomiting, dizziness, insomnia, dry mouth, and diarrhea. The bupropion component of Contrave increases the risk of suicidal thoughts. Contrave can cause seizures and increase blood pressure and heart rate and must not be used in patients with poorly controlled hypertension. Contrave should not be used in patients with eating disorders (e.g., bulimia or anorexia nervosa), in those on opioids or treatments for opioid dependence, or in those experiencing acute opiate withdrawal or undergoing discontinuation of alcohol, benzodiazepines, barbiturates, and antiepileptic drugs. Contrave is contraindicated in pregnancy, uncontrolled hypertension, seizure disorder, eating disorder, use of other bupropion-containing products, chronic opioid use, and use within 14 days of taking monamine oxidase inhibitors. The US FDA requested the following postmarketing studies for Contrave: assessment of cardiovascular risk, efficacy, safety, and clinical pharmacology studies in children; toxicity studies in young animals with a focus on growth, development, behavior, learning, and memory; investigation of the effect of Contrave on cardiac conduction; clinical trials to evaluate the dosing of Contrave in patients with hepatic or renal impairment; and a clinical trial to evaluate interactions between Contrave and other drugs. The LIGHT clinical trial, which assessed cardiovascular outcomes in 8910 patients with overweight/obesity at increased cardiovascular risk randomized to Contrave versus placebo, was terminated early due to a protocol breach when interim study data was prematurely released to the public [109]. The interim analyses demonstrated possible reduction in cardiovascular risk with Contrave, but subsequent data analysis suggested an increase in cardiovascular events in the Contrave treatment group. The final analysis was performed with 64% of the originally planned end points and found that the primary outcome (time to first MACE) occurred in 2.7 versus 2.8% in Contrave versus placebo groups with HR 0.95 (95% CI 0.65–1.38). These results cannot be definitively interpreted; hence, the effect of Contrave on cardiovascular risk remains unknown.

Phentermine/Topiramate

The combination of phentermine and topiramate is marketed as an extended-release formulation (Qsymia), as phentermine (3.75, 7.5, or 15 mg) combined with topiramate (23, 46, or 92 mg) [6, 46]. A dose titration period of 2 weeks is recommended for Qsymia, starting at the lowest combination dose. Phentermine stimulates norepinephrine levels in the hypothalamus which has been linked to appetite suppression. Topiramate stimulates γ-aminobutyric acid (GABA) receptor activity, but it is unclear if this is directly involved in appetite suppression and weight loss. The safety and efficacy of Qsymia were evaluated in two randomized, placebo-controlled trials that included about 3700 obese

or overweight patients with or without weight-related diseases treated for 1 year. The participants received lifestyle intervention consisting of a reduced calorie diet and regular physical activity. In the EQUIP study, phentermine/topiramate was administered in adults ≤70 years of age and with a BMI ≥35 kg/m² [6]. The CONQUER study [46] examined the effects of Qsymia in adults ≤70 years, with a BMI of 27–45 kg/m², and two or more of the following conditions: hypertension, hypertriglyceridemia, abnormal glucose metabolism (impaired fasting glucose, impaired glucose tolerance, or type 2 diabetes), or waist circumference ≥40 in. in men or ≥35 in. in women. Results from these studies showed that after 1 year of treatment, there was a mean weight loss of 6.6% and 8.6% with phentermine 7.5 mg / topiramate 46 mg and phentermine 15 mg / topiramate 92 mg, respectively, over placebo treatment. About 62% and 69% of the participants lost at least 5% of their body weight with the recommended dose and highest doses of Qsymia compared with 20% of placebo-treated patients. Extension of the CONQUER study for a second year, i.e., SEQUEL study, resulted in significant weight loss [47]. Qsymia treatment resulted in significant improvements in blood pressure, and glucose and lipid levels [6, 46, 47], and these changes were related to the degree of weight loss.

The most common side effects of Qsymia are paresthesia, dizziness, altered taste sensation, dry mouth, insomnia, and constipation. Qsymia is contraindicated in pregnancy. Because topiramate has been associated with fetal oral clefts, a negative pregnancy test is required before treatment is initiated. A pregnancy test must be done every month, and effective contraception is required during Qsymia treatment. If a patient becomes pregnant while taking Qsymia, the drug should be discontinued immediately. Qsymia is contraindicated in patients with glaucoma, hyperthyroidism, recent monoamine oxidase inhibitor (MAOI) therapy (within 14 days), or hypersensitivity to topiramate or phentermine. The US FDA approved Qsymia in 2012 with a Risk Evaluation and Mitigation Strategy (REMS), consisting of safety information for prescribers and patients, prescriber training, and pharmacy certification. The REMS is aimed toward educating prescribers and patients about the increased risk of birth defects associated with first trimester exposure to Qsymia, the requirement for pregnancy prevention, and the discontinuation of therapy if pregnancy occurs. Qsymia is only dispensed through specially certified pharmacies, and the manufacturer is required to conduct postmarketing studies, including a long-term cardiovascular outcome trial to assess the risk for major cardiovascular events.

Orlistat

Orlistat (tetrahydrolipstatin) inhibits pancreatic lipase thereby reducing intestinal digestion of fat. Orlistat was approved by the US FDA in 1999 as a prescription drug, and in 2007 as an over-the-counter product for weight loss. Orlistat is available as a prescribed dose of 120 mg three times daily before meals (Xenical) or over-the-counter dose of 60 mg three times daily (Alli). Orlistat decreases body weight in a dose-dependent manner. A 4-year double-blind, randomized, placebo-controlled trial showed that orlistat treatment resulted in more than 11% reduction below the baseline weight compared to 6% in the placebo group [141]. Orlistat treatment attenuates weight regain and the progression of glucose intolerance to diabetes. Orlistat is effective in adolescents [21]. A meta-analysis of orlistat clinical trials showed that orlistat reduced body weight by -5.70 ± 7.28 kg compared to -2.40 ± 6.99 kg in the placebo group [129]. Orlistat has been shown to reduce the diabetes incidence [141] and lower HbA_{1c} by 0.43% in patients with type 2 diabetes [67]. A meta-analysis also reported that orlistat significantly reduces blood pressure and LDL [76]. The side effects of orlistat are related to blockade of triglyceride digestion in the intestine, which causes steatorrhea associated with abdominal discomfort or pain, flatulence, and oily stools. Orlistat can decrease the absorption of fat-soluble vitamins; therefore, patients require multivitamin supplementation. Very rarely orlistat therapy has been associated with liver toxicity, but the etiology is unclear [70]. Modest weight loss and undesirable side effect profile may limit the widespread use of orlistat as a long-term weight loss medication.

Other Weight Loss Medications

Benzphetamine, diethylpropion, phendimetrazine, and phentermine are sympathomimetic drugs approved by the US FDA for short-term weight loss treatment, i.e., 12 weeks [3, 78, 130]. Phentermine and diethylpropion are classified by the US DEA as schedule IV drugs, and benzphetamine and phendimetrazine are classified as schedule III drugs (). Phentermine was approved in 1959 for short-term treatment, and studies have demonstrated a modest dose-related weight loss in phentermine-treated patients [3, 78, 130]. The side effects of the sympathomimetic drugs include insomnia, nervousness, dry mouth, tachycardia, and elevated blood pressure. These drugs should not be prescribed to patients with a history of cardiovascular disease.

Lorcaserin is a serotonin-2C receptor (5HTR-2C) agonist which decreases food intake and body weight [138]. Lorcaserin was effective for weight loss, but it was voluntarily withdrawn from the US market in 2020 due to clinical trial data showing an increased occurrence of cancer.

Treatment of Diabetes

Obesity is closely linked to type 2 diabetes in regard to etiology, pathogenesis, and management [38]. Several drugs used for the treatment of diabetes produce weight gain, e.g., insulin, sulfonylurea drugs (glipizide and glibenclamide), and thiazolidinediones (rosiglitazone and pioglitazone) (Table 3). Therefore, it is important to use medications that are weight neutral or cause weight loss [16]. Table 3 lists diabetes medications that confer additional benefits in other components of metabolic syndrome and thus are preferable agents in individualized treatment strategies for patients with type 2 diabetes and metabolic comorbidities.

Metformin

Metformin is a biguanide that enters hepatocytes via SLC22A1 transporter, acts on mitochondrial complex 1 to reduce ATP production, activates AMPK, and also inhibits glucagon signaling.

Table 3 Effects of medications on body weight

Disease	Drugs associated with weight gain	Drugs that are weight neutral or cause weight loss
Type 2 diabetes	Insulin Sulfonylureas Glitinides Thiazolidinediones	*Weight neutral* Acarbose Miglitol DPP-4 inhibitors *Weight loss* Metformin GLP-1 receptor agonists GLP-1/GIP dual receptor agonist SGLT-2 inhibitors
Hypertension	Alpha-blocker Beta-blocker	Angiotension-conversting enzyme (ACE) inhibitors Angiotensin receptor blockers (ARB) Calcium channel blockers
Depression	Citalopram Escitalopram Fluvoxamine Lithium Tricyclic antidepressants Monoamine oxidase inhibitors Mirtazapine Paroxetine Venlafaxine	Bupropion Nefazodone Fluoxetine Sertraline
Psychosis	Clozapine Risperidone Olanzapine Quetiapine	Ziprasidone Aripiprazole
Epilepsy	Valproate Carbamazepine Gabapentin	Zonisamide Topiramate Lamotrigine

The net effect of metformin is to increase hepatic insulin sensitivity, reduce hepatic glucose production, and inhibit fatty acid synthesis. Metformin may cause weight loss. For example, in the Diabetes Prevention Program, the participants receiving metformin lost more weight than placebo (2.9 vs 0.42 kg), and the weight loss persisted for 8 years of follow-up [37]. Bushe et al. [17] reported that metformin may prevent weight gain and metabolic syndrome during treatment with antipsychotic drugs. Metformin used as a monotherapy has been shown to reduce HbA$_{1c}$ by nearly 1%, which is comparable to or better than other diabetes drugs including sulfonylureas, SGLT-2 inhibitors, and DPP-4 inhibitors in a meta-analysis [142]. Compared to sulfonylureas, metformin treatment was associated with reduced cardiovascular mortality [94]. The most common side effects are gastrointestinal symptoms including diarrhea, nausea, and abdominal discomfort, which can be attenuated by taking the medication with food. Given the glycemic efficacy, low cost, low risk of hypoglycemia or weight gain, and overall tolerability, metformin is often considered initial therapy for most patients with newly diagnosed type 2 diabetes. Lactic acidosis is a rare but serious side effect of metformin. Conditions that increase the risk of developing lactic acidosis include excessive alcohol intake, heart failure, impaired kidney function, and liver disease. Metformin treatment is associated with vitamin B$_{12}$ deficiency, especially in patients receiving a higher dose, longer treatment duration, or in those with preexisting vitamin B$_{12}$ deficiency. Therefore, patients should be monitored periodically and vitamin B$_{12}$ deficiency treated based on current clinical guidelines.

GLP-1 Receptor Agonists

Incretin hormones are released by the enteroendocrine cells in response to nutrients and have insulinotropic action on pancreatic beta cells. Two incretin hormones have been identified – glucose-dependent insulinotropic polypeptide (GIP) and glucagon-like peptide-1 (GLP-1). GIP is produced by K-cells in the duodenum and upper jejunum while GLP-1 is produced by L-cells located throughout the intestine, with higher abundance in the ileum and colon. Incretin hormones are released after ingestion of nutrients and potentiate insulin secretion in response to hyperglycemia, hence glucose-dependent insulin release. In a healthy individual, GIP and GLP-1 levels increase in response to oral glucose intake, but not intravenous glucose infusion. Additionally, GIP stimulates glucagon secretion while

GLP-1 inhibits glucagon release [102]. GLP-1 receptor agonists stimulate insulin secretion, inhibit glucagon secretion, slow gastric emptying, and reduce food intake [56]. Because endogenous GLP-1 is rapidly inactivated by dipeptidyl peptidase-4 enzyme, synthetic GLP-1 receptor agonists with prolonged action have been developed for treatment of type 2 diabetes [95]. In a meta-analysis, injectable GLP-1 receptor agonists (liraglutide, semaglutide, and dulaglutide) reduced HbA_{1c} by 1.29–1.48% while oral semaglutide reduced HbA_{1c} by 1.10% [142]. Additionally, liraglutide (LEADER; [92]), injectable semaglutide (SUSTAIN-6; [93]), and dulaglutide (REWIND; [49]) have been shown to significantly reduce the composite outcome major adverse cardiovascular events (MACE) compared to placebo in randomized controlled trials in patients with type 2 diabetes and either established or at-risk for atherosclerotic cardiovascular disease (ASCVD). Oral semaglutide (PIONEER-6; [65]), once-weekly exenatide (EXSCEL; [61]), and lixisenatide (ELIXA; [114]) have been shown to be noninferior, but not superior, to placebo in reducing MACE. The mechanisms by which GLP-1 receptor agonists reduce cardiovascular events are incompletely understood but are postulated to be due to the improvement in multiple cardiovascular risk factors including glycemic control, weight, blood pressure, and lipid profile, along with direct effects on the cardiovascular system such as improvement in inflammation, endothelial function, and progression of atherosclerosis [104].

GLP-1/GIP Dual Receptor Agonist

Tirzepatide is the first dual GIP/GLP-1 receptor coagonist approved by the US FDA for the treatment of type 2 diabetes in 2022. Tirzepatide is administered as a once-weekly injection (brand name Mounjaro), with a starting dose of 2.5 mg, up-titrated every 4 weeks to a maximum dose of 15 mg. Tirzepatide is a 39-amino-acid-modified peptide with a C20 fatty acid moiety that enables albumin binding and prolongs the half-life. Tirzepatide lowers blood glucose by enhancing glucose-dependent insulin secretion and reducing glucagon levels. Tirzepatide was studied as a monotherapy in a 40-week randomized double-blind trial with 478 adults with type 2 diabetes and inadequate glycemic control with diet and exercise only and reduced HbA_{1c} by 1.7% (SURPASS-1, [126]). When studied as an add-on agent to metformin, Mounjaro 15 mg reduced HbA_{1c} by 2.3%, compared to 1.86% with semaglutide 1 mg, with a treatment difference of 0.45% (SURPASS-2, [44]). Furthermore, tirzepatide demonstrated superior HbA_{1c} reduction along with lower risk of hypoglycemia compared to long-acting insulin degludec and glargine (SURPASS-3, [90]; SURPASS-4, [36]). A meta-analysis of all randomized control trials of tirzepatide in patients with type 2 diabetes found a mean HbA_{1c} reduction of 2.06% with tirzpeatide 15 mg compared to placebo, and a mean HbA_{1c} reduction of 0.92% when compared to GLP-1 receptor agonists (one trial with dulaglutide [43] and one trial with semaglutide [44]) [73]. There was also dose-dependent reduction in body weight with tirzepatide 15 mg treatment, resulting in an average weight loss of 9.36 kg compared to placebo, and 7.16 kg additional weight loss compared to GLP-1 receptor agonists. A study comparing tirzepatide versus dulaglutide in patients with type 2 diabetes on cardiovascular outcomes is ongoing and expected to be completed by 2024 (SURPASS CVOT; [98]). The adverse effects of tirzepatide are similar to those of GLP-1 receptor agonists, with gastrointestinal adverse reactions (nausea, diarrhea, and decreased appetite) being the most frequent. From the two clinical trials that compared tirzepatide to GLP-1 receptor agonists (semaglutide, dulaglutide), the odds of gastrointestinal side effects were similar, except for higher odds for diarrhea with tirzepatide 10 mg. In comparison with GLP-1 receptor agonists, more participants receiving tirzepatide 15 mg discontinued treatment due to adverse effects whereas no differences in treatment discontinuation were evident for lower doses of tirzepatide, i.e., 5 mg or 10 mg. [73].

SGLT-2 Inhibitors

The kidney regulates blood glucose through reabsorption of glucose from the glomerular filtrate via SGLT-1 and SGLT-2. SGLT-2 inhibitors block 90% of glucose reabsorption in the proximal tubule of the nephron, leading to urinary glucose excretion and reduction in blood glucose levels [34]. The US FDA approved SGLT-2 inhibitors, i.e., canagliflozin, empagliflozin, and dapagliflozin, for diabetes treatment. In addition to lowering glucose levels [89], SGLT-2 inhibitor treatment results in loss of calories in the urine and weight loss [40]. SGLT-2 inhibitors may decrease blood pressure [41], increase HDL cholesterol, and decrease triglyceride levels [11, 103, 125]. SGLT-2 inhibitors may also decrease serum uric acid levels [89], suggesting multiple benefits in the metabolic syndrome.

A meta-analysis found that SGLT-2 inhibitors decreased HbA_{1c} by an average of 0.8–1.0% in drug-naïve patients with type 2 diabetes [142] and decreased body weight by 1.82–1.92 kg [143]. Notably, SGLT-2 inhibitors exhibited the most potent blood pressure-lowering effects among diabetic medications, with an average reduction in systolic blood pressure 2.34–3.38 mmHg and in diastolic blood pressure 1.42–1.68 mmHg [143]. SGLT-2 inhibitors have been found to improve cardiovascular and renal outcomes in patients with type 2 diabetes in several large-scale randomized controlled trials. Empagliflozin and canagliflozin were found to reduce the MACE in patients with type 2 diabetes and existing cardiovascular disease and reduced heart failure hospitalization in the subgroup of patients with heart failure (EMPA-REG OUTCOME, [158]; CANVAS, [106]). Dapagliflozin was found to be noninferior to placebo with respect to reduction in MACE and reduced the rate of cardiovascular death or hospitalization for heart failure in patients with type 2 diabetes (DECLARE-TIMI 58, [154]). One notable difference was that in the dapagliflozin trial, only 40% of the study population had established ASCVD and the rest had multiple risk factors for ASCVD, while in the empagliflozin and canagliflozin trials, 65–99% of the study population had prior ASCVD. For renal outcomes, canagliflozin was studied in patients with type 2 diabetes and albuminuric kidney disease and found to reduce progression of renal disease or death from renal or cardiovascular cause (CREDENCE, [113]). Dapagliflozin was studied in patients with albuminuric kidney disease with or without diabetes (67.5%

with type 2 diabetes), and found to reduce progression of chronic kidney disease or death from renal or cardiovascular cause (DAPA-CKD, [58]).

Treatment of Atherogenic Dyslipidemia

Statins are competitive inhibitors of hydroxymethylglutaryl (HMG) coA reductase, which is the rate-limiting step in cholesterol biosynthesis. Statins are effective in reducing total and LDL cholesterol levels [22]. High-intensity statin therapy typically decreased LDL cholesterol by ≥50% while moderate-intensity statin therapy can achieve 30–49% reductions in LDL cholesterol [71]. Additionally, statin therapy can lower triglycerides by 20–30% [71], with up to 50% reduction in patients with hypertriglyceridemia with high-intensity statin such as atorvastatin and rosuvastatin [64]. The role of statins in reducing cardiovascular risk is well established. Prospective studies such as COMETS (COmparative study with rosuvastatin in subjects with METabolic Syndrome) and MERCURY I (Measuring Effective Reductions in Cholesterol Using Rosuvastatin TherapY I) showed that statins improved atherogenic dyslipidemia in patients with metabolic syndrome [139, 140]. A meta-analysis showed that statin therapy reduced the risk of cardiovascular disease (Cholesterol Treatment Trialists [27]). Statin treatment consistently reduces cardiovascular and all-cause mortality in patients at high risk of cardiovascular disease [85, 117]. Statins also reduce oxidative stress and inflammation, improve endothelial function, and decrease cardiovascular morbidity [51, 87, 97]. Statin therapy has been associated with insulin resistance [72, 116, 132]. However, the risk of statin-mediated insulin resistance should be balanced against the benefits in reducing cardiovascular risks [88].

Proprotein convertase subtilisin/kexin type 9 (PCSK9) is a serine protease produced in the liver, binds to the LDL receptor on the surface of hepatocytes, and degrades the LDL receptor, leading to higher plasma LDL levels. There are currently two classes of drugs that target PCSK9: (1) PCSK9 inhibitors (monoclonal antibodies) evolocumab and alirocumab, administered as a subcutaneous injection every 2–4 weeks; and (2) PCSK9-small interfering RNA molecules (siRNA) inclisiran, administered as a subcutaneous injection every 6 months. PCSK9 inhibitors reduce LDL cholesterol levels by 50–60% in patients already on statin therapy [15]. Inclisiran reduces LDL cholesterol levels by approximately 50% in statin-treated patients with ASCVD [121]. In the FOURIER (Further Cardiovascular Outcomes Research with PCSK9 Inhibition in Subjects With Elevated Risk) study, 27,564 patients with established ASCVD who were receiving maximum tolerated statin therapy but still had LDL levels ≥70 mg/dL or non-HDL cholesterol ≥100 mg/dL were randomized to evolocumab versus placebo [131]. After a median follow-up of 2.2 years, evolocumab reduced LDL levels by 59% and significantly reduced the MACE. In the ODYSSEY OUTCOMES (Evaluation of Cardiovascular Outcomes After an Acute Coronary Syndrome During Treatment with Alirocumab) study, 18,942 patients with a recent acute coronary syndrome on maximum tolerated statin therapy but still having LDL levels ≥70 mg/dL or non-HDL cholesterol ≥100 mg/dL or apolipoprotein B level of ≥80 mg/dL were randomized to alirocumab versus placebo [134]. After a median follow-up of 2.8 years, alirocumab significantly reduced the composite end point of death from coronary heart disease, nonfatal myocardial infarction, fatal or nonfatal ischemic stroke, or unstable angina requiring hospitalization. A randomized clinical trial assessing cardiovascular outcomes of inclisiran is ongoing (ORION-4, NCT03705234).

Bempedoic acid is a novel LDL-lowering agent that inhibits ATP citrate lyase, an enzyme upstream of HMG CoA reductase. Bempedoic acid is used to treat adults with heterozygous familial hypercholesterolemia or established ASCVD who require additional LDL lowering despite maximum tolerated statin therapy. The CLEAR Harmony trial showed that bempedoic acid reduced LDL levels by 16.5% compared to placebo in statin-treated patients with LDL cholesterol ≥70 mg/dL [120]. In patients who were statin-intolerant and had a previous

cardiovascular event or at high risk for a cardiovascular event, bempedoic acid reduced LDL levels by 21% and significantly reduced the four-point composite MACE compared to placebo after a median follow-up of 3.4 years [110].

Ezetimibe inhibits cholesterol absorption at the intestinal brush border and has been shown to reduce LDL cholesterol by 17% [81]. Combining statin with ezetimibe has been shown to provide further reduction in LDL cholesterol levels and improvement in cardiovascular outcomes in IMPROVE-IT (IMProved Reduction in Outcomes: Vytorin Efficacy International Trial). The addition of ezetimibe to simvastatin led to a 6.4% relative benefit and 2% absolute reduction in the MACE in patients who had been hospitalized for an acute coronary syndrome within the preceding 10 days [18].

Omega-3 fatty acids, which primarily compose of eicosapentaenoic acid (EPA) and docosahexaenoic acid (DHA), have been shown to reduce triglyceride levels by ~20–50% [137]. However, omega-3 fatty acids may also mildly increase LDL cholesterol, which may be more pronounced with DHA than EPA [68]. Randomized controlled trials have yielded discordant results on the effects of omega-3 fatty acids on cardiovascular outcomes, likely due to differences in study design. In REDUCE-IT (Reduction of Cardiovascular Events with Icosapent Ethyl-Intervention Trial), 8179 patients with known ASCVD or diabetes with an additional risk factor and who were already on statin therapy with LDL levels <100 mg/dL and triglyceride levels >135 mg/dL were randomized to either 4 g/day of icosapent ethyl, which is a purified form of EPA, or placebo with mineral oil [14]. The study found that icosapent ethyl reduced the MACE by 25% after a median of 4.9 years, which corresponded to a number needed to treat of 21. However, the STRENGTH (Statin Residual Risk Reduction with Epanova in High Cardiovascular Risk Patients with Hypertriglyceridemia) trial randomized 13,078 statin-treated patients with high cardiovascular risk, hypertriglyceridemia, and low HDL to either 4 g per day of carboxylic acid formulation of EPA and DHA or placebo with corn oil and found no difference in the MACE

[107]. A meta-analysis of 38 randomized controlled trials of omega-3 fatty acids showed greater reduction in cardiovascular mortality and outcomes with EPA monotherapy than EPA + DHA [75]. Overall, the mixed findings on omega-3 fatty acids and cardiovascular outcomes may be explained by differences in the dosing and formulation of omega-3 fatty acids, the achieved EPA levels, or placebo agents [118].

Fibrates are useful for the treatment of hypertriglyceridemia and low HDL cholesterol levels. Fibrates modulate peroxisome proliferator-activated receptor α (PPAR-α) and reduce triglycerides [4, 80] and increase HDL cholesterol [111]. Fibrates also modulate fibrinogen, IL-1, IL-6, and hsCRP levels [74, 155]. Fenofibrate decreases fibrinolysis inhibitor levels and improves endothelial function in patients with metabolic syndrome [77]. Before the widespread use of statins, an earlier study found fibrates as a monotherapy to be effective in secondary prevention of cardiovascular disease [128]. However, the FIELD (Fenofibrate Intervention and Event Lowering in Diabetes) study showed that fenofibrate did not significantly reduce the risk of coronary events in patients with type 2 diabetes not taking statin therapy at study entry [74]. Furthermore, several randomized controlled trials have shown that fibrates were not effective in reducing cardiovascular events or mortality as an add-on therapy to statins. In the ACCORD-Lipid (The Action to Control Cardiovascular Risk in Diabetes) trial, 5518 patients with type 2 diabetes who were already on simvastatin were randomized to either fenofibrate or placebo. After a median follow-up of 4.7 years, no significant differences in nonfatal myocardial infarction, nonfatal stroke, or cardiovascular mortality were found [1]. The PROMINENT (PEmafibrate to Reduce Cardiovascular OutcoMes by Reducing Triglycerides IN patiENts With diabetes) trial randomized about 10,000 patients with type 2 diabetes with triglyceride levels 200–499 mg/dL, HDL levels ≤40 mg/dL, and LDL levels of ≤100 mg/dL, to either pemafibrate 0.4 mg/day or placebo [29]. After a median follow-up of 3.4 years, there were no differences in the incidence of cardiovascular events between treatment arms, even though pemafibrate lowered triglyceride levels, VLDL cholesterol, remnant cholesterol, and apolipoprotein C-III levels. Notably, there was an increase in plasma LDL cholesterol and apolipoprotein B levels, with no overall change in non-HDL cholesterol and total cholesterol levels. This is because reduction in triglyceride levels by pemafibrate is mediated by increased conversion of triglyceride-rich lipoprotein remnants to LDL rather than by hepatic removal [50]. There are ongoing trials investigating drugs that use alternative pathways to lower triglycerides levels such as inhibition of apolipoprotein C-III and angiopoietin-like 3 proteins, both of which are known inhibitors of lipoprotein lipase-mediated lipolysis but also may play a role in hepatic clearance of triglyceride-rich lipoproteins [50, 52].

Treatment of Hypertension

The pathogenesis of hypertension in the metabolic syndrome is thought to be mediated by various factors including activation of the sympathetic nervous system (SNS), increased renal tubular sodium reabsorption, and dysregulation of the renin-angiotensin-aldosterone system (RAAS). Thiazide diuretics are the first-line agent in the treatment of hypertension within the general population [5, 24]. However, thiazides tend to raise blood glucose levels and may convert prediabetes to diabetes [7, 57, 119].

The RAAS is functionally linked to insulin resistance and endothelial dysfunction in patients with the metabolic syndrome and obesity-related hypertension [59]. Angiotensin II inhibits insulin signaling, induces oxidative stress, and exacerbates hyperglycemia and atherogenesis [135]. In contrast, ACE inhibitors reduce blood pressure as well as glucose levels, inflammation, oxidative stress, and endothelial dysfunction [23, 91]. An analysis with Cardiovascular Health Study showed that RAAS blocking agents reduced cardiovascular events in patients with metabolic syndrome [159]. In the prospective, multicenter, double-blind TROPHY study, patients with obesity and hypertension were treated with hydrochlorothiazide (12.5, 25, or 50 mg) or lisinopril (10, 20, or 40 mg), with a target diastolic blood pressure less than 90 mmHg. About 60% of the patients with obesity receiving lisinopril achieved the blood pressure goal compared to 43% of patients treated with hydrochlorothiazide (HCTZ), and the patients receiving HCTZ had significantly higher plasma glucose and lower plasma potassium levels compared to lisinopril treatment [122]. Treatment with irbesartan alone or in combination with HCTZ was more effective in decreasing blood pressure and also led to improvements in HDL cholesterol, triglyceride levels, fasting blood glucose, and waist circumference in both men and women [79]. To determine whether RAAS inhibition had beneficial metabolic effects, a clinical study compared HCTZ monotherapy, valsartan monotherapy, or HCTZ/valsartan combination therapy in patients with metabolic syndrome. The results showed patients on HCTZ therapy had increased HbA_{1c} or triglyceride levels, while those on valsartan alone or valsartan/HCTZ combination had a favorable metabolic outcome [157]. A subanalysis of patients with diabetes in the Captopril Prevention Project (CAPPP) revealed that ACE inhibitor treatment reduced the total and cardiovascular mortality risk and the risk of fatal and nonfatal myocardial infarction compared to diuretic/beta-blocker treatment [108].

Calcium channel blockers can be given alone or in combination with an ACE inhibitor or ARB for hypertension treatment. In the ACCOMPLISH clinical trial, the patients on HCTZ/benazepril had a higher incidence of cardiovascular morbidity than patients on amlodipine/benazepril [12, 13]. However, a subanalysis of patients classified as normal weight, overweight, and obese based on BMI criteria found no difference in the rates of the primary cardiac end point between obese patients taking HCTZ versus amlodipine [151].

The use of beta-blockers for hypertension treatment has been associated with the development of glucose intolerance, dyslipidemia, and weight gain [124]. Older beta-blockers, e.g., propranolol, metoprolol, and atenolol, act via beta-1 and beta-2 adrenergic receptors to regulate cardiac and vascular responses and metabolism [33]. The International Verapamil-Trandolapril Study (INVEST), the Losartan Intervention for Endpoint Study (LIFE), and the Atherosclerosis Risk in Communities Study (ARIC) all showed higher rates of diabetes in patients treated with older beta-blockers, e.g., atenolol, compared to other medications [28, 55, 112]. Newer beta-blockers have an additive alpha-adrenergic receptor-blocking component (e.g., carvedilol, labetalol) or increased nitric oxide synthesis (e.g., carvedilol, nebivolol) that promotes vasodilation. These beta-blockers often have neutral or favorable effects on body weight compared to older beta-blockers [123].

Future Therapeutic Targets

Tirzepatide (GLP-1/GIP Dual Agonist)

Tirzepatide is under expedited review with the FDA for treatment of obesity [39]. Tirzepatide is a dual GLP-1/GIP agonist that induces weight loss by reducing food intake via central pathways. Additionally, tirzepatide delays gastric emptying. The SURMOUNT-1 trial compared tirzpatide to placebo in about 2500 patients with obesity or overweight with one weight-related complication but without diabetes [69]. At 72 weeks (including a 20-week dose escalation period), tirzepatide induced a mean weight loss of 15%, 19.5%, and 20.9% at 5 mg, 10 mg, and 15 mg doses, respectively, compared to 3.1% with placebo. Impressively, 91% of participants who received tirzepatide 15 mg achieved a mean weight reduction of 5% or more and 57% of participants on tirzepatide 15 mg achieved a mean weight reduction of 20% or more. Tirzepatide also significantly reduced blood pressure and improved lipid profiles. In patients with type 2 diabetes, tirzepatide 15 mg monotherapy reduced body weight by 11%, compared to 0.9% with placebo after 40 weeks [126]. Furthermore, tirzepatide at any dose (8.5% weight loss with 5 mg, 11.0% weight loss with 10 mg, and 13.0% weight loss with 15 mg) resulted in greater weight loss compared to semaglutide 1.0 mg (6.7% weight loss) after 40 weeks in patients with type 2 diabetes on metformin background therapy [44]. Tirzepatide is being studied in several phase 3 trials in patients with obesity and obesity-related comorbidities for weight loss and weight loss maintenance (SURMOUNT-2, NCT04657003; SURMOUNT-3, NCT04657016; and SURMOUNT-4, NCT04660643) and phase 2 trials for the treatment of obesity-related complications including nonalcoholic steatohepatitis (SYNERGY-NASH, NCT0416673), heart failure with preserved ejection fraction (SUMMIT, NCT04847557), chronic kidney disease (TREASURE-CKD, NCT05536804), obstructive sleep apnea (SURMOUNT-OSA, NCT05412004), and overall morbidity and mortality (SURMOUNT-MMO, NCT05556512).

Glucagon Agonist

Glucagon agonist is being investigated as a potential weight loss target, as glucagon increases energy expenditure, reduces food intake, and has lipolytic effects on the liver. However, given the potential hyperglycemic effects of glucagon, glucagon agonists are being studied as a dual agonist with GLP-1 or as a triple agonist with GLP-1 and GIP. Several coagonists are in development for the treatment of obesity, diabetes, and nonalcoholic steatohepatitis. Cotadutide (glucagon/GLP-1 receptor dual agonist) has been studied in phase 2 clinical trials in patients with type 2 diabetes and overweight/obesity and reduced weight by 5% compared to 3.4% with liraglutide 1.8 mg after 14 weeks, with ad hoc analyses demonstrating improvement in lipid and liver profiles [101]. There are other glucagon/GLP-1 receptor coagonists under various stages of investigation [19]. LY3437943, a novel triple GIP, GLP-1, and glucagon receptor agonist, has been studied in a phase 1b trial in patients with type 2 diabetes and found to have an acceptable safety profile, reduced HbA1c by 1.2% at all doses, and reduced weight in a dose-dependent fashion by up to 8.96 kg after 12 weeks [145].

Amylin Analogue

Amylin is cosecreted with insulin from pancreatic beta cells in response to food intake and suppresses postprandial glucagon. Pramlintide was FDA approved in 2005 as an adjunctive therapy to insulin in patients with type 1 and type 2 diabetes, but this first-generation amylin analogue does not promote significant weight loss. Because amylin increases satiety signals in the brain and also delays gastric emptying, a novel amylin analogue has been developed as a potential therapy for weight management [35]. Cagrilintide is a long-acting once-weekly injectable amylin analogue and has been studied as a monotherapy in a phase 2 trial for weight loss and found to reduce weight by 10.8% at 4.5 mg dose versus 9.0% with liraglutide 3.0 mg versus 3% with placebo after 26 weeks [86]. The combination of cagrilintide (a long-acting amylin analogue) and semaglutide is currently being studied in a phase 3 trial for weight loss in patients with obesity and type 2 diabetes (REDEFINE 2, NCT05394519).

Other Medications in Development

Other novel classes of pharmacotherapy for obesity include a neuropeptide Y2 receptor (Y2R) agonist, which inhibits food intake by central action in the hypothalamus, in combination with semaglutide (Phase II trial, NCT04969939), oxytocin (Phase II trial, NCT03043053), ARD-101, a taste receptor activator (Phase II trial, NCT0521441), ERX1000, a leptin sensitizer (Phase I trial, NCT 04890873), and others [20].

Conclusion

Weight management using diet, increased physical activity, and behavioral modification is essential for patients with the metabolic syndrome. Weight loss enhances insulin sensitivity, cardiopulmonary function, and overall health status. Medications approved by the US FDA for chronic treatment of obesity include orlistat, extended-release phentermine/topiramate, sustained release bupropion/naltrexone, and glucagon-like peptide-1 (GLP-1) agonists including liraglutide and semaglutide. In patients with type 2 diabetes, drugs that induce weight loss or are weight neutral such as metformin, GLP-1 agonists, GIP/GLP-1 dual agonist, and SGLT-2 inhibitors are preferred and may confer additional cardiovascular benefit. Treatment of atherogenic dyslipidemia includes using medications such as statins, PCSK9 inhibitors, ezetimibe, and bempedoic acid to lower LDL cholesterol and omega-3 fatty acids and fibrates to lower triglycerides. RAAS and calcium channel blockers are effective for treatment of hypertension and reduction of cardiovascular risk. As much as possible, physicians managing patients with obesity or metabolic syndrome should avoid prescribing medications for hypertension, dyslipidemia, and other diseases that increase body weight and predispose to adverse metabolic outcomes.

Cross-References

▶ Adipokines and Metabolism
▶ Bariatric Surgery
▶ Diet and Obesity
▶ Diet, Exercise, and Behavior Therapy
▶ Overview of Metabolic Syndrome
▶ Prevention and Treatment of Obesity in Children
▶ Principles of Energy Homeostasis

References

1. ACCORD Study Group. Effects of combination lipid therapy in type 2 diabetes mellitus. N Engl J Med. 2010;362:1563–74. https://doi.org/10.1056/NEJMOA1001282.
2. Adams TD, Stroup AM, Gress RE, et al. Cancer incidence and mortality after gastric bypass surgery. Obesity. 2009;17(4):796–802. https://doi.org/10.1038/oby.2008.610.
3. Addy C, Rosko JP, Li S, et al. Pharmacokinetics, safety, and tolerability of phentermine in healthy participants receiving taranabant, a novel cannabinoid-1 receptor (CB1R) inverse agonist. J Clin Pharmacol. 2009;49:1228–38.
4. Aguilar-Salinas CA, Fanghanel-Salmon G, Meza E, et al. Ciprofibrate versus gemfibrozil in the treatment of mixed hyperlipidemias: an open-label, multicenter study. Metab Clin Exp. 2001;50(6):729–33.
5. ALLHAT Officers and Coordinators for the ALLHAT Collaborative Research Group. The Antihypertensive and Lipid-Lowering Treatment to Prevent Heart Attack Trial. Major outcomes in high-risk hypertensive patients randomized to angiotensin-converting enzyme inhibitor or calcium channel blocker vs diuretic: the Antihypertensive and Lipid-Lowering Treatment to Prevent Heart Attack Trial (ALLHAT). JAMA. 2002;288(23):2981–2997. Erratum in: JAMA. 2004; 291(18):2196. JAMA 2003 Jan 8;289(2):178.
6. Allison DB, Gadde KM, Garvey WT, et al. Controlled-release phentermine/topiramate in severely obese adults: a randomized controlled trial (EQUIP). Obesity. 2012;20(2):330–42. https://doi.org/10.1038/oby.2011.330.
7. Amery A, Berthaux P, Bulpitt C, et al. Glucose intolerance during diuretic therapy: results of trial by the European working party on hypertension in the elderly. Lancet. 1978;1(8066):681–3.
8. Apovian CM, Aronne L, Rubino D, et al. A randomized, phase 3 trial of naltrexone SR/bupropion SR on weight and obesity-related risk factors (COR-II). Obesity. 2013;21:935–43. https://doi.org/10.1002/oby.20309.
9. Apovian CM, Aronne LJ, Bessesen DH, et al. Pharmacological management of obesity: an Endocrine Society clinical practice guideline. J Clin Endocrinol Metab. 2015;100:342–62.
10. Astrup A, Rössner S, Van Gaal L, et al. Effects of liraglutide in the treatment of obesity: a randomised, double-blind, placebo-controlled study. Lancet. 2009;374(9701):1606–16.
11. Bailey CJ, Gross JL, Pieters A, et al. Effect of dapagliflozin in patients with type 2 diabetes who have inadequate glycaemic control with metformin: a randomised, double-blind, placebo-controlled trial. Lancet. 2010;375(9733):2223–33. https://doi.org/10.1016/S0140-6736(10)60407-2.
12. Bakris GL, Sarafidis PA, Weir MR, et al. Renal outcomes with different fixed-dose combination therapies in patients with hypertension at high risk for cardiovascular events (ACCOMPLISH): a pre-specified secondary analysis of a randomised controlled trial. Lancet. 2010;375(9721):1173–81. https://doi.org/10.1016/S0140-6736(09)62100-0.
13. Bakris G, Briasoulis A, Dahlof B, et al. Comparison of benazepril plus amlodipine or hydrochlorothiazide in high-risk patients with hypertension and coronary artery disease. Am J Cardiol. 2013;112(2):255–9. https://doi.org/10.1016/j.amjcard.2013.03.026.
14. Bhatt DL, Steg PG, Miller M, et al. Cardiovascular risk reduction with icosapent ethyl for hypertriglyceridemia. N Engl J Med. 2019;380:11–22. https://doi.org/10.1056/NEJMoa1812792.
15. Blom DJ, Hala T, Bolognese M, et al. A 52-week placebo-controlled trial of evolocumab in hyperlipidemia. N Engl J Med. 2014;370:1809–19. https://doi.org/10.1056/NEJMoa1316222.

16. Bray GA, Ryan DH. Medical therapy for the patient with obesity. Circulation. 2012;125(13):1695–703. https://doi.org/10.1161/CIRCULATIONAHA.111. 026567.

17. Bushe CJ, Bradley AJ, Doshi S, et al. Changes in weight and metabolic parameters during treatment with antipsychotics and metformin: do the data inform as to potential guideline development? A systematic review of clinical studies. Int J Clin Pract. 2009;63(12):1743–61. https://doi.org/10.1111/j. 1742-1241.2009.02224.x.

18. Cannon CP, Blazing MA, Giugliano RP, et al. Ezetimibe added to statin therapy after acute coronary syndromes. N Engl J Med. 2015;372:2387–97. https://doi.org/10.1056/NEJMoa1410489.

19. Capozzi ME, D'Alessio DA, Campbell JE. The past, present, and future physiology and pharmacology of glucagon. Cell Metab. 2022;34(11):1654–74. https://doi.org/10.1016/j.cmet.2022.10.001.

20. Chakhtoura M, Haber R, Ghezzawi M, et al. Pharmacotherapy of obesity: an update on the available medications and drugs under investigation. eClinicalMedicine. 2023;58:101882. https://doi.org/10.1016/J.ECLINM.2023.101882.

21. Chanoine JP, Hampl S, Jensen C, et al. Effect of orlistat on weight and body composition in obese adolescents: a randomized controlled trial. JAMA. 2005;293(23):2873–83. https://doi.org/10.1001/jama.293.23.2873.

22. Charlton-Menys V, Durrington PN. Human cholesterol metabolism and therapeutic molecules. Exp Physiol. 2008;93(1):27–42. https://doi.org/10.1113/expphysiol.2007.035147.

23. Chin BS, Langford NJ, Nuttall SL, et al. Antioxidative properties of beta-blockers and angiotensin-converting enzyme inhibitors in congestive heart failure. Eur J Heart Fail. 2003;5(2):171–4.

24. Chobanian AV, Bakris GL, Black HR, et al. National Heart, Lung, and Blood Institute Joint National Committee on prevention, detection, evaluation, and treatment of high blood pressure; national high blood pressure education program coordinating committee. The seventh report of the joint national committee on prevention, detection, evaluation and treatment of high blood pressure: the JNC 7 report. JAMA. 2003;289(19):2560–72.

25. Christensen R, Bartels EM, Astrup A, et al. Effect of weight reduction in obese patients diagnosed with knee osteoarthritis: a systematic review and meta-analysis. Ann Rheum Dis. 2007;66(4):433–9. https://doi.org/10.1136/ard.2006.065904.

26. Cohen RV, Pinheiro JC, Schiavon CA, et al. Effects of gastric bypass surgery in patients with type 2 diabetes and only mild obesity. Diabetes Care. 2012;35(7): 1420–8. https://doi.org/10.2337/dc11-2289.

27. Cholesterol Treatment Trialists Collaborators, Mihaylova B, Emberson J, et al. The effects of lowering LDL cholesterol with statin therapy in people at low risk of vascular disease: meta-analysis of individual data from 27 randomised trials. Lancet. 2012;380(9841):581–90. https://doi.org/10.1016/S0140-6736(12)60367-5.

28. Dahlof B, Devereux RB, Kjeldsen SE, et al. Cardiovascular morbidity and mortality in the Losartan intervention for endpoint reduction in hypertension study (LIFE): a randomised trial against atenolol. Lancet. 2002;359(9311):995–1003. https://doi.org/10.1016/S0140-6736(02)08089-3.

29. Das Pradhan A, Glynn RJ, Fruchart JC, et al. Triglyceride lowering with pemafibrate to reduce cardiovascular risk. N Engl J Med. 2022;387:1923–34. https://doi.org/10.1056/NEJMoa2210645.

30. Davies MJ, Bergenstal R, Bode B, et al. Efficacy of liraglutide for weight loss among patients with type 2 diabetes: the SCALE diabetes randomized clinical trial. JAMA. 2015;314(7):687–99. https://doi.org/10.1001/jama.2015.9676.

31. Davies MJ, Aronne LJ, Caterson ID, et al. Liraglutide and cardiovascular outcomes in adults with overweight or obesity: a post hoc analysis from SCALE randomized controlled trials. Diabetes Obes Metab. 2018;20 (3):734–9. https://doi.org/10.1111/dom.13125.

32. Davies M, Færch L, Jappesen OK, et al. Semaglutide 2.4 mg once a week in adults with overweight or obesity, and type 2 diabetes (STEP 2): a randomized, double-blind, double-dummy, placebo-controlled, phase 3 trial. Lancet. 2021;397:971–84. https://doi.org/10.1016/S0140-6736(21)00213-0.

33. Deedwania P. Hypertension, dyslipidemia, and insulin resistance in patients with diabetes mellitus or the cardiometabolic syndrome: benefits of vasodilating beta-blockers. J Clin Hypertens. 2011;13(1):52–9. https://doi.org/10.1111/j.1751-7176.2010.00386.x.

34. DeFronzo RA, Davidson JA, Del Prato S. The role of the kidneys in glucose homeostasis: a new path towards normalizing glycaemia. Diabetes Obes Metab. 2012;14(1):5–14. https://doi.org/10.1111/j. 1463-1326.2011.01511.x.

35. Dehestani B, Stratford NR, le Roux CW. Amylin as a future obesity treatment. J Obes Metab Syndr. 2021;30 (4):320–5. https://doi.org/10.7570/jomes21071.

36. Del Prato S, Kahn SE, Pavo I, et al. Tirzepatide versus insulin glargine in type 2 diabetes and increased cardiovascular risk (SURPASS-4): a randomised, open-label, parallel-group, multicentre, phase 3 trial. Lancet. 2021;398:1811–24. https://doi.org/10.1016/S0140-6736(21)02188-7.

37. Diabetes Prevention Program Research Group. Long-term safety, tolerability, and weight loss associated with metformin in the diabetes prevention program outcomes study. Diabetes Care. 2012;35(4):731–7. https://doi.org/10.2337/dc11-1299.

38. Diabetes Prevention Program Research Group, Knowler WC, Fowler SE, et al. 10-year follow-up of diabetes incidence and weight loss in the diabetes prevention program outcomes study. Lancet. 2009;374(9702):1677–86. https://doi.org/10.1016/S0140-6736(09)61457-4.

39. Eli Lilly and Company. Lilly receives U.S. FDA Fast Track designation for tirzepatide for the treatment of adults with obesity, or overweight with weight-related comorbidities; 2022. https://investor.lilly.com/news-releases/news-release-details/lilly-receives-us-fda-fast-track-designation-tirzepatide. Accessed 15 April 2023.

40. Ferrannini E, Solini A. SGLT2 inhibition in diabetes mellitus: rationale and clinical prospects. Nat Rev Endocrinol. 2012;8(8):495–502. https://doi.org/10.1038/nrendo.2011.243.

41. Ferrannini E, Ramos SJ, Salsali A, et al. Dapagliflozin monotherapy in type 2 diabetic patients with inadequate glycemic control by diet and exercise: a randomized, double-blind, placebo-controlled, phase 3 trial. Diabetes Care. 2010;33(10):2217–24. https://doi.org/10.2337/dc10-0612.

42. Fransen M. Dietary weight loss and exercise for obese adults with knee osteoarthritis: modest weight loss targets, mild exercise, modest effects. Arthritis Rheum. 2004;50(5):1366–9. https://doi.org/10.1002/art.20257.

43. Frías JP, Nauck MA, Van J, et al. Efficacy and safety of LY3298176, a novel dual GIP and GLP-1 receptor agonist, in patients with type 2 diabetes: a randomised, placebo-controlled and active comparator-controlled phase 2 trial. Lancet. 2018;392:2180–93. https://doi.org/10.1016/S0140-6736(18)32260-8.

44. Frías JP, Davies MJ, Rosenstock J, et al. Tirzepatide versus semaglutide once weekly in patients with type 2 diabetes. N Engl J Med. 2021;385:503–15. https://doi.org/10.1056/NEJMoa2107519.

45. Friedrichsen M, Breitschaft A, Tadayon S, et al. The effect of semaglutide 2.4 mg once weekly on energy intake, appetite, control of eating, and gastric emptying in adults with obesity. Diabetes Obes Metab. 2021;23(3):754–62. https://doi.org/10.1111/dom.14280.

46. Gadde KM, Allison DB, Ryan DH, et al. Effects of low-dose, controlled-release, phentermine plus topiramate combination on weight and associated comorbidities in overweight and obese adults (CONQUER): a randomised, placebo-controlled, phase 3 trial. Lancet. 2011;377(9774):1341–52. https://doi.org/10.1016/S0140-6736(11)60205-5.

47. Garvey WT, Ryan DH, Look M, et al. Two-year sustained weight loss and metabolic benefits with controlled-release phentermine/topiramate in obese and overweight adults (SEQUEL): a randomized, placebo-controlled, phase 3 extension study. Am J Clin Nutr. 2012;95(2):297–308. https://doi.org/10.3945/ajcn.111.024927.

48. Garvey WT, Batterham RL, Bhatta M, et al. Two-year effects of semaglutide in adults with overweight or obesity: the STEP 5 trial. Nat Med. 2022;28(10):2083–91. https://doi.org/10.1038/s41591-022-02026-4.

49. Gerstein HC, Colhoun HM, Dagenais GR, et al. Dulaglutide and cardiovascular outcomes in type 2 diabetes (REWIND): a double-blind, randomised placebo-controlled trial. Lancet. 2019;394:121–30. https://doi.org/10.1016/S0140-6736(19)31149-3.

50. Ginsberg HN, Packard CJ, Chapman MJ, et al. Triglyceride-rich lipoproteins and their remnants: metabolic insights, role in atherosclerotic cardiovascular disease, and emerging therapeutic strategies-a consensus statement from the European Atherosclerosis Society. Eur Heart J. 2021;42(47):4791–806. https://doi.org/10.1093/eurheartj/ehab551.

51. Goff DC Jr, Lloyd-Jones DM, Bennett G, et al. 2013 ACC/AHA guideline on the assessment of cardiovascular risk: a report of the American College of Cardiology/American Heart Association Task Force on Practice Guidelines. Circulation. 2014;129(25 Suppl 2):S49–73. https://doi.org/10.1161/01.cir.0000437741.48606.98.

52. Gordts PLSM, Nock R, Son NH, et al. ApoC-III inhibits clearance of triglyceride-rich lipoproteins through LDL family receptors. J Clin Invest. 2016;126(8):2855–66. https://doi.org/10.1172/JCI86610.

53. Greenway FL, Whitehouse MJ, Guttadauria M, et al. Rational design of a combination medication for the treatment of obesity. Obesity. 2009;17(1):30–9. https://doi.org/10.1038/oby.2008.461.

54. Greenway FL, Fujioka K, Plodkowski RA, for the COR-I Study Group, et al. Effect of naltrexone plus bupropion on weight loss in overweight and obese adults (COR-I): a multicenter, randomised, double-blind, placebo-controlled, phase 3 trial. Lancet. 2010;376:595–605.

55. Gress TW, Nieto FJ, Shahar E, et al. Hypertension and antihypertensive therapy as risk factors for type 2 diabetes mellitus. Atherosclerosis risk in communities study. N Engl J Med. 2000;342(13):905–12. https://doi.org/10.1056/NEJM200003303421301.

56. Gutzwiller JP, Drewe J, Goke B, et al. Glucagon-like peptide-1 promotes satiety and reduces food intake in patients with diabetes mellitus type 2. Am J Phys. 1999;276(5 Pt 2):R1541–4.

57. Harper R, Ennis CN, Heaney AP, et al. A comparison of the effects of low and conventional dose thiazide diuretic on insulin action in hypertensive patients with NIDDM. Diabetologia. 1995;38(7):853–9.

58. Heerspink HJL, Stefánsson BV, Correa-Rotter R, et al. Dapagliflozin in patients with chronic kidney disease. N Engl J Med. 2020;383:1436–46. https://doi.org/10.1056/NEJMoa2024816.

59. Henriksen EJ, Prasannarong M. The role of the renin-angiotensin system in the development of insulin resistance in skeletal muscle. Mol Cell Endocrinol. 2013;378(1–2):15–22. https://doi.org/10.1016/j.mce.2012.04.011.

60. Hollander P, Gupta AK, Plodkowski R, et al. Effects of naltrexone sustained-release/bupropion sustained-release combination therapy on body weight and glycemic parameters in overweight and obese patients with type 2 diabetes. Diabetes Care. 2013;36:4022–9. https://doi.org/10.2337/dc13-0234.

61. Holman RR, Bethel MA, Mentz RJ, et al. Effects of once-weekly exenatide on cardiovascular outcomes

in type 2 diabetes. N Engl J Med. 2017;377:1228–39. https://doi.org/10.1056/NEJMoa1612917.

62. Huang MH, Chen CH, Chen TW, et al. The effects of weight reduction on the rehabilitation of patients with knee osteoarthritis and obesity. Arthritis Care Res. 2000;13(6):398–405.

63. Huang MA, Greenson JK, Chao C, et al. One-year intense nutritional counseling results in histological improvement in patients with non-alcoholic steatohepatitis: a pilot study. Am J Gastroenterol. 2005;100(5):1072–81. https://doi.org/10.1111/j.1572-0241.2005.41334.x.

64. Hunninghake DB, Stein EA, Bays HE, et al. Rosuvastatin improves the atherogenic and atheroprotective lipid profiles in patients with hyper-triglyceridemia. Coron Artery Dis. 2004;15(2):115–23. https://doi.org/10.1097/00019501-200403000-00008.

65. Husain M, Birkenfeld AL, Donsmark M, et al. Oral semaglutide and cardiovascular outcomes in patients with type 2 diabetes. N Engl J Med. 2019;381:841–51. https://doi.org/10.1056/NEJMoa1901118.

66. Ilanne-Parikka P, Eriksson JG, Lindstrom J, et al. Effect of lifestyle intervention on the occurrence of metabolic syndrome and its components in the Finnish Diabetes Prevention Study. Diabetes Care. 2008;31(4):805–7. https://doi.org/10.2337/dc07-1117.

67. Jacob S, Rabbia M, Meier MK, et al. Orlistat 120 mg improves glycaemic control in type 2 diabetic patients with or without concurrent weight loss. Diabetes Obes Metab. 2009;11(4):361–71. https://doi.org/10.1111/j.1463-1326.2008.00970.x.

68. Jacobson TA, Glickstein SB, Rowe JD, et al. Effects of eicosapentaenoic acid and docosahexaenoic acid on low-density lipoprotein cholesterol and other lipids: a review. J Clin Lipidol. 2012;6(1):5–18. https://doi.org/10.1016/j.jacl.2011.10.018.

69. Jastreboff AM, Aronne LJ, Ahmad NN, et al. Tirzepatide once weekly for the treatment of obesity. N Engl J Med. 2022;387:205–16. https://doi.org/10.1056/NEJMoa2206038.

70. Jensen MD, Ryan DH, Apovian CM, et al. 2013 AHA/ACC/TOS guideline for the management of over-weight and obesity in adults: a report of the American College of Cardiology/American Heart Association Task Force on Practice Guidelines and The Obesity Society. Circulation. 2014;129(25 Suppl 2):S102–38. https://doi.org/10.1161/01.cir.0000437739.71477.ee.

71. Jones PH, Davidson MH, Stein EA, et al. Comparison of the efficacy and safety of rosuvastatin versus ator-vastatin, simvastatin, and pravastatin across doses (STELLAR Trial). Am J Cardiol. 2003;92:152–60. https://doi.org/10.1016/S0002-9149(03)00530-7.

72. Kanda M, Satoh K, Ichihara K. Effects of atorvastatin and pravastatin on glucose tolerance in diabetic rats mildly induced by streptozotocin. Biol Pharm Bull. 2003;26(12):1681–4.

73. Karagiannis T, Avgerinos I, Liako A, et al. Management of type 2 diabetes with the dual GIP/GLP-1 receptor agonist tirzepatide: a systematic review and meta-analysis. Diabetologia. 2022;65:1251–61. https://doi.org/10.1007/s00125-022-05715-4.

74. Keech A, Simes RJ, Barter P, et al. Effects of long-term fenofibrate therapy on cardiovascular events in 9795 people with type 2 diabetes mellitus (the FIELD study): randomised controlled trial. Lancet. 2005;366 (9500):1849–61. https://doi.org/10.1016/S0140-6736(05)67667-2.

75. Khan SU, Lone AN, Khan MS, et al. Effect of omega-3 fatty acids on cardiovascular outcomes: a systematic review and meta-analysis. EClinicalMedicine. 2021;38:100997. https://doi.org/10.1016/j.eclinm.2021.100997.

76. Khera R, Pandey A, Chander AK. Effects of weight-loss medications on cardiometabolic risk profiles: a systematic review and network meta-analysis. Gas-troenterology. 2018;154:1309–1319.e7. https://doi.org/10.1053/j.gastro.2017.12.024.

77. Kilicarslan A, Yavuz B, Guven GS, et al. Fenofibrate improves endothelial function and decreases thrombin-activatable fibrinolysis inhibitor concentra-tion in metabolic syndrome. Blood Coagul Fibrinoly-sis. 2008;19(4):310–4. https://doi.org/10.1097/MBC.0b013e3283009c69.

78. Kim KK, Cho H-J, Kang J-C, et al. Effects on weight reduction and safety of short-term phentermine administration in Korean obese people. Yonsei Med J. 2006;47:614–25.

79. Kintscher U, Bramlage P, Paar WD, et al. Irbesartan for the treatment of hypertension in patients with the metabolic syndrome: a sub analysis of the treat to target post authorization survey. Prospective observa-tional, two armed study in 14,200 patients. Cardiovasc Diabetol. 2007;6:12. https://doi.org/10.1186/1475-2840-6-12.

80. Klosiewicz-Latoszek L, Szostak WB. Comparative studies on the influence of different fibrates on serum lipoproteins in endogenous hyperlipoproteinaemia. Eur J Clin Pharmacol. 1991;40(1):33–41.

81. Knopp RH, Gitter H, Truitt T, et al. Effects of ezetimibe, a new cholesterol absorption inhibitor, on plasma lipids in patients with primary hypercholes-terolemia. Eur Heart J. 2003;24(8):729–41. https://doi.org/10.1016/s0195-668x(02)00807-2.

82. Knudsen LB, Lau J. The discovery and development of liraglutide and semaglutide. Front Endocrinol. 2019;10:155. https://doi.org/10.3389/fendo.2019.00155.

83. Kosiborod MN, Bhatta M, Davies M, et al. Semaglutide improves cardiometabolic risk factors in adults with overweight or obesity: STEP 1 and 4 exploratory analyses. Diabetes Obes Metab. 2023;25(2):468–78. https://doi.org/10.1111/dom.14890.

84. Kuna ST, Reboussin DM, Borradaile KE, et al. Long-term effect of weight loss on obstructive sleep apnea severity in obese patients with type 2 diabetes. Sleep. 2013;36(5):641–649A. https://doi.org/10.5665/sleep.2618.

85. LaRosa JC, Grundy SM, Waters DD, et al. Intensive lipid lowering with atorvastatin in patients with stable coronary disease. N Engl J Med. 2005;352(14):1425–35. https://doi.org/10.1056/NEJMoa050461.

86. Lau DCW, Erichsen L, Francisco AM, et al. Once-weekly cagrilintide for weight management in people with overweight and obesity: a multicentre, randomised, double-blind, placebo-controlled and active-controlled, dose-finding phase 2 trial. Lancet. 2021;398(10317):2160–72. https://doi.org/10.1016/S0140-6736(21)01751-7.

87. Liao JK. Beyond lipid lowering: the role of statins in vascular protection. Int J Cardiol. 2002;86(1):5–18.

88. Lim S, Sakuma I, Quon MJ, et al. Potentially important considerations in choosing specific statin treatments to reduce overall morbidity and mortality. Int J Cardiol. 2013;167(5):1696–702. https://doi.org/10.1016/j.ijcard.2012.10.037.

89. List JF, Woo V, Morales E, et al. Sodium-glucose cotransport inhibition with dapagliflozin in type 2 diabetes. Diabetes Care. 2009;32(4):650–7. https://doi.org/10.2337/dc08-1863.

90. Ludvik B, Giorgino F, Jódar E, et al. Once-weekly tirzepatide versus once-daily insulin degludec as add-on to metformin with or without SGLT2 inhibitors in patients with type 2 diabetes (SURPASS-3): a randomised, open-label, parallel-group, phase 3 trial. Lancet. 2021;398:583–98. https://doi.org/10.1016/S0140-6736(21)01443-4.

91. Manabe S, Okura T, Watanabe S, et al. Effects of angiotensin II receptor blockade with valsartan on pro-inflammatory cytokines in patients with essential hypertension. J Cardiovasc Pharmacol. 2005;46(6):735–9.

92. Marso SP, Daniels GH, Brown-Frandsen K, et al. Liraglutide and cardiovascular outcomes in type 2 diabetes. N Engl J Med. 2016a;375:311–22. https://doi.org/10.1056/NEJMoa1603827.

93. Marso SP, Bain SC, Consoli A, et al. Semaglutide and cardiovascular outcomes in patients with type 2 diabetes. N Engl J Med. 2016b;375:1834–44. https://doi.org/10.1056/NEJMoa1607141.

94. Maruthur NM, Tseng E, Hutfless S, et al. Diabetes medications as monotherapy or metformin-based combination therapy for type 2 diabetes. □Ann. Intern Med. 2016;164:740–51. https://doi.org/10.7326/M15-2650.

95. Meier JJ. GLP-1 receptor agonists for individualized treatment of type 2 diabetes mellitus. Nat Rev Endocrinol. 2012;8(12):728–42. https://doi.org/10.1038/nrendo.2012.140.

96. Messier SP, Loeser RF, Miller GD, et al. Exercise and dietary weight loss in overweight and obese older adults with knee osteoarthritis: the arthritis, diet, and activity promotion trial. Arthritis Rheum. 2004;50(5):1501–10. https://doi.org/10.1002/art.20256.

97. Meyer-Sabellek W, Brasch H. Atherosclerosis, inflammation, leukocyte function and the effect of statins. J Hypertens. 2006;24(12):2349–51. https://doi.org/10.1097/HJH.0b013e3280113648.

98. Min T, Bain SC. The role of tirzepatide, dual GIP and GLP-1 receptor agonist, in the management of type 2 diabetes: the SURPASS clinical trials. Diabetes Ther. 2021;12(1):143–57. https://doi.org/10.1007/s13300-020-00981-0.

99. Mingrone G, Panunzi S, De Gaetano A, et al. Bariatric surgery versus conventional medical therapy for type 2 diabetes. N Engl J Med. 2012;366(17):1577–85. https://doi.org/10.1056/NEJMoa1200111.

100. Moon S, Lee J, Chung HS, et al. Efficacy and safety of the new appetite suppressant, liraglutide: a meta-analysis of randomized controlled trials. Endocrinol Metab. 2021;36:647–60. https://doi.org/10.3803/EnM.2020.934.

101. Nahra R, Wang T, Gadde KM, et al. Effects of Cotadutide on metabolic and hepatic parameters in adults with overweight or obesity and type 2 diabetes: a 54-week randomized phase 2b study. Diabetes Care. 2021;44(6):1433–42. https://doi.org/10.2337/dc20-2151.

102. Nauck MA, Meier JJ. The incretin effect in healthy individuals and those with type 2 diabetes: physiology, pathophysiology, and response to therapeutic interventions. Lancet Diabetes Endocrinol. 2016;4:525–36. https://doi.org/10.1016/S2213-8587(15)00482-9.

103. Nauck MA, Del Prato S, Meier JJ, et al. Dapagliflozin versus glipizide as add-on therapy in patients with type 2 diabetes who have inadequate glycemic control with metformin: a randomized, 52-week, double-blind, active-controlled noninferiority trial. Diabetes Care. 2011;34(9):2015–22. https://doi.org/10.2337/dc11-0606.

104. Nauck MA, Meier JJ, Cavender MA, et al. Cardiovascular actions and clinical outcomes with glucagon-like peptide-1 receptor agonists and dipeptidyl peptidase-4 inhibitors. Circulation. 2017;136:849–70. https://doi.org/10.1161/CIRCULATIONAHA.117.028136.

105. Nauck MA, Quast DR, Wefers J, et al. GLP-1 receptor agonists in the treatment of type 2 diabetes – state-of-the-art. Mol Metab. 2021;46:101102. https://doi.org/10.1016/j.molmet.2020.101102.

106. Neal B, Perkovic V, Mahaffey KW, et al. Canagliflozin and cardiovascular and renal events in type 2 diabetes. N Engl J Med. 2017;377:644–57. https://doi.org/10.1056/NEJMoa1611925.

107. Nicholls SJ, Lincoff AM, Garcia M, et al. Effect of high-dose omega-3 fatty acids vs corn oil on major adverse cardiovascular events in patients at high cardiovascular risk: the STRENGTH randomized clinical trial. JAMA. 2020;324(22):2268–80. https://doi.org/10.1001/jama.2020.22258.

108. Niskanen L, Hedner T, Hansson L. et al; CAPPP Group. Reduced cardiovascular morbidity and mortality in hypertensive diabetic patients on first-line therapy with an ACE inhibitor compared with a diuretic/beta-blocker-based treatment regimen: a

subanalysis of the Captopril Prevention Project. Diabetes Care. 2001;24(12):2091–6.

109. Nissen SE, Wolski KE, Prcela L, et al. Effect of naltrexone-bupropion on major adverse cardiovascular events in overweight and obese patients with cardiovascular risk factors: a randomized clinical trial. JAMA. 2016;315(10):990–1004. https://doi.org/10.1001/jama.2016.1558.

110. Nissen SE, Lincoff AM, Brennan D, et al. Bempedoic acid and cardiovascular outcomes in statin-intolerant patients. N Engl J Med. 2023;388(15):1353–64. https://doi.org/10.1056/NEJMoa2215024.

111. Packard KA, Backes JM, Lenz TL, et al. Comparison of gemfibrozil and fenofibrate in patients with dyslipidemic coronary heart disease. Pharmacotherapy. 2002;22(12):1527–32.

112. Pepine CJ, Handberg EM, Cooper-DeHoff RM, et al. A calcium antagonist vs a non-calcium antagonist hypertension treatment strategy for patients with coronary artery disease. The International Verapamil-Trandolapril Study (INVEST): a randomized controlled trial. JAMA. 2003;290(21):2805–16. https://doi.org/10.1001/jama.290.21.2805.

113. Perkovic V, Jardine MJ, Neal B, et al. Canagliflozin and renal outcomes in type 2 diabetes and nephropathy. N Engl J Med. 2019;380:2295–306. https://doi.org/10.1056/NEJMoa1811744.

114. Pfeffer MA, Claggett B, Diaz R, et al. Lixisenatide in patients with type 2 diabetes and acute coronary syndrome. N Engl J Med. 2015;373:2247–57. https://doi.org/10.1056/NEJMoa1509225.

115. Pi-Sunyer X, Astrup A, Fujioka K, et al. A randomized, controlled trial of 3.0 mg of liraglutide in weight management. N Engl J Med. 2015;373:11–22. https://doi.org/10.1056/NEJMoa1411892.

116. Preiss D, Seshasai SR, Welsh P, et al. Risk of incident diabetes with intensive-dose compared with moderate-dose statin therapy: a meta-analysis. JAMA. 2011;305(24):2556–64. https://doi.org/10.1001/jama.2011.860.

117. Pyorala K, Ballantyne CM, Gumbiner B, et al. Reduction of cardiovascular events by simvastatin in non-diabetic coronary heart disease patients with and without the metabolic syndrome: subgroup analyses of the Scandinavian Simvastatin Survival Study (4S). Diabetes Care. 2004;27(7):1735–40.

118. Quispe R, Sweeney T, Varma B, et al. Recent updates in hypertriglyceridemia management for cardiovascular disease prevention. Curr Atheroscler Rep. 2022;24(10):767–78. https://doi.org/10.1007/s11883-022-01052-4.

119. Rapoport MI, Hurd HF. Thiazide-induced glucose intolerance treated with potassium. Arch Intern Med. 1964;113:405–8.

120. Ray KK, Bays HE, Catapano AL, et al. Safety and efficacy of bempedoic acid to reduce LDL cholesterol. N Engl J Med. 2019;380:1022–32. https://doi.org/10.1056/NEJMoa1803917.

121. Ray KK, Wright RS, Kallend D, et al. Two phase 3 trials of inclisiran in patients with elevated LDL cholesterol. N Engl J Med. 2020;382:1507–19. https://doi.org/10.1056/NEJMoa1912387.

122. Reisin E, Jack AV. Obesity and hypertension: mechanisms, cardio-renal consequences, and therapeutic approaches. Med Clin North Am. 2009;93(3):733–51. https://doi.org/10.1016/j.mcna.2009.02.010.

123. Reisin E, Owen J. Treatment: special conditions. Metabolic syndrome: obesity and the hypertension connection. J Am Soc Hypertens. 2015;9(2):156–9. https://doi.org/10.1016/j.jash.2014.12.015. quiz 160

124. Ripley TL, Saseen JJ. Beta-blockers: a review of their pharmacological and physiological diversity in hypertension. Ann Pharmacother. 2014;48(6):723–33. https://doi.org/10.1177/1060028013519591.

125. Rosenstock J, Aggarwal N, Polidori D, et al. Dose-ranging effects of canagliflozin, a sodium-glucose cotransporter 2 inhibitor, as add-on to metformin in subjects with type 2 diabetes. Diabetes Care. 2012;35(6):1232–8. https://doi.org/10.2337/dc11-1926.

126. Rosenstock J, Wysham C, Frías JP, et al. Efficacy and safety of a novel dual GIP and GLP-1 receptor agonist tirzepatide in patients with type 2 diabetes (SURPASS-1): a double-blind, randomised, phase 3 trial. Lancet. 2021;398:143–55. https://doi.org/10.1016/S0140-6736(21)01324-6.

127. Rubino DM, Greenway FL, Khalid U, et al. Effect of weekly subcutaneous semaglutide vs daily liraglutide on body weight in adults with overweight or obesity without diabetes: the STEP 8 randomized clinical trial. JAMA. 2022;327(2):138–50. https://doi.org/10.1001/jama.2021.23619.

128. Rubins HB, Robins SJ, Collins D, et al. Gemfibrozil for the secondary prevention of coronary heart disease in men with low levels of high-density lipoprotein cholesterol. N Engl J Med. 1999;341(6):410–8. https://doi.org/10.1056/NEJM199908053410604.

129. Rucker D, Padwal R, Li SK, et al. Long term pharmacotherapy for obesity and overweight: updated meta-analysis. BMJ. 2007;335(7631):1194–9. https://doi.org/10.1136/bmj.39385.413113.25.

130. Ryan D, Peterson C, Troupin B, et al. Weight loss at 6 months with VI-0521 (PHEN/TPM combination) treatment. Obes Facts. 2010;3:139–46.

131. Sabatine MS, Giugliano RP, Keech AC, et al. Evolocumab and clinical outcomes in patients with cardiovascular disease. N Engl J Med. 2017;376:1713–22. https://doi.org/10.1056/NEJMoa1615664.

132. Sattar N, Preiss D, Murray HM, et al. Statins and risk of incident diabetes: a collaborative meta-analysis of randomised statin trials. Lancet. 2010;375(9716):735–42. https://doi.org/10.1016/S0140-6736(09)61965-6.

133. Schauer PR, Kashyap SR, Wolski K, et al. Bariatric surgery versus intensive medical therapy in obese patients with diabetes. N Engl J Med. 2012;366(17):1567–76. https://doi.org/10.1056/NEJMoa1200225.

134. Schwartz GG, Steg PG, Szarek M, et al. Alirocumab and cardiovascular outcomes after acute coronary syndrome. N Engl J Med. 2018;379:2097–107. https://doi.org/10.1056/NEJMoa1801174.

135. Shatanawi A, Romero MJ, Iddings JA, et al. Angiotensin II-induced vascular endothelial dysfunction through RhoA/Rho kinase/p38 mitogen-activated protein kinase/arginase pathway. Am J Physiol Cell Physiol. 2011;300(5):C1181–92. https://doi.org/10.1152/ajpcell.00328.2010.

136. Sjostrom L, Gummesson A, Sjostrom CD, et al. Effects of bariatric surgery on cancer incidence in obese patients in Sweden (Swedish Obese Subjects Study): a prospective, controlled intervention trial. Lancet Oncol. 2009;10(7):653–62. https://doi.org/10.1016/S1470-2045(09)70159-7.

137. Skulas-Ray AC, Wilson PWF, Harris WS, et al. Omega-3 fatty acids for the management of hypertriglyceridemia: a science advisory from the American Heart Association. Circulation. 2019;140:e673–91. https://doi.org/10.1161/CIR.0000000000000709.

138. Smith SR, Weissman NJ, Anderson CM, et al. Multicenter, placebo-controlled trial of lorcaserin for weight management. N Engl J Med. 2010;363(3):245–56. https://doi.org/10.1056/NEJMoa0909809.

139. Stalenhoef AF, Ballantyne CM, Sarti C, et al. A comparative study with rosuvastatin in subjects with metabolic syndrome: results of the COMETS study. Eur Heart J. 2005;26(24):2664–72. https://doi.org/10.1093/eurheartj/ehi482.

140. Stender S, Schuster H, Barter P, MERCURY I Study Group, et al. Comparison of rosuvastatin with atorvastatin, simvastatin and pravastatin in achieving cholesterol goals and improving plasma lipids in hypercholesterolaemic patients with or without the metabolic syndrome in the MERCURY I trial. Diabetes Obes Metab. 2005;7(4):430–8. https://doi.org/10.1111/j.1463-1326.2004.00450.x.

141. Torgerson JS, Hauptman J, Boldrin MN, et al. XENical in the prevention of diabetes in obese subjects (XENDOS) study: a randomized study of orlistat as an adjunct to lifestyle changes for the prevention of type 2 diabetes in obese patients. Diabetes Care. 2004;27(1):155–61.

142. Tsapas A, Avgerinos I, Karagiannis T, et al. Comparative effectiveness of glucose-lowering drugs for type 2 diabetes. Ann Intern Med. 2020;173:278–86. https://doi.org/10.7326/M20-0864.

143. Tsapas A, Karagiannis T, Kakotrichi P, et al. Comparative efficacy of glucose-lowering medications on body weight and blood pressure in patients with type 2 diabetes: a systematic review and network meta-analysis. Diabetes Obes Metab. 2021;23:2116–24. https://doi.org/10.1111/dom.14451.

144. Ueno T, Sugawara H, Sujaku K, et al. Therapeutic effects of restricted diet and exercise in obese patients with fatty liver. J Hepatol. 1997;27(1):103–7.

145. Urva S, Coskun T, Loh MT, et al. LY3437943, a novel triple GIP, GLP-1, and glucagon receptor agonist in people with type 2 diabetes: a phase 1b, multicentre, double-blind, placebo-controlled, randomised, multiple-ascending dose trial. Lancet. 2022;400:1869–81. https://doi.org/10.1016/S0140-6736(22)02033-5.

146. van Gool CH, Penninx BW, Kempen GI, et al. Effects of exercise adherence on physical function among overweight older adults with knee osteoarthritis. Arthritis Rheum. 2005;53(1):24–32. https://doi.org/10.1002/art.20902.

147. Wadden TA, Foreyt JP, Foster GD, et al. Weight loss with naltrexoneSR/bupropion SR combination therapy as an adjunct to behavior modification: the COR-BMOD trial. Obesity. 2011;19:110–20.

148. Wadden TA, Hollander P, Klein S, et al. Weight maintenance and additional weight loss with liraglutide after low-calorie-diet-induced weight loss: the SCALE Maintenance randomized study. Int J Obes (Lond). 2013;37(11):1443–1451. https://doi.org/10.1038/ijo.2013.120. Epub 2013 Jul 1. Erratum in: Int J Obes (Lond). 2015;39(1):187; Int J Obes (Lond). 2015;39(1):187; Int J Obes (Lond). 2013;37(11):1514.

149. Wadden TA, Bailey TS, Billings LK, et al. Effect of subcutaneous semaglutide vs placebo as an adjunct to intensive behavioral therapy on body weight in adults with overweight or obesity: the STEP 3 randomized clinical trial. JAMA. 2021;325(14):1403–13. https://doi.org/10.1001/jama.2021.1831.

150. Wannamethee SG, Shaper AG, Walker M. Overweight and obesity and weight change in middle aged men: impact on cardiovascular disease and diabetes. J Epidemiol Community Health. 2005;59(2):134–9. https://doi.org/10.1136/jech.2003.015651.

151. Weber MA, Jamerson K, Bakris GL, et al. Effects of body size and hypertension treatments on cardiovascular event rates: subanalysis of the ACCOMPLISH randomised controlled trial. Lancet. 2013;381(9866):537–45. https://doi.org/10.1016/S0140-6736(12)61343-9.

152. Weghuber D, Barrett T, Barrientos-Pérez M, et al. Once-weekly semaglutide in adolescents with obesity. N Engl J Med. 2022;387:2245–57. https://doi.org/10.1056/NEJMoa2208601.

153. Wilding JPH, Batterham RL, Calanna S, et al. Once-weekly semaglutide in adults with overweight or obesity. N Engl J Med. 2021;384:989–1002. https://doi.org/10.1056/NEJMoa2032183.

154. Wiviott ZD, Raz I, Bonaca M, et al. Dapagliflozin and cardiovascular outcomes in type 2 diabetes. N Engl J Med. 2019;24(380):347–57. https://doi.org/10.1056/NEJMoa1812389.

155. Zambon A, Gervois P, Pauletto P, et al. Modulation of hepatic inflammatory risk markers of cardiovascular diseases by PPAR-alpha activators: clinical and experimental evidence. Arterioscler Thromb Vasc

Biol. 2006;26(5):977–86. https://doi.org/10.1161/01. ATV.0000204327.96431.9a.

156. Zanella MT, Uehara MH, Ribeiro AB, et al. Orlistat and cardiovascular risk profile in hypertensive patients with metabolic syndrome: the ARCOS study. Arq Bras Endocrinol Metabol. 2006;50(2): 368–76. S0004-27302006000200023

157. Zappe DH, Sowers JR, Hsueh WA, et al. Metabolic and antihypertensive effects of combined angiotensin receptor blocker and diuretic therapy in prediabetic hypertensive patients with the cardiometabolic

syndrome. J Clin Hypertens. 2008;10(12):894–903. https://doi.org/10.1111/j.1751-7176.2008.00054.x.

158. Zinman B, Wanner C, Lachin J, et al. Empagliflozin, cardiovascular outcomes, and mortality in type 2 diabetes. N Engl J Med. 2015;373:2117–28. https://doi.org/10.1056/NEJMoa1504720.

159. Zreikat HH, Harpe SE, Slattum PW, et al. Effect of Renin-Angiotensin system inhibition on cardiovascular events in older hypertensive patients with metabolic syndrome. Metab Clin Exp. 2014;63(3):392–9. https://doi.org/10.1016/j.metabol.2013.11.006.

Bariatric Surgery

39

Rexford S. Ahima and Hyeong-Kyu Park

Contents

Abstract

Bariatric surgery is the most effective and durable treatment for obesity. This chapter will describe the historic and current bariatric surgical procedures; outcome data focusing on weight loss, diabetes, and other obesity-related diseases; complications; and putative mechanisms underlying the effects of bariatric surgery on body weight and metabolism.

R. S. Ahima (✉)
Department of Medicine, Division of Endocrinology, Diabetes and Metabolism, Johns Hopkins University School of Medicine, Baltimore, MD, USA
e-mail: ahima@jhmi.edu

H.-K. Park
Department of Internal Medicine, Soonchunhyang University College of Medicine, Seoul, South Korea

Keywords

Bariatric surgery · Cardiovascular · Diabetes · Hypertension · Lipids · Metabolism · Obesity

Introduction

Obesity is a major public health problem worldwide [1, 2]. Studies have shown that bariatric surgery is the most effective and durable treatment for individuals with severe obesity and those at the highest risk for obesity-related comorbidity and mortality [3–5]. The use of bariatric surgery as a treatment for obesity has increased due to various factors: (i) the prevalence of obesity in the adult population is very high and has doubled over the past three decades, and the prevalence of severe obesity (class III; body mass index [BMI] > 40) has quadrupled [6]; (ii) obesity-related comorbidities have led to more severely obese patients seeking bariatric surgery treatment; and (iii) behavioral and pharmacologic treatments of obesity may be successful in the short-term but do not translate into longer-term weight loss in most patients [7]. Other factors that have contributed to the increasing use of bariatric procedures include laparoscopic techniques that have improved safety and decreased the length of hospital stays [8–10], increased information concerning the efficacy and safety of bariatric procedures among patients and physicians, media coverage of celebrity patients who have undergone bariatric surgery, and coverage of costs by insurance companies and other health-care payers [11].

Bariatric Procedures

Jejunoileal bypass surgery (JBS) was described in the 1960s–1970s as a method for weight loss. Massive weight loss was accomplished in patients undergoing this procedure in which a short bowel was created by bypassing >90% of the small intestine and creating a long blind loop (Fig. 1). Because 90–95% of the total small intestine is excluded from nutrients absorption as a result of end-to-end or end-to-side connections of intestinal segment, the JBS resulted in severe malabsorption and other systemic complications. The procedure was abandoned due to severe perioperative and long-term complications including hypokalemia, hypocalcemia, hypomagnesemia, liver failure, and kidney stones.

These problems with intestinal bypass led to the development of gastric partitioning procedures designed to decrease the reservoir for ingested food, thereby reducing energy intake [12]. Gastric partitioning was done by applying a double-row stapling across the upper stomach and leaving a gap in the staple lines to allow passage of nutrients into the body of the stomach. Unfortunately, the failure rate of gastric partitioning was very high due to disruption of the staple line or dilation of the connection between the upper and lower gastric compartments, abrogating the retention of food in the upper compartment.

The vertical banded gastroplasty (VBG) procedure was developed to address the problems of

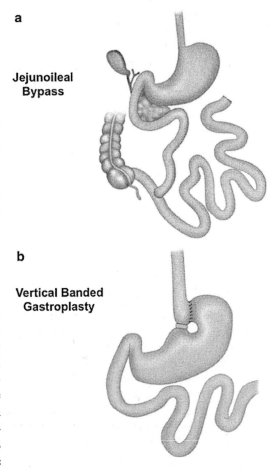

Fig. 1 Jejunoileal bypass and vertical banded gastroplasty. (**a**) Jejunoileal bypass; (**b**) vertical banded gastroplasty. (Figures are reproduced from [154, 155], with the permission of Elsevier Publishers)

gastric partitioning (Fig. 1). The stomach was partitioned with staples, and the opening (stoma) between the upper gastric pouch and body of the stomach was reinforced with a band of prosthetic mesh or a silicon rubber tubing to prevent dilation of the stoma [13]. VBG was the main bariatric procedure in the 1980s, but its use declined due to failure to achieve or maintain weight loss, intractable vomiting and gastroesophageal reflux disease (GERD), band erosion into the stomach, and stricture formation in some patients.

The gastric bypass procedure was developed in the 1970s and initially involved a horizontal partitioning of the upper stomach to create a small gastric pouch and gastrojejunostomy to

a

Roux-en-Y
Gastric Bypass

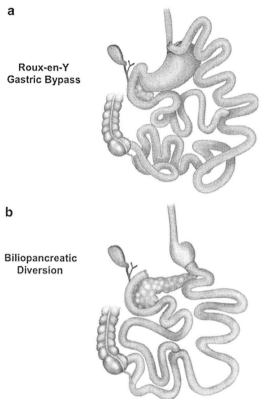

b

Biliopancreatic
Diversion

a

Adjustable
Gastric Banding

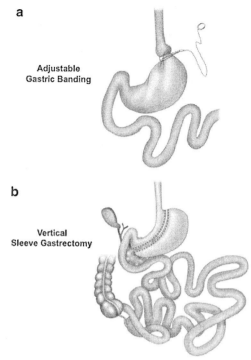

b

Vertical
Sleeve Gastrectomy

Fig. 3 Adjustable gastric banding and vertical sleeve gastrectomy. (**a**) Adjustable gastric banding; (**b**) vertical sleeve gastrectomy. (Figures are reproduced from [154, 155], with the permission of Elsevier Publishers)

Fig. 2 Roux-en-Y gastric bypass and biliopancreatic diversion. (**a**) Roux-en-Y gastric bypass; (**b**) biliopancreatic diversion. (Figures are reproduced from [154, 155], with the permission of Elsevier Publishers)

establish gastrointestinal outflow. However, the latter was soon replaced with a Roux-en-Y reconstruction (RYGB) due to a high incidence of bile reflux associated with the loop procedure [14]. In the current procedure, the size of the gastric pouch is 20–30 mL capacity, an alimentary limb, i.e., jejunal Roux-en-Y limb, is anastomosed to the stomach, and the biliopancreatic limb drains bile and pancreatic secretions to the jejunojejunostomy where the mixing of ingested food and digestive juices occurs (Fig. 2).

The biliopancreatic diversion (BPD) was developed as a method for inducing malabsorption and weight loss but avoiding the intestinal stasis by maintaining the flow of bile and pancreatic juice. Malabsorption is thought to be related to the length of the common channel, varying from 50 cm to 125 cm above the ileocecal valve, and the original procedure was combined with a subtotal gastrectomy. BPD has been modified by adding a duodenal switch procedure [15–17].

Adjustable gastric banding (AGB) procedures are often done using a laparoscopic approach (LAGB) [18]. A saline-filled collar is placed around the upper stomach 1–2 cm below the gastroesophageal junction, creating an upper gastric pouch whose volume can be adjusted by modifying the amount of saline injected into a subcutaneous port linked to a balloon (Fig. 3).

Vertical sleeve gastrectomy (VSG) was introduced as a first-stage procedure in extremely obese patients, or those at high operative risk, undergoing duodenal switch or biliopancreatic diversion procedures [19]. VSG was found to lead to profound weight loss and has emerged as a stand-alone procedure [20]. VSG involves the removal of 80% or more of the stomach including the fundus and greater curvature and preserving the pylorus (Fig. 3) [20, 21].

Clinical Indications for Bariatric Surgery

Obesity is associated with increased morbidity and mortality. Unfortunately, current medical treatment does not achieve sustained weight loss or improve obesity-related comorbidities, including T2DM, hypertension, NAFLD, and cardiovascular diseases in the majority of patients. The results of clinical trials have demonstrated potent effects of bariatric procedures to induce sustained weight loss and improve or normalize obesity-related comorbidities, including T2DM [22–24]. The most commonly performed bariatric procedures are VSG and RYGB [25]. BPD with or without duodenal switch is rarely performed [26]. Patient selection for bariatric surgery is based mainly on the BMI, i.e., those with a BMI of at least $35 \mathrm{kg/m}^2$ or at least $30 \mathrm{~kg/m}^2$ and obesity-associated comorbidity (Table 1) [27, 28]. Several studies have shown that bariatric surgery improves metabolic and other disease outcomes in patients with BMI $30–35 \mathrm{~kg/m}^2$ [29–35].

Table 2 shows examples of retrospective and prospective studies in large cohorts of patients. Long-term follow-up in the Swedish Obese Study (SOS) showed that the incidence of T2DM was halved at 10 years [22]. After 6 years of follow-up, 62% of RYGB patients had a glycosylated hemoglobin (HbA1c) <6.5%, a fasting glucose <7 mmol/L, and did not require antidiabetic therapy [36]. Retrospective data at 9 years demonstrated that >65% of T2DM patients did not require therapy after RYGB [37]. However, it is important to note that the participants in these studies were not enrolled specifically to examine the question of T2DM remission with bariatric surgery [36–38]. The metabolic phenotypes of participants and T2DM duration may confound the clinical outcomes of bariatric surgery. A longer duration of T2DM, higher HbA1c levels, use of insulin therapy, and reduced weight loss after bariatric surgery are all associated with failure of T2DM remission following RYGB and VSG procedures [39].

Few randomized controlled trials (RCT) have compared the effects of bariatric procedures and medical therapy (Table 2) [49, 50, 52]. Over a 2-year period in patients with BMI $30–40 \mathrm{~kg/m}^2$ and a duration of T2DM less than 2 years, AGB resulted in >70% of T2DM patients achieving a HbA1c of <6.2% compared to <15% in patients receiving medical therapy [52]. Weight loss was significantly greater in the AGB T2DM patients compared to the medical therapy group. Glycemic responses to RYGB or BPD or medical therapy have been compared in patients with BMI $\geq 35 \mathrm{~kg/m}^2$ and T2DM duration of at least 5 years. The results showed that 95% of BPD T2DM patients achieved HbA1c $\leq 6.5\%$ compared to 75% of RYGB and none of the medically treated T2D patients after 2-year follow-up [50]. The medical therapy patients lost 5% of their baseline weight compared with 30% in the RYGB and BPD patients. Schauer et al. examined the effects of intensive medical therapy versus RYGB or VSG in obese patients with a mean BMI $> 35 \mathrm{~kg/m}^2$ and T2D duration of 8 years [49]. The HbA1c target of 6% was achieved by 42% of the RYGB patients, 37% of the VSG patients, and 12% of the medical therapy patients. These data are exciting, but the sample sizes are relatively small, and previous studies have shown that glycemic control tends to worsen at 2 years after bariatric surgery [22, 29]. Therefore, longer follow-up studies in larger cohorts are needed to evaluate whether the benefits of bariatric surgery in T2DM can be sustained over longer periods.

The effects of bariatric surgery on microvascular complications of T2DM have been studied. Bariatric surgery decreased kidney damage in T2DM over 5 years follow-up as measured by albumin/creatinine ratio [53]. RYGB improved kidney function as measured by the glomerular filtration rate (GFR) [54], creatinine clearance, and urinary cystatin C/creatinine ratio [55]. Furthermore, RYGB decreased proteinuria for up to 2 years in patients with T2DM [56].

In addition to improving glycemia, bariatric surgery affects other components of the metabolic syndrome, i.e., waist circumference, dyslipidemia, and hypertension [22, 57, 58]. After 10 years, bariatric surgery decreased the rates of hypertension and hypertriglyceridemia and increased HDL cholesterol levels, compared to a matched control group [22]. These changes may decrease

Table 1 Indications, contraindications, and preoperative assessment of bariatric patients

Indications	Contraindications	Preoperative assessment
• Adults with BMI $\geq$ 35 kg/m^2 without comorbid illness • Adults with BMI $\geq$30 kg/m^2 with at least one serious comorbidity (e.g., type 2 diabetes, obstructive sleep apnea, obesity hypoventilation syndrome, GERD, NAFLD, debilitating arthritis)	• Bariatric procedures should not be performed solely for diabetes or lipid treatment or for cardiovascular risk reduction independent of BMI parameters • Psychiatric disorders: bulimia, untreated major depression or psychosis, or binge eating disorders • Inability to understand the type and risks of bariatric procedure and the behavioral changes that are necessary for effective weight loss •Inability to comply with long-term management, e.g., vitamin replacement, and postoperative follow-up • Current alcohol or drug abuse • Severe cardiac disease • Severe coagulopathy	• Comprehensive assessment by a medical specialist, dietitian, psychologist or psychiatrist, nurse specialist, and bariatric surgeon • Psychological assessment (i) to determine whether the patient is able and willing to make lifestyle changes needed for long-term weight; (ii) to identify bipolar disorder, major depression, or antisocial personality disorder, which should be treated in order to improve compliance and weight loss outcome • Diet and eating behavior (total calories, food portions, diet composition, binge eating, grazing, overeating, nighttime eating, stress-related eating) • Physical activity (exercise and non-exercise) • Previous attempts at weight loss (diet, lifestyle modification, medication, bariatric procedures, success, or failure) • Substance abuse (past and present) • Life stressors (e.g., loss of job, discord at home, divorce, bereavement); coping skills, family and social support • Motivation and expectations (extent of weight loss and health goals) • Medical assessment: history and physical examination to evaluate comorbid diseases, e.g., hypertension, diabetes, obstructive sleep apnea, hyperlipidemia, coronary artery disease, NAFLD • Laboratory tests: plasma chemistry, HbA1c, blood count, hemoglobin. TSH, polysomnography, abdominal ultrasound, and cardiac stress test if needed

cardiovascular mortality [23]. Some reports indicate that bariatric surgery may decrease cardiovascular risk in patients with a BMI < 35 kg/m^2 by reducing blood pressure and improving glucose and lipid metabolism [59, 60]. However, others have reported inconsistent effects of bariatric surgery on lipid profiles [61].

Complications of Bariatric Surgery

Although bariatric procedures are effective for weight loss, there are adverse consequences besides typical complications resulting from abdominal surgery (Table 3). As with any

Table 2 Long-term outcome studies (retrospective or prospective)

[22, 23, 40–42]	Prospective observational study, Swedish Obese Subjects Study (SOS), duration 10–20 years, compared 2010 surgical cases (13% RYGB; 19% banding; 68% VBG) vs. 2037 matched controls. Bariatric surgery reduced overall mortality, T2DM myocardial infarction, stroke, and cancer
[43]	Retrospective observational study in Utah, USA, mean duration 7.1 years, compared 7925 RYGB cases vs. 7925 weight-matched controls. Bariatric surgery reduced mortality rates (all-cause, cardiovascular, and T2DM)
[36]	Prospective observational study in Utah, USA, duration 6 years, compared 418 RYGB cases vs. 417 patients seeking bariatric surgery but who did not undergo surgery vs. 321 population-based matched controls. RYGB group lost more weight and had greater T2DM remission rates compared to control groups. Bariatric surgery was associated with greater improvements in blood pressure, cholesterol, and quality of life
[44, 45]	Retrospective observational studies in 6.7 years, in the US Department of Veterans Affairs patients, compared 847 surgical cases vs. 847 matched controls. Bariatric surgery was associated with reduced mortality in unadjusted analysis
[46]	Prospective observational study, Longitudinal Assessment of Bariatric Surgery, USA, duration 3–5 years, studied 2458 bariatric surgery cases (70.7% RYGB vs. 24.8% AGB vs. 5% other procedures). Weight loss and remission of T2DM, dyslipidemia, and hypertension were significantly greater in RYGB compared with AGB
[47]	Retrospective observational study in a Health Maintenance Organization Network in the USA, median duration 3.1 years, studied 4434 RYGB cases with T2DM. 68% of patients had T2DM remission within 5 years after RYGB, but 35.1% of patients with T2DM remission redeveloped T2DM within 5 years
[48]	Prospective observation study, Michigan Bariatric Surgery Collaborative, USA, 3 years duration, studied 8847–35,477 bariatric surgery patients. Complication rates: AGB < VSG < RYGB. Weight loss: RYGB > VSG > AGB

(continued)

Table 2 (continued)

Randomized control trials	
[49]	Stampede I Trial; Cleveland Clinic, USA; 1 year duration; unblinded RCT in 150 patients; BMI, 27–43 with T2DM, randomized to medical therapy vs. medical therapy +RYGB vs. medical therapy+VSG. The primary end point of HbA1c $\leq$ 6.0% was achieved in 12% medical group, 42% RYGB, and 37% VSG. Excess weight loss was 13% in medical group, 88% in RYGB, and 81% in VSG. Serious adverse events occurred in 9% of medical group, 22% RYGB, and 8% VSG
[50]	Teaching hospital in Italy; 2 years duration, unblinded RCT in 80 patients; BMI > 35; T2DM duration $\geq$ 5 years; HbA1c $\geq$ 7.0%; randomized to medical therapy vs. RYBG vs. BPD. The primary end points of FPG < 100 mg/dL and HbA1c < 6.5% were achieved in 75% RYGB and 95% BPD. Bariatric surgery patients discontinued diabetes medications within 15 days after surgery
[51]	Diabetes Surgery Study; four teaching hospitals in the USA and Taiwan; 1-year duration; unblinded RCT in 120 patients with HbA1c $\geq$ 8.0%; BMI 30.0–39.9; C-peptide >1.0 ng/mL; T2DM duration $\geq$ 6 months; patients randomized to intensive medical treatment vs. medical treatment + RYGB. The primary end points of HbA1c < 7.0%, LDL cholesterol < 100 mg/dL, and systolic blood pressure < 130 mmHg were achieved by 49% RYGB and 19% medical patients. RYGB required less medications and lost 26.1% body weight, compared with 7.9% in the medical group. Serious adverse events requiring hospitalization (22 cases) occurred in RYGB

treatment, patients and clinicians must carefully balance the benefits of bariatric surgery against long-term potential complications, such as dumping syndrome, severe hypoglycemia, gastroesophageal reflux (GERD) , and nutritional deficiencies.

(i) *Dumping syndrome* has been reported after RYGB and other bariatric procedures involving partial gastrectomy and/or vagotomy. The prevalence of dumping syndrome may be as high as 40% in RYGB patients

Table 3 Complications of bariatric procedures

Bariatric procedure	Complications
Gastric bypass surgery	Gastric remnant distension
	Stomal stenosis
	Marginal ulcer
	Cholelithiasis
	Internal hernia
	Ventral (incisional hernia)
	Dumping syndrome
	Severe hypoglycemia
	Malodorous flatulence
	Change in bowel movement
	Nutritional deficiencies
Sleeve gastrectomy	Stenosis
	Gastric leakage
	GERD
Gastric banding	Band slippage or erosion
	Port blockage or infection
	Stomal obstruction
	Esophageal dilation
	Esophagitis
	Hiatal hernia
Vertical banded gastroplasty	Staple line disruption
	Erosion of mesh band
	Obstruction
	GERD
	Vomiting
Biliopancreatic diversion/ jejunoileal bypass	Severe malabsorption
	Electrolyte imbalance
	Impaired renal function
	Impaired liver function

[62]. Studies have also reported that up to 40% of VSG patients develop symptoms of dumping syndrome 6–12 months after the procedure [63, 64]. Early dumping is characterized by gastrointestinal symptoms (abdominal pain, bloating, nausea, diarrhea, and borborygmi) and vasomotor symptoms (flushing, palpitations, sweating, dizziness), occurring soon after meal ingestion. Early dumping is thought to be triggered by a rapid passage of hyperosmolar nutrients into the small bowel and a shift of fluids from the circulation into the gastrointestinal tract. Gut peptides, including vasoactive intestinal peptide, peptide YY, pancreatic polypeptide, and neurotensin, may mediate the symptoms of early dumping. Late dumping occurs 1–3 h after a meal and is often characterized by mild hypoglycemia, associated with hunger sensation, palpitations, and sweating. Late dumping has been linked to rapid gastric emptying after bariatric surgery, which increases glucose in the intestinal lumen, triggers insulin release, and induces mild hypoglycemia [65].

Dumping syndrome is evaluated using symptom-based questionnaires, e.g., Sigstad's score or Arts' dumping questionnaire [63, 65, 66]. Patients with dumping syndrome are instructed to ingest small frequent meals, avoid sugars, and limit drinking with meals [65]. Food additives such as pectin may increase food viscosity, slow gastric emptying, and reduce the frequency of dumping symptoms.

(ii) *Severe hypoglycemia* may develop after RYGB and pose major safety risks. Unlike mild hypoglycemia associated with late dumping, a more severe hypoglycemia associated with loss of consciousness, seizures, and accidents is rare and occurs 1–3 years after RYGB. Hypoglycemic symptoms are classified as autonomic, e.g., palpitations, lightheadedness, and sweating, or neuroglycopenic, e.g., confusion, seizure, and loss of consciousness. The prevalence of severe hypoglycemia is uncertain due to underreporting, but documented cases of severe hypoglycemia occur in 0.2–1% of gastric bypass patients [67]. The diagnosis is established by confirming that symptoms are directly related to hypoglycemia and associated with venous blood glucose values <70 mg/dL (3.9 mmol/L) and inappropriately elevated plasma insulin levels. Unlike insulinoma, post-RYGB hypoglycemia is not associated with fasting hyperinsulinemia [68].

The etiology of post-RYGB hyperinsulinemic hypoglycemia is not well understood. It has been postulated that a rapid emptying of the gastric pouch triggers a rapid and excessive rise in glucose, which triggers insulin secretion, and subsequently rapidly suppresses glucose levels. A potential candidate mediator of post-RYGB hyperinsulinemic hypoglycemia is GLP-1, an incretin that is markedly increased postprandially after RYGB [69]. To test the role of GLP-1, Salehi et al. performed studies in controls and two groups of post-RYGB patients: those with severe recurrent hypoglycemia, defined as neuroglycopenia with documented glucose levels <50 mg/dL (2.8 mmol/L), or asymptomatic post-RYGB patients [70]. The patients with a history of hypoglycemia had lower postprandial glucose nadir, as well as higher glucose-stimulated insulin secretion in response to a meal tolerance test. Using tracer methods, the investigators found that hypoglycemic patients had increased rate of glucose appearance after meals compared with controls, while hepatic glucose production was not different in the two groups. As expected, blockade of exendin$_{9-39}$ decreased insulin levels and increased the fasting and postprandial plasma glucose concentrations in control and RYGB patients. Notably, the ability of exendin$_{9-39}$ to increase glycemia and suppress insulin secretion was much greater in RYGB patients prone to hypoglycemia than in RYGB patients without hypoglycemia [70]. These data suggest that GLP-1 is an important contributor to insulin secretion and hypoglycemia in post-RYGB patients with neuroglycopenia.

Given the marked individual variability in the incidence of post-RYGB hypoglycemia, it is possible that genetic differences in GLP-1 receptor-mediated signaling pathways or other modifiers of GLP-1 signaling effects on insulin and glucose are also important. Differences in insulin sensitivity from other mechanisms could alter the risk of insulin-induced hypoglycemia. Also, inadequate liver glycogen stores and impaired secretion of glucagon and other counter-regulatory hormones may predispose to hypoglycemia [71]. Other factors, including gut microbiota [72], bile acid composition [73], and intestinal adaptation [74], could influence brain-gut-liver interactions, resulting in differences in susceptibility to post-RYGB hypoglycemia [75]. Pancreatic islet hyperplasia has been observed in the few pathologic specimens available from patients with post-RYGB hypoglycemia, but it is unclear whether this is adaptive or plays a causal role in hypoglycemia [76–78].

Therapeutic approaches to post-RYGB hypoglycemia include nutrition therapy aimed at reducing sugars and glycemic index carbohydrates [79] and premeal treatment with acarbose, an alpha-glucosidase inhibitor [80], which attenuates rapid postprandial glucose surges and insulin secretion. Continuous glucose monitoring may be necessary in patients with hypoglycemia unawareness [81]. In case the hypoglycemic episodes do not improve in response to changes in diet and acarbose treatment, octreotide can be administered to decrease the secretions of incretins and insulin [82]. Other treatment options include diazoxide or calcium channel blockers to reduce insulin secretion [83, 84]. Gastric restriction surgery or placement of a gastrostomy tube into the bypassed duodenum may be used to alter intestinal nutrient loading and decrease the frequency of hypoglycemic episodes [85, 86]. In rare cases, partial pancreatectomy may be necessary for patients with life-threatening neuroglycopenia [76, 77].

(iii) *Gastroesophageal reflux* has been associated with bariatric surgery. Most studies show improvement of GERD after RYGB surgery [87, 88]. RYGB decreases lower esophageal sphincter pressure, esophageal contractile amplitude, and acid exposure [89, 90]. However, there are variable effects of VBG and ABG on GERD [87, 91–93]. Sleeve gastrectomy increased GERD symptoms in some patients, while others had no symptoms [33, 94, 95]. VSG may increase intragastric pressure leading to postprandial regurgitation [96]. A large study has suggested a less favorable outcome of VSG patients with preexisting GERD symptoms [97].

(iv) *Malnutrition.* Bariatric surgery reduces food intake in the postoperative period, and this may be associated with poor intake of micronutrients, which predisposes to further deficiencies. Preexisting micronutrient deficiencies can exacerbate postoperative deficiencies; hence, weight loss management prior to bariatric surgery should include adequate supplementation of micronutrients [98–100]. The type of bariatric procedure is also a factor in determining nutritional deficiencies. Since AGB is mainly restrictive, it does not predispose to malabsorption. VSG is also less frequently associated with nutritional deficiencies. In contrast, BPD carries the highest risk for nutritional deficiencies [98, 99]. RYGB causes fat and protein malabsorption. Fat malabsorption after RYGB is related to the length of the common intestinal channel, which determines the contact of nutrients with digestive enzymes. A longer biliopancreatic limb in RYGB promotes bacterial overgrowth and decreases fat digestion [99].

Malabsorption should be suspected after bariatric surgery if patients develop abdominal symptoms, e.g., persistent diarrhea, distension, flatulence, and discomfort, or general symptoms, e.g., excessive weight loss, anemia, night blindness, xerophthalmia, peripheral neuropathy, fatigue, amenorrhea, or impotence [99]. Recommended screening tests include blood cell count, lipids, albumin, alkaline phosphatase, calcium, phosphorus, magnesium, zinc, iron, ferritin, prothrombin time, serum vitamin A, parathyroid hormone, serum vitamin D, folic acid, and vitamin B_{12}, preoperatively, and 3-month, and 6-month intervals for 2 years, and then annually, after malabsorptive procedures, e.g., BPD and RYGB [99, 100]. Dietary adjustments are needed in the early postoperative period with protein supplementations (60 g) to avoid loss of body protein [98, 100]. For RYBG, more than 1 g/kg of the ideal body weight/day is the recommended long-term protein intake. In addition, patients who undergo malabsorptive bariatric procedures should receive multivitamin supplements with double the daily recommended doses or more, containing 18 mg of elemental iron and 400 ug of folic acid, as well as vitamin A, copper, and zinc. A daily intake of 2 g of calcium, 1000 ug of vitamin B12, and 1000–2000 IU of vitamin D orally is recommended after malabsorptive bariatric procedures [100]. Specific micronutrient deficiencies resulting from bariatric surgery are discussed next.

Vitamin B_1 (thiamine) deficiency has been reported in 29% of bariatric patients [98–100] and may lead to serious neurological manifestations. Vomiting, poor food intake, and lack of vitamin supplement intake are all predisposing factors [101]. Rarely, intravenous glucose administration may trigger acute thiamine deficiency, characterized by Wernicke's encephalopathy, peripheral neuropathy, nystagmus, and ocular palsy. This can be avoided by prophylactically administering thiamine 100 mg intravenously when starting intravenous fluids in at-risk patients. Symptomatic thiamine deficiency with neurological signs is treated with 100–500 mg thiamine daily administered intravenously. Prophylactic daily intake of a multivitamin preparation with 3 mg of thiamine is recommended after malabsorptive procedures, i.e., BPD and RYGB, and this is increased to 50 mg thiamine daily in patients at risk for Wernicke's encephalopathy [100].

Vitamin B12 deficiency may occur in 18% of patients or more presenting for bariatric surgery. Measurement of serum methylmalonic acid concentrations is a more sensitive marker for vitamin B12 deficiency. Factors predisposing to vitamin B12 deficiency include reduced intake of meat, diminished contact of food and gastric acid, and decreased intrinsic factor levels. Vitamin B12 deficiency leads to megaloblastic anemia, myelopathy, and neuropathy. A prophylactic oral vitamin B12 dose of 500 ug daily or more after bariatric surgery is recommended [100]. Weekly intramuscular injection of 1000 ug for 8 weeks may be necessary for severe vitamin B12 deficiency, and daily intramuscular administrations and lifelong monthly injections are recommended for patients with neurological deficits. Folate deficiency can occur after gastric bypass surgery and lead to megaloblastic anemia. Folate deficiency is prevented with oral intake of 1 mg of folate daily. Patients with proven folate deficiency should be treated with 5 mg daily.

Vitamin D deficiency has been reported in 25–75% of bariatric patients [98, 99]. Vitamin D deficiency decreases intestinal calcium absorption, which is also reduced by reduced gastric acidity as a result of bypassing the duodenum. Clinical manifestations of vitamin D deficiency include osteopenia, osteoporosis, and osteomalacia. Measurements of calcium, vitamin D, and parathyroid hormone levels and postoperative bone mineral density may be indicated after bariatric surgery [102]. Vitamin D intake of 800–2000 IU of cholecalciferol (vitamin D3) is recommended postoperatively. In case of deficiencies, administration of 50,000 IU of ergocalciferol (vitamin D2) weekly, either orally or intramuscularly for 8 weeks, is recommended. In patients with decreased gastric acid secretion, calcium citrate may be better absorbed at doses of up to 2 g daily [100].

Vitamin A deficiency may occur in 11% of bariatric patients [100]. The symptoms include dry eyes and impaired night vision. Confirmed cases of vitamin A deficiency should be treated with doses of 10,000–25,000 IU of vitamin A daily until clinical improvement is noted.

Iron deficiency occurs in 5–44% of bariatric patients. Factors predisposing to iron deficiency include reduced meat intake and diminished gastric acid and intestinal absorption [98, 99]. An oral dose of 35–100 ug of elemental iron is recommended for prevention, and oral supplementation of 300 ug elemental iron daily is sufficient for iron deficiency anemia treatment. If the latter fails, an intravenous iron administration should be given. Zinc deficiency may occur in about 30% of patients prior to bariatric surgery. In cases of zinc deficiency, the recommended dose is 60 mg of elemental zinc given orally twice a day. Zinc treatment may deplete copper stores; hence, the doses of these trace metals need careful adjustments. Copper deficiency is present in up to 18% of patients after bariatric surgery [100] and leads to anemia, leucopenia, neuropathy, and myelopathy. Copper deficiency is treated with 1 week of 6 mg of elemental copper orally daily, then a week of 4 mg daily, and then 2 mg daily as the maintenance dose [100].

Mechanisms of Bariatric Surgery

Weight loss from diet, exercise, and drug therapy is accompanied by a decrease in energy expenditure that makes it difficult to sustain the reduced body weight over long periods [103]. In contrast to conventional weight loss therapies, bariatric procedures produce sustained weight loss [4]. Bariatric surgery decreases food intake, alters taste perception, blunts hedonic responses to food, and prevents the fall in energy expenditure associated with weight loss [5]. Studies in bariatric patients and animal models have provided new insights into gut and central nervous systems' pathways underlying the effects of bariatric procedures on hunger, eating, satiety, and metabolism.

A popular theory is that bariatric surgery causes weight loss by restricting gastric volume and inducing satiety signals [104]. Consistent with this hypothesis, malfunction of LAGB leads to weight regain [105, 106]. Contrary to this theory, weight loss after VSG is slightly less in comparison to RYGB, and yet the stomach volume in VSG is significantly larger than in RYGB [107]. Gastric dilatation following VSG does not affect weight loss in humans, and VSG-mediated weight loss in rats is not dependent on the stomach size [108]. Gastric emptying has been suggested as a mechanism for bariatric surgery-mediated weight loss by altering nutrient, endocrine, and neural signaling in the upper intestine. Enteroendocrine cells are stimulated by increased nutrient delivery and signal via vagal afferent nerves to the brain stem to regulate gastric emptying [109].

Structural changes in the gastrointestinal tract following RYGB, VSG, and AGB may differentially alter gastric emptying and delivery of nutrients to enteroendocrine cells in the intestine, leading to changes in feeding and glucose and lipid metabolism [5]. However, this view is not supported by various studies. LAGB may increase the rate of gastric emptying above the restriction but does not affect total gastric emptying rate, and there is no significant association of gastric emptying, satiety, or weight loss after LAGB [110, 111]. The rate of emptying of the gastric pouch may be delayed in RYGB despite the absence of a pylorus; however, the intestinal transit time is increased [112, 113]. VSG increases gastric emptying as well as intestinal transit time [114, 115], arguing against a causal role of gastric emptying in weight loss.

Another explanation for the dramatic effects of gastric bypass surgery is based on gut hormones. Postprandial GLP-1 levels are markedly increased after RYGB or VSG surgery, but the evidence for a causal link between GLP-1 and weight loss and glucose homeostasis is variable [115]. Administration of a GLP-1 receptor antagonist is well known to attenuate the insulin response to a mixed nutrient liquid meal [116]; however, GLP-1 receptor antagonists do not consistently alter glucose tolerance or insulin sensitivity in patients undergoing RYGB or VSG [117, 118]. Moreover, mice lacking GLP-1 receptor exhibit weight loss and improved glucose tolerance after bariatric surgery similar to normal mice [119, 120]. Furthermore, the weight loss effect of long-acting GLP-1 agonists is much less compared to RYGB and VSG procedures [121, 122].

The level of peptide YY (PYY), a gut hormone that inhibits feeding and increases insulin sensitivity [123], is increased after gastric bypass surgery and has been linked to weight loss [117, 124, 125]. Plasma PYY levels are increased during weight regain in RYGB patients [126], and RYGB-induced weight loss is blunted in PYY knockout mice [127]. Ghrelin is produced mainly in the stomach and has been proposed as a mediator of gastric bypass surgery. Ghrelin levels decrease after VSG [128–130]. In contrast, some reports indicate a reduction in ghrelin levels after RYGB [131], while others show no change in ghrelin [132]. However, ghrelin-deficient mice responded appropriately in weight loss and showed similar improvement in glucose tolerance after VSG,

raising doubts about a causal role of ghrelin in the response to gastric bypass surgery [133].

Bile acids have been implicated in the effects of gastric bypass surgery. Primary bile acids are produced in the liver through oxidation of cholesterol and conjugated with a glycine or taurine to form bile salt that serves as a detergent for lipid hydrolysis. Primary bile acids are also secreted into the intestine and undergo dehydroxylation to form secondary bile acids, which are then conjugated to form bile salts. Bile acids enhance digestion and absorption of lipids and signal via membrane and nuclear receptors in the intestine and liver to regulate lipid and glucose metabolism [134–136]. Studies show that RYGB results in higher plasma bile acid levels compared to AGB [137]. An increase in circulating bile acids and bile salts after RYGB induces weight loss, improves glucose tolerance, and increases GLP-1 secretion [138]. In rodents, ileal interposition surgery increases bile acid levels, improves glucose tolerance, and increases GLP-1 secretion [139].

FXR, a nuclear transcription factor that binds bile acids, has been suggested as a mediator of weight loss after bariatric surgery [140]. Mice lacking FXR display less weight loss after VSG and also increase their food intake to compensate for weight loss [141]. Bile acids also bind to TGR5 (also known as G protein-coupled bile acid receptor 1, GPBAR1), and activation of TGR5 by bile acid increases GLP-1 [142]. These mediators provide plausible functional connections between TGR5 signal pathways and metabolic effects of bariatric surgery.

The gut microbiota are responsive to changes in body weight and dietary composition [143]. Studies indicate that gastric bypass surgery results in a significant change in the composition of the gut microbiome [144]. RYGB changes the gut microbiome of obese individuals to patterns seen in normal weight individuals [145, 146]. Germ-free mice fed the microbiota from RYGB mice are resistant to obesity [72]. The gut microbiota are correlated with bile acid levels in RYGB mice and may require FXR signaling to produce weight loss and improvement in glucose metabolism [147].

Neuronal circuits in the hypothalamus control feeding and energy expenditure [148]. The arcuate nucleus (ARC) contains pro-opiomelanocortin (POMC)-producing neurons that produce α-MSH, a peptide whose role is to inhibit food intake and decrease body weight via melanocortin 4 (MC4) receptor (MC4R). Neurons expressing neuropeptide Y (NPY) and agouti-related peptide (AGRP) are also present in ARC. AGRP is a competitive antagonist/inverse agonist of MC4R. AGRP blocks the action of α-MSH, resulting in stimulation of feeding and weight gain. POMC and NPY/AGRP neurons project to the paraventricular nucleus (PVN), a key center for integration of metabolic signals mediating feeding, energy expenditure, and neuroendocrine function [149]. Studies show that expression of POMC, AGRP, and NPY in the hypothalamus is not different in VSG versus sham-operated obese rats [150]. RYGB induces weight loss in individuals with loss-of-function mutations in MC4R [151]. Individuals with MC4R mutations may or may not be susceptible to LAGB failure [152] [153]. It is likely that other hypothalamic or extra-hypothalamic circuits involved in the regulation of hunger, satiety, and hedonic aspects of feeding are involved in body weight reduction following RYGB and VSG.

Conclusion

Bariatric procedures have evolved over many decades. RYGB and VSG have consistently proven to be the most effective long-term treatment for obesity. Despite evidence showing excellent outcomes with current bariatric procedures, many patients with obesity and obesity-related comorbidities who are eligible for bariatric surgery do not pursue this treatment, partly because of a lack of awareness and understanding of bariatric procedures, poor accessibility especially in underserved communities, and high cost of the surgery and medical follow-up care. A bariatric surgery program based on a multidisciplinary approach will lead to better medical and quality-of-life outcomes for patients. Patients with obesity and obesity-related diseases should have a comprehensive discussion with practitioners about the benefits and risks related to bariatric surgery, and the final decision should be guided by patient's preferences for long-term weight management. Primary care physicians have an important role in initiating the conversation with patients about the treatment of obesity, eligibility for bariatric surgery, referral to specialists for evaluation and treatment, as well as providing long-term follow-up care. There is an important need for ongoing research into the pathophysiology of obesity and related diseases, mechanisms mediating the effects of bariatric surgery, and increased efforts to better inform patients, providers, healthcare payors, policymakers, and the general public about the health impact and socioeconomic consequences of obesity.

Cross-References

▷ Body Composition Assessment
▷ Brain Regulation of Feeding and Energy Homeostasis
▷ Carbohydrate, Protein, and Fat Metabolism in Obesity
▷ Diet, Exercise, and Behavior Therapy
▷ Gut Hormones and Metabolic Syndrome
▷ Gut Microbiome, Obesity, and Metabolic Syndrome
▷ Insulin Resistance in Obesity
▷ Overview of Metabolic Syndrome
▷ Pharmacotherapy of Obesity and Metabolic Syndrome

References

1. Shields M, Carroll MD, Ogden CL. Adult obesity prevalence in Canada and the United States. NCHS Data Brief. 2011;56:1–8.
2. Lobstein T, Brinsden H. Symposium report: the prevention of obesity and NCDs: challenges and opportunities for governments. Obes Rev. 2014;15:630–9.
3. Kraschnewski JL, Boan J, Esposito J, Sherwood NE, Lehman EB, Kephart DK, et al. Long-term weight loss maintenance in the United States. Int J Obes. 2010;34:1644–54.
4. Bray GA. Lifestyle and pharmacological approaches to weight loss: efficacy and safety. J Clin Endocrinol Metab. 2008;93:S81–8.

5. Sandoval D. Bariatric surgeries: beyond restriction and malabsorption. Int J Obes. 2011;35(Suppl 3): S45–9.

6. Sturm R. Increases in morbid obesity in the USA: 2000–2005. Public Health. 2007;121:492–6.

7. Vetter ML, Faulconbridge LF, Webb VL, Wadden TA. Behavioral and pharmacologic therapies for obesity. Nat Rev Endocrinol. 2010;6:578–88.

8. Santry HP, Gillen DL, Lauderdale DS. Trends in bariatric surgical procedures. JAMA. 2005;294:1909–17.

9. Reoch J, Mottillo S, Shimony A, Filion KB, Christou NV, Joseph L, et al. Safety of laparoscopic vs open bariatric surgery: a systematic review and meta-analysis. Arch Surg. 2011;146:1314–22.

10. Lo Menzo E, Szomstein S, Rosenthal RJ. Changing trends in bariatric surgery. Scand J Surg. 2015;104: 18–23.

11. Linkov F, Bovbjerg DH, Freese KE, Ramanathan R, Eid GM, Gourash W. Bariatric surgery interest around the world: what Google trends can teach us. Surg Obes Relat Dis. 2014;10:533–8.

12. Pace WG, Martin EW Jr, Tetirick T, Fabri PJ, Carey LC. Gastric partitioning for morbid obesity. Ann Surg. 1979;190:392–400.

13. Mason EE. Vertical banded gastroplasty for obesity. Arch Surg. 1982;117:701–6.

14. Griffen WO Jr, Young VL, Stevenson CC. A prospective comparison of gastric and jejunoileal bypass procedures for morbid obesity. Ann Surg. 1977;186:500–9.

15. Scopinaro N, Gianetta E, Civalleri D, Bonalumi U, Bachi V. Bilio-pancreatic bypass for obesity: II. Initial experience in man. Br J Surg. 1979;66:618–20.

16. Marceau P, Biron S, Bourque RA, Potvin M, Hould FS, Simard S. Biliopancreatic diversion with a new type of gastrectomy. Obes Surg. 1993;3:29–35.

17. Hess DS, Hess DW. Biliopancreatic diversion with a duodenal switch. Obes Surg. 1998;8:267–82.

18. Belachew M, Legrand MJ, Defechereux TH, Burtheret MP, Jacquet N. Laparoscopic adjustable silicone gastric banding in the treatment of morbid obesity. A preliminary report. Surg Endosc. 1994;8: 1354–6.

19. Frezza EE. Laparoscopic vertical sleeve gastrectomy for morbid obesity. The future procedure of choice? Surg Today. 2007;37:275–81.

20. Gluck B, Movitz B, Jansma S, Gluck J, Laskowski K. Laparoscopic sleeve gastrectomy is a safe and effective bariatric procedure for the lower BMI (35.0–43.0 kg/m2) population. Obes Surg. 2011;21: 1168–71.

21. Brethauer SA. Sleeve gastrectomy. Surg Clin North Am. 2011;91(1265–79):ix.

22. Sjöström L, Lindroos AK, Peltonen M, Torgerson J, Bouchard C, Carlsson B, et al. Lifestyle, diabetes, and cardiovascular risk factors 10 years after bariatric surgery. N Engl J Med. 2004;351:2683–93.

23. Sjöström L, Peltonen M, Jacobson P, Sjöström CD, Karason K, Wedel H, et al. Bariatric surgery and long-term cardiovascular events. JAMA. 2012;307:56–65.

24. Chakravarty PD, McLaughlin E, Whittaker D, Byrne E, Cowan E, Xu K, et al. Comparison of laparoscopic adjustable gastric banding (LAGB) with other bariatric procedures; a systematic review of the randomised controlled trials. Surgeon. 2012;10: 172–82.

25. Buchwald H, Oien DM. Metabolic/bariatric surgery worldwide 2011. Obes Surg. 2013;23:427–36.

26. Smith BR, Schauer P, Nguyen NT. Surgical approaches to the treatment of obesity: bariatric surgery. Med Clin North Am. 2011;95:1009–30.

27. Centre for Public Health Excellence at N, National Collaborating Centre for Primary C. National Institute for Health and Clinical Excellence: Guidance. Obesity: the prevention, identification, assessment and management of overweight and obesity in adults and children. London: National Institute for Health and Clinical Excellence (UK). Copyright © 2006, National Institute for Health and Clinical Excellence; 2006.

28. NIH conference. Gastrointestinal surgery for severe obesity. Consensus Development Conference Panel. Ann Intern Med. 1991;115:956–61.

29. Dixon JB, Zimmet P, Alberti KG, Rubino F. Bariatric surgery: an IDF statement for obese type 2 diabetes. Diabet Med. 2011;28:628–42.

30. Chondronikola M, Harris LL, Klein S. Bariatric surgery and type 2 diabetes: are there weight loss-independent therapeutic effects of upper gastrointestinal bypass? J Intern Med. 2016;280:476–86.

31. Coleman KJ, Wellman R, Fitzpatrick SL, Conroy MB, Hlavin C, Lewis KH, et al. Comparative safety and effectiveness of Roux-en-Y gastric bypass and sleeve gastrectomy for weight loss and type 2 diabetes across race and ethnicity in the PCORnet bariatric study cohort. JAMA Surg. 2022;157:897–906.

32. Yoshino M, Kayser BD, Yoshino J, Stein RI, Reeds D, Eagon JC, et al. Effects of diet versus gastric bypass on metabolic function in diabetes. N Engl J Med. 2020;383:721–32.

33. Salminen P, Grönroos S, Helmiö M, Hurme S, Juuti A, Juusela R, et al. Effect of laparoscopic sleeve gastrectomy vs Roux-en-Y gastric bypass on weight loss, comorbidities, and reflux at 10 years in adult patients with obesity: the SLEEVEPASS randomized clinical trial. JAMA Surg. 2022;157:656–66.

34. Howard R, Chao GF, Yang J, Thumma JR, Arterburn DE, Telem DA, et al. Medication use for obesity-related comorbidities after sleeve gastrectomy or gastric bypass. JAMA Surg. 2022;157:248–56.

35. Patoulias D, Papadopoulos C, Doumas M. The role of bariatric surgery in prevention of kidney disease progression in moderately obese patients with type 2 diabetes. JAMA Surg. 2021;156:204.

36. Adams TD, Davidson LE, Litwin SE, Kolotkin RL, LaMonte MJ, Pendleton RC, et al. Health benefits of gastric bypass surgery after 6 years. JAMA. 2012;308:1122–31.

37. MacDonald KG Jr, Long SD, Swanson MS, Brown BM, Morris P, Dohm GL, et al. The gastric bypass

operation reduces the progression and mortality of non-insulin-dependent diabetes mellitus. J Gastrointest Surg. 1997;1:213–20; discussion 20.

38. Pournaras DJ, Aasheim ET, Søvik TT, Andrews R, Mahon D, Welbourn R, et al. Effect of the definition of type II diabetes remission in the evaluation of bariatric surgery for metabolic disorders. Br J Surg. 2012;99:100–3.

39. Jiménez A, Casamitjana R, Flores L, Viaplana J, Corcelles R, Lacy A, et al. Long-term effects of sleeve gastrectomy and Roux-en-Y gastric bypass surgery on type 2 diabetes mellitus in morbidly obese subjects. Ann Surg. 2012;256:1023–9.

40. Sjöström L, Narbro K, Sjöström CD, Karason K, Larsson B, Wedel H, et al. Effects of bariatric surgery on mortality in Swedish obese subjects. N Engl J Med. 2007;357:741–52.

41. Sjöström L, Gummesson A, Sjöström CD, Narbro K, Peltonen M, Wedel H, et al. Effects of bariatric surgery on cancer incidence in obese patients in Sweden (Swedish obese subjects study): a prospective, controlled intervention trial. Lancet Oncol. 2009;10:653–62.

42. Carlsson LM, Peltonen M, Ahlin S, Anveden Å, Bouchard C, Carlsson B, et al. Bariatric surgery and prevention of type 2 diabetes in Swedish obese subjects. N Engl J Med. 2012;367:695–704.

43. Adams TD, Gress RE, Smith SC, Halverson RC, Simper SC, Rosamond WD, et al. Long-term mortality after gastric bypass surgery. N Engl J Med. 2007;357:753–61.

44. Maciejewski ML, Livingston EH, Smith VA, Kavee AL, Kahwati LC, Henderson WG, et al. Survival among high-risk patients after bariatric surgery. JAMA. 2011;305:2419–26.

45. Maciejewski ML, Livingston EH, Smith VA, Kahwati LC, Henderson WG, Arterburn DE. Health expenditures among high-risk patients after gastric bypass and matched controls. Arch Surg. 2012;147:633–40.

46. Courcoulas AP, Christian NJ, Belle SH, Berk PD, Flum DR, Garcia L, et al. Weight change and health outcomes at 3 years after bariatric surgery among individuals with severe obesity. JAMA. 2013;310:2416–25.

47. Arterburn DE, Bogart A, Sherwood NE, Sidney S, Coleman KJ, Haneuse S, et al. A multisite study of long-term remission and relapse of type 2 diabetes mellitus following gastric bypass. Obes Surg. 2013;23:93–102.

48. Carlin AM, Zeni TM, English WJ, Hawasli AA, Genaw JA, Krause KR, et al. The comparative effectiveness of sleeve gastrectomy, gastric bypass, and adjustable gastric banding procedures for the treatment of morbid obesity. Ann Surg. 2013;257:791–7.

49. Schauer PR, Kashyap SR, Wolski K, Brethauer SA, Kirwan JP, Pothier CE, et al. Bariatric surgery versus intensive medical therapy in obese patients with diabetes. N Engl J Med. 2012;366:1567–76.

50. Mingrone G, Panunzi S, De Gaetano A, Guidone C, Iaconelli A, Leccesi L, et al. Bariatric surgery versus conventional medical therapy for type 2 diabetes. N Engl J Med. 2012;366:1577–85.

51. Ikramuddin S, Korner J, Lee WJ, Connett JE, Inabnet WB, Billington CJ, et al. Roux-en-Y gastric bypass vs intensive medical management for the control of type 2 diabetes, hypertension, and hyperlipidemia: the diabetes surgery study randomized clinical trial. JAMA. 2013;309:2240–9.

52. Dixon JB, O'Brien PE, Playfair J, Chapman L, Schachter LM, Skinner S, et al. Adjustable gastric banding and conventional therapy for type 2 diabetes: a randomized controlled trial. JAMA. 2008;299:316–23.

53. Heneghan HM, Cetin D, Navaneethan SD, Orzech N, Brethauer SA, Schauer PR. Effects of bariatric surgery on diabetic nephropathy after 5 years of follow-up. Surg Obes Relat Dis. 2013;9:7–14.

54. Navaneethan SD, Yehnert H. Bariatric surgery and progression of chronic kidney disease. Surg Obes Relat Dis. 2009;5:662–5.

55. Saliba J, Kasim NR, Tamboli RA, Isbell JM, Marks P, Feurer ID, et al. Roux-en-Y gastric bypass reverses renal glomerular but not tubular abnormalities in excessively obese diabetics. Surgery. 2010;147:282–7.

56. Amor A, Jiménez A, Moizé V, Ibarzabal A, Flores L, Lacy AM, et al. Weight loss independently predicts urinary albumin excretion normalization in morbidly obese type 2 diabetic patients undergoing bariatric surgery. Surg Endosc. 2013;27:2046–51.

57. Picot J, Jones J, Colquitt JL, Gospodarevskaya E, Loveman E, Baxter L, et al. The clinical effectiveness and cost-effectiveness of bariatric (weight loss) surgery for obesity: a systematic review and economic evaluation. Health Technol Assess. 2009;13:1–190, 215–357, iii–iv.

58. Buchwald H, Avidor Y, Braunwald E, Jensen MD, Pories W, Fahrbach K, et al. Bariatric surgery: a systematic review and meta-analysis. JAMA. 2004;292:1724–37.

59. Shah SS, Todkar JS, Shah PS, Cummings DE. Diabetes remission and reduced cardiovascular risk after gastric bypass in Asian Indians with body mass index <35 kg/m(2). Surg Obes Relat Dis. 2010;6:332–8.

60. Sjöholm K, Anveden A, Peltonen M, Jacobson P, Romeo S, Svensson PA, et al. Evaluation of current eligibility criteria for bariatric surgery: diabetes prevention and risk factor changes in the Swedish obese subjects (SOS) study. Diabetes Care. 2013;36:1335–40.

61. Li Q, Chen L, Yang Z, Ye Z, Huang Y, He M, et al. Metabolic effects of bariatric surgery in type 2 diabetic patients with body mass index < 35 kg/m2. Diabetes Obes Metab. 2012;14:262–70.

62. Banerjee A, Ding Y, Mikami DJ, Needleman BJ. The role of dumping syndrome in weight loss after gastric bypass surgery. Surg Endosc. 2013;27:1573–8.

63. Tzovaras G, Papamargaritis D, Sioka E, Zachari E, Baloyiannis I, Zacharoulis D, et al. Symptoms

suggestive of dumping syndrome after provocation in patients after laparoscopic sleeve gastrectomy. Obes Surg. 2012;22:23–8.

64. Papamargaritis D, Koukoulis G, Sioka E, Zachari E, Bargiota A, Zacharoulis D, et al. Dumping symptoms and incidence of hypoglycaemia after provocation test at 6 and 12 months after laparoscopic sleeve gastrectomy. Obes Surg. 2012;22:1600–6.

65. Tack J, Arts J, Caenepeel P, De Wulf D, Bisschops R. Pathophysiology, diagnosis and management of postoperative dumping syndrome. Nat Rev Gastroenterol Hepatol. 2009;6:583–90.

66. Arts J, Caenepeel P, Bisschops R, Dewulf D, Holvoet L, Piessevaux H, et al. Efficacy of the long-acting repeatable formulation of the somatostatin analogue octreotide in postoperative dumping. Clin Gastroenterol Hepatol. 2009;7:432–7.

67. Marsk R, Jonas E, Rasmussen F, Näslund E. Nationwide cohort study of post-gastric bypass hypoglycaemia including 5,040 patients undergoing surgery for obesity in 1986–2006 in Sweden. Diabetologia. 2010;53:2307–11.

68. Mala T. Postprandial hyperinsulinemic hypoglycemia after gastric bypass surgical treatment. Surg Obes Relat Dis. 2014;10:1220–5.

69. Goldfine AB, Mun EC, Devine E, Bernier R, Baz-Hecht M, Jones DB, et al. Patients with neuroglycopenia after gastric bypass surgery have exaggerated incretin and insulin secretory responses to a mixed meal. J Clin Endocrinol Metab. 2007;92: 4678–85.

70. Salehi M, Prigeon RL, D'Alessio DA. Gastric bypass surgery enhances glucagon-like peptide 1-stimulated postprandial insulin secretion in humans. Diabetes. 2011;60:2308–14.

71. Laferrère B, Reilly D, Arias S, Swerdlow N, Gorroochurn P, Bawa B, et al. Differential metabolic impact of gastric bypass surgery versus dietary intervention in obese diabetic subjects despite identical weight loss. Sci Transl Med. 2011;3:80re2.

72. Liou AP, Paziuk M, Luevano JM Jr, Machineni S, Turnbaugh PJ, Kaplan LM. Conserved shifts in the gut microbiota due to gastric bypass reduce host weight and adiposity. Sci Transl Med. 2013;5:178ra41.

73. Patti ME, Houten SM, Bianco AC, Bernier R, Larsen PR, Holst JJ, et al. Serum bile acids are higher in humans with prior gastric bypass: potential contribution to improved glucose and lipid metabolism. Obesity (Silver Spring). 2009;17:1671–7.

74. Hansen CF, Bueter M, Theis N, Lutz T, Paulsen S, Dalbøge LS, et al. Hypertrophy dependent doubling of L-cells in Roux-en-Y gastric bypass operated rats. PLoS One. 2013;8:e65696.

75. Müssig K, Staiger H, Machicao F, Häring HU, Fritsche A. Genetic variants affecting incretin sensitivity and incretin secretion. Diabetologia. 2010;53: 2289–97.

76. Service GJ, Thompson GB, Service FJ, Andrews JC, Collazo-Clavell ML, Lloyd RV. Hyperinsulinemic hypoglycemia with nesidioblastosis after gastric-bypass surgery. N Engl J Med. 2005;353:249–54.

77. Patti ME, McMahon G, Mun EC, Bitton A, Holst JJ, Goldsmith J, et al. Severe hypoglycaemia post-gastric bypass requiring partial pancreatectomy: evidence for inappropriate insulin secretion and pancreatic islet hyperplasia. Diabetologia. 2005;48:2236–40.

78. Meier JJ, Butler AE, Galasso R, Butler PC. Hyperinsulinemic hypoglycemia after gastric bypass surgery is not accompanied by islet hyperplasia or increased beta-cell turnover. Diabetes Care. 2006;29:1554–9.

79. Kellogg TA, Bantle JP, Leslie DB, Redmond JB, Slusarek B, Swan T, et al. Postgastric bypass hyperinsulinemic hypoglycemia syndrome: characterization and response to a modified diet. Surg Obes Relat Dis. 2008;4:492–9.

80. Valderas JP, Ahuad J, Rubio L, Escalona M, Pollak F, Maiz A. Acarbose improves hypoglycaemia following gastric bypass surgery without increasing glucagon-like peptide 1 levels. Obes Surg. 2012;22: 582–6.

81. Halperin F, Patti ME, Skow M, Bajwa M, Goldfine AB. Continuous glucose monitoring for evaluation of glycemic excursions after gastric bypass. J Obes. 2011;2011:869536.

82. Myint KS, Greenfield JR, Farooqi IS, Henning E, Holst JJ, Finer N. Prolonged successful therapy for hyperinsulinaemic hypoglycaemia after gastric bypass: the pathophysiological role of GLP1 and its response to a somatostatin analogue. Eur J Endocrinol. 2012;166:951–5.

83. Spanakis E, Gragnoli C. Successful medical management of status post-Roux-en-Y-gastric-bypass hyperinsulinemic hypoglycemia. Obes Surg. 2009;19: 1333–4.

84. Moreira RO, Moreira RB, Machado NA, Gonçalves TB, Coutinho WF. Post-prandial hypoglycemia after bariatric surgery: pharmacological treatment with verapamil and acarbose. Obes Surg. 2008;18: 1618–21.

85. Fernández-Esparrach G, Lautz DB, Thompson CC. Peroral endoscopic anastomotic reduction improves intractable dumping syndrome in Roux-en-Y gastric bypass patients. Surg Obes Relat Dis. 2010;6:36–40.

86. McLaughlin T, Peck M, Holst J, Deacon C. Reversible hyperinsulinemic hypoglycemia after gastric bypass: a consequence of altered nutrient delivery. J Clin Endocrinol Metab. 2010;95:1851–5.

87. De Groot NL, Burgerhart JS, Van De Meeberg PC, de Vries DR, Smout AJ, Siersema PD. Systematic review: the effects of conservative and surgical treatment for obesity on gastro-oesophageal reflux disease. Aliment Pharmacol Ther. 2009;30:1091–102.

88. Tai CM, Lee YC, Wu MS, Chang CY, Lee CT, Huang CK, et al. The effect of Roux-en-Y gastric bypass on gastroesophageal reflux disease in morbidly obese Chinese patients. Obes Surg. 2009;19:565–70.

89. Madalosso CA, Gurski RR, Callegari-Jacques SM, Navarini D, Thiesen V, Fornari F. The impact of gastric bypass on gastroesophageal reflux disease in patients with morbid obesity: a prospective study based on the Montreal consensus. Ann Surg. 2010;251:244–8.

90. Herbella FA, Vicentine FP, Del Grande JC, Patti MG. Postprandial proximal gastric acid pocket and gastric pressure in patients after gastric surgery. Neurogastroenterol Motil. 2011;23:52–5, e4.

91. Di Francesco V, Baggio E, Mastromauro M, Zoico E, Stefenelli N, Zamboni M, et al. Obesity and gastro-esophageal acid reflux: physiopathological mechanisms and role of gastric bariatric surgery. Obes Surg. 2004;14:1095–102.

92. Angrisani L, Iovino P, Lorenzo M, Santoro T, Sabbatini F, Claar E, et al. Treatment of morbid obesity and gastroesophageal reflux with hiatal hernia by lap-band. Obes Surg. 1999;9:396–8.

93. de Jong JR, van Ramshorst B, Timmer R, Gooszen HG, Smout AJ. The influence of laparoscopic adjustable gastric banding on gastroesophageal reflux. Obes Surg. 2004;14:399–406.

94. Chiu S, Birch DW, Shi X, Sharma AM, Karmali S. Effect of sleeve gastrectomy on gastroesophageal reflux disease: a systematic review. Surg Obes Relat Dis. 2011;7:510–5.

95. Mahawar KK, Jennings N, Balupuri S, Small PK. Sleeve gastrectomy and gastro-oesophageal reflux disease: a complex relationship. Obes Surg. 2013;23:987–91.

96. Del Genio G, Tolone S, Limongelli P, Brusciano L, D'Alessandro A, Docimo G, et al. Sleeve gastrectomy and development of "de novo" gastroesophageal reflux. Obes Surg. 2014;24:71–7.

97. DuPree CE, Blair K, Steele SR, Martin MJ. Laparoscopic sleeve gastrectomy in patients with preexisting gastroesophageal reflux disease: a national analysis. JAMA Surg. 2014;149:328–34.

98. Saltzman E, Karl JP. Nutrient deficiencies after gastric bypass surgery. Annu Rev Nutr. 2013;33:183–203.

99. Hammer HF. Medical complications of bariatric surgery: focus on malabsorption and dumping syndrome. Dig Dis. 2012;30:182–6.

100. Levinson R, Silverman JB, Catella JG, Rybak I, Jolin H, Isom K. Pharmacotherapy prevention and management of nutritional deficiencies post Roux-en-Y gastric bypass. Obes Surg. 2013;23:992–1000.

101. Galvin R, Bråthen G, Ivashynka A, Hillbom M, Tanasescu R, Leone MA. EFNS guidelines for diagnosis, therapy and prevention of Wernicke encephalopathy. Eur J Neurol. 2010;17:1408–18.

102. Heber D, Greenway FL, Kaplan LM, Livingston E, Salvador J, Still C. Endocrine and nutritional management of the post-bariatric surgery patient: an endocrine society clinical practice guideline. J Clin Endocrinol Metab. 2010;95:4823–43.

103. Schwartz A, Doucet E. Relative changes in resting energy expenditure during weight loss: a systematic review. Obes Rev. 2010;11:531–47.

104. Stefater MA, Wilson-Pérez HE, Chambers AP, Sandoval DA, Seeley RJ. All bariatric surgeries are not created equal: insights from mechanistic comparisons. Endocr Rev. 2012;33:595–622.

105. Suter M, Calmes JM, Paroz A, Giusti V. A 10-year experience with laparoscopic gastric banding for morbid obesity: high long-term complication and failure rates. Obes Surg. 2006;16:829–35.

106. Boza C, Gamboa C, Perez G, Crovari F, Escalona A, Pimentel F, et al. Laparoscopic adjustable gastric banding (LAGB): surgical results and 5-year follow-up. Surg Endosc. 2011;25:292–7.

107. Chapman AE, Kiroff G, Game P, Foster B, O'Brien P, Ham J, et al. Laparoscopic adjustable gastric banding in the treatment of obesity: a systematic literature review. Surgery. 2004;135:326–51.

108. Abu-Jaish W, Rosenthal RJ. Sleeve gastrectomy: a new surgical approach for morbid obesity. Expert Rev Gastroenterol Hepatol. 2010;4:101–19.

109. Cummings DE, Overduin J, Foster-Schubert KE. Gastric bypass for obesity: mechanisms of weight loss and diabetes resolution. J Clin Endocrinol Metab. 2004;89:2608–15.

110. Burton PR, Yap K, Brown WA, Laurie C, O'Donnell M, Hebbard G, et al. Changes in satiety, supra- and infraband transit, and gastric emptying following laparoscopic adjustable gastric banding: a prospective follow-up study. Obes Surg. 2011;21:217–23.

111. Usinger L, Hansen KB, Kristiansen VB, Larsen S, Holst JJ, Knop FK. Gastric emptying of orally administered glucose solutions and incretin hormone responses are unaffected by laparoscopic adjustable gastric banding. Obes Surg. 2011;21:625–32.

112. Suzuki S, Ramos EJ, Goncalves CG, Chen C, Meguid MM. Changes in GI hormones and their effect on gastric emptying and transit times after Roux-en-Y gastric bypass in rat model. Surgery. 2005;138:283–90.

113. Dirksen C, Damgaard M, Bojsen-Møller KN, Jørgensen NB, Kielgast U, Jacobsen SH, et al. Fast pouch emptying, delayed small intestinal transit, and exaggerated gut hormone responses after Roux-en-Y gastric bypass. Neurogastroenterol Motil. 2013;25:346–e255.

114. Shah S, Shah P, Todkar J, Gagner M, Sonar S, Solav S. Prospective controlled study of effect of laparoscopic sleeve gastrectomy on small bowel transit time and gastric emptying half-time in morbidly obese patients with type 2 diabetes mellitus. Surg Obes Relat Dis. 2010;6:152–7.

115. Melissas J, Leventi A, Klinaki I, Perisinakis K, Koukouraki S, de Bree E, et al. Alterations of global gastrointestinal motility after sleeve gastrectomy: a prospective study. Ann Surg. 2013;258:976–82.

116. Johnson KM, Farmer T, Schurr K, Patrick Donahue E, Farmer B, Neal D, et al. Endogenously released GLP-1 is not sufficient to alter postprandial glucose regulation in the dog. Endocrine. 2011;39:229–34.

117. Chambers AP, Jessen L, Ryan KK, Sisley S, Wilson-Pérez HE, Stefater MA, et al. Weight-independent changes in blood glucose homeostasis after gastric bypass or vertical sleeve gastrectomy in rats. Gastroenterology. 2011;141:950–8.

118. Jørgensen NB, Dirksen C, Bojsen-Møller KN, Jacobsen SH, Worm D, Hansen DL, et al. Exaggerated glucagon-like peptide 1 response is important for improved β-cell function and glucose tolerance after Roux-en-Y gastric bypass in patients with type 2 diabetes. Diabetes. 2013;62:3044–52.

119. Wilson-Pérez HE, Chambers AP, Ryan KK, Li B, Sandoval DA, Stoffers D, et al. Vertical sleeve gastrectomy is effective in two genetic mouse models of glucagon-like peptide 1 receptor deficiency. Diabetes. 2013;62:2380–5.

120. Mokadem M, Zechner JF, Margolskee RF, Drucker DJ, Aguirre V. Effects of Roux-en-Y gastric bypass on energy and glucose homeostasis are preserved in two mouse models of functional glucagon-like peptide-1 deficiency. Mol Metab. 2014;3:191–201.

121. Fujishima Y, Maeda N, Inoue K, Kashine S, Nishizawa H, Hirata A, et al. Efficacy of liraglutide, a glucagon-like peptide-1 (GLP-1) analogue, on body weight, eating behavior, and glycemic control, in Japanese obese type 2 diabetes. Cardiovasc Diabetol. 2012;11:107.

122. Jiménez A, Mari A, Casamitjana R, Lacy A, Ferrannini E, Vidal J. GLP-1 and glucose tolerance after sleeve gastrectomy in morbidly obese subjects with type 2 diabetes. Diabetes. 2014;63:3372–7.

123. Vrang N, Madsen AN, Tang-Christensen M, Hansen G, Larsen PJ. PYY(3–36) reduces food intake and body weight and improves insulin sensitivity in rodent models of diet-induced obesity. Am J Physiol Regul Integr Comp Physiol. 2006;291:R367–75.

124. Peterli R, Wölnerhanssen B, Peters T, Devaux N, Kern B, Christoffel-Courtin C, et al. Improvement in glucose metabolism after bariatric surgery: comparison of laparoscopic Roux-en-Y gastric bypass and laparoscopic sleeve gastrectomy: a prospective randomized trial. Ann Surg. 2009;250:234–41.

125. Shin AC, Zheng H, Townsend RL, Sigalet DL, Berthoud HR. Meal-induced hormone responses in a rat model of Roux-en-Y gastric bypass surgery. Endocrinology. 2010;151:1588–97.

126. Meguid MM, Glade MJ, Middleton FA. Weight regain after Roux-en-Y: a significant 20% complication related to PYY. Nutrition. 2008;24:832–42.

127. Chandarana K, Gelegen C, Karra E, Choudhury AI, Drew ME, Fauveau V, et al. Diet and gastrointestinal bypass-induced weight loss: the roles of ghrelin and peptide YY. Diabetes. 2011;60:810–8.

128. Basso N, Capoccia D, Rizzello M, Abbatini F, Mariani P, Maglio C, et al. First-phase insulin secretion, insulin sensitivity, ghrelin, GLP-1, and PYY changes 72 h after sleeve gastrectomy in obese diabetic patients: the gastric hypothesis. Surg Endosc. 2011;25:3540–50.

129. Bohdjalian A, Langer FB, Shakeri-Leidenmühler S, Gfrerer L, Ludvik B, Zacherl J, et al. Sleeve gastrectomy as sole and definitive bariatric procedure: 5-year results for weight loss and ghrelin. Obes Surg. 2010;20:535–40.

130. Wang Y, Liu J. Plasma ghrelin modulation in gastric band operation and sleeve gastrectomy. Obes Surg. 2009;19:357–62.

131. Cummings DE, Weigle DS, Frayo RS, Breen PA, Ma MK, Dellinger EP, et al. Plasma ghrelin levels after diet-induced weight loss or gastric bypass surgery. N Engl J Med. 2002;346:1623–30.

132. Tymitz K, Engel A, McDonough S, Hendy MP, Kerlakian G. Changes in ghrelin levels following bariatric surgery: review of the literature. Obes Surg. 2011;21:125–30.

133. Chambers AP, Kirchner H, Wilson-Perez HE, Willency JA, Hale JE, Gaylinn BD, et al. The effects of vertical sleeve gastrectomy in rodents are ghrelin independent. Gastroenterology. 2013;144:50–2.e5.

134. Parks DJ, Blanchard SG, Bledsoe RK, Chandra G, Consler TG, Kliewer SA, et al. Bile acids: natural ligands for an orphan nuclear receptor. Science. 1999;284:1365–8.

135. Kohli R, Kirby M, Setchell KD, Jha P, Klustaitis K, Woollett LA, et al. Intestinal adaptation after ileal interposition surgery increases bile acid recycling and protects against obesity-related comorbidities. Am J Physiol Gastrointest Liver Physiol. 2010;299: G652–60.

136. Cummings BP, Strader AD, Stanhope KL, Graham JL, Lee J, Raybould HE, et al. Ileal interposition surgery improves glucose and lipid metabolism and delays diabetes onset in the UCD-T2DM rat. Gastroenterology. 2010;138:2437–46, 46.e1.

137. Kohli R, Bradley D, Setchell KD, Eagon JC, Abumrad N, Klein S. Weight loss induced by Roux-en-Y gastric bypass but not laparoscopic adjustable gastric banding increases circulating bile acids. J Clin Endocrinol Metab. 2013;98:E708–12.

138. Kohli R, Setchell KD, Kirby M, Myronovych A, Ryan KK, Ibrahim SH, et al. A surgical model in male obese rats uncovers protective effects of bile acids post-bariatric surgery. Endocrinology. 2013;154:2341–51.

139. Strader AD, Vahl TP, Jandacek RJ, Woods SC, D'Alessio DA, Seeley RJ. Weight loss through ileal transposition is accompanied by increased ileal hormone secretion and synthesis in rats. Am J Physiol Endocrinol Metab. 2005;288:E447–53.

140. Kuipers F, Groen AK. FXR: the key to benefits in bariatric surgery? Nat Med. 2014;20:337–8.

141. Ryan KK, Tremaroli V, Clemmensen C, Kovatcheva-Datchary P, Myronovych A, Karns R, et al. FXR is a molecular target for the effects of vertical sleeve gastrectomy. Nature. 2014;509:183–8.

142. Thomas C, Gioiello A, Noriega L, Strehle A, Oury J, Rizzo G, et al. TGR5-mediated bile acid sensing controls glucose homeostasis. Cell Metab. 2009;10: 167–77.

143. Karlsson F, Tremaroli V, Nielsen J, Bäckhed F. Assessing the human gut microbiota in metabolic diseases. Diabetes. 2013;62:3341–9.

144. Sweeney TE, Morton JM. The human gut microbiome: a review of the effect of obesity and surgically induced weight loss. JAMA Surg. 2013;148:563–9.

145. Zhang H, DiBaise JK, Zuccolo A, Kudrna D, Braidotti M, Yu Y, et al. Human gut microbiota in obesity and after gastric bypass. Proc Natl Acad Sci U S A. 2009;106:2365–70.

146. Li JV, Ashrafian H, Bueter M, Kinross J, Sands C, le Roux CW, et al. Metabolic surgery profoundly influences gut microbial-host metabolic cross-talk. Gut. 2011;60:1214–23.

147. Lutz TA, Bueter M. Physiological mechanisms behind Roux-en-Y gastric bypass surgery. Dig Surg. 2014;31:13–24.

148. Blouet C, Schwartz GJ. Hypothalamic nutrient sensing in the control of energy homeostasis. Behav Brain Res. 2010;209:1–12.

149. Kim JD, Leyva S, Diano S. Hormonal regulation of the hypothalamic melanocortin system. Front Physiol. 2014;5:480.

150. Stefater MA, Pérez-Tilve D, Chambers AP, Wilson-Pérez HE, Sandoval DA, Berger J, et al. Sleeve gastrectomy induces loss of weight and fat mass in obese rats, but does not affect leptin sensitivity. Gastroenterology. 2010;138:2426–36, 36.e1–3.

151. Aslan IR, Campos GM, Calton MA, Evans DS, Merriman RB, Vaisse C. Weight loss after Roux-en-Y gastric bypass in obese patients heterozygous for MC4R mutations. Obes Surg. 2011;21:930–4.

152. Elkhenini HF, New JP, Syed AA. Five-year outcome of bariatric surgery in a patient with melanocortin-4 receptor mutation. Clin Obes. 2014;4:121–4.

153. Valette M, Poitou C, Le Beyec J, Bouillot JL, Clement K, Czernichow S. Melanocortin-4 receptor mutations and polymorphisms do not affect weight loss after bariatric surgery. PLoS One. 2012;7: e48221.

154. Elder KA, Wolfe BM. Bariatric surgery: a review of procedures and outcomes. Gastroenterology. 2007;132: 2253–71.

155. Ahima RS, Sabri A. Bariatric surgery: metabolic benefits beyond weight loss. Gastroenterology. 2011;141: 793–5.

Prevention and Treatment of Obesity in Children

40

Talia A. Hitt, Katie L. Wasserstein, Sara N. Malina, and
Sheela N. Magge

Contents

T. A. Hitt (✉) · K. L. Wasserstein · S. N. Malina ·
S. N. Magge (✉)
Division of Endocrinology and Diabetes, Department of
Pediatrics, Johns Hopkins University School of Medicine,
Baltimore, MD, USA
e-mail: thitt2@jhmi.edu; kwasser4@jhmi.edu;
smalina1@jhu.edu; smagge3@jhmi.edu

© Springer Nature Switzerland AG 2023
R. S. Ahima (ed.), *Metabolic Syndrome*,
https://doi.org/10.1007/978-3-031-40116-9_51

Abstract

Pediatric obesity, defined in the USA as body mass index ≥95th percentile on the pediatric growth charts for age and sex, has been rising over the last several decades, currently affecting almost 20% of children and adolescents aged 2–19 years in the USA. Obesity is heritable, and both monogenic and polygenic obesity syndromes exist that should be considered if early onset obesity younger than age 5 years, hyperphagia, and/or dysmorphic features are present. Excess adiposity occurs when energy intake exceeds energy expenditure, due to poor nutrition or maladaptive eating behaviors, minimal physical activity, and high sedentary behavior. In children, numerous risk factors including the antenatal and postnatal environment, home and school environment, and social determinants of health contribute to the development of childhood obesity. Several comorbid conditions and complications occur with increased prevalence in the setting of childhood obesity, with many contributing to increased cardiometabolic risk. Pediatric obesity treatment should include intensive health behavior and lifestyle treatment, early consideration of anti-obesity medications, and in some circumstances, bariatric surgery. Obesity prevention, early efforts to reduce excess adiposity, and management of obesity's comorbidities and complications are essential to prevent cardiometabolic disease early in life.

Keywords

Pediatric · Obesity · Metabolic Syndrome · Diabetes · Youth-onset Type 2 diabetes · Nonalcoholic fatty liver disease · Lifestyle modification · Bariatric surgery

Introduction

Obesity in children is a global epidemic and contributes to increased morbidity and health care costs, with current estimates stating that a 10-year old child with obesity leads to $19,000 more in lifetime medical costs in the USA compared to a child without obesity [1]. Children with overweight or obesity at young ages are more likely to have obesity later in life, and a longer duration and earlier onset of obesity is associated with higher cardiometabolic morbidity [2, 3]. It is essential that health care providers be familiar with the risk factors, prevention strategies, comorbidities, and complications of excess adiposity during childhood, and that

they be skilled in patient assessment and effective treatment.

Pediatric obesity care also requires particular considerations and sensitivity for the potentially harmful aspects of addressing obesity in children and adolescents. Children and families with obesity experience weight stigma and bias that can negatively affect their mental health [4]. Multiple groups have also cited concerns over obesity treatment increasing the risk for eating disorders, although this relationship is uncertain, and obesity treatment may even reduce the risk of eating disorders in youth with obesity [4]. Physicians can be a source of weight bias and stigma for this population and there is a risk that parents will feel blame. Clinicians should be mindful of non-stigmatizing approaches to addressing childhood obesity, including asking permission to discuss a child's BMI or weight and using neutral words and person-first language.

Definition of Pediatric Obesity

Obesity, a measure of excess adiposity, can be quantified in different ways [5]. The ideal way to measure obesity would be percentage body fat, but methods for its quantification (such as densitometry or skin-fold thickness) are impractical for wide-scale use [5]. Instead, obesity is commonly defined using body mass index (BMI = weight in kilograms/height in meters^2) [4]. In adults, overweight is defined by a BMI 25–29.9 kg/m^2 and obesity by a BMI $\geq$30 kg/m^2, definitions which have been shown to be associated with health risks [5].

In pediatric medicine, sex-specific growth charts are utilized to monitor children's growth compared to age and sex-based standards. Several definitions have been proposed for pediatric obesity. In the USA, the Centers for Disease Control and Prevention (CDC) uses percentiles on the CDC sex-specific growth charts for ages 2–19 years to define pediatric obesity: overweight is defined as BMI $\geq$85th to <95th percentile for sex and age, and obesity is defined as BMI $\geq$95th percentile for sex and age [4, 6]. The US definitions of pediatric overweight and obesity have high specificity (overweight: 86.1–98.8%; obesity: 96.3–100%) but lower sensitivity (overweight: 4.3–75%; obesity: 14.3–60%) compared with percentage body fat from densitometry or skin-fold thickness [7].

Globally, the World Health Organization (WHO) utilizes separate growth charts, and for children 5–19 years of age, pediatric overweight is defined as BMI >1 standard deviation (SD) above the WHO growth standard median, and pediatric obesity is defined as BMI >2SD above the WHO growth standard median [8]. The WHO definition of pediatric obesity is equivalent to a CDC BMI >98th percentile [9]. For youth <5 years of age, WHO uses weight-for-height curves and defines overweight as weight-for-height >2SD above the WHO growth standard median and obesity as weight-for-height >3SD above the WHO growth standard median [8]. A third definition for pediatric obesity was proposed using BMI by the International Obesity Task Force: using reference charts created from 97,876 boys and 94,851 girls from international data, BMI percentile lines were drawn that pass through the adult overweight (BMI ≥ 25 kg/m^2) and obesity (BMI ≥ 30 kg/m^2) cut-points at 18 years of age [5]. The International Obesity Task Force definition of pediatric obesity is more stringent than the CDC's or WHO's, as a BMI of 30 kg/m^2 at age 18 years is equivalent to about the 99th percentile [5].

Due to the high prevalence and severity of pediatric obesity, additional growth charts and definitions have been created to further characterize the severity of pediatric obesity. Severe obesity growth charts have utilized the percentage of the 95th percentile for high BMIs and the USA defines severe obesity as ≥ 120th percentile of the 95th percentile for age and sex or a BMI ≥ 35 kg/m^2, whichever is lower for age and sex [4]. Severe obesity is further broken down into class 2 obesity (≥ 120th percentile to <140th percentile of the 95th percentile or BMI 35–40 kg/m^2, whichever is lower for age and sex) and class 3 obesity (≥ 140th percentile of the 95th percentile or BMI ≥ 40 kg/m^2, whichever is lower for age and sex) [4]. Recently in 2022, new extended growth charts were developed by

the CDC to aid in monitoring of obesity in clinical settings and clinical trials, as use of BMI z-score is not sufficient due to the compression of z-scores at extremely high or low values [10].

Other anthropometric markers that indicate central adiposity, including waist circumference, waist-hip ratio and waist-height ratio, may be more indicative of high cardiometabolic risk, particularly as BMI can represent both muscle and fat [11]. Waist circumference >94 cm in men and >80 cm in women is associated with increased cardiometabolic risk [11]. In pediatric populations, various studies have created percentiles and standard deviations for waist circumference for different racial and ethnic groups, but there is no standard definition for all children based on age and sex [11]. Waist-hip ratio (waist circumference divided by hip circumference) ≥ 0.9 in males and ≥ 0.85 in females is also associated with increased cardiometabolic risk, yet is less correlated with body fat content than other measures [11]. Waist-height ratio (waist circumference divided by height) using a cut-off of >0.5 is the most universal marker of central obesity as it is associated with increased cardiometabolic risk in multiple populations and uses the same cut-off for children and adult populations [11, 12].

Prevalence and Epidemiology

The prevalence of pediatric obesity has grown significantly in the past several decades. The CDC data show the prevalence of pediatric obesity in the USA from 2017 to 2020 among children aged 2–19 years is 19.7%, affecting about 14.4 million children [4, 13], a prevalence that has more than tripled from 5% in 1963 [4]. In comparison, obesity prevalence in 1988–1994 was much lower: 7.2% in children aged 2–5 years, 11.3% among children 6–11 years, and 10.5% among adolescents 12–19 years [14]. The prevalence of 2–19 year old children with severe obesity was 7.9% in 2015–2016 (increased from 4.9% in 1999–2000) [15]. The rate of BMI rise among US youth aged 2–19 years also doubled during the COVID-19 pandemic compared to 2 years pre-pandemic [16]. Globally, the prevalence of pediatric obesity among children aged 5–19 years has grown from <1% in 1975 to 6% of females and 8% of males in 2016, a total of 124 million children worldwide [8]. The World Obesity Federation predicted that the number of children and adolescents aged 5–19 years with obesity will increase to 206 million by 2025 and 254 million by 2030 [17]. Pediatric obesity has also been increasing in low- and middle-income countries, and despite a later onset in rise of pediatric obesity, these countries often have a rapid increase in prevalence [18].

Pediatric obesity in the USA disproportionately affects ethnic and racial minorities. In the CDC data from 2017 to 2020, the highest prevalence of pediatric obesity within the USA is among Hispanic youth (26.2%), followed by those from non-Hispanic Black (24.8%), non-Hispanic White (16.6%), and non-Hispanic Asian ancestry (9.0%) [13]. Indian Health Service data from 2015 shows that youth of American Indian (18.5%) and Alaska Native ancestry (29.7%) also have high rates of obesity [19]. There is not an overall difference in pediatric obesity between sexes (females: 18.5%, males: 20.9%); however, males have a higher prevalence among certain groups, including children aged 6–11 years, non-Hispanic Asian youth, and children and adolescents living with a family income >350% of the federal poverty level [13]. Conversely, females have higher rates of obesity among non-Hispanic Black youth [13]. Obesity rates overall increase with age (12.7% for children 2–5 years, 20.7% 6–11 years, 22.2% 12–19 years) [13] and current estimates predict that 57% of current adolescents will be obese by age 35 years [20]. Obesity rates are also associated with lower socioeconomic status, including lower family income and lower parental education level [4, 13, 21].

Of note, early onset obesity predicts later obesity. In a 2014 longitudinal study of kindergarten children, it was revealed that 5-year old children who were overweight were four times as likely to be obese in adolescence compared to peers with normal BMI [22]. The high significance of childhood obesity is compounded as several studies have also shown that youth who are overweight

or obese have increased risk of being overweight or obese as adults [3]. The prevalence of adulthood severe obesity is highest in individuals who had childhood obesity (56%) or severe obesity in childhood (80%), compared to those with normal BMI in childhood (6%) [23].

Etiology and Risk Factors

Obesity develops due to an energy imbalance in which energy intake exceeds energy expenditure. A number of processes may contribute to the development of childhood obesity including genetic, epigenetic, environmental, and social factors (Fig. 1) [4, 24].

Obesity Genetics and Associated Disorders

Obesity is highly heritable with studies estimating 40–70% genetic contribution to the risk of developing obesity [4]. Twin studies have shown 77% heritability, and 32 genetic loci have been found to contribute to obesity risk [4, 25]. Youth who have been adopted demonstrate the obesity risk of their biological parents rather than adoptive parents [25]. However, monogenic or polygenic disorders that cause early childhood obesity by affecting processes that regulate energy intake, energy expenditure, or energy storage are rare: only about 7% of children with obesity have an identifiable genetic cause [26]. These monogenic or polygenic causes of obesity are characterized by early onset of severe obesity (younger than age 5 years) and hyperphagia [4].

The most common monogenic cause of severe obesity in children (2–5%) is a heterozygous mutation in *MCR4* (encoding the melanocortin 4 receptor), which affects the leptin-melanocortin system, an anorexic neural pathway that acts to reduce food intake [4, 25, 27]. Other monogenic obesity disorders associated with hyperphagia include leptin deficiency, leptin receptor deficiency, pro-opiomelanocortin (POMC) deficiency, prohormone convertase 1/3 deficiency, and *SRC1* deficiency (reduces leptin-induced *POMC* expression) [4].

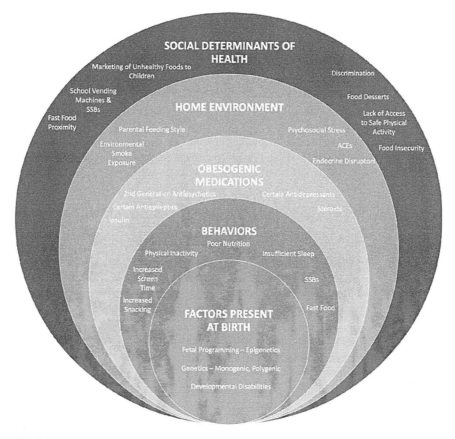

Fig. 1 Major risk factors for pediatric obesity, modeled after Bronfenbrenner's Ecological Theory [24]. *SSBs* sugary sweetened beverages, *ACEs* adverse childhood experiences

Leptin is a hormone produced by adipocytes that acts on neurons in the acuate nucleus of the hypothalamus [25]. Leptin inhibits feeding by stimulating POMC and suppressing NPY and AGRP [25]. Leptin and leptin receptor deficiencies are rare, occurring in children from consanguineous families, who demonstrate severe hyperphagia, rapid weight gain in early infancy, immune dysfunction, central hypogonadism, and growth hormone insufficiency [4, 25]. MC4R deficiency is associated with hyperphagia, early onset obesity, increased linear growth, and low blood pressure [4, 26]. POMC deficiency similarly has early onset childhood obesity, but as POMC is also the precursor for adrenocorticotropin hormone (ACTH), which regulates cortisol production, and α-MSH, which stimulates skin and hair pigmentation, POMC deficiency causes secondary adrenal insufficiency, pale skin color, and red hair in white

individuals [25]. Prohormone convertase-1/3 deficiency post-translationally modifies many substrates in addition to POMC, so the phenotype of the early onset obesity disorder also includes features of small bowel enteropathy, hypoglycemia (due to impaired insulin processing), as well as cortisol deficiency (due to lack of ACTH processing) [4, 25].

Polygenic obesity syndromes are associated with developmental delay and/or dysmorphic features. Prader-Willi syndrome, occurring when the paternally inherited chromosome 15q11.2-q12 is lost due to a mutation or imprinting defect, is characterized by failure to thrive due to hypotonia and poor feeding in the newborn period, followed by hyperphagia and rapid onset of obesity in early childhood [4, 26]. Prader-Willi syndrome also causes intellectual disability, impulsive behavior, short stature, small hands and feet, and hypothalamic hypogonadism [4, 25]. Albright's hereditary osteodystrophy, due to a dominant mutation in the *GNAS1* (which encodes the Gsα protein involved in signaling of several G-protein coupled receptors), has clinical features of obesity, short stature, round face, brachydactyly, and subcutaneous ossifications (called pseudopseudohypoparathyroidism if paternally inherited) and can lead to resistance of multiple hormones if maternally inherited (called pseudohypoparathyroidism type 1a) [4, 25]. Rare autosomal recessive syndromes associated with childhood obesity include Bardet-Biedl syndrome (associated with intellectual disability, dysmorphic extremities, hypogonadism, renal abnormalities or impairment, and retinopathy) and Alström syndrome (associated with short stature, type 2 diabetes, and pulmonary, hepatic, and renal impairments) [4, 26]. Youth with Down syndrome also have high rates of overweight or obesity (64%) and higher rates of dyslipidemia and prediabetes compared to normal developing youth [28]. A more detailed discussion of genetic syndromes associated with obesity is beyond the scope of this chapter, and additional information can be found in the 2023 American Academy of Pediatrics guidelines on pediatric obesity [4].

Other disorders during childhood can cause or contribute to the development of childhood obesity. Endocrine disorders, such as those causing excess glucocorticoid (Cushing syndrome), growth hormone deficiency, or hypothyroidism can be an underlying etiology of childhood obesity [4]. Youth with hypothalamic lesions, such as craniopharyngioma, a tumor located in the hypothalamic/pituitary region, have hyperphagia in >50% of patients and subsequent hypothalamic obesity [29]. Children with special health care needs and disabilities are 27–59% more likely to be obese than their peers, possibly related to reduced physical activity, altered diet (such as due to impulsive eating or sensory issues), use of obesogenic medications, and/or limited appropriate preventive medical and school-based programs [4, 30]. Among common developmental disorders, children with an autism spectrum disorder (ASD) have a 41% greater risk of obesity in childhood than peers without an ASD [31], and children with attention-deficit/hyperactivity disorder (ADHD) have a 40% higher prevalence of obesity compared to peers without ADHD [32].

Fetal Development, Intrapartum, and Infant Risk Factors

The antenatal environment plays a prominent role in the risk of developing obesity in childhood. Infants born small-for-gestational age (SGA) (<2500 g) with intrauterine growth restriction (IUGR) have increased rates of developing obesity and aspects of metabolic syndrome including insulin resistance and type 2 diabetes [4, 9]. Barker and Hales developed the "thrifty phenotype" or "mismatch" hypothesis to explain this association, which states that poor nutrition in the antenatal environment leads to permanent fetal adaptations in glucose-insulin metabolism promoting fat storage, which are then maladapted to the postnatal environment with abundant high-calorie food [9, 33, 34]. This thrifty phenotype leads to obesity and insulin resistance in childhood [9, 33, 34]. Infants born large-for-gestational age (LGA) (>4000 g), typically associated with maternal gestational diabetes or maternal obesity, also have higher risk of developing obesity and metabolic syndrome [4, 35]. The "early life hypernutrition hypothesis" proposes that maternal obesity and chronic hyperglycemia exposes a fetus to increased glucose levels leading to increased fetal insulin production, which drives fetal adipose growth [9, 36]. Maternal insulin resistance, even without hyperglycemia, can lead to hypertriglyceridemia which is proposed to also lead to macrosomia in the fetus [37]. Antibiotic use in pregnancy has been associated with increased infant birth weight and risk of future childhood obesity. Cesarean delivery is also associated with increased risk of developing childhood overweight or obesity [38]. Both of these risk factors are proposed to be related to altered infant microbiome [38]. Premature infant birth also contributes a higher risk of developing childhood obesity, although underlying mechanisms are not well understood [4].

Epigenetic changes are proposed to be underlying the obesogenic relationships with several antenatal factors. Studies in neonates have shown that neonatal epigenetic markers explain more than a quarter of the variance in childhood fat mass [4, 39]. Epigenetic changes alter gene expression and are also heritable, thereby affecting future generations [40]. Additional parental factors that are proposed to lead to epigenetic changes predisposing children to obesity include maternal psychosocial stress during pregnancy, maternal or paternal obesity pre-pregnancy, and maternal excessive weight gain during pregnancy (defined by the National Academy of Medicine as >18 kg gain for women with underweight pre-pregnancy BMI, >16 kg for women with normal pre-pregnancy BMI, >11.5 kg for women with overweight pre-pregnancy BMI, or >9 kg for women with obesity) [4, 38]. Studies on maternal obesity have shown that adolescents born to mothers following bariatric surgery have lower risk for obesity than their siblings born to mothers prior to bariatric surgery [41]. Maternal obesity in pregnancy is proposed to affect pathways regulating appetite, glucose metabolism, cardiovascular regulation, and the hypothalamic-pituitary-adrenal axis [4]. Maternal smoking is also related to an increased risk for childhood obesity in a dose-dependent manner, although a mechanism has not yet been established [42].

Nutrition, weight gain, and other exposures in the early postnatal or infancy period can also affect the risk of developing childhood obesity. Rapid weight gain after birth within the first 2 years of life is associated with an overall 3.6 higher odds of developing obesity, with higher odds of developing childhood obesity than adulthood obesity [43]. Several studies examining breastfeeding have shown a decreased risk of developing childhood obesity in breastfed infants, possibly due to a better ability of a breastfed infant to regulate their intake, or to a slower weight gain in breastfed infants, although the research to date is inconsistent [4]. The introduction of solid food before 4 months, use of high-protein formula, high intake of sugar-sweetened beverages (SSBs) before 2 years of age, and inappropriate bottle-feeding practices including overfeeding, over-concentrating formula, placing infants in bed with a bottle, adding cereal to a bottle, or

delayed transition to sippy cups, have all been associated with increased risk for childhood obesity, although some of these risk factors are under debate [4, 38, 44]. Early use of antibiotic therapy, within the first 2 years of life, is an additional risk factor for developing childhood obesity proposed to be related to alterations of the gut microbiome, especially with repeated antibiotic use, antibiotic use occurring in the first 6 months of life, or with broad-spectrum antibiotics [4]. Youth with pediatric obesity have an altered gut microbiome with high levels of *Firmicutes* and low levels of *Bacteroidetes* populations [45].

Behavioral Factors

The behavioral factors that contribute to the development of pediatric obesity relate to excess energy intake and/or reduced energy expenditure. Diets that are nutrient-poor and energy-dense with high-fat and SSBs increase the risk for obesity [26]. SSBs are one aspect of poorly nutritive energy intake that is highly associated with increased BMI in randomized controlled trials and with childhood obesity in numerous cross-sectional studies [46]. The National Health and Nutrition Examination Survey from 2003 to 2004 revealed that for US children and adolescents 2–18 years of age, about 40% of children's daily energy intake is from nutrient-poor solid fat and sugars [47]. SSBs intake has also doubled in adolescents since 1965 [26]. Aspects of eating habits that contribute to childhood obesity include large portion sizes, snacking on processed foods, eating outside the home and eating fast food, as well as factors relating to eating style such as eating fast, eating in the absence of hunger, high enjoyment in food, low regulation in response to satiety, and less restrained eating [4]. Low physical activity levels increases the risk for childhood obesity and are common among US youth: data from the 2016–2017 National Survey of Children's Health demonstrate that only 23% of US children aged 6–17 years meet the recommended physical activity of ≥60 min per day [48]. Sedentary time has been associated with increased risk for childhood obesity and is related to screen time (television, video games, computers, and mobile phone use, e.g., texting), which has a dose–response effect on childhood adiposity with >2 h per day associated with a 42% higher risk of childhood obesity [4, 26, 49]. Only 33% of US youth aged 6–17 years meet the recommended ≤2 h of screen time per day [48]. Short sleep duration is an additional risk factor that is associated with increased childhood obesity: a meta-analysis showed this relationship is dose–dependent, and for every 1 h/day increase in sleep duration the risk of overweight or obesity decreases by 21% [50].

Obesogenic Medications

Several medications can contribute to iatrogenic obesity and alternatives should be strongly considered when appropriate in youth with obesity. Obesogenic medications used in pediatric medicine include steroids, second-generation atypical antipsychotics (risperidone, dozapine, quetiapine, olanzapine, and aripiprazole), insulin, tricyclic antidepressants, antihistamines, and several anti-epileptic medications (carbamazepine, gabapentin, pregabalin, valproate, and vigabatrin) [4, 51]. An in-depth discussion of all obesogenic medications and alternatives in pediatric medicine is beyond the scope of this chapter, but can be found in Sweeney et al. [51] and the 2023 American Academy of Pediatric guidelines on pediatric obesity [4, 51].

Home Environment

Parental feeding styles are influential in children's feeding behaviors – longitudinal and cross-sectional studies have demonstrated that parental restrictive and controlled feeding are associated with increased child eating in the absence of hunger and reduced child self- regulation of food intake, whereas parental responsiveness to child feeding cues of hunger and satiety is protective [4, 52]. Household organization factors, such as routines and limit setting, are also protective against childhood obesity [53]. Endocrine-disrupting chemicals, such as bisphenol A, poly-fluoroalkyl, and phthalates, present in numerous household products and occasionally in infant supplies, are associated with a higher risk of childhood obesity when exposed during the antenatal, infancy, or childhood phases [4]. Tobacco smoke exposure is also a risk factor for higher BMI in children [4, 54].

Stress is a frequently proposed contributor to obesity risk, both parental stress in the antenatal environment, as well as the child's own psychosocial stress [4]. Adverse childhood experiences (ACEs), experiences in childhood that cause toxic stress, can include abuse of all types; parental household disruptions due to divorce, death, or incarceration; or exposure to substances abuse, mental illness, or economic insecurity [4]. Exposure to four or more ACEs is associated with an increased risk for childhood obesity [55]. Psychosocial stress may contribute to obesity due to maladaptive coping strategies such as eating in the absence of hunger, impulsive and binge eating, decreased physical activity, increased sedentary behavior, and poor sleep [4].

Social Determinants of Health

Outside the home environment, children are exposed to varied social determinants of health, environmental conditions that can affect health. One ubiquitous risk factor for childhood obesity is unhealthy food marketing to children, including food or drinks embedded in different forms of media, which lead to poor nonnutritive food choices and eating behaviors [4, 56]. Additional school-related factors can include access to vending machines, fast food, SSBs, and other nonnutritive food options [57].

Lower socioeconomic status has a negative impact on obesity, particularly in early childhood as subsequent upward mobility does not have different future obesity risk than individuals with chronic childhood poverty [58]. Additionally, youth without early childhood poverty who then have downward mobility do not have an increased risk of obesity [58]. Youth from lower socioeconomic status households may live in under-resourced environments with reduced access to high-quality, affordable nutrition and safe outdoor spaces for physical activity, as well as reduced access to quality health care [4]. Food insecurity is more prevalent in areas with higher poverty, and families with food insecurity have lower access to fresh fruits and vegetables and higher rates of fast food and SSB intake, as well as obesogenic eating patterns [4, 59]. These communities also have exposure to chronic stress, racism, and discrimination, which have been shown to lead to higher pediatric obesity rates [4].

The Role of Body Fat Distribution

The BMI may not be sufficient to identify all individuals with increased cardiometabolic risk. Body fat is stored in different compartments with the majority of fat in the subcutaneous depot, but additional fat is deposited intra-abdominally (visceral fat) and can be present within insulin-responsive organs such as the muscle and liver [60]. Visceral and ectopic adiposity are associated with cardiometabolic abnormalities in adults and are sometimes termed "metabolically unhealthy fat" [60–62]. A cross-sectional study on body composition in healthy pediatric and adult populations demonstrated that children and adolescents have lower amounts of visceral fat compared with adults, and visceral fat starts to increase in puberty [61]. Sex differences have been shown in visceral fat accumulation: boys have higher visceral fat than girls, especially during and after puberty, despite girls having higher overall total body fat [63]. Visceral fat differences are also seen between groups from differing ancestry with higher visceral fat in youth of South Asian descent compared to children of white European ancestry, and lower visceral fat in youth from African American ancestry compared to those from white European ancestry or Hispanic descent [63]. Associations between body fat depots and cardiometabolic traits are present only after puberty and with lower associations in pediatric compared to young adult populations [61]. Despite the lower amount of visceral fat in pediatric populations than adults, several studies have revealed that adolescents with obesity who have a higher ratio of visceral

fat to subcutaneous fat and presence of intrahepatic fat have increased insulin resistance and other abnormal cardiometabolic markers [60, 62–64].

Body fat distribution is proposed to affect the secretion of adipokine and inflammatory cytokines as well as free fatty acid flux [60]. Leptin signals fat mass to the brain leading to appetite suppression, but most people with obesity have leptin resistance [25, 60]. Adiponectin levels are inversely related to adiposity and adiponectin has beneficial effects on glucose homeostasis, inflammation, and atherogenesis [60]. Inflammatory cytokines secreted by fat tissue that contribute to cardiometabolic risk are also elevated in children with obesity [60].

Comorbidities and Complications of Pediatric Obesity

Several co-occurring disorders are associated with pediatric obesity (see Table 1 for detailed information on common comorbidities and complications), many of which are well-known cardiovascular disease risk factors [4, 65–93]. Metabolic syndrome is a common comorbidity and despite varying specific diagnostic criteria in pediatrics, it generally includes the clustering of at least three out of five metabolic risk factors: central obesity (measured by waist circumference and indicative of degree of visceral fat), abnormal glucose tolerance, hypertriglyceridemia, low high-density lipoprotein, and elevated blood pressure [65]. Metabolic syndrome increases in prevalence from 0% to 4% in children with normal BMI to 14.5% to 35% in children with obesity [4, 94]. Hypertension (when defined as ≥95th percentile systolic or diastolic blood pressure for age, sex, and height) prevalence increases from about 1% to 14% in youth with normal BMI to 4% to 30% in youth with obesity, and prevalence increases with age [94]. Prediabetes occurs in approximately 20% of children with obesity [4]. Abnormal glucose is highest in youth with class 3 severe obesity (37.5%) and type 2 diabetes is more prevalent in children with obesity or severe obesity compared to children with normal or overweight BMI [94].

Table 1 Common comorbidities and complications of pediatric obesity

Comorbidity or complication	Diagnostic criteria	Symptoms	Clinical findings	Workup	Treatment
Metabolic syndrome	Varying criteria that typically includes central obesity, glucose intolerance, hypertension, and dyslipidemia (high TG and low HDL-C) [65, 70, 71]	Central obesity [65]	Glucose intolerance, hypertension, dyslipidemia (high TG and low HDL-C), acanthosis nigricans [65, 66] Peaks during puberty [71]	BMI and waist circumference, blood pressure, fasting lipid profile, fasting serum glucose, and HbA1c [65]	Lifestyle changes (diet, exercise, weight loss) Severe dyslipidemia: statins Severe hypertension: antihypertensive drugs Bariatric surgery in some cases [65, 70]
Hypertension	Stage 1 hypertension: 1–12 years: ≥95th to <95th + 12 mm Hg or 130/80–139/89 (lower) ≥13 years: 130–139/80–89 Sage 2 hypertension: 1–12 years: ≥95th + 12 mm Hg or ≥140/90 (lower) >13 years: ≥140/90 [67, 69]	Uncommon to have symptoms, but in hypertensive crisis can have headache, nausea, vomiting, blurring of vision, or increased anxiety [68]	Elevated blood pressure [69]	Urinalysis, electrolyte panel, and creatinine with an estimated glomerular filtration rate calculation [67, 69]	Lifestyle changes (low sodium intake and high potassium diet and exercise) Antihypertensive drugs for children who remain hypertensive despite lifestyle modification therapy, symptomatic hypertension, or hypertension associated with chronic kidney disease or diabetes (ACEi, angiotensin receptor blockers, calcium channel blockers, and diuretics) [67, 69]
Dyslipidemia	TC >170 mg/dL LDL-C >110 mg/dL Non-HDL-C >120 mg/dL TG >75 mg/dL for age 0–9 years, > 90 mg/dL for age 10–19 years HDL-C <45 mg/dL [90]	Typically asymptomatic, significantly elevated TG increases risk for pancreatitis (symptoms: significant abdominal pain, nausea, vomiting) [89]	Cholesterol depositions rare in children but can occur in tendons, skin (xanthelasma), and cornea (arcus) Elevated TC, elevated LDL-C, elevated non-HDL-C, elevated TG, and/or low HDL-C [89]	Fasting lipid profile [89]	Dietary changes (low saturated fat and cholesterol intake) and can consider plant sterol or stanol, weight reduction therapy If lifestyle modification fails, statin therapy or niacin to lower LDL-C and TG; bile acid binding agents or ezetimibe to lower LDL-C; fibrates or omega 3 ethyl esters to lower TG [89]

Prediabetes/type 2 diabetes	Prediabetes is diagnosed with 1 or more of the following [91]: HbA1c 5.7–6.4% Fasting BG 100–125 mg/dL 2-H BG from OGTT 140–199 mg/dL Diabetes is diagnosed with 2 or more of the following (if unequivocal hyperglycemia is not present) [91]: HbA1c ≥6.5% Fasting BG ≥126 mg/dL 2-H BG from OGTT ≥200 mg/dL Random BG ≥200 mg/dL if combined with symptoms of hyperglycemia	Polyuria, polydipsia, nocturia, variable weight loss, candidal infections, secondary enuresis [91] Can present in diabetic ketoacidosis with or without hyperosmolar features or hyperosmolar hyperglycemic non-ketoacidosis [91, 92]	Acanthosis nigricans [91]	HbA1c, fasting BG, 2-h BG on OGTT [91]	Prediabetes [92]: Lifestyle changes (diet, exercise, weight loss) Diabetes: Lifestyle changes (diet, exercise, weight loss) Metformin, insulin, GLP1-agonist Bariatric surgery in certain cases
Non-alcoholic fatty liver disease (NAFLD)	Liver biopsy with histologic evidence of at least 5% hepatic steatosis (could also show hepatocyte ballooning, inflammation and/or fibrosis) [72–74]	Typically asymptomatic; symptoms can include abdominal pain, fatigue, irritability, headaches, and difficulty concentrating [72–74]	Elevated ALT levels in the absence of other causes of liver injury, acanthosis nigricans, enlarged liver upon palpation [72–74] Peaks before puberty [93]	ALT level (NAFLD more likely with higher ALT levels >80 U/l) or splenomegaly and AST/ALT >1, liver biopsy, labs to rule out other causes of liver steatosis (such as chronic exposure to steatogenic agents, hereditary metabolic conditions, and viral hepatitis) [72–74]	Lifestyle changes (diet, exercise, weight loss) [72–74]
Obstructive sleep apnea	Symptoms of sleep apnea Polysomnography demonstrates one or more of the following:	Frequent snoring, gasps or labored breathing during sleep, disturbed sleep, daytime sleepiness,	Tonsillar hypertrophy, adenoidal facies, micro- or retrognathia, high-arched palate, elevated blood	Nocturnal polysomnography (apnea-hypopnea index of ≥1/h); pulse oximetry if	Leukotriene inhibitors (montelukast), intranasal steroid treatment,

(continued)

Table 1 (continued)

Comorbidity or complication	Diagnostic criteria	Symptoms	Clinical findings	Workup	Treatment
	≥1 obstructive or mixed apneas/hour of sleep a pattern of obstructive hypoventilation (25% of total sleep time with hypercapnia) arterial oxygen desaturation with snoring, flattening of the inspiratory nasal pressure waveform, and/or paradoxical thoracoabdominal motion [76]	inattention and/or learning problems, nocturnal enuresis, headaches [75, 95]	pressure [75, 76] Peaks between 2 and 8 years [75]	polysomnography is unavailable [75, 76]	adenotonsillectomy, CPAP [75, 76]
Idiopathic intracranial hypertension (IIH)	LP opening pressure >28 cm H_2O or >25 cm H_2O if the child is not obese and not sedated [77]	Persistent headaches often associated with nausea or vomiting, pulsatile tinnitus, binocular horizontal diplopia, visual changes or loss [77]	Papilledema (bilateral optic nerve swelling), normal neuroimaging (except signs of raised intracranial pressure), elevated LP pressure Peaks between 12 and 17 years [77]	Optic nerve assessment, neuroimaging (MRI), LP [77]	Acetazolamide, topiramate, furosemide, bariatric surgery (if the patient has other complications), shunting, optic nerve sheath fenestration, venous sinus stenting [77]
Polycystic ovary syndrome	Irregular menses or oligomenorrhea 2 years post-menarche Evidence of hyperandrogenism (biochemical and/or clinical) [78–80]	Irregular or missed menses (oligo- or amenorrhea), clinical hyperandrogenism including acne, hirsutism (excessive dark hair on the face, chest, and back) and/or male-pattern baldness or alopecia [78–80]	Biologic hyperandrogenism (elevated testosterone concentration), insulin resistance or hyperinsulinemia, acanthosis nigricans [78–80]	Physical assessment for signs of hyperandrogenism (use modified Ferriman-Gallwey score) or insulin resistance Laboratory assessment for diagnosis: free and total testosterone, dehydroepiandrosterone sulfate Additional labs to assess differential diagnoses:	Lifestyle changes (diet, exercise, weight loss), combined oral contraceptive, antiandrogens, insulin-sensitizing agents (metformin) [78–80]

Comorbidity	Definition	Signs and symptoms	Clinical findings	Diagnostic assessment	Management
Cholelithiasis	Gallstones [81, 82]	Often asymptomatic, symptoms can include icterus, abdominal pain, nausea, vomiting, and a positive Murphy's sign [81]	Gallstones [81, 82]	17-OH progesterone, LH-to-FSH ratio. Screen for thyroid disease, T2DM, hyperprolactinemia, and hyperlipidemia [78–80]. Liver, gallbladder, and biliary tract ultrasonography. Laboratory assessment: complete blood count, differential tests, Coombs test, reticulocyte count, hemoglobin electrophoresis, G6PD test, liver functional tests, amylase, lipase and copper serum levels, Wilson's disease diagnostic tests, as well as sweat and stool exams [82]	If symptomatic, cholecystectomy. If asymptomatic, conservative management (wait-and-see) [82]
Slipped capital femoral epiphysis	Displacement of the capital femoral epiphysis from the femoral neck through the physeal plate [83]	Limping, hip, groin, thigh, or knee pain [83]	External rotation with passive hip flexion, limitation of internal rotation and antalgic gait 8–15 years old, usually during the adolescent growth spurt [83]	Bilateral hip radiography (anteroposterior and frog-leg lateral views) [83]	In situ screw fixation, postoperative rehabilitation [83]
Blount disease	Varus deformity of the tibia [84]	Leg pain, abnormal gait with bowing of the lower legs, and leg-length discrepancy [84]	Asymmetric tibia vara, tibial torsion, and procurvatum. Infantile: 2–5 years of age. Adolescent: > 10 (84)	Long-leg anteroposterior radiographs, MRI [84]	Brace, graded growth (hemiepiphysiodesis), re-alignment osteotomy [84]
Depression	Use of the DSM-5 as depressed mood or loss of interest for at least 2 weeks, accompanied by 4 additional symptoms [85]	Anhedonia (loss of interest or pleasure), insomnia or hypersomnia, changes in appetite or weight (decreased or increased), poor concentration, fatigue,	N/A	Universal screening for depression in children 12–18 years with PHQ-9. Assessment for other signs and symptoms of psychopathology (anxiety,	CBT, interpersonal psychotherapy, and SSRIs such as fluoxetine and escitalopram [85]

(continued)

Table 1 (continued)

Comorbidity or complication	Diagnostic criteria	Symptoms	Clinical findings	Workup	Treatment
		mania, and psychosis), history of alcohol and substance use, evaluation for general medical conditions [85]			
Anxiety (general anxiety disorder)	Use of the DSM-5 criteria, which requires that the excessive worry persists for more than 6 months, is difficult to control, and is accompanied by at least one symptom [88]	Restlessness, edginess, difficulty concentrating, irritability, muscle aches or soreness, difficulty falling or staying asleep, fatigue [88]	N/A	Use of the Screen for Child Anxiety Related Disorders tool [88]	Psychoeducation of the parent/caregiver and child, behavior therapy (most commonly CBT), and medication in severe cases (most commonly SSRIs, SNRIs, benzodiazepines, and typical anxiolytics) [88]

TG triglycerides, *HDL-C* high-density lipoprotein cholesterol, *BMI* body-mass index, *HbA1c* hemoglobin A1c, *ACEi* angiotensin-converting enzyme inhibitors, *TC* total cholesterol, *LDL-C* low-density lipoprotein cholesterol, *BG* blood glucose, *OGTT* oral glucose tolerance test, *GLP-1 agonist* glucagon-like peptide-1 receptor agonist, *ALT* alanine aminotransferase, *AST* aspartate aminotransferase, *CPAP* continuous positive airway pressure, *LP* lumbar puncture, *MRI* magnetic resonance imaging, *LH* luteinizing hormone, *FSH* follicle-stimulating hormone, *T2DM* type 2 diabetes mellitus, *G6PD* Glucose-6-phosphate dehydrogenase deficiency, *DSM-5* diagnostic and statistical manual of mental disorders, *PHQ-9* patient health questionnaire 9, *CBT* cognitive behavioral therapy, *SSRI* selective serotonin-reuptake inhibitor, *SNRI* serotonin and norepinephrine reuptake inhibitor

Nonalcoholic fatty liver disease (NAFLD) is another disorder highly associated with abnormal glucose tolerance and insulin resistance [73]. Children with NAFLD have 14x increased risk of developing future severe liver disease compared to youth without NAFLD [73]. One meta-analysis reported that NAFLD was found in 34% of children seen in pediatric obesity clinics [96]. NAFLD can potentially be indicated by an elevated alanine aminotransferase (ALT) – several studies have shown higher odds of elevated ALT in children with obesity compared to children with normal BMI, and some studies showed ALT increases in children with obesity with increasing severity of obesity [94]. Pediatric NAFLD is more frequent in males compared to females, increases in prevalence with increasing age, and is prevalent in children of Hispanic descent [4]. In those youth who develop type 2 diabetes or NAFLD, studies have revealed that both of these disorders in pediatric populations seem to be more aggressive than in adults with comparable BMI [4].

Dyslipidemia with elevated low-density lipoprotein cholesterol also occurs in children with increased prevalence as BMI increases, an association more prominent in males compared to females [94]. Additional comorbidities that are associated with childhood and adolescent obesity include obstructive sleep apnea (occurs in 45% of children with obesity compared to 9% of children without obesity) [97], idiopathic intracranial hypertension (increased incidence by 3.5× for adolescent and adult women with obesity compared to women without obesity) [98], polycystic ovary syndrome, cholelithiasis, orthopedic disorders (slipped capital femoral epiphysis (SCFE) and Blount disease), and psychiatric conditions (particularly depression and anxiety) [4, 94] (see Table 1) [65–93].

Secondary to the increased cardiometabolic risk factors with childhood obesity, long-term consequences of childhood obesity include cardiovascular disease, stroke, and premature mortality [99]. Atherosclerotic cardiovascular disease is noted in children with obesity, especially in those with concurrent metabolic syndrome [62]. Other cardiovascular abnormalities that are noted in childhood obesity include increased aging of vascular structures and arterial stiffness, as measured by carotid-femoral pulse wave velocity, augmentation index, or carotid intima-media thickness [62].

Clinical Patient Evaluation

Pediatric clinicians should be familiar with the unique aspects of patient evaluation and assessment for children with overweight and obesity in order to recognize comorbidities and complications and provide personalized prevention and treatment guidance for families. In a primary care setting, weight, height, and BMI status should be monitored to facilitate early identification of overweight and obesity. When addressing obesity in children, providers should be sensitive to non-stigmatizing approaches in order to facilitate a supportive and trusting relationship with the patient and their family.

Medical History

In the medical history-taking of a child with obesity, it is beneficial to obtain information about the weight gain trajectory (including review of the growth chart) and identification of any prenatal to childhood risk factors that may have contributed [4]. Open-ended questions can help in getting a patient's narrative, which allows assessment of patient and family readiness to change behavior and prior attempts at obesity treatment. Particular focus should be spent on determining a detailed diet (with sensitivity to cultural norms) as well as physical activity, and several tools can be utilized, including 24-h food recalls, food diaries, pedometers, and smartphone apps [4]. Dietary history and assessment of eating habits should also include screening for disordered eating behaviors and other mental health disorders (such as depression, anxiety, and ADHD) [4]. A family history should include genetic obesity syndromes, obesity-related comorbidities and complications, and a history of bariatric surgery to assess the severity of obesity in family members [4]. Clinicians should get a detailed medication history to determine if obesogenic medications have been used. Providers should also spend some time on a detailed social history and assessment of social determinant of health barriers (such as food insecurity, lack of safe outdoor spaces, etc.).

Physical Exam

A physical exam for children with obesity should include several aspects that will assess for genetic causes, comorbidities, and complications. These include vital signs (hypertension), fundoscopic exam (papilledema), oral exam (tonsillar hypertrophy consistent with obstructive sleep apnea), neck exam (thyroid goiter), chest and back exam (gynecomastia, cervicodorsal hump), abdominal exam (hepatomegaly), genitourinary exam (penile length with depression of suprapubic fat pad), skin exam (acanthosis nigricans, acne, hirsutism, striae, and skin infections), and an extensive musculoskeletal exam (proximal muscle wasting, abnormal gait, spinal curvature, knee or hip pain characteristic of SCFE, or genu varum/valgum) [100]. Assessment of the heart and lungs can reveal tachypnea, dyspnea, or tachycardia, which along with decreased strength and flexibility on musculoskeletal exam may be signs of decreased physical activity tolerance [4]. Growth assessments should also pay special attention to growth velocity – obesity typically has an early onset of height velocity increases, although falling height percentiles can suggest obesity secondary to endocrine disorders (growth hormone or thyroid deficiency, Cushing syndrome) or genetic syndromes that lead to childhood obesity [100]. Of note, after children have completed most of linear growth, the height growth is no longer helpful.

Assessment

The American Academy of Pediatrics 2023 Guidelines on Pediatric Obesity recommend universal laboratory testing for all children ≥10 years with obesity to screen for common comorbidities and complications including a fasting lipid panel (dyslipidemia); hemoglobin A1c, fasting blood glucose or oral glucose tolerance (prediabetes

and type 2 diabetes); and ALT (NAFLD) [4]. These universal lab tests for pediatric obesity should be repeated every 2 years or sooner based on clinical findings and assessment for risk factors [4]. Dyslipidemia screening should also be considered in children aged 2–9 years with obesity and sent in all children and adolescents regardless of BMI at age 9–11 years and 17–21 years [4, 86]. Based on history and physical exam features, additional laboratory or imaging tests may be an important next step to evaluate for other comorbidities and complications (see Table 1 for a detailed description of typical symptoms, clinical findings, work-up, diagnostic criteria, and treatment of obesity-related comorbidities and complications found in pediatric populations) [4, 65–93]. History or physical exam signs of potential endocrine etiologies (low linear growth velocity for age, sex, and pubertal stage in a growing child; goiter indicating thyroid disease; violaceous striae, proximal muscle wasting, full facies, cervicodorsal hump, and hypertension indicating Cushing syndrome; or microphallus) should prompt an endocrine work-up [4]. Additionally, genetic testing for monogenic or polygenic disorders associated with obesity should be considered in patients with early-onset severe obesity (particularly before age 5 years), history of extreme hyperphagia, unexplained global developmental delay, dysmorphic features, skeletal anomalies, ophthalmic abnormalities, and/or other features distinctive for particular syndromes [4, 101].

Prevention of Pediatric Obesity

As there are numerous risk factors for the development of pediatric obesity, prevention methods should be utilized from pregnancy through adolescence (detailed in Fig. 2) [4, 38, 42]. Antenatal risk factors for childhood obesity can be mitigated in part by a healthy BMI pre-pregnancy as well as avoidance of excessive pregnancy weight gain and gestational diabetes through a healthy diet and exercise [4, 38]. Pregnant women should also have minimal antibiotic and nicotine exposure [38, 42]. During infancy, several additional practices should be considered to prevent rapid weight gain during the first 2 years of life and

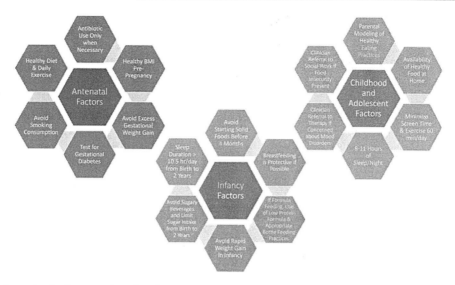

Fig. 2 Strategies for the prevention of pediatric obesity from the antenatal period through adolescence. *BMI* body-mass index

future childhood obesity including breastfeeding if able, appropriate bottle-feeding practices, low protein-formula, avoidance of SSBs, adequate sleep, and solid food start after 4 months of age [38]. Actions to prevent childhood obesity past infancy should be implemented in the home environment (e.g., responsive parenting of feeding patterns, household availability of healthy food, and reduced frequency of eating outside the home) [4]. In addition, children and adolescents can implement preventive behaviors including reduction of sedentary behavior and increase in physical activity, adequate sleep, and healthy nutrition [4]. Obstetricians and pediatricians should provide counseling on these topics during routine prenatal and well-child visits for mothers, children/adolescents, and their families; they should identify and address modifiable behavioral and home-related obesity risk factors early, as well as screen for potential socioeconomic and psychiatric contributors to childhood obesity, and address these factors if present.

Treatment of Pediatric Obesity

Lifestyle modification is an essential element of all obesity treatment to reduce ongoing behavioral risk factors for obesity. The recommended lifestyle changes for youth by the American Academy of Pediatrics and other major organizations include elimination of SSBs, minimal screen time (no use under 18 months, 1 h/day for youth 2–5 years, and ≤2 h/day for older children), aerobic exercise for 60 min daily with muscle and bone strengthening exercises at least 3 days per week, adequate sleep (9–12 h/night for children 6–12 years, and 8–10 h/night for adolescents 13–17 years), and use of the US Department of Agriculture's MyPlate to organize a healthy diet (which emphasizes nutrient dense low-calorie foods and low amounts of added sugar and concentrated fat) [4, 48, 102]. Other important behavioral strategies include avoidance of smoking and alcohol for teenagers, and stress management [62]. Motivational interviewing by clinicians is a critical aspect of assisting patients and their families to make behavioral changes by partnering with the patient or family to identify areas for change and make goals that are feasible [4]. It is also important for clinicians to screen for unhealthy disordered eating or extreme weight-control behaviors, and encourage healthier options in order to prevent the development of eating disorders in children and adolescents [103].

As these strategies have limited success by themselves, the American Academy of Pediatrics recommends early referral for children 2–18 years of age to intensive health behavior and lifestyle treatment (IHBLT) programs that consist of at least 26 h of in-person, family-based counseling on health behavior strategies to treat pediatric obesity over a period of 3–12 months [4]. IHBLT of ≥26 h has led to BMI reductions (mean reduction in BMI z-score: −0.2) in 75% of programs studied; IHBLT of ≥52 h within 3–12 months leads to even further BMI improvement (mean reduction in BMI z-score: −0.3) and reduction in cardiometabolic comorbidities [4]. IHBLT is more successful when physical activity or physical therapy is included in the program rather than counseling about physical activity alone [4]. Nutrition counseling that includes meal preparation or food tastings are effective to increase the palate of a child with obesity [4]. IHBLT programs can also address mental health and parenting skills [4]. Despite IHBLT being a cornerstone of the American Academy of Pediatrics recommendations for children with obesity, it leads to about 1–3% BMI reduction alone, and is less successful in families who are not engaged (overall attrition: 40%) or have socioeconomic stressors (attrition in low-income families: 60%) [4, 62].

Since IHBLT programs and behavioral therapies are not always successful for BMI reduction, several obesity medications are now available and recommended for youth with obesity. The American Academy of Pediatrics recommends offering obesity pharmacotherapy for youth ≥12 years and considering medication for youth 8–11 years (see Table 2 for detailed descriptions of available medications used for pediatric obesity) [4, 104–124]. Until recently, orlistat was the only medication approved by the US Food & Drug Administration (2003) for treatment of pediatric obesity; it acts to block fat absorption in the gastrointestinal (GI) tract [4, 106]. Orlistat has low tolerability with significant GI side effects, and is therefore infrequently prescribed [4, 106]. In 2020, the first glucagon-like peptide-1 (GLP-1) receptor agonist to be approved for use with pediatric obesity was liraglutide, a daily subcutaneous injection medication [4, 107]. Since then, a second GLP-1 agonist medication, semaglutide, was approved in 2022 as a weekly injection [4, 105]. These GLP-1 agonists are successful in reducing BMI in pediatric randomized controlled trials (reduction by −0.22 BMI standard deviation at 56 weeks for liraglutide, reduction in BMI by 16.1% at 68 weeks for semaglutide) and act by slowing gastric emptying and decreasing hunger [4, 105, 107] (see Table 2 for complete list including contraindications) [104–124]. A combination of phentermine and topiramate was a recently approved medication for the treatment of pediatric obesity (2022) with a 8–10% BMI decrease by 56 weeks in a pediatric randomized controlled trial [104]. Phentermine and topiramate alone have also been prescribed off-label for youth with obesity – phentermine acts to inhibit serotonin and dopamine reuptake, which reduces appetite, and topiramate also works to suppress appetite by an unknown mechanism [4]. Metformin has also been used off-label as a treatment for pediatric obesity outside of its primary indication for type 2 diabetes, particularly to prevent weight gain in youth on atypical antipsychotic medications [4], but has not shown significant BMI decreases for adolescents in general (two randomized studies in adolescents show a BMI reduction of 1 kg/m^2 although a third of studies on metformin show no benefit) [4, 114, 115]. For youth 6 years and older with monogenic or polygenic disorders associated with early onset severe obesity, setmelanotide, a melanocortin 4 receptor agonist was approved in 2020 for POMC deficiency, prohormone convertase 1/3 deficiency (PCSK1 deficiency), or leptin receptor deficiency and in 2022 for Bardet-Biedl syndrome [4, 110, 111].

Youth with severe obesity may also benefit significantly from bariatric surgery. The American Academy of Pediatrics recommends considering referral to pediatric bariatric surgery programs at age ≥13 years (and can be considered at younger ages) for youth who qualify for bariatric surgery: class II obesity with a significant comorbidity (e.g., youth-onset type 2 diabetes, obstructive sleep apnea, idiopathic intracranial hypertension, SCFE, Blount's disease) or class III obesity [4, 125]. The bariatric surgery types performed in adolescents include laparoscopic Roux-en-Y gastric bypass and vertical sleeve gastrectomy, although vertical sleeve gastrectomy is most well tolerated [4, 62]. The pivotal trial assessing bariatric surgery in adolescents is the Teen-Longitudinal Assessment

Table 2 Drug treatment of obesity in children and adolescents

Drug (brand name)	FDA approval + administration	Study outcomes	Side effects	Monitoring	Contraindications and guidelines
Orlistat (Alli (OTC), Xenical)	2003 for long-term treatment of obesity in children 12+ [116] Oral, 3× daily	RCT with 539 obese adolescents: Primary: average BMI decrease 0.55 kg/m² after 1 year, compared to BMI increase of 0.31 with placebo; Secondary: average loss of 1.33 cm in waist circumference [106]	≥5% experienced: oily spotting, flatus with discharge, fecal urgency, fatty/oily stool, oily evacuation, increased defecation, fecal incontinence (GI adverse events experienced by 9–50% of participants in RCT) Less common: cholelithiasis [116]	Monitor levels of fat-soluble vitamins (encourage multivitamin), monitor for symptoms of liver dysfunction (anorexia, pruritus, jaundice, dark urine, light-colored stools, right upper quadrant pain) and obtain ALT/AST if present, monitor kidney function [116]	Pregnancy, chronic malabsorption syndrome, cholestasis, hypersensitivity Should avoid if patient taking following drugs: cyclosporine, anticoagulants, amiodarone Generally low tolerability, good for constipation [116]
Liraglutide (Saxenda)	2020, children 12+, >60 kg, BMI >95th%tile [117] Subcutaneous injection, daily	RCT with 251 obese adolescents: Primary: estimated treatment difference in BMI SDS of −0.22 at 56 weeks; Secondary: did not improve CVD risk factors [107]	>5% experienced: nausea, vomiting, diarrhea, hypoglycemia, gastroenteritis, dizziness, pyrexia Less common: abdominal discomfort, constipation, dyslipidemia, fatigue, cough, depression, dyspepsia, pain in extremity, injection site pain, flatulence, increased blood creatine kinase, increased lipase, rash, acute pancreatitis [117]	Monitor blood glucose, especially in individuals with T2DM; monitor heart rate at intervals consistent with clinical practice, risk of increased heartrate; monitor for changes in behavior/mood, especially depression and suicidal ideation [117]	Personal or family history of MTC or MEN2, hypersensitivity to ingredients, pregnancy Should be cautious of use in populations with kidney disease Avoid in patients with history of/active suicidal ideation Patients with a history of pancreatitis may be at higher risk of developing pancreatitis [117]
Semaglutide (Wegovy)	2022, children 12+, BMI >95th%ile [118] Subcutaneous injection, weekly	RCT with 201 obese adolescents: Primary: Median decrease in BMI of 16.1% at 68 weeks; Secondary: median loss of 12.7 cm waist	≥3% experienced: Nausea, vomiting, diarrhea, headache, abdominal pain, nasopharyngitis, dizziness, gastroenteritis, constipation, GERD, sinusitis, UTI,	Monitor blood glucose prior to initiation and during treatment in both patients with and without T2DM, especially if patient is taking insulin secretagogue; check	Family history of MTC or MEN2, hypersensitivity to ingredients Avoid in patients with history of suicide attempts or active suicidal ideation

(continued)

Table 2 (continued)

Drug (brand name)	FDA approval + administration	Study outcomes	Side effects	Monitoring	Contraindications and guidelines
		circumference, improvement in blood pressure, HbA1c, lipid profile, and ALT [105]	ligament sprain, anxiety, hair loss, cholelithiasis, eructation, influenza, rash, urticaria. Less common: acute pancreatitis, acute gallbladder disease, hypoglycemia (in patients with and without T2DM), acute kidney injury, increased heart rate, hypotension, syncope, appendicitis, injection site reactions [118]	heart rate at regular intervals; monitor renal function, especially during dose escalation; monitor for depression, suicidal thoughts, and behaviors [118]	Patients with a history of pancreatitis may be at higher risk of developing pancreatitis [118]
Setmelanotide (Imcivree)	2020: patients 6 years or older with monogenic/syndromic obesity due to POMC, PCSK1, or LEPR deficiency, as determined by genetic testing demonstrating pathogenic variants. 2022: patients 6 years or older with BBS [119] Subcutaneous injection, daily	POMC: 80% of patients achieved weight loss of at least 10% at 52 weeks [111] LEPR: 46% of patients achieved weight loss of at least 10% at 52 weeks [111] POMC, PCSK1, LEPR heterozygous (not separated by gene): 34.3% of patients achieved weight loss of at least 5% at 12 weeks [124] BBS: 32.3% of patients achieved weight loss of at least 10% at 52 weeks of treatment (RCT) [110]	>20% experienced: skin hyperpigmentation, injection site reactions, nausea, headache, diarrhea, abdominal pain, vomiting, depression, spontaneous penile erection [119]	For POMC, PCSK1, or LR deficiency: assess weight loss at 12–16 weeks of treatment – if <5% loss of BMI, discontinue treatment For BBS: assess weight loss at 1 year of treatment – if <5% loss of BMI, discontinue treatment Monitor for signs of depression and suicidal ideation and changes to skin pigmentation Advise patients to seek medical attention if they experience a penile erection lasting more than 4 h [119]	No contraindications Should not be used in neonates or infants [119]

Phentermine (Adipex-P)	1959, short-term (<12 weeks) use in children over 16, BMI >30 or BMI >27 + comorbidity [120] Oral, daily	Retrospective chart review of 299 adolescents: phentermine was associated with a greater % decrease in BMI than standard of care alone [112] Phentermine was associated with greater percent decrease in BMI among long-term users after 12+ months of use compared to reference group after 24 months [113]	Primary pulmonary hypertension, regurgitant valvular disease, palpitation, tachycardia, elevated blood pressure, restlessness and other CNS symptoms, gastrointestinal disturbances, impotence [120]	Monitor for symptoms of primary pulmonary hypertension: dyspnea, angina, syncope, edema of lower extremities [120]	History of cardiovascular disease, use of MAOI, hyperthyroidism, glaucoma, agitated states, history of drug abuse, pregnancy, nursing, hypersensitivity to ingredients Patients should take in the morning to limit risk of insomnia [120]
Topiramate (Topamax)	1999 for treatment of epilepsy in children 2+ and migraine prevention in children 12+; used off-label for treatment of pediatric obesity [121] Oral, daily	Primary: weight loss of at least 5% achieved by 67% of subjects taking highest dose; Secondary: significant improvements in blood pressure and glycemic markers [108] Another study showed no difference in BMI change between topiramate and placebo [109]	$\geq$10% experienced: fever Less common: paresthesia, psychiatric/cognitive problems, fatigue, dizziness, eye problems, oligohydrosis and hyperthermia, metabolic acidosis, decreased bone mineral density, kidney stones [121]	Can result in decreased growth velocity – monitor pediatric patients' growth; monitor for decreased sweating and increased body temperature; serial measurements of bicarbonate are recommended to monitor for metabolic acidosis; monitor for depression and suicidal ideation [121]	No contraindications Decreased efficacy of oral contraceptives, especially when used at high doses [121]
Combination phentermine and topiramate (Qsymia)	2022, children 12+ with BMI >95th%ile [122] Oral, daily *Schedule 4 controlled substance	Primary: 8–10.4% decrease in BMI at 56 weeks (depending on dosing); Secondary: 20.72% decrease in triglycerides and 8.75% increase in HDL-C No significant change in BP or glycemic markers [104]	> 5% experienced: depression, dizziness, arthralgia, influenza, ligament sprain, insomnia Less common: Slowing of linear growth, decreased bone mineral density, kidney stones [122]	Negative pregnancy test prior to starting and monthly in patients able to become pregnant; obtain blood chemistry profile including bicarbonate, creatinine, and potassium, as well as glucose for patients with T2DM, before initiation and periodically during treatment; resting heart rate; suicidal ideation [122]	Pregnancy, kidney stones, MAOI use, glaucoma, hyperthyroidism, hypersensitivity to ingredients Should avoid in patients with end-stage renal disease, severe hepatic impairment, history of depression/other mood disorder Helpful for migraines May increase sensitivity to alcohol [122]

(continued)

Table 2 (continued)

Drug (brand name)	FDA approval + administration	Study outcomes	Side effects	Monitoring	Contraindications and guidelines
Metformin	1994 for treatment of T2DM, used off-label for treatment of pediatric obesity [123] Oral, 2x daily	Studies include: 1. RCT with 39 obese adolescents: Primary (XR): average BMI decrease 0.9 kg/m² at 48 weeks; Secondary: no effect observed on body composition or glycemic measures [114] 2. RCT of 100 severely obese children: Primary: average BMI decrease of 1.09 kg/m² at 6 months; Secondary: improved fasting glucose and HOMA-IR [115]	≥5% experienced: diarrhea, nausea/vomiting, flatulence, asthenia, indigestion, abdominal discomfort, headache, vitamin B12 deficiency [123]	Monitor patients taking concomitant carbonic anhydrase inhibitors for signs of lactic acidosis Monitor for hypoglycemia, especially in patients taking insulin or insulin secretagogue [123]	Severe renal impairment, hypersensitivity to ingredients, metabolic acidosis (acute or chronic) First-line therapy for T2DM in children and adults Used off label in PCOS Particularly helpful for weight gain associated with atypical anti-psychotic medication [123]

RCT randomized-controlled trial, *BMI* body mass index, *ALT* alanine aminotransferase, *AST* aspartate aminotransferase, *CVD* cardiovascular disease, *T2DM* type 2 diabetes mellitus, *MTC* medullary thyroid cancer, *MEN2* multiple endocrine neoplasia type 2, *HbA1c* hemoglobin A1c, *GERD* gastroesophageal reflux disease, *UTI* urinary tract infection, *POMC* proopiomelanocortin, *PCSK1* proprotein convertase subtilisin/kexin type 1, *LEPR* leptin receptor, *BBS* Bardet-Biedl syndrome, *MAOI* monoamine oxidase inhibitor, *CNS* central nervous system, *HDL-C* high-density lipoprotein cholesterol, *BP* blood pressure, *HOMA-IR* homeostatic model assessment for insulin resistance, *PCOS* polycystic ovary syndrome

of Bariatric Surgery (Teen-LABS) study, which followed 242 adolescent who underwent bariatric surgery [126, 127]. Teen-LABS and other studies have revealed that these procedures are relatively safe and lead to significant and sustained improvements in BMI and obesity-related comorbidities [4, 62, 125–127]. There is a risk for long-term micronutrient deficiencies following bariatric surgery as well as a need for repeated procedures (13–25% of patients after 5 years) and other post-procedure complications [4]. Clinicians should refer to multidisciplinary programs that include an experienced pediatric bariatric surgeon, a dietician, a behavioral specialist, and a medical advisor [4, 125].

Conclusions

Pediatric obesity is a growing epidemic with numerous modifiable and non-modifiable risk factors and limited but growing effective treatment options. Knowledge gaps remain in the understanding of individual characteristics that predispose youth to significant obesity-related comorbidities and severe cardiovascular long-term consequences of pediatric obesity. Further research is also needed to identify effective therapies for children at younger ages. In addition, future studies to understand which individual characteristics relate to specific treatment effects could lead to more personalized approaches to treatment of pediatric obesity, matching the individual and family to the optimal treatment options.

References

1. Finkelstein EA, Graham WC, Malhotra R. Lifetime direct medical costs of childhood obesity. Pediatrics. 2014;133(5):854–62.
2. Zamrazilova H, Weiss R, Hainer V, Aldhoon-Hainerova I. Cardiometabolic health in obese adolescents is related to length of obesity exposure: a pilot study. J Clin Endocrinol Metab. 2016;101(8):3088–95.
3. Singh AS, Mulder C, Twisk JW, van Mechelen W, Chinapaw MJ. Tracking of childhood overweight into adulthood: a systematic review of the literature. Obes Rev. 2008;9(5):474–88.
4. Hampl SE, Hassink SG, Skinner AC, Armstrong SC, Barlow SE, Bolling CF, et al. Clinical practice guideline for the evaluation and treatment of children and adolescents with obesity. Pediatrics. 2023;151(2)
5. Cole TJ, Bellizzi MC, Flegal KM, Dietz WH. Establishing a standard definition for child overweight and obesity worldwide: international survey. BMJ. 2000;320(7244):1240–3.
6. Barlow SE, Dietz WH. Obesity evaluation and treatment: expert Committee recommendations. The Maternal and Child Health Bureau, Health Resources and Services Administration and the Department of Health and Human Services. Pediatrics. 1998;102(3): E29.
7. Malina RM, Katzmarzyk PT. Validity of the body mass index as an indicator of the risk and presence of overweight in adolescents. Am J Clin Nutr. 1999;70(1):131S–6S.
8. Obesity and Overweight Fact Sheet. 2021. Available from https://www.who.int/news-room/fact-sheets/detail/obesity-and-overweight
9. Lakshman R, Elks CE, Ong KK. Childhood obesity. Circulation. 2012;126(14):1770–9.
10. Hales CM, Freedman DS, Akinbami L, Wei R, Ogden CL. Evaluation of alternative body mass index (BMI) metrics to monitor weight status in children and adolescents with extremely high BMI using CDC BMI-for-age growth charts. Vital Health Stat. 2022;197:1–42.
11. Baioumi AYAA. Comparing measures of obesity: waist circumference, waist-hip, and waist-height ratios. In: Watson RR, editor. Nutrition in the prevention and treatment of abdominal obesity. 2nd ed. Academic Press; 2019. p. 29–40.
12. McCarthy HD, Ashwell M. A study of central fatness using waist-to-height ratios in UK children and adolescents over two decades supports the simple message – 'keep your waist circumference to less than half your height'. Int J Obes. 2006;30(6):988–92.
13. Stierman B, Afful J, Carroll MD, Chen T-C, Davy O, Fink S, Fryar CD, Gu Q, Hales CM, Hughes JP, Ostchega Y, Storandt RJ, Akinbami LJ. National health and nutrition examination survey 2017–March 2020 prepandemic data files development of files and prevalence estimates for selected health outcomes [06/14/2021]. Available from https://stacks.cdc.gov/view/cdc/106273
14. Ogden CL, Carroll MD, Lawman HG, Fryar CD, Kruszon-Moran D, Kit BK, et al. Trends in obesity prevalence among children and adolescents in the United States, 1988–1994 through 2013–2014. JAMA. 2016;315(21):2292–9.
15. Ogden CL, Fryar CD, Martin CB, Freedman DS, Carroll MD, Gu Q, et al. Trends in obesity prevalence by race and Hispanic origin-1999–2000 to 2017–2018. JAMA. 2020;324(12):1208–10.
16. Lange SJ, Kompaniyets L, Freedman DS, Kraus EM, Porter R, Dnp, et al. Longitudinal trends in body mass index before and during the COVID-19 pandemic

among persons aged 2-19 years – United States, 2018–2020. MMWR Morb Mortal Wkly Rep. 2021;70(37):1278–83.

17. Lobstein TaB H. Atlas of childhood obesity. London: World Obesity Federation; 2019.

18. Lobstein T, Jackson-Leach R, Moodie ML, Hall KD, Gortmaker SL, Swinburn BA, et al. Child and adolescent obesity: part of a bigger picture. Lancet. 2015;385(9986):2510–20.

19. Bullock A, Sheff K, Moore K, Manson S. Obesity and overweight in American Indian and Alaska native children, 2006–2015. Am J Public Health. 2017;107 (9):1502–7.

20. Ward ZJ, Long MW, Resch SC, Giles CM, Cradock AL, Gortmaker SL. Simulation of growth trajectories of childhood obesity into adulthood. N Engl J Med. 2017;377(22):2145–53.

21. Vazquez CE, Cubbin C. Socioeconomic status and childhood obesity: a review of literature from the past decade to inform intervention research. Curr Obes Rep. 2020;9(4):562–70.

22. Cunningham SA, Kramer MR, Narayan KM. Incidence of childhood obesity in the United States. N Engl J Med. 2014;370(5):403–11.

23. Woo JG, Zhang N, Fenchel M, Jacobs DR Jr, Hu T, Urbina EM, et al. Prediction of adult class II/III obesity from childhood BMI: the i3C consortium. Int J Obes. 2020;44(5):1164–72.

24. Bronfenbrenner U. Ecological systems theory (1992). In: Making human beings human: bioecological perspectives on human development, vol. 2005. Thousand Oaks: Sage Publications Ltd. p. 106–73.

25. Farooqi IS, O'Rahilly S. The genetics of obesity in humans. In: Feingold KR, Anawalt B, Blackman MR, Boyce A, Chrousos G, Corpas E, et al., editors. Endotext; 2000.

26. Styne DM, Arslanian SA, Connor EL, Farooqi IS, Murad MH, Silverstein JH, et al. Pediatric obesity-assessment, treatment, and prevention: an endocrine society clinical practice guideline. J Clin Endocrinol Metab. 2017;102(3):709–57.

27. Vaisse C, Clement K, Durand E, Hercberg S, Guy-Grand B, Froguel P. Melanocortin-4 receptor mutations are a frequent and heterogeneous cause of morbid obesity. J Clin Invest. 2000;106(2):253–62.

28. Magge SN, Zemel BS, Pipan ME, Gidding SS, Kelly A. Cardiometabolic risk and body composition in youth with down syndrome. Pediatrics. 2019;144(2)

29. Heymsfield SB, Avena NM, Baier L, Brantley P, Bray GA, Burnett LC, et al. Hyperphagia: current concepts and future directions proceedings of the 2nd international conference on hyperphagia. Obesity (Silver Spring). 2014;22(Suppl 1):S1–S17.

30. Bandini L, Danielson M, Esposito LE, Foley JT, Fox MH, Frey GC, et al. Obesity in children with developmental and/or physical disabilities. Disabil Health J. 2015;8(3):309–16.

31. Kahathuduwa CN, West BD, Blume J, Dharavath N, Moustaid-Moussa N, Mastergeorge A. The risk of

overweight and obesity in children with autism spectrum disorders: a systematic review and meta-analysis. Obes Rev. 2019;20(12):1667–79.

32. Cortese S, Moreira-Maia CR, St Fleur D, Morcillo-Penalver C, Rohde LA, Faraone SV. Association between ADHD and obesity: a systematic review and meta-analysis. Am J Psychiatry. 2016;173(1): 34–43.

33. Hales CN, Barker DJ. The thrifty phenotype hypothesis. Br Med Bull. 2001;60:5–20.

34. Calkins K, Devaskar SU. Fetal origins of adult disease. Curr Probl Pediatr Adolesc Health Care. 2011;41(6):158–76.

35. Boney CM, Verma A, Tucker R, Vohr BR. Metabolic syndrome in childhood: association with birth weight, maternal obesity, and gestational diabetes mellitus. Pediatrics. 2005;115(3):e290–6.

36. Catalano PM, Thomas A, Huston-Presley L, Amini SB. Phenotype of infants of mothers with gestational diabetes. Diabetes Care. 2007;30(Suppl 2):S156–60.

37. Heerwagen MJ, Miller MR, Barbour LA, Friedman JE. Maternal obesity and fetal metabolic programming: a fertile epigenetic soil. Am J Physiol Regul Integr Comp Physiol. 2010;299(3):R711–22.

38. Larque E, Labayen I, Flodmark CE, Lissau I, Czernin S, Moreno LA, et al. From conception to infancy – early risk factors for childhood obesity. Nat Rev Endocrinol. 2019;15(8):456–78.

39. Godfrey KM, Sheppard A, Gluckman PD, Lillycrop KA, Burdge GC, McLean C, et al. Epigenetic gene promoter methylation at birth is associated with child's later adiposity. Diabetes. 2011;60(5):1528–34.

40. Devaskar SU, Thamotharan M. Metabolic programming in the pathogenesis of insulin resistance. Rev Endocr Metab Disord. 2007;8(2):105–13.

41. Smith J, Cianflone K, Biron S, Hould FS, Lebel S, Marceau S, et al. Effects of maternal surgical weight loss in mothers on intergenerational transmission of obesity. J Clin Endocrinol Metab. 2009;94(11): 4275–83.

42. von Kries R, Toschke AM, Koletzko B, Slikker W Jr. Maternal smoking during pregnancy and childhood obesity. Am J Epidemiol. 2002;156(10): 954–61.

43. Zheng M, Lamb KE, Grimes C, Laws R, Bolton K, Ong KK, et al. Rapid weight gain during infancy and subsequent adiposity: a systematic review and meta-analysis of evidence. Obes Rev. 2018;19(3):321–32.

44. Woo Baidal JA, Locks LM, Cheng ER, Blake-Lamb TL, Perkins ME, Taveras EM. Risk factors for childhood obesity in the first 1,000 days: a systematic review. Am J Prev Med. 2016;50(6):761–79.

45. Riva A, Borgo F, Lassandro C, Verduci E, Morace G, Borghi E, et al. Pediatric obesity is associated with an altered gut microbiota and discordant shifts in firmicutes populations. Environ Microbiol. 2017;19 (1):95–105.

46. Luger M, Lafontan M, Bes-Rastrollo M, Winzer E, Yumuk V, Farpour-Lambert N. Sugar-sweetened

beverages and weight gain in children and adults: a systematic review from 2013 to 2015 and a comparison with previous studies. Obes Facts. 2017;10(6): 674–93.

47. Reedy J, Krebs-Smith SM. Dietary sources of energy, solid fats, and added sugars among children and adolescents in the United States. J Am Diet Assoc. 2010;110(10):1477–84.

48. Friel CP, Duran AT, Shechter A, Diaz KM. U.-S. children meeting physical activity, screen time, and sleep guidelines. Am J Prev Med. 2020;59(4): 513–21.

49. Poorolajal J, Sahraei F, Mohamdadi Y, Doosti-Irani A, Moradi L. Behavioral factors influencing childhood obesity: a systematic review and meta-analysis. Obes Res Clin Pract. 2020;14(2):109–18.

50. Ruan H, Xun P, Cai W, He K, Tang Q. Habitual sleep duration and risk of childhood obesity: systematic review and dose-response meta-analysis of prospective cohort studies. Sci Rep. 2015;5:16160.

51. Sweeney B, Kelly AS, San Giovanni CB, Kelsey MM, Skelton JA. Clinical approaches to minimize iatrogenic weight gain in children and adolescents. Clin Obes. 2021;11(1):e12417.

52. Kral TVE, Moore RH, Chittams J, Jones E, O'Malley L, Fisher JO. Identifying behavioral phenotypes for childhood obesity. Appetite. 2018;127: 87–96.

53. Bates CR, Buscemi J, Nicholson LM, Cory M, Jagpal A, Bohnert AM. Links between the organization of the family home environment and child obesity: a systematic review. Obes Rev. 2018;19(5): 716–27.

54. Nadhiroh SR, Djokosujono K, Utari DM. The association between secondhand smoke exposure and growth outcomes of children: a systematic literature review. Tob Induc Dis. 2020;18:12.

55. Burke NJ, Hellman JL, Scott BG, Weems CF, Carrion VG. The impact of adverse childhood experiences on an urban pediatric population. Child Abuse Negl. 2011;35(6):408–13.

56. Villegas-Navas V, Montero-Simo MJ, Araque-Padilla RA. The effects of foods embedded in entertainment media on children's food choices and food intake: a systematic review and meta-analyses. Nutrients. 2020;12(4)

57. Kakarala M, Keast DR, Hoerr S. Schoolchildren's consumption of competitive foods and beverages, excluding a la carte. J Sch Health. 2010;80(9):429–35; quiz 61–3

58. Li M, Mustillo S, Anderson J. Childhood poverty dynamics and adulthood overweight/obesity: unpacking the black box of childhood. Soc Sci Res. 2018;76:92–104.

59. Lee J, Kubik MY, Fulkerson JA. Diet quality and fruit, vegetable, and sugar-sweetened beverage consumption by household food insecurity among 8- to 12-year-old children during summer months. J Acad Nutr Diet. 2019;119(10):1695–702.

60. Weiss R, Bremer AA, Lustig RH. What is metabolic syndrome, and why are children getting it? Ann N Y Acad Sci. 2013;1281(1):123–40.

61. Hubers M, Geisler C, Plachta-Danielzik S, Muller MJ. Association between individual fat depots and cardio-metabolic traits in normal- and overweight children, adolescents and adults. Nutr Diabetes. 2017;7(5):e267.

62. Chung ST, Krenek A, Magge SN. Childhood obesity and cardiovascular Disease risk. Curr Atheroscler Rep. 2023;

63. Staiano AE, Katzmarzyk PT. Ethnic and sex differences in body fat and visceral and subcutaneous adiposity in children and adolescents. Int J Obes. 2012;36(10):1261–9.

64. Taksali SE, Caprio S, Dziura J, Dufour S, Cali AM, Goodman TR, et al. High visceral and low abdominal subcutaneous fat stores in the obese adolescent: a determinant of an adverse metabolic phenotype. Diabetes. 2008;57(2):367–71.

65. Magge SN, Goodman E, Armstrong SC, Committee On N, Section On E, Section OO. The metabolic syndrome in children and adolescents: shifting the focus to cardiometabolic risk factor clustering. Pediatrics. 2017;140(2)

66. Skinner AC, Perrin EM, Moss LA, Skelton JA. Cardiometabolic risks and severity of obesity in children and young adults. N Engl J Med. 2015;373 (14):1307–17.

67. Guzman-Limon M, Samuels J. Pediatric hypertension: diagnosis, evaluation, and treatment. Pediatr Clin N Am. 2019;66(1):45–57.

68. Seeman T, Hamdani G, Mitsnefes M. Hypertensive crisis in children and adolescents. Pediatr Nephrol. 2019;34(12):2523–37.

69. Flynn JT, Kaelber DC, Baker-Smith CM, Blowey D, Carroll AE, Daniels SR, et al. Clinical practice guideline for screening and management of high blood pressure in children and adolescents. Pediatrics. 2017;140(3)

70. Bussler S, Penke M, Flemming G, Elhassan YS, Kratzsch J, Sergeyev E, et al. Novel insights in the metabolic syndrome in childhood and adolescence. Horm Res Paediatr. 2017;88(3–4):181–93.

71. Wan Mahmud Sabri WMN, Mohamed RZ, Yaacob NM, Hussain S. Prevalence of metabolic syndrome and its associated risk factors in pediatric obesity. J ASEAN Fed Endocr Soc. 2022;37(1):24–30.

72. Nobili V, Alisi A, Valenti L, Miele L, Feldstein AE, Alkhouri N. NAFLD in children: new genes, new diagnostic modalities and new drugs. Nat Rev Gastroenterol Hepatol. 2019;16(9):517–30.

73. Shah J, Okubote T, Alkhouri N. Overview of updated practice guidelines for pediatric nonalcoholic fatty liver Disease. Gastroenterol Hepatol (NY). 2018;14 (7):407–14.

74. Vos MB, Abrams SH, Barlow SE, Caprio S, Daniels SR, Kohli R, et al. NASPGHAN clinical practice guideline for the diagnosis and treatment of

nonalcoholic fatty liver disease in children: recommendations from the expert Committee on NAFLD (ECON) and the North American Society of Pediatric Gastroenterology, Hepatology and Nutrition (NASPGHAN). J Pediatr Gastroenterol Nutr. 2017;64(2):319–34.

75. Gouthro K, Slowik JM. Pediatric obstructive sleep Apnea. Treasure Island: StatPearls; 2023.

76. Bitners AC, Arens R. Evaluation and management of children with obstructive sleep apnea syndrome. Lung. 2020;198(2):257–70.

77. Malem A, Sheth T, Muthusamy B. Paediatric idiopathic intracranial hypertension (IIH) – a review. Life (Basel). 2021;11(7)

78. Trent M, Gordon CM. Diagnosis and management of polycystic ovary syndrome in adolescents. Pediatrics. 2020;145(Suppl 2):S210–S8.

79. Ibanez L, Oberfield SE, Witchel S, Auchus RJ, Chang RJ, Codner E, et al. An international consortium update: pathophysiology, diagnosis, and treatment of polycystic ovarian syndrome in adolescence. Horm Res Paediatr. 2017;88(6):371–95.

80. Bremer AA. Polycystic ovary syndrome in the pediatric population. Metab Syndr Relat Disord. 2010;8(5):375–94.

81. Zdanowicz K, Daniluk J, Lebensztejn DM, Daniluk U. The etiology of cholelithiasis in children and adolescents – a literature review. Int J Mol Sci. 2022;23(21)

82. Karami H, Kianifar HR, Karami S. Cholelithiasis in children: a diagnostic and therapeutic approach. J Pediatr Rev. 2017;5(1)

83. Peck DM, Voss LM, Voss TT. Slipped capital femoral epiphysis: diagnosis and management. Am Fam Physician. 2017;95(12):779–84.

84. De Leucio A. Blount disease. Treasure Island: StatPearls; 2023.

85. Miller L, Campo JV. Depression in adolescents. N Engl J Med. 2021;385(5):445–9.

86. Expert Panel on Integrated Guidelines for Cardiovascular H, Risk Reduction in C, Adolescents, National Heart L, Blood I. Expert panel on integrated guidelines for cardiovascular health and risk reduction in children and adolescents: summary report. Pediatrics. 2011;128 Suppl 5(Suppl 5):S213–56.

87. Witchel SF, Oberfield S, Rosenfield RL, Codner E, Bonny A, Ibanez L, et al. The diagnosis of polycystic ovary syndrome during adolescence. Horm Res Paediatr. 2015;

88. Doyle MM. Anxiety disorders in children. Pediatr Rev. 2022;43(11):618–30.

89. Gujral J, Gupta J. Pediatric dyslipidemia. Treasure Island: StatPearls; 2023.

90. Stewart J, McCallin T, Martinez J, Chacko S, Yusuf S. Hyperlipidemia. Pediatr Rev. 2020;41(8):393–402.

91. ElSayed NA, Aleppo G, Aroda VR, Bannuru RR, Brown FM, Bruemmer D, et al. 2. Classification and diagnosis of diabetes: standards of care in diabetes-2023. Diabetes Care. 2023;46(Suppl 1): S19–40.

92. ElSayed NA, Aleppo G, Aroda VR, Bannuru RR, Brown FM, Bruemmer D, et al. 14. Children and adolescents: standards of care in diabetes-2023. Diabetes Care. 2023;46(Suppl 1):S230–S53.

93. Suzuki A, Abdelmalek MF, Schwimmer JB, Lavine JE, Scheimann AO, Unalp-Arida A, et al. Association between puberty and features of nonalcoholic fatty liver disease. Clin Gastroenterol Hepatol. 2012;10(7): 786–94.

94. Skinner AC, Staiano AE, Armstrong SC, Barkin SL, Hassink SG, Moore JE, et al. Appraisal of clinical care practices for child obesity treatment. Part II: Comorbidities. Pediatrics. 2023;151(2)

95. Bitners AC, Sin S, Agrawal S, Lee S, Udupa JK, Tong Y, et al. Effect of sleep on upper airway dynamics in obese adolescents with obstructive sleep apnea syndrome. Sleep. 2020;43(10)

96. Anderson EL, Howe LD, Jones HE, Higgins JP, Lawlor DA, Fraser A. The prevalence of non-alcoholic fatty liver disease in children and adolescents: a systematic review and meta-analysis. PLoS One. 2015;10(10):e0140908.

97. Andersen IG, Holm JC, Homoe P. Obstructive sleep apnea in children and adolescents with and without obesity. Eur Arch Otorhinolaryngol. 2019;276(3): 871–8.

98. Kilgore KP, Lee MS, Leavitt JA, Mokri B, Hodge DO, Frank RD, et al. Re-evaluating the incidence of idiopathic intracranial hypertension in an era of increasing obesity. Ophthalmology. 2017;124(5): 697–700.

99. Styne DM, Arslanian SA, Connor EL, Farooqi IS, Murad MH, Silverstein JH, et al. Response to letter: "pediatric obesity-assessment, treatment, and prevention: an endocrine society clinical practice guideline". J Clin Endocrinol Metab. 2017;102(6):2123–4.

100. Armstrong S, Lazorick S, Hampl S, Skelton JA, Wood C, Collier D, et al. Physical examination findings among children and adolescents with obesity: an evidence-based review. Pediatrics. 2016;137(2): e20151766.

101. Miclea D, Alkhzouz C, Bucerzan S, Grigorescu-Sido P. Genetic testing in pediatric endocrine pathology. Med Pharm Rep. 2021;94(Suppl 1):S15–S8.

102. Lobelo F, Muth ND, Hanson S, Nemeth BA, Council On Sports M, Fitness, et al. Physical activity assessment and counseling in pediatric clinical settings. Pediatrics. 2020;145(3)

103. Hornberger LL, Lane MA, Committee OA. Identification and management of eating disorders in children and adolescents. Pediatrics. 2021;147(1)

104. Kelly AS, Bensignor MO, Hsia DS, Shoemaker AH, Shih W, Peterson C, et al. Phentermine/topiramate for the treatment of adolescent obesity. NEJM Evid. 2022;1(6)

105. Weghuber D, Barrett T, Barrientos-Perez M, Gies I, Hesse D, Jeppesen OK, et al. Once-weekly semaglutide in adolescents with obesity. N Engl J Med. 2022;387(24):2245–57.

106. Chanoine JP, Hampl S, Jensen C, Boldrin M, Hauptman J. Effect of orlistat on weight and body composition in obese adolescents: a randomized controlled trial. JAMA. 2005;293(23):2873–83.

107. Kelly AS, Auerbach P, Barrientos-Perez M, Gies I, Hale PM, Marcus C, et al. A randomized, controlled trial of Liraglutide for adolescents with obesity. N Engl J Med. 2020;382(22):2117–28.

108. Wilding J, Van Gaal L, Rissanen A, Vercruysse F, Fitchet M, Group O-S. A randomized double-blind placebo-controlled study of the long-term efficacy and safety of topiramate in the treatment of obese subjects. Int J Obes Relat Metab Disord. 2004;28(11):1399–410.

109. Fox CK, Kaizer AM, Rudser KD, Nathan BM, Gross AC, Sunni M, et al. Meal replacements followed by topiramate for the treatment of adolescent severe obesity: a pilot randomized controlled trial. Obesity (Silver Spring). 2016;24(12):2553–61.

110. Haqq AM, Chung WK, Dollfus H, Haws RM, Martos-Moreno GA, Poitou C, et al. Efficacy and safety of setmelanotide, a melanocortin-4 receptor agonist, in patients with Bardet-Biedl syndrome and Alstrom syndrome: a multicentre, randomised, double-blind, placebo-controlled, phase 3 trial with an open-label period. Lancet Diabetes Endocrinol. 2022;10(12):859–68.

111. Clement K, van den Akker E, Argente J, Bahm A, Chung WK, Connors H, et al. Efficacy and safety of setmelanotide, an MC4R agonist, in individuals with severe obesity due to LEPR or POMC deficiency: single-arm, open-label, multicentre, phase 3 trials. Lancet Diabetes Endocrinol. 2020;8(12):960–70.

112. Ryder JR, Kaizer A, Rudser KD, Gross A, Kelly AS, Fox CK. Effect of phentermine on weight reduction in a pediatric weight management clinic. Int J Obes. 2017;41(1):90–3.

113. Lewis KH, Fischer H, Ard J, Barton L, Bessesen DH, Daley MF, et al. Safety and effectiveness of longer-term phentermine use: clinical outcomes from an electronic health record cohort. Obesity (Silver Spring). 2019;27(4):591–602.

114. Wilson DM, Abrams SH, Aye T, Lee PD, Lenders C, Lustig RH, et al. Metformin extended release treatment of adolescent obesity: a 48-week randomized, double-blind, placebo-controlled trial with 48-week follow-up. Arch Pediatr Adolesc Med. 2010;164(2):116–23.

115. Yanovski JA, Krakoff J, Salaita CG, McDuffie JR, Kozlosky M, Sebring NG, et al. Effects of metformin on body weight and body composition in obese insulin resistant children: a randomized clinical trial. Diabetes. 2011;60(2):477–85.

116. Cheplapharm. Xenical (orlistat) [package insert]. U.S. Food and Drug Administration website. https://www.accessdata.fda.gov/drugsatfda_docs/label/2012/020766s029lbl.pdf. Revised January 2012.

117. Novo Nordisk. Saxenda (liraglutide) [package insert]. U.S. Food and Drug Administration website. https://www.accessdata.fda.gov/drugsatfda_docs/label/2020/206321s012s013s014lbl.pdf. Revised December 2020.

118. Novo Nordisk. Wegovy (semaglutide) [package insert]. U.S. Food and Drug Administration website. https://www.accessdata.fda.gov/drugsatfda_docs/label/2022/215256s005lbl.pdf. Revised December 2022.

119. Rhythm Pharmaceuticals. Imcivree (setmelanotide) [package insert]. U.S. Food and Drug Administration website. https://www.accessdata.fda.gov/drugsatfda_docs/label/2022/213793s001lbl.pdf. Revised June 2022.

120. Teva. Adipex-P (phentermine) [package insert]. U.S. Food and Drug Administration website Revised January 2012.

121. Janssen Pharmaceuticals. Topamax (topiramate) [package insert]. U.S. Food and Drug Administration website. https://www.accessdata.fda.gov/drugsatfda_docs/label/2012/085128s065lbl.pdf. Revised October 2012.

122. Vivus Medical. Qsymia (phentermine and topiramate) [package insert]. U.S. Food and Drug Administration website. https://www.accessdata.fda.gov/drugsatfda_docs/label/2022/022580s021lbl.pdf. Revised June 2022.

123. Merck Pharmaceuticals. Glucophage (metformin) [package insert]. U.S. Food and Drug Administration website. https://www.accessdata.fda.gov/drugsatfda_docs/label/2000/21202lbl.pdf. Revised October 2000.

124. Farooqi S, Miller JL, Ohayon O, Yuan G, Stewart M, Scimia C, et al. Effects of setmelanotide in patients with POMC, PCSK1, or LEPR heterozygous deficiency obesity in a phase 2 study. J Endocr Soc. 2021;5(Supplement_1):A669–A70.

125. Pratt JSA, Browne A, Browne NT, Bruzoni M, Cohen M, Desai A, et al. ASMBS pediatric metabolic and bariatric surgery guidelines, 2018. Surg Obes Relat Dis. 2018;14(7):882–901.

126. Inge TH, Courcoulas AP, Jenkins TM, Michalsky MP, Helmrath MA, Brandt ML, et al. Weight loss and health status 3 years after bariatric surgery in adolescents. N Engl J Med. 2016;374(2):113–23.

127. Inge TH, Courcoulas AP, Jenkins TM, Michalsky MP, Brandt ML, Xanthakos SA, et al. Five-year outcomes of gastric bypass in adolescents as compared with adults. N Engl J Med. 2019;380(22):2136–45.

Global, National, and Community Obesity Prevention Programs

41

Regien Biesma and Mark Hanson

Contents

Abstract

Although some high-income countries have managed to flatten the rate of increase in their (already high) obesity rates, no country in the world has been able to reverse the obesity epidemic. Obesity prevention is not an easy task because it requires multiple population-wide policy interventions targeted at global, national, and community settings. Public health strategies must be comprehensive and multisectoral and range from improving individual behavior to modifying the obesogenic environment, from promoting an individual responsibility to changing health policy, and from targeting adults to adopting a life-course approach. The latter approach has recently been recognized in global strategies as critical to curb the obesity prevention. It stresses the importance of early intervention during the life

R. Biesma (✉)
Department of Epidemiology and Public Health Medicine, Royal College of Surgeons in Ireland, Dublin, Ireland
e-mail: Rbiesma@rcsi.ie

M. Hanson
Institute of Developmental Sciences, Faculty of Medicine, University of Southampton, Southampton, UK
e-mail: m.hanson@soton.ac.uk

© Springer Nature Switzerland AG 2023
R. S. Ahima (ed.), *Metabolic Syndrome*,
https://doi.org/10.1007/978-3-031-40116-9_47

cycle to preventing obesity in the population. Interventions targeting the preconception period aim to assist parents-to-be in the best shape as possible, preferably resulting in women with a healthy prepregnancy BMI, lower gestational weight gain, and postpartum weight retention. Interventions in the postnatal phase aim to ensure the provision of sufficient and nutritious food to infants, children and adolescents to promote healthy growth. Comprehensive food policies are needed to create an enabling environment for infants and children so that they can acquire healthy food preferences and targeted actions to enable disadvantaged populations to overcome barriers to meeting healthy preferences. We argue that a focus on these so-called early life risk factors is essential in obesity prevention and could be the missing link in stopping the vicious cycle of obesity begetting obesity.

Keywords

Early life · Life course · Prevention strategies · Obesity

Introduction

Obesity is now one of the most important public health threats worldwide and is a major risk factor of noncommunicable diseases (NCDs) [101]. The worldwide prevalence of obesity has more than doubled since 1980, with 1.9 billion adults aged 18 years and older overweight in 2014 [102]. A particular concern is childhood obesity. More and more children are becoming obese, especially in low- and middle-income countries, and these children are more likely to stay obese in adult life [63].

The obesity epidemic is a complex multifactorial health problem, affecting society as well as individuals, and single, isolated interventions are unlikely to work [100]. Interventions need to address behavioral, cultural, social, political, economic, environmental, and physiological factors and their interrelationships throughout the life course. Governments, health-care organizations, schools, work settings, neighborhoods, communities, individuals, and families need to work together to create an environment where the healthy option is the default choice [29]. Prevention starting early in life, even before birth, is likely to be the most cost-effective and feasible approach for many countries [4, 19, 34, 62]. This chapter provides an overview of promising strategies for obesity prevention at global, national, and community levels. First, we outline the life-course approach with a focus on early prevention of obesity. Then, we describe the guiding principles for the development of a global NCD prevention strategy, followed by national approaches for population-based obesity prevention. In the last section we will look at community-based interventions in early life.

Life-Course Approach

Evidence is accumulating that obesity should be prevented using a life-course approach, beginning in early life and continuing throughout every stage of the life course [30, 41, 68, 91]. Perez-Escamilla and Kac [68] described two evidence-based cycles that help to understand the need for an early focus of the life-course approach [68]. The first cycle in the life-course approach is the "maternal" cycle when prepregnancy overweight (especially primiparous) women are more likely to gain and retain excessive weight during pregnancy and after delivery. The second or "offspring" cycle indicates that the children of prepregnancy overweight women have an increased risk for storing excessive fat themselves, especially if the mother gained excessive weight during pregnancy, and the infant is not (exclusively) breastfed for the first 6 months and is introduced early to solids and sugar-sweetened beverages. Such infants are then more likely to grow rapidly in the first year of life, which in itself is an important risk factor for the development of obesity in early childhood. If during the toddler and preschool period exposure to an obesogenic environment is continued, the child is more likely to remain overweight or obese during the primary school and adolescent years and indeed as an adult.

Socioeconomic status (SES) is an important mediator in this intergenerational cycle. Young low-SES mothers are less likely to breastfeed, and if they do, for a shorter duration, they are more likely to start early with formula and cow's

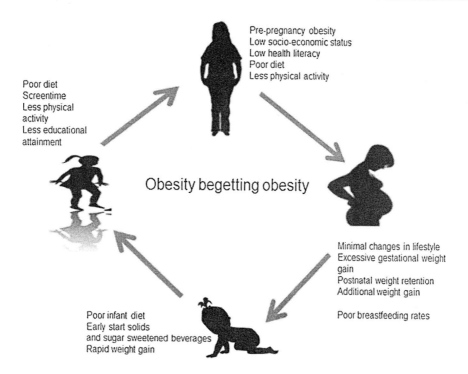

Fig. 1 Life-course approach to obesity

milk consumption [71]. These mothers are more likely to be overweight and obese and less likely to adhere to lifestyle guidelines. This all implies a vicious cycle of "obesity begetting obesity": a girl born to an overweight or obese low-SES mother is very likely that she herself will enter her first pregnancy being overweight and obese (see Fig. 1). The pattern of "obesity begetting obesity" in low-SES mothers has been mostly apparent in high-income countries but is now rapidly emerging in low- and middle-income countries affected by globalization, urbanization, and economic development. These countries are now faced with a double burden of over- and undernutrition which both have major implications for the obesity epidemic [6, 68].

Obesity: A Global Problem Requires a Global Strategy

There are several reasons why a global view of obesity prevention is helpful. The first is that obesity is genuinely a global problem, because the prevalence of overweight and obesity is static or increasing in every country so far examined. National, regional, and global trends in body mass index (BMI) since 1980, from systematic analysis of health examination surveys and epidemiological studies with 960 country-years and 9.1 million participants from 199 countries and territories, showed large variations in the rates of overweight and obesity globally. 19 countries showed a nonsignificant decrease since 1980 while at the other extreme, the mean BMI increased at the rate of 2.0 kg/m^2 per decade over this period in adults over the age of 20 years [27]. The global trend between 1980 and 2008 was 0.4 kg/m^2. Recent analyses have indicated the impact of these trends and emphasized the need for global action [64].

A second reason is that the increase in overweight and obesity is associated with increases in NCDs in every country. However, these global trends mask substantial regional differences in risk. Some Asian populations show large increases in prevalence of NCDs such as metabolic syndrome at much lower levels of BMI or waist-hip ratio than Caucasian populations [59]. Asian Americans have greater prevalence of metabolic syndrome despite lower BMI [59]. In part, this appears to be due to greater abdominal fat and less skeletal muscle in the former, constituting two risk factors for type 2 diabetes which starts in early development (the "thin-fat" Indian baby syndrome) [52]. A further complication is that, at a similar BMI, ethnic groups in the same country can show different patterns of disease [36].

A third reason is that both basic and clinical research indicate that there are fundamental developmental reasons for the increase in obesity globally. They include the effects of "mismatch" which occurs when aspects of the developmental environment such as nutrition, which induce adaptive changes in the phenotype of the offspring, are not met by similar aspects in the postnatal environment [33]. The changes in body composition and physiological control mechanisms in individuals exposed to a poor nutritional level prenatally leave them "mismatched," i.e., unprepared to meet the challenges of the contemporary, urban obesogenic environment. This mismatch is an important feature of populations going through socioeconomic and nutritional transitions and of vulnerable groups such as economic migrants and ethnic minority groups [24, 49]. The underlying mechanisms are beginning to be elucidated [43], revealing how the human species appears to have evolved a propensity to deposit body fat during prenatal development, perhaps to protect brain growth postnatally [51]. The fact that these processes appear to be common to members of our species to different degrees in different settings and that their operation may be identified in early life through the use of biomarkers (especially epigenetic changes) [35] provides a mechanistic basis for believing that global interventions may be feasible.

Need for Early Life Interventions Now Recognized in Global NCD Strategies

These insights have become clearer over the first decade of the twenty-first century. The greater health problem posed by NCDs than by communicable disease, accidents, and other causes of mortality in both men and women globally was not identified in the Millennium Development Goals (MDGs), despite some related to maternal and child health. Nonetheless, the challenge posed by obesity and associated NCDs, in particular in developing countries and other deprived populations, was clearly evident from the Global Strategy for the Prevention and Control of NCDs 2000 and the Global Strategy on Diet, Physical Activity, and Health 2004 [98]. In 2008, the need for population-based prevention and a multisectoral approach as being vital to addressing rising levels of noncommunicable diseases was translated into concrete action in the World Health Organization (World Health Organization) Action Plan for the Global Strategy for the Prevention and Control of NCDs 2008–2013 [99] and endorsed at the Sixty-First World Health Assembly in May 2008. In September 2011, the High-Level Meeting of the United Nations General Assembly convened a summit to address the issue, resulting in the Political Declaration of the Prevention and Control of Noncommunicable Diseases of September 2011. There are several new elements in the UNGA Political Declaration, of which one of the most striking refers to the need to recognize the part played by early developmental origins of conditions such as obesity in the problem. Phrased in this way, it is clear that interventions can share common elements globally and that a life-course approach is needed to take them forward. This theme is very much taken up in subsequent World Health Organization recommendations, for example, the Global Action Plan for the Prevention and Control of NCDs 2013–2020 [99]. This Action Plan identified life-course approach as an overarching principle and recognized that interventions in early life often offer the best chance for primary prevention.

In parallel, a range of nongovernmental organizations (NGOs), civil society organizations (CSOs), and other organizations have produced reports on the global obesity crisis, for example, the International Obesity Task Force (IOTF) [85] and the US Institute of Medicine (IOM) [48]. These draw attention to the multifactorial basis for the epidemic, from international, national, societal, community, family, and personal components, each of which has to be addressed simultaneously, albeit with differing emphases in different countries, if the problem is to be effectively addressed. A picture therefore emerges of a truly integrated approach to the problem across both temporal (life course) and spatial (from personal to public) domains. The economic benefits of intervention have been calculated [22] and make a strong case for interventions. This is strengthened still further by the clear perception that obesity and associated NCDs are associated with social inequalities in health [58] and thus raise rights and ethical issues.

The life-course aspect of obesity prevention focuses attention on starting early, for example, in childhood. In 2014, The Director-General of World Health Organization established a Commission on Ending Childhood Obesity (ECHO), which has met several times, consulted widely, and aims to report in mid-2016. The Commission's Interim Report in 2015 identified key issues including the need to tackle the obesogenic environment in which children and adolescents grow and develop and the importance of a life-course approach to address the risk factors for childhood obesity [103]. One of the thorny issues with which the ECHO Commission will have to engage, as will the architects and actors of the SDGs at all levels, is the role of the private sector, especially the food companies. The global multinational food companies have been pilloried repeatedly, "big food" being likened to "big pharma" in terms of conflicts of interest [7, 86]. Many proposals to restrict their influence through legislation, taxation of unhealthy products, have been made [17], although questions have been raised about whether such fiscal measures may merely widen inequalities in health [83] and they may not be compatible with trade agreements, UN member state financial policies, etc. Some successes in this respect have been achieved (e.g., Mexico's soft drink tax has been effective in reducing soda consumption and in turn had an effect on the rate of obesity). It seems likely that a more inclusive approach to collaboration to address the problem with "as appropriate" the private sector as suggested in the UNGA Political Declaration of 2011 will be needed. New frameworks for public-private partnerships with the food industry, to provide transparency and control of conflicts of interest, are now being discussed [1].

National Obesity Prevention: Focusing on the Obesogenic Environment

Traditionally, public health strategies to promote healthy lifestyles have targeted the individual [8]. However, recently this paradigm is shifting toward the environment in which individuals make choices on food consumption and physical activity. Creating supportive environments requires the use of policy instruments, such as laws and regulations, taxation and subsidies, and advocacy to the public and private sector and other jurisdictions [100]. They involve shifting the responsibility of healthy behavior from individual to the national level and typically target the so-called social determinants of health [5].

Although there are several key players in obesity prevention at the national level, such as the government, the private sector, and civil society/nongovernmental organizations (NGOs), governments generally lead and drive policy changes [100]. Ministries of Health play a leading role in developing and implementing health policies and bringing together other ministries, the private sector, health professional bodies, academics, and NGOs that are needed to effectively address obesity and NCD risk in subpopulations [87]. However, the determinants of obesity are complex, and a key challenge for governments is to make the most appropriate and effective mix of multiple policy-based obesity prevention interventions, across different settings, levels, and sectors. Strategies are usually combined so as to complement each other.

National Policies for Obesity Prevention

There are different public health strategies for risk reduction available at the national level. These are usually categorized as (i) "upstream" policies which are broad social and economic conditions (socio-ecological approach) that are indirectly influencing population behavior, (ii) "midstream" or behavioral policies which are directly influencing population behaviors, and (iii) "downstream" policies which support health service and clinical interventions (typically individual based) [76]. The upstream (socio-ecological) approach aims to influence the underlying determinants of health in society and represents the greatest potential for obesity prevention by creating environments that support healthy diets and physical activity [17, 23, 77]. This approach is in line with Geoffrey Rose's original idea of "population-based prevention approaches" which focus on changing the contextual conditions of risk rather than the individual risk per se [75]. Upstream policies target the food environments, physical activity environments, and the broader socioeconomic environments (such as taxation, employment, education, housing, and welfare) and can improve outcomes across all socioeconomic groups, both adults and children, and often with greater cost-effectiveness than individual interventions [100].

The midstream policy approach aims at influencing directly the behavior of subpopulations to improve eating and physical activity. In order to influence behavior directly, interventions need to take place in settings where people eat and/or can be physically active, such as schools, workplaces, households, hospitals, prisons, and military establishments [84]. Government policy instruments to influence behavior directly are almost exclusively based on education- and campaign-based programs. Downstream policy approaches supporting health services and medical interventions are predominantly focused on obesity management rather than prevention. These are typically individual based rather than population based. Both downstream investments (individualized health care) and upstream investments (high-level policy and legislation) are both needed to alter obesogenic environments by providing incentives for healthy eating and physical activity [92]. In addition, integrated healthy living strategies (healthy eating, active living, and mental health) are needed to address common risk factors associated with obesity and related chronic diseases [28]. In the next section, we will focus on population-based prevention strategies with specific emphasis on childhood and discuss the most important "upstream" and "midstream" interventions: policies influencing the food environment, policies influencing physical activity environment, and social marketing campaigns.

Population-Wide Policies Influencing the Food Environment

The aim of these policies is to alter the food environment so that the *healthy choice will become the easy choice*. They are based on national nutrition guidelines, food selection guides, and policies relating to breastfeeding and infant nutrition [48, 100]. For example, the Institute of Medicine (IOM) in the United States offers detailed recommendations, strategies, and action steps for implementation by key stakeholders and sectors for accelerating progress in obesity prevention [48]. Evidence suggests that a number of policy interventions in food environments are cost-effective and have the potential to prevent obesity in the population [53]. These are related to combined efforts to reduce unhealthy food and beverage options and to increase the availability and reduce the prices of healthier food and beverage options [96]. Examples are regulations to reduce food marketing to children, "nutrition labeling" to encourage consumers to make healthy food choices, and increased taxation on obesogenic food and price subsidies or production incentives for foods that are encouraged [13, 98, 100].

Hawkes, Smith, et al. [44] went one step further and claimed that food policies could be more effective and sustainable in preventing obesity if focused on the interaction between human food preferences and the early life environment in which those preferences are learned, expressed, and reassessed [44]. Comprehensive food policies are needed that create an enabling environment for infants and children to learn healthy food preferences and targeted actions that enable disadvantaged populations to overcome barriers to meeting healthy preferences. This is an important addition to the literature as antenatal and infant determinants of appetite and food preference persist through adult life [3, 9, 18]. It is well known that unhealthy behavior is highly habitual, evolves in early life, and, once established, is not easy to change. Again, this suggests that the most effective time to instigate new interventions to prevent obesity is early in life, before appetite control, food preference, and fat cell number are established, to make sure that *the healthy choice* is not the easy choice but also *the preferred choice* [44].

Population-Wide Policies Influencing Physical Activity Environment

Physical activity is important for healthy growth and development of young children. It is recommended that children and adults accumulate at least 60 min of moderate to vigorous physical activity every day [100]. National policies should include the encouragement of physical activity in early life as it can help reduce stunting and encourage healthy linear growth.

Furthermore, there is a need for multifaceted physical activity policies to increase active and safe methods of transport, to encourage physical activity in school settings, and to provide sport and recreation facilities available for all [100]. A Cochrane systematic review found that school-based physical activity interventions can be effective in increasing duration of physical activity, reducing time per day spent watching television, and increasing physical fitness levels of children [21]. The evidence also suggested that children exposed to school-based physical activity interventions are approximately three times more likely to engage in moderate to vigorous physical activity during the school day than those not exposed. These are discussed further in the section on community-based interventions.

Mass Media or Social Marketing Campaigns

Mass media or social marketing campaigns are tools, based on commercial marketing approaches, to increase awareness and change attitudes toward diet and physical activity of the whole population [38]. It is an important task of the government to use effective social marketing campaigns to motivate individuals to adopt healthy lifestyles and create healthy environments, such as educating children about selecting healthy food [37]. An example is the use of national health brands or logos to assist consumers in making healthy food choices. However, evidence is limited on the (long-term) effect of social marketing campaigns promoting healthy diets [50, 54], and some have argued that social marketing campaigns focusing on the undesirability of obesity can be harmful [71].

It has been suggested that the promotion of a single simple message with frequent exposure to increase, for example, the consumption of low-fat milk or to promote regular physical activity is most effective [77]. Until recently, social marketing campaigns have primarily aimed to influence individual behavior (also called the "downstream approach"), but recently this has shifted toward targeting the environment as the means to bringing about desired change (the "upstream approach") [46]. Some have argued that social marketing campaigns should first consider the social determinants of health before attempting to persuade individuals to change their behavior [76].

Community Obesity Prevention: Focusing on the Child, Families, and Communities

Community-based interventions are multicomponent interventions and programs, typically tailored to the local environment. Community-based interventions have been demonstrated to be successful when applied in multiple childhood settings, including home, schools, and neighborhoods. First, we discuss community-based obesity prevention interventions targeting the maternal cycle followed by interventions aimed at the offspring cycle.

Obesity Prevention Via Addressing Maternal Factors

Maternal obesity has become a major public health issue worldwide and affects health of both the mother and her offspring [16]. Maternal obesity may result from prepregnancy obesity or excessive weight gain. High prepregnancy BMI increases the risk of gestational diabetes mellitus (GDM) and type 2 diabetes in women [14], while excessive weight gain increases the risk of fetal macrosomia, maternal overweight, and postpartum weight retention [78]. During the postpartum period, postpartum weight retention and additional weight gain increase the risk of becoming obese [79]. Moreover, children who are exposed to an intrauterine environment of maternal hyperglycemia are at increased risk of developing obesity later in life [16, 26, 94]. This suggests that pregnancy is a key period in shaping a healthy future of mothers and their children. However, it has not been easy to influence health-related behavior in pregnant women effectively. There is the widespread social belief that pregnant women should "eat for two" and rest physically [16]. On the other hand, pregnancy is a time when behavior can be challenged as a woman is more likely to improve her lifestyle for her baby's health [47].

Socioeconomic inequalities play an important role in this scenario, with the highest prevalence rates of obesity among low-SES mothers and their children [45]. Nutrition knowledge is poorest in low-SES mothers and affects intake of fruit and vegetables and overall diet quality [10]. This suggests that tailored interventions may be needed to improve maternal literacy in lower socioeconomic groups.

Pregnancy Interventions

Women who gain excessive weight during pregnancy are more likely to retain and gain weight after delivery, creating a vicious circle of increasing body weight and obesity [55]. To date, evidence on the effective pregnancy interventions on dietary habits, physical activity, and gestational weight gain has been limited and inconsistent [66]. Some dietary and lifestyle interventions in pregnancy have been found to reduce total gestational weight gain and long-term postpartum weight retention [2, 39]. Specific components of these successful interventions were weight monitoring, setting weight goals, education counseling, and physical activity settings [82, 89].

Furthermore, there has been some success with antenatal lifestyle interventions in preventing excessive gestational weight gain in overweight/obese women and reducing the risk of GDM [70]. However, it has been suggested that interventions in overweight/obese women need to be more intense than in normal-weight women and involve frequent contact and emphasis on caloric restriction [89]. This may limit the possibility of such labor-intensive and costly interventions being implemented at wider, national scale.

Preconception Interventions

Many young adults do not realize that their body weight and lifestyle during the reproductive years affect their future health and that of their children (Krummel 2007). Targeting lifestyles of adolescents and young couples before they become pregnant to reduce prepregnancy BMI would perhaps be the ideal intervention [12, 41]. To date, there are few preconception interventions. Pregnancies are often unplanned, and even women who are planning to conceive often do not contact a health professional [12]. As a result, it is difficult to target women before conception.

Focusing interventions on adolescents and young couples would require the promotion of health literacy for reducing risks of obesity and NCDs for the mother and her child(dren), such as the importance of appropriate weight gain before and during pregnancy and breastfeeding [41]. It is well known that parents with low literacy have less health knowledge and are more likely to negatively affect their children's health compared with parents with higher literacy [20]. Renkert and Nutbeam defined maternal health literacy as "the cognitive and social skills that determine the motivation and ability of women to gain access to, understand, and use information in ways that promote and maintain their health and that of their children" [72]. A systematic review on interventions to improve health literacy and child health outcomes found that education classes, clearly written instructions, and counseling for parents improved health outcomes in their children [20]. In improving a woman's ability and motivation to adhere to health recommendations for herself and her child, it is critical to address barriers to change, such as time limitations, social pressure, and a perceived lack of control [41]. It is therefore important in intervention design to incorporate components to tackle barriers to adhere and improve attendance [42].

Postpartum Interventions

An additional approach to interventions targeting couples before pregnancy would be to target maternal weight after delivery [12]. It is known that women in the highest BMI category are more likely to retain weight and to be insufficiently active postpartum, especially if they were less active before pregnancy, had more gestational weight gain, worked greater hours, and reported lack of childcare as a barrier [67]. Clearly it is difficult to help mothers with young children to improve aspects of their behavior.

Indeed, the number of experimental interventions for promoting physical activity and healthy eating among new mothers is limited, and attrition is very high in most of the interventions [42]. Effective intervention components targeted toward mothers aimed to promote lifestyle change including nutrition advice sessions, use of peer educators and strategies to promote targeted food choice by reducing costs, and those to overcome barriers to physical activity and healthy eating. It seems that, in particular for intervening in the postpartum period, it is essential to address the key barriers to postpartum weight loss, such as locality, childcare provision, and including the whole family in goal setting and behavior change [91].

Interventions to Promote Breastfeeding and Delay Introduction of Solid Foods

The health benefits of breastfeeding for both mother and child are well documented. Babies who are not breastfed exclusively for at least 4 months are more likely to suffer health problems, such as gastroenteritis, and develop obesity. Despite that, many women chose to formula-feed their babies. The reasons are likely to be sociocultural and may include attitudes of family and close friends, attitudes towards breastfeeding in public, and employment practices [80]. Helping and supporting women to initiate and prolong breastfeeding is therefore critical. There are a number of global strategies aimed at enabling mothers to breastfeed babies, such as the World Health Organization/UNICEF *International Code of Marketing of Breast-Milk Substitutes* [97] and the *Baby-Friendly Hospital Initiative* (BFHI) [104]. However, breastfeeding initiation rates are still relatively low, especially in low social class,

income, and education levels and among overweight and obese women [12]. Interventions that have shown to have an impact on breastfeeding rates typically included needs-based and informal peer support in the antenatal and postnatal period [15, 25]. Peer support can also help mothers to breastfeed for longer. Furthermore, there is evidence of a positive association between antenatal care and breastfeeding among low-SES women. It seems that interventions to improve health literacy and attitudes are key to helping mothers among all population groups to make informed choices about breastfeeding and infant feeding practices.

Obesity Prevention in Children

Home Settings

The home and family environment have the most important and lasting influence on the development of children's health in general and eating and lifestyles in particular [31]. Parental weight has been found one of the most robust predictors of child's weight [69]. Parents determine their child's lifestyle and parenting and home life, especially in early childhood [56]. Parenting style, parental role modeling, family lifestyle, responsive feeding, infant feeding, use of food for non-nutritional purposes, exposure to television, and sleeping habits are all risk factors in the home environment that increase the risk of childhood obesity [32, 74]. Young children are dependent on parents and caregivers for food, and parents' choices on when to eat, responses to children's indication of hunger or distress, the context in which eating happens, and foods and portion sizes influence children's early learning about food and eating [11].

Surprisingly, few interventions have been developed that address general parenting in the prevention of childhood obesity [31]. These interventions provide evidence that suggests that the promotion of authoritative parenting is an effective strategy for the prevention and management of childhood obesity. There is some evidence that suggests that interventions promoting authoritative parenting (high demandingness, high responsiveness) are effective in improving weight-related outcomes in children [91].

Other home- and family-based interventions have been shown to be effective in affecting child weight status. These have focused on engaging with parents to support activities in the home setting to encourage healthy eating, more physical exercise, and less screen time [93]. Several studies found evidence for the association between pressure and child eating and preferences. Generally, children who are *rewarded* for eating certain types of food, such as vegetables, would eat more of that food but had a decreased preference for it. On the other hand, *pressuring* children to eat certain types of food would lead to eating less of it and having a lower preference for it [65].

Preschool Settings

Given that early childhood is a period where children are developing food preferences and behavior and activity behavior, interventions and strategies to promote active living, motor development, and healthy eating should start as early as possible [40]. Preschool settings (nurseries, day care, kindergarten, preschools) provide excellent access to the young child and their families to help attain and maintain a healthy lifestyle. Even though physical activity guidelines for the preschool years in several countries are inconsistent, preschoolers (aged 3–5 years) should accumulate at least 60 min of physical activity at any intensity spread throughout the day [81]. This would include any activity which gets them moving, such as climbing stairs or moving around the house, playing outside and exploring the environment, and crawling, walking, running, or dancing.

However, evidence of effectiveness of obesity prevention programs at this early life stage is limited [28, 93]. A systematic review and meta-analysis on the prevention of overweight and obesity in young children conducted in 2010 [60] identified prevention programs aimed to promote healthy eating, physical activity, and reduced television viewing among preschool children. Some focused on health education or training or had a component on physical activity, while three of the preschool interventions included an educational component for parents. However, the included interventions were not able to prove an effect on weight gain or BMI, while some small effects were observed in dietary or physical activity behavior. It has been suggested that growth velocity or rapid weight gain (identified by crossing BMI centiles) [90] or the timing of adiposity rebound [95] could be better indicators of overweight and obesity in children [60].

School Settings

Schools are critical settings for obesity prevention programs as they can help to establish lifelong healthy habits in school-aged children [28]. Schools can play a particularly critical role by establishing a safe and supportive environment with policies and practices that support healthy behaviors such as school lunch programs. Schools also provide opportunities for students to learn about and practice healthy eating and physical activity behaviors (health education). A Cochrane systematic review of 55 published interventions found strong evidence for the effect of child obesity prevention programs on the relative reduction of BMI, especially in 6- to 12-year-old children [93]. These included the following promising strategies and policies: include healthy eating, physical activity, and body image integrated into regular curriculum; include more sessions for physical activity/ fundamental movement skills throughout the school week; create an environment and culture that support children eating nutritious foods and being active throughout each day; provide professional development and capacity building activities for teachers to implement health promotion strategies and activities; and educate parents in the importance of continuing these activities at home [93].

Challenges in Obesity Prevention

Even though governments are prioritizing actions to tackle obesity and NCDs, there has been insufficient progress worldwide. Obesity prevalence rates have reached a plateau in some high-income countries but are still alarmingly high. Low- and middle-income countries are catching up rapidly and are faced with a double burden of under- and overnutrition. Obesity is a complex and multifactorial problem that requires a comprehensive and multisectoral approach, but all too often the debate around obesity prevention is based on polarizing and seemingly opposing approaches [73] such as:

- Individual behavior versus an obesogenic environment
- Lack of physical activity versus unhealthy diets
- Prevention versus treatment
- Government regulation versus industry self-regulation
- Treatment versus prevention
- Children versus adults
- Undernutrition versus overnutrition

Simplifying the problem into dichotomizing approaches will not reduce obesity at the population level. Firstly, most implemented obesity prevention strategies have targeted individual behavior rather than the wider environment in a more holistic way as part of a response to the current dominant political climate of free markets and individualism [88]. Secondly, preventive interventions aimed at children require a large investment in both time and resources, and the resulting health gains may not become apparent for decades [53]. For politicians, the electoral cycle is short, and there are limited resources for competing policy priorities [57]. Thirdly, the ultra-processed food industry has been very successful in blocking government-led regulatory and fiscal measures to modify the obesogenic environment [53].

Obesity prevention has been challenging not only because of these problems in trying to understand its causes and solutions to obesity but also because of the lack of evidence on what policy actions are effective, sustainable, and feasible [73]. This has made it difficult for national policymakers in the obesity field to invest in the best possible package of interventions to reverse the obesity epidemic [61]. There has been insufficient recognition of the early origins of obesity and the life-course trajectory which is established during development: both research and prevention strategies should focus more on these concepts.

Summary

There is a broad range of population-level actions that governments and other organizations can take to prevent childhood obesity. A comprehensive childhood obesity prevention strategy will incorporate a variety of approaches across a range of areas that may include social marketing, obesogenic environments, government policy, legislative and fiscal measures, and wider community approaches. The concept that obesity preventions should be based on a life-course approach with an emphasis on early life is relatively new [43]. There is now extensive evidence that the mother's diet and body composition before and during pregnancy and that of her child in the first few years of postnatal life are related to increased adiposity in childhood, setting up a trajectory of risk which can be tracked into adulthood [91]. Interventions aimed very early in the life course offer most potential for reducing obesity prevalence by focusing on the early, plastic phases of development.

Cross-References

▷ Diet, Exercise, and Behavior Therapy
▷ Prevention and Treatment of Obesity in Children
▷ Social and Community Networks and Obesity
▷ The Built Environment and Metabolic Syndrome

References

1. Alexander N, Rowe S, Brackett RE, et al. Achieving a transparent, actionable framework for public-private partnerships for food and nutrition research. Am J Clin Nutr. 2015;101(6):1359–63. Epub 2015/06/03.
2. Asbee SM, Jenkins TR, Butler JR, et al. Preventing excessive weight gain during pregnancy through dietary and lifestyle counseling: a randomized controlled

trial. Obstet Gynecol. 2009;113(2 Pt 1):305–12. Epub 2009/01/22.

3. Bachmanov AA, Inoue M, Ji H, et al. Glutamate taste and appetite in laboratory mice: physiologic and genetic analyses. Am J Clin Nutr. 2009;90(3): 756S–63S. Epub 2009/07/03.

4. Baidal JA, Taveras EM. Childhood obesity: shifting the focus to early prevention. Arch Pediatr Adolesc Med. 2012;166(12):1179–81.

5. Bambra C, Gibson M, Sowden A, et al. Tackling the wider social determinants of health and health inequalities: evidence from systematic reviews. J Epidemiol Community Health. 2009;64(4): 284–91. Epub 2009/08/21.

6. Barker DJ, Gluckman PD, Godfrey KM, et al. Fetal nutrition and cardiovascular disease in adult life. Lancet. 1993;341(8850):938–41. Epub 1993/04/10.

7. Beaglehole R, Bonita R, Alleyne G, et al. UN high-level meeting on non-communicable diseases: addressing four questions. Lancet. 2011;378(9789): 449–55. Epub 2011/06/15.

8. Belay B, Dietz WH. Obesity prevention and control: from clinical tools to public health strategies. Acad Pediatr. 2009;9(5):291–2. Epub 2009/09/19.

9. Belsky DW. Appetite for prevention: genetics and developmental epidemiology join forces in obesity research. JAMA Pediatr. 2014;168(4):309–11. Epub 2014/02/19.

10. Beydoun MA, Wang Y. Do nutrition knowledge and beliefs modify the association of socio-economic factors and diet quality among US adults? Prev Med. 2008;46(2):145–53. Epub 2007/08/19.

11. Birch LL, Ventura AK. Preventing childhood obesity: what works? Int J Obes. 2009;33(Suppl 1):S74–81. Epub 2009/04/14.

12. Birdsall KM, Vyas S, Khazaezadeh N, et al. Maternal obesity: a review of interventions. Int J Clin Pract. 2009;63(3):494–507. Epub 2009/02/19.

13. Bodker M, Pisinger C, Toft U, et al. The Danish fat tax-effects on consumption patterns and risk of ischaemic heart disease. Prev Med. 2015;77:200–3. Epub 2015/05/20.

14. Boney CM, Verma A, Tucker R, et al. Metabolic syndrome in childhood: association with birth weight, maternal obesity, and gestational diabetes mellitus. Pediatrics. 2005;115(3):e290–6. Epub 2005/03/03.

15. Britton C, McCormick FM, Renfrew MJ, Wade A, King SE. Support for breastfeeding mothers. Cochrane Database Syst Rev. 2007;(1):CD001141. Epub 2007/01/27.

16. Catalano PM, Ehrenberg HM. The short- and long-term implications of maternal obesity on the mother and her offspring. BJOG. 2006;113(10):1126–33. Epub 2006/07/11.

17. Cecchini M, Sassi F, Lauer JA, et al. Tackling of unhealthy diets, physical inactivity, and obesity: health effects and cost-effectiveness. Lancet. 2010;376(9754):1775–84. Epub 2010/11/16.

18. Cripps RL, Martin-Gronert MS, Ozanne SE. Fetal and perinatal programming of appetite. Clin Sci (London, England: 1979). 2005;109(1):1–11. Epub 2005/06/22.

19. Darnton-Hill I, Nishida C, James WP. A life course approach to diet, nutrition and the prevention of chronic diseases. Public Health Nutr. 2004;7 (1A):101–21.

20. DeWalt DA, Hink A. Health literacy and child health outcomes: a systematic review of the literature. Pediatrics. 2009;124(Suppl 3):S265–74. Epub 2009/11/05.

21. Dobbins M, De Corby K, Robeson P, Husson H, Tirilis D. School-based physical activity programs for promoting physical activity and fitness in children and adolescents aged 6–18. Cochrane Database Syst Rev. 2009;(1):CD007651. Epub 2009/01/23.

22. Dobbs R, Sawers C, Thompson F, et al. Overcoming obesity: an initial economic analysis. Washington, DC: Mckinsey Global Institute; 2014.

23. Dobe M. Hypertension: the prevention paradox. Indian J Public Health. 2013;57(1):1–3. Epub 2013/ 05/08.

24. Drewnowski A, Popkin BM. The nutrition transition: new trends in the global diet. Nutr Rev. 1997;55(2): 31–43.

25. Dyson L, Renfrew MJ, McFadden A, et al. Policy and public health recommendations to promote the initiation and duration of breast-feeding in developed country settings. Public Health Nutr. 2009;13(1): 137–44. Epub 2009/08/19.

26. Ferrara A. Increasing prevalence of gestational diabetes mellitus: a public health perspective. Diabetes Care. 2007;30(Suppl 2):S141–6. Epub 2007/07/13.

27. Finucane MM, Stevens GA, Cowan MJ, et al. National, regional, and global trends in body-mass index since 1980: systematic analysis of health examination surveys and epidemiological studies with 960 country-years and 9.1 million participants. Lancet. 2011;377(9765):557–67. Epub 2011/02/08.

28. Flynn MA, McNeil DA, Maloff B, et al. Reducing obesity and related chronic disease risk in children and youth: a synthesis of evidence with "best practice" recommendations. Obes Rev. 2006;7(Suppl 1):7–66. Epub 2005/12/24.

29. Friel S, Chopra M, Satcher D. Unequal weight: equity oriented policy responses to the global obesity epidemic. BMJ. 2007;335(7632):1241–3. (Clinical research ed).

30. Garmendia ML, Corvalan C, Uauy R. Assessing the public health impact of developmental origins of health and disease (DOHaD) nutrition interventions. Ann Nutr Metab. 2014;64(3–4):226–30.

31. Gerards SM, Sleddens EF, Dagnelie PC, et al. Interventions addressing general parenting to prevent or treat childhood obesity. IJPO. 2011;6(2–2):e28–45. Epub 2011/06/11.

32. Gillman MW, Ludwig DS. How early should obesity prevention start? N Engl J Med. 2013;369(23): 2173–5.

33. Gluckman P, Hanson M. Mismatch. Why our world no longer fits our bodies. Oxford: Oxford University Press; 2006.

34. Gluckman PD, Hanson MA. Developmental and epigenetic pathways to obesity: an evolutionary-developmental perspective. Int J Obes. 2008;32 (Suppl 7):S62–71. Epub 2009/01/16.

35. Godfrey KM, Lillycrop KA, Burdge GC, et al. Epigenetic mechanisms and the mismatch concept of the developmental origins of health and disease. Pediatr Res. 2007;61(5 Pt 2):5R–10R. Epub 2007/04/07.

36. Goff LM, Griffin BA, Lovegrove JA, et al. Ethnic differences in beta-cell function, dietary intake and expression of the metabolic syndrome among UK adults of south Asian, black African-Caribbean and white-European origin at high risk of metabolic syndrome. Diab Vasc Dis Res. 2013;10(4):315–23. Epub 2013/01/05.

37. Gortmaker SL, Swinburn BA, Levy D, et al. Changing the future of obesity: science, policy, and action. Lancet. 2011;378(9793):838–47. Epub 2011/08/30.

38. Grier SA, Kumanyika S. Targeted marketing and public health. Annu Rev Public Health. 2010;31: 349–69. Epub 2010/01/15.

39. Guelinckx I, Devlieger R, Vansant G. Pregnancies complicated by obesity: clinical approach and nutritional management. Verh K Acad Geneeskd Belg. 2010;72(5–6):253–76. Epub 2010/01/01.

40. Hanson MA, Fall CH, Robinson S, et al. Early life nutrition and lifelong health. London: BMA Board of Science; 2009.

41. Hanson MA, Gluckman PD, Ma RCW, et al. Early life opportunities for prevention of diabetes in low and middle income countries. BMC Public Health. 2012;12(1):1025.

42. Hartman MA, Hosper K, Stronks K. Targeting physical activity and nutrition interventions towards mothers with young children: a review on components that contribute to attendance and effectiveness. Public Health Nutr. 2011;14(8):1364–81. Epub 2010/07/17.

43. Haugen G, Hanson M, Kiserud T, et al. Fetal liver-sparing cardiovascular adaptations linked to mother's slimness and diet. Circ Res. 2005;96(1):12–4. Epub 2004/12/04.

44. Hawkes C, Smith TG, Jewell J, et al. Smart food policies for obesity prevention. Lancet. 2015;385(9985):2410–21. Epub 2015/02/24.

45. Hedley AA, Ogden CL, Johnson CL, et al. Prevalence of overweight and obesity among US children, adolescents, and adults, 1999–2002. JAMA. 2004;291(23):2847–50. Epub 2004/06/17.

46. Henley N, Raffin S. Social marketing to prevent childhood obesity. In: Waters E, Swinburn B, Seidell J, Uauy R, editors. Preventing childhood obesity- evidence policy and practice. Hoboken: Wiley-Blackwell; 2010.

47. Inskip HM, Crozier SR, Godfrey KM, et al. Women's compliance with nutrition and lifestyle recommendations before pregnancy: general population cohort study. BMJ. 2009;338:b481. Epub 2009/02/14.

48. Institute of Medicine. Accelerating progress in obesity prevention: solving the weight of the nation. Washington, DC: National Academies Press; 2012.

49. Kalhan R, Puthawala K, Agarwal S, et al. Altered lipid profile, leptin, insulin, and anthropometry in offspring of South Asian immigrants in the United States. Metab Clin Exp. 2001;50(10):1197–202. Epub 2001/10/05.

50. Kremers S, Reubsaet A, Martens M, et al. Systematic prevention of overweight and obesity in adults: a qualitative and quantitative literature analysis. Obes Rev. 2010;11(5):371–9. Epub 2009/06/23.

51. Kuzawa CW, Hallal PC, Adair L, et al. Birth weight, postnatal weight gain, and adult body composition in five low and middle income countries. Am J Hum Biol. 2011;24(1):5–13. Epub 2011/11/29.

52. Lakshmi S, Metcalf B, Joglekar C, et al. Differences in body composition and metabolic status between white U.K. and Asian Indian children (EarlyBird 24 and the Pune Maternal Nutrition Study). Pediatr Obes. 2012;7(5):347–54. Epub 2012/09/04.

53. Lehnert T, Sonntag D, Konnopka A, et al. The long-term cost-effectiveness of obesity prevention interventions: systematic literature review. Obes Rev. 2012;13(6):537–53. Epub 2012/01/19.

54. Lemmens VE, Oenema A, Klepp KI, et al. A systematic review of the evidence regarding efficacy of obesity prevention interventions among adults. Obes Rev. 2008;9(5):446–55. Epub 2008/02/27.

55. Linne Y. Effects of obesity on women's reproduction and complications during pregnancy. Obes Rev. 2004;5(3):137–43. Epub 2004/07/13.

56. Lloyd AB, Lubans DR, Plotnikoff RC, et al. Maternal and paternal parenting practices and their influence on children's adiposity, screen-time, diet and physical activity. Appetite. 2014;79:149–57. Epub 2014/04/23.

57. Lobstein T, Brinsden H. Symposium report: the prevention of obesity and NCDs: challenges and opportunities for governments. Obes Rev. 2014;15(8): 630–9. Epub 2014/06/04.

58. Marmot M. Social determinants of health inequalities. Lancet. 2005;365(9464):1099–104. Epub 2005/03/23.

59. McKeigue PM, Shah B, Marmot MG. Relation of central obesity and insulin resistance with high diabetes prevalence and cardiovascular risk in South Asians. Lancet. 1991;337(8738):382–6. Epub 1991/02/16.

60. Monasta L, Batty GD, Macaluso A, et al. Interventions for the prevention of overweight and obesity in preschool children: a systematic review of randomized controlled trials. Obes Rev. 2011;12(5):e107–18. Epub 2010/06/26.

61. Mongeau L. Curbing the obesity epidemic: the need for policy action in a risk-balanced, orchestrated,

comprehensive strategy. Int J Public Health. 2008;53(6):320–1. Epub 2008/12/30.

62. Muller MJ, Asbeck I, Mast M, et al. Prevention of obesity–more than an intention. Concept and first results of the Kiel Obesity Prevention Study (KOPS). Int J Obes Relat Metab Disord. 2001;25 (Suppl 1):S66–74. Epub 2001/07/24.

63. Nader PR, O'Brien M, Houts R, et al. Identifying risk for obesity in early childhood. Pediatrics. 2006;118(3):e594–601.

64. Ng M, Fleming T, Robinson M, et al. Global, regional, and national prevalence of overweight and obesity in children and adults during 1980–2013: a systematic analysis for the Global Burden of Disease Study 2013. Lancet. 2014;384(9945):766–81.

65. Ogden J, Reynolds R, Smith A. Expanding the concept of parental control: a role for overt and covert control in children's snacking behaviour? Appetite. 2006;47(1):100–6. Epub 2006/05/10.

66. Oteng-Ntim E, Pheasant H, Khazaezadeh N, et al. Developing a community-based maternal obesity intervention: a qualitative study of service providers' views. BJOG. 2010;117(13):1651–5. Epub 2010/12/04.

67. Pereira MA, Rifas-Shiman SL, Kleinman KP, et al. Predictors of change in physical activity during and after pregnancy: project viva. Am J Prev Med. 2007;32(4):312–9. Epub 2007/03/27.

68. Perez-Escamilla R, Kac G. Childhood obesity prevention: a life-course framework. Int J Obes. 2013;Suppl 3(Suppl 1):S3–5. Epub 2014/07/16.

69. Perez-Pastor EM, Metcalf BS, Hosking J, et al. Assortative weight gain in mother-daughter and father-son pairs: an emerging source of childhood obesity. Longitudinal study of trios (EarlyBird 43). Int J Obes. 2009;33(7):727–35. Epub 2009/05/13.

70. Poston L, Harthoorn LF, Van Der Beek EM. Obesity in pregnancy: implications for the mother and lifelong health of the child. A consensus statement. Pediatr Res. 2010;69(2):175–80. Epub 2010/11/16.

71. Puhl RM, Luedicke J, Depierre JA. Parental concerns about weight-based victimization in youth. Child Obes. 2013;9(6):540–8. Epub 2013/10/24.

72. Renkert S, Nutbeam D. Opportunities to improve maternal health literacy through antenatal education: an exploratory study. Health Promot Int. 2001;16(4):381–8.

73. Roberto CA, Swinburn B, Hawkes C, et al. Patchy progress on obesity prevention: emerging examples, entrenched barriers, and new thinking. Lancet. 2015;385(9985):2400–9. Epub 2015/02/24.

74. Robinson SM, Crozier SR, Harvey NC, et al. Modifiable early-life risk factors for childhood adiposity and overweight: an analysis of their combined impact and potential for prevention. Am J Clin Nutr. 2015;101(2):368–75. Epub 2015/02/04.

75. Rose G. The strategy of preventive medicine. New York: Oxford University Press; 1994.

76. Sacks G, Swinburn BA, Lawrence MA. A systematic policy approach to changing the food system and physical activity environments to prevent obesity. Aust NZ Health Policy. 2008;5:13. Epub 2008/06/07.

77. Sacks G, Swinburn B, Lawrence M. Obesity Policy Action framework and analysis grids for a comprehensive policy approach to reducing obesity. Obes Rev. 2009;10(1):76–86. Epub 2008/09/03.

78. Scholl TO, Chen X. Insulin and the "thrifty" woman: the influence of insulin during pregnancy on gestational weight gain and postpartum weight retention. Matern Child Health J. 2002;6(4):255–61. Epub 2003/01/07.

79. Siega-Riz AM, Viswanathan M, Moos MK, et al. A systematic review of outcomes of maternal weight gain according to the Institute of Medicine recommendations: birthweight, fetal growth, and postpartum weight retention. Am J Obstet Gynecol. 2009;201(4):339.e1–339.e14. Epub 2009/10/01.

80. Sikorski J, Renfrew MJ, Pindoria S, Wade A. Support for breastfeeding mothers. Cochrane Database Syst Rev. 2002;(1):CD001141. Epub 2002/03/01.

81. Skouteris H, Dell'Aquila D, Baur LA, et al. Physical activity guidelines for preschoolers: a call for research to inform public health policy. Med J Aust. 2012;196(3):174–7. Epub 2012/02/22.

82. Streuling I, Beyerlein A, von Kries R. Can gestational weight gain be modified by increasing physical activity and diet counseling? A meta-analysis of interventional trials. Am J Clin Nutr. 2010;92(4):678–87. Epub 2010/07/30.

83. Swinburn BA. Obesity prevention: the role of policies, laws and regulations. Aust NZ Health Policy. 2008;5:12. Epub 2008/06/07.

84. Swinburn B, Egger G, Raza F. Dissecting obesogenic environments: the development and application of a framework for identifying and prioritizing environmental interventions for obesity. Prev Med. 1999;29 (6 Pt 1):563–70. Epub 1999/12/22.

85. Swinburn B, Gill T, Kumanyika S. Obesity prevention: a proposed framework for translating evidence into action. Obes Rev. 2005;6(1):23–33. Epub 2005/01/19.

86. Swinburn BA, Sacks G, Hall KD, et al. The global obesity pandemic: shaped by global drivers and local environments. Lancet. 2011;378(9793):804–14. Epub 2011/08/30.

87. Swinburn B, Vandevijvere S, Kraak V, et al. Monitoring and benchmarking government policies and actions to improve the healthiness of food environments: a proposed Government Healthy Food Environment Policy Index. Obes Rev. 2013;14(Suppl 1):24–37. Epub 2013/10/23.

88. Swinburn B, Kraak V, Rutter H, et al. Strengthening of accountability systems to create healthy food environments and reduce global obesity. Lancet. 2015;385(9986):2534–45. Epub 2015/02/24.

89. Tanentsapf I, Heitmann BL, Adegboye AR. Systematic review of clinical trials on dietary interventions to

prevent excessive weight gain during pregnancy among normal weight, overweight and obese women. BMC Pregnancy Childbirth. 2011;11:81. Epub 2011/10/28.

90. Taveras EM, Rifas-Shiman SL, Sherry B, et al. Crossing growth percentiles in infancy and risk of obesity in childhood. Arch Pediatr Adolesc Med. 2011;165(11):993–8. Epub 2011/11/09.

91. Uauy R, Caleyachetty R, Swinburn B. Childhood obesity prevention overview. In: Waters E, Swinburn B, Seidell J, Uauy R, editors. Preventing childhood obesity- evidence policy and practice. Oxford: Wiley-Blackwell; 2010.

92. Walls HL, Peeters A, Proietto J, et al. Public health campaigns and obesity – a critique. BMC Public Health. 2011;11:136.

93. Waters E, de Silva-Sanigorski A, Hall BJ, Brown T, Campbell KJ, Gao Y, et al. Interventions for preventing obesity in children. Cochrane Database Syst Rev. 2011;12:CD001871. Epub 2011/12/14.

94. Whitaker RC. Predicting preschooler obesity at birth: the role of maternal obesity in early pregnancy. Pediatrics. 2004;114(1):e29–36. Epub 2004/07/03.

95. Whitaker RC, Pepe MS, Wright JA, et al. Early adiposity rebound and the risk of adult obesity. Pediatrics. 1998;101(3):E5. Epub 1998/03/11.

96. Williams SL, Mummery KW. Characteristics of consumers using "better for you" front-of-pack food labelling schemes – an example from the Australian Heart Foundation Tick. Public Health Nutr. 2013;16(12):2265–72. Epub 2012/11/28.

97. World Health Organization. International code of marketing of breast-milk substitutes. Geneva: World Health Organization; 1981.

98. World Health Organization. Global strategy on diet, physical activity and health. Geneva: World Health Organization; 2004.

99. World Health Organization. 2008–2013 action plan for the global strategy for the prevention and control of noncommunicable diseases. Geneva: World Health Organization; 2008.

100. World Health Organization. Population-based approaches to childhood obesity prevention. Geneva: World Health Organization; 2012.

101. World Health Organization. Global status report on noncommunicable diseases. Geneva: World Health Organization; 2014a.

102. World Health Organization. Childhood overweight and obesity. http://www.who.int/dietphysicalactivity/childhood/en/; 2014b [cited 2014 13 November].

103. World Health Organization. Interim report of the commission on ending childhood obesity. Geneva: World Health Organization; 2015.

104. World Health Organization, UNICEF. Baby-friendly hospital initiative (BFHI). Geneva: World Health Organization; 1991.

Index

© Springer Nature Switzerland AG 2023
R. S. Ahima (ed.), *Metabolic Syndrome*,
https://doi.org/10.1007/978-3-031-40116-9